So engaging ... so inviting ... so up-to-the-minute ...

An Invitation to Health, Eleventh Edition

gives your students the tools they need to explore, experience, and better understand the benefits of a healthy lifestyle!

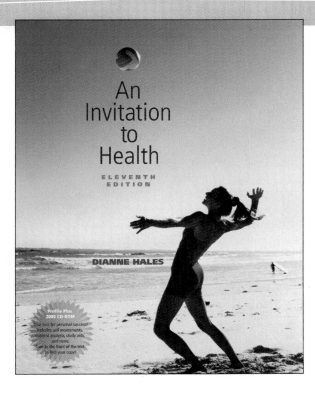

Dianne Hales is unmatched in her ability to inform, inspire change, and convey how attainable a healthy lifestyle can be. Hales presents the latest research, information, and recommendations related to health and wellness, using an engaging writing style that allows her to present extensive research that addresses those health- and wellness-related issues that affect your students— now and in the future. Hales illustrates the concepts and ideas your students will need to master in order to make responsible health decisions in their daily lives.

The Eleventh Edition expands upon the strengths of its predecessors by introducing a new emphasis on behavior change and prevention—the cornerstones of optimal health and wellness. It also includes new information and changes based on the input of over 40 instructors who reviewed the text.

An Invitation to Health, Eleventh Edition is complemented in every chapter by vivid, up-to-date examples and effective pedagogy. And, as you review this text, you'll see how *connected* the book is to **Profile Plus 2005 CD-ROM** and the other technology tools that accompany your adoption. This new Eleventh Edition of Dianne Hales' highly praised text truly stands above the rest!

Your quick tour of this outstanding book starts here! Turn the page ▷▷▷►►►

Preview

THOMSON
✳
WADSWORTH™

The Eleventh Edition works chapter-by-chapter with the text-specific Profile Plus® 2005 CD-ROM to help students take control of their personal health and lifestyle habits

Profile Plus 2005 is one of the most powerful, easy-to-use software packages available, drawing your students into a world of multimedia and online learning. With intuitive navigation and actual video demonstrations, **Profile Plus 2005** is an invaluable tool that lets students generate a personalized profile that allows them to:

■ conduct self assessments and record their current state of wellness and physical health
■ create and implement a Behavior Change Plan
■ track and analyze their nutritional intake
■ test their comprehension of the key concepts discussed in each chapter of the text
■ email their results and completed assessments to their instructor
■ track the types and quantities of exercises they have performed
■ consider an 'exercise prescription' for ways to integrate an exercise program into their lives

When combined with Hales' Eleventh Edition, this valuable tool is the ideal solution to get your students excited, motivated, and involved in achieving their own lifelong health and well being. Your students will find it an easy transition from the book to the CD-ROM as they study and explore the possibilities for behavior change.

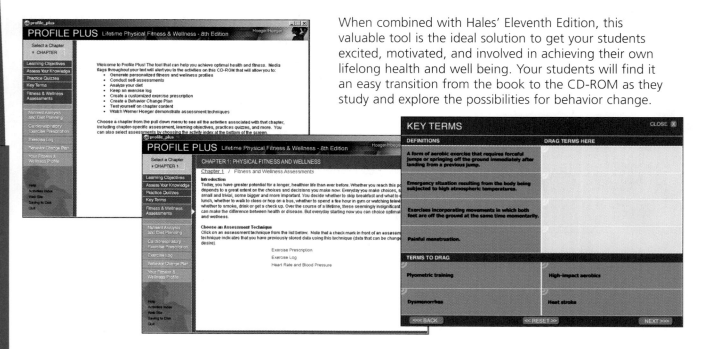

In the Eleventh Edition, **Profile Plus 2005** activities help link the chapter content to the CD-ROM, and end-of-chapter suggested activities prompt students to take full advantage of this study and enrichment tool.

▼▼▼

Profile Plus

Assess your current fitness levels and begin planning for a fitter future with these activities on your Profile Plus CD-ROM:

Profile Plus

• Exercise Prescription
• Exercise Log
• Cardiovascular Risk
• Cardiorespiratory Endurance

Profile Plus

• Skill-Related Fitness
• Muscular Strength and Endurance Test
• Heart Rate and Blood Pressure

The Profile Plus® 2005 CD-ROM includes so many features:

- The **"Behavior Change Plan"** allows students to write down their goals and electronically track them. This gives them the power to do a side-by-side "before-and-after" comparison to see how their behavior has changed and what it will mean for them as they move forward.

- **"Making This Chapter Work for You"** features include 10 review questions that allow students to test themselves on key fitness and wellness concepts covered in the CD-ROM and in the text. Answers and page references are included at the end of each quiz, and the results can be printed or e-mailed to the instructor.

- **More foods!** The "Nutrition Analysis and Diet Planning" section is now easier to navigate and includes approximately 6,000 foods from the USDA database, allowing easier and more accurate assessment of the student's daily intakes.

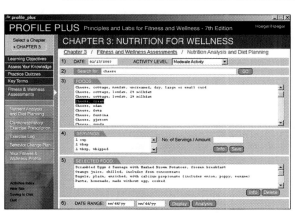

- **"Learning Objectives"** now match Hales' chapter-by-chapter learning objectives, better linking the Eleventh Edition to the CD-ROM.

- **Ideal for all learning types**. Considered the most motivating, entertaining, easy-to-use, and useful CD-ROM on the market, it includes videos, interactive exercises, explanations, definitions, personal logs, and more.

- A **"Fitness and Wellness Profile"** compiles the information from all completed assessments and generates a personalized report.

- An **"Exercise Log"** allows students to track their physical activities, such as step aerobics or walking, and monitor such measurements as one's heart rate, duration of exercise, and calories burned.

- A **"Cardiorespiratory Exercise Prescription"** provides students with suggested fitness goals.

- **"Practice Quizzes"** allow students to review core concepts on the CD-ROM and in the text. Answers and page references are included at the end of each quiz, and can be printed or e-mailed.

For a demonstration, visit the Thomson Wadsworth **Health, Fitness, & Wellness Resource Center** at http://health.wadsworth.com.

With a new emphasis on behavior change, Dianne Hales includes new features, new topics, new research in every chapter . . .

Dianne Hales is known for the way she speaks *with* students—not at them. Throughout the Eleventh Edition, Hales points out to students that health is not a subject that students must memorize, but one to be both learned and lived. Hales' text—with its renewed emphasis on behavior change and prevention—is the perfect tool to help students acquire the skills they need to protect their well being and prevent serious health problems.

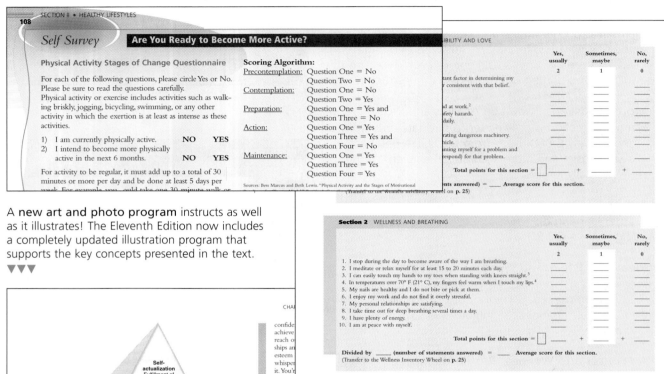

Self Survey — Are You Ready to Become More Active?

Physical Activity Stages of Change Questionnaire

For each of the following questions, please circle Yes or No. Please be sure to read the questions carefully.
Physical activity or exercise includes activities such as walking briskly, jogging, bicycling, swimming, or any other activity in which the exertion is at least as intense as these activities.

1) I am currently physically active.   NO   YES
2) I intend to become more physically active in the next 6 months.   NO   YES

For activity to be regular, it must add up to a total of 30 minutes or more per day and be done at least 5 days per week. For example, you could take one 30-minute walk or...

Scoring Algorithm:
Precontemplation: Question One = No
Question Two = No
Contemplation: Question One = No
Question Two = Yes
Preparation: Question One = Yes and
Question Three = No
Action: Question One = Yes and
Question Three = Yes and
Question Four = No
Maintenance: Question One = Yes
Question Three = Yes
Question Four = Yes

Sources: Bess Marcus and Beth Lewis. "Physical Activity and the Stages of Motivational

...IBILITY AND LOVE

	Yes, usually	Sometimes, maybe	No, rarely
	2	1	0
...tant factor in determining my ...r consistent with that belief.	___	___	___
...d at work.[2]	___	___	___
...fety hazards.	___	___	___
...daily.	___	___	___
...rating dangerous machinery.	___	___	___
...hicle.	___	___	___
...ming myself for a problem and ...espond) for that problem.	___	___	___

Total points for this section = ☐ ___ + ___ + ___

...nts answered) = ___ Average score for this section.
(Transfer to the wellness inventory wheel on p. 25)

Section 2 WELLNESS AND BREATHING

	Yes, usually	Sometimes, maybe	No, rarely
	2	1	0
1. I stop during the day to become aware of the way I am breathing.	___	___	___
2. I meditate or relax myself for at least 15 to 20 minutes each day.	___	___	___
3. I can easily touch my hands to my toes when standing with knees straight.[3]	___	___	___
4. In temperatures over 70° F (21° C), my fingers feel warm when I touch my lips.[4]	___	___	___
5. My nails are healthy and I do not bite or pick at them.	___	___	___
6. I enjoy my work and do not find it overly stressful.	___	___	___
7. My personal relationships are satisfying.	___	___	___
8. I take time out for deep breathing several times a day.	___	___	___
9. I have plenty of energy.	___	___	___
10. I am at peace with myself.	___	___	___

Total points for this section = ☐ ___ + ___ + ___

Divided by ___ **(number of statements answered)** = ___ **Average score for this section.**
(Transfer to the Wellness Inventory Wheel on **p. 25**)

A **new art and photo program** instructs as well as it illustrates! The Eleventh Edition now includes a completely updated illustration program that supports the key concepts presented in the text.
▼▼▼

Self-actualization
Fulfillment of one's potential

Self-esteem
Respect for self, respect of others

Love and affection
Ability to give and receive affection; feeling of belonging

Safety-security
Ability to protect oneself from harm

Physiological needs
Fulfillment of needs for food, water, shelter, sleep, sexual expression

Figure 2-1 THE MASLOW PYRAMID
To attain the highest level of psychological health, you must first satisfy your needs for safety and security, love and affection, and self-esteem.

Source: A. Maslow. *Motivation and Personality*, 3rd ed., © 1997. Reprinted by permission of Pearson Education, Inc.

that you can live in accordance with your beliefs. To do so, follow these steps:

1. Carefully consider the consequences of each choice.
2. Choose freely from among all the options.
3. Publicly affirm your values by sharing them with others.
4. Act out your values.

Values clarification is not a once-in-a-lifetime task, but an ongoing process of sorting out what matters most to you. If you believe in protecting the environment, do you shut off lights, or walk rather than drive, in order to conserve energy? Do you vote for political candidates who support environmental protection? Do you recycle newspapers, bottles, and cans? Values are more than ideals we'd like to attain; they should be reflected in the way we live day by day.

Boosting Self-Esteem

Each of us wants and needs to feel significant as a human being with unique talents, abilities, and roles in life. A sense

CHAP...

confide...
achieve...
reach o...
ships an...
esteem...
whisper...
it. You'r...
Sel...
external factors like wealth or beauty, but on what you believe about yourself. It's not something you're born with; self-esteem develops over time. It's also not something anyone else can give to you, although those around you can either help boost or diminish your self-esteem.

The seeds of self-esteem are planted in childhood when parents provide the assurance and appreciation youngsters need to push themselves toward new accomplishments: crawling, walking, forming words and sentences, learning control over their bladder and bowels.

Adults, too, must consider themselves worthy of love, friendship, and success if they are to be loved, to make friends, and to achieve their goals. Low self-esteem is more common in people who have been abused as children and in those with psychiatric disorders, including depression, anxiety, alcoholism, and drug dependence. Feeling a lack of love and encouragement as a child can also lead to poor self-esteem. Adults

Self-esteem, which is based on what you believe about yourself, tends to increase when you experience success.

▲▲▲
Beginning in Chapter 1, "An Invitation to Health for the 21st Century," Hales introduces and explains the concept of behavior change, including the stages and progress of making healthy changes. Discussion of **behavior change** is woven throughout the book's narrative, and a new feature, **Your Health Change Plan**, appears in every chapter, to give students practical help in changing health behaviors. Some of the topics explored in this feature include, "Your Health Change Plan for Responsible Drinking," and "Your Health Change Plan for Personal Safety on Campus."

... all designed to get students engaged and motivated!

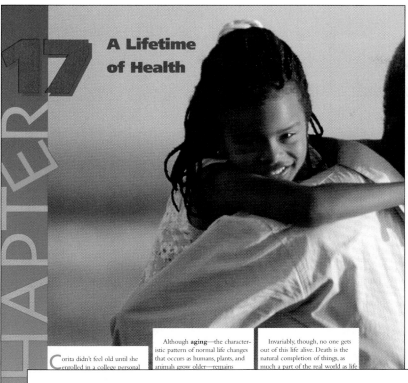

CHAPTER 17

A Lifetime of Health

Corita didn't feel old until she enrolled in a college personal

Although **aging**—the characteristic pattern of normal life changes that occurs as humans, plants, and animals grow older—remains

Invariably, though, no one gets out of this life alive. Death is the natural completion of things, as much a part of the real world as life

◄◄◄

In response to reviewer recommendations, Hales now includes an entirely new Chapter 17, "A Lifetime of Health." This chapter includes in-depth coverage of important topics like the aging brain, sexuality and aging, near death experiences, preparing for a medical crisis and end of life, grief's effects on health, and more.

Chapter by chapter, Hales includes so much **new information on the latest topics in health!** For example, you'll find the most recent information and research on topics such as:

- alternative food guides
- daily energy requirements
- cohabitation
- sexual activity of college students
- the future of contraceptives
- early influences of drug use
- alcohol and smoking and gender
- evidence-based medicine
- West Nile Virus and new infectious threats
- health care and college students
- and much more

◄◄◄   ▼▼▼

---

your life so full that you worry about coming apart at the seams. One thing is for certain: You're not alone.

After a steady surge upward in the 1990s, the percentage of students who say they are "frequently overwhelmed by all they have to do" has declined from the peak of 30.7 percent in 1999 to 26.8 percent in 2002. However, women are twice as likely to report stress as men.[16] (See the X & Y Files: "Men, Women, and Stress.") According to surveys of students at colleges and universities around the country and the world, stressors are remarkably similar. Among the most common are:

:: Test pressures.
:: Financial problems.
:: Frustrations, such as delays in reaching goals.
:: Problems in friendships and dating relationships.
:: Daily hassles.
:: Academic failure.
:: Pressures as a result of competition, deadlines, and the like.
:: Changes, which may be unpleasant, disruptive, or too frequent.
:: Losses, whether caused by the breakup of a relationship or the death of a loved one.

Many students bring complex psychological problems with them to campus, including learning disabilities and mood disorders like depression and anxiety. "Students arrive with the underpinnings of problems that are brought out by the stress of campus life," says one counselor. Some have grown

up in broken homes and bear the scars of family troubles. Others fall into the same patterns of alcohol abuse that they observed for years in their families or suffer lingering emotional scars from childhood physical or sexual abuse.

Students Under Stress

Almost a third of freshmen feel overwhelmed by all they have to do at the beginning of the academic year; by the year's end, 44 percent feel overwhelmed.[17] In a recent study of students at three universities, underclassmen were most vulnerable to negative life events, perhaps because they lacked experience in coping with stressful situations. Freshmen had the highest levels of depression; sophomores had the most anger and hostility. Seniors may handle life's challenges better because [...] nisms. In the [...] problems squa[...] younger stude[...] instance, by tr[...]

First-gen[...] ents never exp[...] encounter mo[...] freshmen who[...] generation stu[...] knowledge of[...] preparation fo[...] college activit[...]

The perc[...] because of str[...] last 15 years.[...]

The first year of college can be overwhelming as you learn your way around the campus, meet new people, and strive to succeed.

Men also report nonconsensual sexual activity. In studies of college-age men, one in four reported at least one incident in which a woman (often a friend or ex-partner) attempted to engage them in unwanted kissing, petting, oral sex, or intercourse.[24]

During adolescence, sexuality develops rapidly. Teens explore different social and intimate relationships as they begin to develop a sexual identity.

Why Don't College Students Practice Safer Sex?

Decades of education about sexual risks has had an impact. More students today are aware of and use safer sex practices—but not consistently. In a survey of 119 American colleges, condom use varied from 32 to 52 percent among unmarried sexually active students.[25] Heterosexual students—male and female—were more likely to say they always used condoms than gay men. Of those engaging in heterosexual sex, 52 percent of men and 43 percent of women reported consistent condom use, compared with 32 percent of men with only male partners.

Researchers explain that the college environment "provides students with a sense of new independence, self-determination, and strong peer pressure to experiment with a variety of sexual behaviors." Yet by engaging in sex with multiple partners and not regularly using condoms, college students in general—and African-American students in particular—put themselves at high risk of contracting HIV and other sexual infections.

In a recent study of African-American undergraduates, male and female students identified barriers to their use of safer sex practices. Negative views of condoms rank first. But the reason men and women don't like condoms is not reduced sensitivity or pleasure, but a sense that not wearing a condom provides a sense of greater intimacy.[26]

New to This Edition

For a full listing of the chapter-by-chapter changes to the Eleventh Edition, visit **http://health.wadsworth.com**

Hales invites students to a happier, healthier, fuller life!

NEW! ▶▶▶

Cutting Edge boxes (formerly called *Genes in Focus*) present fascinating discussions of state-of-the-science research. In these boxes, you'll find topics such as, "Magnets for the Brain," and "Anti-Nicotine Vaccination."

NEW! ▼▼▼

Fact or Fiction boxes get students thinking about provocative issues. These features present accurate information on newsworthy topics, such as, "Is Heart Disease Just for Older People?" and "Echinacea Can Help Fight the Common Cold."

THE CUTTING EDGE

Magnets for the Brain

A new treatment for serious mental illness involv[es] an invisible force: magnetic energy. By directing magnetic waves toward specific regions of the br[ain], psychiatrists have brought relief to patients suffe[ring] from severe disorders.

Magnetic stimulation, produced by an electri[c] coil shaped like a figure 8 placed over the brain, [has] led to improvement in some individuals with maj[or] depression who had not improved with medicatio[n]. In small studies, magnetic energy also has quiete[d] the imaginary voices heard by some patients with schizophrenia. Side effects include headaches and feeling lightheaded for a few minutes after the procedure.

"Patients find magnetic therapy to be a signifi[cant] relief from often debilitating symptoms," sa[id] psychiatrist Ralph Hoffman, M.D., of Yale University, who is studying this approach, "But this is still at the level of research, as opposed to something patients can call up and get."

Source: Lauren Marangelli et al. "Psychopharmacology and Electroconvulsive Therapy," *Textbook of Clinical Psychiatry* (4th edition). Washington, D.C.: American Psychiatric Publishing, Inc., 2003. Hoffman, Ralph, et al. "Transcranial Magnetic Stimulation of Left Temporoparietal Cortex and Medication-Resistant Auditory Hallucinations," *Archives of General Psychiatry,* January 2003; Vol. 60, p. 49.

The Bottom Line: ▼ De-stress Your Life

College is a perfect time to learn and practice the art of stress reduction. You can start applying the techniques and concepts outlined in this chapter immediately. You may want to begin by doing some relaxation or awareness exercises. They can give you the peace of mind you need to focus more effectively on larger issues, goals, and decisions.

You needn't see stress as a problem to solve on your own. Reach out to others. As you build friendships and intimate relationships, you may find that some irritating problems are easier to put into perspective. Don't be afraid to laugh at yourself and to look for the comic or absurd aspects of a situation. In addition, you might try some simple approaches that can help boost your stress resistance and reslience, including the following:

:: **Focusing.** Take a strain inventory of your body every day to determine where things aren't feeling quite right. Ask yourself, "What's keeping me from feeling

NEW! ▲▲▲

Bottom Line sections conclude each chapter on an upbeat note. These features allow students to focus on practical behavior changes, such as. "Smart Sex," and "Living Drug Free."

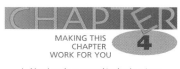

FACT OR FICTION?

The Internet and e-mail have transformed the way patients use the health-care system.

Fiction: Although many people use the Internet for health information, very few report a significant impact on their health-care decisions. In a national survey, more than 90 percent of those who looked up health information online said the Internet had no impact on the number of times they called or visited a doctor. Only 6 percent used e-mail to contact a health-care professional; 5 percent or fewer used the Internet to obtain prescriptions.

Source: Laurence Baker et al. "Use of the Internet and E-Mail for Health Care Information." *Journal of the American Medical Association,* Vol. 289, No. 18, May 14, 2003, p. 2400.

▶▶▶

Making This Chapter Work for You study features review important chapter material in a format of 10 multiple-choice questions per chapter. **NEW!** These questions are also located on the **accompanying Profile Plus 2005 CD-ROM,** and include answers and page references for easy review. In addition, students can email their responses to their instructor.

CHAPTER 4

MAKING THIS CHAPTER WORK FOR YOU

1. Mary Ann takes a step aerobics class three times a week. Which component of physical fitness does her exercise routine emphasize?
   a. muscular strength and endurance
   b. flexibility
   c. cardiorespiratory fitness
   d. body composition
2. The benefits of regular physical activity include:
   a. decreased bone mass.
   b. lowered risk of shin splints.
   c. enhanced immune response.
   d. altered sleep patterns.
3. To motivate yourself to stick to an exercise program:
   a. Watch professional athletic competitions.
   b. Set a long-term goal, then break it down into short-term goals that can be achieved in a few months.
   c. Keep a detailed record of all the times that you avoided working out.
   d. Join an expensive health club so that you feel pressured to get your money's worth.
4. Which of the following best describes the primary benefit of aerobic exercise?
   a. It improves cardiorespiratory endurance.
   b. It helps condition your muscles, enabling them to work efficiently and reliably.
   c. It can enhance weight loss.
   d. It increases the range of motion of your joints.
5. An aerobic workout may consist of
   a. 5 minutes of brisk walking, 30 minutes of flexibility exercises, 5 minutes of brisk walking.
   b. 15 minutes of resistance exercises followed by 10 minutes of stretching.
   c. 10 minutes of sprints, 5 minutes of slow jogging, 5 minutes of stretching, and 10 minutes of sprints.
   d. 5 minutes of stretching, 5 minutes of brisk walking, 45 minutes of jogging, 5 minutes of slow walking, 5 minutes of stretching.
6. Which statement is true about isometric, isotonic, and isokinetic exercises?
   a. Isokinetic exercises usually involves pushing on an object, isotonic exercises involve pulling on an object, and isotonic exercises involve lifting an object.
   b. Isometric and isokinetic exercises can be done with free weights, but isotonic exercises require special resistance machines.
   c. Weight lifting is an isotonic exercise, pushing against the wall is an isometric exercise, and isokinetic exercises require special machines that move muscles through their range of motion.
   d. Isotonic exercises are much more effective at contracting muscles than isometric or isokinetic.
7. A regular flexibility program provides which of the following benefits?
   a. stronger heart and lungs
   b. relief of muscle strain and soreness
   c. increased strength and endurance
   d. increased bone mass and leaner muscles
8. Body composition estimates can be obtained with which of the following methods?
   a. skinfold fat weighing
   b. bioelectrical impedance analysis
   c. biofeedback analysis
   d. basal metabolic rate measurement
9. Which nutrient is the most important during exercise and exertion?
   a. water
   b. carbohydrates
   c. fat
   d. protein
10. Which of the following precautions could help prevent a serious sports injury from occurring?
    a. Wear swimming goggles when doing laps to decrease the irritating effects of chlorine.
    b. Wear knee pads when cycling to prevent knee gashes if you fall off your bicycle.
    c. To eliminate persistent muscle soreness, increase the frequency and/or time period of your workout.
    d. Wear a helmet, wrist guards, and knee pads when inline skating to help prevent fractures and head injuries.

Answers to these questions can be found on page 652.

The Eleventh Edition is packed with information, advice, research, and recommendations—leading students toward the first step of personal responsibility

Dianne Hales updated and revised every chapter in **An Invitation to Health, Eleventh Edition** in order to make it the ultimate learning tool—one that can serve as an "owner's manual" to students' minds and bodies. In doing so, Hales helps students learn to make better decisions, to assume responsibility, and to create and follow a healthy lifestyle, and most of all, to live what they learn!

◄◄◄
A **Wellness Inventory** begins the text that allows students to evaluate and assess their current state of wellness before exploring various topics related to healthy living. The "Wellness Inventory" is also available on the Hales Book Companion Web Site (http://health.wadsworth.com) so students can pre-test and post-test their personal understanding of the dimensions of wellness.

WELLNESS INVENTORY

WHAT IS WELLNESS?*

BY JOHN W. TRAVIS M.D.

The Joy of Fitness

▲▲▲
In Chapter 4, **"The Joy of Fitness,"** students will find a table of why college students exercise or don't exercise, new information on the toll of inactivity, updated statistics on the benefits of exercise, expanded coverage of sports safety (including temperature considerations), and a new section on FIT guidelines for cardiovascular exercise, strength, and flexibility.

◄◄◄
In Chapters 8, **"Personal Sexuality,"** and 9, **"Reproductive Choices,"** the author presents the latest information on the availability of emergency contraceptives, the contraceptive ring, and the contraceptive patch.

Personal Sexuality

Proven Features

7

▶▶▶

Self Survey sections are integrated throughout the text and allow students to assess their own state of health and relate chapter material to their own lives. Some of the topics presented in the **Self Survey** sections include, "How Much Do You Know About Sex?" "Are You Ready to Become More Active?" and "Check Your Cholesterol and Heart Disease IQ."

▶▶▶

Your Health Change Plan features follow each survey and provide specific guidelines on implementing necessary changes.

Hales includes new information on topics that resonate with students, such as the toll of college drinking, binge drinking, tobacco use on campus, and how sexually active college students are. Additionally, the redesigned **Student Snapshot** features report recent data on the health, habits, and concerns of today's college students. These features reveal a compelling view of campus behaviors—representing all types of students in an eye-catching, thought-provoking format. Examples include "Campus Couch Potatoes," "Behind Closed Doors on Campus," and "Do Students Want Marijuana Legalized?" ▼▼▼

▲▲▲

This edition of **An Invitation to Health** offers even more features designed to intrigue and involve your students. For instance, **The Savvy Consumer** feature offers specific advice on getting the best possible health care and services and information, whether students are interested in spotting nutrition misinformation or evaluating the risks of contraceptives.

The most up-to-date health research is presented in the Eleventh Edition, along with the fundamental background students need to understand and apply these findings. Research on college students (and college-age individuals) appears in every chapter, and is indicated with a **Student Research** icon—a feature designed to help students recognize how relevant health topics are to their everyday lives.

... and help them take charge of their own well-being

the X & Y file — *Gender Differences and Physical Fitness*

Men and women benefit equally from physical activity and exercise. Nevertheless, the components of physical fitness do have gender differences. Many are related to size. On average, men are 10 to 15 percent bigger than women, with roughly twice the percentage of muscle mass and half the percentage of body fat. Overall, men are about 30 percent stronger, particularly above the waist. They have more sweat glands and a greater maximum oxygen uptake. A man's bigger heart pumps more blood with each beat. His larger lungs take in 10 to 20 percent more oxygen. His longer legs cover more distance with each stride. If a man jogs along at 50 percent of his capacity, a woman has to push to 73 percent of hers to keep up.

Women have a higher percentage of body fat than men, and more is distributed around the hips and thighs; men carry more body fat around the waist and stomach. The average woman has a smaller heart, a lower percent-age of slow twitch muscle fibers, and a smaller volume than a man. Because women have a lower concentration of red blood cells, their bodies are less effective at transporting oxygen to their working muscles during exercise.

Even though training produces the same relative increases for both genders, a woman's maximum oxygen intake remains about 25 to 30 percent lower than that of an equally well-conditioned man. In elite athletes, the gender difference is smaller: 8 to 12 percent. Because the angle of the upper leg bone (femur) to the pelvis is greater in a woman, her legs are less efficient at running.

In some endurance events, such as ultramarathon running and long-distance swimming, female anatomy and physiology may have some aerobic advantages. The longer a race—on land, water, or ice—the better women perform. In an analysis of world-record times in running, swimming, and speed skating, researchers at Northeastern University observed that in all three sports the superiority of men's performances diminished with increasing distance.

	Female	Male
Percent fat	27%	15%
Lean body mass	107.8 pounds	134.2 pounds
Blood volume	4.5-5 liters	5-6 liters
Maximum oxygen consumption	3-3.5 liters per minute	5.5-5.9 liters per minute

◄◄◄
The **X & Y Files** are boxes that focus on topics related to gender differences in health, such as "Why Men and Women Drink," "Diseases that Discriminate," and "Gender Differences and Physical Fitness."

Strategies for Change appear throughout the book and provide practical, checklist-style behavioral change strategies for achieving better health. Some of the topics you'll find in this feature include, "How to Spot a Dangerous Weight Loss Program," "How to Say No to Sex," and "How to Talk with Your Doctor."
▼▼▼

STRATEGIES FOR CHANGE

How to Talk with Your Doctor

■ Prepare in advance. Write down your questions, organize them in a logical fashion, and select the top ten queries you want answered. Make a copy of all your questions to review and leave with your doctor.

■ Ask about a "question hour." Many health-care practitioners set aside a specific time of day for patients with call-in questions. Find out if your college health center offers this service. Does a nurse field all calls? Can you get specific advice?

■ Go online. Many doctors' offices answer queries by e-mail. Ask your doctor if you can e-mail follow-up questions or progress reports on how you're feeling.

■ Interrupt the interrupter. If you're having difficulty explaining what's wrong, say so. If your doctor tries to put words in your mouth, say, "Please just listen so I can tell you the whole story without getting sidetracked."

STRATEGIES FOR PREVENTION

Taking Care of Your Mouth

■ Brush your teeth every morning and every night. Oral bacteria reach their highest count during sleep because fluids in the mouth accumulate. Nighttime cleaning reduces the bacterial population; morning cleaning lets you reduce the buildup.

■ Use a toothpaste that has the American Dental Association (ADA) seal of acceptance and a toothbrush with soft, rounded bristles. Replace your toothbrush every three months.

■ Hold the brush at a 45-degree angle from your gums. Pay particular attention to the space between your teeth and gums, especially on the inside, toward your tongue. Brush for two to five minutes. Don't brush too vigorously. If you scrub as hard as you can, you may damage your teeth and gums. Abrasion—a problem for more than half of American adults—erodes tooth surfaces, weakens teeth, and increases sensitivity to hot and cold foods.

■ Because brushing can't reach plaque and food trapped between teeth, daily flossing is essential. Using waxed or unwaxed floss, start behind the upper and lower molars at one side of your mouth and work toward the other side.

■ See your dentist twice a year for routine cleaning and examination. To find a dentist, call a local dental school, which may have a public clinic, or check with your county dental society. Ask for information regarding fees, hours, and after-hour emergency service. Your dentist should take a complete medical history from you and update it every six months, examine your mouth for signs of cancer, and thoroughly outline all treatment options.

■ Make sure that everyone who works on the inside of your mouth wears a mask and rubber gloves to reduce the risk of disease transmission (that is, bacterial and viral infections, such as hepatitis, herpes, and HIV).

■ Check your family's dental insurance coverage. Many dental plans cover all costs for regular six-month checkups and cleanings and a percentage of the costs for fillings, gum treatment, root canals, and so on.

◄◄◄
Strategies for Prevention boxes provide effective, practical checklists for preventing health problems and reducing health risks. Just some of the topics discussed in this feature include, "Natural Ways to Bolster Immunity," "Taking Care of Your Mouth," and "Lowering the Risk of Diabetes."

Hales has taken great care to

update and expand the coverage of **diversity in health,** which is integrated throughout every chapter. The book's diversity topics include mental health, dietary diversity, and cancer risks for minority men and women. An **icon** indicates where issues related to race, class, and gender are covered.

Proven Features

With an emphasis on critical thinking and the resources to expand learning, the Eleventh Edition gets students assessing the material and relating it to their own lives!

▶▶▶

Sites and Bytes boxes include updated interactive Web sites and InfoTrac® College Edition activities, encouraging students to use these resources for additional information and learning. Hales urges students to explore issues and organizations such as "The Transtheoretical Model," "National Institute of Mental Health," and "Prevention of Smoking and Tobacco Control."

Sites and Bytes

Just Move.
www.justmove.org
At this website sponsored by the American Heart Association, after a free registration, you can access an interactive exercise diary where you can keep track of your own exercise progress. In addition, an information resource called My Fitness provides recommendations for optimizing your exercise program to match your lifestyle, as well as a list of health and fitness resources.

Sites and Bytes

Georgia State University's Exercise and Physical Fitness Page
www.gsu.edu/~wwwfit
Sponsored by the Department of Kinesiology and Health at Georgia State University, this site features a series of links containing research-based exercise and fitness information, including how to get started on an exercise program and stay with it, aerobic exercises, strength training, flexibility, nutrition, and body composition.

Sites and Bytes

Health A to Z
www.healthatoz.com/healthatoz/
Atoz/hl/fit/demo/excerdemo.html
This website has animated models showing the proper technique for various exercises. The site also has a "Getting Started" section that has tips and short workouts good for the heart.

InfoTrac College Edition

 Activity
Suminski, Richard R., et al. "Physical Activity Among Ethnically Diverse College Students" *Journal of American College Health,* Volume 51, No. 2, September 2002, p. 75(6).
1. What is the relationship between ethnicity and gender differences on

InfoTrac College Edition

the rates of physical activity in college students?
2. What factors influence physical activity patterns among college students?
3. Describe some of the explanations for the relatively low levels of physical activity seen in women.

InfoTrac College Edition

You can find additional readings related to fitness with InfoTrac College Edition, an online library of more than 900 journals and publications. Follow the instructions for accessing InfoTrac that were packaged with your textbook; then search for articles using a keyword search.

For addition links, resources, and suggested readings on InfoTrac, visit our Health & Wellness Resource Center at **http://health.wadsworth.com**.

▶▶▶

Critical Thinking questions ask students to consider some applications of the chapter's coverage or weigh in on a health-related controversy.

Critical Thinking

1. Allison knows that exercise is good for her health, but she figures she can keep her weight down by dieting and worry about her heart and health when she gets older. "I look good. I feel okay. Why should I bother exercising?" she asks. What would you reply?
2. When he started working out, Jeff simply wanted to stay in shape. But he felt so pleased with the way his body looked and responded that he kept doing more. Now he runs 10 miles a day (longer on weekends), lifts weights, works out on

Critical Thinking

exercise equipment almost every day, and plays racquetball or squash whenever he gets a chance. Is Jeff getting too much of a good thing? Is there any danger in his fitness program? What would be a more reasonable approach?
3. Your younger brother Andre is hoping to get a starting position on his high school football team. Practices began in July. You are aware that a couple of other players have suffered heat-related incidences, but according to Andre,

Critical Thinking

these players just weren't tough enough. What can you do to help your brother protect his health?
4. Although anabolic steroids have been banned for use by athletes in certain competitions, other performance-enhancing supplements are used routinely to provide a competitive advantage. Do you believe that most athletes use such substances routinely? Do you think that athletes should be able to use these substances without intervention or regulation? Why or why not?

Key Terms conclude each chapter and highlight the most important terms discussed in the chapter. Page references are also included to make it easier for students to quickly turn to the page where the term is being presented.

 After watching the CNN video segment, discuss the following question. What are the behavioral strategies for getting a good nights sleep?

CNN Today Video icons appear at the end of each chapter and include suggested video segments and discussion questions that relate to chapter material. For instance, students are asked to discuss the positive and negative aspects of a new drug rehabilitation Web community that gives people an anonymous alternative to the traditional therapies available. Another example, "Sizing Up Fast Foods," asks students to discuss alternatives to portion sizes in fast food restaurants. *See page 13 for a description of the CNN Videos available with your adoption.*

These valuable resources are FREE with your adoption of the Eleventh Edition

The Profile Plus® 2005 CD-ROM is automatically packaged with the text! See pages 2–3 for details

InfoTrac® College Edition

. . . automatically packaged with the text

http://www.infotrac-college.com

Give your students anytime, anywhere access to reliable resources with **InfoTrac College Edition,** the online library! This fully searchable database offers more than 20 years' worth of full-text articles from almost 5,000 diverse sources, such as academic journals, newsletters, and up-to-the-minute periodicals including *Time, Newsweek, Science, Forbes,* and *USA Today,* as well as a host of health and physical fitness publications. This incredible depth and breadth of material—available 24 hours a day from any computer with Internet access—makes conducting research so easy, your students will want to use it to enhance their work in every course! And, incorporating **InfoTrac College Edition** is easy as well—references to this virtual library are built into Hales' text. Both adopters and their students receive unlimited access for four months.

NEW! Students now have instant access to critical thinking and paper writing tools through *InfoWrite.*

Book Companion Web Site

Accessible via http://health.wadsworth.com

When you adopt Hales' text, you and your students will have access to a rich array of teaching and learning resources you won't find anywhere else. This outstanding site features both student and instructor resources for this text, including instructor downloads, student quizzing, Web links, suggested online readings, student activities, flashcards, and a comprehensive glossary—as well as other resources, Microsoft® *PowerPoint®* presentations, and more for instructors. You can access the Book Companion Web Site via the Wadsworth Health Web Site.

Health, Fitness, and Wellness Internet Explorer

. . . automatically packaged with the text

0-534-58963-4

This handy trifold contains listings of relevant Web sites related to Health and Fitness and Wellness.

Choose to package access to one of these useful online resources with the text!

Health and Wellness Resource Center
http://www.gale.com/health

Gale's **Health and Wellness Resource Center** is a new comprehensive Web site that provides easy-to-find answers to health questions. It is made up of hundreds of the best medical journals, pamphlets and reference materials available—delivered to your screen via customizable search features.

Opposing Viewpoints Resource Center
http://www.gale.com/OpposingViewpoints

Newly available from Thomson Wadsworth, this online center allows you to expose your students to all sides of today's most compelling issues! The **Opposing Viewpoints Resource Center** draws on Greenhaven Press' acclaimed social issues series, as well as core reference content from other Gale and Macmillan Reference USA sources. The result is a dynamic online library of current event topics—the facts as well as the arguments of each topic's proponents and detractors.

For you and your students...

WebTutor™ ToolBox on WebCT and Blackboard
On WebCT packaged with the text 0-534-59277-5
On Blackboard packaged with the text 0-534-59250-3

WebTutor ToolBox is preloaded with content and available via pincode when packaged with **Invitation to Health, Eleventh Edition**. WebTutor ToolBox pairs all the content of the text's rich Book Companion Web Site with all the sophisticated course management functionality of a WebCT or Blackboard product. You can assign materials (including online quizzes) and have the results flow automatically to your gradebook. Students only have access to student resources on the Web site. Instructors can enter a pincode for access to password-protected Instructor Resources.

For more information, contact your Thomson Wadsworth representative or call 800-423-0563.

Thought-provoking videos launch dynamic lectures!

CNN® Today Video Series
. . . short clips to launch your lectures

Health and Wellness
Volume I 0-534-54625-0
Volume II 0-534-55526-8
Volume III 0-534-57787-3
Volume IV 0-534-63573-3

Fitness and Wellness
Volume I 0-534-58975-8
Volume II 0-534-57838-1

New! CNN Today Video:
Health and Wellness
Volume IV CD-ROM
0-534-64486-4

Launch your lectures with riveting footage from CNN, the world's leading 24-hour global news television network. **CNN Videos** allow you to integrate the newsgathering and programming power of CNN into your classroom to show students the relevance of course topics to their everyday lives.

Wadsworth Health, Fitness, and Wellness Video Library

A comprehensive library of videos! Topics include weight management and fitness, AIDS, sexual communication, peer pressure, compulsive and addictive behaviors, and the relationship between alcohol and violence. Contact your Thomson Wadsworth representative for a detailed list of video options for your course.

Trigger Video Series
Fitness 0-534-36233-8
Stress 0-534-34832-7

Designed to promote or "trigger" classroom discussion on a variety of important topics. These videos contain five 8-10 minute clips, followed by questions for answer or discussion, and material appropriate to the chapters in Hales' text.

Relaxation: A Personal Guide to Stress Management
0-534-58928-6

Covering the causes, symptoms, and effects of stress, this 30-minute video helps students develop lifelong strategies for stress management. Experts explain relaxation techniques and guide students through progressive relaxation, guided imagery, breathing, and physical activity.

Contact your Thomson Wadsworth representative for a detailed list of video options for your course.

Electronic and print resources to help you do what you do best—teach!

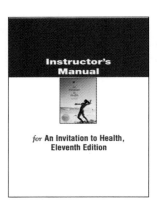

Instructor's Manual
0-534-63565-2

The Instructor's Manual provides chapter outlines, suggested Web sites, classroom activities and teaching strategies, discussion questions, transparency masters and more.

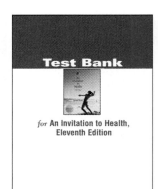

Test Bank
0-534-63562-8

Includes true/false, multiple-choice, short-answer, and essay questions for each chapter of the text. Questions also vary based on level of difficulty. The same questions are available in an electronic format in the ExamView Computerized Testing.

Multimedia Manager CD-ROM for *An Invitation to Health, Eleventh Edition*
0-534-63564-4

This impressive instructor resource is a dual-platform presentation CD-ROM that includes illustrations, photographs, a text-specific Microsoft® *PowerPoint®* slide presentation, as well as electronic versions of our instructional materials such as the Instructor's Manual and Test Bank and digital video from our CNN Today Video Series.

ExamView® Computerized Testing
. . . including online testing!
0-534-63567-9

Create, deliver, and customize tests and study guides (both print and online) in minutes with this easy-to-use assessment and tutorial system. ExamView offers both a *Quick Test Wizard* and an *Online Test Wizard* that guide you step-by step through the process of creating tests.

Transparency Acetates
0-534-63561-X

More than 100 transparency acetates are available with this text, consisting of art from the text as well as supplementary outlines.

Package one of these useful tools with the text!

These resources are FREE when you choose to package one with the text!

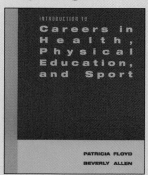

Careers in Health, Physical Education, and Sport
0-534-60785-3
Packaged with the text 0-534-21771-0
This is the essential careers manual for Health, Physical Education, and sport majors interested in pursuing a position in their chosen field of study. It takes them through the complicated process of picking the type of careers they want to pursue, how to prepare for the transition into the working world, and insight to different types of career paths, education requirements, and reasonable salary expectations. The supplement explains the differences in credentials found in the field and testing requirements for certain professions.

Wellness Worksheets
0-534-57788-1
Packaged with the text 0-534-21897-0
Contains additional, detachable self-assessments that students can use to evaluate their own health behaviors and knowledge.

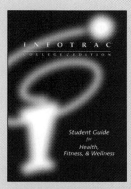

InfoTrac® College Edition Student Guide for Health and Wellness
0-534-24733-4 • Packaged with the text 0-534-21816-4
Unique to Thomson Wadsworth and free to students. This guide provides instructions on ways to use get the most out of InfoTrac® College Edition.

Integrative Medicine: The Mind-Body Connection, Second Edition
0-534-58271-0 • Packaged with the text 0-534-21834-2
by John Janowiak, Appalachian State University
This brief guide explains the relationship between Western medical practice and more traditional therapies, and traces the evolution of integrative medicine. Also provided is a detailed list of Internet resources, a comprehensive list of herbs and their interactions, and more.

Journey to Health Telecourse Guide for *An Invitation to Health, Eleventh Edition*
0-534-63574-1
Packaged with the text 0-534-27616-4
To accompany the "Journey to Health" telecourse produced by DALLAS TeleLearning of the LeCroy Center for Educational Telecommunications. The **Journey to Health** course explores health in its broadest sense. Students are encouraged to use critical thinking and problem solving skills to develop their own healthy lifestyle using the most current information in the health and wellness field. The telecourse components consist of 26 half-hour video programs, the Hales **An Invitation to Health** text, the student telecourse guide, a faculty manual, and text-specific teaching and learning tools, including testing. To learn more about the course, visit http://telelearning.dcccd.edu.

Study Guide
0-534-63563-6
Packaged with the text 0-534-21861-X

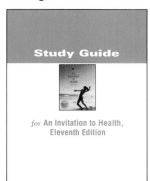

The **Study Guide** is an excellent aid to students' understanding of the text! It contains learning objectives, key terms, chapter review questions, and a detailed practice text for each chapter.

Dianne Hales
MS, Columbia University

Dianne Hales is a successful health, fitness, and wellness author of several higher education textbooks, including **An Invitation to Health, Brief Third Edition,** and **An Invitation to Fitness and Wellness, First Edition**, both published by Thomson Wadsworth.

Dianne is also an accomplished journalist and trade author, having written **Just Like a Woman** (Bantam, 2000), as well as **Caring for the Mind** (Bantam, 1996), and **The Mind Mood Pill Book** (Bantam, 2001). She is a contributing author to **Parade** Magazine and writes regularly for many national publications.

Her success is due in large part to her extensive research into the latest developments in health, fitness, and wellness. Her engaging writing style, vivid examples, and creative pedagogy are highly effective in capturing and keeping students' interest. In her role as a journalist, Dianne interviews leading health, fitness and wellness researchers/experts and incorporates their insights into her textbooks.

Dianne Hales is one of the few journalists to be honored with national awards for excellence in writing by both the *American Psychiatric Association* and the *American Psychological Association*. Her writing awards include an **EMMA** (Exceptional Media Merit Award) for health reporting from the *National Women's Political Caucus* and Radcliffe College.

An

Invitation

to

Health

www.wadsworth.com

wadsworth.com is the World Wide Web site for Wadsworth and is your direct source to dozens of online resources.

At *wadsworth.com* you can find out about supplements, demonstration software, and student resources. You can also send email to many of our authors and preview new publications and exciting new technologies.

wadsworth.com
Changing the way the world learns®

An
Invitation
to
Health

ELEVENTH EDITION

DIANNE HALES

THOMSON
—————
WADSWORTH

Australia • Canada • Mexico • Singapore • Spain
United Kingdom • United States

Publisher: Peter Marshall
Executive Editor: Nedah Rose
Assistant Editor: Andrea Kesterke
Editorial Assistant: Sarah Lowe
Technology Project Manager: Travis Metz
Marketing Manager: Jennifer Somerville
Marketing Assistant: Melanie Banfield
Advertising Project Manager: Shemika Britt
Project Manager, Editorial Production: Sandra Craig
Creative Director: Rob Hugel
Print/Media Buyer: Barbara Britton

Permissions Editor: Joohee Lee
Development Editor: Pat Brewer
Production: The Book Company
Text and Cover Designer: Norman Baugher
Photo Researcher: Myrna Engler
Copy Editor: Heidi Marschner
Illustrator: Hans Neuhart, EIG
Cover Image: Lenz / Zefa
Compositor: Parkwood Composition Service
Printer: Quebecor World / Dubuque

Printed in the United States of America
1 2 3 4 5 6 7 08 07 06 05 04

For more information about our products, contact us at:
Thomson Learning Academic Resource Center
1-800-423-0563
For permission to use material from this text or product, submit a request online at http://www.thomsonrights.com
Any additional questions about permissions can be submitted by email to **thomsonrights@thomson.com**.

Library of Congress Control Number: 2003111918

Student Edition: ISBN 0-534-63558-X

Instructor's Edition: ISBN 0-534-63566-0

Thomson Wadsworth
10 Davis Drive
Belmont, CA 94002-3098
USA

Asia
Thomson Learning
5 Shenton Way #01-01
UIC Building
Singapore 068808

Australia/New Zealand
Thomson Learning
102 Dodds Street
Southbank, Victoria 3006
Australia

Canada
Nelson
1120 Birchmount Road
Toronto, Ontario M1K 5G4
Canada

Europe/Middle East/Africa
Thomson Learning
High Holborn House
50/51 Bedford Row
London WC1R 4LR
United Kingdom

Latin America
Thomson Learning
Seneca, 53
Colonia Polanco
11560 Mexico D.F.
Mexico

Spain/Portugal
Paraninfo
Calle Magallanes, 25
28015 Madrid, Spain

To my husband, Bob,

and my daughter, Julia,

who make every

day an invitation to joy.

BRIEF CONTENTS

CONTENTS

SECTION II
Healthy Lifestyles 101

CHAPTER 4
The Joy of Fitness 102

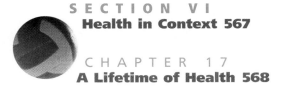

To the Student

This textbook is an invitation to you—an invitation to a healthier, happier, fuller life. Every day you make choices that can affect both how long and how well you live. The knowledge you acquire in this course will help you make better choices, ones that will have a direct impact on how you look, feel, and function—now and for decades to come.

Perhaps you are in good health and think you know all you need to know about how to take care of yourself. If so, take a minute and ask yourself some questions:

:: How well do you understand yourself? Are you able to cope with emotional upsets and crises? Do you often feel stressed out?

:: How nutritiously do you eat? Are you always going on—and off—diets?

:: Do you exercise regularly?

:: How solid and supportive are your relationships with others? Are you conscientious about birth control and safe-sex practices?

:: Do you occasionally get drunk or high? Do you smoke?

:: Are you a savvy health-care consumer? Do you know how to evaluate medical products and health professionals?

:: How much do you know about complementary and alternative medicine?

:: If you need health care, do you know where you'd turn or how you'd pay?

:: What do you know about your risk for infectious diseases, heart problems, cancer, or other serious illnesses?

:: Have you taken steps to ensure your personal safety at home, on campus, and on the streets?

:: What can you do to live a long and healthy life?

:: What are you doing today to prevent physical, psychological, social, and environmental problems in the future?

As you consider these questions, chances are there are some aspects of health you haven't considered before—and others you feel you don't have to worry about for years. Yet the choices you make and the actions you take now will have a dramatic impact on your future.

Your health is your personal responsibility. Over time, your priorities and needs will inevitably change, but the connections between various dimensions of your well-being will remain the same: The state of your mind will affect the state of your body, and vice versa. The values that guide you through today can keep you mentally, physically, and spiritually healthy throughout your lifetime. Your ability to cope with stress will influence your decisions about alcohol and drug use. Your commitment to honest, respectful relationships will affect the nature of your sexual involvements. Your eating and exercise habits will determine whether you develop a host of medical problems.

An Invitation to Health, 11th Edition, is packed with information, advice, recommendations, and research, and provides the first step in taking full charge of your own well-being. An important theme of this book is prevention. Ultimately, the power of prevention belongs to you—and it's a lot easier than you might think. You could simply add a walk or workout to your daily routine. You could snack on fruit instead of high-fat foods. You could cut back on alcohol. You could buckle your seat belt whenever you get in a car. These things may not seem like a big deal now, yet they could make a crucial difference in determining how active and fulfilling the rest of your life will be.

Knowledge alone can't assure you a lifetime of well-being. The rest depends on you. The skills you acquire, the habits you form, the choices you make, the ways you live day by day will all shape your health and your future. You cannot simply read this book and study health the way you study French or chemistry. You must decide to make it part of your daily life.

This is our invitation to you.

—*Dianne Hales*

To the Instructor

The only constant in life is change. The same is true for *An Invitation to Health*. A great deal has changed over the lifetime of this book—in medical research, in the field of health, on college and university campuses, in the nation and the world. What has not changed is the commitment we share to prepare students to make informed, thoughtful choices that will help them live longer, healthier, happier, fuller lives.

For more than twenty years, it has been my privilege to work closely with health educators around the country toward this goal. *An Invitation to Health* contains the insights, perspectives, and wisdom of many people. Each edition has been enriched by what we've learned before. In this eleventh edition, much has changed—but the essentials remain the same.

As I point out to students, health—unlike physics or history—is not a subject that they must memorize and master, but one to be both learned and lived. Often for the first time in their lives, students in a university health class become aware of the importance of personal responsibility for their health and acquire the skills they need to protect their well-being and prevent serious health problems.

By its very nature, health is an interactive course. Every topic of every lecture prompts questions. Every week brings health news that students are eager to discuss and debate. This edition of *An Invitation to Health* offers

even more features designed to intrigue and involve your students. Every chapter begins with a campus-based vignette illustrating the relevance of the material to a student's life. Every chapter incorporates research on col-

lege students or college-age individuals; these findings are highlighted by an icon. In addition, the redesigned "Student Snapshot" feature reports recent data on the health, habits, and concerns of today's college students.

As always, this edition defines health in the broadest sense of the word—not as an entity in itself but as a process of discovering, using, and protecting all possible resources within the individual, family, community, and environment. It presents the most recent, state-of-the-science information on medical research, along with the fundamental background students need to understand and apply these findings. Some chapters, such as those on drugs, alcohol, and infectious diseases have been rewritten to present the latest information and insight into what stu-

dents should know and can do to protect their health. I've also updated and expanded the coverage of diversity in health, which is integrated throughout every chapter and highlighted by another icon.

As I tell students, *An Invitation to Health* can serve as an owner's manual to their bodies and minds. By using this book and taking your course, they can acquire a special type of power—the power to make good decisions, to assume responsibility, and to create and follow a healthy lifestyle. This textbook is our invitation to them to live what they learn and make the most of their health and of their lives.

This textbook also is an invitation to you as an instructor. I invite you to share your passion for education and to enter into a partnership with the editorial team at Wadsworth. We welcome your feedback and suggestions. Please let us hear from you at health.wadsworth.com. I personally look forward to working with you toward our shared goal of preparing a new generation for a healthful future.

◼ Overview of the Eleventh Edition: A Commitment to Change

The keystone of this edition is behavioral change. This new emphasis reflects the growing recognition of the need for improving health behaviors and instructing students in the best ways to make healthy changes both now and in the future.

While every edition of *An Invitation to Health* has included strategies and tools for change, the eleventh edition greatly expands this material. Chapter 1 introduces students to the latest insights into behavioral change, including how people change, the stages of change, and change processes. Every chapter provides practical application of these theories in a new feature, "Your Health Change Plan." Each "Plan" follows the chapter health survey so students can recognize the behaviors they need to change and implement changes successfully. Examples include "Your Health Change Plan for Stress Management" (Chapter 3), "Your Health Change Plan for Responsible Drinking" (Chapter 11), "Your Health Change Plan for Protecting Yourself from Medical Mistakes and Misdeeds" (Chapter 16), and "Your Health Change Plan for Personal Safety on Campus" (Chapter 19).

Although your students may not be aware of it, this textbook works to promote change in indirect as well as direct ways. Simply reading the text and taking a health course can have a significant impact. One reason is what psychologists call the *exposure effect*. The more that individuals see, hear, or read about a topic, the more positively they view it. Because of the sheer quantity of information your students receive in the classroom and in their readings, they will want to heed at least some of the suggestions for change.

Once they do, another law of influence kicks in: the consistency principle. Students begin to see themselves as individuals who have control over their actions and who can change the way they think and behave. Without any conscious effort, their commitment to change grows, and the process of change takes on a momentum of its own.

The eleventh edition includes many other changes in its content and organization. It introduces one new chapter, "A Lifetime of Health" (Chapter 17). Developed in response to reviewer recommendations, this chapter provides in-depth coverage of midlife, theories of aging, the aging brain, challenges of age, preparing for medical crises, near-death experiences, the process of dying, and grief's effects on health.

The entire section on the use, misuse, and abuse of drugs, alcohol, and tobacco has been extensively revised and rewritten to reflect the most recent trends, particularly those affecting college students. In fact, every single chapter has been updated with the most current research, including dozens of citations from 2003. Chapter 5,

"Personal Nutrition," includes the most recent nutritional guidelines from the federal government. Chapter 14, "Keeping Your Heart Healthy," provides the new guidelines on heart risk factors, including information on prehypertension and the stages of hypertension.

In addition to "Your Health Change Plan," new features in this edition include "Fact or Fiction?", included in every chapter, which asks students to respond to a provocative statement about a common health belief or misconception. Also in every chapter are new "Bottom Line" sections which provide a positive summary of practical behavioral changes for students to implement. "Cutting Edge" boxes, which replace the "Genes in Focus" boxes in each section, convey late-breaking reports from all areas of research in health.

In addition, we've retained, updated, and enhanced other popular features, including the chapter "FAQs," "Self-Surveys," "Strategies for Change" / "Strategies for Prevention," "The X & Y Files," "Student Snapshots," and "Savvy Consumer" sections.

Because the health sciences advance so rapidly, all of the chapters have been updated with the most current research, including hundreds of citations published in 2002 and 2003 and incorporating the latest available statistics. The majority come from primary sources, including professional books, medical, health, and mental health journals, health education periodicals, scientific meetings, federal agencies and consensus panels, publications from research laboratories and universities, and personal interviews with specialists in a number of fields. In addition, "Sites & Bytes" presents reliable Internet addresses where students can turn for additional information and a suggested reading from InfoTrac® College Edition, an online library of literally hundreds of academic journals and popular periodicals.

Following is a chapter-by-chapter listing of some of the key topics that have been added, expanded, or revised for the eleventh edition:

Chapter 1: An Invitation to Health

- New section: Can Prayer Heal?
- Totally updated section: Students Health, with new subsections:
  Health Problems on Campus
  Unhealthy Habits
  Risky Behaviors
  Do Healthy Behaviors Have an Effect on Academic Performance?
- Fact or Fiction?
- The Cutting Edge: Into the Future
- Your Health Change Plan: How to Make a Change
- The Bottom Line: Ten Small Changes to Improve Your Health

Chapter 2: Psychological Health

- New section: Could Prayer Be Good Medicine?
- New Self-Survey: The Well-Being Scale
- Your Health Change Plan for Psychological Wellness

- New section: Mental Health on Campus
- Updated section: Depressive Disorders, with a new subsection: Minor Depression
- The Cutting Edge: Magnets for the Brain
- Fact or Fiction?
- Updated Section: Suicide
- The Bottom Line: The Keys to Psychological Wellness

Chapter 3: Personal Stress Management

- Updated section: Stress on Campus
- Updated section: Violence and Terrorism
- Fact or Fiction?
- Your Health Change Plan for Stress Management
- The Bottom Line: De-stress Your Life

Chapter 4: The Joy of Fitness

- New section: The Inactivity Epidemic
- New section: The Campus Couch Potato Crisis
- New Student Snapshot: Campus Couch Potatoes
- New Self-Survey: Are You Ready to Become More Active?
- Your Health Change Plan for Physical Fitness
- New section: The Principles of Exercise
- Completely revised section: How Much Exercise Is Enough?
- New figure on target heart rate
- Borg Rating of Perceived Exertion
- Fact or Fiction?
- The Bottom Line: Fitness for Life

Chapter 5: Personal Nutrition

- New section: Should I Choose Salmon, Steak—or Soy?
- Your Health Change Plan for Better Nutrition
- New section: Does the Pyramid Need Rebuilding?
- New section: Alternative Food Guides
- Fact or Fiction?
- The Cutting Edge: A New Pyramid?
- The Bottom Line: A Lifetime of Healthy Eating

Chapter 6: Eating Patterns and Problems

- New Student Snapshot: Body Dissatisfaction in African-American and White Students
- New section: The Anatomy of Appetite
- New Self-Survey: Are you ready to lose weight?
- Your Health Change Plan for Weight Loss
- Completely revised section: A Practical Guide to Weight Loss
- Fact or Fiction?
- New section: Which Diets Are Safe and Effective?
- The Bottom Line: Healthy Weight Management for Life

Chapter 7: Communication and Relationships

- Your Health Change Plan for Better Communication
- New section: Can Relationships Be Bad for You?
- New Strategies for Change: Coping with Unhealthy Relationships
- Fact or Fiction?
- The Bottom Line: Building Better Relationships

Chapter 8: Personal Sexuality
- Your Health Change Plan for Responsible Sexuality
- New Student Snapshot: Behind Closed Doors on Campus
- New section: Why Don't College Students Practice Safer Sex?
- New X & Y File: The Other Sex
- Fact or Fiction?
- The Bottom Line: Smarter Sex

Chapter 9: Reproductive Choices
- Your Health Change Plan for Choosing a Contraceptive
- New Student Snapshot: Condoms on Campus
- The Cutting Edge: Future Contraceptives
- New section: Essure
- Fact or Fiction?
- The Bottom Line: Reproductive Health

Chapter 10: Drug Use, Misuse, and Abuse
- Your Health Change Plan for Recognizing Substance Abuse
- New section: The Psychology of Vulnerability
- Fact or Fiction?
- New Student Snapshot: Do Students Want Marijuana Legalized?
- New section: Khat
- The Bottom Line: Living Drug-Free

Chapter 11: Alcohol Use, Misuse, and Abuse
- New section: Weight and Waists
- New section: Breast Cancer
- New section: Teen Drinking
- New section: Why do Students Binge?
- Fact or Fiction?
- New Student Snapshot: The Consequences of College Drinking
- New section: Alcohol and Gender
- New X & Y File: Why Men and Women Drink
- Your Health Change Plan for Responsible Drinking
- The Bottom Line: Taking Charge of Your Alcohol Use

Chapter 12: Tobacco Use, Misuse, and Abuse
- Updated section: Health Effects of Cigarette Smoking
- Fact or Fiction?
- Your Health Change Plan for Kicking the Habit
- New Student Snapshot: Smoke-free Housing
- New X & Y File: Which Gender Finds It Harder to Quit?
- New section: "Big Tobacco"
- Updated section: Quitting
- New section: Nicotine Inhaler
- The Cutting Edge: An Anti-Nicotine Vaccine
- The Bottom Line: Living Smoke-Free

Chapter 13: Preventing Infectious Diseases
- New section: Autoimmune Disorders
- New X & Y File: Diseases That Discriminate
- Fact or Fiction?

- New Savvy Consumer: Before You Get a Tattoo
- New section: New Infectious Threats, including new subsections on SARS, Bioterror Infections, Anthrax and Smallpox
- New Student Snapshot: Unsafe Sex on Campus
- New Self-Survey: How Much Do You Know About STIs?
- The Bottom Line: The Best Defense

Chapter 14: Keeping Your Heart Healthy
- Fact or Fiction?
- New Student Snapshot: How Students Rate Their Heart Disease Risk
- Your Health Change Plan for Lowering Heart Disease Risk
- The Cutting Edge: The Big Chill
- The Bottom Line: Heart-Smart Strategies for Life

Chapter 15: Lowering Your Risk of Cancer and Other Major Diseases
- New section: How Cancer Begins
- New X & Y File: 2003 Data on Cancer Cases and Deaths
- Your Health Change Plan for Early Detection of Cancer
- Fact or Fiction?
- Updated sections on diabetes, asthma, and lower back pain
- The Bottom Line: Protecting Yourself from Cancer and Major Illnesses

Chapter 16: Health-Care Consumerism and Complementary/Alternative Medicine
- New section: Health Care and the College Student
- New Student Snapshot: Health Beliefs of Students Born in the USA, China, and India
- Fact or Fiction?
- New section: Evidence-Based Medicine
- Your Health Change Plan for Protecting Yourself from Medical Mistakes and Misdeeds
- New Savvy Consumer: Spotting Health Hoaxes
- New section: Evidence-Based CAM
- The Bottom Line: Taking Charge of Your Health Care

Chapter 17: A Lifetime of Health
- Expanded chapter with coverage of Living in an Aging Society, Successful Aging, The Challenges of Age
- Fact or Fiction?
- The Cutting Edge: Time in a Bottle?
- New Self-Survey: What Is Your Aging IQ?
- Your Health Change Plan for Preparing for a Medical Crisis in an Aging Relative
- New Savvy Consumer: Alternative Treatments for Menopausal Symptoms
- The Bottom Line: Living Long and Well

Chapter 18: Staying Safe: Preventing Injury, Violence, and Victimization
- New Student Snapshot: Risky Driving

- Fact or Fiction?
- New Self-Survey: How Safe Is Your School?
- Your Health Change Plan for Personal Safety on Campus
- Updated section: Sexual Harassment
- The Bottom Line: Helping the Victims of Violence

Chapter 19: Working Toward a Healthy Environment

- Updated section: What Is Global Warming?
- Fact or Fiction?
- Your Health Change Plan for Protecting the Planet
- The Bottom Line: Taking Care of Mother Earth

Features and Pedagogy

Chapter Opening Vignettes engage students with stories and experiences to further stimulate their interest in the chapter content. These practical vignettes mirror the information, advice, and recommendations of the text.

Cutting Edge reports headline-making news from different fields of medical research. Examples include "Magnets for the Brain" (Chapter 2), "A New Pyramid?" (Chapter 5), and "An Anti-Nicotine Vaccine" (Chapter 12).

Fact or Fiction? boxes are designed to highlight controversies and myths about health, engage students' curiosity, and provide accurate information. Among the statements that students must decide are true or not are: "Couples who live together usually get married" (Chapter 9), "Most college students are not engaging in frequent, casual sex" (Chapter 10), and "Echinacea can help fight the common cold" (Chapter 13).

The Bottom Line ends each chapter on a positive, practical note by providing ways in which students can apply what they've learned to their daily lives. Examples include "Healthy Weight Management for Life" (Chapter 6), "Smart Sex" (Chapter 8), and "Living Drug-Free" (Chapter 10).

FAQ—Frequently Asked Questions appear at the beginning of each chapter, immediately engaging students with questions such as "How can I change a bad health habit?" (Chapter 1), "How did we get so fat?" (Chapter 6) and "How sexually active are college students?" (Chapter 8). Page references are included after each question, and each corresponding heading is marked with an icon, signaling that the answer can be found there.

Student Snapshot, a popular feature that appears in every chapter, presents eye-catching data on college populations. Topics include student stress levels, campus couch potatoes, whether students want marijuana legalized, condoms on campus, and the consequences of college drinking. Campus data have been completely revised for this edition.

X & Y Files are found throughout the text and present scientific findings on health-related differences between men and women. Much of this truly ground-breaking research has shattered stereotypes about sex and gender and challenged the traditional assumption that women are essentially smaller, shorter, rounder versions of men. Among the topics covered: differences in nutritional needs; why men and women drink; differences in physical fitness and eating patterns and why women live longer than men.

Self Surveys appear in every chapter and allow students to assess themselves on various aspects of health. Examples: "Is Something Wrong?" (Ch 2), "Stress Scale" (Ch 3), "Are You at Risk for Cancer?" (Ch 15), "Are You a Savvy Medical Consumer?" (Ch 16).

Strategies for Change appear throughout the text and provide practical, checklist-format behavioral change strategies for achieving better health.

Strategies for Prevention appear throughout the text and provide effective, checklist-format strategies for preventing health problems and reducing health risks.

Savvy Consumer focuses on consumer-related health topics and provides guidelines for critical thinking about health care and services. Topics include "Don't Fall for the Muscle Hustle (Chapter 4) and "Before You Get A Tattoo" (Chapter 13).

Sites & Bytes presents engaging and reliable Internet resources. Every chapter includes three websites relevant to chapter topics (along with descriptions of each) and a suggested reading from the InfoTrac College Edition online library—a terrific way to have students research topics on the Internet from *trusted and credible* sources. Moreover, students can go to **http://health.wadsworth.com** to find link updates, over 500 additional health-related links (researched by a health professor), and additional suggested readings on InfoTrac, complete with review/discussion questions.

The Wellness Inventory is a self-inventory at the end of Chapter 1. It allows students to assess and rate their lifestyles in various areas of wellness, providing a useful springboard for deciding which areas they would like to pay special attention to and improve.

Hales Health Almanac appears at the end of the text and includes a full-page Contract for Change; resources related to finding health information on the Internet; a comprehensive, completely updated health directory of contact information for various health organizations; what to do in an emergency; a consumer's guide to medical tests; and tables for counting calories and fat in specific foods.

In addition:

- *Learning Objectives* open each chapter and outline the most essential information for students.
- *Key Terms* are boldfaced when they first appear in the chapter and are listed at the end of each chapter with page references. They are also defined in the Glossary at the end of the book.
- *Integrated Coverage of Diversity* related to race and ethnicity is highlighted with an icon throughout each chapter.
- *Integrated Coverage of Student Research* is highlighted with an icon throughout each chapter.
- *Critical Thinking* questions are included at the end of each chapter and ask the students to consider some

applications of the chapter's coverage, or weigh in on a health-related controversy.

- *CNN Video Discussion Question,* included at the end of each chapter, is designed to work in conjunction with the video of CNN health clips that has been developed with this edition. The CNN health video is complimentary with adoption of this textbook.
- *Making This Chapter Work for You.* This end-of-chapter section both summarizes key content and tests students' understanding and knowledge with multiple-choice questions.

Ancillary Package

Instructor's Manual   The Instructor's Manual provides chapter outlines, learning objectives, classroom handouts, discussion questions, a video list, a resource integration guide, and more.

Test Bank   The test bank for the new edition contains a variety of questions to test students' understanding and comprehension of the text. It contains at least 75 questions per chapter, with 50 multiple-choice questions, 20 fill-in-the-blank questions, and 5 essay questions.

ExamView® Computerized Testing   Create, deliver, and customize the thorough Test Bank in minutes with this easy-to-use assessment and tutorial system. *ExamView* offers both a *Quick Test Wizard* and an *Online Test Wizard* that guide you step-by-step through the process of creating tests, while it allows you to see the test you are creating on the screen exactly as it will print or display online. You can build tests of up to 250 questions using up to 12 question types. Using *ExamView's* complete word-processing capabilities, you can enter an unlimited number of new questions or edit existing questions.

Multimedia Manager for Health, Fitness, and Wellness: A Microsoft® PowerPoint® Link Tool This comprehensive CD-ROM contains more than 100 PowerPoint slides, featuring text art.

Transparency Acetates   More than 100 transparency acetates of art taken from the text enhance lectures and provide visual support in the classroom.

WebTutor™ Toolbox   *WebTutor Toolbox's* text-specific content allows instructors to create and manage a personal website! *WebTutor Toolbox's* course management tool gives you the ability to provide virtual office hours, post syllabi, set up threaded discussions, track student progress with the quizzing material, and much more. For students, *WebTutor Toolbox* offers real-time access to a full array of study tools, including chapter outlines, summaries, learning objectives, glossary flashcards (with audio), practice quizzes, web links, *InfoTrac® College Edition* exercises, animations, and videos.

Study Guide   The Study Guide is an excellent aid to the student's understanding of the text. It contains learning objectives, key terms, chapter review questions, and a detailed practice test for each chapter.

InfoTrac College Edition Student Guide for Health   This 24-page booklet offers detailed guidance for students on how to use the *InfoTrac® College Edition* database. Includes log-in help, a complete search tips "cheat sheet," and a topic list of key word search terms for health, fitness, and wellness. Available FREE when packaged with the text. The text also features InfoTrac Activities for each chapter that challenge the student to critically read articles and studies relating to key topics in the chapters. These activities help guide students through the vast database and answer questions relating to specific articles.

Telecourse Study Guide   For use with the Dallas County Community College Telecourse, the telecourse guide contains a brief summary of each lesson, followed by learning objectives, study assignments for the text and video, key terms, a list of the experts interviewed with their affiliations, video focus points, individual health plan assignments, enrichment opportunities, and practice tests with page-referenced answers.

Health, Fitness, and Wellness Internet Explorer A handy full-color trifold brochure contains dozens of useful health, fitness, and wellness Internet links.

Personal Daily Log   The Personal Daily Log contains an exercise pyramid, study and exercise tips, a goal setting worksheet, cardiorespiratory exercise record form, strength training record form, a daily nutrition diary, helpful Internet links, and more.

Wellness Worksheets   These detachable self-assessments and wellness worksheets are handy, easy to use, and make a terrific bundle item.

Careers in Health, Physical Education, and Sport   This is the essential manual for majors who are interested in pursuing a position in their chosen field. It guides them through the complicated process of picking the type of career they want to pursue, suggests how to prepare for the transition into the working world, and offers information about different career paths, education requirements, and reasonable salary expectations. The supplement also describes the differences in credentials found in the field and testing requirements for certain professions.

Integrative Medicine: The Mind-Body Prescription   This interesting supplement, written by Dr. John Janowiak from Appalachian State University, explains the relationship between Western medical practice and more traditional therapies. The supplement explains the evolution of integrative medicine, provides a detailed list of Internet resources, a comprehensive list of herbs and their interactions, and more.

Profile Plus 2005   The most comprehensive software pack available with any health textbook, *Profile Plus* allows students to generate personalized fitness and wellness profiles, conduct self-assessments, analyze their diets, tailor exercise prescriptions to their individual needs, keep an exercise log, and much more.

Diet Analysis 6.0   This unique assessment tool provides students with experience in the estimation and analysis of dietary patterns and practices. It allows students to track their food intake for up to seven days and to create a personal dietary profile based on height, weight, age, gender, and activity level. *Diet Analysis Plus* calculates Dietary Reference Intakes, goal percentages, and actual percentages of essential nutrients, vitamins, and minerals. Comprehensive dietary data is displayed in attractive, easy-to-read reports that enhance learning. Students can view data as a bar graph or spreadsheet, in Food Pyramid form, or as a Nutrition Fact Panel Report. They can then identify dietary habits, correct nutritional deficiencies, and truly appreciate the impact of nutrient dense foods.

http://health.wadsworth.com   When you adopt *An Invitation to Health,* Eleventh Edition, you and your students will have access to a rich array of teaching and learning resources that you won't find anywhere else. This outstanding site features both student resources for the text, including quizzes, web links, suggested online readings, and discussion forums, and instructor resources, including downloadable supplementary resources and multimedia presentation slides. You will also find an online catalog of Wadsworth's health, fitness, wellness, and physical education books and supplements.

CNN Today: Health and Wellness Video, Volumes I, II and III.   A Wadsworth exclusive—updated yearly!

An exclusive agreement between Wadsworth Group and Turner Learning! Launch your lectures with riveting footage from CNN, the world's leading 24-hour global news television network. The *CNN Today: Health and Wellness* videos allow you to integrate the newsgathering and programming power of CNN into the classroom to show students the relevance of course topics to their everyday lives. The videos include news clips correlated directly with the Hales text and cover such topics as the role of vegetables in cancer prevention, abuse of Ritalin on college campuses, gambling addiction, and stress and the immune system.

Relaxation: A Guide to Personal Stress Management   This 30-minute video shows students how to manage their stress and what is a healthy stress level in their life. Experts explain relaxation techniques and guide the student through progressive relaxation, guided imagery, breathing, and physical activity.

Trigger Video Series: Fitness   This 60-minute video focuses on changing concepts of fitness, contains five 8–10 minute clips followed by questions for answer or discussion, and material appropriate to the fitness chapters in the text.

Trigger Video Series: Stress   This 60-minute video focuses on stress, contains five 8–10 minute clips followed by questions for answer or discussion, and material appropriate to the text chapters concerning stress and its positive and negative effects on health.

◼ Acknowledgments

Eleven editions of a textbook mean hundreds of contributors to thank. I remain deeply indebted to all the instructors, students, reviewers, editors, artists, and others who have made this project so successful and so satisfying for so long. I have learned a great deal from all of you, and I am grateful.

One of the joys of writing *An Invitation to Health* is the opportunity to work with a team I consider the very best of the best in textbook publishing. Pete Marshall once again brought full enthusiasm, creativity, and support to this edition. April Lemons, the former health editor, imbued it with her characteristic vision and insight. Nedah Rose, the new health editor, picked up the baton and ran with it. Never for a moment did I doubt that *Invitation* would be in very good hands.

My deepest thanks go to Pat Brewer, the developmental editor on this edition, whose contributions always extend far beyond the demands of duty. I consider her a partner, co-conspirator, and friend. Once again I have come to think of Dusty Friedman of The Book Company as a worker of miracles and other marvels. Sandra Craig, Project Manager, Editorial Production of Wadsworth, has guided us all with wisdom and unfailing professionalism.

My thanks extend to Jennifer Somerville, Marketing Manager, for her enthusiastic support, to Shemika Britt for her work on the promotional materials, and to Andrea Kesterke, who guides the ancillaries. Thanks also to Norman Baugher for our new design and cover and Hans Neuhart for art and to Myrna Engler, for her work on photos and permissions.

To one and all I extend my appreciation and admiration. Finally, I would like to thank the reviewers whose input has been so valuable through these many editions. For the eleventh edition, I thank, the following for their comments and helpful assistance:

Peggy L. Chin, University of Connecticut
Melinda K. Everman, The Ohio State University
Terri Langford, University of Central Florida
David G. Lorenzi, West Liberty State College
Jerry Mayo, Hendrix College
John W. Munson, University of Wisconsin—Stevens Point
Pamela Rost, Buffalo State College
Behjat Sharif, California State University—Los Angeles
Martin L. Wood, Ball State University

For their help as reviewers or focus group participants from previous editions, I want to thank the following:

Ghulam Aasef, Kaskaskia College
Andrea Abercrombie, Clemson University
Judy Baker, East Carolina University
Marcia Ball, James Madison University
Jeremy Barnes, Southeast Missouri State University
Rick Barnes, East Carolina University
Lois Beach, SUNY-Plattsburg
Betsy Bergen, Kansas State University
Nancy Bessette, Saddleback College
Carol Biddington, California University of Pennsylvania
David Black, Purdue University

Jill M. Black, Cleveland State University
Cynthia Pike Blocksom, Cincinnati Health Department
James Brik, Willamette University
Mitchell Brodsky, York College
Jodi Broodkins-Fisher, University of Utah
James G. Bryant, Jr., Western Carolina University
Marsha Campos, Modesto Junior College
Richard Capriccioso, University of Phoenix
James Lester Carter, Montana State University
Patti Cost, Weber State University
Maxine Davis, Eastern Washington University
Lori Dewald, Shippensburg University of Pennsylvania
Julie Dietz, Eastern Illinois University
Robert Dollinger, Florida International University
Gary English, Ithaca College
Michael Felts, East Carolina University
Kathie C. Garbe, Kennesaw State College
Gail Gates, Oklahoma State University
Dawn Graff-Haight, Portland State University
Carolyn Gray, New Mexico State University
Mary Gress, Lorain County Community College
Janet Grochowski, University of St. Thomas
Stephen Haynie, College of William and Mary
Ron Heinrichs, Central Missouri State University
Michael Hoadley University of South Dakota
Harold Horne, University of Illinois at Springfield
Linda L. Howard, Idaho State University
Kim Hyatt, Weber State University
Dee Jacobsen, Southeastern Louisiana University
John Janowiak, Appalachian State University
Peggy Jarnigan, Rollins College
Jim Johnson, Northwest Missouri State University
Chester S. Jones, University of Arkansas
Herb Jones, Ball State University
Jane Jones, University of Wisconsin, Stevens Point
Lorraine J. Jones, Muncie, Indiana
Becky Kennedy-Koch, Ohio State University
Mark J. Kittleson, Southern Illinois University
Darlene Kluka, University of Central Oklahoma
Debra A. Krummel, West Virginia University
Roland Lamarine, California State University, Chico
David Langford, University of Maryland, Baltimore County
Beth Lanning, Baylor University
Norbert Lindskog, Harold Washington College
Loretta Liptak, Youngstown State University
S. Jack Loughton, Weber State University
Rick Madson, Palm Beach Community College
Ashok Malik, College of San Mateo
Michele P. Mannion, Temple University
Jessica Middlebrooks, University of Georgia
Esther Moe, Oregon Health Sciences University
Kris Moline, Lourdes College
Richard Morris, Rollins College
Anne O'Donnell, Santa Rosa Junior College
Randy M. Page, University of Idaho

Carolyn P. Parks, University of North Carolina
Anthony V. Parrillo, East Carolina University
Miguel Perez, University of North Texas
Pamela Pinahs-Schultz, Carroll College
Rosanne Poole, Tallahassee Community College
Janet Reis, University of Illinois at Urbana-Champaign
Sadie Sanders, University of Florida
Steven Sansone, Chemeketa Community College
Debra Secord, Coastline College
Andrew Shim, Southwestern College
Steve Singleton, Wayne State University
Larry Smith, Scottsdale Community College
Teresa Snow, Georgia Institute of Technology
Carl A. Stockton, Radford University
Linda Stonecipher, Western Oregon State College
Emogene Johnson Vaughn, Norfolk State University
David M. White, East Carolina University
Sabina White, University of California—Santa Barbara
Robert Wilson, University of Minnesota
Roy Wohl, Washburn University
Martin L. Wood, Ball State University

About the Author

Dianne Hales, a contributing editor for *Parade,* has written more than 2,000 articles for national publications. Her trade books include *Just Like a Woman: How Gender Science Is Redefining What Makes Us Female* and the award-winning compendium of mental health information, *Caring for the Mind: The Comprehensive Guide to Mental Health.* Dianne Hales is one of the few journalists to be honored with national awards for excellence in magazine writing by both the American Psychiatric Association and the American Psychological Association. She also has won the EMMA (Exceptional Media Merit Award) for health reporting from the National Women's Political Caucus and Radcliffe College, and numerous writing awards from various organizations, including the Arthritis Foundation, California Psychiatric Society, CHAAD (Children and Adults with Attention-Deficit Disorders), Council for the Advancement of Scientific Education, National Easter Seal Society, and the New York City Public Library.

SECTION I

TAKING CHARGE OF YOUR HEALTH

HEALTH may be a science; living is an art. The principles that can help you understand the science and practice the art are simple and timeless and form the basic premise of this book: You have more control over your life and well-being than does anything or anyone else. Through the decisions you make and the habits you develop, you can influence how well—and perhaps how long—you will live. This section defines health and wellness and provides the information you need to take charge of your well-being now and in the years to come.

© Gary Buss/Taxi/Getty Images

1

An Invitation to Health for the Twenty-First Century

How are you?" You may hear that question dozens of times each day. "Fine," you answer, without thinking. But how often do you ask yourself how you *really* are? How do you feel about yourself and your life? Are you under pressure to get good grades? Are you eating well and exercising regularly? Do you have close friends with whom to share your triumphs and traumas? If you choose to be sexually active, what do you do to prevent unwanted pregnancy or sexually transmitted illnesses? Do you smoke or use drugs? How much do you drink? Are you taking steps to prevent major illnesses? Do you get regular health check-ups? Are you aware of safety and environmental threats to your health? How are you going to make the most of your life? What do you hope to accomplish before you die?

This book asks these questions and many more. It is a book about you: your mind and your body, your spirit and your social ties, your needs and your wants, your past and your potential. It will help you explore options, discover possibilities, and find new ways to make your life worthwhile.

This book is also about living in a human body, thinking with a human mind, responding to a world of ideas and experiences with a human spirit. You are designed to move, to think, to act—to stretch yourself in every way. If you don't make the most of what you are, you risk never discovering what you might become.

Health involves more than physical well-being. It is a state of body, mind, and spirit that must be viewed within the context of community, society, and environment.

By providing the information and understanding you need to take care of your own health, *An Invitation to Health* can help you live more fully, more happily, and more healthfully. It also goes beyond the basis of health maintenance. Its primary themes—prevention of health problems, protection from health threats, and promotion of the health of others—can establish the basis for good health now and in the future.

The invitation to health that we extend to every reader is one offer you literally cannot afford to refuse: The quality of your life depends on it.

© Zephyr Picture/Index Stock Imagery

After studying the material in this chapter, you should be able to:

- **Identify and describe** the components of health and how they relate to total wellness.
- **Describe** how gender, race, and ethnicity can influence health and access to health care.

- **List** the factors that influence the development of health behaviors.
- **Discuss** the principles and goals of prevention, and **differentiate** prevention from protection.
- **Create** a complete plan to change or develop a health behavior.

✴ Health and Wellness

By simplest definition, **health** means being sound in body, mind, and spirit. The World Health Organization defines health as "not merely the absence of disease or infirmity," but "a state of complete physical, mental, and social well-being."[1] Health is the process of discovering, using, and protecting all the resources within our bodies, minds, spirits, families, communities, and environment.

Health has many components: physical, psychological, spiritual, social, intellectual, and environmental. This book takes a *holistic* approach, one that looks at health and the individual as a whole, rather than part by part. Your own definition of health may include different elements, but chances are you and your classmates agree that it includes at least some of the following:

:: A positive, optimistic outlook.

:: A sense of control over stress and worries; time to relax.

:: Energy and vitality; freedom from pain or serious illness.

:: Supportive friends and family, and a nurturing intimate relationship with someone you love.

:: A personally satisfying job.

:: A clean environment.

Wellness can be defined as purposeful, enjoyable living or, more specifically, a deliberate lifestyle choice characterized by personal responsibility and optimal enhancement of physical, mental, and spiritual health. Wellness means more than not being sick; it means taking steps to prevent illness and to lead a richer, more balanced, and more satisfying life.

Although physical well-being is essential to health, the term *wellness,* as used by health professionals, has a broader meaning. To understand how the concepts of wellness and health fit together, think of an automobile transmission: Having a disease (illness) is like being in reverse; absence of disease (health) puts you in neutral; positive health changes (wellness) push you into forward motion. When your entire lifestyle is based on health-enhancing behaviors, you're in high gear and going at top speed—and you've achieved total wellness.

Health is the process of discovering, using, and protecting all the resources within our bodies, minds, spirits, families, communities, and environment.

John Travis, M.D., has created a Wellness Inventory for you to assess yourself in 12 areas—we will come back to the Wellness Wheel when we talk about changing behaviors later in the chapter. Dr. Travis compares the various levels of wellness to an iceberg (see Figure 1-1). Only about one-tenth of the mass of an iceberg is visible—the rest is submerged. Your current state of health is like the tip of the iceberg, the part that shows.

"To understand all that creates and supports your current state of health," says Travis, "you have to look 'underwater.'" The first hidden level—the "lifestyle/behavioral" level—consists of what you eat, how active you are, how you manage stress, and how you protect yourself from hazards. Below this level is the "cultural/psychological/motivational" level, the often invisible influences that lead us to choose a certain lifestyle. The foundation of the iceberg is the "spiritual/being/meaning" realm, which encompasses issues such as your reason for being, the meaning of your life, and your place in the universe. "Ultimately," says Travis, "this realm determines whether the tip of the iceberg, representing your state of health, is one of disease or wellness."[2]

In wellness, health, and sickness, there is considerable overlap of the functions of the mind, body, and spirit. As scientists have shown again and again in recent decades, psychological factors play a major role in enhancing physical well-being and preventing illness, but they can also trigger, worsen, or prolong physical symptoms. Similarly, almost every medical illness affects people psychologically as well as physically.

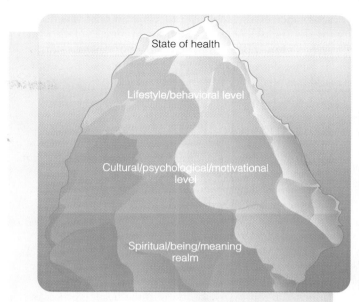

Figure 1-1 ICEBERG MODEL OF WELLNESS

Like an iceberg, only a small part of your total wellness is visible: your current state of health. Just as important are hidden dimensions, including lifestyle habits, cultural and psychological factors, and the realm of spiritual meaning and being.

Source: Reprinted with permission, Wellness Workbook, Travis & Ryan, Ten Speed Press, Berkeley, CA. © 1981, 1988 by John W. Travis, M.D. <www.thewellspring.com>

Physical Health

The various states of good and ill physical health can be viewed as points on a continuum (see Figure 1-2). At one end is early and needless death; at the other is optimal wellness, in which you feel and perform at your very best. In the middle, individuals are neither sick enough to need medical attention nor well enough to live each day with zest and vigor. For the sake of optimal physical health, we must take positive steps away from illness and toward well-being. We must feed our bodies nutritiously, exercise them regularly, avoid harmful behaviors and substances, watch out for early signs of sickness, and protect ourselves from accidents.

Psychological Health

Like physical well-being, psychological health is more than the absence of problems or illness. Psychological health refers to both our emotional and mental states—that is, to our feelings and our thoughts. It involves awareness and

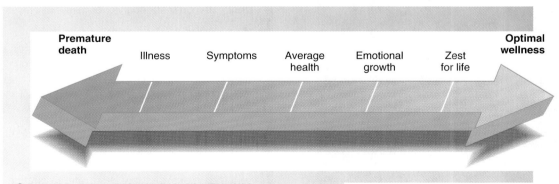

Figure 1-2 WELLNESS-ILLNESS CONTINUUM

acceptance of a wide range of feelings in oneself and others, the ability to express emotions, to function independently, and to cope with the challenges of daily stressors. (Chapter 2 provides more information on psychological health.)

Spiritual Health

Spiritually healthy individuals identify their own basic purpose in life; learn how to experience love, joy, peace, and fulfillment; and help themselves and others achieve their full potential. As they devote themselves to others' needs more than their own, their spiritual development produces a sense of greater meaning in their lives.

Prayer, a spiritual practice of millions, is the most commonly used form of complementary and alternative medicine. However, only in recent years has science launched rigorous investigations of the healing power of prayer. Dr. Dale Matthews of Georgetown University, author of *The Faith Factor,* estimates that about 75 percent of studies of spirituality have confirmed health benefits.[3]

Can Prayer Heal?

In dozens of studies, even when age, health, habits, demographics and other factors are considered, individuals who pray regularly and attend religious services stay healthier and live longer than those who rarely or never do.[4] Petitionary prayer—praying directly to a higher power—affects both the quality and quantity of life, says Dr. Harold Koenig, director of Duke University's Center for the Study of Religion/Spirituality and Health. "It boosts morale, lowers agitation, loneliness, and life dissatisfaction and enhances ability to cope in men, women, the elderly, the young, the healthy, and the sick."[5]

People who pray regularly have significantly lower blood pressure and stronger immune systems than the less religious, says Dr. Koenig. They're also less prone to alcoholism, less likely to smoke heavily, and are hospitalized less often. Studies at several medical centers have shown that prayer and faith speed recovery from depression, alcoholism, hip surgery, drug addiction, stroke, rheumatoid arthritis, heart attacks, and bypass surgery.[6] Science cannot explain the physiological mechanisms for what happens in human beings when they pray, but in cultures around the world throughout recorded history when people or their loved ones are sick, they pray.

Scientists also are trying to determine the impact of prayer for others—called "intercessory prayer" or distant healing. At nine medical centers around the country, 750 patients with potentially life-threatening heart problems are participating in the Mantra project. The names of half have been given to prayer groups around the world—including Carmelite nuns, Buddhist monks, and Evangelical congregations—who pray for their recovery. The final results will show if others' prayers reduce symptoms and lower the risk of heart attacks and other complications.

Findings from earlier intercessory prayer investigations have been mixed. In two studies—in San Francisco and in Kansas City—patients in coronary care units who were prayed for by strangers had lower complication rates. But a similar study at the Mayo Clinic found "no significant effect on medical outcomes," including death and compli-

Prayer provides physical health benefits as well as spiritual health benefits.

© SW Production/Index Stock Imagery

STRATEGIES FOR CHANGE

Enhancing Spiritual Health

If you are religious
Deepen your spiritual commitment through prayer, more frequent church attendance, or joining a prayer group.

If you are not religious
Keep an open mind about the value of religion or spirituality. Consider visiting a church or synagogue. Read the writings of inspired people of deep faith, such as Rabbi Harold Kushner and Rev. Martin Luther King.

If you are not ready to consider religion
Try nonreligious meditation or relaxation training. In decades of research, Dr. Herbert Benson of Harvard University has shown that focusing the mind on a single sound or image can slow heart rate, respiration, and brain waves; relax muscles; and lower stress-rated hormones—responses similar to those induced by prayer. (See Chapter 3.)

cations. A review of 23 studies concluded only that "the evidence thus far merits further study."

Will science ever be able to prove the power of prayer? No one is certain. "While I personally believe that God heals people in supernatural ways, I don't think science can shape a study to prove it," says Duke's Dr. Koenig. "But we now know enough, based on solid scientific research, to recommend prayer, much like exercise and diet, as one of the best and most cost-effective ways of protecting and enhancing health."

Social Health

Social health refers to the ability to interact effectively with other people and the social environment, to develop satisfying interpersonal relationships, and to fulfill social roles. It involves participating in and contributing to your community, living in harmony with fellow human beings, developing positive interdependent relationships with others (discussed in Chapter 7), and practicing healthy sexual behaviors.

In times of crisis, social connections provide comfort and support. Even in tranquil times, social isolation increases the risk of sickness and mortality. In a landmark study of 4,725 men and women in Alameda County, California, death rates were twice as high for loners as for those with strong social ties. In other studies, social isolation greatly increased the risk of dying of a heart attack. Heart attack patients have a better chance of long-term survival if they believe they have adequate help in performing daily tasks from family and friends. People with spouses, friends, and a rich social network may outlive isolated loners by as much as 30 years.

Health educators are placing greater emphasis on social health in its broadest sense as they expand the tradi-

Humans are social beings, and social interactions enhance good health.

tional individualistic concept of health to include the complex interrelationships between one person's health and the health of the community and environment. This change in perspective has given rise to a new emphasis on **health promotion** (discussed later in this chapter), which enhances health by building knowledge and skills among individuals and modifying their environment to foster healthier lifestyles.

Intellectual Health

Your brain is the only one of your organs capable of self-awareness. Every day you use your mind to gather, process, and act on information; to think through your values; to make decisions, set goals, and figure out how to handle a problem or challenge. Intellectual health refers to your ability to think and learn from life experience, your openness to new ideas, and your capacity to question and evaluate information. Throughout your life, you'll use your critical thinking skills, including your ability to evaluate health information, to safeguard your well-being.

Environmental Health

You live in a physical and social setting that can affect every aspect of your health. Environmental health refers to the impact your world has on your well-being. It means protecting yourself from dangers in the air, water, and soil, and in products you use—and also working to preserve the environment itself. (Chapter 19 offers a thorough discussion of environmental health.)

The State of Our Health

Americans are living longer and healthier lives than ever before in history. Life expectancy has reached a new high of 77.2 years, increasing for both men and women and blacks and whites. The gender gap between male and female life expectancies has narrowed to 5.4 years.[7] The age-adjusted death rate has hit an all-time low of 855 deaths per 100,000 people, with declines in mortality from stroke, heart disease, cancer, and accidents.[8]

Yet, as discussed in Chapter 16, other developed nations outrank the United States on various measures of well-being, including lower infant mortality rates and even longer life expectancies. This is not the case throughout the world, where major risk factors, such as malnutrition, poor water, and inadequate sanitation, endanger the lives of millions.[9]

 Both the developed and developing world share one common health risk: obesity. For the first time in history, more than half of the people on the planet—seven in ten of the Dutch and Spanish, two in three Americans and Canadians, and one in two Britons, Germans, and Italians—are overweight or obese. According to the International Obesity Task Force, more than 115 million people in developing countries suffer from obesity-related problems.[10] Other global threats include smoking, sexually transmitted infections (STIs), and new agents of infection, such as the deadly SARS virus (discussed in Chapter 13).

Many factors can and do affect health, including genetics, race, education, and socioeconomic status. One long ignored by medical science is whether a person is male or female. As discussed in "The X&Y File" on page 9, biological sex determines different risk factors for certain health conditions, diseases, or treatments, while gender influences different exposures to certain risks and different treatment-seeking patterns. For example, more women develop melanoma, a potentially fatal skin cancer, but more men die of melanoma. Women's thinner, fairer skin—a sex-related difference—may increase their risk from sun exposure, but men may have higher mortality rates because of gender differences in behaviors such as willingness to wear sunscreen and reluctance to seek medical attention.[11]

Healthy People 2010

Healthy People 2010 is the prevention agenda for the nation. Every decade the federal government identifies the most significant preventable threats to health and creates leading indicators that assess the health of Americans. Its first goal is to help individuals of all ages increase life expectancy *and* improve their quality of life. Its second goal is to eliminate health disparities among different segments of the population.

Among the specific goals of Healthy People 2010 are:

:: **Reduce the prevalence of cigarette smoking** among adults to 12 percent from the current 23.4 percent.

:: **Reduce the number of new cancer cases** as well as the illnesses, disability, and death caused by cancer.

:: **Promote the health of people with disabilities,** prevent secondary conditions, and eliminate disparities between people with and without disabilities in the U.S. population.

:: **Reduce foodborne illnesses.**

:: **Reduce the proportion of obese children and adolescents** from 11 percent to 5 percent.

:: **Reduce the number of adolescents and adults** using illegal substances.

:: **Reduce the number of adults** engaging in binge drinking.[12]

Diversity and Health

We live in the most diverse nation on Earth, one that is becoming increasingly diverse. For society, this variety can be both enriching and divisive. Tolerance and acceptance of others have always been part of the American creed. By working together, Americans have created a country that remains, to those outside our borders, a symbol of opportunity. Yet members of different ethnic groups still have to struggle against discrimination.

Today, in this country's third century, all Americans still aren't equal in their access to health care. Poverty remains a major barrier to quality health care for minorities. Without adequate insurance or the ability to pay, many cannot afford the tests and treatments that could prevent illness or overcome it at the earliest possible stages.

As public health experts explore the links between race, culture, and health, they are moving beyond any narrow definition of *minority* to the broader concept of *underserved,* a group made up of many cultures that also includes the homeless, rural Americans, and women. Special problems also exist for illegal immigrants, who often live in extreme poverty; perform difficult, hazardous jobs; and have little or no access to health services. Even when they desperately need medical care, they may be so fearful of deportation that they do not seek help.

Diversity poses special challenges in health care. Racial and ethnic minority communities have a disproportionately high burden of disability from inadequately treated mental health problems and illnesses.[13] In some cultures, physicians are seen as less effective than other healers, who are believed to cure illness caused by bad karma or evil spirits. American physicians, trained to believe that high-tech medicine is best, may not understand or appreciate traditional healing practices. In many communities, innovative programs have begun to educate patients from other cultures about the American health-care system, as well as to educate American health-care providers about the beliefs and health practices of their diverse patients.

✒ Can Race Affect Health?

Different racial and ethnic groups often face different health risks. Consider the following statistics:

:: The infant mortality rate for African-American babies remains higher than for white babies.

:: Life expectancy for African Americans, though increasing, is six years lower than for whites.

:: African Americans have higher rates of high blood pressure (hypertension), develop this problem earlier in life, suffer more severe hypertension, and have higher rates of strokes and hypertension-related deaths than whites. Cardiovascular risk is higher in minority than white youth.

the X & Y file   *Do Sex and Gender Matter?*

"Sex does matter. It matters in ways that we did not expect. Undoubtedly, it also matters in ways that we have not begun to imagine." This was the conclusion of the Institute of Medicine Committee on Understanding the Biology of Sex and Gender Differences in the first significant review of the status of sex and gender differences in biomedical research.

Sex, the committee stated, is "a classification, generally as male or female, according to the reproductive organs and functions that derive from the chromosomal complement." *Gender* refers to "a person's self-representation as male or female, or how that person is responded to by social institutions on the basis of the individual's gender presentation." Rooted in biology, gender is shaped by environment and experience.

In animals other than humans, sex alone influences the prevalence and severity of a broad range of diseases, disorders, and conditions. In human beings, gender also matters. The experience of being male or female in a par-

ticular culture and society can and does have an effect on physical and psychological well-being. In fact, sex and gender may have a greater impact than any other variable on how our bodies function, how long we live, and the symptoms, course, and treatment of the diseases that strike us.

This realization is both new and revolutionary. For centuries, scientists based biological theories solely on a male model and viewed women as shorter, smaller, and rounder versions of men. Even modern medicine is based on the assumption that, except for their reproductive organs, both sexes are biologically interchangeable. We now know that this simply isn't so. Sex begins in the womb, but sex and gender differences affect behavior, perception, and health throughout life.

Recognition of these gender differences is transforming medical research and practice. A new science called *gender-specific medicine* is replacing one-size-fits-all health care with new definitions of what is normal in both men and women, more complex concepts of disease, more precise diagnostic tests, and more effective treatments.

He:

- averages 12 breaths a minute
- has lower core body temperature
- has a slower heart rate
- has more oxygen-rich hemoglobin in his blood
- is more sensitive to sound
- produces twice as much saliva
- has a 10 percent larger brain
- is 10 times more likely to have attention deficit disorder
- as a teen, has an attention span of 5 minutes
- is more likely to be physically active
- is more prone to lethal diseases, including heart attacks, cancer, and liver failure
- is five times more likely to become an alcoholic
- has a life expectancy of 74.4 years

She:

- averages 9 breaths a minute
- has higher core body temperature
- has a faster heart rate
- has higher levels of protective immunoglobulin in her blood
- is more sensitive to light
- takes twice as long to process food
- has more neurons in certain brain regions
- is twice as likely to have an eating disorder
- as a teen, has an attention span of 20 minutes
- is more likely to be overweight
- is more vulnerable to chronic diseases, like arthritis and autoimmune disorders, and age-related conditions like osteoporosis
- is twice as likely to develop depression
- has a life expectancy of 77.2 years

:: African Americans have higher rates of glaucoma, systemic lupus erythematosus, liver disease, and kidney failure than whites.

:: The death rate for heart disease among middle-aged black women is 150 percent higher than among white

women the same age. Among those with diabetes, the death rate is 134 percent higher than for white female diabetics.

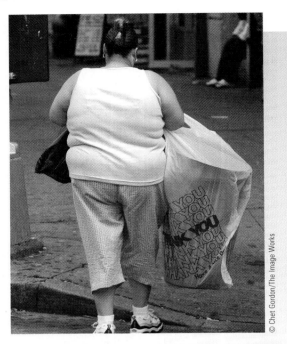

Both genetic and environmental factors have contributed to the increase in diabetes among the Pima tribe. Half of all Pima adults have diabetes.

:: Of all black women diagnosed with breast cancer, 37 percent are younger than 50—compared with 22 percent of white women.

:: Women of Filipino, Hawaiian, Indian-Pakistani, Mexican, South and Central American, and Puerto Rican descent are 20 to 260 percent more likely to be diagnosed with late-stage breast cancer than white women.[14]

:: Caucasians are prone to osteoporosis (progressive weakening of bone tissue); cystic fibrosis; skin cancer; and phenylketonuria (PKU), a metabolic disorder that can lead to mental retardation.

:: Women with Chinese or Hispanic backgrounds face a significantly greater risk of developing diabetes during pregnancy than African Americans or whites.

:: Asians and Asian Americans metabolize some medications faster than whites and thus require much smaller doses.

:: Hispanics have higher rates of death from diabetes and infectious and parasitic diseases than African Americans or whites.

:: Native Americans have the highest rate of diabetes in the world. Among the Pima Indians, half of all adults have diabetes.

:: Native Hawaiian women have a higher rate of breast cancer than women from other racial and ethnic groups.

:: Native Americans, including those indigenous to Alaska, are more likely to die young than the population as a whole, primarily as a result of accidental injuries, cirrhosis of the liver, homicide, pneumonia, and the complications of diabetes.[15]

:: The suicide rate among American Indians and Alaska natives is 50 percent higher than the national rate. The rates of co-occurring mental illness and substance abuse (especially alcohol) are also higher among Native American youth and adults.[16]

:: Disproportionate numbers of African Americans are among the groups most vulnerable to mental illness: the homeless, the incarcerated, those in the child welfare system, and the victims of trauma.

Are these increased susceptibilities the result of genetics, an unhealthy lifestyle, lack of access to health services, poverty or the stress of living with discrimination? It is hard to say precisely. Certainly, poverty presents a major barrier to seeking preventive care and getting timely and effective treatment.

In some cases, both genetic and environmental factors may play a role. Take, for example, the high rates of diabetes among the Pima Indians. Until 50 years ago, these Native Americans were not notably obese or prone to diabetes. After World War II, the tribe started trading handmade baskets for lard and flour. Their lifestyle became more sedentary, and their diet, higher in fats. In addition, researchers have discovered that many Pima Indians have an inherited resistance to insulin that increases their susceptibility to diabetes. The combination of a hereditary predisposition and environmental factors may explain why the Pimas now have epidemic levels of diabetes.

Health-care providers often fail to recognize racial health risks, in part because the discussion of ethnicity in health is politically controversial. Yet recognition of different health needs and risks is the first step toward overcoming the health problems of many Americans.

Closing the Minority Health Gap

In the words of a National Institutes of Health (NIH) report, minorities have carried "an unequal burden with respect to disease and disability, resulting in a lower life expectancy." Each year minorities in the United States—African Americans, Hispanics, Asian Americans, Pacific Islanders, Native Americans, and other groups—experience as many as 75,000 more deaths than they would if they lived under the same health conditions as the white population.

But race itself isn't the primary reason for the health problems faced by minorities in the United States. Poverty is. One in three Hispanics under age 65 has no health insurance.[17] According to public health experts, low income may account for one-third of the racial differences in death rates for middle-aged African-American adults. High blood pressure, high cholesterol, obesity, diabetes, and smoking are responsible for another third. The final third has been blamed on "unexplained factors," which may well include poor access to health care and the stress of living in a society in which skin color remains a major barrier to equality.

When African Americans receive the same cancer treatments as whites, they are equally likely to survive. In a study of nearly 3,400 colon cancer patients, white and black patients treated with surgery and chemotherapy had virtually the same five-year survival rates. In past studies, African Americans were less likely to survive for five years than whites. When blacks and whites have equal access to quality health care, perhaps some of the racial-based differences in overall health will also be reduced.

NIH has established an Office of Research on Minority Health (ORMH) with the goal of "closing the gap that currently exists between the health of minorities and the majority population." Funds have been provided for research and prevention efforts aimed at improving minority health. Some researchers focus on prenatal care to improve survival rates. Others are educating minority youths about HIV infection and AIDS.

Student Health

As one of the nation's 15.7 million undergraduate or graduate students, you belong to one of the most diverse groups in America. A quarter of all 18- to 24-year-olds in the United States are enrolled at one of the nation's 3,800 colleges and universities. Two in five college students are age 25 or older. The number of undergraduates age 35 or older has tripled since 1970 to a total of 2.95 million.[18]

The majority of college students are in the physical prime of life. As young, healthy adults, they are statistically less likely to develop life-threatening illnesses than older men and women. But contrary to what they may believe, they are not invincible. College students can and do develop a wide range of illnesses, ranging from allergies (which afflict more than half of undergraduates[19]) to potentially deadly cancers and heart conditions. However, the top killer of undergraduates is not disease but injury—unintentional, mainly motor vehicle accidents, and intentional, mainly suicide.

College students, who have a greater tendency to worry in general, worry less about health than older adults.[20] In fact, researchers describe them as having "an optimism bias," tending to underestimate their health risks. As noted in Chapter 14, about two-thirds of those surveyed at a large state university rate their risk of heart disease as lower or much lower than their peers—regardless of their family history or lifestyles.[21]

In a survey of 1,283 Houston-area community college students, even smokers were optimistic—unrealistically so—about their risk of health problems. Over half of the current smokers believed that their health was better than the average same-age smoker's health, and 19 percent believed that their health was better than that of the same-age nonsmoker. Virtually all the smokers perceived that their health was either not at all or only slightly affected by smoking. Almost half thought that quitting would bring either no benefit or only minor benefit to their health.[22]

Students, usually covered by parental or school policies, don't have to concern themselves with paying for health care should they need it. However, the majority say they worry about getting and paying for health insurance after graduation. Those older than age 25 express the greatest concerns.[23] (See Fact or Fiction: "Many students worry. . . .")

Health Problems on Campus

College itself can seem hazardous to health. Dormitories have proven to be breeding grounds for serious infectious diseases, such as meningitis and Group B streptococcus[24] (discussed in Chapter 13). Secondhand smoke can present a long-term threat to smokers' roommates. Binge drinking imperils not only the drinkers but those in their immediate environment, including anyone on the road if an intoxicated student gets behind the wheel of a car.[25] However, most health problems on campus stem from unhealthy habits or risky behaviors.

FACT OR FICTION?

Many students worry about health insurance coverage after they graduate.

Fact: In a survey of 425 college and graduate students, 86 percent said they're concerned about going without health insurance after graduation. About one-third of them are unsure as to whether they will be able to obtain coverage because of its costs and their uncertainty about finding jobs. The majority of students are currently covered under their parents' health insurance plan, a school/university plan or an employer's plan. Students typically lose eligibility for health coverage under their parents' plan once they graduate. Nearly 40 percent of college graduates have no health insurance at some point during their first year following graduation.

Source: "College Students Concerned About Lack of Health Coverage After Graduation." *Health & Medicine Week*, August 4, 2003, p. 287.

Unhealthy Habits

Often on their own for the first time, college students leave behind their family's ways of eating, sleeping, and relaxing and develop new habits and routines—usually not healthier ones. Many simply don't get enough sleep or keep irregular schedules that throw their sleep patterns off kilter.[26] Often it seems that there aren't enough hours in the day for all the things undergraduates need or want to do—study, socialize, pursue extracurricular activities, surf the Internet, work at part-time jobs, participate in community service. Sleeping less, juggling more, students can quickly end up exhausted—and at greater risk for colds, flus, digestive problems, and other maladies.

Poor sleep can be both a symptom and a cause of stress, which, as discussed in Chapter 3, is especially common among freshmen. More undergraduates are seeking psychological counseling to deal with the strain they feel as well as mental disorders such as anxiety and depression.[27]

 In a Canadian survey, college students reported more distress than the general Canadian population and than same-age peers not enrolled in college.[28] Nearly a third of more than 7,500 undergraduates surveyed had significantly elevated psychological distress—women more than men, younger students more than upperclassmen.

Students who endure harassment or abuse of any sort are more likely to report health-related symptoms. Those most at risk include minority students as well as gay, lesbian, and bisexual undergraduates.[29]

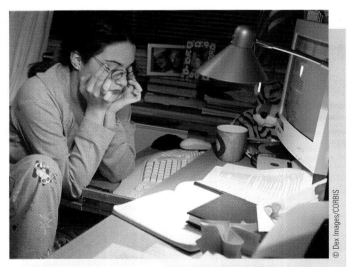

Unhealthy habits often become routine for college students—and may make them more susceptible to health problems both in the short and long term.

Nutrition habits also change during college. As discussed in Chapter 5, the majority of freshmen say their diet has changed for the worse. During their first year, students often gain a few pounds (although less than the notorious "freshman 15"). In a survey of undergraduates from six college campuses, more women than men worried about weight and health.[30] Eating disorders are more common among women, particularly those who become vegetarians in college.[31]

Students also become more sedentary in college, as they log more hours in classes and in front of computers. In one survey at a Midwestern university, 53 percent of the women and 40.3 percent of the men had not engaged in vigorous physical activity in the preceding month.[32] The combination of a high-fat diet and a sedentary lifestyle in college can set the stage for the development of health problems that include obesity, diabetes, metabolic syndrome, heart disease, and certain cancers.

Risky Behaviors

Risky behaviors are not new or unusual on campus, but today's students face different—and often deadlier—risks than undergraduates did a generation ago. Now as then, many students are sexually active, but these days there are more and more serious sexually transmitted infections (STIs) on campus. Despite awareness of these dangers, almost three in four students report that they have engaged in unprotected sex.[33] (See Student Snapshots: "Risks Students Take.") Of those who have had unprotected sex, about two-thirds said they didn't believe they were at risk of STIs.

Although smoking has declined nationwide, according to the National Household Survey on Drug Abuse, college-age young adults have the highest percentage of smokers.[34] The more and the longer they smoke, the more these young men and women boost their risks of heart disease, respiratory problems, several types of cancer, and a shortened lifespan.[35]

Drinking also has long been part of college life, and despite the efforts across U.S. college campuses to curb alcohol abuse, two out of five students engage in binge drinking—consumption of five or more drinks at a single session for men, four for women.[36] Heavy drinking increases the likelihood of other risky behaviors, such as smoking cigarettes, using drugs, or having multiple sexual partners.[37] According to new research, genes may increase the likelihood of dangerous drinking in college students. Those with a short variant of the gene that transports the brain chemical serotonin consume more alcohol per occasion, drink more often to get drunk, and are more likely to binge drink than others.[38]

In a recent survey of substance use on college campuses, 56 percent of undergraduates reported that they had smoked marijuana; approximately one-fifth reported using

Student Snapshot — **Health Risks Students Take**

Undergraduates who say they've...

- engaged in unprotected sex — **73%**
- smoked marijuana — **56%**
- had more than 4 or 5 drinks at a time (binge-drinking) — **40%**
- driven after drinking — **34%**

Sources: www.adolescenthealth.org; M. Eisenberg and H. Wechsler. "Substance Use Behaviors Among College Students with Same-Sex and Opposite-Sex Experience: Results from a National Study." *Addictive Behaviors,* Vol. 28, No. 6, 2003, p. 899; Elissa Weitzman, et al. "Taking Up Binge Drinking in College: The Influences of Person, Social Group, and Environment." *Journal of Adolescent Health,* Vol. 32, No. 1, January 2003, p. 26; M. J. Paschall. "College Attendance and Risk-Related Driving Behavior in a National Sample of Young Adults." *Journal of Studies of Alcohol,* Vol. 64, No. 1, January 2003, p. 43.

pot within the previous month.[39] In general, drug use has remained steady in recent years with one exception—a doubling of ecstasy use on campus, although the percentage of students who use ecstasy is small.[40]

Some behaviors are riskier than students realize. "Body art"—piercings and tattoos—may seem harmless, but health officials warn of hidden risks, including Hepatitis B and C infection and transmission of HIV (See Chapter 13). In a survey of undergraduates at a university in New York, 51 percent reported body piercings and 23 percent had gotten tattoos. Almost one in five—17 percent—who had had a body part pierced reported medical complications. Bacterial infection was the most common, following by bleeding and injury or tearing at the site. Eighteen percent of the students' piercings and 4 percent of tattoos were removed.[41]

College-age men are more likely than women to engage in risk-taking behaviors—to use drugs and alcohol; to engage in risky sexual behaviors, such as having multiple partners and having sex while under the influence of alcohol; and to drive dangerously. Men also are more likely to be hospitalized for injuries and to commit suicide. Three-fourths of the deaths in the 15- to 24-year age range are men.[42]

Although women are less frequently victims of crime than men, they perceive themselves at higher risk—with reason. According to the Department of Justice, almost half of violence against women occurs between the ages of 16 and 24 years. As many as one-third of college women are sexually assaulted during their college careers.[43] Female

undergraduates are twice as likely to be stalked as women in the general population; as many as one in eight is stalked each year.[44]

Health Benefits of Education

Despite potential health risks, the great majority of students not only survive college but, simply by acquiring more years of schooling, increase their chances of a long and healthful life. Many risk factors for disease—including high blood pressure, elevated cholesterol, and cigarette smoking—decline steadily as education increases, regardless of how much money people make. Education may be good for the body as well as the mind by influencing lifestyle behaviors, problem-solving abilities, and values. People who earn college degrees gain positive attitudes about the benefits of healthy living, learn how to gain access to preventive health services, join peer groups that promote healthy behavior, and develop higher self-esteem and greater control over their lives.

Do Healthy Behaviors Have an Effect on Academic Performance?

In a study of 200 students living in on-campus residence halls at a large private university, researchers weighed the impact of various health-related variables on first-year students' grade point averages (GPAs). Variables associated with higher grades included female gender, age, studying spiritually oriented material, eating breakfast, and using a planner to organize time. Students with lower GPAs were more likely to stay up and wake up later on weekdays and weekends, sleep more on weekend nights, and work longer hours.

In its National College Health Assessment, the American College Health Association found the conditions that most affect a student's grade or class attendance are stress, depression, sleep problems, family concerns, and time spent on the Internet.[45] The academic performance of African Americans has improved, with most students getting average grades and some excelling. However Caucasian students typically get better grades. One reason may be higher stress levels for minority students at predominantly white universities. (See Chapter 3 for a discussion of minority stress.) Caucasian students also report feeling more parental pressure to get good grades.[46]

❖ How People Change

Nothing is certain in life except change. Every day ushers in changes large and small, but the changes that matter most are those we make ourselves. In recent decades behavioral scientists have dissected the process of how people change, mapping the stages of change and identifying the components of successful change.

The Wellness Wheel on page 25 can help identify areas of your life that could use some attention—and change. The following sections, along with "Your Health Change Plan: How to Make a Change," describe some of the steps that can help you make changes for the better.

Understanding Health Behavior

Your choices and behaviors affect how long and how well you live. Nearly half of all deaths in the United States are linked to behaviors such as tobacco use, improper diet, abuse of alcohol and other drugs, use of firearms, motor vehicle accidents, risky sexual practices, and lack of exercise.

If you would like to improve one health behavior, you have to realize that change isn't easy. As Savvy Consumer: "Too Good to Be True?" points out, there are no easy answers or quick solutions. Between 40 and 80 percent of those who try to kick bad health habits lapse back into their unhealthy ways within six weeks. To make lasting beneficial changes, you have to understand the three types of influences that shape behavior: predisposing, enabling, and reinforcing factors (Figure 1-3).

Predisposing Factors

Predisposing factors include knowledge, attitudes, beliefs, values, and perceptions. Unfortunately, knowledge isn't enough to cause most people to change their behavior; for example, people fully aware of the grim consequences of smoking often continue to puff away. Nor is attitude—one's likes and dislikes—sufficient; an individual may dislike the smell and taste of cigarettes but continue to smoke regardless.

Beliefs are more powerful than knowledge and attitudes, and researchers report that people are most likely to change health behavior if they hold three beliefs:

:: **Susceptibility.** They acknowledge that they are at risk for the negative consequences of their behavior.

:: **Severity.** They believe that they may pay a very high price if they don't make a change.

:: **Benefits.** They believe that the proposed change will be advantageous to their health.

There can be a gap between stated and actual beliefs, however. Young adults may say they recognize the very real dangers of casual, careless sex in this day and age. Yet, rather than act in accordance with these statements, they may impulsively engage in unprotected sex with individuals whose health status and histories they do not know. The reason: Like young people everywhere and in every time, they feel invulnerable, that nothing bad can or will happen to them, that if there were a real danger, they would somehow know it. Often it's not until something happens—a former lover may admit to having a sexually transmitted infection—that their behaviors become consistent with their stated beliefs.

Young people, especially young men, are the greatest risk takers, a fact reflected in their high rates of auto accidents, binge drinking, drug use, and pathological gambling. The death rates for injuries related to swimming, boating, driving, cycling, and even crossing the street are higher in college-age men than women.

The value or importance we give to health also plays a major role in changing behavior. Many people aren't concerned about their health just for the sake of being healthy. Usually they want to look or feel better, be more productive or competitive, or behave more independently. They're more likely to change, and to stick with a change, if they can see that the health benefits also enhance other important aspects of their lives.

Perceptions are the way we see things from our unique perspective; they vary greatly with age. As a student, you may not think that living a few hours longer is a significant gain; as you grow older, however, you may prize every additional second.

Savvy Consumer

TOO GOOD TO BE TRUE?

Almost every week you're likely to come across a commercial or an ad for a new health product that promises better sleep, more energy, clearer skin, firmer muscles, lower weight, brighter moods, longer life—or all of these combined. As the Savvy Consumer throughout this book points out, you can't believe every promise you read or hear. Keep these general guidelines in mind the next time you come across a health claim:

- If it sounds too good to be true, it probably is. If a magic pill could really trim off excess pounds or banish wrinkles, the world would be filled with thin people with unlined skin. Look around and you'll realize that's not the case.

- Look for objective evaluations. If you're watching an infomercial for a treatment or technique, you can be sure that the enthusiastic endorsements have been skillfully scripted and rehearsed. Even ads that claim to be presenting the science behind a new breakthrough are really sales pitches in disguise.

- Consider the sources. Research findings from carefully controlled scientific studies are reviewed by leading experts in the field and published in scholarly journals. Just because someone has conducted a study doesn't mean it was a valid scientific investigation.

- Check credentials. Anyone can claim to be a scientist or a health expert. Find out if advocates of any type of therapy have legitimate degrees from recognized institutions and are fully licensed in their fields.

- Do your own research. Check with your doctor or with the student health center. Go to the library or do some online research to gather as much information as you can.

Enabling Factors

Enabling factors include skills, resources, accessible facilities, and physical and mental capacities. Before you initiate a change, assess the means available to reach your goal. No matter how motivated you are, you'll become frustrated if you keep encountering obstacles. That's why breaking a task or goal down into step-by-step strategies is so important in behavioral change.

Reinforcing Factors

Reinforcing factors may be praise from family and friends, rewards from teachers or parents, or encouragement and recognition for meeting a goal. Although these help a great deal in the short run, lasting change depends not on external rewards, but on an internal commitment and sense of achievement. To make a difference, reinforcement must come from within.

A decision to change a health behavior should stem from a permanent, personal goal, not from a desire to please or impress someone else. If you lose weight for the homecoming dance, you're almost sure to regain pounds afterward. But if you shed extra pounds because you want to feel better about yourself or get into shape, you're far more likely to keep off the weight.

Stages of Change

According to the transtheoretical model of change, developed by psychologist James Prochaska, individuals progress through a sequence of stages as they make a change. Certain activities and experiences, called change processes, can help individuals progress through these stages.[47] (See Figure 1-4.)

1. **Precontemplation**
   Whether or not they're aware of a problem behavior, people in this stage have no intention of making a change in the next six months. Busy college students in good health, for instance, might never think about getting more exercise.

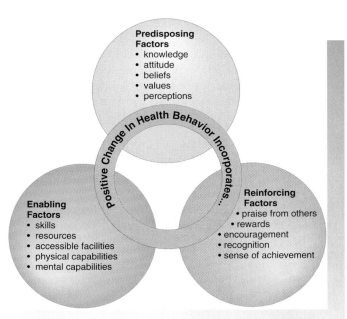

Figure 1-3 FACTORS THAT SHAPE POSITIVE BEHAVIOR

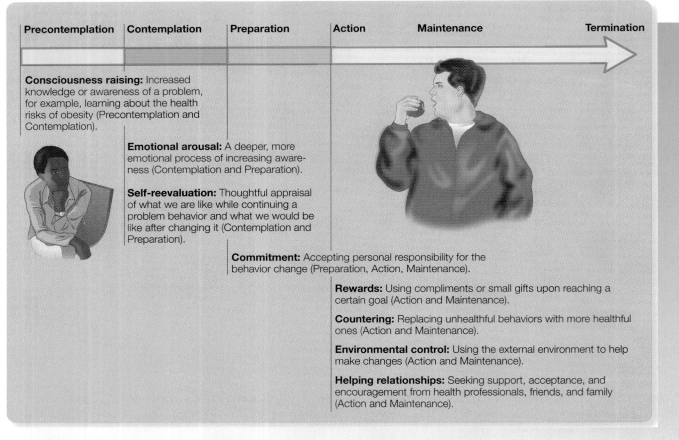

Figure 1-4 THE STAGES OF CHANGE AND SOME CHANGE PROCESSES

These change processes can help you progress through the stages of change. Each can be used through more than one stage.

Source: John Petrocelli. "Processes and Stages of Change: Counseling with the Transtheoretical Model of Change." *Journal of Counseling and Development,* Vol. 8, No. 1, Winter 2002, p. 22.

2. **Contemplation**

Individuals in this stage are aware they have a problem behavior and are considering changing it within the next six months. However, they may be torn between the positives of the new behavior and the amount of energy, time, and other resources required to change. Students in a health course, for instance, may start thinking about exercising but struggle to balance potential benefits with the effort of getting up early to jog or go to the gym.[48]

3. **Preparation**

People in this stage intend to change a problem behavior within the next month. Some focus on a master plan. For instance, they might look into fitness classes, gyms, or other options for working out. Others might start by making small changes, such as walking to classes rather than taking a campus shuttle bus.

4. **Action**

People in this stage are modifying their behavior according to their plan. For instance, they might be jogging or working out at the gym three times a week.

5. **Maintenance**

In this stage, individuals have continued to work at changing their behavior and have avoided relapse for at least six months. New exercisers are likely to stop during the first three to six months. One reason that researchers have identified: the temptation to not exercise.

6. **Termination**

While it may take two to five years, a behavior becomes so deeply ingrained that a person can't imagine abandoning it. More than eight in ten college seniors who exercised regularly remain as active, or even more active, after graduation.[49]

 As research on college students has shown, attitudes and feelings are related to stages of change. Smokers who believe that continuing to smoke would have only a minor or no impact on their health remain in the precontemplation stage; those with respiratory symptoms move on to contemplation and preparation.[50] In a study at Ohio State University, researchers classified student heavy drinkers according to the stages of change: Nearly two-thirds of the "pre-contemplators" continued to drink heavily and had no intention of changing their behavior. In the maintenance stage, students drank an average of one alcoholic drink a month even though they felt that heavy drinking was the norm on their campus.[51]

The Process of Change

"The process of changing from what you are to what you would like to become can be either arduous and frustrating or easy and rewarding," observes Stan Goldberg, Ph.D., who has spent 25 years researching how people change. Because change can be frightening, he encourages individuals to examine the consequences of both sticking with the status quo and switching to the desired behavior.[52]

Some people find it helpful to sign a contract, a written agreement in which they make a commitment to change, with their partner, parent, or health educator. Spelling out what they intend to do, and why, underscores the seriousness of what they're trying to accomplish (see Figure 1-5).

Above all else, change depends on the belief that you can and will succeed. In his research on **self-efficacy,** psychologist Albert Bandura of Stanford University found that the individuals most likely to reach a goal are those who believe they can. The more strongly they feel that they can and will change their behavior, the more energy and persistence they put into making the change. Other researchers have linked positive health change with optimism. Individuals who see themselves as optimists may underestimate their susceptibility to problems, such as hypertension, because they always expect things to turn out well. Individuals who perceive themselves as susceptible—that is, who anticipate potentially negative consequences—may be more cautious.

Another crucial factor is **locus of control.** If you believe that your actions will make a difference in your health, your locus of control is internal. If you believe that external forces or factors play a greater role, your locus of control is external. Individuals with an external locus of control for health are less likely to seek preventive health care, are less optimistic about early treatment, rate their own health as poorer, and spend more time in bed because of illness than those with an internal locus of control.

Reinforcements—either positive (a reward) or negative (a punishment)—also can play a role. If you decide to set up a regular exercise program, for instance, you might reward yourself with a new sweat suit if you stick to it for three months or you might punish yourself for skipping a day by doing an extra ten minutes of exercises the following day.

Social and cultural **norms**—behaviors that are expected, accepted, or supported by a group—can make change much harder if they're constantly working against a person's best intentions. You may resolve to eat less, for instance, yet your mother may keep offering you home-made fudge and brownies because your family's norm is to show love by making and offering delicious treats. Or you might decide to drink less, yet your friends' norm may be to equate drinking with having a good time.

If you're aware of the norms that influence your behavior, you can devise strategies either to change them (by encouraging your friends to dance more and drink less at parties, for example) or adapt to them (having just a bite of your mother's sweets). Another option is to develop relationships with people who share your goals and whose norms can reinforce your behavior.

Your **self-talk**—the messages you send yourself—also can play a role. In recent decades, mental health professionals have recognized the conscious use of positive self-talk as a powerful force for changing the way individuals think, feel, and behave. "We have a choice about how we think," explains psychologist Martin Seligman, Ph.D., author of *Learned Optimism.* As he notes, by learning to challenge automatic negative thoughts that enter our brains and asserting our own statements of self-worth, we can transform ourselves into optimists who see what's right rather than pessimists forever focusing on what's wrong. "Optimism is a learned set of skills," Seligman contends. "Once learned, these skills persist because they feel so good to use. And reality is usually on our side."[53]

How Can I Change a Bad Health Habit?

Change is never easy—even if it's done for the best possible reasons. When you decide to change a behavior, you have to give up something familiar and easy for something new and challenging. Change always involves risk—and the prospect of rewards.

Researchers have identified various approaches that people use to make beneficial changes. In the moral model, you take responsibility for a problem (such as smoking) and its solution; success depends on adequate motivation, while failure is seen as a sign of character weakness. In the enlightenment model, you submit to strict discipline to correct a problem; this is the approach used in Alcoholics Anonymous. The behavioral model involves rewarding yourself when you make positive changes. The medical model sees the behavior as caused by forces beyond your control (a genetic predisposition to being overweight, for example) and employs an expert to provide advice or treatment. For many people, the most effective approach is the compensatory model, which doesn't assign blame but puts responsibility on individuals to acquire whatever skills or power they need to overcome their problems.

Figure 1-5 SAMPLE HEALTH-CHANGE CONTRACT

My Contract For Change

Date: _____

Personal Goal: _____

Motivating Factors: _____

Change(s) I Promise to Make to Reach This Goal: ____

Plan for Making This Change: _____

Start Date: _____

Assessment Plan: _____

If I Need Help: _____

Target Date for Reaching Goal: _____

Reward for Achieving Goal: _____

Penalty for Failing to Achieve Goal: _____

Signed: _____

Witnessed By: _____

Before they reach the stage where they can and do take action to change, most people go through a process comparable to religious conversion. First they reach a level of accumulated unhappiness that makes them ready for change. Then they have a moment of truth that makes them want to change. One pregnant woman, for instance, felt her unborn baby quiver when she drank a beer and swore never to drink again. As people change their behavior, they change their lifestyles and identities as well. Ex-smokers, for instance, may start an aggressive exercise program, make new friends at the track or gym, and participate in new types of activities, like racquetball games or fun runs.

Assessing Risks

As discussed earlier in this chapter, young people face a host of risks, from the danger of being the victim of violence to the hazards of self-destructive behaviors like drinking and using illegal drugs. At any age, the greatest health threats stem from high-risk behaviors—smoking, excessive drinking, not getting enough exercise, eating too many high-fat foods, and not getting regular medical checkups, to name just a few. That's why changing unhealthy habits is the best way to reduce risks and prevent health problems.

Environmental health risks are the subject of newspaper headlines. Every year brings calls of alarm about a new hazard to health: electromagnetic radiation, fluoride in drinking water, hair dyes, silicone implants, radon, lead. Often the public response is panic. Consumers picket and protest. Individuals arrange for elaborate testing. Yet how do we know whether or not alleged health risks are acceptable? Some key factors to consider:

:: **Are there possible benefits?** Advantages—such as the high salary paid for working with toxic chemicals or radioactive materials—may make some risks seem worth taking.

:: **Is the risk voluntary?** All of us tend to accept risks that we freely choose to take, such as playing a sport that could lead to injuries, as opposed to risks imposed on us, such as threats of terrorism.

:: **Is the risk fair?** The risk of skin cancer affects us all. We may worry about it and take action to protect ourselves and our planet, but we don't resent it the way we resent living with the risk of violence because the only housing we can afford is in a high-crime area.

:: **Are there alternatives?** As consumers, we may become upset about cancer-causing pesticides or food additives when we learn about safer chemicals or methods of preservation.

:: **Are lives saved or lost?** Our thinking about risks often depends on how they're presented. For instance, if we're told that a new drug may kill 1 out of every 100 people, we react differently than if we're told that it may save the lives of 99 percent of those who use it.

Making Decisions

Every day you make decisions that have immediate and long-term effects on your health. You decide what to eat, whether to drink or smoke, when to exercise, and how to cope with a sudden crisis. Beyond these daily matters, you decide when to see a doctor, what kind of doctor, and with what sense of urgency. You decide what to tell your doctor and whether to follow the advice given, whether to keep up your immunizations, whether to have a prescription filled and comply with the medication instructions, and whether to seek further help or a second opinion. The entire process of maintaining or restoring health depends on your decisions; it cannot start or continue without them.

The small decisions of everyday life—what to eat, where to go, when to study—are straightforward choices. Larger decisions—which major to choose, what to do about a dead-end relationship, how to handle an awkward work situation—are more challenging. However, if you think of decision making as a process, you can break down even the most difficult choices into manageable steps:

STRATEGIES FOR PREVENTION

Setting Realistic Goals

Here's a framework for setting goals and objectives, the crucial preliminary step for prevention:

■ Determine your goal or objective. Define it in words and on paper. Then test your definition against your own value system. Can you attain your goal and still be the person you want to be?

■ Think in terms of evolution, not revolution. Revolutionary changes only inspire counterrevolutions. If you want to change the way you eat, start by changing just one meal a week.

■ Identify your resources. Do you have the knowledge, skills, finances, time—whatever it takes? Find out from others who know. Be sure you're ready for the next step.

■ Systematically analyze barriers. How can missing resources be acquired? Identify and select alternative plans. List solutions for any obstacles you foresee.

■ Choose a plan. Think it through, step by step, trying to anticipate what might go wrong and why.

:: **Set priorities.** Rather than getting bogged down in details, step back and look at the big picture. What matters most to you? What would you like to accomplish in the next week, month, year? Look at the decision you're about to make in the context of your values and goals.

:: **Inform yourself.** The more you know—about a person, a position, a place, a project—the better you'll be able to evaluate it. Gathering information may involve formal research, such as an online or library search for relevant data, or informal conversations with teachers, counselors, family members, or friends.

:: **Consider all your options.** Most complex decisions don't involve simple either-or alternatives. List as many options you can think of, along with the advantages and disadvantages of each.

:: **Tune in to your gut feelings.** After you've gotten the facts and analyzed them, listen to your intuition. While it's not infallible, your sixth sense can provide valuable feedback. If something just doesn't feel right, try to figure out why. Are there any fears you haven't dealt with? Do you have doubts about taking a certain path?

:: **Consider a worst-case scenario.** When you've come close to a final decision, imagine what will happen if everything goes wrong—the workload becomes overwhelming, your partner betrays your trust, your

expectations turn out to be unrealistic. If you can live with the worst consequences of a decision, you're probably making the right choice.

✖ A New Era in Health Education

In the past, health education focused on individual change. Today many educators are using a new framework in which behavior change occurs within the context of the entire environment of a person's life. Its primary themes—prevention of health problems and protection from health threats—can establish the basis for good health now and in the future.

The Power of Prevention

No medical treatment, however successful or sophisticated, can compare with the power of **prevention.** Two out of every three deaths and one in three hospitalizations in the United States could be prevented by changes in six main risk factors: tobacco use, alcohol abuse, accidents, high

© Michael Keller/Index Stock Imagery

The most effective single step you can take to prevent hypertension is to learn your own blood pressure.

blood pressure, obesity, and gaps in screening and primary health care. Preventive efforts have already proved helpful in increasing physical activity, quitting smoking, reducing dietary fat, preventing sexually transmitted infections and unwanted pregnancy, reducing intolerance and violence, and avoiding alcohol and drug abuse. Prevention remains the best weapon against cancer and heart disease.[54]

Prevention can take many forms. Primary or before-the-fact prevention efforts might seek to reduce stressors and increase support to prevent problems in healthy people. Consumer education, for instance, provides guidance about how to change our lifestyle to prevent problems and enhance well-being. Other preventive programs identify people at risk and empower them with information and support so they can avoid potential problems. Prevention efforts may target an entire community and try to educate all of its members about the dangers of alcohol abuse or environmental hazards, or they may zero in on a particular group (for instance, seminars on safer sex practices offered to teens) or an individual (one-on-one counseling about substance abuse).

In the past, physicians did not routinely incorporate prevention into their professional practices. Instead, consumers played the role of Humpty-Dumpty: As long as they sat quietly on the wall, they were ignored. When they fell, the medical equivalents of all the king's horses and all the king's men came running to put them back together again. Often, however, even the best these professionals could provide was still too little, too late.

But times have changed. Medical schools are providing more training in preventive care. A growing number of studies have demonstrated that prevention saves not only money but also productivity, health, and lives. As many as 50 to 80 percent of the deaths caused by cardiovascular disease, strokes, and cancer could be avoided or delayed by preventive measures. Eliminating smoking could prevent more than 300,000 deaths each year, for instance, while changes in diet could prevent 35 percent of unnecessary deaths from heart disease.

The Potential of Protection

There is a great deal of overlap between prevention and **protection.** Some people might think of immunizations (discussed in Chapter 13) as a way of preventing illness; others see them as a form of protection against dangerous diseases. In many ways, protection picks up where prevention leaves off. You can prevent STIs or unwanted pregnancy by abstaining from sex. But if you decide to engage in potentially risky sexual activities, you can protect yourself with condoms and spermicides (discussed in Chapter 9). Similarly, you can prevent many automobile accidents by not driving when road conditions are hazardous. But if you do have to drive, you can protect yourself by wearing a seat belt and using defensive driving techniques (discussed in Chapter 18).

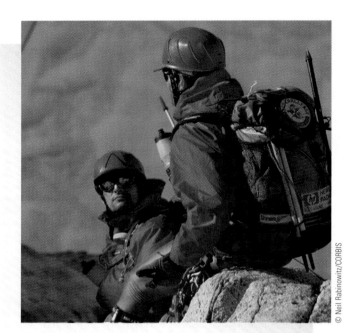

Wearing a helmet can protect rock-climbers from serious injury.

The very concept of protection implies some degree of risk—immediate and direct (for instance, the risk of intentional injury from an assailant or unintentional harm from a fire) or long-term and indirect (such as the risk of heart disease and cancer as a result of smoking). To know how best to protect yourself, you have to be able to realistically assess risks.

Colleges and universities take varied steps to protect students' well-being. These range from offering vaccination against meningitis to banning alcohol at athletic and social events. Reliable health-related information also can make a difference. Although the majority of college students report receiving some health information, only 6 percent in one recent survey had information on a comprehensive range of health topics. Full-time, single students between ages 18 and 25 are most likely to receive health information.

Students who are black, Hispanic, or belong to another racial or ethnic group are more likely than white students to have received information from campus sources.[55]

According to a survey of 1,200 Americans between the ages of 15 and 24, school is their number-one source for health information, followed by parents and doctors.

The Promise of Promotion

If the best defense is a good offense, health promotion represents the ultimate form of prevention and protection. The World Health Organization defines health promotion as the process of enabling people to improve and increase control over their health. Other health specialists define it as "a science and an art devoted to helping people achieve a state of optimal health."

Health promotion programs emphasize health-enhancing behaviors, such as exercising regularly; eating nutritious foods; managing stress well; avoiding tobacco, excess alcohol, and drugs; forming fulfilling relationships with friends; living in a community with clean air; and having purpose in life. They may focus on risk avoidance, such as staying out of the sun at midday, and risk reduction, such as using sunscreen.

 One of the best examples of how effective health promotion can be is the dramatic reduction in smoking among young African Americans. In the past, black male teenagers started smoking earlier and in much greater numbers than white adolescents. But the African-American community began to send messages to its youth. Some people whitewashed billboards advertising cigarettes. Black musicians, athletes, and celebrities stopped using cigarettes in a public, glamorized way. Most powerful of all were the messages sent from teen to teen: that smoking was a bad, uncool habit that exploited the African-American community. As discussed in Chapter 12, African-American adolescents now smoke much less than white teens.

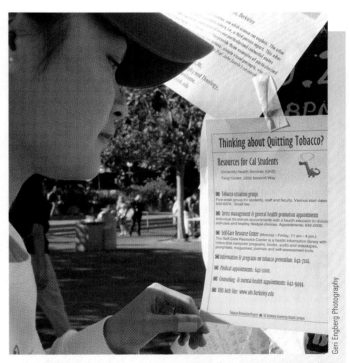

Health promotion helps to give people control over their own health, for instance, by informing them about responsible sexual behavior.

Peer counseling—support offered by one student to another—has proven effective in many areas, from awareness of the dangers of casual, unprotected sex to education about what constitutes sexual harassment and coercion. However, often it's not enough to provide information and focus on an individual's responsibility to practice safer sex, eat less fat, exercise regularly, or stop a dangerous behavior. The reality is that all health decisions are made within the complex context of culture and community.

Increasingly, health educators are realizing that overemphasizing individual responsibility sets people up to fail and, with repeated failures, to blame themselves, even in circumstances beyond their control. A college student, for instance, may decide to eat more nutritiously. However, if the only available choices are high-fat foods in vending machines and campus cafeterias, all the good intentions and willpower in the world won't lead to success.

 Students tend to support college's efforts at health promotion. In a survey of 10,904 undergraduates at 119 colleges and universities, over three-quarters of students favored smoke-free policies for all college buildings, residences, and dining areas, while seven in ten supported prohibiting tobacco advertising and sponsorship of campus social events. More than half favored prohibiting tobacco sales on campus and supported smoke-free campus bars. All policies had more support among nonsmokers than smokers, but smokers who intended to quit also voiced their support.[56]

Many health promotion efforts look beyond the campus to make the same opportunities for nutritious food, leisure, exercise, and support open to others. To develop social responsibility in students, they encourage volunteering at community centers, homeless shelters, nursing homes, environmental agencies, and advocacy groups. Their goal is to help students define health, not only in terms of their own behaviors and well-being, but also in terms of what they can do to reach out and help others in the broader community make healthier choices and changes. Students are stepping up to this challenge, with record numbers participating in community service.[57] (See Fact or Fiction?: "Today's college students . . .")

The Bottom Line: ▼
Ten Small Changes to Improve Your Health

Change always begins with a single step. Use this course as an opportunity to zero in on at least one less-than-healthful behavior and improve it. Here are some suggestions:

:: **Use seat belts.** In the last decade seat belts have saved more than 40,000 lives and prevented millions of injuries.

:: **Eat an extra fruit or vegetable every day.** Adding more fruit and vegetables to your diet can improve your digestion and lower your risk of several cancers.

:: **Get enough sleep.** A good night's rest provides the energy you need to make it through the following day.

:: **Take regular stress breaks.** A few quiet minutes spent stretching, looking out the window, or simply letting yourself unwind are good for body and soul.

:: **Lose a pound.** If you're overweight, you may not think a pound will make a difference, but it's a step in the right direction.

:: **If you're a woman, examine your breasts regularly.** Get in the habit of performing a breast self-examination every month after your period (when breasts are least swollen or tender).

:: **If you're a man, examine your testicles regularly.** These simple self-exams can spot the early signs of cancer when they're most likely to be cured.

:: **Get physical.** Just a little exercise will do some good. A regular workout schedule will be good for your heart, lungs, muscles, bones—even your mood.

:: **Drink more water.** Eight glasses a day are what you need to replenish lost fluids, prevent constipation, and keep your digestive system working efficiently.

:: **Do a good deed.** Caring for others is a wonderful way to care for your own soul and connect with others.

FACT OR FICTION?

Today's college students perform less community service than in the past.

Fiction: Record numbers of undergraduates are engaging in campus-based service initiatives and in "service-learning" opportunities as part of their course work. In a recent survey of students at 504 colleges and universities, an average of one in three reported doing some form of community service. More than half of the schools surveyed noted an increase in student involvement in community service. "The fact that a third of college and university students are engaged in community service belies the common image of students as cynical and self-involved," says Elizabeth Hollander, executive director of Campus Compact, which conducted the survey.

Source: "Survey Reveals Record Numbers of Students Involved in Service." *Black Issues in Higher Education,* Vol. 20, No. 10, July 3, 2003, p. 12.

THE CUTTING EDGE

Into the Future

Cloning. Deciphering the human genome. Painless diagnostic tests. Technology that enables the blind to see, the deaf to hear, the paralyzed to walk. Robotic limbs. Bloodless surgery. Once these were the stuff of science fiction. Today they are realities of modern medicine. What will the future bring? Technology is evolving daily, and within decades the current "state-of-the-art" treatments may seem as primitive and old-fashioned as therapies from the turn of the 20th century.

One of the most exciting scientific frontiers has been genetic research. The completion of the mapping of the human genome sequence in 2001 was a milestone in biological science. So much progress has since been made in the new science of "genomics" that geneticists describe themselves as "swimming in a rapidly rising sea of data." Analysis of that data will point the way to new possibilities in screening, diagnosing, and treating diseases.

In their quest for new cures for deadly or disabling diseases, scientists have ventured into uncharted and highly controversial territory. The ethics of cloning, whether of animals or of human embryos, and the use of embryonic stem cells (which have the potential to grow into any type of cell, such as muscle, bone, or skin) have stirred passionate debate among legislators, scientists, religious leaders, and patient advocacy groups. Gene therapy, which replaces defective genes with normal ones, also has come under attack after the deaths of volunteers in experimental programs. The federal government has restricted funding for certain types of research and has set up a panel of doctors, lawyers, and ethicists to advise the president on stem cells, cloning, and other challenging research issues.

Without doubt medical advances will touch your life. If injured, you may recover more rapidly because of them. If you develop a serious illness, you may be spared life-threatening complications. Your children will be more likely to be born and to grow up healthy and strong. You may remain active and healthy for decades longer than your great-grandparents. But despite the promise of medical breakthroughs, your future well-being remains in your hands. Your choices, your habits, your lifestyle, your vigilance ultimately will decide how long and how healthfully you will live.

WHAT IS WELLNESS?*

BY JOHN W. TRAVIS M.D.

MOST of us think in terms of illness, and assume that the absence of illness indicates wellness. There are actually many degrees of wellness, just as there are many degrees of illness. The Wellness Inventory is designed to stir up your thinking about many areas of wellness.

While people often lack physical symptoms, they may still be bored, depressed, tense, anxious, or generally unhappy with their lives. Such emotional states often set the stage for physical and mental disease. Even cancer may be brought on through the lowering of the body's resistance from excessive stress. These same emotional states can also lead to abuse of the body through smoking, overdrinking, and overeating. Such behaviors are usually substitutes for other, more basic human needs such as recognition from others, a more stimulating environment, caring and affection

*Abridged from the Wellness Index in *The Wellness Workbook,* Travis & Ryan, Ten Speed Press, 1988. Used with the permission of John W. Travis, M.D. www.thewellspring.com.

from friends, and greater self-acceptance.

Wellness is not a static state. High-level wellness involves giving good care to your physical self, using your mind constructively, expressing your emotions effectively, being creatively involved with those around you, and being concerned about your physical, psychological and spiritual environments.

◼ Instructions

Set aside a half hour for yourself in a quiet place where you will not be disturbed while taking the Inventory. Record your responses to each statement in the columns to the right where:

2 = **Yes, usually**
1 = **Sometimes, maybe**
0 = **No, rarely**

Select the answer that best indicates how true the statement is for you presently.

After you have responded to all the appropriate statements in each section, compute your average score for that section and transfer it to the corresponding box provided around the Wellness Inventory Wheel on page 25. Your completed Wheel will give you a clear presentation of the balance you have given to the many dimensions of your life.

You will find some of the statements are really two in one. We do this to show an important relationship between the two parts—usually an awareness of an issue, combined with an action based on that awareness. Mentally average your score for the two parts of the question.

Each statement describes what we believe to be a wellness attribute. Because much wellness information is subjective and "unprovable" by current scientific methods, you (and possibly other authorities as well), may not agree with our conclusions. Many of the statements have further explanation in a footnote. We ask only that you keep an open mind until you have studied available information, then decide.

This questionnaire was designed to educate more than to test. All statements are worded so that you can easily tell what we think are wellness attributes (which also makes it easy to "cheat" on your score). This means there can be no trick questions to test your honesty or consistency—the higher your score, the greater you believe your wellness to be. Full responsibility is placed on you to answer each statement as honestly as possible. It's not your score but what you learn about yourself that is most important.

If you decide that a statement does not apply to you, or you don't want to answer it, you can skip it and not be penalized in your score.

Transfer your average score from each section to the corresponding box around the Wheel. Then graph your score by drawing a curved line between the "spokes" that define each segment. (Use the scale provided—beginning at the center with 0.0 and reaching 2.0 at the circumference.) Last, fill in the corresponding amount of each wedge-shaped segment, using different colors if possible.

⚫ Your Health Change Plan: How to Make a Change

When you have completed the Wellness Inventory, study your wheel's shape and balance. How smoothly would it roll? What does it tell you? Are there any surprises in it? How does it feel to you? What don't you like about it? What do you like about it?

We recommend that you use colored pens to go back over the questions, noting the ones on which your scores were low and choosing some areas on which you are interested in working. It is easy to overwhelm yourself by taking on too many areas at once. Ignore, for now, those of lower priority to you. Remember, if you don't enjoy at least some aspects of the changes you are making, they probably won't last.

Here are some guidelines to help you as you change

:: Get support from friends, but don't expect them to supply all the reinforcement you need. You may join a group of overweight individuals and rely on their encouragement to stick to your diet. That's a great way to get going; but in the long run, your own commitment to losing weight has got to be strong enough to help you keep eating right and light.

:: Focus on the immediate rewards of your new behavior. You may stop smoking so that you'll live longer, but take note of every other benefit it brings you—more stamina, less coughing, more spending money, no more stale tobacco taste in your mouth.

:: Remind yourself of past successes you've had in making changes. Give yourself pep talks, commending yourself on how well you've done so far and how well you'll continue to do. This will boost your self-confidence.

:: Reward yourself regularly. Plan a pleasant reward as an incentive for every week you stick to your new behavior—sleeping in on a Saturday morning, going out with some friends, or spending a sunny afternoon outdoors. Small, regular rewards are more effective in keeping up motivation than one big reward that won't come for many months.

:: Expect and accept some relapses. The greatest rate of relapse occurs in the first few weeks after making a behavior change. During this critical time, get as much support as you can. In addition, work hard on self-motivation, reminding yourself daily of what you have to gain by sticking with your new health habit.

Sample Questions

	Yes, usually	Sometimes, maybe	No, rarely
	2	1	0
1. I am an adventurous thinker.	✔		
2. I have no expectations, yet look to the future optimistically.		✔	
3. I am a nonsmoker.	✔		
4. I love long, hot baths.			✔

Total points for this section = 5 | 4 + 1 + 0

Divided by 4 (number of statements answered) = 1.3 Average score for this section.

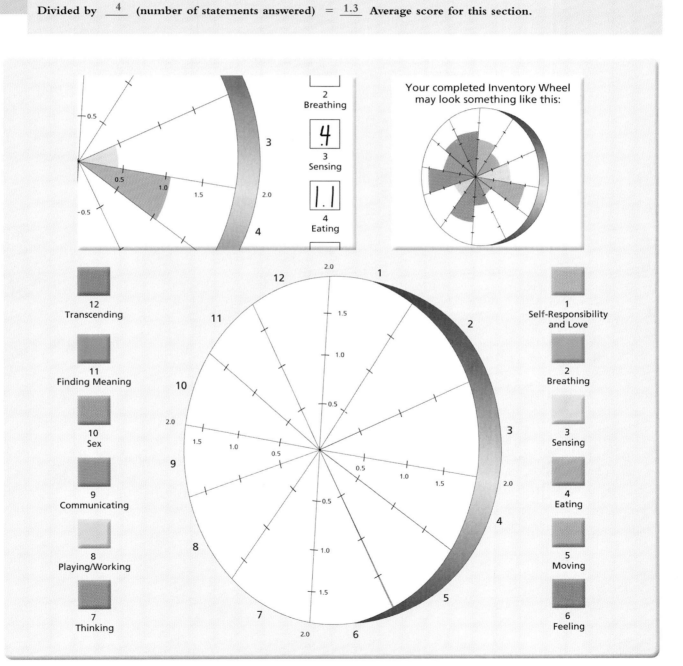

Your completed Inventory Wheel may look something like this:

2 Breathing

3 Sensing

4 Eating

12 Transcending
11 Finding Meaning
10 Sex
9 Communicating
8 Playing/Working
7 Thinking

1 Self-Responsibility and Love
2 Breathing
3 Sensing
4 Eating
5 Moving
6 Feeling

Section 1 WELLNESS, SELF-RESPONSIBILITY AND LOVE

	Yes, usually	Sometimes, maybe	No, rarely
	2	1	0
1. I believe how I live my life is an important factor in determining my state of health, and I live it in a manner consistent with that belief.			
2. I vote regularly.[1]			
3. I feel financially secure.			
4. I conserve materials/energy at home and at work.[2]			
5. I protect my living area from fire and safety hazards.			
6. I use dental floss and a soft toothbrush daily.			
7. I am a nonsmoker.			
8. I am always sober when driving or operating dangerous machinery.			
9. I wear a safety belt when I ride in a vehicle.			
10. I understand the difference between blaming myself for a problem and simply taking responsibility (ability to respond) for that problem.			

Total points for this section = ☐ _____ + _____ + _____

Divided by ____ (number of statements answered) = ____ Average score for this section.
(Transfer to the Wellness Inventory Wheel on **p. 25**)

Section 2 WELLNESS AND BREATHING

	Yes, usually	Sometimes, maybe	No, rarely
	2	1	0
1. I stop during the day to become aware of the way I am breathing.			
2. I meditate or relax myself for at least 15 to 20 minutes each day.			
3. I can easily touch my hands to my toes when standing with knees straight.[3]			
4. In temperatures over 70° F (21° C), my fingers feel warm when I touch my lips.[4]			
5. My nails are healthy and I do not bite or pick at them.			
6. I enjoy my work and do not find it overly stressful.			
7. My personal relationships are satisfying.			
8. I take time out for deep breathing several times a day.			
9. I have plenty of energy.			
10. I am at peace with myself.			

Total points for this section = ☐ _____ + _____ + _____

Divided by _____ (number of statements answered) = ____ Average score for this section.
(Transfer to the Wellness Inventory Wheel on **p. 25**)

---

[1] Voting is a simple measure of your willingness to participate in the social system, which ultimately impacts your state of health.

[2] Besides recycling glass, paper, aluminum, and other recyclables, if you purchase products that are reusable rather than disposable, and are packaged with a minimum of material, you will reduce the drain of resources and the toxic load on the environment caused by the disposal of wastes.

[3] A lack of spinal flexibility is usually a symptom of chronic muscle tension as well as indicative of a poor balance of physical activities.

[4] If your hand temperature is below 85° F (30° C) in a warm room, you're cutting off circulation to your hands via an overactive sympathetic nervous system. You can learn to warm your hands with biofeedback and to thereby better relax.

Section 3 WELLNESS AND SENSING

	Yes, usually 2	Sometimes, maybe 1	No, rarely 0
1. My place of work has mostly natural lighting or full-spectrum fluorescent lighting.[5]	___	___	___
2. I avoid extremely noisy areas or wear protective ear covers.[6]	___	___	___
3. I take long walks, hikes, or other outings to actively explore my surroundings.	___	___	___
4. I give myself presents, treats, or nurture myself in other ways.	___	___	___
5. I enjoy getting, and can acknowledge, compliments and recognition from others.	___	___	___
6. It is easy for me to give sincere compliments and recognition to other people.	___	___	___
7. At times I like to be alone.	___	___	___
8. I enjoy touching or hugging other people.[7]	___	___	___
9. I enjoy being touched or hugged by others.[8]	___	___	___
10. I get and enjoy backrubs or massages.	___	___	___

Total points for this section = ☐ ___ + ___ + ___

Divided by ___ **(number of statements answered)** = ___ **Average score for this section.**
(Transfer to the Wellness Inventory Wheel on **p. 25**)

Section 4 WELLNESS AND EATING

	Yes, usually 2	Sometimes, maybe 1	No, rarely 0
1. I am aware of the difference between refined carbohydrates and complex carbohydrates and eat a majority of the latter.[9]	___	___	
2. I think my diet is well balanced and wholesome.	___	___	
3. I drink fewer than five alcoholic drinks per week.	___	___	
4. I drink fewer than two cups of coffee or black (nonherbal) tea per day.[10]	___	___	
5. I drink fewer than five soft drinks per week.[11]	___	___	
6. I add little or no salt to my food.[12]	___	___	
7. I read the labels for the ingredients of all processed foods I buy and I inquire as to the level of toxic chemicals used in production of fresh foods—choosing the purest available to me.	___	___	
8. I eat at least two raw fruits or vegetables each day.	___	___	
9. I have a good appetite and am within 15% of my ideal weight.	___	___	
10. I can tell the difference between "stomach hunger" and "mouth hunger," and I don't stuff myself when I am experiencing only "mouth hunger."[13]	___	___	___

Total points for this section = ☐ ___ + ___ + ___

Divided by ___ **(number of statements answered)** = ___ **Average score for this section.**
(Transfer to the Wellness Inventory Wheel on **p. 25**)

[5] Full-spectrum light, like sunlight, contains many different wavelengths. Most eye-glasses, and the glass windows in your home or car, block the "near" ultraviolet light needed by your body. Special bulbs and lenses are available.

[6] Loud noises that leave your ears ringing cause irreversible and cumulative nerve damage over time. Ear plugs/muffs, obtained in sporting goods stores, should be worn around power saws, heavy equipment, and rock concerts!

[7,8] Long recognized by hospitals as therapeutic, touch can be a powerful preventative as well.

[9] Refined carbohydrates (white flour, sugar, white rice, alcohol, and others) are burned up by the body very quickly and contain no minerals or vitamins. Complex carbohydrates (fruits and vegetables) burn evenly and provide the bulk of dietary nutrients.

[10] Coffee and nonherbal teas contain stimulants that, when overused, abuse your body's adrenal glands.

[11] Besides caffeine, the empty calories in these chemical brews may cause a sugar "crash" shortly after drinking. Artificially sweetened ones may be worse. Consider the other nutrients you won't be getting, and the prices!

[12] In addition to having a presumed connection with high blood pressure, the salting of foods during cooking draws out minerals, which are lost when the water is poured off.

[13] Stomach hunger is a signal that your body needs food. Mouth hunger is a signal that it needs something else (attention/acknowledgement), which you are not getting, so it asks for food, a readily available "substitute."

Section 5 WELLNESS AND MOVING

	Yes, usually	Sometimes, maybe	No, rarely
	2	1	0
1. I climb stairs rather than ride elevators.[14]	_____	_____	_____
2. My daily activities include moderate physical effort.[15]	_____	_____	_____
3. My daily activities include vigorous physical effort.[16]	_____	_____	_____
4. I run at least 1 mile three times a week (or equivalent aerobic exercise).[17]	_____	_____	_____
5. I run at least 3 miles three times a week (or equivalent aerobic exercise).	_____	_____	_____
6. I do some form of stretching/limbering exercise for 10 to 20 minutes at least three times per week.[18]	_____	_____	_____
7. I do some form of stretching/limbering exercise for 10 to 20 minutes at least six times per week.	_____	_____	_____
8. I enjoy exploring new and effective ways of caring for myself through the movement of my body.	_____	_____	_____
9. I enjoy stretching, moving, and exerting my body.	_____	_____	_____
10. I am aware of and respond to messages from my body about its needs for movement.	_____	_____	_____

Total points for this section = ☐ _____ + _____ + _____

Divided by _____ (number of statements answered) = _____ **Average score for this section.**
(Transfer to the Wellness Inventory Wheel on **p. 25**)

Section 6 WELLNESS AND FEELING

	Yes, usually	Sometimes, maybe	No, rarely
	2	1	0
1. I am able to feel and express my anger in ways that solve problems, rather than swallow anger or store it up.[19]	_____	_____	_____
2. I allow myself to experience a full range of emotions and find constructive ways to express them.	_____	_____	_____
3. I am able to say "no" to people without feeling guilty.	_____	_____	_____
4. I laugh often and easily.	_____	_____	_____
5. I feel OK about crying and allow myself to do so when appropriate.[20]	_____	_____	_____
6. I listen to and consider others' criticisms of me rather than react defensively.	_____	_____	_____
7. I have at least five close friends.	_____	_____	_____
8. I like myself and look forward to the rest of my life.	_____	_____	_____
9. I easily express concern, love and warmth to those I care about.	_____	_____	_____
10. I can ask for help when needed.	_____	_____	_____

Total points for this section = ☐ _____ + _____ + _____

Divided by _____ (number of statements answered) = _____ **Average score for this section.**
(Transfer to the Wellness Inventory Wheel on **p. 25**)

---

[14] If a long elevator ride is necessary, try getting off five flights below your destination. Urge building managers to keep stair doors unlocked.

[15] Moderate = rearing young children, gardening, scrubbing floors, brisk walking, and so on.

[16] Vigorous = heavy construction work, farming, moving heavy objects by hand, and so on.

[17] An aerobic exercise (like running) should keep your heart rate at about 60% of its maximum (120–150 bpm) for 12–20 minutes. Brisk walking for 20 minutes every day can produce effects similar to aerobic exercise.

[18] The stretching of muscles is important for maintaining maximum flexibility of joints and ligaments. It feels good, too.

[19] Learning to take charge of your emotions and using them to solve problems can prevent disease, improve communications, and increase your self-awareness. Suppressing emotions or using them to manipulate others is destructive to all.

[20] Crying over a loss relieves the body of pent-up feelings. In our culture males often have a difficult time allowing themselves to cry, while females may have learned to cry when angry, using tears as a means of manipulation.

Section 7 WELLNESS AND THINKING

	Yes, usually	Sometimes, maybe	No, rarely
	2	**1**	**0**
1. I am in charge of the subject matter and the emotional content of my thoughts, and am satisfied with what I choose to think about.[21]	_____	_____	_____
2. I am aware that I make judgments wherein I think I am "right" and others are "wrong."[22]	_____	_____	_____
3. It is easy for me to concentrate.	_____	_____	_____
4. I am conscious of changes (such as breathing pattern, muscle tension, skin moisture, and so on) in my body in response to certain thoughts.[23]	_____	_____	_____
5. I notice my perceptions of the world are colored by my thoughts at the time.[24]	_____	_____	_____
6. I am aware that my thoughts are influenced by my environment.	_____	_____	_____
7. I use my thoughts and attitudes to make my reality more life-affirming.[25]	_____	_____	_____
8. Rather than worry about a problem when I can do nothing about it, I temporarily shelve it and get on with the matters at hand.	_____	_____	_____
9. I approach life with the attitude that no problem is too big to confront, and some mysteries aren't meant to be solved.	_____	_____	_____
10. I use my creative powers in many aspects of my life.	_____	_____	_____

Total points for this section = ☐ _____ + _____ + _____

Divided by _____ **(number of statements answered)** = _____ **Average score for this section.**
(Transfer to the Wellness Inventory Wheel on **p. 25**)

Section 8 WELLNESS AND PLAYING/WORKING

	Yes, usually	Sometimes, maybe	No, rarely
	2	**1**	**0**
1. I enjoy expressing myself through art, dance, music, drama, sports, or other activities, and make time to do so.	_____	_____	_____
2. I regularly exercise my creativity "muscles."	_____	_____	_____
3. I enjoy spending time without planned or structured activities and make the effort to do so.	_____	_____	_____
4. I can make much of my work into play.	_____	_____	_____
5. At times I allow myself to do nothing.[26]	_____	_____	_____
6. At times I can sleep late without feeling guilty.	_____	_____	_____
7. The work I do is rewarding to me.	_____	_____	_____
8. I am proud of my accomplishments.	_____	_____	_____
9. I am playful and the people around me support my playfulness.	_____	_____	_____
10. I have at least one activity, hobby, or sport that I enjoy regularly but do not feel compelled to do.	_____	_____	_____

Total points for this section = ☐ _____ + _____ + _____

Divided by _____ **(number of statements answered)** = _____ **Average score for this section.**
(Transfer to the Wellness Inventory Wheel on **p. 25**)

---

[21] When you are unconscious of the content of your thoughts, they are more likely to control you. Observing them objectively develops self-awareness and strengthens your ability to take charge.

[22] Rather than trying to completely stop yourself from judging, you can observe your judgments as efforts by your ego to avoid getting on with life and hiding behind "right/wrong" game playing.

[23] Both biofeedback and the field of psycho-neuro-immunology have shown the connections between the mind, nervous system and body. The more you become consciously aware of that connection, the greater responsibility you can take for your health.

[24] Being aware of your internal distortion of perceptions can allow you to step back and reassess a situation more objectively.

[25] Honesty, tempered with care and concern, clears out many negative thoughts that can clutter up your mind, thus making your reality more fun. "Positive thinking" without honesty and truthfulness can backfire by suppressing valid concerns that must be addressed.

[26] Doing "nothing" can give us access to the more creative and nonverbal aspects of our being, so from another perspective, doing nothing becomes doing much more.

Section 9 WELLNESS AND COMMUNICATING

	Yes, usually	Sometimes, maybe	No, rarely
	2	**1**	**0**
1. In conversation I can introduce a difficult topic and stay with it until I've gotten a satisfactory response from the other person.	____	____	____
2. I enjoy silence.	____	____	____
3. I am truthful and caring in my communications with others.	____	____	____
4. I assert myself (in a nonattacking manner) in an effort to be heard, rather than be passively resentful of others with whom I don't agree.[27]	____	____	____
5. I readily acknowledge my mistakes, apologizing for them if appropriate.	____	____	____
6. I am aware of my negative judgments of others and accept them as simply judgments—not necessarily truth.[28]	____	____	____
7. I am a good listener.	____	____	____
8. I am able to listen to people without interrupting them or finishing their sentences for them.	____	____	____
9. I can let go of my mental "labels" (for example, this is good, that is wrong) and judgmental attitudes about events in my life and see them in light of what they offer me.	____	____	____
10. I am aware when I play psychological "games" with those around me and work to be truthful and direct in my communications.[29]	____	____	____

Total points for this section = [ ] ____ + ____ + ____

Divided by ____ **(number of statements answered)** = ____ **Average score for this section.**
(Transfer to the Wellness Inventory Wheel on **p. 25**)

Section 10 WELLNESS AND SEX

	Yes, usually	Sometimes, maybe	No, rarely
	2	**1**	**0**
1. I feel comfortable touching and exploring my body.	____	____	____
2. I think it's OK to masturbate if one chooses to do so.	____	____	____
3. My sexual education is adequate.	____	____	____
4. I feel good about the degree of closeness I have with men.	____	____	____
5. I feel good about the degree of closeness I have with women.	____	____	____
6. I am content with my level of sexual activity.[30]	____	____	____
7. I fully experience the many stages of lovemaking rather than focus only on orgasm.[31]	____	____	____
8. I desire to grow closer to some other people.	____	____	____
9. I am aware of the difference between needing someone and loving someone.	____	____	____
10. I am able to love others without dominating or being dominated by them.	____	____	____

Total points for this section = [ ] ____ + ____ + ____

Divided by ____ **(number of statements answered)** = ____ **Average score for this section.**
(Transfer to the Wellness Inventory Wheel on **p. 25**)

---

[27] Attacking others rarely accomplishes your goals in the long run. Persisting in your convictions without using force is more effective and usually solves the problem without creating new ones.

[28] It is important to recognize that our internal judgments of others are based on personal biases that often have little objective basis.

[29] Psychological games, defined by Eric Berne in *Games People Play,* are complex unconscious manipulations that result in the players getting negative attention and feeling bad about themselves.

[30] Including the choice to have no sexual activity.

[31] A common problem for many people is an overemphasis on performance and orgasm, rather than on enjoying a close sensual feeling with their partner whether or not they experience orgasm.

Section 11 WELLNESS AND FINDING MEANING

	Yes, usually	Sometimes, maybe	No, rarely
	2	1	0
1. I believe my life has direction and meaning.	_____	_____	_____
2. My life is exciting and challenging.	_____	_____	_____
3. I have goals in my life.	_____	_____	_____
4. I am achieving my goals.	_____	_____	_____
5. I look forward to the future as an opportunity for further growth.	_____	_____	_____
6. I am able to talk about the death of someone close to me.	_____	_____	_____
7. I am able to talk about my own death with family and friends.	_____	_____	_____
8. I am prepared for my death.	_____	_____	_____
9. I see my death as a step in my evolution.[32]	_____	_____	_____
10. My daily life is a source of pleasure to me.	_____	_____	_____

Total points for this section = ☐ _____ + _____ + _____

Divided by _____ **(number of statements answered)** = _____ **Average score for this section.**
(Transfer to the Wellness Inventory Wheel on **p. 25**)

This portion of the Inventory goes beyond the scope of most generally accepted "scientific" principles and express-es the values and beliefs of the authors. It is intended to stimulate interest in these areas. If you have strong beliefs to the contrary, you can skip the questions or make up your own.

Section 12 WELLNESS AND TRANSCENDING

	Yes, usually	Sometimes, maybe	No, rarely
	2	1	0
1. I perceive problems as opportunities for growth.	_____	_____	_____
2. I experience synchronistic events in my life (frequent "coincidences" seeming to have no cause–effect relationship).[33]	_____	_____	_____
3. I believe there are dimensions of reality beyond verbal description or human comprehension.	_____	_____	_____
4. At times I experience confusion and paradox in my search for understanding of the dimensions referred to above.	_____	_____	_____
5. The concept of god has personal definition and meaning to me.	_____	_____	_____
6. I experience a sense of wonder when I contemplate the universe.	_____	_____	_____
7. I have abundant expectancy rather than specific expectations.	_____	_____	_____
8. I allow others their beliefs without pressuring them to accept mine.	_____	_____	_____
9. I use the messages interpreted from my dreams.	_____	_____	_____
10. I enjoy practicing a spiritual discipline or allowing time to sense the presence of a greater force in guiding my passage through life.	_____	_____	_____

Total points for this section = ☐ _____ + _____ + _____

Divided by _____ **(number of statements answered)** = _____ **Average score for this section.**
(Transfer to the Wellness Inventory Wheel on **p. 25**)

[32] Seeing your death as a stage of growth and preparing yourself consciously is an important part of finding meaning in your life.

[33] Modern physics reveals that the idea of cause and effect may be as limited as Newton's theory of a mechanical universe. It suggests that we must expand our view to see that everything in the universe is connected to everything else. (Synchronicity describes that experience.)

After watching the CNN video segment, discuss the following question. Why is taking the stairs a healthier alternative than riding an elevator?

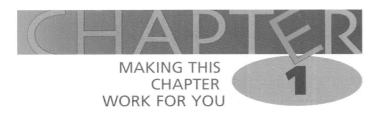

MAKING THIS CHAPTER WORK FOR YOU

1

1. The components of health include all of the following *except*
   a. supportive friends and family.
   b. a well-paying job.
   c. energy and vitality.
   d. a clean environment.

2. Wellness is defined as
   a. purposeful, enjoyable living, characterized by personal responsibility and enhancement of physical, mental, and spiritual health.
   b. a state of complete physical, mental, and social well-being.
   c. attitudes and beliefs that contribute to a healthy state of mind.
   d. the absence of physical or mental illness.

3. Which of the following statements about the dimensions of health are true?
   a. Spirituality provides solace and comfort for those who are severely ill, but it has no health benefits.
   b. The people who reflect the highest levels of social health are usually among the most popular individuals in a group and are often thought of as the life of the party.
   c. Intellectual health refers to one's academic abilities.
   d. Optimal physical health requires a nutritious diet, regular exercise, avoidance of harmful behaviors and substances, and self-protection from accidents.

4. The goals of the *Healthy People 2010* initiative include all of the following *except*
   a. reduce the proportion of obese adults and children in the population.
   b. decrease the number of teens using illegal substances.
   c. increase the number of adults engaging in daily vigorous physical activity for 30 minutes per occasion.
   d. reduce the percentage of teens and adults who report smoking cigarettes in the past month.

5. Health risks faced by different ethnic and racial groups include all of the following *except:*
   a. Whites have higher rates of hypertension, lupus, liver disease, and kidney failure than African Americans.
   b. Native Hawaiian women have a higher rate of breast cancer than women from other racial and ethnic groups.
   c. Infant mortality is higher for African-American babies than for white babies.
   d. Chinese and Hispanic women are at greater risk of developing diabetes during pregnancy than African-American and white women.

6. Which of the following health hazards faced by college students can be avoided?
   a. binge drinking
   b. unprotected sex
   c. smoking
   d. all of the above

7. The development of health behaviors is influenced by all of the following *except*
   a. reinforcing factors, which involve external recognition for achieving a goal.
   b. preexisting health factors, which take into account the individual's current position on the wellness continuum.
   c. predisposing factors, which include knowledge, attitudes, and beliefs.
   d. enabling factors, which are related to an individual's skills and capabilities to make behavior changes.

8. If you want to change unhealthy behavior, which of the following strategies is *least* likely to promote success?
   a. Believe that you can make the change.
   b. Reward yourself regularly.
   c. During self-talks, remind yourself about all your faults.
   d. Accept that you are in control of your health.

9. According to the stages of change in the transtheoretical model of change, which statement is *incorrect*?
   a. In the maintenance stage, individuals have avoided relapse for six months.
   b. In the contemplation stage, individuals are considering changing a problem behavior in the next six months.
   c. In the action stage, individuals are actually modifying their behavior according to their plan.
   d. In the preparation stage, individuals intend to change a problem behavior in the next six months.

10. Which of the following statements is *incorrect?*
    a. Prevention involves specific actions that an individual can take when participating in risky behavior to prevent health threats.
    b. You can prevent health problems by educating yourself about them and then avoiding the risky behavior that may cause them.
    c. An example of a preventive measure is to avoid driving in icy, snowy conditions, and an example of a protective measure is to put chains on your tires.
    d. In assessing risks, two questions to ask are: Is the risk voluntary? Are there alternatives?

Answers to these questions can be found on page 652.

Critical Thinking

1. What is the definition of health according to the text? Does your personal definition differ from this? If so, in what ways? How would you have defined health before reading this chapter?

2. Talk to classmates from different racial or ethnic backgrounds than yours about their culture's health attitudes. Ask them what is considered healthy behavior in their culture. For example, is having a good appetite a sign of health? What kinds of self-care practices did their parents and grandparents use to treat colds, fevers, rashes, and other health problems? What are their attitudes about the health-care system?

3. Where are you on the wellness–illness continuum? What variables might affect your place on the scale? What do you consider your optimum state of health to be?

4. In what ways would you like to change your present lifestyle? What steps could you take to make those changes?

Profile Plus

Get on the road to wellness by participating in the following activities on your Profile Plus CD-ROM:

- Wellness Inventory
- Life Expectancy and Physiological Age Prediction Questionnaire

- Self-Evaluation and Behavioral Objectives for the Future
- Behavior Change Plan.

Sites & Bytes

Healthy People 2010
www.healthypeople.gov

Healthy People 2010 is a statement of national health objectives designed to identify the most significant preventable causes of acute and chronic illnesses and accidents, and to establish national goals to reduce these threats to health.

LiveWell Health Risk Appraisal
http://wellness.uwsp.edu/Health_Service/services/livewell

This comprehensive site sponsored by the National Wellness Institute features a series of self-assessment surveys composed of questions in a variety of wellness dimensions, including physical fitness, nutrition, self-care, drugs, emotional health, and spiritual wellness.

Selfgrowth.com
www.selfgrowth.com

This site is an online guide to self-help, self-improvement, and personal growth, featuring information on psychology, dieting, recovery, relationships, health and fitness, natural medicine, and spiritual development. An online IQ test, daily and weekly newsletters, and links to more than 4,000 websites are included.

InfoTrac College Edition

Activity

Haber, David. "Wellness General of the United States: A Creative Approach to Promote Family and Community Health." *Family and Community Health,* Vol. 25, No. 3, October 2002, p. 71(12).

1. According to the author, what is the definition of health promotion and primary prevention? Provide an example of secondary and tertiary prevention strategies.

2. What are some of the reasons for changing the title of the chief United States medical officer from "Surgeon General" to "Wellness General"?

3. According to the author, what are three ways to increase the utilization of prevention services in the United States?

InfoTrac College Edition

You can find additional readings relating to personal health with InfoTrac College Edition, an online library of more than 900 journals and publications. Follow the instructions for accessing InfoTrac that were packaged with your textbook; then search for articles using a keyword search.

For additional links, resources, and suggested readings on InfoTrac College Edition, visit our Health & Wellness Resource Center at **http://health.wadsworth.com**.

Key Terms

The terms listed are used on the page indicated. Definitions of the terms are in the Glossary at the end of this book.

health 4
health promotion 7
locus of control 17
norms 17

prevention 19
protection 20
reinforcement 17

self-efficacy 17
self-talk 17
wellness 4

References

1. "Constitution of the World Health Organization." *Chronicle of the World Health Organization.* Geneva, Switzerland: WHO, 1947.
2. Travis, John. Personal interview.
3. Mathews, Dale. Personal interview.
4. Hales, Dianne. "Can Prayer Really Heal?" *Parade,* March 23, 2003, p. 4.
5. Koenig, Harold. Personal interview.
6. Hales, "Can Prayer Really Heal?"
7. "Annual Mortality Report: Life Expectancy Increase." *Public Health Reports,* Vol. 118, No. 3, May–June 2003, p. 275.
8. Centers for Disease Control and Prevention, www.cdc.gov/nchs.
9. "Tackling Major Risk Factors Simultaneously Key to Improving Global Health." *Canadian Chemical News,* Vol. 55, No. 7, July–August 2003, p. 24.
10. International Obesity Task Force (IOTF). "Controlling the Global Obesity Epidemic," www.iotf.org.
11. "Sex vs. Gender Matters in Health Promotion and Disease Prevention." *Women's Health Weekly,* September 11, 2003, p. 50.
12. Healthy People 2010, www.healthypeople.gov.
13. *Mental Health: Culture, Race, and Ethnicity.* Washington, DC: Office of the Surgeon General, August 2001. www.surgeongeneral.gov/library/mentalhealth/cre/

14. "Treatments, Outcomes Differ Widely Among Women of Different Races, Ethnicities." *Women's Health Weekly,* February 13, 2003, p. 14.
15. McCollum, David, et al. "Outcomes and Toxicity in African-American and Caucasian Patients in a Randomized Adjuvant Chemotherapy Trial for Colon Cancer." *Journal of the National Cancer Institute,* Vol. 94, August 7, 2002, p. 1160.
16. United States Department of Health and Human Services.
17. *Mental Health: Culture, Race, and Ethnicity.*
18. National Center for Education Statistics. Office of Educational Improvement. U.S. Department of Statistics. http://nces.ed.gov.
19. Howland, Jonathan, et al. "Prevalence of Allergy Symptoms and Associated Medication Use in a Sample of College Seniors." *Journal of American College Health,* Vol. 51, No. 2, September 2002, p. 67.
20. Hunt, S., et al. "Worry and Use of Coping Strategies Among Older and Younger Adults." *Journal of Anxiety Disorders,* Vol. 17, No. 5, 2003, pp. 547–560.
21. Green, John, et al. "Heart Disease Risk Perception in College Men and Women." *Journal of American College Health,* Vol. 51, No. 5, March 2003, p. 207.

22. Prokhorov, A., et al. "Self-Reported Health Status, Health Vulnerability, and Smoking Behavior in College Students: Implications for Intervention." *Nicotine and Tobacco Research,* Vol. 5, No. 4, August 2003, p. 545.
23. "College Students Concerned About Lack of Health Coverage After Graduation." *Health and Medicine Week,* August 4, 2003, p. 287.
24. Manning, S., et al. "Group B Streptococcus Acquisition Among College Students Living in a Single Dormitory." *Annals of Epidemiology,* Vol. 13, No. 8, September 2003, p. 582.
25. Keeling, Richard. "Is College Dangerous?" *Journal of American College Health,* Vol. 50, No. 2, September 2001, p. 53.
26. Engle-Friedman, M., et al. "The Effect of Sleep Loss on Next Day Effort." *Journal of Sleep Research,* Vol. 12, No. 2, June 2003, p. 113.
27. Benton, Sherry, et al. "Changes in Counseling Center Client Problems Across 13 Years." *Professional Psychology: Research and Practice,* Vol. 34, No. 1, January 2003, p. 66.
28. Adlaf, Edward, et al. "The Prevalence of Elevated Psychological Distress Among Canadian Undergraduates: Findings from the 1998 Canadian Campus Survey." *Journal of American College Health,* Vol. 50, No. 2, September 2001, p. 67.

References

29. Bowen, Anne, and Martin Bourgeois. "Attitudes Toward Lesbian, Gay, and Bisexual College Students." *Journal of American College Health,* Vol. 50, No. 2, September 2001, p. 91.

30. Rozin, P., et al. "Food and Life, Pleasure and Worry, Among American College Students: Gender Differences and Regional Similarities." *Journal of Personality and Social Psychology,* Vol. 85, No. 1, July 2003, p. 132.

31. Klopp, S., et al. "Self-Reported Vegetarianism May Be a Marker for College Women at Risk for Disordered Eating." *Journal of the American Dietetic Association,* Vol. 103, No. 6, June 2003, p. 745.

32. Suminski, Richard. "Physical Activity Among Ethnically Diverse College Students." *Journal of American College Health,* Vol. 51, September 2002, p. 75.

33. The Society for Adolescent Medicine, www.adolescenthealth.org.

34. National Household Survey on Drug Abuse. *The NHSDA Report: Cigarette Brand Preferences,* U.S. Department of Health and Human Services, July 11, 2003.

35. Parmet, Sharon. "Smoking and the Heart." *Journal of the American Medical Association,* Vol. 290, No. 1, July 2, 2003, p. 146.

36. Gruenewald, Paul, et al. "Understanding College Drinking: Assessing Dose Response from Survey Self-Reports." *Journal of Studies on Alcohol,* Vol. 64, No. 4, July 2003, p. 500.

37. Weitzman, Elissa, et al. "Taking Up Binge Drinking in College: The Influences of Person, Social Group, and Environment." *Journal of Adolescent Health,* Vol. 32, No. 1, January 2003, p. 26.

38. "Gene Variant May Influence College Drinking Behaviors." *Alcoholism and Drug Abuse Weekly,* Vol. 15, No. 33, September 1, 2003, p. 8.

39. Eisenberg, M., and H. Wechsler. "Substance Use Behaviors Among College Students with Same-Sex and Opposite-Sex Experience: Results from a National Study." *Addictive Behaviors,* Vol. 28, No. 6, 2003, p. 899.

40. Yacoubian, George, et al. "Correlates of Ecstasy Use Among Students Surveyed Through the 1997 College Alcohol Study." *Journal of Drug Education,* Vol. 33, No. 1, January 2003, p. 61.

41. Mayers, L. B., et al. "Tattooing and Body Piercing." *Pediatrics,* Vol. 111, May 2003, p. 1126.

42. Davies, Jon, et al. "Identifying Male College Students' Perceived Health Needs, Barriers to Seeking Help, and Recommendations to Help Men Adopt Healthier Lifestyles." *Journal of American College Health,* Vol. 48, No. 5, May 2000.

43. Hughes, Patricia, et al. "Self-Defense and Martial Arts Evaluation for College Women: Preliminary Validation of Perceptions of Dangerous Situations Scale." *Research Quarterly for Exercise and Sport,* Vol. 74, No. 2, June 2003, p. 153.

44. Dye, M. L., and K. E. Davis. "Stalking and Psychological Abuse: Common Factors and Relationship-Specific Characteristics." *Violence and Victims,* Vol. 18, No. 2, April 2003, p. 163.

45. Swinford, Paula. "Advancing the Health of Students: A Rationale for College Health Programs." *Journal of American College Health,* Vol. 50, No. 6, May 2002, p. 261.

46. Walker, Katrina, and Tammy Satterwhite. "Academic Performance Among African American and Caucasian College Students: Is the Family Still Important?" *College Student Journal,* Vol. 36, No. 1, March 2002, p. 113.

47. Petrocelli, John. "Processes and Stages of Change: Counseling with the Transtheoretical Model of Change." *Journal of Counseling and Development,* Vol. 80, No. 1, Winter 2002, p. 22.

48. Wallace, L., and J. Buckworth. "Longitudinal Shifts in Exercise Stages of Change in College Students." *Journal of Sports Medicine and Physical Fitness,* Vol. 43, No. 2, June 2003, p. 209.

49. Sparling, Phillip, and Teresa Snow. "Physical Activity Patterns in Recent College Alumni," *Research Quarterly for Exercise and Sport,* Vol. 73, No. 2, June 2002, p. 200.

50. Prokhorov et al., "Self-Reported Health Status, Health Vulnerability, and Smoking Behavior in College Students."

51. Steinman, K. J. "College Students' Early Cessation from Episodic Heavy Drinking: Prevalence and Correlates." *Journal of American College Health,* Vol. 51, No. 5, March 2003, p. 197.

52. Goldberg, Stan. "The 10 Rules of Change." *Psychology Today,* Vol. 35, No. 5, September–October 2002, p. 38.

53. Martin Seligman, personal interview.

54. Berchuck, Andres. "An Ounce of Cancer Prevention Really is Worth a Pound of Cure." *Contemporary OB/GYN,* Vol. 48, No. 8, August 2003, p. 8.

55. Brener, Nancy, and Vani Gowda. "U.S. College Students' Reports of Receiving Health Information on College Campuses." *Journal of American College Health,* Vol. 49, No. 5, March 2001, p. 223.

56. Halperin, A. C., and N. A. Rigotti. "U.S. Public Universities' Compliance with Recommended Tobacco-Control Policies." *Journal of American College Health,* Vol. 51, No. 5, March 2003, p. 181.

57. "Survey Reveals Record Numbers of Students Involved in Service." *Black Issues in Higher Education,* Vol. 20, No. 10, July 3, 2003, p. 12.

Psychological Health

CHAPTER 2

For years, Travis put on his "happy face" around his friends and family. Popular and athletic in high school, he never let anyone know how desperately unhappy he actually felt. "Whatever I was doing during the day, nothing was on my mind more than wanting to die," he recalls. On a perfectly ordinary day in his senior year, Travis tried to kill himself with an overdose of pills. Rushed to a hospital, Travis recovered, resumed his studies, and entered college. By the middle of his freshman year, he was struggling once more with feelings of hopelessness. This time he realized what was happening and sought help from a therapist. "I thought college was supposed to be the happiest time of your life," he said. "What went wrong?"

This is a question many young people might ask. Although youth can seem a golden time, when body and mind glow with potential, the process of becoming an adult is a challenging one in every culture and country. Psychological health can make the difference between facing this challenge with optimism and confidence or feeling overwhelmed by expectations and responsibilities.

This isn't always easy. At some point in life, one of every three people develops an emotional disorder. Young adulthood—the years from the late teens to the mid-twenties—is a time when many serious disorders, including bipolar illness (manic depression) and schizophrenia, often develop. The saddest fact is not that so many feel so bad, but that so few realize they can feel better. Only one of every five men and women who could use treatment ever seeks help. Yet 80 to 90 percent of those treated for psychological problems recover, most within a few months.

By learning about psychological disorders, you may be able to recognize early warning signals in yourself or your loved ones so you can deal with potential difficulties or seek professional help for more serious problems.

After studying the material in this chapter, you should be able to:

- **Identify** the characteristics of emotional, mental, and spiritual health.

- **Discuss** the concepts of emotional and spiritual intelligence.

- **Describe** the values and other self-esteem components of psychological health.

- **Identify** effective coping strategies that promote positive attitudes and actions.

- **Explain** the differences between mental health and mental illness and **list** some effects of mental illness on physical health.

- **List** the key structures of the brain and **describe** the role of neurons in communication within the brain.

- **Describe** the major mental illnesses and the characteristic symptoms of each type.

- **Discuss** some of the factors that may lead to suicide as well as strategies for prevention.

- **Describe** the treatment options available for those with psychological problems.

© Marac Romanelli/The Image Bank/Getty Images

◼ What Is Psychological Health?

Unlike physical health, psychological well-being cannot be measured, tested, X-rayed, or dissected. Yet psychologically healthy men and women generally share certain characteristics: They value themselves and strive toward happiness and fulfillment. They establish and maintain close relationships with others. They accept the limitations as well as the possibilities that life has to offer. And they feel a sense of meaning and purpose that makes the gestures of living worth the effort required.

Psychological health encompasses both our emotional and mental states—that is, our feelings and our thoughts. **Emotional health** generally refers to feelings and moods, both of which are discussed later in this chapter. Characteristics of emotionally healthy persons, identified in an analysis of major studies of emotional wellness, include the following:

:: Determination and effort to be healthy.

:: Flexibility and adaptability to a variety of circumstances.

:: Development of a sense of meaning and affirmation of life.

:: An understanding that the self is not the center of the universe.

:: Compassion for others.

:: The ability to be unselfish in serving or relating to others.

:: Increased depth and satisfaction in intimate relationships.

:: A sense of control over the mind and body that enables the person to make health-enhancing choices and decisions.[1]

Mental health describes our ability to perceive reality as it is, to respond to its challenges, and to develop rational strategies for living. The mentally healthy person doesn't try to avoid conflicts and distress but can cope with life's transitions, traumas, and losses in a way that allows for emotional stability and growth. The characteristics of mental health include:

:: The ability to function and carry out responsibilities.

:: The ability to form relationships.

:: Realistic perceptions of the motivations of others.

:: Rational, logical thought processes.

:: The ability to adapt to change and to cope with adversity.[2]

There is considerable overlap between psychological and **spiritual health,** which involves our ability to identify our basic purpose in life and to experience the fulfillment of achieving our full potential. In one recent study, more than half of individuals with mental disorders, including

Psychologically healthy people have compassion for others and are able to form strong and deep relationships. They can adapt to a variety of circumstances and strive to achieve their full potential.

© Tom Stewart/CORBIS

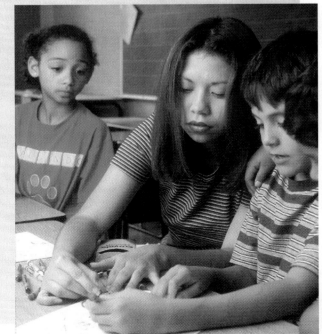

© Bob Daemmrich Photography

depression, turned to spiritual readings or practices to increase calmness, find inner strength and meaning, improve self-awareness, and increase their sense of well-being.[3] Religious support has also been shown to help lower depression and increase life satisfaction beyond the benefits of social support from friends and family.[4]

In addition, **culture** helps to define psychological health. In one culture, men and women may express feelings with great intensity, shouting in joy or wailing in grief, while in another culture such behavior might be considered abnormal or unhealthy. In our diverse society, many cultural influences affect Americans' sense of who they are, where they came from, and what they believe. Cultural rituals help bring people together, strengthen their bonds, reinforce the values and beliefs they share, and provide a sense of belonging, meaning, and purpose.

Emotional Intelligence

A person's "IQ"—or intelligence quotient—was once considered the leading predictor of achievement. However, psychologists have determined that another "way of knowing," dubbed **emotional intelligence,** makes an even greater difference in a person's personal and professional success. In his international best-seller on what some call "EQ" (for emotional quotient), psychologist Daniel Goleman identified five components of emotional intelligence: self-awareness, altruism, personal motivation, empathy, and the ability to love and be loved by friends, partners, and family members. People who possess high emotional intelligence are the people who truly succeed in work as well as play, building flourishing careers and lasting, meaningful relationships.[5]

Men and women, who vary more in the intensity of their emotional experiences than in the nature of their emotions, are equally capable of cultivating greater emotional intelligence. Emotional intelligence isn't fixed at birth, nor is it the same as intuition. Among the emotional competencies that most benefit students are focusing on clear, manageable goals and identifying and understanding emotions rather than relying on "gut" feelings.

Spiritual Intelligence

Mental health professionals have recognized the power of **spiritual intelligence,** which some define as "the capacity to sense, understand, and tap into the highest parts of ourselves, others, and the world around us." Spiritual intelligence, unlike spirituality, does not center on the worship of a God above, but on the discovery of a wisdom within. All of us are born with the potential to develop spiritual intelligence, but relatively few do.

STRATEGIES FOR CHANGE

Tapping into Spiritual Strength

If you are religious:

- Deepen your spiritual commitment through prayer or more frequent attendance at a house of worship.

- Join a prayer or religious reading group.

- Read scriptures or inspirational literature.

If you are not religious:

- Build silence and solitude into your daily life. Even a few stolen moments in the early morning or evening hours can help.

- Spend time in nature. A walk on the beach, a stroll through a park, or simply looking up at the night sky helps put our mostly man-made problems into perspective.

- Keep company with the wise—either in person or through their words. Their insight can enable us to examine serious issues.

- Reflect on the nature of life and death: Life is precious. Death is certain. While life involves difficulties, these can be transcended rather than avoided.

- Practice spiritual values. Spiritual intelligence is not a spectator sport. Rather than just contemplating kindness and honesty, we have to live them as best we can.

Could Prayer Be Good Medicine?

Hundreds of scientific studies are investigating the healing power of prayer and spirituality. With funding from the National Institutes of Health, investigators at Johns Hopkins Medical Center are studying prayer groups of women with breast cancer. At the University of Pennsylvania, neuroradiologists are documenting changes in brain scans of meditating monks and praying nuns. At Baptist Memorial Hospital in Memphis, patients are receiving an intensive "prayer intervention" prior to undergoing bypass surgery.[6]

"We are not out to prove that a deity exists," says Diane Becker, Ph.D., of Johns Hopkins University, recipient of two NIH grants for research on therapeutic prayer. "We are trying to see whether prayer has meaning to people that translates into biology and affects a disease process."[7]

Medical acceptance has grown along with solid scientific data on prayer's impact, says Dale Matthews, M.D., of Georgetown University, author of *The Faith Factor,* who estimates that about 75 percent of studies of spirituality have confirmed health benefits. "If prayer were available in pill form," he notes, "no pharmacy could stock enough of it."[8]

Even when age, health, habits, demographics, and other factors are considered, individuals who pray regularly and attend religious services stay healthier and live longer than those who rarely or never do. They have significantly lower blood pressure and stronger immune systems than the less religious, are less prone to alcoholism, less likely to smoke heavily, and are hospitalized less often. In studies at several medical centers, prayer and faith have speeded recovery from depression, alcoholism, hip surgery, drug addiction, stroke, rheumatoid arthritis, heart attacks, and bypass surgery.[9]

How does prayer do these things? Some scientists speculate that prayer may foster a state of peace and calm that could lead to beneficial changes in the cardiovascular and immune systems. Sophisticated brain imaging techniques have shown that prayer and meditation cause changes in blood flow in particular regions of the brain that may lead to lower blood pressure, slower heart rate, decreased anxiety, and an enhanced sense of well-being.

❖ The Science of Positive Psychology

Psychology, a field that traditionally concentrated on what goes wrong in our lives and in our minds, has shifted its focus to the study of human strengths, virtues, and positive emotions.[10] The three pillars of positive psychology are the study of positive emotions, such as hope and trust; positive traits, such as wisdom and courage; and positive institutions, such as strong families and democracy.

According to psychologist Martin Seligman, Ph.D., the "father" of positive psychology, everyone, regardless of genes or fate, can achieve a happy, gratifying, meaningful life. The goal is not simply to feel good momentarily or to avoid bad experiences, but to build positive strengths and virtues that enable us to find meaning and purpose in life.[11]

"Psychology is not just the study of weakness and damage," Seligman argues, "it is also the study of strength and virtue. Treatment is not just fixing what is broken, it is nurturing what is best within ourselves."[12] The traits that may well protect us from physical and mental illness include courage, optimism, hope, interpersonal skills, a work ethic, responsibility, future-mindedness, honesty, and perseverance.

Knowing Your Needs

Newborns are unable to survive on their own. They depend on others for the satisfaction of their physical needs for food, shelter, warmth, and protection, as well as their less tangible emotional needs. In growing to maturity, children take on more responsibility and become more independent. No one, however, becomes totally self-sufficient. As adults, we easily recognize our basic physical needs, but we often fail to acknowledge our emotional needs. Yet they, too, must be met if we are to be as fulfilled as possible.

The humanist theorist Abraham Maslow believed that human needs are the motivating factors in personality development. First, we must satisfy basic physiological needs, such as those for food, shelter, and sleep. Only then can we pursue fulfillment of our higher needs—for safety and security, love and affection, and self-esteem. Few individuals reach the state of **self-actualization,** in which one functions at the highest possible level and derives the greatest possible satisfaction from life. (See Figure 2-1 on page 43.)

Clarifying Your Values

Your **values** are the criteria by which you evaluate things, people, events, and yourself; they represent what's most important to you. In a world of almost dizzying complexity, values can provide guidelines for making decisions that are right for you. If understood and applied, they help give life meaning and structure.

Social psychologist Milton Rokeach distinguished between two types of values. *Instrumental* values represent ways of thinking and acting that we hold important, such as being loving or loyal. *Terminal* values represent goals, achievements, or ideal states that we strive toward, such as happiness. Instrumental and terminal values form the basis for your attitudes and your behavior.

There can be a large discrepancy between what people say they value and what their actions indicate about their values. That's why it's important to clarify your own values, making sure you understand what you believe so

STRATEGIES FOR CHANGE

Being True to Yourself

■ Take the tombstone test: What would you like to have written on your tombstone? In other words, how would you like to be remembered? Your honest answer should tell you, very succinctly, what you value most.

■ Describe yourself, as you are today, in a brief sentence. Ask friends or family members for their descriptions of you. How would you have to change to become the person you want to be remembered as?

■ Try the adjective test: Choose three adjectives that you'd like to see associated with your reputation. Then list what you've done or can do to earn such descriptions.

Self Survey **Well-Being Scale**

Part I

The following questions contain statements and their opposites. Notice that the statements extend from one extreme to the other. Where would you place yourself on this scale? Place a circle on the number that is most true for you at this time. Do not put your circles between numbers.

Life Purpose and Satisfaction

1. During most of the day,
   my energy level is   very low   1 2 3 4 5 6 7   very high

2. As a whole, my life seems   dull   1 2 3 4 5 6 7   vibrant

3. My daily activities are   not a source of satisfaction   1 2 3 4 5 6 7   a source of satisfaction

4. I have come to expect that
   every day will be   exactly the same   1 2 3 4 5 6 7   new and different

5. When I think deeply
   about life   I do not feel there is any purpose to it   1 2 3 4 5 6 7   I feel there is a purpose to it

6. I feel that my life so far has   not been productive   1 2 3 4 5 6 7   been productive

7. I feel that the work*
   I am doing   is of no value   1 2 3 4 5 6 7   is of great value

8. I wish I were different
   than who I am.   agree strongly   1 2 3 4 5 6 7   disagree strongly

9. At this time, I have   no clearly defined goals for my life   1 2 3 4 5 6 7   clearly defined goals for my life

10. When sad things happen
    to me or other people   I cannot feel positive about life   1 2 3 4 5 6 7   I continue to feel positive about life

11. When I think about what I
    have done with my life, I feel   worthless   1 2 3 4 5 6 7   worthwhile

12. My present life   does not satisfy me   1 2 3 4 5 6 7   satisfies me

13. I feel joy in my heart   never   1 2 3 4 5 6 7   all the time

14. I feel trapped by the
    circumstances of my life.   agree strongly   1 2 3 4 5 6 7   disagree strongly

15. When I think about my past   I feel many regrets   1 2 3 4 5 6 7   I feel no regrets

16. Deep inside myself   I do not feel loved   1 2 3 4 5 6 7   I feel loved

17. When I think about the
    problems that I have   I do not feel hopeful about solving them   1 2 3 4 5 6 7   I feel very hopeful about solving them

*The definition of work is not limited to income-producing jobs. It includes childcare, housework, studies, and volunteer services.

Part II

Self-Confidence During Stress (answer according to how you feel during stressful times)

1. When there is a great deal of
   pressure being placed on me   I get tense   1 2 3 4 5 6 7   I remain calm

2. I react to problems and difficulties   with a great deal of frustration   1 2 3 4 5 6 7   with no frustration

3. In a difficult situation, I am confident
   that I will receive the help that I need.   disagree strongly   1 2 3 4 5 6 7   agree strongly

4. I experience anxiety   all the time   1 2 3 4 5 6 7   never

5. When I have made a mistake   I feel extreme dislike for myself   1 2 3 4 5 6 7   I continue to like myself

6. I find myself worrying that
   something bad is going to happen
   to me or those I love   all the time   1 2 3 4 5 6 7   never

7. In a stressful situation   I cannot concentrate easily   1 2 3 4 5 6 7   I can concentrate easily

(Continued)

Self Survey

Well-Being Scale (continued)

8. I am fearful	all the time	1 2 3 4 5 6 7	never
9. When I need to stand up for myself	I cannot do it	1 2 3 4 5 6 7	I can do it easily
10. I feel less than adequate in most situations	agree strongly	1 2 3 4 5 6 7	disagree strongly
11. During times of stress, I feel isolated and alone.	agree strongly	1 2 3 4 5 6 7	disagree strongly
12. In really difficult situations	I feel unable to respond in positive ways	1 2 3 4 5 6 7	I feel able to respond in positive ways
13. When I need to relax	I experience no peace— only thoughts and worries	1 2 3 4 5 6 7	I experience a peacefulness— free of thoughts and worries
14. When I am frightened	I panic	1 2 3 4 5 6 7	I remain calm
15. I worry about the future	all the time	1 2 3 4 5 6 7	never

Scoring

The number you circled is your score for that question. Add your scores in each of the two sections and divide each sum by the number of questions in the section.

:: Life Purpose and Satisfaction: _____ ÷ 17 = ___.__

:: Self-Confidence During Stress: ___ ÷ 15 = ___.__

:: Combined Well-Being:

(add scores for both) _____ ÷ 32 = ___.__

Each score should range between 1.00 and 7.00 and may include decimals (for example 5.15).

Interpretation:

VERY LOW: 1.00 TO 2.49
MEDIUM LOW: 2.50 TO 3.99
MEDIUM HIGH: 4.00 TO 5.49
VERY HIGH: 5.50 TO 7.00

These scores reflect the strength with which you feel these positive emotions. Do they make sense to you? Review each scale and each question in each scale. Your score on each item gives you information about the emotions and areas in your life where your psychological resources are strong, as well as the areas where strength needs to be developed.

If you notice a large difference between the LPS and SCDS scores, use this information to recognize which central attitudes and aspects of your life most need strengthening. If your scores on both scales are very low, talk with a counselor or a friend about how you are feeling about yourself and your life.

Source: © 1989. Jared Kass. *Inventory of Positive Psychological Attitudes.* The Well-Being Scale is the self-test version of the Inventory of Positive Psychological Attitudes (IPPA-32) developed by Dr. Jared D. Kass. Reprinted with author's permission. For information, contact: Dr. Jared Kass, Division of Counseling and Psychology, Graduate School of Arts and Social Sciences, Lesley College, Cambridge, MA 02138.

Your Health Change Plan

for Psychological Wellness

Just as you can improve your physical well-being, you can enhance the state of your mind. Here are some suggestions:

:: Recognize and express your feelings. Pent-up emotions tend to fester inside, building into anger or depression.

:: Don't brood. Rather than merely mulling over a problem, try to find solutions that are positive and useful.

:: Take one step at a time. As long as you're taking some action to solve a problem, you can take pride in your ability to cope.

:: Spend more time doing those activities you know you do best. For example, if you are a good cook, prepare a meal for someone.

:: Separate what you do, especially any mistakes you make, from who you are. Instead of saying, "I'm so stupid," tell yourself, "That wasn't the smartest move I ever made, but I'll learn from it."

:: Use affirmations, positive statements that help reinforce the most positive aspects of your personality and experience. Every day, you might say, "I am a loving, caring person," or "I am honest and open in expressing my feelings." Write some affirmations of your own on index cards and flip through them occasionally.

:: List the things you would like to have or experience. Construct the statements as if you were already enjoying the situations you list, beginning each sentence with "I am." For example, "I am feeling great about doing well in my classes."

:: When your internal critic—the negative inner voice we all have—starts putting you down, force yourself to think of a situation that you handled well.

:: Set a limit on self-pity. Tell yourself, "I'm going to feel sorry for myself this morning, but this afternoon, I've got to get on with my life."

:: Volunteer. A third of Americans—some 89 million people—give of themselves through volunteer work. By doing the same, you may feel better too.

:: Exercise. In various studies around the world, physical exertion ranks as one of the best ways to change a bad mood, raise energy, and reduce tension.

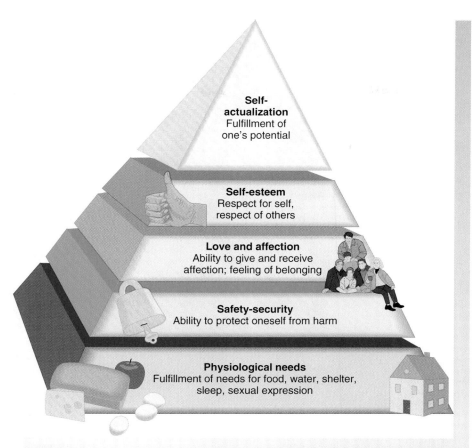

Figure 2-1 THE MASLOW PYRAMID

To attain the highest level of psychological health, you must first satisfy your needs for safety and security, love and affection, and self-esteem.

Source: A. Maslow. *Motivation and Personality,* 3rd ed., © 1997. Reprinted by permission of Pearson Education, Inc.

that you can live in accordance with your beliefs. To do so, follow these steps:

1. Carefully consider the consequences of each choice.
2. Choose freely from among all the options.
3. Publicly affirm your values by sharing them with others.
4. Act out your values.

Values clarification is not a once-in-a-lifetime task, but an ongoing process of sorting out what matters most to you. If you believe in protecting the environment, do you shut off lights, or walk rather than drive, in order to conserve energy? Do you vote for political candidates who support environmental protection? Do you recycle newspapers, bottles, and cans? Values are more than ideals we'd like to attain; they should be reflected in the way we live day by day.

Boosting Self-Esteem

Each of us wants and needs to feel significant as a human being with unique talents, abilities, and roles in life. A sense of **self-esteem,** of belief or pride in ourselves, gives us confidence to dare to attempt to achieve at school or work and to reach out to others to form friendships and close relationships. Self-esteem is the little voice that whispers, "You're worth it. You can do it. You're okay."

Self-esteem is based, not on external factors like wealth or beauty, but on what you believe about yourself. It's not something you're born with; self-esteem develops over time. It's also not something anyone else can give to you, although those around you can either help boost or diminish your self-esteem.

The seeds of self-esteem are planted in childhood when parents provide the assurance and appreciation youngsters need to push themselves toward new accomplishments: crawling, walking, forming words and sentences, learning control over their bladder and bowels.

Adults, too, must consider themselves worthy of love, friendship, and success if they are to be loved, to make friends, and to achieve their goals. Low self-esteem is more common in people who have been abused as children and in those with psychiatric disorders, including depression, anxiety, alcoholism, and drug dependence. Feeling a lack of love and encouragement as a child can also lead to poor self-esteem. Adults

Self-esteem, which is based on what you believe about yourself, tends to increase when you experience success.

© 2000 Bob Torrez/Stone/Getty Images

with poor self-esteem may unconsciously enter relationships that reinforce their self-perceptions and may prefer and even seek out people who think poorly of them.

One of the most useful techniques for bolstering self-esteem and achieving your goals is developing the habit of positive thinking and talking. While negative observations, such as constant criticisms or reminders of the most minor of faults, can undermine self-image, positive affirmations—compliments, kudos, encouragements—have proven effective in enhancing self-esteem and psychological well-being. Individuals who fight off negative thoughts fare better psychologically than those who collapse when a setback occurs or who rely on others to make them feel better.

 Self-esteem has proven to be one of the best predictors of college adjustment. Students with high self-esteem report better personal, emotional, social, and academic adjustment.[13] However, true self-esteem requires an honest sense of your own worth. In a study of college students, psychology professors followed self-enhancers who began their freshman year with an inflated sense of their own academic ability. These students expected to get much higher college grades than might be predicted based on their high school grades and test scores. While they felt confident and happy for a while, they did no better academically and were no more likely to graduate than their realistic or self-deprecating peers. In fact, the short-term benefits of their self-illusions took a toll over the long term: Their self-esteem and interest in school declined with each passing year.[14]

Managing Your Moods

Feelings come and go within minutes. A **mood** is a more sustained emotional state that colors our view of the world for hours or days. According to surveys by psychologist Randy Larsen, of the University of Michigan, bad moods descend upon us an average of three out of every ten days. "A few people—about 2 percent—are happy just about every day," he says. "About 5 percent report bad moods four out of every five days."[15]

There are gender differences in mood management: Men typically try to distract themselves (a partially successful strategy) or use alcohol or drugs (an ineffective tactic). Women are more likely to talk to someone (which can help) or to ruminate on why they feel bad (which doesn't help). Learning effective mood-boosting, mood-regulating strategies can help both men and women pull themselves up and out of an emotional slump.

The most effective way to banish a sad or bad mood is by changing what caused it in the first place—if you can figure out what made you upset and why. "Most bad moods are caused by loss or failure in work or intimate relationships," says Larsen. "The questions to ask are: What

Giving and getting support from others is fundamental to good psychological health.

can I do to fix the failure? What can I do to remedy the loss? Is there anything under my control that I can change? If there is, take action and solve it." Rewrite the report. Ask to take a make-up exam. Apologize to the friend whose feelings you hurt. Tell your parents you feel bad about the argument you had.

If there's nothing you can do, accept what happened and focus on doing things differently next time. "In our studies, resolving to try harder actually was as effective in improving mood as taking action in the present," says Larsen. You also can try to think about what happened in a different way and put a positive spin on it. This technique, known as *cognitive reappraisal,* or "reframing," helps you look at a setback in a new light: What lessons did it teach you? What would you have done differently? Could there be a silver lining or hidden benefit?

If you can't identify or resolve the problem responsible for your emotional funk, the next-best solution is to concentrate on altering your negative feelings. For example, try setting a quick, achievable goal that can boost your spirits with a small success. Clean out a drawer; sort through the piles of paper on your desk; send an e-mail or instant message to an old friend.

Another good option is to get moving. In studies of mood regulation, exercise consistently ranks as the single most effective strategy for banishing bad feelings. Numerous studies have confirmed that aerobic workouts, such as walking or jogging, significantly improve mood. Even nonaerobic exercise, such as weight lifting, can boost spirits; improve sleep and appetite; reduce anxiety, irritability, and anger; and produce feelings of mastery and accomplishment.

Taking your mind off your troubles, rather than mulling over what's wrong, is one of the most often used mood boosters, but it's only partly successful. Simple distractions—watching television, for instance, or reading—work only temporarily. Activities that engage the imagination, on the other hand, seem to have more lasting effects. Listening to music, for instance, is one of the most popular and effective ways of distracting people from their troubles and changing their bad moods.

How Can I Find Happiness?

A joke, a chocolate, a compliment, or a back rub can make us happy—briefly. The more such happy moments we experience, the more pleasant life feels. But according to positive psychologist Martin Seligman, picture-perfect Hollywood happiness represents the lowest level of gratification. The second category is the good life, which consists of applying core virtues and character strengths daily in relationships, studies, work, and leisure. The third and highest is the meaningful life, in which individuals commit their abilities to the service of some larger purpose.[16]

Many factors influence individual happiness, including genetics. Research on twins raised separately and apart suggests that each of us may have an innate "set point" for happiness, just as we may have a set point for body weight (discussed in Chapter 6). Although a set point may fluctuate, it rarely changes radically.

 Having an unhappy childhood does not doom anyone to a lifetime of misery, but it does increase the likelihood of unhappiness in adulthood. In a study of community college students, the vast majority reported a

happy or very happy childhood. Only 9 percent of these students were unhappy as adults. About two-thirds of those reporting unhappy or very unhappy childhoods reported that they were unhappy or very unhappy adults. The risk of having an unhappy adulthood was two and a half time greater for those who'd been unhappy as children.

Life events, such as illness, unemployment, or marriage, can have a temporary impact on happiness.[17] In general people react to events, whether positive or negative, but quickly adapt back to baseline levels of subjective well-being. Setbacks, such as being laid off, and achievements, such as being promoted, lose their impact on happiness levels in less than three months.[18] However, a 15-year longitudinal study of the impact of marital transitions on more than 24,000 individuals found significant individual differences. A major loss, such as the death of a loved one, can continue to undermine happiness for many years.[19]

Age, health, and wealth have different and often surprising effects on happiness. (See "Fact or Fiction?") Life satisfaction goes up slightly with age, and emotions become less intense and more stable. Good health is not a prerequisite for happiness. Even seriously ill cancer patients differ only slightly in life satisfaction from healthier people.

 Education, intelligence, gender, and race do not matter much for happiness. African Americans and Hispanics in the United States have lower rates of depression than white Americans, but they do not report greater happiness. Neither gender is clearly happier, but in different studies women are both happier and sadder than men. Religious people rank as somewhat happier and more satisfied with life than nonreligious ones. Relationships are key to happiness among undergraduates. In a survey of 222 college students, psychologists found that the "happiest" 10 percent, as determined by six different rating scales, shared one distinctive characteristic: a rich and fulfilling social life. Almost all are involved in a romantic relationship as well as in rewarding friendships. The happiest students spent the least time alone, and their friends rated them as highest on good relationships.[20]

The best predictors of happiness are the characteristics of good psychological health: high self-esteem, optimism, extroversion, and a sense of being in control. In addition to these four key traits, happy people are more likely to have healthy and fit bodies; realistic goals and expectations; supportive friendships; an intimate, sexually warm marriage; and a faith that provides support, purpose, and acceptance.

Becoming Optimistic

The dictionary defines **optimism** as "an inclination to anticipate the best possible outcome." For various reasons—because they believe in themselves, because they trust in a higher power, because they feel lucky—optimists

---

FACT OR FICTION? ???????????????

"People who are wealthy, healthy, or lucky are happier than others."

Fiction: Rich people are, on average, only slightly happier than poor ones. Individuals with life-threatening illnesses or serious disabilities are not unhappier than the rest of the population. In general, major events—a thrill like winning the lottery or a setback like losing a job—lose their impact on happiness within a few months.

What does make a difference? Love and faith. Married people consistently rank as happier than single or divorced ones. And religious people are usually happier than nonreligious ones.

Source: Martin Seligman. *Authentic Happiness.* New York: Free Press, 2002.

expect positive experiences from life. When bad things happen, they tend to see setbacks or losses as specific, temporary incidents. In their eyes, a disappointment is "one of those things" that happens every once in a while, rather than the latest in a long string of disasters. And rather than blaming themselves ("I always mess things up," pessimists might say), optimists look at all the different factors that may have caused the problem.

Individuals aren't born optimistic or pessimistic; in fact, researchers have documented changes over time in the ways that individuals view the world and what they expect to experience in the future. The key is disputing the automatic negative thoughts that flood our brains and choosing to believe in our own possibilities.

 Positive psychologist Martin Seligman provides "optimism training" to freshmen at the University of Pennsylvania. According to his follow-up data, those trained to look on the bright side suffered fewer illnesses throughout college than those who did not.[21] Optimism may even help people live longer, healthier lives. In a forty-year Mayo Clinic study the longevity of optimists was 19 percent greater compared to pessimists. On average, people with positive attitudes regarding aging live about 7.5 years longer.[22]

Looking on the Light Side

Humor, which enables us to express fears and negative feelings without causing distress to ourselves or others, is one of the healthiest ways of coping with life's ups and downs. Laughter stimulates the heart, alters brain wave patterns and breathing rhythms, reduces perceptions of pain, decreases stress-related hormones, and strengthens the immune system. In psychotherapy, humor helps channel negative emotions toward a positive effect. Even in cases of critical or fatal illnesses, humor can relieve pain and help people live with greater joy until they die.

Happiness and optimism go hand in hand. Small rewards can keep spirits high and remind you that you are special.

STRATEGIES FOR CHANGE

How to Be Happy

- Make time for yourself. It's impossible to meet the needs of others without recognizing and fulfilling your own.

- Invest yourself in closeness. Give your loved ones the gift of your time and caring.

- Work hard at what you like. Search for challenges that satisfy your need to do something meaningful.

- Be upbeat. If you always look for what's wrong about yourself or your life, you'll find it—and feel even worse.

- Organize but stay loose. Be ready to seize an unexpected opportunity to try something different.

Joking and laughing are ways of expressing honest emotions, of overcoming dread and doubt, and of connecting with others. They also can defuse rage. After all, it's almost impossible to stay angry when you're laughing. To tickle your funny bone, try keeping a file of favorite cartoons or jokes. Go to a comedy club instead of a movie. And when you see or hear something that makes you laugh out loud, don't keep it to yourself—multiply the mirth by sharing it with a friend.

Loving and Being Loved

"One can live magnificently in this world if one knows how to work and how to love, to work for the person one loves and to love one's work," Leo Tolstoy wrote. You may not think of love as a basic need like food and rest, but it is essential for both physical and psychological well-being.

Mounting evidence suggests that people who lack love and commitment are at high risk for a host of illnesses, including infections, heart disease, and cancer. "Love and intimacy are at the root of what makes us sick and what makes us well," says cardiologist Dean Ornish, author of *Love & Survival: The Scientific Basis for the Healing Power of Intimacy.* "No other factor in medicine—not diet, not smoking, not exercise—has a greater impact."[23]

Doing Good

Altruism—helping or giving to others—enhances self-esteem, relieves physical and mental stress, and protects psychological well-being. Hans Selye, the father of stress research, described cooperation with others for the self's sake as altruistic egotism, whereby we satisfy our own needs while helping others satisfy theirs. This concept is essentially an updated version of the golden rule: Do unto others as you would have them do unto you. The important difference is that you earn your neighbor's love and help by offering them love and help.

Volunteerism helps those who give as well as those who receive. People involved in community organizations, for instance, consistently report a surge of well-being called *helper's high,* which they describe as a unique sense of calmness, warmth, and enhanced self-worth. College students who provided community service as part of a semester-long course reported changes in attitude (including a decreased tendency to blame people for their misfortunes), self-esteem (primarily a belief that they can make a difference), and behavior (a greater commitment to do more volunteer work).

The options for giving of yourself are limitless: Volunteer to serve a meal at a homeless shelter. Collect donations for a charity auction. Teach in an illiteracy program. Perform the simplest act of charity: Pray for others.

❖ Feeling in Control

Although no one has absolute control over destiny, we can do a great deal to control how we think, feel, and behave. By assessing our life situations realistically, we can make plans and preparations that allow us to make the most of our circumstances. By doing so, we gain a sense of mastery. In nationwide surveys, Americans who feel in control of their lives report greater psychological well-being than

You may not have complete control over your destiny, but you can control how you respond to challenges. Even under the most difficult of circumstances, individuals can gain a sense of mastery.

those who do not, as well as extraordinarily positive feelings of happiness.

Developing Autonomy

One goal that many people strive for is **autonomy,** or independence. Both family and society influence our ability to grow toward independence. Autonomous individuals are true to themselves. As they weigh the pros and cons of any decision, whether it's using or refusing drugs or choosing a major or career, they base their judgment on their own values, not those of others. Their ability to draw on internal resources and cope with challenges has a positive impact on both their psychological well-being and their physical health, including recovery from illness.

Those who've achieved autonomy may seek the opinions of others, but they do not allow their decisions to be dictated by external influences. For autonomous individuals, their **locus of control**—that is, where they view control as originating—is *internal* (from within themselves) rather than *external* (from others).

Asserting Yourself

Being **assertive** means recognizing your feelings and making your needs and desires clear to others. Unlike aggression, a far less healthy means of expression, assertiveness

STRATEGIES FOR CHANGE

How to Assert Yourself

▪ Use "I" statements to explain your feelings. This allows you to take ownership of your opinions and feelings without putting down others for how they feel and think.

▪ Listen to and acknowledge what the other person says. After you speak, find out if the other person understands your position. Ask how he or she feels about what you've said.

▪ Be direct and specific. Describe the problem as you see it, using neutral language rather than assigning blame. Also suggest a specific solution, but make it clear that you'd like the lines of communication and negotiation to remain open.

▪ Don't think you have to be obnoxious in order to be assertive. It's most effective to state your needs and preferences without any sarcasm or hostility.

usually works. You can change a situation you don't like by communicating your feelings and thoughts in nonprovocative words, by focusing on specifics, and by making sure you're talking with the person who is directly responsible.

Becoming assertive isn't always easy. Many people have learned to cope by being passive and not communicating their feelings or opinions. Sooner or later they become so irritated, frustrated, or overwhelmed that they explode in an outburst—which they think of as being assertive. However, such behavior is so distasteful to them that they'd rather be passive. But assertiveness doesn't mean screaming or telling someone off. You can communicate your wishes calmly and clearly. Assertiveness is a behavior that respects your rights and the rights of other people even when you disagree.

Even at its mildest, assertiveness can make you feel better about yourself and your life. The reason: When you speak up or take action, you're in the pilot seat. And that's always much less stressful than taking a back seat and trying to hang on for dear life.

✖ Connecting with Others

At every age, people who feel connected to others tend to be healthier physically and psychologically.[24] College students are no exception: Those who have a supportive, readily available network of relationships are less psychologically distressed and more satisfied with life. (See Chapter 7 for a comprehensive discussion of communication, friendship, and intimacy.)

The opposite of *connectedness* is **social isolation,** a major risk factor for illness and early death. Individuals with few social contacts face two to four times the mortality rate of others. The reason may be that their social isolation weakens the body's ability to ward off disease. Medical students with higher-than-average scores on a loneliness scale had lower levels of protective immune cells. The end of a long-term relationship—through separation, divorce, or death—also dampens immunity.

It is part of our nature as mammals and as human beings to crave relationships. But invariably we end up alone at times. Solitude is not without its own quiet joys— time for introspection, self-assessment, learning from the past, and looking toward the future. Each of us can cultivate the joy of our company, of being alone without crossing the line and becoming lonely.

Overcoming Loneliness

More so than many other countries, we are a nation of loners. Recent trends—longer work hours, busy family schedules, frequent moves, high divorce rates—have created even more lonely people. Only 23 percent of Americans say they're never lonely. Loneliest of all are those who are divorced, separated, or widowed and those who live alone

or solely with children. Among single adults who have never been married, 42 percent feel lonely at least sometimes. However, loneliness is most likely to cause emotional distress when it is chronic rather than episodic.

To combat loneliness, people may join groups, fling themselves into projects and activities, or surround themselves with superficial acquaintances. Others avoid the effort of trying to connect, sometimes limiting most of their personal interactions to chat groups on the Internet.

The true keys to overcoming loneliness are developing resources to fulfill our own potential and learning to reach out to others. In this way, loneliness can become a means to personal growth and discovery.

Race and gender also affect the experience of loneliness. In a study of 100 African-American undergraduates, having a best friend was the most important factor in low levels of emotional loneliness in men and high levels of feeling in control in women. Some studies have found that men are lonelier than women. Others find no gender differences in loneliness, but researchers note that men may be more hesitant than women to admit that they're lonely.

In cross-cultural studies, married people of all ages generally report less loneliness than single individuals and than unmarried individuals living together. In most nations, having children has little or no effect on how lonely people feel. Even in middle and old age, the childless are not more vulnerable to loneliness or depression. Widowed and divorced men and women report higher levels of loneliness and depression than married people, regardless of whether they have children.

Loneliness also affects positive health practices among college students. Those who do not have a network of supportive relationships report feeling a sense of utter aloneness, of living in a barren environment, of feeling empty and hollow, and of frequently experiencing boredom and aimlessness. These students also feel least motivated to take the best possible care of their minds and bodies.

Facing Social Anxiety

Many people are uncomfortable meeting strangers or speaking or performing in public. In some surveys, as many as 40 percent of people describe themselves as shy, or socially anxious. Some shy people—an estimated 10 to 15 percent of children—are born with a predisposition to shyness. Others become shy because they don't learn proper social responses or because they experience rejection or shame.

Social anxiety often becomes a problem in late adolescence. Students may develop symptoms when they go to a party or are called on in class. Some experience symptoms

Social situations can be extremely uncomfortable if you suffer from social anxiety. But over time you can overcome shyness by learning how to interact with others.

when they try to perform any sort of action in the presence of others, even such everyday activities as eating in public, using a public restroom, or writing a check. About 7 percent of the population could be diagnosed with a severe form of social anxiety, called **social phobia,** in which individuals typically fear and avoid various social situations. Adolescents and young adults with severe social anxiety are at increased risk of major depression.[25] Phobias are discussed later in this chapter. The key difference between these problems and normal shyness and self-consciousness is the degree of distress and impairment that individuals experience.

If you're shy, you can overcome much of your social apprehensiveness on your own, in much the same way as you might set out to stop smoking or lose weight. For example, you can improve your social skills by pushing yourself to introduce yourself to a stranger at a party or to chat about the weather or the food selections with the person next to you in a cafeteria line. Gradually you'll acquire a sense of social timing and a verbal ease that will take the worry out of close encounters with others.

Those with more disabling social anxiety may do best with professional guidance, which has proven highly effective. One common technique used by experts is role playing, in which individuals act out situations that normally produce butterflies in the stomach, such as returning a defective product to a store or calling for a date. With practice and time, most individuals are able to emerge

from the walls that shyness has built around them and take pleasure in interacting with others.

◙ Understanding Mental Health

Mentally healthy individuals value themselves, perceive reality as it is, accept their limitations and possibilities, carry out their responsibilities, establish and maintain close relationships, pursue work that suits their talent and training, and feel a sense of fulfillment that makes the efforts of daily living worthwhile. (See Figure 2-2.)

According to research conducted by the World Health Organization (WHO), mental disorders affect 400 million people around the world, and these numbers will surge even higher in the coming decades. In its first-ever official report on mental health, the Office of the U.S. Surgeon General called for increased efforts to recognize, treat, and prevent mental disorders. "We now realize that, just as things can go wrong with the heart, the lungs, the kidneys, and the liver, things can also go wrong with the human brain," the report states. "A person cannot be truly healthy overall without mental health."[26]

▣ What Is a Mental Disorder?

While lay people may speak of "nervous breakdowns" or "insanity," these are not scientific terms. The U.S. government's official definition states that a serious mental illness

Figure 2-2 THE MENTALLY HEALTHY INDIVIDUAL
Mental well-being is a combination of many factors.

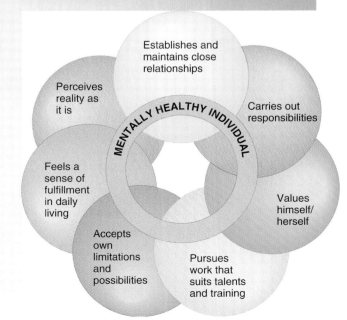

is "a diagnosable mental, behavioral, or emotional disorder that interferes with one or more major activities in life, like dressing, eating, or working." According to the U.S. Surgeon General, one in five Americans experiences a mental disorder in the course of a year.

The mental health profession's standard for diagnosing a mental disorder is the pattern of symptoms, or diagnostic criteria, spelled out for the almost 300 disorders in the American Psychiatric Association's *Diagnostic and Statistical Manual,* 4th edition (DSM-IV). Psychiatrists define a **mental disorder** as "a clinically significant behavioral or psychological syndrome or pattern that occurs in an individual and that is associated with present distress (a painful symptom) or disability (impairment in one or more important areas of functioning) or with a significantly increased risk of suffering death, pain, disability, or an important loss of freedom."[27]

Does Mental Health Affect Physical Health?

Mental disorders affect not just the mind but also the body. **Anxiety** can lead to intensified asthmatic reactions, skin conditions, and digestive disorders. Stress can play a role in hypertension, heart attacks, sudden cardiac death, and immune disorders in the young as well as in older individuals.[28]

Depression has increasingly been recognized as a serious risk factor for physical illness. According to a recent review of large-scale studies on depression, of more than 36,000 men and women, depressed individuals were 1.5 to 4 times more likely to develop heart problems.[29] In still-unknown ways, depression may increase risk factors for heart disease, such as high blood pressure, and for premature death.[30] Together, depression and heart disease worsen a patient's prognosis more than either condition alone.[31]

Depressed individuals are more likely to suffer heart attacks and chest pain than others and to die of heart disease. Between 15 to 20 percent of patients experience major depression following a heart attack, and the incidence of depression is three times higher in people with heart disease than in the general public.[32] Since depression can and often does recur, physicians now view it as a chronic illness with lifelong implications for mental and physical health.

By some estimates, as many as 60 percent of those who seek help from physicians suffer primarily from a psychological problem. Treating mental health problems leads not only to improved health but also to lower health-care costs. Psychiatric treatment reduces hospitalizations, cuts medical expenses, and reduces work disability.

Mental Health on Campus

About 15 percent of students seek counseling during college. The percentage of students feeling depressed or overwhelmed by all they have to do rises during the freshman year.[33] Undergraduates are more likely to seek psychological counseling as they progress through college. (See Figure 2-3.) Those with A and B averages are more likely to seek help than those with averages of C or below.[34]

In one survey, anxiety and fears were the most severe problems that women reported, followed by academic worries such as grades. For men, academics ranked before anxiety. Depression rated third for both genders. Students who do not seek on-campus counseling report different difficulties: academics, career decisions, and finances. About half of students who turn to college counselors for help had previously received psychological care.[35]

The emotional difficulties of college students have become more complex and more severe than in the past. In one national survey more than 80 percent of directors of counseling centers reported an increase in the number of students with serious psychological disorders.[36]

According to a Kansas State study of students who sought counseling over a 13-year period, the percentage of students with depression doubled, as did the percentage with suicidal thoughts. Among students who sought counseling prior to 1994, trouble with dating and other relationships were reported most frequently. Beginning in 1996, stress and anxiety became more common than relationship difficulties. (See Student Snapshot: "Why Students Seek Psychological Help.")[37]

Figure 2-3 WHEN STUDENTS SEEK COUNSELING
The percentage of students seeking counseling increases from freshman to senior year. Data are based on the number of students who sought help at a university counseling center over a 13-year period.

Source: Sherry Benton, et al. "Changes in Counseling Center Client Problems Across 13 Years," *Professional Psychology: Research and Practice,* Vol. 34, No. 1, January 2003, p. 66.

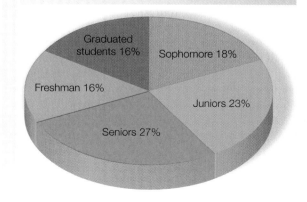

Student Snapshot — Why Students Seek Psychological Help

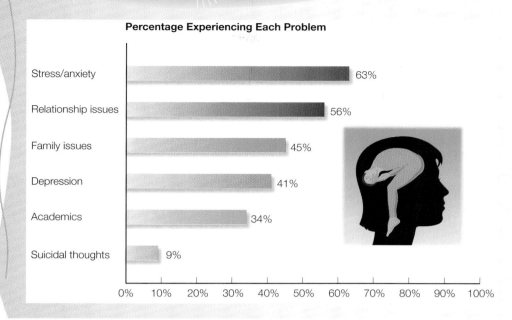

Percentage Experiencing Each Problem

Problem	Percentage
Stress/anxiety	63%
Relationship issues	56%
Family issues	45%
Depression	41%
Academics	34%
Suicidal thoughts	9%

0%   10%   20%   30%   40%   50%   60%   70%   80%   90%   100%

Source: Sherry Benton, et al. "Changes in Counseling Center Client Problems Across 13 Years," *Professional Psychology: Research and Practice*, Vol. 34, No. 1, January 2003, p. 66.

Of the 19 types of problems the counselors reported, 14 increased significantly during the 13 years studied. These include depression, stress/anxiety, personality disorders, suicidal thoughts, grief, developmental issues (such as severe homesickness), and struggles with academic skills. "Situational" problems, triggered by some immediate event, almost tripled. Problems with substance abuse and eating disorders, as well as chronic mental illnesses, remained steady.

College women are twice as likely as men to say that they frequently feel overwhelmed (35.2 percent versus 16.4 percent). More women than men (8.1 percent versus 5.8 percent) report feelings of depression.[38]

 "Religiosity"—a term used for various spiritual practices—may protect individuals against symptoms of depression. In one study, researchers assessed religiosity and symptoms of depression in 105 intercollegiate athletes at a public university in the Southeast. The greater the athletes' intrinsic religiosity, the less likely they were to suffer depressive symptoms.

"Perhaps intrinsic religious beliefs provide a sense of hope and security that protect against distressing events," the researchers speculated. "It may also be that uncondi-tional love by one's God provides a stable sense of self worth" that buffers against stress.[39]

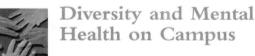

Diversity and Mental Health on Campus

College students have traditionally been viewed as psychologically troubled. Studies in the 1970s and 1980s concluded that half to three-quarters of students might have "significant emotional difficulties," while a smaller number—estimated from 10 to 40 percent—suffered more serious "psychological impairment." Many predicted that as campuses became more diverse in ethnicity and gender, rates of mental disorders would rise.

More recent studies of ethnic and gender differences challenged this assumption. The few that have looked into ethnic variations yielded conflicting or inconclusive results: Some found no differences; others suggested higher rates of depression among Korean and South Asian students. Studies comparing male and female students have also been inconclusive. Some reported higher rates of depression and anxiety in women; others showed no difference.

The Brain: The Last Frontier

The brain has intrigued scientists for centuries, but only recently have its explorers made dramatic progress in unraveling its mysteries. Leaders in **neuropsychiatry**—the field that brings together the study of the brain and the mind—remind us that 95 percent of what is known about brain anatomy, chemistry, and physiology has been learned in the last decade. These discoveries have reshaped our understanding of the organ that is central to our identity and well-being and have fostered great hope for more effective therapies for the more than 1,000 disorders—psychiatric and neurologic—that affect the brain and nervous system.

Inside the Brain

Each human brain contains hundreds of billions of nerve cells, or **neurons,** and support cells called **glia.** Most are present at birth, when the brain weighs less than a pound. In the first six years of life—the period when we acquire more knowledge more rapidly than ever again—the brain

reaches its full weight of about 3 pounds (see Figure 2-4). From birth, male and female brains differ in a variety of ways. (See The X & Y Files: "Are Men's and Women's Brains Different?")

The neurons are the basic working units of the brain. Like snowflakes, no two are exactly the same. Each consists of a cell body containing the **nucleus;** a long fiber, called the **axon,** which can range from less than an inch to several feet in length; an **axon terminal,** or ending; and multiple branching fibers called **dendrites.** (See Figure 2-5.) The glia serve as the scaffolding for the brain, separate the brain from the bloodstream, assist in the growth of neurons, speed up the transmission of nerve impulses, and engulf and digest damaged neurons.

As the master control center for the body, the brain is constantly receiving information from the senses and relaying messages to various parts of the body. Some of these messages travel through the spinal cord, which extends from the neck about two-thirds of the way down the backbone. Other signals are carried by nerves that connect the brain directly with certain parts of the body.

Historically, scientists have focused on the anatomy or structures of the brain in their attempts to understand how it functions and why it sometimes malfunctions. Modern neuropsychiatrists have shifted much of their attention to biochemical processes within the brain, particularly those involved in communication between neurons.

Communication Within the Brain

Neurons "talk" with each other by means of electrical and chemical processes (see Figure 2-5). An electric charge, or impulse, travels along an axon to the terminal, where packets of chemicals called **neurotransmitters** are stored. When released, these messengers flow out of the axon terminal and cross a **synapse,** a specialized site at which the axon terminal of one neuron comes extremely close to a dendrite from another neuron. On the surface of the dendrite are **receptors,** protein molecules designed to bind with neurotransmitters. It takes only about a tenthousandth of a second

Figure 2-4 THE BRAIN

The three major parts of the brain are the cerebrum, cerebellum, and brainstem. The cerebrum is divided into two hemispheres—the left, which regulates the right side of the body, and the right, which regulates the left side of the body. The cerebellum plays the major role in coordinating movement, balance, and posture. The brainstem contains centers that control breathing, blood pressure, heart rate, and other physiological functions.

Cerebral cortex
Frontal lobe
Corpus callosum
Hypothalamus (part of the limbic system)
Pituitary gland
Brainstem { Midbrain, Pons, Medulla }
Spinal cord
Parietal lobe
①
Occipital lobe
Thalamus (part of the limbic system)
③
Cerebellum
②
Central canal of spinal cord
① Cerebrum
② Medulla
③ Cerebellum

the XY file *Are Men's and Women's Brains Different?*

"The brain is not an organ of sex," the pioneering feminist and economist Charlotte Perkins Gilman declared in 1898. "[We might] as well speak of the female liver." These days, gender scientists do indeed speak of the female liver, describing it as one of the most gender-distinctive organs. What then of the brain? Consider these recent findings:

:: **Men's brains are bigger; women use more neurons.** Overall, a woman's brain, like her body, is 10 to 15 percent smaller than a man's, yet the regions dedicated to higher cognitive functions such as language are more densely packed with neurons—and women use more of them. When a male puts his mind to work, neurons turn on in highly specific areas. When females set their minds on similar tasks, cells light up all over the brain.

:: **Male and female brains perceive light and sound differently.** A man's eyes are more sensitive to bright light and retain their ability to see well at long distances longer in life. A woman hears a much broader range of sounds, and her hearing remains sharper longer.

:: **The female brain responds more intensely to emotion.** According to neuroimaging studies, the genders respond differently to emotions, especially sad-

ness, which activates, or turns on, neurons in an area eight times larger in women than men.

:: **Male and female brains age in different ways.** The male brain loses tissue at almost three times the rate of the female brain. Because of this gender difference, the all-important frontal lobes, which are larger in men in youth and early adulthood, reach approximately the same size in men and women by the time they reach their forties. Other parts of men's brains—including the corpus callosum and the left hemisphere—also atrophy more rapidly.

:: **Neither gender's brain is "better."** Intelligence per se appears equal in both. The greatest gender differences appear both at the top and bottom of the intelligence scales. Men outnumber women both as geniuses and as morons. Nevertheless, more than half the time, regardless of the type of test, most women and men perform more or less equally—even though they may well take different routes to arrive at the same answers. Cognitive skills show greater variability both among women and among men than between the genders. The best evaluation may have come from essayist Samuel Johnson. When asked whether women or men are more intelligent, he responded, "Which man? Which woman?"

Figure 2-5 THE NEURON, THE BASIC WORKING UNIT OF THE BRAIN
Neurotransmitters released across the synapse transmit the chemical nerve impulse from one neuron to another.

Nucleus

Axon terminal

Dendrite

Nerve impulse

Presynaptic nuron

Axon

Postsynaptic nuron

Receptors

Transmitted nerve impulse

Approaching nerve impulse

Synaptic vesicles (containing neurotransmitters)

Released neurotransmitter molecules

© Secchi-Lecaque/Roussel-UCLA/CNRI/Photo Researchers, Inc.

Neuron, magnified 3100 times.

for a neurotransmitter and a receptor to come together. Neurotransmitters that do not connect with receptors may remain in the synapse until they are reabsorbed by the cell that produced them—a process called **reuptake**—or broken down by enzymes.

A malfunction in the release of a neurotransmitter, in its reuptake or elimination, or in the receptors or secondary messengers may result in abnormalities in thinking, feeling, or behavior. Some of the most promising and exciting research in neuropsychiatry is focusing on correcting such malfunctions. The neurotransmitter serotonin and its receptors have been shown to affect mood, sleep, behavior, appetite, memory, learning, sexuality, and aggression and to play a role in several mental disorders. The discovery of a possible link between low levels of serotonin and some cases of major depression has led to the development of more precisely targeted **antidepressant** medications that boost serotonin to normal levels.

The Role of Sleep

You stay up late cramming for a final. You drive through the night to visit a friend at another campus. You get up for an early class during the week but stay in bed until noon on weekends. And you wonder: "Why am I so tired?" The answer: You're not getting enough sleep.

Whenever we fail to get adequate sleep, we accumulate what researchers call a *sleep debt*. With each night of too little rest, our body's need for sleep grows until it becomes irresistible. The only solution to sleep debt is the obvious one: paying it back. Individuals who add an hour or two to their nightly sleep time are more alert, more productive, and less likely to have accidents. And because sleepy people tend to be irritable and edgy, those who get more rest also tend to be happier, healthier, and easier to get along with.

The Night Shift

We spend a third of our lives sleeping—more time than we spend working, loving, or playing. Although sleepers may look quiet and seem unresponsive to the world around them, their brains and bodies are going through a series of profound changes. Scientists differentiate between certain periods of the night when the eyes dart rapidly back and forth beneath closed lids, called **rapid-eye-movement (REM) sleep,** and quieter, non-REM sleep stages. Most adults spend 20 to 25 percent of the night in REM sleep, when our most vivid dreaming takes place.

Each night as you fall asleep, you go through the same sequence of sleep stages: Your body begins to slow down, and muscular tension decreases. As you enter stage 1 of non-REM sleep, your brain waves become smaller, pinched, and irregular. Mundane thoughts flit through your mind; if awakened from this twilight zone, you might deny having slept at all. As you enter stage 2, your brain waves become larger, with occasional bursts of activity. Your eyes become unresponsive, so that even if your eyelids were gently lifted, you wouldn't see. In stage 3, your brain waves are much slower and about five times larger than in stage 1. In stage 4, the most profound state of unconsciousness, your brain waves form a slow, jagged pattern; and you would be very difficult to arouse. (See Figure 2-6.)

The full journey to the depths of tranquility takes more than an hour. Then you begin your ascent—not to consciousness but to REM sleep. The muscles of your middle ear vibrate. Your brain waves resemble the patterns of waking more than of deep sleep. The muscles of your face, limbs, and trunk are slack. Your pulse and breathing quicken, and your brain temperature and blood flow increase. Your eyes dart back and forth. If wakened, you're likely to report a fantasylike dream.

Your body repeats this sequence four or five times a night. In an eight-hour night's rest, you spend two hours in REM sleep; over the course of a lifetime, you'll spend five or six years dreaming and three times that amount in the quieter stages of sleep.

Figure 2-6 A SLEEP CYCLE
During the first hour or so, sleep becomes deeper; then the level ascends to a period of REM sleep (indicated by thick bars). The sleep cycle is repeated, with some variations, throughout the night.

How Much Sleep Do I Need?

According to a national poll, 69 percent of Americans experience frequent sleep problems. About two-thirds of adults average less than seven hours of sleep a night.[40]

No formula can say how long a good night's sleep should be. Normal sleep times range from five to ten hours; the average is seven and a half. About one or two people in a hundred can get by with just five hours; another small minority needs twice that amount. Each of us seems to have an innate sleep *appetite* that is as much a part of our genetic programming as hair color and skin tone.

To figure out your sleep needs, keep your wake-up time the same every morning and vary your bedtime. Are you groggy after six hours of shut-eye? Does an extra hour give you more stamina? What about an extra two hours? Since too much sleep can make you feel sluggish, don't assume that more is always better. Listen to your body's signals, and adjust your sleep schedule to suit them.

Getting Enough Sleep

Although sleep needs vary from person to person, physicians have recognized "problem sleepiness" as a threat to health and safety. Its effects are insidious, however, and often neither the individuals nor their doctors realize that problem sleepiness is undermining emotional and physical health.

About 5 percent of Americans suffer from persistent insomnia. Medications can help in the short run but lose their effectiveness over time and interfere, to varying degrees, with the normal stages of sleep. One of the most promising alternatives is cognitive-behavior training (CBT), which combines cognitive therapy with specific strategies to improve sleep habits, such as avoiding daytime naps and limiting time in bed.

Chronic Fatigue Syndrome (CFS)

The characteristic symptom of this complex problem is profound, disabling fatigue that lasts at least six months and occurs along with a variety of symptoms, such as loss of appetite, nausea, drenching night sweats, headache, joint pain, aching or stiff muscles, and impaired memory or concentration. Although estimates vary, chronic fatigue syndrome may affect up to 3 percent of the population, primarily young, white, successful women.

The causes of CFS remain unknown, and researchers theorize that several biological and psychological factors may work together to trigger the illness. Doctors diagnose CFS by ruling out other conditions, including depression.

Cognitive-behavior therapy (discussed later in this chapter) and a progressive aerobic exercise program have proven especially effective in relieving fatigue and other symptoms of CFS. Controlled studies have found no benefit from alternative remedies, such as megavitamins, herbal supplements, and special diets.[41]

STRATEGIES FOR CHANGE

How to Sleep Like a Baby

- Keep regular hours for going to bed and getting up in the morning. Stay as close as possible to this schedule on weekends as well as weekdays.

- Develop a sleep ritual—such as stretching, meditation, yoga, prayer, or reading a not-too-thrilling novel—to ease the transition from wakefulness to sleep.

- Don't drink coffee late in the day. The effects of caffeine can linger for up to eight hours. And don't smoke. Nicotine is an even more powerful stimulant—and sleep saboteur—than caffeine.

- Don't rely on alcohol to get to sleep. Alcohol disrupts normal sleep stages, so you won't sleep as deeply or as restfully as you normally would.

- Don't nap during the day if you're having problems sleeping through the night.

▚ Anxiety Disorders

Anxiety disorders may involve inordinate fears of certain objects or situations **(phobias)**, episodes of sudden, inexplicable terror **(panic attacks)**, chronic distress **(generalized anxiety disorder, or GAD)**, or persistent, disturbing thoughts and behaviors **(obsessive-compulsive disorder)**. Over a lifetime, according to the National Comorbidity Survey, as many as one in four Americans may experience an anxiety disorder. Only one of every four of these individuals is ever correctly diagnosed and treated. Yet most who do get treatment, even for severe and disabling problems, improve dramatically.[42]

Phobias

Phobias—the most prevalent type of anxiety disorder—are out-of-the-ordinary, irrational, intense, persistent fears of certain objects or situations. About two million Americans develop such acute terror that they go to extremes to avoid whatever it is that they fear, even though they realize that these feelings are excessive or unreasonable. The most common phobias involve animals, particularly dogs, snakes, insects, and mice; the sight of blood; closed spaces *(claustrophobia)*; heights *(acrophobia)*; air travel and being in places or situations from which they perceive it would be difficult or embarrassing to escape *(agoraphobia)*.

Although various medications have been tried, none is effective by itself in relieving phobias. The best approach is behavior therapy, which consists of gradual, systematic exposure to the feared object (a process called *systematic desensitization*). Numerous studies have proven that exposure—especially in-vivo exposure, in which individuals are exposed to the actual source of their fear rather than simply imagining it—is highly effective. Medical hypnosis—the use of induction of an altered state of consciousness—also can help.

The characteristic symptoms of a phobia include:

:: Excessive or unreasonable fear of a specific object or situation.

:: Immediate, invariable anxiety when exposed to the object or situation.

:: Recognition that the fear is excessive or unreasonable.

:: Avoidance of the feared object or situation or enduring it only with intense anxiety or distress.

:: Inability to function as usual at school or work or in social relationships because of the phobia.

Panic Attacks and Panic Disorder

Individuals who have had panic attacks describe them as the most frightening experiences of their lives. Without reason or warning, their hearts race wildly. They may become light-headed or dizzy. Because they can't catch their breath, they may start breathing rapidly and hyperventilate. Parts of their bodies, such as their fingers or toes, may tingle or feel numb. Worst of all is the terrible sense that something horrible is about to happen: that they will die, lose their minds, or have a heart attack. Most attacks reach peak intensity within ten minutes. Afterward, individuals live in dread of another one. In the course of a lifetime, your risk of having a single panic attack is 7.2 percent.

Panic disorder develops when attacks recur or apprehension about them becomes so intense that individuals cannot function normally. Full-blown panic disorder occurs in about 1.6 percent of all adults in the course of a lifetime and usually develops before age 30. Women are more than twice as likely as men to experience panic attacks, although no one knows why. Parents, siblings, and children of individuals with panic disorders also are more likely to develop them than are others.

The two primary treatments for panic disorder are (1) cognitive-behavior therapy, which teaches specific strategies for coping with symptoms like rapid breathing, and (2) medication. Treatment helps as many as 90 percent of those with panic disorder either improve significantly or recover completely, usually within six to eight weeks. Individuals who receive cognitive-behavior therapy as well as medication are less likely to suffer relapses than those taking medication alone and often can learn to control their symptoms without drugs.[43]

Generalized Anxiety Disorder

About 10 million adults in the United States suffer from a generalized anxiety disorder (GAD), excessive or unrealistic apprehension that causes physical symptoms and lasts for six months or longer. It usually starts when people are in their twenties. Unlike fear, which helps us recognize and avoid real danger, GAD is an irrational or unwarranted response to harmless objects or situations of exaggerated danger. The most common symptoms are faster heart rate, sweating, increased blood pressure, muscle aches, intestinal pains, irritability, sleep problems, and difficulty concentrating.[44]

Chronically anxious individuals worry—not just some of the time, and not just about the stresses and strains of ordinary life—but constantly, about almost everything: their health, families, finances, marriages, potential dangers. Treatment for GAD may consist of a combination of psychotherapy, behavioral therapy, and antianxiety drugs.

Obsessive-Compulsive Disorder

As many as 1 in 40 Americans has a type of anxiety called obsessive-compulsive disorder (OCD). Some of these individuals suffer only from an *obsession,* a recurring idea, thought, or image that they realize, at least initially, is senseless. The most common obsessions are repetitive thoughts of violence (e.g., killing a child), contamination (becoming infected by shaking hands), and doubt (wondering whether one has performed some act, such as having hurt someone in a traffic accident). Most people with OCD also suffer from a compulsion, repetitive behavior performed according to certain rules or in a stereotyped fashion. The most common compulsions involve handwashing, cleaning, hoarding useless items, counting, or checking (for example, making sure dozens of times that a door is locked).

Individuals with OCD realize that their thoughts or behaviors are bizarre, but they cannot resist or control them. Eventually, the obsessions or compulsions consume a

Worry is a normal part of daily life, but individuals with generalized anxiety disorder worry constantly about everything and anything that might go wrong.

great deal of time and significantly interfere with normal routine, job functioning, or usual social activities or relationships with others. A young woman who must follow a very rigid dressing routine may always be late for class, for example; a student who must count each letter of the alphabet as he types may not be able to complete a term paper.

OCD is believed to have biological roots. It may be a result of gene abnormalities, head injury, or even an autoimmune reaction after childhood infection with strep bacteria. Treatment may consist of cognitive therapy to correct irrational assumptions, behavioral techniques such as progressively limiting the amount of time someone obsessed with cleanliness can spend washing and scrubbing, and medication. About 70 to 80 percent of those with OCD improve with treatment.

Depressive Disorders

Depression, the world's most common mental ailment, affects the brain, the mind, and the body in complex ways. An estimated 16.2 percent of adults experience depression at some point in their lives, according to a recent national survey. After a single episode, the risk of a recurrence, or second episode, is about 50 percent. After a third, the risk of a fourth is about 90 percent.[45] Stress-related events may trigger half of all depressive episodes; great trauma in childhood can increase vulnerability to depression later in life.[46]

Depression has become so widespread that the U.S. Preventive Services Task Force is encouraging physicians to screen all their adult patients for this disorder.[47] Public attitudes also have changed. According to the National Mental Health Association, 55 percent of Americans recognize depression as an illness—up from 38 percent in 1991. Almost half of all Americans have a family member, close friend, or both who has been diagnosed with depression.[48] Of the most common reasons for patient visits to family physicians, depression ranks 11th; anxiety, 17th.

 An estimated 15 to 40 percent of college-age men and women (18- to 24-year-olds) may develop depression.[49] Women have two to three times the rates of depression as men and also are likely to experience other psychiatric conditions at the same time. Women are more likely than men to report "atypical" symptoms such as oversleeping and overeating. They account for 80 percent of cases of seasonal affective disorder.[50]

Comparing everyday "blues" to a **depressive disorder** is like comparing a cold to pneumonia. Major depression can destroy a person's joy for living. Food, friends, sex, or any form of pleasure no longer appeals. It is impossible to concentrate on work and responsibilities. Unable to escape a sense of utter hopelessness, depressed individuals may fight back tears throughout the day and toss and turn through long, empty nights. Thoughts of death or suicide may push into their minds.

Why Are So Many Young People Depressed?

Once young people were considered immune to sadness. Now mental health professionals know better. An estimated 5 to 10 percent of American teenagers suffer from a serious depressive disorder; girls are twice as susceptible as boys. Prior to puberty, girls and boys are equally likely to develop depression. Even preschoolers can develop symptoms of depression, such as irritability, sadness, and withdrawal.[51]

The risks of depression in the young are high. Four in ten depressed adolescents think about killing themselves; two in ten actually try to do so. Every year an estimated 11 to 13 in every 100,000 teens take their own lives, twice as many as the number who die from all natural causes combined.

"Depression is the most common emotional problem in adolescence and the single greatest risk factor for teen suicide," says child psychiatrist Peter Jensen, M.D., director for the Center for the Advancement of Children's Mental Health at Columbia University, who notes that depression rates have been rising over the last half century. "Teens born in the 1980s are more likely to develop depression than those who were born in the 1970s, whose rate of depression is higher than for those born in the 1960s."[52]

No one knows the reason for this steady surge in sadness, but experts point to the breakdown of families, the

Factors that can contribute to the development of depression during the college years include stressful events, poor academic performance, loneliness, and relationship problems.

© David Young-Wolff/PhotoEdit

pressures of the information age, and increased isolation. "Social environment doesn't cause depression," explains psychiatrist John March, M.D., of Duke University, who is heading a nationwide study of therapies for teen depression. "But environmental stress can bring out depression in people who are susceptible. Depression is more than teenage angst. It is an illness of the central nervous system that is common, impairing, and lethal."[53]

A family history of depression greatly increases a young person's vulnerability. In one recent study of high school students diagnosed with depression, family members of depressed adolescents had much higher rates of major depression.[54] A mother's anxiety and depression during early childhood can increase the risk that adolescents will develop symptoms of anxiety and depression.[55] However, the strongest predictor of depression is cigarette smoking. Depressed teens may smoke because they think smoking will make them feel better, but nicotine alters brain chemistry and actually worsens symptoms of depression.

 In a study of 649 college students, those who experienced greater levels of adversity in childhood are more likely to develop depression early in life. Students who were male, nonwhite, and had parents with less than a college education reported significantly more challenges in early life.[56]

Depression can be hard to recognize in the young. Many depressed teens don't look or act sad. Rather than crying, they may snap grouchily at parents or burst into angry tirades. Some turn to alcohol or drugs in hopes of feeling better; others become depressed after they start abusing these substances. As they drop out of activities and pull away from friends, depressed teens spend more time alone. Their schoolwork suffers, and many are labeled as underachievers. Those whose anger explodes in public are branded as troublemakers.

Only in the last decade have researchers in mental health specifically studied treatments for teen depression. They now know that 60 to 75 percent of teenagers—the same percentage as adults—respond to treatment with the medications called SSRIs (a group of antidepressants that includes Prozac and Paxil). The use of these antidepressants in children and teenagers has increased three- to five-fold in recent years. Older antidepressants called tricyclics, once the mainstay of treatment for adults, are not effective in adolescents. Some therapies are as effective as the SSRIs—particularly an approach called cognitive behavior therapy (CBT), which focuses on teaching new ways to deal with stress and sadness, such as changing unrealistic or highly negative ways of thinking.

Minor Depression

Minor depression is a common disorder that is often unrecognized and untreated, affecting about 7.5 percent of Americans during their lifetime. Its symptoms are the same

STRATEGIES FOR PREVENTION

Recognizing the Signs of Teen Depression

- Mood changes, including feeling sad, irritable, or cranky; being easily angered; or having difficulty getting along with family members

- Loss of interest in hobbies, sports, or social activities

- Lack of enjoyment even when involved in an activity they used to enjoy

- Changes in sleep patterns, such as difficulty falling asleep or staying asleep

- Changes in appetite; gaining or losing a lot of weight

- Changes in energy levels, such as feeling tired a lot of the time, moving more slowly, or being physically restless or agitated

- School difficulties, including problems concentrating or a decline in grades

- Personal criticism, such as saying they can't do anything right or blaming themselves for things that are not really their fault

- Self-harm, including thoughts or conversations about hurting themselves

as those of major depression, but less severe and fewer in number. They include either a depressed mood most of the day, nearly every day, or diminished interest or pleasure in daily activities.

Psychotherapy is remarkably effective for mild depression. In more serious cases, antidepressant medication can lead to dramatic improvement in 40 to 80 percent of depressed patients.

Exercise also is a good way to both prevent and treat psychological problems. Several studies have shown that exercise effectively lifts mild to moderate depression.

The National Institutes of Health has launched a major clinical study to determine if a conventional antidepressant or the herbal supplement St. John's wort (discussed later in this chapter) helps individuals with minor depression.[57]

Major Depression

The simplest definition of **major depression** is sadness that does not end. The incidence of major depression has soared over the last two decades, especially among young adults.

Paul Avis/Getty Image

Depression and suicidal thoughts are closely linked. If you know someone who is severely depressed, offer help and comfort during difficult times.

Major depressive disorder affects an estimated 4.9 to 17.9 percent of the population in the course of a lifetime. About 20 to 30 percent of these individuals suffer at least one relapse.[58]

The characteristic symptoms of major depression include:

:: Feeling depressed, sad, empty, discouraged, tearful.

:: Loss of interest or pleasure in once-enjoyable activities.

:: Eating more or less than usual and either gaining or losing weight.

:: Having trouble sleeping or sleeping much more than usual.

:: Feeling slowed down or restless and unable to sit still.

:: Lack of energy.

:: Feeling helpless, hopeless, worthless, inadequate.

:: Difficulty concentrating, forgetfulness.

:: Difficulty thinking clearly or making decisions.

:: Persistent thoughts of death or suicide.

:: Withdrawal from others, lack of interest in sex.

:: Physical symptoms (headaches, digestive problems, aches and pains).

As many as half of major depressive episodes are not recognized because the symptoms are "masked." Rather than feeling sad or depressed, individuals may experience low energy, insomnia, difficulty concentrating, and physical symptoms. An episode of major depression can trigger a relapse in individuals with substance abuse problems.[59]

Most cases of major depression can be treated successfully, usually with psychotherapy, medication, or both. Psychotherapy alone works in more than half of mild-to-moderate episodes of major depression. Psychotherapy helps individuals pinpoint the life problems that contribute to their depression, identify negative or distorted thinking patterns, explore behaviors that contribute to depression, and regain a sense of control and pleasure in life. Two specific psychotherapies—cognitive-behavior therapy and interpersonal therapy (described later in this chapter)—have proved as helpful as antidepressant drugs, although they take longer than medication to achieve results.

Antidepressants help about 70 percent of individuals feel better within six to ten weeks. According to long-term studies, treatment should continue for at least nine months after a single acute episode of depression, longer for chronic or recurrent depression. The two most bothersome side effects—reported by some patients taking some antidepressants—are weight gain and sexual dysfunction.[60]

The genders differ in their responses to depression treatments. In one study, premenopausal women responded much more favorably to sertraline (Zoloft), an SSRI, than to a tricyclic antidepressant. In men, the opposite was true. Postmenopausal women responded equally to both types of medication. Other studies have disputed these findings.[61]

Exercise also helps. In a study of 150 individuals diagnosed with major depression, one group was assigned to four months of walking, jogging, or cycling; another took antidepressant medication; and a third both exercised and took medication. At the end of four months, all had improved significantly. Six months later, the exercisers were in better shape physically and mentally—and much less likely to have suffered a relapse. At ten months, the chance of a patient still being depressed was reduced by 50 percent for every 50 minutes of current weekly exercise. In older adults, low-intensity exercise that included weight training improved overall mood more than just aerobic exercise.[62]

For individuals who cannot take antidepressant medications because of medical problems, or who do not improve with psychotherapy or drugs, *electroconvulsive therapy* (ECT)—the administration of a controlled electrical current through electrodes attached to the scalp—remains the safest and most effective treatment. About 50 percent of depressed individuals who do not get better with antidepressant medication and psychotherapy improve after ECT. Experimental new techniques are using electrical and magnetic stimulation to treat depression. [See The Cutting Edge: "Magnets for the Brain," p. 60]

Bipolar Disorder (Manic Depression)

Bipolar disorder, or manic depression, consists of mood swings that may take individuals from *manic* states of feeling euphoric and energetic to depressive states of utter despair. In episodes of full mania, they may become so impulsive and out of touch with reality that they endanger their careers, relationships, health, or even survival. One percent of the population—about 2 million American adults—suffer from this serious but treatable disorder, which affects both genders and all races equally.

The characteristic symptoms of bipolar disorder include:

:: Mood swings (from happy to miserable, optimistic to despairing, and so on)

:: Changes in thinking (thoughts speeding through one's mind, unrealistic self-confidence, difficulty concentrating, delusions, hallucinations)

:: Changes in behavior (sudden immersion in plans and projects, talking very rapidly and much more than usual, excessive spending, impaired judgment, impulsive sexual involvement)

:: Changes in physical condition (less need for sleep, increased energy, fewer health complaints than usual).

During "manic" periods, individuals may make grandiose plans or take dangerous risks. But they often plunge from this highest of highs to a horrible low depressive episode, in which they may feel sad, hopeless, and helpless, and develop other symptoms of major depression. The risk of suicide is very real.

Professional therapy is essential in treating bipolar disorders. Mood-stabilizing medications are the keystone of treatment, although psychotherapy plays a critical role in helping individuals understand their illness and rebuild their lives. Most individuals continue taking medication indefinitely after remission of their symptoms because the risk of recurrence is high.

Suicide

Suicide is not in itself a psychiatric disorder, but it can be the tragic consequence of emotional and psychological problems. Every year 30,000 Americans—among them many young people who seem to have "everything to live for"—commit suicide. An estimated 752,000 attempt to take their own lives; there may be 4.5 million suicide "survivors" in the U.S.[63]

The suicide rate for African-American and Caucasian men peaks between ages 20 and 40. It rises again after age 65 among white men and after age 75 among blacks. In general, whites are at highest risk for suicide, followed by Native Americans, African Americans, Hispanic Americans, and Asian Americans. Internationally, suicide rates are highest in Germany, Scandinavia, Eastern Europe, and Japan, average in the United States, Canada, and Great Britain, and low in Italy, Spain, and Ireland.[64]

Depressed teens are more likely to attempt suicide—and to die. "In psychological interviews after a teen suicide, we see that the warning signs were there," child psychiatrist Madelyn Gould, M.D., of Columbia University, notes, "but no one realized the underlying problem was depression."[65] Stresses that may contribute to the soaring suicide rates among the young are psychological problems, mental disorders, drug abuse, school pressures, social difficulties, concern and confusion about sexual orientation, and family problems.

At all ages, men commit suicide three times more frequently than women, but women attempt suicide much more often than men. (See Table 2-1.) Elderly men are ten times more likely to take their own lives than older women. (See Fact or Fiction?) Native Americans have a suicide rate five times higher than that of the general population.

TABLE 2-1	Suicide Risk	
	Who attempts suicide?	**Who completes suicide?**
Sex	Female	Male
Age	Under 35	Under 20 or over 60
Means	Less deadly, such as wrist slashing	More deadly, such as a gun
Circumstances	High chance of rescue	Low chance of rescue

Source: Tapu Carroll-Ghosh et al. "Suicide," *Textbook of Clinical Psychiatry* (4th edition). Washington, D.C.: American Psychiatric Publishing, Inc., 2003.

FACT OR FICTION? ????????????

"Young people are most likely to kill themselves."

Fiction: Despite what many believe, Americans between the ages of 15 and 24 have the lowest suicide rate (13 per 100,000), while white men in their eighties have the highest (63.1 per 100,000).

Source: Tapu Carroll-Ghosh et al. "Suicide," *Textbook of Clinical Psychiatry* (4th edition). Washington, D.C.: American Psychiatric Publishing, Inc., 2003.

 Suicide is the third leading cause of death among children and adolescents 10 to 19 years old in the United States. The age-adjusted death rate for suicide has decreased in recent years, but the death rate for suicide among children 10 to 14 years old has doubled. Although black youths have historically had lower suicide rates than whites, the gap between suicide rates for black and white youths has narrowed.[66] Among all young people under age 25, firearms-related deaths account for 67 percent of suicides.

Among the factors that increase the likelihood of teen suicide are a previous suicide attempt, violence (either as victim or perpetrator), and use of alcohol or marijuana. For girls, medical symptoms, having a friend attempt or complete suicide, illicit drug use, and a history of mental health problems also increase the risk. Among boys, risk factors include carrying a weapon at school, same-sex romantic attraction, a family history of suicide or suicide attempts, easy household access to guns, skipping school, and being held back or skipping a grade.

About 20 percent of teenagers seriously consider suicide; a much smaller number actually attempt to take their own lives. Talking to a counselor at a suicide hot line may help a young person deal with feelings of despondency.

Researchers also have identified factors that protect young people from suicide. Number one for both boys and girls was feeling connected to their parents and family. For girls, emotional well-being was also protective; grade point average was an additional protective factor for boys. High parental expectations for their child's school achievement, more people living in the household, and religiosity were protective for some of the boys, but not for the girls. Availability of counseling services at school and parental presence at key times during the day were protective for some of the girls, but not for the boys.

Suicide is also the third leading cause of death among college-aged Americans. Males in this age group have a suicide rate six times greater than that of females.[67] Participation in sports seems to have a protective effect and decreases the odds of suicide among male and female college students.[68]

Suicide is not inevitable. Appropriate treatment can help as many as 70 to 80 percent of those at risk for suicide. Among young people, early recognition and treatment for depressive disorders and alcohol and drug use could save thousands of lives each year.

What Leads to Suicide?

Researchers have looked for explanations for suicide by studying everything from phases of the moon to seasons (suicides peak in the spring and early summer) to birth order in the family. They have found no conclusive answers. A constellation of influences—mental disorders, personality traits, biologic and genetic vulnerability, medical illness, and psychosocial stressors—may combine in ways that lower an individual's threshold of vulnerability. The risk of suicide is higher in people who live in cities, are single, have a low income, or are unemployed. No one factor in itself may ever explain fully why a person chooses death.

Mental Disorders

More than 95 percent of those who commit suicide have a mental disorder. Two in particular—depression and alcoholism—account for two-thirds of all suicides. Suicide also is a risk for those with other disorders, including schizophrenia, posttraumatic stress disorder, and personality disorders.[69]

Among patients diagnosed with a mental disorder, the average fatality risk is 2 percent for depressed patients outside of hospitals, 4 percent for depressed patients in hospitals, and 6 percent for hospitalized patients diagnosed as suicidal. These figures are five or six times the rate in the general population.[70]

Substance Abuse

Many of those who commit suicide drink beforehand, and their use of alcohol may lower their inhibitions. Since alcohol itself is a depressant, it can intensify the despondency suicidal individuals are already feeling. Alcoholics who attempt suicide often have other risk factors, including major depression, poor social support, serious medical illness, and unemployment. Drugs of abuse also can alter thinking and lower inhibitions against suicide.

Hopelessness

The sense of utter hopelessness and helplessness may be the most common contributing factor in suicide. When hope dies, individuals view every experience in negative terms and come to expect the worst possible outcomes for their problems. Given this way of thinking, suicide often seems a reasonable response to a life seen as not worth living.

Family History

One of every four people who attempt suicide has a family member who also tried to commit suicide. While a family history of suicide is not in itself considered a predictor of suicide, two mental disorders that can lead to suicide—depression and bipolar disorder (manic depression)—do run in families.

Physical Illness

People who commit suicide are likely to be ill or to believe that they are. About 5 percent actually have a serious physical disorder, such as AIDS or cancer. While suicide may seem to be a decision rationally arrived at in persons with serious or fatal illness, this may not be the case. Depression, not uncommon in such instances, can warp judgment. When the depression is treated, the person may no longer have suicidal intentions.

More than 80 percent of those who commit suicide have seen a physician about a medical complaint within the six months preceding suicide. To help general physicians identify people at risk of suicide, researchers at Johns Hopkins University developed a set of four crucial questions:

:: Have you ever had a period of two weeks or more when you had trouble falling asleep, staying asleep, waking up too early, or sleeping too much?

:: Have you ever had two weeks or more during which you felt sad, blue, depressed or when you lost interest and pleasure in things you usually cared about or enjoyed?

:: Has there been a period of two weeks or more when you felt worthless, sinful, or guilty?

:: Has there ever been a period of time when you felt that life was hopeless?

STRATEGIES FOR PREVENTION

If You Start Thinking About Suicide

At some point, the thought of ending it all—the disappointments, problems, bad feelings—may cross your mind. This experience isn't unusual. But if the idea of taking your life persists or intensifies, you should respond as you would to other warnings of potential threats to your health—by getting the help you need:

■ Talk to a mental health professional. If you have a therapist, call immediately. If not, call a suicide hot line.

■ Find someone you can trust and talk honestly about what you're feeling. If you suffer from depression or another mental disorder, educate trusted friends or relatives about your condition so they are prepared if called upon to help.

■ Write down your more uplifting thoughts. Even if you are despondent, you can help yourself by taking the time to retrieve some more positive thoughts or memories. A simple record of your hopes for the future and the people you value in your life can remind you of why your own life is worth continuing.

■ Avoid drugs and alcohol. Most suicides are the results of sudden, uncontrolled impulses, and drugs and alcohol can make it harder to resist these destructive urges.

■ Go to the hospital. Hospitalization can sometimes be the best way to protect your health and safety.

Anyone who answers yes to these questions should be referred immediately to a mental health professional.

Brain Chemistry

Investigators have found abnormalities in the brain chemistry of individuals who complete suicide, especially low levels of a metabolite of the neurotransmitter serotonin. There are indications that individuals with a deficiency in this substance may have as much as a ten times greater risk of committing suicide than those with higher levels.

Access to Guns

For individuals already facing a combination of predisposing factors, access to a means of committing suicide, particularly to guns, can add to the risk. Unlike other methods of suicide, guns almost always work. States with stricter gun-control laws have much lower rates of suicides than states with more lenient laws. Health professionals are urging parents whose children undergo psychological treatment or assessment to remove all weapons from their homes and to make sure their youngsters do not have access to potentially lethal medications or to alcohol.

Other Factors

Individuals who kill themselves often have gone through more major life crises—job changes, births, financial reversals, divorce, retirement—in the previous six months, compared with others. Long-standing, intense conflict with family members or other important people may add to the danger. In some cases, suicide may be an act of revenge that offers the person a sense of control—however temporary or illusory. For example, a husband whose wife has had an affair may rationalize that he can get back at her, and have the final word, by killing himself. Others may feel that, by rejecting life, they are rejecting a partner or parent who abandoned or betrayed them.

Suicide Prevention

If someone you know has talked about suicide, behaved unpredictably, or suddenly emerged from a severe depression into a calm, settled state of mind, don't rule out the possibility that he or she may attempt suicide.

:: Encourage your friend to talk. Ask concerned questions. Listen attentively. Show that you take the person's feelings seriously and truly care.

:: Don't offer trite reassurances. List reasons to go on living, try to analyze the person's motives, or try to shock or challenge him or her.

:: Suggest solutions or alternatives to problems. Make plans. Encourage positive action, such as getting away for a while to gain a better perspective on a problem.

:: Don't be afraid to ask whether your friend has considered suicide. The opportunity to talk about thoughts of suicide may be an enormous relief, and—contrary to a long-standing myth—will not fix the idea of suicide more firmly in a person's mind.

:: Don't think that people who talk about killing themselves never carry out their threat. Most individuals who commit suicide give definite indications of their intent to die.[71]

❖ Attention Disorders

Estimates of the percentage of children and adolescents who develop **attention deficit/hyperactivity disorder (ADHD)** by age 19 range from 7.4 to 16 percent.[72] As many as two-thirds of children with ADHD continue to face major challenges as adults.

Its causes are complex and include genetic and biological factors, including differences within the brain.

Sophisticated brain scanning techniques show anatomical differences in the brains of girls, boys, and adults with ADHD, as well as differences in brain wave activity and neurochemical function that controls mood, thoughts, and impulses.

If one family member has been diagnosed with ADHD, there is a 25 to 35 percent chance that at least one other family member will have it. Other contributing causes include prenatal use of alcohol, tobacco, and cocaine; delivery complications, which may alter brain development; and postnatal problems, such as meningitis, encephalitis, chronic lead exposure, or severe head trauma.

The diagnosis of ADHD in childhood remains controversial. Some critics charge that children with a variety of temperaments, neurological delays, and behavioral difficulties are being lumped together and labeled as being hyperactive or attention-disordered. Others feel that attention disorders are still under-diagnosed, especially in girls, who tend to develop a type of ADHD primarily characterized by inability to concentrate.[73]

Three times as many boys as girls are affected by ADHD, but that gap is closing as medical professionals recognize more subtle symptoms in girls, who tend to be less hyperactive, less defiant and more compliant, and often are dismissed as flighty or disorganized. Often the self-esteem of girls with ADHD suffers as they encounter academic problems in school, and they may develop depression, eating disorders, anxiety disorders, or other emotional problems.[74]

Women's reproductive hormones may also affect ADHD. ADHD symptoms often get worse just before menstrual periods as estrogen drops and seem to worsen as women enter menopause, another time of low estrogen. Many women are first diagnosed during perimenopause when their mood swings and distractibility become worse.

One-half to two-thirds of youngsters with ADHD do not outgrow their restless, reckless ways at puberty. In all, 1 to 2 percent of adult men and women—at least 5 million Americans—have problems sustaining attention or controlling their movements and impulses.

Adults with ADHD have one or more of three primary symptoms: hyperactivity, impulsivity, and distractibility. Rather than scooting around a room, they may tap their fingers or jiggle their feet. Some appear calm and organized but cannot concentrate long enough to finish reading a paragraph or follow a list of directions. Others, on a whim, go on buying sprees or take wild dares.

 An estimated 1 percent of college students have an attention disorder that can have a significant impact on their academic performance. At one midwestern university, for instance, the counseling service estimates that students with attention disorders have an average GPA of 2.4, compared to a university average mean of 3.1.

No specific test can detect attention disorders, and diagnosis, based on the patient's history and a therapist's interview, can be difficult. Adults with ADHD may take the same medications that children do—stimulant drugs that, paradoxically, can aid concentration and reduce restlessness. Recent studies have shown that long-term use of stimulants does not lead to substance abuse by teenagers or young adults.[75]

New medications, including the first non-stimulant drug for ADHD, directly target neurotransmitters such as dopamine and norepinephrine. Some antidepressants are effective in treating adult ADHD and may be an alternative to stimulants. Medication often makes it possible for adults with ADHD to benefit from other treatments, such as psychotherapy, general counseling, vocational rehabilitation, and academic tutoring.

⚫ Schizophrenia

Schizophrenia, one of the most debilitating mental disorders, profoundly impairs an individual's sense of reality. As the National Institute of Mental Health (NIMH) puts it, schizophrenia, which is characterized by abnormalities in brain structure and chemistry, destroys "the inner unity of the mind" and weakens "the will and drive that constitute our essential character." It affects every aspect of psychological functioning, including the ways in which people think, feel, view themselves, and relate to others.

The symptoms of schizophrenia include:

:: Hallucinations.

:: Delusions.

:: Inability to think in a logical manner.

:: Talking in rambling or incoherent ways.

:: Making odd or purposeless movements or not moving at all.

:: Repeating others' words or mimicking their gestures.

:: Showing few, if any, feelings; responding with inappropriate emotions.

:: Lacking will or motivation to complete a task or accomplish something.

:: Functioning at a much lower level than in the past at work, in interpersonal relations, or in taking care of themselves.

Individuals with schizophrenia may hear, see, or feel things that do not exist—a voice telling them to jump from a bridge, a statue crying tears of blood, a spaceship beaming a light upon them. Frightened and vulnerable, they may devote all their energy to warding off the demons within. Unable to take care of themselves, they may look messy and disheveled. They often move in unusual ways, such as rocking or pacing, or repeat certain gestures again and again. They may believe that someone or something, such as the devil, is putting thoughts into their heads or controlling their actions. Some think they are reincarnations of Christ or Napoleon. About a third attempt to take their own lives, often in response to a command they hear inside their heads. Researchers have identified early markers of

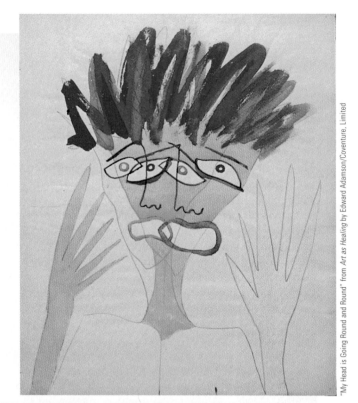

"My Head is Going Round and Round." **This drawing by a patient suffering from schizophrenia expresses the anxiety and agitation that may occur with this brain abnormality.**

"My Head is Going Round and Round" from *Art as Healing* by Edward Adamson/Coventure, Limited

schizophrenia, including impaired social skills, intellectual ability, and capacity for organization.[76]

Schizophrenia is one of the leading causes of disability among young adults. The mean age for schizophrenia to develop is 21.4 years for men and 26.8 years for women.[77] Although symptoms do not occur until then, they are almost certainly the result of a failure in brain development that occurs very early in life. The underlying defect is probably present before birth. Schizophrenia has a strong genetic basis and is not the result of upbringing, social conditions, or traumatic experiences.[78]

Multiple genes may contribute to susceptibility to schizophrenia, particularly the rare but severe form that begins in childhood, but many other factors also are involved.[79]

One-half to 1 percent of the population—about 1 in every 150 people—suffers from this disorder. Danish researchers have found that children born during late winter or in urban areas appear to be at greater risk of schizophrenia, possibly because their mothers were more likely to contract a viral infection during pregnancy that could have affected the developing fetal brain. Retroviruses (discussed in Chapter 13) also may play a role. About half have a history of substance abuse or dependence, including alcoholism. According to NIMH's epidemiological data, the total lifetime prevalence for schizophrenia in the United States ranges from 1 to 1.9 percent. This means that between 2.5 million and 4.75 million Americans may have schizophrenia at any one time.

Schizophrenia typically consists of several stages. During the *prodromal phase,* a period ranging from months to years, individuals withdraw from social interactions, pay less attention to keeping clean or dressing appropriately, or act in peculiar ways. In the acute, or *active phase,* individuals develop "positive symptoms." They may experience delusions and become convinced that space aliens have taken control of their bodies or hallucinate and hear voices mocking them. Some talk nonstop, rambling on without making any clear point; others repeatedly shake their heads, tap their feet, or assume odd postures or positions. After positive symptoms subside, individuals enter the *residual phase,* which is characterized by "negative symptoms," such as general apathy, flattened emotions, or inappropriate emotional reactions (for example, laughing when someone is hurt).

For the vast majority of individuals with schizophrenia, antipsychotic drugs are the foundation of treatment. They make most people with schizophrenia feel more comfortable and in control of themselves, help organize chaotic thinking, and reduce or eliminate delusions or hallucinations, allowing fuller participation in normal activities. Those who do not improve significantly on medication almost invariably do even worse without it.

Nearly one-third of individuals given conventional antipsychotics continue to have residual symptoms, such as apathy. In the past, little, if anything, could be done to relieve these negative symptoms. However, new "atypical" antipsychotics, such as Abilify (aripiprazole) and Zyprexa (olanzapine), can relieve such symptoms and help individuals who do not improve with standard medications or who develop intolerable side effects. They are less likely to cause abnormal body movements, such as muscle spasms and restless pacing.

Some individuals with schizophrenia recover completely. However, many thousands—perhaps as many as 200,000—live on the street or in homeless shelters.

⚫ Overcoming Problems of the Mind

Mental illness costs our society an estimated $150 billion a year in lost work time and productivity, employee turnover, disability payments, and death. Yet many Americans do not have access to mental health services, nor do they have insurance for such services. Despite the fact that treatments for mental disorders have a higher success rate than those for many other diseases, employers often restrict mental health benefits. HMOs and health insurance plans are much more likely to limit psychotherapy visits and psychiatric hospitalizations than treatments for medical illnesses.

Even when cost is not a barrier, many people do not seek treatment because they see psychological problems as a sign of weakness rather than illness. They also may not realize that scientifically proven therapies can bring relief, often in a matter of weeks or months.

Because an individual's perception of a problem is "culture-specific"—that is, influenced by his or her cultural, social, and religious beliefs—immigrants to the United States may treat symptoms of psychological distress in different ways. For instance, Asian-American college students tend to seek medical care for physical symptoms, such as aches, pains, or sleep problems, but forgo counseling for a mental disorder, because it is more appropriate in their native cultures to do so.

📞 Where Can I Turn for Help?

As a student, your best contact for identifying local services may be your health education instructor or department. The health instructors can tell you about general and mental health counseling available on campus, school-based support groups, community-based programs, and special emergency services. On campus, you can also turn to the student health services or the office of the dean of student services or student affairs.

Within the community, you may be able to get help through the city or county health department and neighborhood health centers. Local hospitals often have special clinics and services; and there are usually local branches of national service organizations, such as United Way or Alcoholics Anonymous, other 12-step programs, and various support groups. You can call the psychiatric or psychological association in your city or state for the names of licensed professionals. (Check the telephone directory for listings.) Your primary physician may also be able to help.

The telephone book is another good resource. Special programs are often listed either by the nature of the service, by the name of the neighborhood or city, or by the name of the sponsoring group. In some places, the city's name may precede a listing: the New York City Suicide Hot Line, for instance. In addition to suicide-prevention programs, other listings usually include crisis intervention, violence prevention, and child-abuse prevention programs; drug-treatment information; shelters for battered women; senior citizen centers; and self-help and counseling services. Many services have special hot lines for coping with emergencies. Others provide information as well as counseling over the phone.

An increasing number of mental health professionals—primarily psychologists and marriage and family therapists—are offering "e-therapy" on the Internet. Online therapy is convenient, discrete, less costly (some therapists charge for their time or the number of questions a client asks), and may be helpful with relationship or work issues. However, there is no regulation of therapists, and mental health professionals warn that online counseling is inadequate for diagnosing or dealing with serious psychological problems.[80]

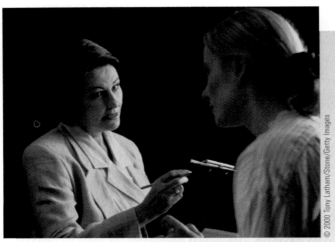

© 2000 Tony Latham/Stone/Getty Images

When choosing a therapist, you should always consider the individual's education, title, and qualifications. Also important are qualities such as compassion and caring.

Types of Therapists

Only professionally trained individuals who have met state licensing requirements are certified as psychiatrists, psychologists, or social workers. Before selecting any of these mental health professionals, be sure to check the person's background and credentials.

Psychiatrists are licensed medical doctors (M.D.) who complete medical school; a year-long internship; and a three-year residency that provides training in various forms of psychotherapy, psychopharmacology, and both outpatient and inpatient treatment of mental disorders. They can prescribe medications and make medical decisions. *Board-certified* psychiatrists have passed oral and written examinations following completion of residency training.

Psychologists complete a graduate program (including clinical training and internships) in human psychology but do not study medicine and cannot prescribe medication. They must be licensed in most states in order to practice independently.

Certified social workers or **licensed clinical social workers (LCSWs)** usually complete a two-year graduate program and have specialized training in helping people with mental problems in addition to conventional social work.

Psychiatric nurses have nursing degrees and have passed a state examination. They usually have special training and experience in mental health care, although no specialty licensing or certification is required.

Marriage and family therapists, licensed in some but not all states, usually have a graduate degree, often in psychology, and at least two years of supervised clinical training in dealing with relationship problems.

Other therapists include pastoral counselors, members of the clergy who offer psychological counseling; hypnotherapists, who use hypnosis for problems such as smok-

ing and obesity; stress-management counselors, who teach relaxation methods; and alcohol and drug counselors, who help individuals with substance abuse problems. Anyone can use these terms to describe themselves professionally, and there are no licensing requirements.

Options for Treatment

The term **psychotherapy** refers to any type of counseling based on the exchange of words in the context of the unique relationship that develops between a mental health professional and a person seeking help. The process of talking and listening can lead to new insight, relief from distressing psychological symptoms, changes in unhealthy or maladaptive behaviors, and more effective ways of dealing with the world.

Both the number of Americans seeking psychotherapy and those treated with a combination of talking therapy and psychiatric medication has increased in the last decade. The use of psychiatric drugs in children and adolescents has increased two to threefold in the last 15 years.[81]

Most mental health professionals today are trained in a variety of psychotherapeutic techniques and tailor their approach to the problem, personality, and needs of each person seeking their help. Because skilled therapists may combine different techniques in the course of therapy, the lines between the various approaches often blur.

Because insurance companies and health-care plans often limit the duration of psychotherapy, many mental health professionals are adopting a *time-limited* format in order to make the most of every session, regardless of the length of treatment. Brief or short-term psychotherapy typically focuses on a central theme, problem, or topic and may continue for several weeks to several months. The individuals most likely to benefit are those who are interested in solving immediate problems rather than changing their characters, who can think in psychological terms, and who are motivated to change.

Psychodynamic Psychotherapy

For the most part, today's mental health professionals base their assessment of individuals on a **psychodynamic** understanding that takes into account the role of early experiences and unconscious influences in *actively* shaping behavior. (This is the *dynamic* in psychodynamic.) Psychodynamic treatments work toward the goal of providing greater insight into problems and bringing about behavioral change. Therapy may be brief, consisting of 12 to 25 sessions, or may continue for several years. According to current thinking, psychotherapy can actually rewire the network of neurons within the brain in ways that ease distress and improve functioning in many areas of daily life.

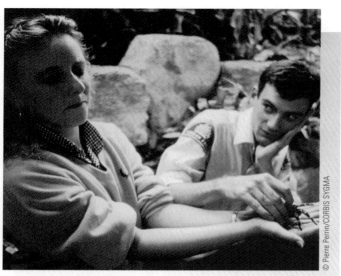

Systematic desensitization is one of the behavior therapies used to treat phobias.

Cognitive-Behavior Therapy

Cognitive-behavior therapy (CBT) focuses on inappropriate or inaccurate thoughts or beliefs to help individuals break out of a distorted way of thinking. The techniques of **cognitive therapy** include identification of an individual's beliefs and attitudes, recognition of negative thought patterns, and education in alternative ways of thinking. Individuals with major depression or anxiety disorders are most likely to benefit, usually in 15 to 25 sessions. However, many of the positive messages used in cognitive therapy can help anyone improve a bad mood or negative outlook.[82]

Behavior therapy strives to substitute healthier ways of behaving for maladaptive patterns used in the past. Its premise is that distressing psychological symptoms, like all behaviors, are learned responses that can be modified or unlearned. Some therapists believe that changing behavior also changes how people think and feel. As they put it, "Change the behavior, and the feelings will follow." Behavior therapies work best for disorders characterized by specific, abnormal patterns of acting—such as alcohol and drug abuse, anxiety disorders, and phobias—and for individuals who want to change bad habits.[83]

Interpersonal Therapy (IPT)

Interpersonal therapy (IPT), originally developed for research into the treatment of major depression, focuses on relationships in order to help individuals deal with unrecognized feelings and needs and improve their communication skills. IPT does not deal with the psychological origins of symptoms but rather concentrates on current problems of getting along with others. The supportive, empathic relationship that is developed with the therapist, who takes an even more active role than in psychodynamic psychotherapy, is the most crucial component of this therapy. The emphasis is on the here and now and on interpersonal—rather than intrapsychic—issues. Individuals with major depression, chronic difficulties developing relationships, chronic mild depression, or bulimia (see Chapter 6 on eating disorders) are most likely to benefit. IPT usually consists of 12 to 16 sessions.

Psychiatric Drug Therapy

Medications that alter brain chemistry and relieve psychiatric symptoms have brought great hope and help to millions of people. Thanks to the recent development of a new generation of more precise and effective **psychiatric drugs,** success rates for treating many common and disabling disorders—depression, panic disorder, schizophrenia, and others—have soared. Often used in conjunction with psychotherapy, sometimes used as the primary treatment, these medications have revolutionized mental health care.

At some point in their lives, about half of all Americans will take a psychiatric drug. The reason may be depression, anxiety, a sleep difficulty, an eating disorder, alcohol or drug dependence, impaired memory, or another disorder that disrupts the intricate chemistry of the brain. (See Savvy Consumer: "What You Need to Know About Mind-Mood Medications.")

Psychiatric drugs are now among the most widely prescribed drugs in the United States. Serotonin-boosting medications, called SSRIs, have become the drugs of choice in treating depression. They also are effective in treating obsessive compulsive disorder, panic disorder, social phobia, posttraumatic stress disorder, premenstrual dysphoric disorder, and generalized anxiety disorder. New agents, such as Remeron (mirtazapine), a "tetracyclic," stimulates the release of both norepinephrine and serotonin. In patients who don't respond, psychiatrists may add another drug to boost the efficacy of the treatment.[84]

Psychiatric medications affect every aspect of a person's physical, mental, and emotional functioning. Some take effect immediately; others take several weeks to relieve symptoms; a few continue to exert their effects even after an individual discontinues their use. When taken appropriately, psychiatric agents can alleviate tremendous suffering and reduce the financial and personal costs of mental illness by lessening the need for hospitalization and by restoring an individual's ability to function normally, to work, and to contribute to society. But they do have side effects and must be used with care.

Alternative Mind-Mood Products

People with serious mental illnesses, including depression and bipolar disorder, often use at least one alternative health care practice, such as yoga or meditation.[85] They

Savvy Consumer

WHAT YOU NEED TO KNOW ABOUT MIND-MOOD MEDICATIONS

Before taking any "psychoactive" drug (one that affects the brain), talk to a qualified health professional. Here are some points to raise:

- What can this medication do for me? What specific symptoms will it relieve? Are there other possible benefits?
- When will I notice a difference? How long does it take for the medicine to have an effect?

- Are there any risks? What about side effects? Do I have to take it before or after eating? Will it affect my ability to study, work, drive, or operate machinery?
- How will I be able to tell if the medication is working? What are the odds that it will help me?
- How long will I have to take medication? Is there any danger that I'll become addicted?
- What if it doesn't help?
- Is there an herbal or natural alternative? If so, has it been studied? What do you know about its possible risks and side effects?

---

also are trying "natural" products, such as herbs and enzymes, that claim to have psychological effects. However, because they are not classified as drugs, these products have not undergone the rigorous scientific testing required of psychiatric medications, and little is known about their safety or efficacy. "Natural" doesn't mean risk-free. Opium and cocaine are "natural" substances that have dramatic and potentially deadly effects on the mind.

St. John's wort (named after St. John the Baptist because the yellow flowers of the *Hypericum perforatum* plant bloom in June, the anniversary month of his execution) has been used to treat anxiety and depression in Europe for many years. Data from clinical studies in the United States do not support the efficacy of St. John's wort for moderate to severe depression. In two carefully controlled studies, the herb did not prove more effective than a placebo. However, St. John's wort remains popular for mild to moderate depression in Europe. A German review of more than two-dozen studies found that St. John's wort was similar in efficacy to standard antidepressants.[86] Side effects include dizziness, abdominal pain and bloating, constipation, nausea, fatigue, and dry mouth. St. John's wort should not be taken in combination with other prescription antidepressants. St. John's wort can lower the efficacy of oral contraceptives and increase the risk of an unwanted pregnancy.[87]

Other substances are widely used despite little or no scientific evaluation of their risks and benefits. Valerian, derived from the root of *Valeriana officinalis,* is taken primarily for insomnia and may help induce sleepiness. Kava, from a pepper tree native to the South Pacific, is thought to have a naturally soothing effect that can relieve anxiety and tension. Gingko biloba, long used in Chinese medicine, is considered a natural brain booster that may improve memory and concentration. However, excessive bleeding and, in rare cases, stroke have been reported with the use of gingko.[88]

Researchers have found a correlation between low levels of S-adenosylmethionine (SAM-e), a naturally occurring compound in human cells that boosts mood-influencing brain chemicals like serotonin, and depression. According to a limited number of small studies, dietary supplements containing SAM-e may enhance the effectiveness of conventional antidepressants. In seven of eight controlled studies since the 1980s, SAM-e has been found more effective than a placebo in treating depression, but its effects are modest, and the methodology used in the studies has been criticized. In some controlled studies in Europe, SAM-e has been shown to be effective as a treatment for arthritic pain and inflammation. Sold as an unregulated dietary supplement, there are no guarantees of the actual contents of SAM-e as purchased in retail stores or on the Internet, nor has it been proven safe for children, nursing or pregnant women, or people with serious medical problems.[89]

The Bottom Line ▼
The Keys to Psychological Wellness

Feeling good does not depend on money, success, recognition, or status. At any age, at any level of education and achievement, regardless of disability or disease, it is possible to find happiness and fulfillment in life. Achieving the highest possible level of psychological well-being, like achieving peak physical well-being, depends primarily on assuming responsibility for yourself.

Like physical health, psychological well-being is not a fixed state of being, but a process. The way you live every day affects how you feel about yourself and your world. Here are some basic guidelines that you can rely on to make the most of the process of living:

:: **Accept yourself.** As a human being, you are, by definition, imperfect. Come to terms with the fact that you are a worthwhile person despite your mistakes.

:: ***Respect yourself.*** Recognize your abilities and talents. Acknowledge your competence and achievements, and take pride in them.

:: ***Trust yourself.*** Learn to listen to the voice within you, and let your intuition be your guide.

:: ***Love yourself.*** Be happy to spend time by yourself. Learn to appreciate your company and to be glad you're you.

:: ***Stretch yourself.*** Be willing to change and grow, to try something new and dare to be vulnerable.

:: ***Look at challenges as opportunities for personal growth.*** "Every problem brings the possibility of a widening of consciousness," psychologist Carl Jung once noted. Put his words to the test.

:: ***Think of not only where but also who you want to be a decade from now.*** The goals you set, the decisions you make, the values you adopt now will determine how you feel about yourself and your life in the future.

After watching the CNN video segment, discuss the following question. What is known about biofeedback in the treatment of Attention Deficit Disorder?

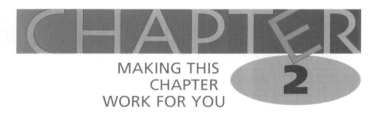

MAKING THIS
CHAPTER
WORK FOR YOU
2

1. Psychological health is influenced by all of the following *except*
   a. spiritual health
   b. physical agility
   c. culture
   d. a firm grasp on reality

2. Emotional intelligence encompasses which of the following components?
   a. creativity, sense of humor, scholastic achievement
   b. integrity, honesty, and perseverance
   c. piety, tolerance, and self-esteem
   d. empathy, self-awareness, and altruism

3. Which of the following activities can contribute to a lasting sense of personal fulfillment?
   a. becoming a Big Sister or Big Brother to a child from an inner city single-parent home
   b. volunteering at a local soup kitchen on Thanksgiving
   c. being a regular participant in an Internet chat room
   d. going on a shopping spree

4. Individuals who have developed a sense of mastery over their lives are
   a. skilled at controlling the actions of others.
   b. usually passive and silent when faced with a situation they don't like.
   c. aware that their locus of control is internal, not external.
   d. aware that their locus of control is external, not internal.

5. A mental disorder can be described as
   a. a condition associated with migraine headaches and narcolepsy.
   b. a condition that is usually caused by severe trauma to the brain.
   c. a behavioral or psychological disorder that impairs an individual's ability to conduct one or more important activities of daily life.
   d. a psychological disorder that is easily controlled with medication and a change in diet.

6. Neurons
   a. transmit information within the brain and throughout the body by means of electrical impulses and chemical messengers.
   b. are specialized support cells that travel through the spinal cord, carrying signals related to movement.
   c. are protein molecules designed to bind with neurotransmitters.
   d. consist of nuclei, dendrites, and glia.

7. Which of the following statements about anxiety disorders is true?
   a. Anxiety disorders are the least prevalent type of mental illness.
   b. An individual suffering from a panic attack may mistake her symptoms for a heart attack.
   c. The primary symptom of obsessive-compulsive disorder is irrational, intense, and persistent fear of a specific object or situation.
   d. Generalized anxiety disorders respond to systematic desensitization behavior therapy.

8. Some characteristic symptoms of major depression are
   a. difficulty concentrating, lack of energy, and eating more than usual.
   b. exaggerated sense of euphoria and energy.
   c. palpitations, sweating, numbness, and tingling sensations.
   d. talking in rambling ways, inability to think in a logical manner, and delusions.

9. A person may be at higher risk of committing suicide if
   a. he is taking antidepressant medication.
   b. he lives in a rural environment and is married.
   c. he has been diagnosed with hyperactivity disorder.
   d. he has lost his job because of alcoholism.

10. Which of the following statements is true?
    a. Individuals with schizophrenia are most likely to benefit from psychodynamic therapy in combination with nutritional supplements.

b. SSRIs are used to treat depression, obsessive-compulsive disorder, and panic disorder.

c. Psychologists are usually trained in a variety of psychotherapeutic techniques and are licensed to prescribe psychiatric medications.

d. Interpersonal therapy focuses on the role of early experiences and unconscious influences in shaping patterns of behavior, such as repeated failed relationships.

Answers to these questions can be found on page 652.

Critical Thinking

1. Would you say that you view life positively or negatively? Would your friends and family agree with your assessment? Ask two of your closest friends for feedback about what they perceive are your typical responses to a problematic situation. Are these indicative of positive attitudes? If not, what could you do to become more psychologically positive?

Critical Thinking

2. Paula went to a therapist when she was feeling depressed and was given a prescription for an antidepressant called fluoxetine (trade name Prozac). Her therapist recommended the drug because it causes fewer side effects than other medications. However, Paula later read in a news magazine that some patients, claiming that Prozac had made them violent or suicidal, had sued the drug's manufacturers. Their suits didn't win in court, but Paula was less certain about taking the prescribed medication. What do you think she should do? How would you weigh the risks and benefits of taking a psychiatric drug?

Critical Thinking

3. Research has indicated that many homeless men and women are in need of outpatient psychiatric care, often because they suffer from chronic mental illnesses or alcoholism. Yet government funding for the mentally ill is inadequate, and homelessness itself can make it difficult, if not impossible, for people to gain access to the care they need. How do you feel when you pass homeless individuals who seem disoriented or out of touch with reality? Who should take responsibility for their welfare? Should they be forced to undergo treatment at psychiatric institutions?

Profile Plus

Take stock of your emotional and mental state with these activities on your Profile Plus CD-ROM:

Profile Plus

- Well Being Scale
- Is Something Wrong?

Profile Plus

Sites and Bytes

National Institute of Mental Health

www.nimh.nih.gov

This professional site features information for the public as well as health practitioners on a variety of mental health topics, including depression, anxiety, ADHD, eating disorders, learning disabilities, posttraumatic stress disorder, and suicide.

Sites and Bytes

American Psychological Association

www.apa.org

This site has information for mental health professionals, students, and the public on a variety of mental health topics, including mind-body medicine. This site also features a help center that provides advice on how to access psychological services and an online literature search.

Sites and Bytes

Psych Central

www.psychcentral.com

Dr. John Grohol's Mental Health Page is a comprehensive site for psychology, support, and mental health issues, with a FAQ section and online mental health resources. The site also features interactive quizzes on eating disorders, depression, mania, obsessive-compulsive disorder, and attention disorders. During free, weekly live chats Dr. Grohol answers mental health and relationship questions online.

InfoTrac College Edition

Activity

Patterson, Karen. "College Students Report More Stress, Depression, Suicidal Thoughts" *Knight Ridder/Tribune News Service,* February 12, 2003, p. K2831.

1. How have mental health problems facing college students changed over the past 12 years?

InfoTrac College Edition

2. Compare and contrast the three most common types of mental health complaints among college women with the mental health symptoms found in college men.

3. How do the psychosocial difficulties that are found in students who visited the college counseling center differ from those of students who did not seek psychological assistance at the college counseling center?

InfoTrac College Edition

You can find additional readings related to psychological health with InfoTrac College Edition, an online library of more than 900 journals and publications. Follow the instructions for accessing InfoTrac College Edition that were packaged with your textbook; then search for articles using a key word search.

For additional links, resources, and suggested readings on InfoTrac College Edition, visit our Health & Wellness Resource Center at **http://health.wadsworth.com**.

Key Terms

The terms listed are used on the page indicated. Definitions of the terms are in the Glossary at the end of this book.

Key Terms

altruism 46
antidepressant 54
anxiety 50
anxiety disorders 55
assertive 47
attention deficit/hyperactivity disorder (ADHD) 63
autonomy 47
axon 52
axon terminal 52
behavior therapy 67
bipolar disorder 59
certified social workers 66
cognitive therapy 67
culture 39
dendrites 52
depression 50
depressive disorders 57
emotional health 38
emotional intelligence 39
generalized anxiety disorder (GAD) 55

Key Terms

glia 52
interpersonal therapy (IPT) 67
licensed clinical social workers (LCSW) 66
locus of control 47
major depression 58
marriage and family therapists 66
mental disorder 50
mental health 38
mood 44
neurons 52
neuropsychiatry 52
neurotransmitters 52
nucleus 52
obsessive-compulsive disorder (OCD) 55
optimism 45
panic attacks 55
panic disorder 56
phobias 55

Key Terms

psychiatric drugs 67
psychiatric nurses 66
psychiatrists 66
psychodynamic 66
psychologists 66
psychotherapy 66
rapid-eye-movement (REM) sleep 54
receptors 52
reuptake 53
schizophrenia 64
self-actualization 40
self-esteem 43
social isolation 48
social phobia 49
spiritual health 38
spiritual intelligence 39
synapse 52
values 40

References

1. Shapiro, Deane, and Roger Walsh. *Beyond Health and Normalcy.* New York: Van Nostrand Reinhold, 1983.
2. Satcher, David. "Executive Summary: A Report of the Surgeon General on Mental Health." *Public Health Reports,* Vol. 115, No. 1, January 2000.

References

3. Russinova, Zlaytka, et al. "Use of Alternative Health Care Practices by Persons with Serious Mental Illness: Perceived Benefits," *American Journal of Public Health,* Vol. 92, March 2003, p. 1600.

References

4. Fiala, William, et al. "The Religious Support Scale," *American Journal of Community Psychology,* Vol. 30, No. 6, December 2002, p. 761.
5. Goleman, Daniel. *Emotional Intelligence.* New York: Bantam Books, 1997.

References

6. Hales, Dianne. "Why Prayer Could Be Good Medicine," *Parade,* March 23, 2003, p. 4.
7. Becker, Diane. Personal interview.
8. Matthews, Dale. Personal interview.
9. Hales, "Why Prayer Could Be Good Medicine."
10. Aspinwall, Lisa, and Ursula Staudinger. *A Psychology of Human Strengths: Fundamental Questions and Future Directions for a Positive Psychology.* Washington, D.C.: American Psychological Association, 2002.
11. Seligman, Martin. *Authentic Happiness.* New York: Free Press, 2002.
12. Seligman, Martin. Personal interview.
13. Hertel, James. "College Students Generational Status: Similarities, Differences, and Factors in College Adjustment." *The Psychological Record,* Vol. 52, No. 1, Winter 2002, p. 3.
14. Robins, Richard, and Jennifer Beer. "Positive Illusions about the Self: Short-term Benefits and Long-term Costs." *Journal of Personality & Social Psychology,* Vol. 80, No. 2, February 2001, p. 340.
15. Larsen, Randy. Personal interview.
16. Seligman, *Authentic Happiness.*
17. Clark, A. E., A. J. Oswald. "A Simple Statistical Method for Measuring How Life Events Affect Happiness," *International Journal of Epidemiology,* Vol. 31, No. 6, December 2002, p. 1139.
18. Seligman, *Authentic Happiness.*
19. Lucas, R. F., et al. "Reexamining Adaptation and the Set Point Model of Happiness: Reactions to Changes in Marital Status," *Journal of Personality and Social Psychology,* Vol. 84, No. 3, March 2003, p. 527.
20. Seligman, *Authentic Happiness.*
21. Ibid.
22. Levy, B. C. E., et al. "Longitudinal Benefit of Positive Self-Perceptions of Aging on Functional Health." *Journals of Gerontology. Series B Psychological Sciences and Social Sciences.* Vol. 57, No. 5, September 2002, pp. 409–417.
23. Ornish, Dean. *Love & Survival: The Scientific Basis for the Healing Power of Intimacy.* New York: HarperCollins, 1999.
24. "What Is the Psychiatric Significance of Loneliness?" *Harvard Mental Health Letter,* Vol. 16, No. 10, April 2000.
25. Lang, Ariel, and Murray Stein. "Social Phobia: Prevalence and Diagnostic Threshold." *Journal of Clinical Psychiatry,* Vol. 62, Suppl. 1, 2001, pp. 5–10.
26. Satcher, David. "Heads Up." *Psychology Today,* May–June 2001, p. 13.
27. *Diagnostic & Statistical Manual IV TR*(electronic), Washington, D.C.: American Psychiatric Publishing, Inc., 2003.

References

28. Ketterer, Mark. "Stress and Early Heart Disease in Young Men," Presentation, American Psychosomatic Society, March 6, 2003.
29. "Mounting Evidence Indicates Heart Disease Link." *Medical Letter on the CDC & FDA,* July 21, 2002, p. 14.
30. Vythilingam, Meena, et al. "Psychotic Depression and Mortality," *American Journal of Psychiatry,* Vol. 160, No. 3, March 2003, p. 425.
31. "Depression Increases Risk of Death," *Women's Health Weekly,* February 27, 2003, p. 1.
32. Strike, P. C., and A. Steptoe. "Depression, Stress, and the Heart," *Heart,* Vol. 88, No. 5, November 2002, p. 441.
33. Bartlett, Thomas. "Freshmen Pay, Mentally and Physically, as They Adjust to Life in College," *Chronicle of Higher Education,* February 1, 2002.
34. Benton, Sherry, et al. "Changes in Counseling Center Client Problems Across 13 Years," *Professional Psychology: Research and Practice,* Vol. 34, No. 1, January 2003, p. 66.
35. Goode, Eric. "More in College Seek Help for Psychological Problems," *New York Times,* February 3, 2003, p. A11.
36. Ibid.
37. Benton et al., "Changes in Counseling Center Client Problems."
38. Engle, Shaena. "College Freshmen Spend Less Time Studying and More Time Surfing the Net, UCLA Survey Reveals," News Release. Higher Educational Research Institute, UCLA, January 27, 2003.
39. Storch, Eric, et al. "Religiosity and Depression in Intercollegiate Athletes," *College Student Journal,* Vol. 36, No. 4, December 2002, p. 526.
40. Neylan, Thomas, et al. "Sleep Disorders," *Textbook of Clinical Psychiatry* (4th edition). Washington, D.C.: American Psychiatric Publishing, Inc., 2003, p. 975.
41. Afari, Niloofar, and Dedra Buchwald. "Chronic Fatigue Syndrome: A Review," *American Journal of Psychiatry,* Vol. 160, No. 2, February 2003, p. 221.
42. Hollander, Eric, Daphne Simeon. "Anxiety Disorders," *Textbook of Clinical Psychiatry* (4th edition). Washington, D.C.: American Psychiatric Publishing, Inc., 2003, p. 543.
43. "CBT May Help Patients Control Panic Disorder." *Mental Health Weekly,* Vol. 12, No. 7, February 18, 2002, p. 7.
44. Hollander and Simeon, "Anxiety Disorders."
45. Kessler, Ronald, et al. "The Epidemiology of Major Depressive Disorder," *Journal of the American Medical Association,* Vol. 289, No. 23, June 18, 2003, p. 3095.

References

46. Turner, Heather, and Melissa Butler. "Direct and Indirect Effects of Childhood Adversity on Depressive Symptoms in Young Adults," *Journal of Youth & Adolescence,* Vol. 32, No. 2, April 2003, p. 89.
47. Torrey, Brian. "USPSTF Depression Screening Recommendations." *American Family Physician,* Vol. 66, No. 12, July 15, 2002, p. 335.
48. "Depression Survey Reveals Dramatic Change in Public Opinion." *Healthcare Review,* Vol. 15, No. 4, April 22, 2002, p. 8.
49. Walling, Anne. "Depression in Young Adults." *American Family Physician,* Vol. 62, No. 1, July 1, 2000.
50. Jancin, Bruce. "When It Comes to Treating Depression, Gender Matters," *Family Practice News,* Vol. 33, No. 2, January 15, 2003, p. 41.
51. Dubin, Julie Weingarden. "More Than a Mood." *Psychology Today,* May–June 2001, p. 26.
52. Jensen, Peter. Personal interview.
53. March, John. Personal interview.
54. "Teenage Depression Shows Family Ties." *Science News,* Vol. 159, No. 1, February 3, 2001, p. 72.
55. Spence, S. H., et al. "Mother's Depression in Early Childhood Increases the Risk of Adolescent Anxiety and Depression," *Evidence-Based Mental Health,* Vol. 6, No. 1, February 2003, p. 15.
56. Turner and Butler, "Direct and Indirect Effects of Childhood Adversity on Depressive Symptoms in Young Adults."
57. Burr, Constance. "Treatment for Minor Depression," National Institutes of Health News Release, March 21, 2003.
58. Rush, John, et al. "Depression, IV," *American Journal of Psychiatry,* Vol. 160, No. 2, p. 237.
59. "Major Depression Related to Course of Substance Dependence," *The Brown University Digest of Addiction Theory and Application,* Vol. 22, No. 1, January 2003, p. 1.
60. Marano, Hara. "How to Take an Antidepressant," *Psychology Today,* January/February 2003, p. 58.
61. Jancin, "When It Comes to Treating Depression, Gender Matters."
62. LeTourneau, Melanie. "Pump Up to Cheer Up." *Psychology Today,* May–June 2001, p. 27.
63. Wetzstein, Cheryl. "Preventing Suicide." *Insight on the News,* Vol. 16, No. 16, May 1, 2000.
64. Carroll-Ghosh, Tapu, et al. "Suicide," *Textbook of Clinical Psychiatry* (4th edition). Washington, D.C.: American Psychiatric Publishing, Inc., 2003, p. 543.

References

65. Gould, Madelyn. Personal interview.
66. Borowsky, Iris, et al. "Adolescent Suicide Attempts: Risks and Protectors." *Pediatrics,* Vol. 107, No. 3, March 2001, p. 485.
67. "Suicide and Suicide Attempts in Adolescents." *Pediatrics,* Vol. 105, No. 4, April 2000.
68. Brown, David, and Curtis Blanton. "Physical Activity, Sports Participation, and Suicidal Behavior Among College Students." *Science in Sports and Exercise,* Vol. 34, No. 7, July 2002, p. 1087.
69. Oquendo, Maria, et al. "Association of Comorbid Posttraumatic Stress Disorder and Major Depression With Greater Risk for Suicidal Behavior," *American Journal of Psychiatry,* Vol. 160, No., 3, March 2003, p. 574.
70. Bostwick, J. M., et al. "Affective Disorders and Suicide Risk: A Reexamination." *American Journal of Psychiatry,* Vol. 157, No. 12, December 2000, p. 1925.
71. Eagles, J. M., et al. "Suicide Prevention: A Study of Patients' Views," *British Journal of Psychiatry,* Vol. 182, No. 3, March 2003, p. 261.
72. Barbaresi, William, et al. "How Common Is Attention-Deficit/Hyperactivity Disorder?" *Journal of the American Academy of Child and Adolescent Psychiatry,* Vol. 42, No. 1, January 2003, p. 40.
73. Popper, Charles, et al. "Disorders Usually First Diagnosed in Infancy, Childhood, or Adolescence," *Textbook of Clinical*

References

Psychiatry (4th edition). Washington, D.C.: American Psychiatric Publishing, Inc., 2003, p. 1047.
74. "ADHD & Women's Health," *National Women's Health Report,* Vol. 25, No. 1, February 2003, p. 1.
75. Barkley R. A., et al. "Does the Treatment of Attention-Deficit/Hyperactivity Disorder with Stimulants Contribute to Drug Use/Abuse? A 13-Year Prospective Study," *Pediatrics,* Vol. 111, No. 1, January 2003, pp. 97–109.
76. Ho, Beng-Choon, et al. "Schizophrenia and Other Psychotic Disorders," *Textbook of Clinical Psychiatry* (4th edition). Washington, D.C.: American Psychiatric Publishing, Inc., 2003, p. 379.
77. Ibid.
78. "How Schizophrenia Develops: New Evidence and New Ideas." *Harvard Mental Health Letter,* Vol. 17, No. 8, February 2001.
79. Jablensky, Assen and Luba Kalaydjieva. "Genetic Epidemiology of Schizophrenia: Phenotypes, Risk Factors, and Reproductive Behavior," *American Journal of Psychiatry,* Vol. 160, No. 3, March 2003, p. 425.
80. "Is the Internet as Good as the Couch?" *Health Data Management,* Vol. 11, No. 2, February 2003, p. 14.
81. Rosack, Jim. "Prescription Data on Youth Raise Important Questions," *Psychiatric News,* Vol. 28, No. 3, February 7, 2003.

References

82. Wright, Jesse, et al. "Cognitive Therapy," *Textbook of Clinical Psychiatry* (4th edition). Washington, D.C.: American Psychiatric Publishing, Inc., 2003, p. 1047.
83. Berkowitz, Robert. "Behavior Therapies," *Textbook of Clinical Psychiatry* (4th edition). Washington, D.C.: American Psychiatric Publishing, Inc., 2003, p. 1047.
84. Ables, Adrienne and Otis Baughmann. "Antidepressants: Update on New Agents and Indications," *American Family Physician,* Vol. 67, No. 3, January 15, 2003, p. 547.
85. Russinova et al., "Use of Alternative Health Care Practices by Persons with Serious Mental Illness."
86. Walsh, Nancy. "St. John's Wort for Depression," *Family Practice News,* Vol. 33, No. 1, January 1, 2003, p. 25.
87. Jancin, "When It Comes to Treating Depression, Gender Matters."
88. "Alternative Therapies for Depression, Diabetes, and Obesity." *Journal of the American Dietetic Association,* Vol. 101, No. 3, March 2001, p. 364.
89. Levy, Sandra. "SAM-e: Good for Liver Disease, Depression, Osteoarthritis?" *Drug Topics,* Vol. 146, No. 2, November 4, 2002, p. 55.

Personal Stress Management

Two months into her freshman year, Maria feels as if a tornado has torn through her life. She is living thousands of miles from her family and the friends who share her culture and ethnic background. Her dormmates range from different to downright difficult. Her professors expect her to read and learn more in a week than in an entire month of high school. After blowing her budget decorating her room, she took on a part-time job—only to end up so exhausted that she dozes off in lectures. Stress? Maria considers it a way of life.

Like Maria, you live with stress every day, whether you're studying for exams, meeting people, facing new experiences, or figuring out how to live on a budget. You're not alone. Everyone, regardless of age, gender, race, or income, has to deal with stress—as an individual and as a member of society.

As researchers have demonstrated time and again, stress has profound effects, both immediate and long-term, on our bodies and minds. While stress alone doesn't cause disease, it triggers molecular changes throughout the body that make us more susceptible to many illnesses. Its impact on the mind is no less significant. The burden of chronic stress can undermine one's ability to cope with day-to-day hassles and can exacerbate psychological problems like depression and anxiety disorders.

Yet stress in itself isn't necessarily bad. What matters most is not the stressful situation itself, but an individual's response to it. By learning to anticipate stressful events, to manage day-to-day hassles, and to prevent stress overload, you can find alternatives to running endlessly on a treadmill of alarm, panic, and exhaustion. As you organize your schedule, find ways to release tension, and build up coping skills, you will begin to experience the sense of control and confidence that makes stress a challenge rather than an ordeal.

© Paul Thomas/The Image Bank/Getty Images

After studying the material in this chapter, you should be able to:

- **Define** stress and stressors and **describe** how the body responds to stress according to the general adaptation syndrome theory.
- **List** the physical changes associated with frequent or severe stress and **discuss** how stress can affect the cardiovascular, immune, and digestive systems.
- **Describe** some personal causes of stress, especially those experienced by students, and **discuss** how their effects can be prevented or minimized.
- **Discuss** the major social issues that can cause stress.
- **Describe** some techniques to help manage stress.
- **Explain** how stressful events can affect psychological health and **describe** the factors contributing to posttraumatic stress disorder.
- **Identify** ways of managing time more efficiently.

75

What Is Stress?

People use the word *stress* in different ways: as an external force that causes a person to become tense or upset, as the internal state of arousal, and as the physical response of the body to various demands. Dr. Hans Selye, a pioneer in studying physiological responses to challenge, defined **stress** as "the nonspecific response of the body to any demand made upon it." In other words, the body reacts to **stressors**—the things that upset or excite us—in the same way, regardless of whether they are positive or negative.

Stress can be acute, episodic, or chronic, depending on the nature of the stressors or external events that cause the stress response. Acute or short-term stressors, which can range from a pop quiz to a bomb threat in a crowded stadium, trigger a brief but intense response to a specific incident. Episodic stressors like monthly bills or quarterly exams cause regular but intermittent elevations in stress levels. Chronic stressors include everything from rush-hour traffic to a learning disability to living with an alcoholic parent or spouse.

Not all stressors are negative. Some of life's happiest moments—births, reunions, weddings—are enormously stressful. We weep with the stress of frustration or loss; we weep, too, with the stress of love and joy. Selye coined the term **eustress** for positive stress in our lives (*eu* is a Greek prefix meaning "good"). Eustress challenges us to grow, adapt, and find creative solutions in our lives. **Distress** refers to the negative effects of stress that can deplete or even destroy life energy. Ideally, the level of stress in our lives should be just high enough to motivate us to satisfy our needs and not so high that it interferes with our ability to reach our fullest potential.

What Causes Stress?

Of the many biological theories of stress, the best known may be the **general adaptation syndrome (GAS),** developed by Hans Selye. He postulated that our bodies constantly strive to maintain a stable and consistent physiological state, called **homeostasis.** Stressors, whether in the form of physical illness or a demanding job, disturb this state and trigger a nonspecific physiological response. The body attempts to restore homeostasis by means of an **adaptive response. Allostasis** describes the body's ability to adapt to constantly changing environments.

Selye's general adaptation syndrome, which describes the body's response to a stressor—whether threatening or exhilarating—consists of three distinct stages:

1. **Alarm.** When a stressor first occurs, the body responds with changes that temporarily lower resistance. Levels of certain hormones may rise; blood pressure may increase (see Figure 3-1). The body quickly makes internal adjustments to cope with the stressor and return to normal activity.

2. **Resistance.** If the stressor continues, the body mobilizes its internal resources to try to sustain homeostasis. For example, if a loved one is seriously hurt in an accident, we initially respond intensely and feel great anxiety. During the subsequent stressful period of

An automobile accident is an acute negative stressor. Getting married is an example of a positive stressor that triggers both joy and apprehension.

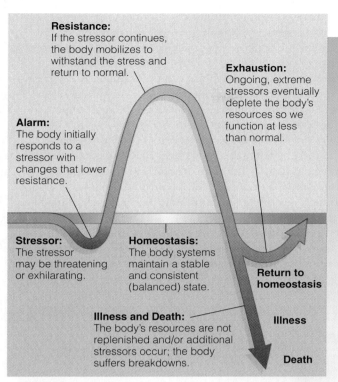

Figure 3-1 GENERAL ADAPTATION SYNDROME (GAS)
The three stages of Hans Selye's GAS are alarm, resistance, exhaustion.

recuperation, we struggle to carry on as normally as possible, but this requires considerable effort.

3. **Exhaustion.** If the stress continues long enough, we cannot keep up our normal functioning. Even a small amount of additional stress at this point can cause a breakdown.

Among the nonbiological theories is the cognitive-transactional model of stress, developed by Richard Lazarus, which looks at the relation between stress and health. As he sees it, stress can have a powerful impact on health. Conversely, health can affect a person's resistance or coping ability. Stress, according to Lazarus, is "neither an environmental stimulus, a characteristic of the person, nor a response, but a relationship between demands and the power to deal with them without unreasonable or destructive costs."[1] Thus, an event may be stressful for one person but not for another, or it may seem stressful on one occasion but not on another. For instance, one student may think of speaking in front of the class as extremely stressful, while another relishes the chance to do so—except on days when he's not well-prepared.

At any age, some of us are more vulnerable to life changes and crises than are others. The stress of growing up in families troubled by alcoholism, drug dependence, or physical, sexual, or psychological abuse may have a lifelong impact—particularly if these problems are not recognized and dealt with. Other early experiences, positive and nega-

tive, also can affect our attitude toward stress—and our resilience to it. Our general outlook on life, whether we're optimistic or pessimistic, can determine whether we expect the worst and feel stressed or anticipate a challenge and feel confident. The when, where, what, how, and why of stressors also affect our reactions. The number and frequency of changes in our lives, along with the time and setting in which they occur, have a great impact on how we'll respond.

Our level of ongoing stress affects our ability to respond to a new day's stressors. Each of us has a breaking point for dealing with stress. A series of too-intense pressures or too-rapid changes can push us closer and closer to that point. That's why it's important to anticipate potential stressors and plan how to deal with them.

Stress experts Thomas Holmes, M.D., and Richard Rahe, M.D., devised a scale to evaluate individual levels of stress and potential for coping, based on *life-change units* that estimate each change's impact. The death of a partner or parent ranks high on the list, but even changing apartments is considered a stressor. People who accumulate more than 300 life-change units in a year are more likely to suffer serious health problems. Scores on the scale, however, represent "potential stress"; the actual impact of the life change depends on the individual's response. (See Self-Survey: "Student Stress Scale," on page 84.)

Holmes has evaluated variations in life events among many groups, including college students, medical students, football players, pregnant women, alcoholics, and heroin addicts. Heroin addicts and alcoholics have the highest totals of life-change units, followed by college students. In general, younger people experience more life changes than do older people; factors such as gender, education, and social class also have a strong impact.[2] Marriage seems to promote greater stability and fewer changes.

If you score high on the Student Stress Scale, think about the reasons your life has been in such turmoil. Of course, some events, such as your parents' divorce or a friend's accident, are beyond your control. Even then, you can respond in ways that may protect you from disease. Review the Health Change Plan at the end of the Self-Survey (p. 84).

Is Stress Hazardous to Physical Health?

These days we've grown accustomed to warning labels advising us of the health risks of substances like alcohol and cigarettes. Medical researchers speculate that another component of twenty-first-century living also warrants a warning: stress.[3] In recent years, an ever-growing number of studies has implicated stress as a culprit in a range of medical problems. While stress itself may not kill, it clearly undermines our ability to stay well.[4]

Stress triggers complex changes in the body's endocrine, or hormone-secreting, system. The scientific field of **psychoneuroimmunology** has been exploring these intricate interconnections. When you confront a stressor, the adrenal glands, two triangle-shaped glands that sit atop the kidneys, respond by producing stress hormones, including catecholamines, cortisol (hydrocortisone), and epinephrine (adrenaline), that speed up heart rate and raise blood pressure and prepare the body to deal with the threat. This "fight-or-flight" response prepares you for quick action: Your heart works harder to pump more blood to your legs and arms. Your muscles tense, your breathing quickens, and your brain becomes extra alert. And because they're nonessential in a crisis, your digestive and immune systems practically shut down (Figure 3-2).

Unlike many other molecules in the body (such as the neurotransmitters that transmit messages in the brain), most stress hormones are water-insoluble, which means that they remain in the bloodstream longer. The effects of neurotransmitters disappear within seconds or milliseconds; stress hormones persist in the blood for hours. Cortisol remains elevated for the longest period and has the most important long-term effects on our health.

Cortisol speeds the conversion of proteins and fats into carbohydrates, the body's basic fuel, so we have the energy to fight or flee from a threat. However, stress increases the amount of time required to clear triglycerides, a type of fat linked to heart disease, from the bloodstream.[5] Thus, cortisol can cause excessive central or abdominal fat, which heightens the risk of diseases such as diabetes, high blood pressure, and stroke. Even slender, premenopausal women faced with increased stress and lacking

Figure 3-2 THE EFFECTS OF STRESS ON THE BODY

Brain becomes more alert.
- Stress hormones can effect memory and cause neurons to atrophy and die.
- Headaches, anxiety, and depression
- Disrupted sleep

Digestive system slows down.
- Mouth ulcers or cold sores

Heart rate increases and blood pressure rises.
- Persistently elevated blood pressure and heart rate can increase potential for blood clotting and risk of stroke or heart attack.

Adrenal glands produce stress hormones.
- Cortisol and other stress hormones can increase central or abdominal fat.
- Cortisol increases glucose production in the liver, causing renal hypertension.

Skin problems such as eczema and psoriasis

Breathing quickens.
- Increased susceptibilty to colds and respiratory infections

Immune system is suppressed.
- Increased susceptibility to infection
- Slower healing

Digestive system slows down.
- Upset stomach

Muscles tense.
- Muscular twitches or nervous tics

Reproductive system
- Menstrual disorders in women
- Impotence and premature ejaculation in men

■ = Immediate response to stress
■ = Effects of cronic or prolonged stress
■ = Other possible effects of chronic stress

good coping skills are more likely to accumulate excess weight around their waists, thereby increasing their risk of heart disease and other health problems.[6]

Figure 3-2 illustrates how persistent or repeated increases in the stress hormones can be hazardous throughout the body. In the brain, stress hormones linked to powerful emotions may help create long-lasting memories of events such as the collapse of the World Trade Center towers. But very prolonged or severe stress can damage the brain's ability to remember and can actually cause brain cells, or neurons, to atrophy and die.

Hundreds of studies over the last 20 years have shown that stress contributes to approximately 80 percent of all major illnesses: cardiovascular disease, cancer, endocrine and metabolic disease, skin rashes, ulcers, ulcerative colitis, emotional disorders, musculoskeletal disease, infectious ailments, premenstrual syndrome (PMS), uterine fibroid cysts, and breast cysts. As many as 75 to 90 percent of visits to physicians are related to stress.

The first signs of stress include muscle tightness, tension headaches, backaches, upset stomach, and sleep disruptions (caused by stress-altered brain-wave activity). Some people feel fatigued, their hearts may race or beat faster than usual at rest, and they may feel tense all the time, easily frustrated and often irritable. Others feel sad; lose their energy, appetite, or sex drive; and develop psychological problems, including depression, anxiety, and panic attacks (Chapter 2). Stress can lead to self-destructive behaviors, such as drinking, drug use, and reckless driving. Some people see such acts as offering an escape from the pressure they feel. Unfortunately, they end up adding to their stress load.

Stress and the Heart

Stress may be the most significant inherited risk factor in people who develop heart disease at a young age. According to behavioral researchers, family transmission of emotional and psychosocial stress, specifically anger in males, greatly increases the likelihood of early heart disease.[7]

In the 1970s, cardiologists Meyer Friedman, M.D., and Ray Rosenman, M.D., compared their patients to individuals of the same age with healthy hearts and developed two general categories: Type A and Type B. Hardworking, aggressive, and competitive, Type A's never have time for all they want to accomplish, even though they usually try to do several tasks at once. Type B's are more relaxed, though not necessarily less ambitious or successful.

The degree of danger associated with Type-A behavior remains controversial. According to a 22-year follow-up study of 3,000 middle-aged men by researchers at the University of California, Berkeley, both smoking and high blood pressure proved to be much greater threats than Type-A behavior with respect to heart attack risk. Of all the personality traits linked with Type-A behavior, the one

that has emerged as most sinister is chronic hostility or cynicism. People who are always mistrustful, angry, and suspicious are twice as likely to suffer blockages of their coronary arteries.

Depression, a mental disorder often linked with stress, clearly affects the prognosis of individuals who suffer heart attacks. (See Chapter 14.) The National Heart, Lung, and Blood Institute currently is studying 2,000 cardiac patients to determine if treating their depression may improve the quality of their lives and their survival odds.

Stress and the Immune System

The powerful chemicals triggered by stress dampen or suppress the immune system—the network of organs, tissues, and white blood cells that defend against disease. Impaired immunity makes the body more susceptible to many diseases, including infections (from the common cold to tuberculosis) and disorders of the immune system itself. It also may interfere with the immune system's ability to respond to inflammation caused by allergic, autoimmune, or cardiovascular illnesses.[8] Research has shown that traumatic stress, such as losing a loved one through death or divorce, can impair immunity for as long as a year.

 Even minor hassles take a toll. Under exam stress, students experience a dip in immune function and a higher rate of infections. Ohio State University researchers found that during exam periods there is a significant drop in the immune cells that normally ward off infection and cancer in medical students.

Scientists have identified what may be an important biological link between stress and the common cold: interleukin-6 (IL-6), a chemical pathway used by the immune system. People under stress who also come into contact with many different groups of people are most vulnerable to infectious diseases like colds and flus.[9]

 Studies of university students and staff in the United States and in Spain have implicated stress and a generally negative outlook as increasing susceptibility to the common cold, even in individuals taking vitamin C and zinc to ward off infection.[10]

 The immune response induced by vaccination is lower in people under stress. In a British study of 60 first-year university students vaccinated against meningitis, those who saw themselves as highly stressed and who felt anxious or under strain produced lower levels of protective antibodies against the disease.[11]

Stress also interferes with the body's ability to heal itself. By inflicting small cuts in volunteers who are then subjected to controlled stressful situations, researchers have shown a significant delay in healing among those under stress.[12]

Stress hormones also may play a role in the progression of breast cancer. In research on women with metastatic breast cancer, psychiatrist David Spiegel of Stanford University correlated variations in cortisol secretion with survival rates. The average survival time of women with normal cortisol patterns (high levels in the early morning and progressively lower concentrations during the day) was significantly longer than that of the women whose cortisol remained high all day (a stress indicator).[13]

Aging seems to compound the negative impact of stress on health. Older adults show even greater immunological impairments associated with stress or depression than younger adults and face a greater risk of illness and death.[14]

 Certain uplifts, including humor and altruism, may buffer the harmful effects of stress. In studies of college students, watching videotapes of comedians bolstered immune function. Students who provided services to others show a temporary boost in immunity.

Stress and the Digestive System

Do you ever get butterflies in your stomach before giving a speech in class or before a big game? The digestive system is, as one psychologist quips, "an important stop on the tension trail." To avoid problems, pay attention to how you eat: Eating on the run, gulping food, or overeating results in poorly chewed foods, an overworked stomach, and increased abdominal pressure. The combination of poor eating habits and stress can add up to real pain in the stomach.

After identifying the bacterium *H. pylori* as a cause of most peptic ulcers, scientists had downplayed the role of stress. However, more recent studies suggest that stress may indeed be a factor. About 80 percent of people carrying the *H. pylori* bacteria do not get ulcers; about 30 percent of patients who do have ulcers test negative for the bacteria. Researchers now contend that stress does contribute to the development of ulcers, hamper their healing, and increase the likelihood of their recurrence.[15]

Good nutrition can help soothe a stressed-out stomach. Complex carbohydrates are an ideal antistress food because they boost the brain's level of the mood-enhancing chemical serotonin. Good sources include broccoli, leafy greens, potatoes, corn, cabbage, spinach, whole-grain breads and pastas, muffins, crackers, and cereals. Leafy vegetables, whole grains, nuts, and seeds also are rich in other important nutrients, including magnesium and vitamin C.

Some simple strategies can help you avoid stress-related stomachaches. Many people experience dry mouth or sweat more under stress. By drinking plenty of water, you replenish lost fluids and prevent dehydration. Fiber-rich foods counteract common stress-related problems, such as cramps and constipation. Do not skip meals. If you do, you're more likely to feel fatigued and irritable.

Be wary of overeating under stress. Some people eat more because they scarf down meals too quickly. Others reach for snacks to calm their nerves or comfort themselves. Watch out for caffeine. Coffee, tea, and cola drinks can make your strained nerves jangle even more. Also avoid sugary snacks. They'll send your blood sugar levels on a roller coaster ride—up one minute, down the next.

Other Stress Symptoms

Stress can affect any organ system in the body, causing painful symptoms or a flare-up of chronic conditions such as asthma. By interfering with our alertness and ability to concentrate, stress also increases the risk of accidents at home, at work, and on the road.

Headaches are one of the most common stress-related conditions. The most common type, tension headache, is caused by involuntary contractions of the scalp, head, and neck muscles. **Migraine headache** is the result of constriction (narrowing), then dilation (widening) of blood vessels within the brain; chemicals leak through the vessel walls, inflame nearby tissues, and send pain signals to the

 brain. Surveys of college women show that Type-A behavior can trigger both types of headache.

Stress also is closely linked to skin conditions. If you break out the week before an exam, you know firsthand that skin can be extremely sensitive to stress. Skin conditions worsened by stress include acne, psoriasis, herpes, hives, and eczema. With acne, increased touching of the face, perhaps while cramming for a test, may be partly responsible. Other factors, such as temperature, humidity, and cosmetics and toiletries, may also play a role.

 ⚉ Stress on Campus

You've probably heard that these are the best years of your life, but being a student—full-time or part-time, in your late teens, early twenties, or later in life—can be extremely stressful. You may feel pressure to perform well to qualify for a good job or graduate school. To meet steep tuition payments, you may have to juggle part-time work and coursework. You may feel stressed about choosing a major, getting along with a difficult roommate, passing a particularly hard course, or living up to your parents' and teachers' expectations. If you're an older student, you may have children, housework, and homework to balance. Your days may seem so busy and your life so full that you worry about coming apart at the seams. One thing is for certain: You're not alone.

After a steady surge upward in the 1990s, the percentage of students who say they are "frequently overwhelmed by all they have to do" has declined from the peak of 30.7 percent in 1999 to 26.8 percent in 2002. However, women are twice as likely to report stress as men.[16] (See the X & Y Files: "Men, Women, and Stress.") According to surveys of students at colleges and universities around the country and the world, stressors are remarkably similar. Among the most common are:

:: Test pressures.

:: Financial problems.

:: Frustrations, such as delays in reaching goals.

:: Problems in friendships and dating relationships.

:: Daily hassles.

:: Academic failure.

:: Pressures as a result of competition, deadlines, and the like.

:: Changes, which may be unpleasant, disruptive, or too frequent.

:: Losses, whether caused by the breakup of a relationship or the death of a loved one.

Many students bring complex psychological problems with them to campus, including learning disabilities and mood disorders like depression and anxiety. "Students arrive with the underpinnings of problems that are brought out by the stress of campus life," says one counselor. Some have grown up in broken homes and bear the scars of family troubles. Others fall into the same patterns of alcohol abuse that they observed for years in their families or suffer lingering emotional scars from childhood physical or sexual abuse.

Students Under Stress

Almost a third of freshmen feel overwhelmed by all they have to do at the beginning of the academic year; by the year's end, 44 percent feel overwhelmed.[17] In a recent study of students at three universities, underclassmen were most vulnerable to negative life events, perhaps because they lacked experience in coping with stressful situations. Freshmen had the highest levels of depression; sophomores had the most anger and hostility. Seniors may handle life's challenges better because they have developed better coping mechanisms. In the study, more seniors reported that they faced problems squarely and took action to resolve them, while younger students were more likely to respond passively, for instance, by trying not to let things bother them.[18]

First-generation college students—those whose parents never experienced at least one full year of college—encounter more difficulties with social adjustment than freshmen whose parents attended college. Second-generation students may have several advantages: more knowledge of college life, greater social support, more preparation for college in high school, a greater focus on college activities, and more financial resources.[19]

The percentage of students seeking psychological help because of stress or anxiety has risen dramatically in the last 15 years.[20] (See Student Snapshot: "Are Students More Stressed Today?") Excessive levels of stress can lead to increased headaches, sleep disturbances, and colds.[21] Students say they react to stress in various ways: physiologically (by sweating, stuttering, trembling, or developing physical symptoms); emotionally (by becoming anxious, fearful, angry, guilty, or depressed); behaviorally (by crying, eating, smoking, being irritable or abusive); or cognitively (by thinking about and analyzing stressful situations and strategies that might be useful in dealing with them).

Social support makes a difference. Students with a truly supportive network of friends and family available to them report greater satisfaction and less psychological distress.[22] In a recent study of

The first year of college can be overwhelming as you learn your way around the campus, meet new people, and strive to succeed.

© Bill Aron/PhotoEdit

the X & Y file *Men, Women, and Stress*

Women, who make up 56 percent of today's college students, also shoulder the majority of the stress load. In a nationwide survey of students in the class of 2005, freshmen women were twice as likely to be anxious as men. More women (36.6 percent) described themselves as "overwhelmed by all I have to do," compared with just 17.4 percent of men. More women than men reported feeling depressed, insecure about their physical and mental health, and worried about paying for college. More men—60.4 percent, compared with 47.7 percent of women—considered themselves above average or in the top 10 percent of people their age in terms of emotional health.

Gender differences in lifestyle may help explain why women feel so stressed. College men, the survey revealed, spend significantly more time doing things that are fun and relaxing: exercising, partying, watching TV, and playing video games. Women, on the other hand, tend to study more, do more volunteer work, and handle more household and child-care chores.

The stress gender gap, which appeared in the mid-1980s, is "one of the ironies of the women's movement," says Alexander Astin of UCLA, founder of the annual American Freshman Survey, which has tracked shifting student attitudes for 35 years. By adding more commitments and responsibilities on top of all the other things they have to cope with, he believes that college women are experiencing an early version of the stress that "super-moms" feel later in life when they pursue a career, care for children, and maintain a household.

So many women complain about fatigue, weight gain, and a decreased interest in sex that doctors have coined a term for this trio: "hurried woman syndrome." The combination of work and marital stress seems particularly intense for women and substantially increases their risk of heart disease.

Where can stressed-out college women turn for support? The best source, according to University of California research, is other women. In general, the social support women offer their friends and relatives seems more effective in reducing the blood-pressure response to stress than that provided by men.

At all ages, women and men tend to respond to stress differently. While males (human and those of other species) react with the classic fight-or-flight response, females under attack try to protect their children and seek help from other females—a strategy dubbed *tend-and-befriend*. When exposed to experimental stress (such as a loud, harsh noise), women show more affection for friends and relatives; men show less. When working mothers studied by psychologists had a bad day, they coped by concentrating on their children when they got home. Stressed-out fathers were more likely to withdraw.

Sources: Linda Sax, et al. *The American Freshman: National Norms for Fall 2002.* Los Angeles: Higher Education Research Institute, UCLA, 2002. "How Women Handle Stress: Is There a Difference?" *Harvard Mental Health Letter,* Vol. 17, No. 10, April 2001. "Women's Response to Stress," *Harvard Women's Health Watch,* Vol. 9, No. 9, May 2002. "Hurried Woman Syndrome." *Family Practice News,* Vol. 33, No. 3, February 1, 2003, p. 48. Bruce Jancin. "Marital, Work Stress Raise Coronary Event Risk in Women." *Family Practice News,* Vol. 32, No. 24, December 15, 2002, p. 32.

university students, those who developed and relied on coping strategies in their leisure time ranked higher in levels of psychological well-being and physical and mental health.[23] In other research, undergraduates with higher levels of social support and self-efficacy reported feeling less stressed and more satisfied with life than others.[24]

Campuses are providing more frontline services than they have in the past, including career-guidance workshops, telephone hot lines, and special social programs for lonely, homesick freshmen. In one study of 128 undergraduates, those who learned relaxation and stress-reduction techniques in a six-week program reported less stress, anxiety, and psychological distress than a control group of students. The participants—who had described themselves as "extremely stressed" before the intervention—also began to increase health-promoting behaviors.[25]

Test Stress

For many students, midterms and final exams are the most stressful times of the year. Studies at various colleges and universities found that the incidence of colds and flu soared during finals. Some students feel the impact of test stress in other ways—headaches, upset stomachs, skin flare-ups, or insomnia.

Test stress affects people in different ways. Sometimes students become so preoccupied with the possibility of failing that they can't concentrate on studying. Others, including many of the best and brightest students, freeze up during tests and can't comprehend multiple-choice questions or write essay answers, even if they know the material.

The students most susceptible to exam stress are those who believe they'll do poorly and who see tests as extremely threatening. Unfortunately, such negative thoughts often become a self-fulfilling prophecy. As they

Student Snapshot — Are Students More Stressed Today?

Percentage of students who sought psychological help for stress and anxiety in three different time periods.

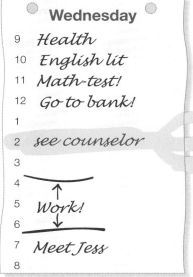

Wednesday

9 *Health*
10 *English lit*
11 *Math-test!*
12 *Go to bank!*
1
2 *see counselor*
3
4
5 *Work!*
6
7 *Meet Jess*
8

1996-2001	63%
1992-1996	62%
1988-1992	36%

Percentage of students who sought psychological help for stress and anxiety

Source: Sherry Benton, et al. "Changes in Counseling Center Client Problems Across 13 Years," *Professional Psychology: Research and Practice*, Vol. 34, No. 1, January 2003, p. 66.

study, these students keep wondering, "What good will studying do? I never do well on tests." As their fear increases, they try harder, pulling all-nighters. Fueled by caffeine, munching on sugary snacks, they become edgy and find it harder and harder to concentrate. By the time

You can take control of your stress responses by practicing relaxation techniques, avoiding cramming, and being positive about your performance on the test.

© Ulrike Welsch

STRATEGIES FOR PREVENTION

Defusing Test Stress

■ *Plan ahead.* A month before finals, map out a study schedule for each course. Set aside a small amount of time every day or every other day to review the course materials.

■ *Be positive.* Picture yourself taking your final exam. Imagine yourself walking into the exam room feeling confident, opening up the test booklet, and seeing questions for which you know the answers.

■ *Take regular breaks.* Get up from your desk, breathe deeply, stretch, and visualize a pleasant scene. You'll feel more refreshed than you would if you chugged another cup of coffee.

■ *Practice.* Some teachers are willing to give practice finals to prepare students for test situations, or you and your friends can test each other.

■ *Talk to other students.* Chances are that many of them share your fears about test taking and may have discovered some helpful techniques of their own. Sometimes talking to your adviser or a counselor can also help.

■ *Be satisfied with doing your best.* You can't expect to ace every test; all you can and should expect is your best effort. Once you've completed the exam, allow yourself the sweet pleasure of relief that it's over.

Self Survey | Student Stress Scale

The Student Stress Scale, an adaptation of Holmes and Rahe's Life Events Scale for college-age adults, provides a rough indication of stress levels and possible health consequences.

In the Student Stress Scale, each event, such as beginning or ending school, is given a score that represents the amount of readjustment a person has to make as a result of the change. In some studies, using similar scales, people with serious illnesses have been found to have high scores.

To determine your stress score, add up the number of points corresponding to the events you have experienced in the past 12 months.

1. Death of a close family member	100	
2. Death of a close friend	73	
3. Divorce of parents	65	
4. Jail term	63	
5. Major personal injury or illness	63	
6. Marriage	58	
7. Getting fired from a job	50	
8. Failing an important course	47	
9. Change in the health of a family member	45	
10. Pregnancy	45	
11. Sex problems	44	
12. Serious argument with a close friend	40	
13. Change in financial status	39	
14. Change of academic major	39	
15. Trouble with parents	39	
16. New girlfriend or boyfriend	37	
17. Increase in workload at school	37	
18. Outstanding personal achievement	36	
19. First quarter/semester in college	36	
20. Change in living conditions	31	
21. Serious argument with an instructor	30	
22. Getting lower grades than expected	29	
23. Change in sleeping habits	29	
24. Change in social activities	29	
25. Change in eating habits	28	
26. Chronic car trouble	26	
27. Change in number of family get-togethers	26	
28. Too many missed classes	25	
29. Changing colleges	24	
30. Dropping more than one class	23	
31. Minor traffic violations	20	
Total Stress Score _____		

Here's how to interpret your score: If your score is 300 or higher, you're at high risk for developing a health problem. If your score is between 150 and 300, you have a 50–50 chance of experiencing a serious health change within two years. If your score is below 150, you have a 1-in-3 chance of a serious health change.

Source: Kathleen Mullen and Gerald Costello. *Health Awareness Through Discovery.*

Your Health Change Plan
for Stress Management

:: **Strive for balance.** Review your commitments and plans, and if necessary, scale down.

:: **Get the facts.** When faced with a change or challenge, seek accurate information, which can bring vague fears down to earth.

:: **Talk with someone you trust.** A friend or a health professional can offer valuable perspective as well as psychological support.

:: **Exercise.** Even when your schedule gets jammed, carve out 20 or 30 minutes several times a week to walk, swim, bicycle, jog, or work out at the gym.

:: **Help others.** One of the most effective ways of dealing with stress is to find people in a worse situation and do something positive for them.

:: **Cultivate hobbies.** Pursuing a personal pleasure can distract you from the stressors in your life and help you relax.

:: **Master a form of relaxation.** Whether you choose meditation, yoga, mindfulness, or another technique, practice it regularly.

of the test, they're nervous wrecks, scarcely able to sit still and focus on the exam.

 Can you do anything to reduce test stress and feel more in control? Absolutely. One way is to defuse stress through relaxation. Students taught relaxation techniques—such as controlled breathing, meditation, progressive relaxation, and guided imagery (visualization)—a month before finals tend to have higher levels of immune cells during the exam period and feel in better control during their tests.

Minorities and Stress

Regardless of your race or ethnic background, college may bring culture shock. You may never have encountered such a degree of diversity in one setting. You probably will meet students with different values, unfamiliar customs, entirely new ways of looking at the world—experiences you may find both stimulating and stressful.

Mental health professionals have long assumed that minority students may feel a double burden of stress. Many undergraduates experience emotional difficulties (see Chapter 2), and researchers have theorized that students from a racial or ethnic minority would be especially likely to develop psychological symptoms, such as anger, anxiety, and depression, as a result of increased stress.

Racism has indeed been shown to be a source of stress that can affect health and well-being.[26] In the past, some African-American students have described predominately white campuses as hostile, alienating, and socially isolating and have reported greater estrangement from the campus community and heightened estrangement in interactions with faculty and peers.[27] However, the generalization that all minority students are more stressed may not be valid.

A recent study conducted at a racially diverse university in a large metropolitan area in the Northeast evaluated 595 freshmen. The study group was made up of both genders and students of various racial and ethnic backgrounds, including Asians, African Americans, and Hispanics.[28] Less than 15 percent of these students—whether Asian, African American, Hispanic, white, or another ethnic minority—reported clinically significant levels of anger, anxiety, and depression, and there was no correlation between these stress-linked symptoms and ethnicity or race.

"Diversity, in and of itself, is unlikely to be related to higher levels of reported psychological symptoms on campus," the researchers concluded, theorizing that minority students "may have developed strengths while growing up within their particular cultures, subcommunities, and families that have often gone unrecognized or unnoted."[29] And some coping mechanisms, especially spirituality, can buffer the negative effects of racism.[30]

All minority students do share some common stressors. In one study of minority freshmen entering a large,

competitive university, Asian, Filipino, African-American, and Native-American students all felt more sensitive and vulnerable to the college social climate, to interpersonal tensions between themselves and nonminority students and faculty, to experiences of actual or perceived racism, and to racist attitudes and discrimination (discussed later in this chapter, under Societal Stressors). Despite scoring above the national average on the SAT, the minority students in this study did not feel accepted as legitimate students and sensed that others viewed them as unworthy beneficiaries of affirmative action initiatives. While most said that overt racism was rare and relatively easy to deal with, they reported subtle pressures that undermined their

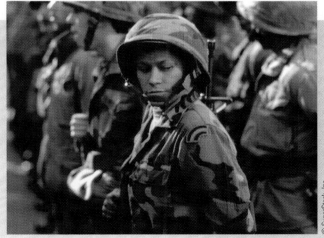

Minority students can often find support services on campus.

academic confidence and their ability to bond with the university. Balancing these stressors, however, was a strong sense of ethnic identity, which helped buffer some stressful effects.

Hispanic students have identified three major types of stressors in their college experiences: academic (related to exam preparation and faculty interaction), social (related to ethnicity and interpersonal competence), and financial (related to their economic situation). Some Asian students who recently immigrated to the United States report feeling ostracized by students of similar ancestry who are second- or third-generation Americans. While they take pride in being truly bicultural and bilingual, the newcomers feel ambivalent about mainstream American culture. "My parents stress the importance of traditions; my friends tell me to get with it and act like an American," says one Asian-born student who has spent five years in the United States. "I feel trapped between cultures."

Other Personal Stressors

At every stage of life, you will encounter challenges and stressors. Among the most common are those related to anger, conflict, work, and overwork.

Why Is Everyone So Angry?

According to the AAA Foundation for Traffic Safety, violent aggressive driving—which some dub "road rage"—has been rising by 7 percent per year.[31] Sideline rage at amateur and professional sporting events has become so widespread that a Pennsylvania midget football game ended in a brawl involving more than 100 coaches, players, parents, and fans.

No one seems immune. Women fly off the handle just as often as men, although they're less likely to get physical. The young and the infamous, including several rappers and musicians sentenced to anger management classes for violent outbursts, may seem more volatile, but ordinary senior citizens have erupted into "line rage" and pushed ahead of others simply because they feel they've "waited long enough" in their lives.

"Everyone everywhere seems to be hotter under the collar these days," observes Sybil Evans, a conflict resolution expert who singles out three primary culprits: time, technology, and tension. "Americans are working longer hours than anyone else in the world. The cell phones and pagers that were supposed to make our lives easier have put us on call 24–7–365. Since we're always running, we're tense and low on patience, and the less patience we have, the less we monitor what we say to people and how we treat them."[32]

Getting a Grip

For years therapists encouraged people to "vent" their anger. However, recent research shows that letting anger out only makes it worse. "Catharsis is worse than useless," says psychology professor Brad Bushman of Iowa State University, whose research has shown that letting anger out makes people more aggressive, not less. "Many people think of anger as the psychological equivalent of the steam in a pressure cooker that has to be released or it will explode. That's not true. People who react by hitting, kicking, screaming, and swearing aren't dealing with the underlying cause of their anger. They just feel more angry."[33]

Over time, temper tantrums sabotage physical health as well as psychological equanimity. By churning out stress hormones, chronic anger revs the body into a state of combat readiness, multiplying the risk for stroke and heart attack—even in healthy individuals. In one study by Duke University researchers, young women with "Jerry-Springer type anger," who tended to slam doors, curse, and throw things in fury, had higher cholesterol levels than those who reacted more calmly.

The first step to dealing with anger is figuring out what's really making you mad. Usually the jammed soda machine is the final straw that unleashes bottled-up fury over a more difficult issue, such as a recent breakup or a domineering parent. Also monitor yourself for early signs of exhaustion and overload. While stress alone doesn't cause a blowup, it makes you more vulnerable to overreacting.

Conflict Resolution

Disagreements are inevitable; disagreeable ways of dealing with them are not. One of the most important skills in any setting—from dormitory floor to staff meeting to corpo-

How you manage your anger has consequences for your health and personal and professional relationships.

© Anthony Redpath/CORBIS

STRATEGIES FOR CHANGE

How to Deal with an Angry Person

- Become an impartial observer. Act as if you were watching someone else's two-year-old have a temper tantrum at the supermarket.

- Stay calm. Letting your emotions loose only adds fuel to fury. Talk quietly and slowly; let the person know you understand that he or she is angry.

- Refuse to engage. Step back to avoid invading his or her space. Retreat further if need be until the person is back in control.

- Find something to agree with. Look for common ground, if only to acknowledge that you're both in a difficult situation.

rate boardroom—is resolving conflicts. The key is to focus on the problem, not the individual. Try to put aside unconscious biases, such as assuming a person is difficult to deal with, or preconceived notions about what others really want. Rather than planning what you might say, focus your attention on what others are saying.

Professionals recommend the following steps:

:: **Listen.** To work through a conflict, you need to understand the other person's point of view. This demands careful listening in a quiet, private setting, away from activity and background noise. If conflict erupts in a public place, move the discussion elsewhere.

:: **Assimilate.** Rather than taking a position and focusing only on defending it, try not to shut yourself off to other possibilities. Keep open the possibility that no one party is completely right or completely wrong. To get a fresh perspective, consider the situation from the "third person." If you were seeing the conflict from the outside, what would you think about the information? Once you've taken in all available information, ask yourself: What do I know now about the overall situation? Has my opinion changed?

:: **Respond.** Especially if another person is responding in anger, give a calm, well-reasoned response. It will help defuse a highly emotional situation. Try to find a common goal that will benefit you both. Restate the other person's position when both of you are finished speaking so you both know you've been heard and understood.

Job Stress

More so than ever, many people find that they are working more and enjoying it less. Many people, including working parents, spend 55 to 60 hours a week on the job. More people are caught up in an exhausting cycle of overwork, which causes stress, which makes work harder, which leads to more stress. Even the workplace itself can contribute to stress. A noisy, open-office environment can increase levels of stress without workers realizing it.[34]

Yet work in itself is not hazardous to health. Attitudes about work and habits related to how we work are the true threats. In fact, a job—stressful or not, enjoyable or not—can be therapeutic.

Workaholism and Burnout

People who become obsessed by their work and careers can turn into *workaholics,* so caught up in racing toward the top that they forget what they're racing toward and why. In some cases they throw themselves into their work to mask or avoid painful feelings or difficulties in their own lives. One consequence is **burnout,** a state of physical, emotional, and mental exhaustion brought on by constant or repeated emotional pressure. Particularly in the helping professions, such as social work or nursing, men and women who've dedicated themselves to others may realize they have nothing left in themselves to give.

Early signs of burnout include exhaustion, sleep problems or nightmares, increased anxiety or nervousness, muscular tension (headaches, backaches, and the like), increased use of alcohol or medication, digestive problems, such as nausea, vomiting, or diarrhea, loss of interest in sex, frequent body aches or pain, quarrels with family or friends, negative feelings about everything, problems concentrating, job mistakes and accidents, and feelings of depression, hopelessness, and helplessness.

Age is the one variable most consistently associated with burnout: Younger employees between ages 30 and 40 report the highest rates. Both men and women are susceptible to burnout. Unmarried individuals, particularly men, seem more prone to burnout than married workers. Single employees who've never been married have higher burnout rates than those who are divorced.

North American workers are more likely to experience burnout than employees in Western Europe. High burnout also has been reported in Japan, Taiwan, and other Asian countries. Certain occupations, particularly the helping professions, such as social work and nursing, have been linked with a greater risk of burnout. However, burnout also is common in teaching, law enforcement, and medicine.

In a study of physicians, researchers found that hard work and fatigue can be countered by job satisfaction. A high sense of accomplishment was associated with an increase in the number of T cells, the white blood cells that protect the body against disease.[35] However, the best way to avoid burnout is learning to cope well with smaller, day-to-day stresses. Then, tiny frustrations won't smolder into a blaze that may be impossible to put out.

Desk Rage

Job stress has intensified into a more intense and dangerous condition that has been dubbed "desk rage." Experts blame corporate downsizing, intense competition, longer hours, economic insecurity, and nonstop electronic communication. "Many employees today have a sense of voiceless overload," says Ken Jacobsen, an expert in workplace distress at the University of Northern Iowa, "Each is doing the job of two or two-and-a-half people, and the demands on them may be completely unrealistic. In the past, there was a belief that if you worked harder or longer, you'd be rewarded. That's no longer the case, and it flies in the face of an employee's sense of fairness."[36]

While rage can smolder in any workplace, it is most likely to reach a boiling point when job responsibilities are ambiguous or unpredictable or when employees think they can't or shouldn't express negative feelings. Many develop physical symptoms, such as insomnia or indigestion, or take up self-destructive habits, like eating or drinking too much.

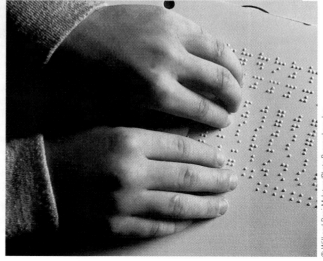

STRATEGIES FOR PREVENTION

Defusing Desk Rage

Desk rage builds in little steps, so you can take it away in little steps. Here are suggestions on how to do so:

- If you sense a problem, monitor the situation for a week. Write down when you're feeling hungry, tired, overloaded. Try to identify the triggers that might cause you to do something you'll later regret.

- Get feedback from friends. An objective person who knows you well can provide a fresh take on a troubling situation.

- If your irritation stems from a coworker, approach him or her in a nonthreatening way. You might say, "Could you hear me out for a few minutes?" To lower the hostility level, start by stating something you have in common, such as "We both want this project to work."

- If you fly off the handle, learn from the experience. Do immediate damage control by apologizing to coworkers and explaining that you've been under stress. Plan what you might do differently the next time someone or something sets you off.

Illness and Disability

Just as the mind can have profound effects on the body, the body can have an enormous impact on our emotions. Whenever we come down with the flu or pull a muscle, we feel under par. When the problem is more serious or persistent—a chronic disease like diabetes, for instance, or a lifelong hearing impairment—the emotional stress of constantly coping with it is even greater.

A common source of stress for college students is a learning disability, which may affect one of every ten Americans. Most learning-disabled have average or above-average intelligence, but they rarely live up to their ability in school. Some have only one area of difficulty, such as reading or math. Others have problems with attention, writing, communicating, reasoning, coordination, and social skills.

Not all students with learning disabilities experience greater stress. In one in-depth study comparing 34 undergraduates with and without learning disabilities, the learning-disabled (LD) students reported significantly fewer college stressors and demonstrated a higher need for achievement. The LD students also scored significantly higher in resiliency and initiative in solving problems and working toward goals.[37]

⬛ Societal Stressors

Not all stressors are personal. Centuries ago the poet John Donne observed that no man is an island. Today, on an increasingly crowded and troubled planet, these words

A blind college student has unique challenges and stressors that sighted students do not.

© Will and Deni McIntyre/Photo Researchers, Inc.

seem truer than ever. Problems such as discrimination and terrorism can no longer be viewed only as economic or political issues. Directly or indirectly, they affect the well-being of all who inhabit the Earth—now and in the future. Even more mundane stressors, such as traffic, can lead to outbursts of anger that have come to be known as "road rage."[38] (This common stress-related response is discussed in Chapter 18.)

Discrimination

Discrimination can take many forms—some as subtle as not being included in a conversation or joke, some as blatant as threats scrawled on a wall, some as violent as brutal beatings and other hate crimes. Because it can be hard to deal with individually, discrimination is a particularly sinister form of stress. By banding together, however, those who experience discrimination can take action to protect themselves, challenge the ignorance and hateful assumptions that fuel bigotry, and promote a healthier environment for all.

In the last decade, there have been reports of increased intolerance among young people and greater tolerance of expressions and acts of hate on college campuses. To counteract this trend, many schools have set up programs and classes to educate students about each other's backgrounds and to acknowledge and celebrate the richness diversity brings to campus life. Educators have called on universities to make campuses less alienating and more culturally and emotionally accessible, with programs and policies targeted not only at minority students but also at the university as a whole.

Violence and Terrorism

The deliberate use of physical force to abuse or injure is a leading killer of young people in the United States—and a potential source of stress in all our lives. Chances are that you or someone you know has been the victim of a violent crime, and awareness of our own vulnerability adds to the stress of daily living.

In the weeks after the September 11, 2001, terrorist attacks in New York and Washington, many Americans reported one or more significant symptoms of psychological distress. In a study of 219 African-American college students shortly after the events of September 11, 2001, many students experienced stress symptoms and distressing thoughts and feelings, including academic problems, concerns about family and friends in the military, and fear about war. Most students were highly distressed by specific attack-related news reports and images. Students in the last years of college and those whose parents were not currently together had the most severe

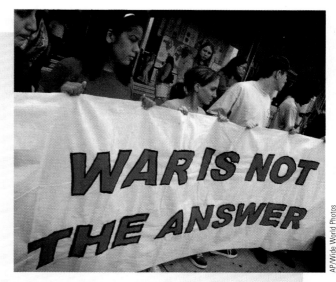

Protest marches are one way in which college students have often responded to national and international crises.

symptoms.[39] Many Americans continue to suffer high stress levels because of the continuing fear of terrorism.[40]

✸ Stress Survival

Sometimes we respond to stress or challenge with self-destructive behaviors, such as drinking or using drugs. These responses can lead to psychological problems, such as anxiety or depression, and physical problems, including psychosomatic illnesses.

Defense mechanisms, such as those described in Table 3-1, are another response to stress. These psychological devices are mental processes that help us cope with personal problems. Such responses are also not the answer to stress—and learning to recognize them in yourself will enable you to deal with your stress in a healthier way.

The key to coping with stress is realizing that your *perception* of and *response* to a stressor are crucial. Changing the way you interpret events or situations—a skill called *reframing*—makes all the difference. An event, such as a move to a new city, is not stressful in itself. A move becomes stressful if you see it as a traumatic upheaval rather than an exciting beginning of a new chapter in your life.

In times of stress, the following simple exercises can stop the stress buildup inside your body and help you regain a sense of calm and control.

:: *Breathing.* Deep breathing relaxes the body and quiets the mind. Draw air deeply into your lungs, allowing your chest to fill with air and your belly to rise and fall. You will feel the muscle tension and stress begin

TABLE 3-1	Common Defense Mechanisms Used to Alleviate Anxiety and Eliminate Conflict
Defense Mechanism	**Example**
Denial: the refusal to accept a painful reality.	You don't accept as true the news that a loved one is seriously ill.
Displacement: the redirection of feelings from their true object to a more acceptable or safer substitute.	Instead of lashing out at a coach or a teacher, you snap at your best friend.
Projection: the attribution of unacceptable feelings or impulses to someone else.	When you want to end a relationship, you project your unhappiness onto your partner.
Rationalization: the substitution of "good," acceptable reasons for the real motivations for our behavior.	You report a classmate who has been mean to you for cheating on an exam and explain that cheating is unfair to other students.
Reaction formation: adopting attitudes and behaviors that are the opposite of what you feel.	You lavishly compliment an acquaintance whom you really despise.
Repression: the way we keep threatening impulses, fantasies, memories, feelings, or wishes from becoming conscious.	You don't "hear" the alarm after a late night, or you "forget" to take out the trash.

to melt away. When you're feeling extremely stressed, try this calming breath: Sit or lie with your back straight and place the tip of your tongue on the roof of your mouth behind your teeth. Exhale completely through the mouth, then inhale through the nose for 4 seconds. Hold the breath for 7 seconds, then exhale audibly through the mouth for 8 seconds. Repeat four times.

:: **Refocusing.** Thinking about a situation you can't change or control only increases the stress you feel. Force your mind to focus on other subjects. If you're stuck in a long line, distract yourself. Check out what other people are buying or imagine what they do for a living. Imagine that you're in a hot shower and a wave of relaxation is washing your stress down the drain.

:: **Serenity breaks.** Build moments of tranquility into your day. For instance, while waiting for your computer to start up or a file to download, look at a photograph of someone you love or a poster of a tropical island. If none is available, close your eyes and visualize a soothing scene, such as walking in a meadow or along a beach.

:: **Stress signals.** Learn to recognize the first signs that your stress load is getting out of hand: Is your back bothering you? Do you have a headache? Do you find yourself speeding or misplacing things? Whenever you spot these early warnings, force yourself to stop and say, "I'm under stress. I need to do something about it."

:: **Reality checks.** To put things into proper perspective, ask yourself: Will I remember what's made me so upset a month from now? If you had to rank this problem on a scale of 1 to 10, with worldwide catastrophe as 10, where would it rate?

:: **Stress inoculation.** Rehearse everyday situations that you find stressful, such as speaking in class. Think of how you might make the situation less tense, for instance, by breathing deeply before you talk or jotting down notes beforehand. Think of these small "doses" of stress as the psychological equivalent of allergy shots: They immunize you so you feel less stressed when bigger challenges come along.[41]

:: **Rx: Laughter.** Humor counters stress by focusing on comic aspects of difficult situations and may, as various studies have shown, lessen harmful effects on the immune system and overall health. However, humor may have different effects on stress in men and women. In a study of 131 undergraduates, humor buffered stress–related physical symptoms in men and women. However, it reduced stress-linked anxiety only in men. The researchers theorized that men may prefer humor as a more appropriate way of expressing emotions such as anxiety, whereas women are more likely to use self-disclosure, that is, to confide in friends.[42]

:: **Spiritual coping.** Saying a prayer under stress is one of the oldest and most effective ways of calming yourself. Other forms of spiritual coping, such as putting trust in God and doing for others (for instance, by volunteering at a shelter for battered women) also can provide a different perspective on daily hassles and stresses.

:: **Sublimation.** This term refers to the redirection of any drives considered unacceptable into socially acceptable channels. Outdoor activity is one of the best ways to reduce stress through sublimation. For instance, if you're furious with a friend who betrayed your trust or frustrated because your boss rejects all of your proposals, you might go for a long run or hike to sublimate your anger.

:: **Exercise.** Regular physical activity can relieve stress, boost energy, lift mood, and keep stress under control.

Savvy Consumer

CAN STRESS-RELIEF PRODUCTS HELP?

You're stressed out, and you see an ad for a product—an oil, candle, cream, herbal tea, pill, or potion—that promises to make all your cares disappear. Should you soak in an aromatic bath, have a massage, try kava, squeeze foam balls? In most cases, you're probably not doing yourself much harm, but you aren't necessarily doing yourself much good either. Keep these considerations in mind:

- Be wary of instant cures. Regardless of the promises on the label, it's unrealistic to expect any magic ingredient or product to make all your problems disappear.

- Focus on stress-reducing behavior, rather than a product. An aromatic candle may not bring instant serenity, but if

you light a candle and meditate, you may indeed feel more at peace. A scented pillow may not be a cure for a stress, but if it helps you get a good night's sleep, you'll cope better the next day.

- Experiment with physical ways to work out stress. Exercise is one of the best ways to lower your stress levels. Try walking, running, swimming, cycling, kick-boxing— anything physical that helps you release tension.

- Don't make matters worse by smoking (the chemicals in cigarettes increase heart rate, blood pressure, and stress hormone), consuming too much caffeine (it speeds up your system for hours), eating snacks high in sugar (it produces a quick high followed by a sudden slump), or turning to drugs or alcohol (they can only add to your stress when their effects wear off.)

- Remember that stress is a matter of attitude. Remind yourself of some basic words of wisdom: Don't sweat the small stuff—and it's all small stuff.

:: *Journaling.* One of the simplest, yet most effective, ways to work through stress is by putting your feelings into words that only you will read. The more honest and open you are as you write, the bet- ter. College students who wrote in their journals about traumatic events felt much better afterward than those who wrote about superficial topics. Focus on intense emotional experiences and "autopsy" them to try to understand why they affected you the way they

did. Rereading and thinking about your notes may reveal the underlying reasons for your response.

 In one study, college students who engaged in an eight-week weight training reported lower stress levels than those who participated in an aerobic dance program.[43]

� What Can Help Me Relax?

Relaxation is the physical and mental state opposite that of stress. Rather than gearing up for fight or flight, our bodies and minds grow calmer and work more smoothly. We're less likely to become frazzled and more capable of staying in control. The most effective relaxation techniques include progressive relaxation, visualization, meditation, mindfulness, and biofeedback.

Progressive relaxation works by intentionally increasing and then decreasing tension in the muscles. While sitting or lying down in a quiet, comfortable setting, you tense and release various muscles, beginning with those of the hand, for instance, and then proceeding to the arms, shoulders, neck, face, scalp, chest, stomach, buttocks, genitals, and so on, down each leg to the toes. Relaxing the muscles can quiet the mind and restore internal balance.

Visualization, or **guided imagery,** involves creating mental pictures that calm you down and focus your mind. Some people use this technique to promote healing when they are ill (see Chapter 16). Visualization skills require

Writing in your journal about feelings and difficulties is a simple and very effective way to help control your stress.

© CORBIS

practice and, in some cases, instruction by qualified health professionals.

Meditation has been practiced in many forms over the ages, from the yogic techniques of the Far East to the Quaker silence of more modern times. Brain scans have shown that meditation activates the sections of the brain in charge of the autonomic nervous system, which governs bodily functions, such as digestion and blood pressure, that we cannot consciously control.[44] Although many studies have documented the benefits of meditation for overall health, it may be particularly helpful for people dealing with stress-related medical conditions such as high blood pressure.

In a study of African Americans with atherosclerosis, or hardening of the arteries, those who meditated showed a marked decrease in the thickness of their artery walls, while the nonmeditators showed an increase. This benefit is particularly important because African Americans are twice as likely to die from cardiovascular disease as are whites.

Meditation helps a person reach a state of relaxation, but with the goal of achieving inner peace and harmony. There is no one right way to meditate, and many people have discovered how to meditate on their own, without even knowing what it is they are doing.

Among college students, meditation has proven especially effective in increasing relaxation. Most forms of meditation have common elements: sitting quietly for 15 to 20 minutes once or twice a day, concentrating on a word or image, and breathing slowly and rhythmically. If you wish to try meditation, it often helps to have someone guide you through your first sessions. Or try tape recording your own voice (with or without favorite music in the background) and playing it back to yourself, freeing yourself to concentrate on the goal of turning the attention within.

STRATEGIES FOR CHANGE

"Mini-relaxation"

Here is a quick deep-breathing exercise from Harvard psychologist Alice Domar:

- Sit upright or lie on your back.

- Place your hand just beneath your navel so you can feel the rise and fall of your belly as you breathe deeply through your nose.

- As you inhale, count slowly, saying to yourself, "one, two, three, four." Exhale slowly, counting back down from four to one.

- Do this for one minute or longer.[45]

Spending time outdoors is a great way to leave behind daily tensions.

Mindfulness is a modern form of an ancient Asian technique that involves maintaining awareness in the present moment. You tune in to each part of your body, scanning from head to toe, noting the slightest sensation. You allow whatever you experience—an itch, an ache, a feeling of warmth—to enter your awareness. Then you open yourself to focus on all the thoughts, sensations, sounds, and feelings that enter your awareness. Mindfulness keeps you in the here-and-now, thinking about what *is* rather than about *what if* or *if only*.

Biofeedback, discussed in Chapter 16, is a method of obtaining feedback, or information, about some physiological activity occurring in the body. An electronic monitor-

Biofeedback training uses electronic monitoring devices to teach conscious control over heart rate, body temperature, and muscle tension. Once the technique is learned, the electronic devices are unnecessary.

ing device attached to the body detects a change in an internal function and communicates it back to the person through a tone, light, or meter. By paying attention to this feedback, most people can gain some control over functions previously thought to be beyond conscious control, such as body temperature, heart rate, muscle tension, and brain waves. Biofeedback training consists of three stages:

1. Developing increased awareness of a body state or function.
2. Gaining control over it.
3. Transferring this control to everyday living without use of the electronic instrument.

The goal of biofeedback for stress reduction is a state of tranquility, usually associated with the brain's production of alpha waves (which are slower and more regular than normal waking waves). After several training sessions, most people can produce alpha waves more or less at will.

▶ Is Stress Hazardous to Psychological Health? ▣◉

Traumatic events (such as a robbery, assault, or sudden death of a loved one) always take a toll on an individual, and it's normal to feel sad, tense, overwhelmed, angry, or incapable of coping with the ordinary demands of daily living. Usually such feelings and behaviors subside with time. The stressful event fades into the past, and those whose lives it has touched adapt to its lasting impact. But sometimes individuals remain extremely distressed and unable to function as they once did. While the majority of individuals who survive a trauma recover, at least a quarter of such individuals later develop serious psychological symptoms.

Posttraumatic Stress Disorder

In the past, **posttraumatic stress disorder (PTSD)** was viewed as a psychological response to out-of-the-ordinary stressors, such as captivity or combat. However, other experiences can also forever change the way people view themselves and their world. Thousands of individuals experience or witness traumatic events, such as fires or floods. Children, in particular, are likely to develop PTSD symptoms when they live through a traumatic event or witness a loved one or friend being assaulted.

 In a study of 649 college students, those who reported more traumatic experiences in childhood were more likely to develop symptoms of depression and to do so at an earlier age.[46]

According to recent research, almost half of car accident victims may develop PTSD. Individuals who were

seriously injured are especially vulnerable.[47] The main symptoms are re-experiencing the traumatic event, avoiding the site of the accident, refraining from driving in weather and road conditions similar to those on the day of the accident, and feeling a general increase in distress.

As shown in a recent Canadian study of 65 women over age 18, sexual abuse during childhood or adolescence can increase vulnerability to PTSD later in life.[48] An episode that repeats the abuse, such as a sexual assault or rape, can trigger an intense reaction as individuals "re-experience" the initial trauma.

 Childhood abuse—physical, sexual, or emotional—can affect student dropout rates. In one study that followed 210 freshmen (aged 17–21 years) for four years, those suffering PTSD symptoms in the second week of their freshman year were less likely to remain enrolled through their senior years. Half of those who'd been sexually abused and 65 percent of those who'd experienced multiple forms of abuse dropped out.[49]

In PTSD, individuals re-experience their terror and helplessness again and again in their dreams or intrusive thoughts. To avoid this psychic pain, they may try to avoid anything associated with the trauma. Some enter a state of emotional numbness and no longer can respond to people and experiences the way they once did, especially when it comes to showing tenderness or affection. Those who've been mugged or raped may be afraid to venture out by themselves.

The sooner trauma survivors receive psychological help, the better they are likely to fare. Often talking about what happened with an empathic person or someone who's shared the experience as soon as possible—preferably before going to sleep on the day of the event—can help an individual begin to deal with what has occurred. Group sessions, ideally beginning soon after the trauma, allow individuals to share views and experiences. Behavioral, cognitive, and psychodynamic therapy (described in Chapter 2) can help individuals suffering PTSD.

Resilience: Bouncing Back from Adversity

Adversity—whether in the form of a traumatic event or chronic stress—has different effects on individuals. Some people never recover and continue on a downward slide that may ultimately prove fatal. Others return, though at different rates, to their prior level of functioning. In recent years researchers have focused their attention on a particularly intriguing group: those people who not only survive stressful experiences but also thrive, that is, who actually surpass their previous level of functioning.

Resilience can take many forms.[50] A father whose child is kidnapped and killed may become a nationwide advocate for victims' rights. A student whose roommate dies in a car crash after a party may campaign for tougher laws against drunk driving. A couple whose premature baby spends weeks in a neonatal intensive care unit may find that their marriage has grown closer and stronger. Even though their experiences were painful, the individuals often look back at them as bringing positive changes into their lives.

Researchers have studied various factors that enable individuals to thrive in the face of adversity. These include:

:: *An optimistic attitude.* Rather than reacting to a stressor simply as a threat, these men and women view stress as a challenge—one they believe they can and will overcome. Researchers have documented that individuals facing various stressors, including serious illness and bereavement, are more likely to report experiencing growth if they have high levels of hope and optimism.

:: *Self-efficacy.* A sense of being in control of one's life can boost health, even in times of great stress.

:: *Stress inoculation.* People who deal well with adversity often have had previous experiences with stress that toughened them in various ways, such as teaching them skills that enhanced their ability to cope and boosting their confidence in their ability to weather a rough patch.

:: *Secure personal relationships.* Individuals who know they can count on the support of their loved ones are more likely to be resilient.

:: *Spirituality or religiousness.* Religious coping may be particularly related to growth and resilience. In particular, two types seem most beneficial: spiritually based religious coping (receiving emotional reassurance and guidance from God) and good-deeds coping (living a better, more spiritual life that includes altruistic acts).

Resilience sometimes means developing new skills simply because, in order to get through the stressful experience, people had to learn something they hadn't known how to do before—for instance, wrangling with insurance companies or other bureaucracies. By mastering such skills, they become more fit to deal with an unpredictable world and develop new flexibility in facing the unknown.

Along with new abilities comes the psychological sense of mastery. "I survived this," an individual may say. "I'll be able to deal with other hard things in the future." Such confidence keeps people actively engaged in the effort to cope and is itself a predictor of eventual success. Stress also can make individuals more aware of the fulfilling aspects of life, and they may become more interested in spiritual pursuits. Certain kinds of stressful experiences also have social consequences. If a person experiencing a traumatic event finds that the significant others in his or her life can be counted on, the result can be a strengthening of their relationship.

Researchers are trying to determine ways in which more people can derive positive benefits from stressful experiences. One important step, they believe, is to encourage people to view a traumatic situation as an opportunity for personal growth, rather than a test of whether or not they "have what it takes" to survive.

Trauma survivors can often find support and comfort from those who have shared the experience.

© AFP/CORBIS

In a study of the life narratives of midlife adults (aged 35–65 years) and college students (aged 18–24), both groups reported greater psychological well-being when the stories of low points and turning points in their lives contained images of redemption and they were able to find benefits and lessons in their experiences of adversity.[51]

Focusing on finding meaning in their experience— what some call "cognitive coping"—can help individuals move beyond initial emotional responses such as anxiety, distress, and confusion. Over time, some people may develop what may be the ultimate "gift" of a stressful experience: wisdom.

Time Management

We live in what some sociologists call hyperculture, a society that moves at warp speed. Information bombards us constantly. The rate of change seems to accelerate every year. Our "time-saving" devices—pagers, cell phones, modems, faxes, palm-sized organizers, laptop computers— have simply extended the boundaries of where and how we work.

As a result, more and more people are suffering from "timesickness," a nerve-racking feeling that life has become little more than an endless to-do list. The best antidote is time management, and hundreds of books, seminars, and experts offer training in making the most of the hours in the day. Yet these well-intentioned methods often fail, and sooner or later most of us find ourselves caught in a time trap.

Poor Time Management

Every day you make dozens of decisions, and the choices you make about how to use your time directly affect your stress level. If you have a big test on Monday and a term paper due Tuesday, you may plan to study all weekend. Then, when you're invited to a party Saturday night, you go. Although you set the alarm for 7:00 A.M. on Sunday, you don't pull yourself out of bed until noon. By the time you start studying, it's 4:00 P.M., and anxiety is building inside you.

How can you tell if you've lost control of your time? The following are telltale symptoms of poor time management:

:: Rushing.

:: Chronic inability to make choices or decisions.

:: Fatigue or listlessness.

:: Constantly missed deadlines.

:: Not enough time for rest or personal relationships.

:: A sense of being overwhelmed by demands and details and having to do what you don't want to do most of the time.

One of the hard lessons of being on your own is that your choices and your actions have consequences. Stress is just one of them. But by thinking ahead, being realistic about your workload, and sticking to your plans, you can gain better control over your time and your stress levels.

How Can I Better Manage My Time?

Time management involves skills that anyone can learn, but they require commitment and practice to make a difference in your life. It may help to know the techniques that other students have found most useful:

:: **Schedule your time.** Use a calendar or planner. Beginning the first week of class, mark down deadlines for each assignment, paper, project, and test scheduled that semester. Develop a daily schedule, listing very specifically what you will do the next day, along with the times. Block out times for working out, eating dinner, calling home, and talking with friends as well as for studying.

:: **Develop a game plan.** Allow at least two nights to study for any major exam. Set aside more time for researching and writing papers. Make sure to allow time to revise and print out a paper—and to deal with emergencies like a computer breakdown. Set daily and weekly goals for every class. When working on a big project, don't neglect your other courses. Whenever possible, try to work ahead in all your classes.

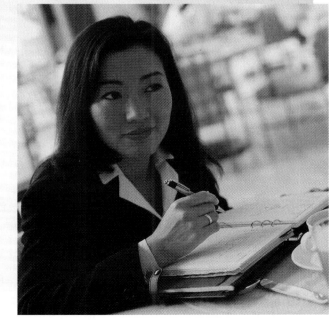

A calendar or planner is an important tool in time management. You can use it to keep track of assignment due dates, class meetings, and other "to do's."

© CORBIS

:: ***Identify time robbers.*** For several days keep a log of what you do and how much time you spend doing it. You may discover that disorganization is eating away at your time or that you have a problem getting started. (See the following section on Overcoming Procrastination.)

:: ***Make the most of classes.*** Read the assignments before class rather than waiting until just before you have a test. By reading ahead of time, you'll make it easier to understand the lectures. Go to class yourself. Your own notes will be more helpful than a friend's or those from a note-taking service. Read your lecture notes at the end of each day or at least at the end of each week.

:: ***Develop an efficient study style.*** Some experts recommend studying for 50 minutes, then breaking for 10 minutes. Small incentives, such as allowing yourself to call or visit a friend during these 10 minutes, can provide the motivation to keep you at the books longer. When you're reading, don't just highlight passages. Instead, write notes or questions to yourself in the margins, which will help you retain more information. Even if you're racing to start a paper, take a few extra minutes to prepare a workable outline. It will be easier to structure your paper when you start writing.

:: ***Focus on the task at hand.*** Rather than worrying about how you did on yesterday's test or how you'll ever finish next week's project, focus intently on whatever you're doing at any given moment. If your mind starts to wander, use any distraction—the sound of the phone ringing or a noise from the hall—as a reminder to stay in the moment.

:: ***Turn elephants into hors d'oeuvres.*** Cut a huge task into smaller chunks so it seems less enormous. For instance, break down your term paper into a series of steps, such as selecting a topic, identifying sources of research information, taking notes, developing an outline, and so on.

:: ***Keep your workspace in order.*** Even if the rest of your room is a shambles, try to keep your desk clear. Piles of papers are distracting, and you can end up wasting lots of time looking for notes you misplaced or an article you have to read by morning. Try to spend the last ten minutes of the day getting your desk in order so you get a fresh start on the new day.

Overcoming Procrastination

 Putting off until tomorrow what should be done today is a habit that creates a great deal of stress for many students. It also takes a surprising toll. In studies with students taking a health psychology course, researchers found that although procrastinating provided short-term benefits, including periods of low stress, the tendency to dawdle had long-term costs, including poorer health and lower grades. Early in the semester, the procrastinators reported

less stress and fewer health problems than students who scored low on procrastination. However, by the end of the semester, procrastinators reported more health-related symptoms, more stress, and more visits to health-care professionals than nonprocrastinators. Students who procrastinate also get poorer grades in courses with many deadlines.[52]

The three most common types of procrastination are: putting off unpleasant things, putting off difficult tasks, and putting off tough decisions. Procrastinators are most likely to delay by wishing they didn't have to do what they must or by telling themselves they "just can't get started," which means they never do.

To get out of the procrastination trap, keep track of the tasks you're most likely to put off, and try to figure out why you don't want to tackle them. Think of alternative ways to get tasks done. If you put off library readings, for instance, is the problem getting to the library or the reading itself? If it's the trip to the library, arrange to walk over with a friend whose company you enjoy.

Develop daily time-management techniques, such as a to-do list. Rank items according to priorities: A, B, C, and schedule your days to make sure the A's get accomplished. Try not to fixate on half-completed projects. Divide large tasks, such as a term paper, into smaller ones, and reward yourself when you complete a part.

Do what you like least first. Once you have it out of the way, you can concentrate on the tasks you enjoy. Build time into your schedule for interruptions, unforeseen problems, and unexpected events, so you aren't constantly racing around. Establish ground rules for meeting your own needs (including getting enough sleep and making time for friends) before saying yes to any activity. Learn to live according to a three-word motto: Just do it!

The Bottom Line: ▼ De-stress Your Life

College is a perfect time to learn and practice the art of stress reduction. You can start applying the techniques and concepts outlined in this chapter immediately. You may want to begin by doing some relaxation or awareness exercises. They can give you the peace of mind you need to focus more effectively on larger issues, goals, and decisions.

You needn't see stress as a problem to solve on your own. Reach out to others. As you build friendships and intimate relationships, you may find that some irritating problems are easier to put into perspective. Don't be afraid to laugh at yourself and to look for the comic or absurd aspects of a situation. In addition, you might try some simple approaches that can help boost your stress resistance and reslience, including the following:

:: ***Focusing.*** Take a strain inventory of your body every day to determine where things aren't feeling quite right. Ask yourself, "What's keeping me from feeling terrific today?" Focusing on problem spots, such as stomach knots or neck tightness, increases your sense of control over stress.

:: **Reconstructing stressful situations.** Think about a recent episode of distress; then write down three ways it could have gone better and three ways it could have gone worse. This should help you see that the situation wasn't as disastrous as it might have been, and help you find ways to cope better in the future.

:: **Self-improvement.** When your life feels out of control, turn to a new challenge. You might try volunteering at a nursing home, going for a long-distance bike trip, or learning a foreign language. As you work toward your new goal, you'll realize that you still can cope and achieve.

If stress continues to be a problem in your life, you may be able to find help through support groups or counseling. Your school may provide counseling services or referrals to mental health professionals; ask your health instructor or the campus health department for this information. Remember that each day of distress robs you of energy, distracts you from life's pleasures, and interferes with achieving your full potential.

 After watching the CNN video segment, discuss the following questions. What is the difference between short-term and long-term stress? How does stress affect your health?

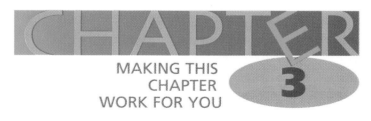

MAKING THIS
CHAPTER
WORK FOR YOU

1. Stress can be defined as
   a. a negative emotional state related to fatigue and similar to depression.
   b. the physiological and psychological response to any event or situation that either upsets or excites us.
   c. the end result of the general adaptation syndrome.
   d. a motivational strategy for making life changes.

2. According to the general adaptation syndrome theory, how does the body typically respond to an acute stressor?
   a. The heart rate slows, blood pressure declines, and eye movement increases.
   b. The body enters a physical state called eustress and then moves into the physical state referred to as distress.

   c. If the stressor is viewed as a positive event, there are no physical changes.
   d. The body demonstrates three stages of change: alarm, resistance, and exhaustion.

3. Over time, increased levels of stress hormones have been shown to increase a person's risk for which of the following conditions?
   a. diabetes, high blood pressure, memory loss, and skin disorders
   b. stress fractures, male pattern baldness, and hypothyroidism
   c. hemophilia, AIDS, and hay fever
   d. none of the above

4. Stress levels in college students
   a. may be high due to stressors such as academic pressures, financial concerns, learning disabilities, and relationship problems.
   b. are usually low because students feel empowered, living independently of their parents.
   c. are typically highest in seniors because their self-esteem diminishes during the college years.
   d. are lower in minority students because they are used to stressors such as a hostile social climate and actual or perceived discrimination.

5. Which of the following statements about anger is true?
   a. The healthiest way to deal with anger is to express the rage.
   b. When confronted by an angry person, you can usually defuse the situation quickly by explaining that he or she is acting immaturely and inappropriately.
   c. Venting anger can adversely affect one's physical health over time.
   d. Statistics show that anger-related public behaviors such as aggressive driving and workplace outbursts have been on the decrease.

6. Which of the following illustrates the defense mechanism of displacement?
   a. You have a beer in the evening after a tough day.
   b. You act as if nothing has happened after you have been laid off from your job.
   c. You start an argument with your sister after being laid off from your job.
   d. You argue with your boss after he lays you off from your job.

7. Which of the following situations is representative of a societal stressor?
   a. Peter has been told that his transfer application has been denied because his transcripts were not sent in by the deadline.
   b. Nia and Kwame find an unsigned note pinned to the door of their new home ordering them to move out or face the consequences.
   c. Kelli's boyfriend drives her car after he had been drinking and has an accident.

d. Joshua, who is the leading basketball player on his college varsity team, has just been diagnosed with diabetes.

8. If you are stuck in a traffic jam, which of the following actions will help reduce your stress level?
   a. deep slow breathing
   b. honking your horn
   c. berating yourself for not taking a different route
   d. getting on your cell phone to reschedule appointments

9. A relaxed peaceful state of being can be achieved with which of the following activities?
   a. an aerobic exercise class

b. playing a computer game
c. meditating for 15 minutes
d. attending a rap concert

10. A person suffering from posttraumatic stress disorder may experience which of the following symptoms?
   a. procrastination
   b. constant thirst
   c. drowsiness
   d. terror-filled dreams

Answers to these questions can be found on page 652.

Critical Thinking

1. What reasons can you think of to account for high stress levels among college students? Consider possible social, cultural, and economic factors that may play a role.

2. Identify three stressful situations in your life and determine whether they are examples of eustress or

distress. Describe both the positive and negative aspects of each situation.

3. Can you think of any ways in which your behavior or attitudes might create stress for others? What changes could you make to avoid doing so?

Critical Thinking

4. What advice might you give an incoming freshman at your school about managing stress in college? What techniques have been most helpful for you in dealing with stress? Suppose that this student is from a different ethnic group than you. What additional suggestions would you have for this student?

Profile Plus

How is stress affecting you? Discover how you respond to stressful situations by participating in the following activities on your Profile Plus CD-ROM:

Profile Plus

• Life Experiences Survey
• Type A Behavior
• The Stress Test

Profile Plus

• Stress Vulnerability Questionnaire
• Hostile Personality Assessment

Sites and Bytes

Stress Assess
http://wellness.uwsp.edu/Health_Service/services/stress

This three-part outline educational tool was developed by the National Wellness Institute at the University of Wisconsin—Steven's Point. Designed to increase your knowledge about stress, this questionnaire features separate evaluations for stress sources, distress symptoms, and stress-balancing strategies.

Sites and Bytes

Family Doctor—Stress: Who Has Time for It?
http://familydoctor.org/teens.html

This site describes signs of stress as well as strategies to cope with stress.

Sites and Bytes

How to Survive Unbearable Stress
www.teachhealth.com

This comprehensive website is written specifically for college students by Steven Burns, M.D. It features the following topics: signs of how to recognize stress, two stress surveys for adults and college students, information on the pathophysiology of stress, the genetics of stress and stress tolerance, and information on how to best manage and even treat stress.

InfoTrac College Edition

Activity

Lee, Richard M., et al. "Social Connectedness, Social Appraisal, and Perceived Stress in College Women and Men" *Journal of Counseling and Development,* Vol. 80, No. 3, Summer 2002, p. 355(7).

InfoTrac College Edition

1. What is the relationship between social connectedness and perceived stress levels in the population of college students studied?

2. What gender differences exist when measuring levels of social connectedness?

InfoTrac College Edition

3. Why does an indirect association between social connectedness and perceived stress seem to be more significant in college women than in college men?

For additional links, resources, and suggested readings on InfoTrac College Edition, visit our Health & Wellness Resource Center at **http://health.wadsworth.com**.

Key Terms

The terms listed are used on the page indicated. Definitions of the terms are in the Glossary at the end of this book.

Key Terms

adaptive response 76
allostasis 76
biofeedback 92
burnout 87
defense mechanisms 89
distress 76
eustress 76
**general adaptation
    syndrome (GAS) 76**

Key Terms

guided imagery 91
homeostasis 76
meditation 92
migraine headache 80
mindfulness 92
**posttraumatic stress
    disorder (PTSD) 93**

Key Terms

progressive relaxation 91
**psychoneuroimmunology
    78**
stress 76
stressors 76
visualization 91

References

1. Lazarus, R., and R. Launier. "Stress-Related Transactions Between Person and Environment" in *Perspectives in Interactional Psychology.* New York: Plenum, 1978.

2. Gadzella, Bernadette. "Student-Life Stress Inventory: Identification of and Reactions to Stressors." *Psychological Reports,* Vol. 74, No. 2, April 1994.

3. Senior, Kathryn. "Should Stress Carry a Health Warning?" *Lancet,* Vol. 357, No. 9250, January 13, 2001, p. 126.

4. Booth, Roger, et al. "The State of the Science: The Best Evidence for the Involvement of Thoughts and Feelings in Physical Health." *Advances in Mind-Body Medicine,* Vol. 17, No. 1, Winter 2001, p. 2.

5. "Stress Makes Fat Linger Longer," *Tufts University Health & Nutrition Letter,* Vol. 20, No. 8, October 2002, p. 1(1).

6. Epel, Elissa. "Can Stress Shape Your Body? Stress and Cortisol Reactivity Among Women with Central Body Fat Distribution." *Yale University, U.S. Dissertation Abstracts International: Section B: The Sciences & Engineering,* Vol. 60, No. 5-B, December 1999, p. 2403.

7. Ketterer, Mark. "Stressed Out Men May Have Inherited Risk for Early Heart Disease," Presentation, American Psychosomatic Society, March 2003.

8. "Psychological Stress May Affect Immune System," *Pain & Central Nervous System Week,* October 14, 2002, p. 6.

9. "Social Sickness," *Vibrant Life,* Vol. 19, No. 1, January–February 2003, p. 7.

10. Takkouche, Bahi, et al. "Stress and Susceptibility to the Common Cold." *Epdiemiology,* Vol. 11, April 2001, p. 345.

11. "Stressful Feelings May Influence Vaccine Effectiveness," *Health & Medicine Week,* December 23, 2002, p. 3.

12. Rubin, Aaron, and Karageanes, Steven. "Stress, Cytokine Changes, and Wound Healing." *Physician and Sportsmedicine,* Vol. 28, No. 5, May 2000, p. 21.

13. Turner-Cobb, Julie, et al. "Social Support and Salivary Cortisol in Women with Metastatic Breast Cancer." *Psychosomatic Medicine,* Vol. 62, No. 3, May–June 2000, p. 337.

14. Kiecolt-Glaser, Janice, and Ronald Glaser. "Stress and Immunity: Age Enhances the Risks." *Current Directions in Psychological Science,* Vol. 10, No. 1, February 2001, p. 18.

15. Senior, "Should Stress Carry a Health Warning?"

16. Engle, Shaena. "College Freshmen Spend Less Time Studying and More Time Surfing the Net, UCLA Survey Reveals," News Release. Higher Educational

Research Institute, UCLA, January 27, 2003.

17. Bartlett, Thomas. "Freshmen Pay, Mentally and Physically, As They Adjust to Life in College." *Chronicle of Higher Education,* February 1, 2002.

18. Jackson, Pamela Braboy, and Montenique Finney. "Negative Life Events and Psychological Distress Among Young Adults." *Social Psychology Quarterly 2002,* Vol. 65, No. 2, p. 186.

19. Hertel, James. "College Students Generational Status: Similarities, Differences, and Factors in College Adjustment." *The Psychological Record,* Vol. 52, No. 1, Winter 2002, p. 3.

20. Benton, Sherry, et al. "Changes in Counseling Center Client Problems Across 13 Years," *Professional Psychology: Research and Practice,* Vol. 34, No. 1, January 2003, p. 66.

21. Deckro, Gloria, et al. "The Evaluation of a Mind/Body Intervention to Reduce Psychological Distress and Perceived Stress in College Students." *Journal of American College Health,* Vol. 50, No. 6, May 2002, p. 281.

22. Hertel, "College Students Generational Status."

23. Iwasaki, Yoshi. "Roles of Leisure in Coping with Stress Among University Students: A Repeated Assessment Field

References

Study," *Anxiety, Stress, & Coping,* Vol. 16, No. 1, March 2003, p. 31.

24. Coffman, Donna and Tammy Gilligan. "Social Support, Stress, and Self-Efficacy: Effects on Students' Satisfaction," *Journal of College Student Retention,* Vol. 4, No. 1, 2002–2003, p. 53.

25. Deckro et al. "The Evaluation of a Mind/Body Intervention."

26. Harrell, Shelly. "A Multidimensional Conceptualization of Racism-Related Stress: Implications for the Well-Being of People of Color." *American Journal of Orthopsychiatry,* Vol. 70, No. 1, January 2000.

27. Launier, Raymond. "Stress Balance and Emotional Life Complexes in Students in a Historically African American College." *Journal of Psychology,* Vol. 131, No. 2, March 1997.

28. Rosenthal, Beth Spenciner, and Arleen Cedeno Schreiner. "Prevalence of Psychological Symptoms Among Undergraduate Students in an Ethnically Diverse Urban Public College." *Journal of American College Health,* Vol. 49, No. 1, July 2000.

29. Ibid.

30. Bowen-Reid, Terra, and Jules Harrell. "Racist Experiences and Health Outcomes: An Examination of Spirituality As a Buffer." *Journal of Black Psychology,* Vol. 28, No. 1, February 2002, p. 18.

31. AAA Foundation for Traffic Safety website. www.aaafts.org

32. Evans, Sybil. Personal interview.

33. Bushman, Brad. Personal interview.

34. Evans, Gary, and Dana Johnson. "Stress and Open-Office Noise." *Journal of Applied Psychology,* Vol. 85, No. 5, October 2000.

35. Bargellinia, Annalisa, et al. "Relation Between Immune Variables and Burnout in a Sample of Physicians." *Occupational and Environmental Medicine,* Vol. 57, July 2000.

36. Jacobsen, Ken. Personal interview.

37. Hall, Cathy, et al. "Motivational and Attitudinal Factors in College Students With and Without Learning Disabilities." *Learning Disability Quarterly,* Vol. 25, No. 1, Spring 2002, p. 79.

38. "Driving-Induced Stress in Urban College Students." *Perceptual and Motor Skills,* Vol. 90, No. 2, April 2000.

39. Murphy, R.T., et al. "Stress Symptoms Among African-American College Students After the September 11, 2001 Terrorist Attacks," *Journal of Nervous and Mental Disorders,* Vol. 191, No. 2, February 2003, p. 108.

40. "Temple University Survey Shows Stress Levels Highest Since 9/11," *Ascribe Higher Education News Service,* February 20, 2003.

41. Saunders, Teri, et al. "The Effect of Stress Inoculation Training on Anxiety and Performance." *Journal of Occupational Health Psychology,* Vol. 1, No. 2, pp. 170–186.

42. Abel, Millicent. "Interaction of Humor and Gender in Moderating Relationships Between Stress and Outcomes." *Journal of Psychology,* Vol. 132, No. 3, May 1998.

43. Bass, M. A., et al. "Comparison of Two Exercise Programs on General Well-Being of College Students," *Psychological Reports,* Vol. 3, No. 2, December 2002, p. 1195.

44. Barbar, Cary. "The Science of Meditation." *Psychology Today,* May–June 2001, p. 54.

45. "Three for 2003: Reducing the Burden of Stress," *Harvard Women's Health Watch,* Vol. 10, No. 5, January 2003, p. 1.

46. Turner, Heather and Melissa Butler. "Direct and Indirect Effects of Childhood Adversity on Depressive Symptoms in Young Adults," *Journal of Youth & Adolescence,* Vol. 32, No. 2, April 2003, p. 89.

47. Schnyder, Ulrich, et al. "Incidence and Prediction of Posttraumatic Stress Disorder Symptoms in Severely Injured Accident Victims." *American Journal of Psychiatry,* Vol. 158, No. 4, April 2001, p. 594.

48. McLean, L. M. and R. Gallop. "Implications of Childhood Sexual Abuse for Adult Borderline Personality Disorder and Complex Posttraumatic Stress Disorder," *American Journal of Psychiatry,* Vol. 160, No. 2, February 2003, p. 369.

49. Duncan, Renae. "Childhood Maltreatment and College Drop-out Rates: Implications for Child Abuse Researchers." *Journal of Interpersonal Violence,* Vol. 15, No. 9, September 2000, p. 987.

50. Lindstroem, Bengt. "The Meaning of Resilience." *International Journal of Adolescent Medicine & Health,* Vol. 13, No. 1, January–March 2001, p. 7.

51. McAdams, Dan, et al. "When Bad Things Turn Good and Good Things Turn Bad: Sequences of Redemption and Contamination in Life Narrative and Their Relation to Psychosocial Adaptation in Midlife Adults and in Students." *Personality & Social Psychology Bulletin,* Vol. 27, No. 4, April 2001, p. 474.

52. Tuchman, Bruce. "Procrastinators." Presentation, American Psychological Association, Chicago, August 22, 2002.

SECTION II

HEALTHY

LIFESTYLES

YOU have enormous influence over your health and vitality. This section provides information about the tools you have at hand to become healthier and feel more energetic throughout your lifetime. By learning how to eat a balanced and varied diet, how to manage your weight, and how to become physically fit, you can get started on a lifelong journey of becoming all you can be. As you take better care of your body today, you'll build the foundation for feeling your best for many tomorrows to come.

© ZEFA/Masterfile

101

The Joy of Fitness

As a boy, Derek never thought about doing anything special to stay physically fit. He loved sports so much that he spent every free moment on a softball field or basketball court. He could sprint faster, jump higher, and hit a ball harder than any of his friends. In high school Derek's life revolved around practices and games. He was a varsity athlete and a regional all-star.

Early in his first year in college, an injury sidelined Derek. Frustrated that he had to sit out the season, he gave up his rigorous training routine. As he became immersed in academics and other activities, Derek stopped going to the gym or working out on his own. Yet he continued to think of himself as an athlete in excellent physical condition. When Derek went home for spring break, he joined his younger brothers on a neighborhood basketball court. While he wasn't surprised that his long shots were off, Derek was

amazed by how quickly he got winded. In fifteen minutes, he was panting for breath. "Getting old," one of his brothers joked. "Getting soft," the other teased.

Often the college years represent a turning point in physical fitness. Like Derek, many students, busy with classes and other commitments, devote less time to physical activity. About four in ten undergraduates do not participate in moderate or vigorous physical activity on a regular basis.[1] Physical

activity drops off even more after graduation, particularly among those who did not exercise regularly in college.[2]

The choices you make and the habits you develop now can affect how long and how well you'll live. As you'll see in this chapter, exercise yields immediate rewards: It boosts energy, improves mood, soothes stress, improves sleep, and makes you look and feel better. In the long term, physical activity slows many of the changes associated with chronological aging, such as loss of calcium and bone density, lowers the risk of serious chronic illnesses, and extends the lifespan.

© Petar Correz/Stone/Getty Images

After studying the material in this chapter, you should be able to:

- **Describe** the components of physical fitness.
- **Discuss** the differences between sedentary and active lifestyles and develop strategies to become more active.
- **Describe** the health benefits of regular physical activity.

- **List** the different forms of cardiorespiratory activities and **describe** their potential health benefits and risks.
- **Explain** the benefits of a muscle training program and **describe** how to design a workout.
- **List** the potential health risks of strength-enhancing drugs and supplements.
- **Define** flexibility and describe the different types of stretching exercises.
- **Define** body mass index (BMI) and **describe** the different methods of estimating body composition.

103

:◖: What Is Physical Fitness?

The simplest, most practical definition of **physical fitness** is the ability to respond to routine physical demands while retaining enough reserve energy to cope with a sudden challenge. You can consider yourself fit if you meet your daily energy needs, can handle unexpected extra demands, have a realistic but positive self-image, and are protecting yourself against potential health problems, such as heart disease.

Fitness is important both for health and for athletic performance. The health-related components of physical fitness, which this chapter emphasizes, include aerobic or cardiorespiratory endurance, muscular strength and endurance, flexibility, and body composition (the ratio of fat and lean body tissue). Athletic performance depends on additional skills, such as agility, coordination, balance, and speed, which vary with specific sports. While many amateur and professional athletes are in superb overall condition, you do not need athletic skills to keep your body operating at maximum capacity throughout life.

Cardiorespiratory fitness refers to the ability of the body to sustain prolonged rhythmic activity. It is achieved through **aerobic exercise**—any activity, such as brisk walking or swimming, in which the amount of oxygen taken into the body is slightly more than, or equal to, the amount of oxygen used by the body. In other words, aerobic exercise involves working out strenuously without pushing to the point of breathlessness.

Muscular fitness has two components: strength and endurance. **Strength** refers to the force within muscles; it is measured by the absolute maximum weight that we can lift, push, or press in one effort. **Endurance** is the ability to perform repeated muscular effort; it is measured by counting how many times you lift, push, or press a given weight. Both are equally important. It's not enough to be able to hoist a shovelful of snow; you've got to be able to keep shoveling until the entire driveway is clear.

Flexibility is the range of motion around specific joints—for example, the stretching you do to touch your toes or twist your torso. Flexibility depends on many factors: your age, gender, and posture; bone spurs; and how fat or muscular you are. As children develop, their flexibility

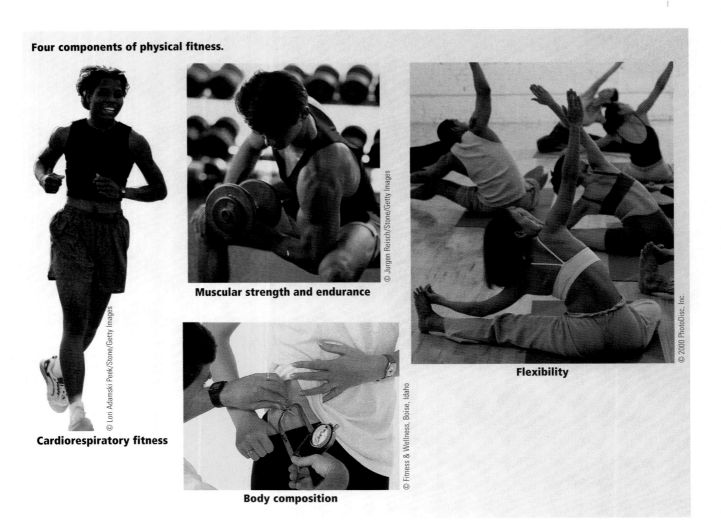

Four components of physical fitness.

Cardiorespiratory fitness
© Lori Adamski Peek/Stone/Getty Images

Muscular strength and endurance
© Jurgen Reisch/Stone/Getty Images

Body composition
© Fitness & Wellness, Boise, Idaho

Flexibility
© 2000 PhotoDisc, Inc.

increases until adolescence. Then a gradual loss of joint mobility begins and continues throughout adult life. Both muscles and connective tissue, such as tendons and ligaments, shorten and become tighter if not used at all or not used through their full range of motion.

Body composition refers to the relative amounts of fat and of lean tissue (bone, muscle, organs, water) in the body. A high proportion of body fat has serious health implications, including increased incidence of heart disease, high blood pressure, diabetes, stroke, gallbladder problems, back and joint problems, and some forms of cancer.

 College-age men average 15 percent body fat; college-age women, 23 percent. On average, women have 11 percent more body fat and 8 percent less muscle mass than men.[3] (See The X&Y Files: "Gender Differences and Physical Fitness.")

Physical **conditioning** (or training) refers to the gradual building up of the body to enhance cardiorespiratory or aerobic fitness, muscular strength and endurance, flexibility, and a healthy body composition.

◨ The Inactivity Epidemic

One in four Americans reports no physical activity at all, according to the CDC. About half exercise occasionally, but not at the levels recommended by the National Center for Chronic Disease Prevention and Health Promotion. Only one in four adults meets the levels of physical activity recommended by federal health officials.[4]

Many factors affect physical activity levels, including geographic location, gender, education, and income. According to the CDC, city-dwellers are more active than country folks: Westerners more active than those in other regions. Men, people with higher education levels, and high-income earners work out more often.[5]

 Ethnicity also correlates with activity levels: 40 percent of the Mexican Americans surveyed by the CDC did not engage in any physical activity in their leisure time, compared with 35 percent of blacks and 18 percent of whites. African-American and Hispanic men and women reported less activity than their white counterparts, even when their income and education were similar.[6]

How do Americans spend most of their leisure time? Watching television. According to a national survey, adult men spend about 29 hours a week watching television; women average 34 hours per week. The more time that individuals spend in front of the TV, the greater their risk of obesity. Compared with other sedentary activities, such as reading, writing, or driving, watching TV lowers metabolic rate so people burn fewer calories. TV viewers are likely to snack as they watch, so they also take in more calories.[7]

The Campus Couch Potato Crisis

 Although most are young and healthy, college students aren't necessarily more active than the general population. About four in ten undergraduates do not participate in moderate or vigorous physical activity on a regular basis. In a survey of 2,837 American students at a public university in the Midwest, 53 percent of the women and 40.3 percent of the men had not engaged in vigorous physical activity during the preceding month.[8]

Mexican-American students, both male and female, and African-American women reported the lowest rates of physical activity. The most physically active men were African American; the most active women, white.[9] (See Student Snapshot: "Campus Couch Potatoes.") Activity levels fall off dramatically during adolescence and young adulthood. By age 19 or 20, the activity level of more than 2,000 African-American girls in one study had dropped 83 percent.[10]

Patterns set in college influence lifelong activity levels. In a survey of 367 alumni who graduated two to ten years previously from a Southern university, more than half (54.8 percent) of those who had exercised regularly in college were even more physically active. The irregular exercisers were more likely to remain at the same or a lower level of activity. The non-exercisers tended to become even less active after graduation.[11]

◨ How Can I Motivate Myself to Get Moving?

Before you move a muscle, you need to be motivated. You may never even have thought about becoming more active. You may be thinking about getting into shape—someday. You may exercise, but not on a regular basis. Or you may have started working out in the last six months.

Each of these statements applies to a different stage of motivational readiness for change, discussed in depth in Chapter 1. In studies on increasing activity in adults, researchers have found that strategies tailored to an individual's stage of readiness for change are effective in boosting motivation and getting people moving.[12] You can evaluate your own level of readiness with the Self-Survey: "Are You Ready to Become More Active?" p. 108.

Both cognitive and behavioral strategies are effective in motivating change. Cognitive strategies, such as learning about the risks of remaining sedentary, typically work best in the preparation stage. Behavioral strategies, such as keeping athletic shoes in the car or in a locker at the gym, are most effective at the action stage.[13] (See "Your Health Change Plan for Physical Fitness," p. 108.)

the XY file *Gender Differences and Physical Fitness*

Men and women benefit equally from physical activity and exercise. Nevertheless, the components of physical fitness do have gender differences. Many are related to size. On average, men are 10 to 15 percent bigger than women, with roughly twice the percentage of muscle mass and half the percentage of body fat. Overall, men are about 30 percent stronger, particularly above the waist. They have more sweat glands and a greater maximum oxygen uptake. A man's bigger heart pumps more blood with each beat. His larger lungs take in 10 to 20 percent more oxygen. His longer legs cover more distance with each stride. If a man jogs along at 50 percent of his capacity, a woman has to push to 73 percent of hers to keep up.

Women have a higher percentage of body fat than men, and more is distributed around the hips and thighs; men carry more body fat around the waist and stomach. The average woman has a smaller heart, a lower percent-

age of slow twitch muscle fibers, and a smaller blood volume than a man. Because women have a lower concentration of red blood cells, their bodies are less effective at transporting oxygen to their working muscles during exercise.

Even though training produces the same relative increases for both genders, a woman's maximum oxygen intake remains about 25 to 30 percent lower than that of an equally well-conditioned man. In elite athletes, the gender difference is smaller: 8 to 12 percent. Because the angle of the upper leg bone (femur) to the pelvis is greater in a woman, her legs are less efficient at running.

In some endurance events, such as ultramarathon running and long-distance swimming, female anatomy and physiology may have some aerobic advantages. The longer a race—on land, water, or ice—the better women perform. In an analysis of world-record times in running, swimming, and speed skating, researchers at Northeastern University observed that in all three sports the superiority of men's performances diminished with increasing distance.

	Female	Male
Percent fat	27%	15%
Lean body mass	107.8 pounds	134.2 pounds
Blood volume	4.5–5 liters	5–6 liters
Maximum oxygen consumption	3–3.5 liters per minute	5.5–5.9 liters per minute

According to research on physical education classes, college students tend to possess one of two types of motivation toward sports and physical activity. "Ego-oriented" youths care about the extrinsic rewards of participation, such as socializing and meeting people. "Task-oriented" young people participate in sports or physical activities for intrinsic reasons, such as an enhanced sense of self-worth.[14]

Looking better and feeling better are two of the strongest motivators that pull college students to their feet. However, there are some gender differences. In a study of 258 college freshmen enrolled in a personal health course, the women were significantly more fit than the men and more health- and appearance-conscious. However, the men placed more value on fitness and expressed greater satisfaction with their appearance.[15] As in other studies, the students—male and female—with a greater sense of self-efficacy and an internal locus of con-

trol placed greater value on health and fitness, were more conscious about living a healthy lifestyle, and were more likely to be actively involved in activities that maintain or enhance fitness.[16]

According to an Ohio State University survey, the "buddy system" gets college men moving. If their friends exercise, they do too. This isn't true for college women, who rely more on family support and encouragement and have fewer friends who exercise.[17]

What keeps you from working out? When that question was posted on a national chat board, students listed a variety of excuses: "Gym membership is too expensive." "I'm not going to run in the snow!" "I don't have enough time." "I don't like the school gym—it stinks, people are trying too hard, and it takes too long to get a machine." "The workout room in my dorm is always crowded."

Student Snapshot — Campus Couch Potatoes

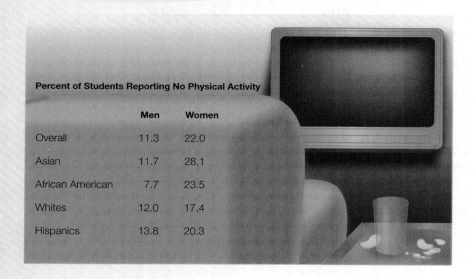

Percent of Students Reporting No Physical Activity

	Men	Women
Overall	11.3	22.0
Asian	11.7	28.1
African American	7.7	23.5
Whites	12.0	17.4
Hispanics	13.8	20.3

Source: Data from Richard Suminski. "Physical Activity Among Ethnically Diverse College Students," *Journal of American College Health*, Vol. 51, September 2002, p. 75.

Others revealed ways they had managed to overcome these barriers and motivate themselves, including:

:: **Sign up for a fitness class,** such as spinning or step-aerobics, so that exercise is built into your weekly schedule.

:: **Go to the gym with friends.** "Even if it's rainy and cold, I know they're waiting for me so I go," one woman explained.

:: **Find a fun workout.** "I love working out when it's something different—like water aerobics, ice skating, or swing dance," said one student.

:: **Use humor.** One student put this sign on the wall: "You think flu season is scary? Wait till bathing suit season hits!"

Find a group of friends who are as interested in physical fitness as you are to help keep your motivation high.

:: **Build activity into your day.** Many students walk to classes or always take the stairs rather than the elevator.

:: **Do double-duty.** Some students read class notes while on a Stairmaster or stationary bicycle. Others listen to audio-cassettes of required reading books as they work out.

 The course in which you're using this text may help you get motivated and moving. In a study that compared college alumni who had taken a health and physical education course with others who had not, those who'd taken the course were more likely to engage in aerobic exercise. Not coincidentally, they also were less likely to smoke and had lower intakes of dietary fat and cholesterol. In another study at a Colorado university, students enrolled in a fitness and wellness course were more likely to participate in regular physical activity when tired, in a bad mood, in bad weather, time-pressured, or unsure of their ability to perform an activity.[18]

Physical Activity and Health

If exercise could be packed into a pill, it would be the single most widely prescribed and beneficial medicine in the nation. Why? Because nothing can do more to help your

Self Survey **Are You Ready to Become More Active?**

Physical Activity Stages of Change Questionnaire

For each of the following questions, please circle Yes or No. Please be sure to read the questions carefully.
Physical activity or exercise includes activities such as walking briskly, jogging, bicycling, swimming, or any other activity in which the exertion is at least as intense as these activities.

1) I am currently physically active. **NO** **YES**
2) I intend to become more physically active in the next 6 months. **NO** **YES**

For activity to be regular, it must add up to a total of 30 minutes or more per day and be done at least 5 days per week. For example, you could take one 30-minute walk or take three 10-minute walks for a daily total of 30 minutes.

3) I currently engage in regular physical activity. **NO** **YES**
4) I have been regularly physically active for the past 6 months. **NO** **YES**

Scoring Algorithm:

Precontemplation:	Question One = No
	Question Two = No
Contemplation:	Question One = No
	Question Two = Yes
Preparation:	Question One = Yes and
	Question Three = No
Action:	Question One = Yes
	Question Three = Yes and
	Question Four = No
Maintenance:	Question One = Yes
	Question Three = Yes
	Question Four = Yes

Sources: Bess Marcus and Beth Lewis. "Physical Activity and the Stages of Motivational Readiness for Change Model," *President's Council on Physical Fitness and Sports Research Digest*, Series 4, No. 1, March 2003, p. 1. H. Marcus and L. J. Forsyth. *Motivating People to Be Physically Active*. Champaign, Il.: Human Kinetics, 2003. Reprinted, by permission, from B. H. Marcus & L. H. Forsyth, 2003, *Motivating People to be Physically Active*, (Champaign, IL: Human Kinetics), 21.

Your Health Change Plan

for Physical Fitness

Once you know your stage of motivational readiness, you can employ the cognitive and behavioral strategies most likely to work for you now. As you progress through the stages of change, you can shift to other approaches. Here are some suggestions:

Precontemplation (not active and not thinking about becoming active)

:: Use this course as an opportunity to learn about the benefits of physical activity, including better mood, lower stress, stronger bones, and a lower risk of cardio-vascular disease.

:: Set a small, reasonable goal that does not involve working up a sweat, such as looking up "exercise, benefits of" in the index of this book and reading the pages cited.

:: List what you see as the cons of physical activity. For example, do you fear it would take time you need for your studies? Think of small changes that don't require time, for instance, standing rather than sitting when talking on the phone, doing stretches while watching television, or taking a quick walk down the hall or up the stairs while waiting for a friend or a class to begin.

:: Identify barriers to physical activity, such as lack of money. Take advantage of your student status, and check out facilities, such as the swimming pool at the

body function at its best (Figure 4-1). With regular activity, your heart muscles become stronger and pump blood more efficiently. Your heart rate and resting pulse slow down. Your blood pressure may drop slightly from its normal level.

Regular physical activity thickens the bones and can slow the loss of calcium that normally occurs with age. Exercise increases flexibility in the joints and improves digestion and elimination. It speeds up metabolism, so the body burns up more calories and body fat decreases. It heightens sensitivity to insulin (a great benefit for diabetics) and may lower the risk of developing diabetes. In addition, exercise enhances clot-dissolving substances in the blood, helping to prevent strokes, heart attacks, and pulmonary

embolisms (clots in the lungs). Regular, vigorous exercise can actually extend the lifespan.[19]

The Toll of Inactivity

Sedentary living is as great a hazard to health as obesity.[20] Inactivity increases all causes of mortality, doubles the risk of cardiovascular diseases, diabetes, and obesity, and increases the risk of colon cancer, high blood pressure, osteoporosis, depression, and anxiety.[21] The combination of physical inactivity and being overweight is responsible for athletic center, or opportunities, such as an intramural soccer team, available to you free (or almost).

Contemplation (not active but thinking about becoming active)

:: Think back to activities you found enjoyable in the past. You might consider inline skating to class or around campus, or plan a hike for a weekend or school break.

:: Determine the types of activity you can realistically fit into your daily schedule. You might join friends for softball every Saturday, or sign up for an evening body-sculpting class.

:: Visualize success. Focus on the person you want to become: How would you look? What would you do differently? Find an image—from a magazine advertisement, for example—and post it where you can see it often.

:: Plan your rewards. Use a technique called shaping, which reinforces progress on the way to a goal. For instance, initially you might reward yourself once you engage in physical activity for 15 minutes a day. After a week, you get the reward only after 20 minutes a day. Over time you increase the number of days you are physically active as well as the number of minutes of activity per day.

:: Reach out for support. Find a friend, family member, or classmate who is willing or able to provide support for being active. Or join an organized martial arts class or an informal team.

Preparation (active but not at recommended levels)

:: Identify specific barriers that limit your activity. If your daily jogs are rained or snowed out, develop a list of indoor alternatives, such as walking stairs or working out to an exercise video.

:: Set specific daily and weekly goals. Your daily goal might begin with 10 or 15 minutes of activity. Your weekly goal might be to try a new activity, such as spinning or a dance class.

:: Divide physical activity over the course of the day with a 10 or 15 minute walk in the morning, another at lunch, and a third at the end of the day.

:: Document your progress. You could use a monthly calendar to keep track of the number of days you've exercised as well as the length of each workout. Or you can keep a more detailed record, noting the types of exercise you do every day, the intensity you work at, the duration of each workout, etc.

Action and Maintenance (active at recommended levels for less than six months)

:: Identify risk factors that might lead to relapse. If vacations or holiday breaks disrupt your routine, make a plan for alternative ways to remain active before you leave campus.

:: Stress proof your fitness program. In crunch times, you may feel you don't have time to spare for exercise. Multiple 10-minute walks during the day may be particularly useful both to keep up your fitness and to relieve stress buildup.

:: Avoid boredom. Think through ways to vary your exercise routine. Take different routes on your walks. Invite different friends to join you. Alternate working with free weights and resistance machines at the gym.

:: Set secondary goals. Once you've reached and maintained your goal for physical activity, set goals related to secondary benefits of exercise, for instance, losing weight or changing your body composition.

---

approximately 300,000 deaths a year. Only cigarette smoking claims more lives.[22]

"Sedentary death syndrome," or SeDS, refers to the lack of physical activity that is expected to lead to 2.5 million premature deaths in the next decade—a greater toll than alcohol, guns, motor vehicles, illicit drug use, and sexually transmitted diseases combined.[23] The economic impact of SeDS is equally staggering: an estimated $1 trillion in health-care bills a year.[24] As a risk factor for heart disease, physical inactivity ranks as high as elevated cholesterol, high blood pressure, or cigarette smoking.[25]

The inactivity epidemic doesn't stop at the border. According to the College of Family Physicians of Canada, an estimated 21,000 Canadians die prematurely every year because of medical problems related to physical inactivity.[26]

Two-thirds of Canadian children and young people are not active enough for optimal growth and development.[27]

The Benefits of Physical Activity

At your next medical checkup, don't be surprised if your doctor "prescribes" something with more potential benefits than any medication: exercise. Increasingly physicians in the United States, Canada, and other countries are writing prescriptions for specific physical activities to motivate patients, particularly sedentary ones, to become more

Improves your mood
and reduces psychological symptoms

Increases your respiratory capacity

Reduces your risk
of heart disease

Improves your digestion and
your fat metabolism

Lowers your body fat and
reduces your weight

Strengthens your bones and
increases joint flexibility

Increases your muscle
strength and tone

Improves your circulation

Figure 4-1 THE BENEFITS OF EXERCISE
Regular physical activity enhances your overall health and helps prevent disease.

active.[28] According to followup studies, brief counseling on exercise by a doctor, coupled with ongoing telephone support, can boost activity levels for at least a year.[29]

What can exercise do for you? Here are some of the proven benefits:

Longer Life

Capacity for exercise has proven a better predictor of whether a man would die in the next few years than other risk factors, such as high blood pressure, high total cholesterol, or smoking.[30] Formerly sedentary people, even the elderly, who begin to exercise live longer, on average, than those who remain inactive.[31]

Protection Against Heart Disease and Certain Cancers

Sedentary people are about twice as likely to die of a heart attack as people who are physically active. (See Chapter 14 for a discussion of heart disease.) As demonstrated in a 20-year study of almost 4,000 men, regular physical activity also makes blood less likely to clot and cause a stroke or heart attack.[32] Exercise itself, even without weight loss, may reduce the risk of developing the pre-diabetic condition called insulin resistance syndrome, which, if untreated, can develop into type 2 diabetes and increase the risk of heart disease.[33]

In addition to its effects on the heart, exercise makes the lungs more efficient. They take in more oxygen, and their vital capacity (ability to take in and expel air) is increased, providing more energy for you to use.

In a study that followed more than 5,000 men and women for more than 20 years, fitness was a strong predictor of cancer death rates for men, but not for women. The fittest men had the lowest cancer death rates. But for women, body weight, as measured by body mass index (BMI), discussed later in this chapter, proved more significant. Cancer deaths were much higher in obese women, that is, those with the highest BMIs.[34]

Recent studies have shown that exercise reduces the risk of colon and rectal cancers, possibly by enhancing digestion and elimination. Fitter men are less likely to die of prostate and colon cancer than others.[35] In a recent study, strenuous exercise proved "moderate" protection against breast cancer, particularly for women who were consistently active throughout their lifetime.[36]

Better Bones

Weak and brittle bones are common among people who don't exercise. **Osteoporosis,** a condition in which bones lose their mineral density and become susceptible to injury, affects a great many older people. Women, in particular, are more vulnerable because their bones are less dense to begin with.

Although scientists had speculated that years of running might break down rather than build up bone density, a recent five-year study found no significant loss of bone density in women master runners after years on the move.[37] Yet not all activities that benefit the heart also help the bones. According to researchers at Johns Hopkins University, neither light-intensity activities, like gardening, nor mild aerobic activities build bone mineral density.[38] What does strengthen bones? Resistance training, such as regular weight lifting.[39]

Enhanced Immunity

Moderate exercise correlates with a reduced number of sick days. Researchers speculate that exercise may enhance immune function by reducing stress hormones like cortisol that can dampen resistance to disease.

In recent studies, women who walked briskly for 35 to 45 minutes five days a week experienced half the number of sick days with cold symptoms as inactive women. While moderate exercise seems to bolster a person's immune system, heavy training may increase the risk of upper respiratory tract infections for endurance athletes.[40]

Brighter Mood

Exercise makes people feel good from the inside out. Exercise boosts mood, increases energy, reduces anxiety, improves concentration and alertness, and enables people to handle stress better. During long workouts, some people experience what is called "runner's high," which may be the result of increased levels of mood-elevating brain chemicals called **endorphins.**

Better Mental Health

Exercise is an effective—but underused—treatment for mild to moderate depression and may help in treating other mental disorders. Regular, moderate exercise, such as walking, running, or lifting weights, three times a week, has proven helpful for depression and anxiety disorders, including panic attacks. In a study of people with major depression, exercise proved as effective as medication in improving mood and also helped prevent relapse.[41]

Lower Weight

Aerobic exercise burns off calories during your workout, because as your body responds to the increased demand from your muscles for nutrients, your metabolic rate rises. Moreover, this surge persists for as long as 12 hours after exercise, so you continue to use up more calories than usual even after you've stopped sweating. Resistance training builds muscle tissue, which burns up more calories throughout the day.

For individuals on a diet, exercise provides extra benefits: A combination of dietary change and moderate to high level intensity of exercise leads to greater weight loss than either alone.[42] Dieters who work out lose more fat than lean muscle tissue, which improves their body com-position. In one study, college age men who started exercising lost abdominal fat, which poses the greatest risk to health.[43] (See Chapter 6 for information on exercise and weight control.)

A More Active Old Age

Exercise slows the changes that are associated with advancing age: loss of lean muscle tissue, increase in body fat, and decrease in work capacity. In addition to lowering the risk of heart disease and stroke, exercise also helps older men and women retain the strength and mobility needed to live independently. Even in old age, exercise boosts strength and stamina, lessens time in wheelchairs, and improves outlook and sense of control.[44]

 ## Benefits for Students

Unlike middle-aged and older individuals, traditional-age college students cite improved fitness as the number-one advantage that exercise offers, followed by improved appearance and muscle tone. But undergraduates who recognize any benefits from exercise are more likely to be physically active than those who focus on barriers to working out.[45] (See Table 4-1.)

TABLE 4-1	Why College Students Exercise—or Don't

 In a sample of 147 graduates, the regular exercisers—92 percent of the men and 63.8 percent of the women—perceived more benefits than those who didn't exercise.

Top Exercise Benefits

1. Exercise increases my level of physical fitness.

2. Exercise improves the way my body looks.

3. My muscle tone is improved with exercise.

4. Exercise gives me a sense of personal accomplishment.

5. Exercise increases my muscle strength.

Top Exercise Barriers

1. Exercise tires me.

2. Exercise is hard work for me.

3. I am fatigued by exercise.

4. Exercising takes too much of my time.

5. My family members do not encourage me to exercise.

Source: Laurie Grubbs and Jason Carter. "The Relationship of Perceived Benefits and Barriers to Reported Exercise Behaviors in College Undergraduates." *Family and Community Health*, Vol. 25, No. 2, July 2002, p. 76.

Will exercise improve your grades? Not necessarily. A study at two Texas universities found that the fittest students didn't necessarily have higher GPAs. However, increasing their level of physical fitness did have a positive impact on the GPAs of the female students.[46]

✖ The Principles of Exercise

Why does exercise work? As you begin working toward fitness, keep these principles of exercise in mind: overload, FITT, reversibility, and specificity.

Overload Principle

The **overload principle** requires a person exercising to provide a greater stress or demand on the body than it's usually accustomed to handling. For any muscle, including the heart, to get stronger, it must work against a greater-than-normal resistance or challenge. To continue to improve, you need further increases in the demands—but not too much too quickly. **Progressive overloading**—gradually increasing physical challenges—provides the benefits of exercise without the risk of injuries.

The FITT Principle

Although slow and gentle activity can enhance basic health, you need to work harder—that is, at a greater intensity—to improve fitness. Whatever exercise you do, there is a level, or threshold, at which fitness begins to improve; a target zone, where you can achieve maximum benefits; and an upper level, at which potential risks outweigh any further benefits. The acronym **FITT** sums up the four dimensions of progressive overload: *frequency* (how often you exercise) *intensity* (how hard), *time* (how long), and *type* (specific activity). (See Table 4-2.)

Frequency

To attain and maintain physical fitness, you need to exercise regularly, but the recommended frequency varies with different types of exercise and with an individual's fitness goals. The minimum frequency recommended by federal health officials is three to five days of cardiovascular or aerobic exercise a week and two to three days of resistance and flexibility training a week.

Intensity

Exercise intensity varies with the type of exercise and with personal goals. To improve cardiovascular fitness, you need to increase your heart rate to a target zone (the level that produces benefits). To develop muscular strength and endurance, you need to increase the amount of weight you lift or the resistance you work against and/or the number of repetitions. For enhanced flexibility, you need to stretch muscles beyond their normal length.

Time (Duration)

The amount of time, or duration, of your workouts is also important, particularly for cardiovascular exercise. In general, experts have found similar health benefits from a single 30-minute session of moderate exercise as from several shorter sessions throughout the day. Duration and intensity are interlinked. If you're exercising at high intensity (biking or running at a brisk pace, for instance), you don't need to exercise as long as when you're working at lower intensity (walking or swimming at a moderate pace). For muscular strength and endurance and for flexibility, duration is defined by the number of sets or repetitions rather than total time.

Type (Specificity)

The **specificity principle** refers to the body's adaptation to a particular type of activity or amount of stress placed upon it. Jogging, for instance, trains the heart and lungs to

TABLE 4-2	Guidelines for Physical Fitness: The FITT Principle		
	Cardiorespiratory	**Strength**	**Flexibility**
	© 2001 PhotoDisc	© David Hanover	© David Hanover
Frequency: Most days of the week. Start with three days and gradually increase frequency.	A minimum of 3 to 5 days per week	2 to 3 days per week	A minimum of 2 to 3 days per week
Intensity: Start at low to moderate intensity and gradually increase to more vigorous efforts over several weeks	60 to 85% of maximum heart rate	Enough to enhance muscle strength and improve body composition	Enough to develop and maintain a full range of motion
Time: 30 to 60 minutes, using a gradual progression	20 to 60 minutes	8 to 12 repetitions of 8 to 10 different exercises (minimum)	4 repetitions of 10 to 30 seconds per muscle group (minimum)
Type of activity: Start with low-impact activities (walking, cycling, low-impact aerobics, water exercise); resistance or weight training; flexibility exercises	Aerobic activity that uses large-muscle groups and can be maintained continuously	Resistance activity that is performed at a controlled speed and through a full range of motion	Stretching activity that uses the major muscle groups

Source: Adapted from American College of Sports Medicine, "Position Stand: The Recommended Quantity and Quality of Exercise for Developing and Maintaining Cardiorespiratory and Muscular Fitness, and Flexibility in Healthy Adults." *Medicine and Science in Sports and Exercise,* Vol. 30, 1998, pp. 975–991; and from Kyle McInnis et al., "Counseling for Physical Activity in Overweight and Obese Patients." *American Family Physician,* Vol. 67, No. 6, March 15, 2003, p. 1254.

work more efficiently and strengthens certain leg muscles. However, it does not build upper body strength or enhance flexibility.

Reversibility Principle

The **principle of reversibility** is the opposite of the overload principle. Just as the body adapts to greater physical demands, it also adjusts to lower levels. If you stop exercising, you can lose as much as 50 percent of your fitness improvements within two months. If you have to curtail your usual exercise routine because of a busy schedule, you can best maintain your fitness by keeping the intensity constant and reducing frequency or duration. The principle of reversibility is aptly summed up by the phrase, "Use it or lose it."

How Much Exercise is Enough?

If you're not exercising at all, some activity is better than none. Simply turning off the television and doing housework or taking a walk can lower your risk of obesity, type 2 diabetes, and other health problems.[47] If sedentary men and women were to burn up just 150 calories a day by walking, gardening, vacuuming, or dancing, they would lower their relative heart attack risk more than veteran exercisers who increase the duration or intensity of their routine. If you've been inactive, start small and gradually increase how long, how hard, or how often you exercise. By varying your activities and breaking them into 15 or 20 minute periods, you may find that it's easier than you expected to spend an hour in motion.[48]

While some activity is good, more is better. Over the years exercise guidelines have changed. In the past, health officials recommended a minimum of twenty minutes of vigorous activity three times a week. More recently, the American College of Sports Medicine, the United States Surgeon General, and Health Canada's Physical Activity Guide to Healthy Active Living has recommended a minimum of 30 to 60 minutes of moderate activity (such as walking at a speed of three to four miles per hour) most days of the week to reduce the risk of cardiovascular disease.[49] In its most recent Dietary Guidelines, the National Academy of Sciences suggests 60 minutes of moderate exercise every day in order to maintain a healthy weight and gain additional health benefits.[50]

As a recent 10-year study confirmed, light to moderate exercise, such as thirty minutes of brisk walking five days a week, may lead to other health benefits but does not prolong life or protect against fatal heart problems. Only vigorous exercise reduced the risk of dying of heart disease and of premature death from other causes.[51]

Cardiorespiratory or Aerobic Fitness

Since physical activity requires more energy, the heart, lungs, and blood vessels have to work harder to deliver more oxygen to the cells. A person with good cardiorespiratory endurance can engage in a physical activity for a long time without becoming fatigued. The heart of a person who isn't in good condition has to pump more often; as a result, it becomes fatigued more easily.

Unlike muscular endurance, which is specific to individual muscles, cardiorespiratory endurance involves the entire body. The exercises that improve cardiorespiratory endurance are referred to as aerobic because the body uses as much, or slightly more, oxygen than it takes in. Aerobic exercise can take many forms, as noted later in this chapter, but all involve working strenuously without pushing to the point of breathlessness.

In **anaerobic exercise,** the amount of oxygen taken in by the body cannot meet the demands of the activity. This quickly creates an oxygen deficit that must be made up later. Anaerobic activities are high in intensity but short in duration, usually lasting only about ten seconds to two minutes. An example is sprinting the quarter-mile, which leaves even the best-trained athletes gasping for air.

In nonaerobic exercise, such as bowling, softball, or doubles tennis, there is frequent rest between activities. Because the body can take in all the oxygen it needs, the heart and lungs really don't get much of a workout.

How Can I Tell If I'm Working Hard Enough?

To be sure you're working hard enough to condition your heart and lungs, but not overdoing it, use your pulse, or heart rate, as a guide. One of the easiest places to feel your pulse is in the carotid artery in your neck. Slightly tilt your head back and to one side. Use your middle finger or forefinger, or both, to feel for your pulse. (Do not use your thumb; it has a beat of its own.) To determine your heart rate, count the number of pulses you feel for 10 seconds and multiply that number by six, or count for 30 seconds and multiply that number by two. Learn to recognize the pulsing of your heart when you're sitting or lying down. This is your **resting heart rate.**

Start taking your pulse during, or immediately after, exercise, when it's much more pronounced than when you're at rest. Three minutes after heavy exercise, take your pulse again. The closer that reading is to your resting heart rate, the better your condition. If it takes a long time for your pulse to recover and return to its resting level, your body's ability to handle physical stress is poor. As you continue working out, however, your pulse will return to normal much more quickly.

You don't want to push yourself to your maximum heart rate, yet you must exercise at about 60 to 85 percent of that maximum to get cardiovascular benefits from your training. This range is called your **target heart rate.** If you don't exercise intensely enough to raise your heart rate at least this high, your heart and lungs won't benefit from the workout. If you push too hard, and exercise at or near your absolute maximum heart rate, you run the risk of placing too great a burden on your heart. Figure 4-2 shows the target heart rate for various ages and activities. Find your age at the bottom of the figure and move up the grid to find your target heart rate for "aerobic workout."

You can also use the following steps to determine your maximum heart rate and target heart rate (in beats per minute):

1. Estimate your maximum heart rate by subtracting your age from 220. So if you are 20, your maximum heart rate is $220 - 20 = 200$ beats per minute.

Figure 4-2 TARGET HEART RATES FOR AGES AND VARIOUS ACTIVITIES
Your maximum heart rate is 220 minus your age.

2. Determine your lower-limit target heart rate by multiplying your maximum heart rate by .6. So if you are 20, your lower-limit target heart rate is 200 × .6 = 120 beats per minute.

3. Determine your upper-limit target heart rate by multiplying your maximum heart rate by .85. If you are 20, your upper-limit target heart range is 200 × .85 = 170.

Your target heart rate range is between your lower and upper limits.

According to the American College of Sports Medicine, for most people exercising at the lower end of the target heart rate range for a long time is more beneficial than exercising at the higher end of the range for a short time.[52] If your goal is losing weight, exercise at 60 to 70 percent of your maximum heart rate in order to burn fat calories. To improve aerobic endurance and strengthen your heart, work at 70 to 80 percent of your maximum heart rate. Competitive athletes may train at 80 to 100 percent of their maximum heart rate.[53] (See Figure 4-2.)

Although many fitness experts still believe that maximum target heart rate, also known as the Karvonen formula, is the best measurement of exercise intensity, others have doubts because many factors, such as caffeine, stress, and lack of sleep, can affect heart rate. According to

research at the University of Colorado, Boulder, the Karvonen formula overestimates maximum heart rate in young adults and underestimates it in older adults. One alternative formula, developed by Hirofumi Tanaka, is:

208 minus 70% of age.

However, Tanaka notes that actual maximum heart rate may vary by as many as 10 beats per minute.[54]

Another option is **Rating of Perceived Exertion (RPE),** a self-assessment scale that rates symptoms of breathlessness and fatigue. The original scale used ratings of 6 to 20. The American College of Sports Medicine revised it to a range of 0 to 10. (See Figure 4-3.) Most exercisers should aim for a perceived exertion of "somewhat hard," the equivalent of about 13 on the original RPE and 4 on the modified scale.

RPE is considered fairly reliable, but about 10 percent of people tend to over- or underestimate their exertion. Your health or physical education instructor can help you learn to match what your body is feeling to the RPE scale. By paying attention to how you feel at different exercise intensities, you can learn how to challenge yourself without risking your safety.

A simple way to gauge how hard you are working during aerobic activity is the "talk test." If you are gasping for air and unable to talk, you have pushed past the aerobic to the anaerobic zone. If you can belt out the national anthem, you're probably not working hard enough. If you can sing "Row, Row, Row Your Boat" but have to take a breath after each word "row," you're probably just where you should be—in the "hard" zone.

Designing an Aerobic Workout

Whatever activity you choose, your aerobic workout should consist of several stages, including a warm-up and a cool-down.

Warm-Up

Just as you don't get in your car and immediately gun your engine to 60 miles per hour, you shouldn't do the same with your body. You need to prepare your cardiorespiratory system for a workout, speed up the blood flow to your lungs, and increase the temperature and elasticity of your muscles and connective tissue to avoid injury.

Start by walking briskly for about 5 minutes. This helps your body make the transition from inactivity to exertion. Follow this general warm-up with about 5 minutes of simple stretches of the muscles you'll be exercising most. Before a jog, for instance, you can stretch the muscles

Original scale

6	No exertion at all
7	Extremely light
8	—
9	Very light
10	—
11	Light
12	—
13	Somewhat hard
14	—
15	Hard
16	—
17	Very hard
18	—
19	Extremely hard
20	Maximal exertion

Modified scale

0	Nothing at all
0.5	Extremely weak (just noticeable)
1	Very weak
2	Weak (light)
3	Moderate
4	—
5	Strong (heavy)
6	—
7	Very strong
8	—
9	—
10	Extremely strong (almost maximum)

Figure 4-3 BORG SCALE FOR RATING OF PERCEIVED EXERTION (RPE)
You can learn to rate your exertion based on this scale.

Source: G. Borg. "Phychophysical Bases of Perceived Exertion." *Medicine and Science in Sports and Exercise,* Vol. 14, No. 5, 2003, pp. 377–381.

in your ankle and the back of your leg by leaning against a wall, with one leg bent and tilted forward and the other straight. Lean forward until you feel the stretch and hold.

Aerobic Activity

The two key components of this part of your workout are intensity and duration. As described in the previous section, you can use your target heart rate range to make sure you are working at the proper intensity. The current recommendation is to keep moving for at least 60 minutes, either in one session or several briefer sessions, each lasting at least 10 minutes.

Cool-Down

After you've pushed your heart rate up to its target level and kept it there for a while, the worst thing you can do is slam on the brakes. If you come to a sudden stop, you put your heart at risk. When you stand or sit immediately after vigorous exercise, blood can pool in your legs. You need to keep moving at a slower pace to ensure an adequate supply

of blood to your heart. Ideally, you should walk for 5 to 10 minutes at a comfortable pace before you end your workout session.

Your Long-Term Plan

One of the most common mistakes people make is to push too hard too fast. Often they end up injured or discouraged and quit entirely. If you are just starting an aerobic program, think of it as a series of phases: beginning, progression, and maintenance:

:: *Beginning (4–6 weeks).* Start slow and low (in intensity). If you're walking, monitor your heart rate and aim for 55 percent of your maximum heart rate. Another good rule of thumb to make sure you're moving at the right pace: If you can sing as you walk, you're going too slow; if you can't talk, you're going too fast.

:: *Progression (16–20 weeks).* Gradually increase the duration and/or intensity of your workouts. For instance, you might add 5 minutes every two weeks to your walking time. You also can gradually pick up your pace, using your target heart rate as your guide. Keep a log of your workouts so you can chart your progress until you reach your goal.

:: *Maintenance (lifelong).* Once you've reached the stage of exercising for an hour every day, you may want to develop a repertoire of aerobic activities you enjoy. Combine or alternate activities to avoid monotony and keep up your enthusiasm. This is called **cross-training.**

Aerobic Interval Training

In aerobic activities, intensity training often is referred to as "interval" training, which intersperses small, manageable bouts of all-out effort with periods of low to moderate exertion. When the body works at its maximum, it quickly moves beyond aerobic to anaerobic and taps glycogen stored in the muscles for fuel. The combustion of this fuel leads to a buildup of lactate in the muscles and fatigue. The body slows down to a lower level of exertion and decreases intensity back into an aerobic training mode. Interval training helps improve overall fitness levels and also burns more calories than exercising at a steady rate.

Aerobic Options

Walking

More men and women are taking to their feet. Some are casualties of high-intensity sports and can no longer withstand the wear and tear of rigorous workouts. Others want to shape up, slim down, or ward off heart disease and other health problems. The good news for all is that walking is good exercise. Walking at least 30 minutes a day at a moderate pace is effective in reducing the risk of heart disease, according to the Women's Health Initiative Observational study of more than 70,000 postmenopausal women.[55]

Recent research has demonstrated the health benefits of walking for both men and women and for both healthy individuals and those with heart disease. One major study of women, the Nurses' Health Study, found that women who walk briskly three hours a week are as well protected from heart disease as women who spend an hour and a half a week in more vigorous activities, such as aerobics or running. Women engaged in either form of exercise had a rate of heart attacks 30 to 40 percent lower than that of sedentary women. The Women's Health Study, a randomized, controlled trial of aspirin and heart disease, found that even walking one hour per week can lower heart disease risk among relatively sedentary women.[56] Walking also protects men's hearts, whether they're healthy or have had heart problems. In a recent British study of 772 men, those who regularly engaged in light exercise, including walking,

had a risk of death that was 58 percent lower than that of their sedentary counterparts.[57]

Walking is good for the brain as well as the body. In a study that followed almost 6,000 women age 65 or older for up to eight years, those who walked regularly were less likely to experience memory loss and other age-related declines in mental function.[58] Another bonus is stress reduction. Since you can do it during a break or at lunchtime, walking builds relaxation into your day.

Treadmills are a good alternative to outdoor walks—and not just in bad weather. They keep you moving at a certain pace, they're easier on the knees, and they allow you to exercise in a climate-controlled, pollution-free environment—a definite plus for many city dwellers. Holding onto the handrails while walking on a treadmill reduces both heart rate and oxygen consumption, so you burn fewer calories. Experts advise slowing the pace if necessary so you can let go of the handrails while working out.[59]

Here are some guidelines for putting your best foot forward:

:: Walk very slowly for 5 minutes, and then do some simple stretches.

:: Maintain good posture. Focus your eyes ahead of you, stand erect, and pull in your stomach.

:: Use the heel-to-toe method of walking. The heel of your leading foot should touch the ground before the ball or toes of that foot do. When you push off with your trailing foot, bend your knee as you raise your heel. You should be able to feel the action in your calf muscles.

:: Pump your arms back and forth to burn 5 to 10 percent more calories and get an upper-body workout as well.

:: End your walk the way you started it—let your pace become more leisurely for the last 5 minutes.

America on the Move, a new campaign to shape up Americans, encourages people to take 2,000 extra steps a day as a way to avoid excess pounds. Walking 2,000 steps burns about 100 calories, or two pounds over a year. The CDC recommends a total of 10,000 steps a day—which should satisfy the goal of 30 minutes of moderate activity.[60]

Jogging and Running

The difference between jogging and running is speed. You should be able to carry on a conversation with someone on a long jog or run; if you're too breathless to talk, you're pushing too hard.

If your goal is to enhance aerobic fitness, long, slow, distance running is best. If you want to improve your speed, try *interval training*—repeated hard runs over a certain distance, with intervals of relaxed jogging in between. Depending on what suits you and what your training goals are, you can vary the distance, duration, and number of fast runs, as well as the time and activity between them.

If you have been sedentary, it's best to launch a walking program before attempting to jog or run. Start by walking for 15 to 20 minutes three times a week at a comfortable pace. Continue at this same level until you no longer feel sore or unduly fatigued the day after exercising. Then increase your walking time to 20 to 25 minutes, speeding up your pace as well.

When you can handle a brisk 25-minute walk, alternate fast walking with slow jogging. Begin each session walking, and gradually increase the amount of time you spend jogging. If you feel breathless while jogging, slow down and walk. Continue to alternate in this manner until you can jog for 10 minutes without stopping. If you gradually increase your jogging time by 1 or 2 minutes with each workout, you'll slowly build up to 20 or 25 minutes per session. For optimal fitness, you should jog at least three times a week.

Here's how to be sure you're running right:

:: Always take time to warm up and to stretch. Warm up with jumping jacks or running in place for 3 to 5 minutes. Spend at least one-fourth of the time that you plan to run on stretching exercises.

:: As you run, keep your back straight and your head up. Run tall, with your buttocks tucked in. Look straight ahead. Hold your arms slightly away from your body. Your elbows should be bent slightly so that your forearms are almost parallel to the ground. Move your arms rhythmically to propel yourself along.

:: Have your heels hit the ground first. Land on your heel, rock forward, and push off the ball of your foot. If this is difficult, try a more flat-footed style.

:: Avoid running on the balls of your feet; this produces soreness in the calves because the muscles must contract for a longer time. To avoid shin splints (a dull ache in the lower shins), stretch regularly to strengthen the shin muscles and to develop greater flexibility in your ankles.

:: Avoid running on hard surfaces and making sudden stops or turns.

Other Aerobic Activities

Because variety is the spice of an active life, many people prefer different forms of aerobic exercise. All can provide many health benefits. Among the popular options:

:: *Swimming.* For aerobic conditioning, you have to swim laps using the freestyle, butterfly, breaststroke, or backstroke. (The sidestroke is too easy.) You must also be a good enough swimmer to keep churning through the water for at least 20 minutes. Your heart will beat more slowly in water than on land, so your heart rate while swimming is not an accurate guide to exercise intensity. You should try to keep up a steady pace that's fast enough to make you feel pleasantly tired, but not completely exhausted, by the time you get out of the pool.

:: *Cycling.* Bicycling, indoors and out, can be an excellent cardiovascular conditioner, as well as an effective way to control weight—provided you aren't just along for the ride. If you coast down too many hills, you'll have to ride longer up hills or on level ground to get a good workout. Half of all bikes now sold in the United States are mountain bikes, sturdy cycles with knobby tires that allow bikers to climb up and zoom down dirt trails and explore places traditional racing bikes couldn't go. An 18-speed bike can make pedaling too easy, however, unless you choose gears carefully. To gain aerobic benefits, mountain bikers have to work hard enough to raise their heart rates to their target zone and keep up that intensity for at least 20 minutes.

:: *Spinning.*™ Spinning is a cardiovascular workout for the whole body that utilizes a special stationary bicycle. Led by an instructor, a group of bikers listens to music, and modifies their individual bike's resistance and their own pace according to the rhythm. An average spinning class lasts 45 minutes and has between 20 and 40 participants.

Unlike an ordinary stationary bike, a spinning bike has a larger saddle area and a heavier flywheel to create greater resistance; the rider, rather than a built-in computer, monitors performance. Introduced in 1987, this indoor cycling program has grown in appeal because it is time efficient and nonimpact, and because people of all ages, skills, and fitness levels can participate in the same class.

Spinning has become a popular option for aerobic exercise because people of different ages, skills, and fitness levels can participate in the same class.

©Jim Cummins/Taxi/Getty Images

:: *Skipping rope.* Essentially a form of stationary jogging with some extra arm action thrown in, skipping rope is excellent as both a heart conditioner and a way of losing weight. Always warm up before starting and cool down afterward. To alleviate boredom, try skipping to music and vary the steps: both feet together, alternating left and right feet, or jumping up and down on one leg.

:: *Aerobic dancing.* This activity combines music with kicking, bending, and jumping. A typical class (you can also dance at home to a video or TV program) consists of stretching exercises and sit-ups, followed by aerobic dances and cool-down exercises. A particular benefit of aerobic dance is that people get enjoyment and stimulation from the music; they're also able to move their bodies without worrying about skill and technique. "Soft," or low-impact, aerobic dancing doesn't put as much strain on the joints as "hard," or high-impact, routines.

:: *Step training or bench aerobics.* "Stepping" combines step, or bench, climbing with music and choreographed movements. Basic equipment consists of a bench 4 to 12 inches high. The fitter you are, the higher the bench—but the higher the bench, the greater the risk of knee injury. Injuries have skyrocketed in recent years as movements and choreography have become more complex and the pace of the music has picked up.

Tugging on supersized rubber stretch cords, which has the same effect as weight training, can increase the benefits of a step workout. In a controlled study, exercisers who added resistance exercises with stretch cords to their step routines showed improvements in aerobic capacity as well as muscle strength and size. A 40-minute step workout is equivalent to running seven miles an hour in terms of oxygen uptake and calories burned.

:: *Stair-climbing.* An estimated 4 million Americans are stepping up to fitness, according to the American Sports Data Institute. You could run up the stairs in an office building or dormitory, but most people use stair-climbing machines available in home models and at gyms and health clubs. On most versions of these machines, exercisers push a pair of pedals up and down, which is much easier on the feet and legs than many other activities.

:: *Inline skating.* Inline skating can increase aerobic endurance and muscular strength, and is less stressful on joints and bones than running or high-impact aerobics. Skaters can adjust the intensity of their workout by varying the terrain. (Obviously, they'll have to work harder while going up hills, and less so on the slide down.) They can also buy special training wheels and weights to increase resistance and make muscles work harder. One caution: Protective gear, including a helmet, knee and elbow pads, and wrist guards, is essential.

:: *Tennis.* As with other sports, tennis can be an aerobic activity—depending on the number of players and their skill level. In general, a singles match requires more continuous exertion than playing doubles. Intermediate to advanced players, who engage in prolonged volleys, experience a more challenging workout than beginners, who spend less time in motion.

⬛ Muscular Strength and Endurance

Although aerobic workouts condition your insides (heart, blood vessels, and lungs), they don't exercise many of the muscles that shape your outsides and provide power when you need it. Strength workouts are important because they enable muscles to work more efficiently and reliably. Conditioned muscles function more smoothly, and contract somewhat more vigorously and with less effort. With exercise, muscle tissue becomes firmer and can withstand much more strain—the result of toughening the sheath protecting the muscle and developing more connective tissue within it (see Figure 4-4).

Muscular strength and endurance are critical for handling everyday burdens, such as cramming a 20-pound suitcase into an overhead luggage bin or hauling a trunk down from the attic. Prolonged exercise prepares the muscles for sustained work by improving the circulation of blood in the tissue. The number of tiny blood vessels, called capillaries, increases by as much as 50 percent in regularly exercised muscles, and existing capillaries open wider so that the total circulation increases by as much as 400 percent, thus providing the muscles with a much greater supply of nutrients. This increase occurs after about 8 to 12 weeks in young persons, but takes longer in older individuals (see Figure 4-4). Inactivity reverses the process, gradually shutting down the extra capillaries that have developed.

FACT OR FICTION????????????????

Sit-ups will flatten your stomach.

Fiction: Sit-ups (crunches) do strengthen abdominal and back muscles, but they don't whittle the waistline. If you have excess "belly fat," you won't be able to see the muscles beneath it, no matter how many sit-ups you do. To lose fat you need to eat fewer calories than you burn. The good news: When you do lose weight, abdominal fat often is the first to go.

Source: www.MayoClinic.com; Fitness and Sport Medicine Center, 2003.

Strength workouts increase circulation

The heart's right half pumps oxygen-poor blood to capillary beds in lungs. There, O_2 diffuses into blood and CO_2 diffuses out. The oxygenated blood flows into the heart's left half where it is then pumped to capillary beds throughout the body.

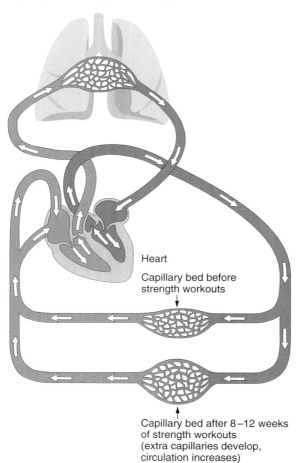

Heart

Capillary bed before strength workouts

Capillary bed after 8–12 weeks of strength workouts (extra capillaries develop, circulation increases)

Strength workouts build muscles

Outer sheath of connective tissue around muscle (toughened by strength workouts)

Bundles of muscle cells surrounded by connective tissue (more connective tissue develops from strength workouts)

Figure 4-4 BENEFITS OF STRENGTH TRAINING ON THE BODY
Strength training in combination with aerobic exercise increases blood circulation and oxygen supply to body tissues and develops muscles.

The latest research on fat-burning shows that the best way to reduce your body fat is to add muscle-strengthening exercise to your workouts. Muscle tissue is your very best calorie-burning tissue, and the more you have, the more calories you burn, even when you are resting. You don't have to become a serious body builder. Using handheld weights (also called *free weights*) two or three times a week is enough. Just be sure you learn how to use them properly because you can tear or strain muscles if you don't practice the proper weight-lifting techniques. As more people have begun to lift weights, injuries have soared.

A balanced workout regimen of muscle building and aerobic exercise does more for you than just burn fat. It gives you more endurance by promoting better distribution of oxygen to your tissues and increasing the blood flow to your heart.

Exercise and Muscles

Your muscles never stay the same. If you don't use them, they atrophy, weaken, or break down. If you use them rigorously and regularly, they grow stronger. The only way to develop muscles is by demanding more of them than you usually do. This is called **overloading.** (Remember the overload principle?) As you train, you have to gradually

You can build up muscular strength and endurance through weight training.

© 2000 PhotoDisc, Inc.

tension remains the same. In an isotonic exercise, the muscle moves a moderate load several times, as in weight lifting or calisthenics. The best isotonic exercise for producing muscular strength involves high resistance and a low number of repetitions. On the other hand, you can develop the greatest flexibility, coordination, and endurance with isotonic exercises that incorporate lower resistance and frequent repetitions.

True **isokinetic** contraction is a constant speed contraction. Isokinetic exercises require special machines that provide resistance to overload muscles throughout the entire range of motion.

increase the number of repetitions or the amount of resistance and work the muscle to temporary fatigue. That's why it's important not to quit when your muscles start to tire. Progressive overload—steadily increasing the stress placed on the body—builds stronger muscles.[61]

You need to exercise differently for strength than for endurance. *To develop strength,* do a few repetitions with heavy loads. As you increase the weight your muscles must move, you increase your strength. *To increase endurance,* you do many more repetitions with lighter loads. If your muscles are weak and you need to gain strength in your upper body, you may have to work for weeks to do a half-dozen regular push-ups. Then you can start building endurance by doing as many push-ups as you can before collapsing in exhaustion.

Muscles can do only two things: contract or relax. As they do so, skeletal muscles either pull on bones or stop pulling on bones. All exercise involves muscles pulling on bones across a joint. The movement that takes place depends on the structure of the joint and the position of the muscle attachments involved.

In an **isometric** contraction, the muscle applies force while maintaining an equal length. The muscle contracts and tries to shorten but cannot overcome the resistance. An example is pushing against an immovable object, like a wall, or tightening an abdominal muscle while sitting. The muscle contracts but there is no movement. Push or pull against the immovable object, with each muscle contraction held for 5 to 8 seconds; repeat five to ten times daily.

An **isotonic** contraction involves movement, but the muscle

Designing a Muscle Workout

A workout with weights should exercise your body's primary muscle groups: the *deltoids* (shoulders), *pectorals* (chest), *triceps* and *biceps* (back and front of upper arms), *quadriceps* and *hamstrings* (front and back of thighs), *gluteus maximus* (buttocks), *trapezius* and *rhomboids* (back), and *abdomen* (see Figure 4-5). Various machines and free-weight routines focus on each muscle group, but the principle is always the same: Muscles contract as you raise and lower a weight, and you repeat the lift-and-lower routine until the muscle group is tired.

A weight training program is made up of **reps** (the single performance, or **repetition,** of an exercise, such as

Figure 4-5 PRIMARY MUSCLE GROUPS
Different exercises can strengthen and stretch different muscle groups.

STRATEGIES FOR PREVENTION

Working with Weights

If you plan to work with free weights, here are some guidelines for using them safely and effectively:

- Don't train alone—for safety's sake. Work with a partner so you can serve as spotters for each other and help motivate each other as well.

- Always warm up and stretch before weight training; also be sure to stretch after training.

- Begin with relatively light weights (50 percent of the maximum you can lift), and increase the load slowly until you find the weight that will cause muscle failure at anywhere from eight to twelve repetitions. (Muscle failure is the point during a workout at which you can no longer perform or complete a repetition through the entire range of motion.)

- In the beginning, don't work at maximum intensity. Increase your level of exertion gradually over two to six weeks to allow your body to adapt to new stress without soreness.

- Always train your entire body, starting with the larger muscle groups. Don't focus only on specific areas, although you may want to concentrate on your weakest muscles.

- Always use proper form. Unnecessary twisting, lurching, lunging, or arching can cause serious injury. Remember, quality matters more than quantity. One properly performed set of lifts can produce a greater increase in strength and muscle mass than many sets of improperly performed lifts.

lifting 50 pounds one time) and **sets** (a *set* number of repetitions of the same movement, such as a set of 20 push-ups). You should allow your breath to return to normal before moving on to each new set. Pushing yourself to the limit builds strength.

Maintaining proper breathing during weight training is crucial. To breathe correctly, inhale when muscles are relaxed, and exhale when you push or lift. Don't ever hold your breath because oxygen flow helps prevent muscle fatigue and injury.

No one type of equipment—free weight or machine—has a clear advantage in terms of building fat-free body mass, enhancing strength and endurance, or improving a sport-specific skill. Each type offers benefits but also has drawbacks.

Free weights offer great versatility for strength training. With dumbbells, for example, you can perform a vari-

ety of exercises to work specific muscle groups, such as the chest and shoulders. Machines, in contrast, are much more limited; most allow only one exercise.

Strength-training machines have several advantages. They ensure correct movement for a lift, which helps protect against injury and prevent cheating when fatigue sets in. They isolate specific muscles, which is good for rehabilitating an injury or strengthening a specific body part. Because they offer high-tech options like varying resistance during the lifting motion, they can tax muscles in ways that a traditional barbell cannot.

Remember that your muscles need sufficient time to recover from a weight-training session. Allow no less than 48 hours, but no more than 96 hours, between training sessions, so your body can recover from the workout and you avoid overtraining. Workouts on consecutive days do more harm than good because the body can't recover that quickly. Two or three 30-minute training sessions a week should be sufficient for building strength and endurance. Strength training twice a week at greater intensity and for a longer duration can be as effective as working out three times a week. However, your muscles will begin to atrophy if you let more than three or four days pass without exercising them. For total fitness, you may want to schedule aerobic workouts for your days off from weight training.

Smoking impairs muscle recovery from exercise, even in a young healthy population of smokers.[62]

What Should I Know About Performance-Boosting Drugs?

They sound too good to be true: dietary supplements or drugs that boost strength and enhance athletic performance. Teenage boys and men in their twenties are the heaviest users. Do these aids work? Or are users endangering their health for an unproven benefit? Here's what we know—and don't know—about the most widely used performance boosters.[63]

Androstenedione

Androstenedione ("andro") is a testosterone precursor normally produced by the adrenal glands and gonads. Manufacturers claim that androstenedione improves testosterone concentration, increases muscular strength and mass, helps reduce body fat, enhances mood, and improves sexual performances. However, most studies contradict these claims and raise serious concerns about potential dangers of long-term use.[64]

In a study of its effects on men between the ages of 19 and 29, androstenedione did not show any effect on muscle strength but did increase concentrations of estrogen, which is associated with breast enlargement and increased risk of cardiovascular disease and pancreatic cancer in men. Androstenedione also raises testosterone above normal levels, which can lead to acne, male pattern baldness, and a decrease in "good" cholesterol. In women, high testosterone levels can also cause increased body hair, deepening of the voice, and other male characteristics.

Androstenedione is banned by the Olympics, the National College Athletic Association, the National Football League, and the men's and women's tennis tours.

Steroids

Anabolic steroids are synthetic derivatives of the male hormone testosterone that promote the growth of skeletal muscle and increase lean body mass. Some athletes and others use anabolic steroids to enhance performance and improve physical appearance.

Taken orally or injected, anabolic steroids are typically used in cycles of weeks or months, rather than continuously. Users take multiple doses over a specific period of time, stop for a period, and start again. In addition, users frequently combine several different types of steroids to maximize their effectiveness while minimizing their negative effects. This practice is known as stacking.

Anabolic steroids have been reported to increase lean muscle mass, strength, and ability to train longer and harder, but they pose serious health hazards, including liver tumors, jaundice (yellowish pigmentation of skin, tissues, and body fluids), fluid retention, high blood pressure, and severe acne. Men may experience shrinking of the testicles, reduced sperm count, infertility, baldness, and development of breasts. Women may experience growth of facial hair, changes in or cessation of the menstrual cycle, enlargement of the clitoris, and deepened voice. In adolescents, steroids may bring about a premature halt in skeletal maturation.

Anabolic steroid abuse may lead to aggression and other psychiatric side effects. Many users report feeling good about themselves while on anabolic steroids, but researchers report that anabolic steroid abuse can cause wild mood swings including manic-like symptoms leading to violent, even homicidal, episodes. Researchers have reported that users may suffer from paranoid jealousy, extreme irritability, delusions, and impaired judgment stemming from feelings of invincibility. Stopping the drugs abruptly can lead to depression.

Creatine

Creatine is an amino acid made by the body and stored predominantly in skeletal muscle. Creatine serves as a reservoir to replenish adenosine triphosphate (ATP), a substance involved in energy production. While some studies show creatine may increase strength and endurance, other effects on the body remain unknown.[65]

Creatine supplements increase muscle stores of the compound, which theoretically allows athletes to work out harder and longer. Athletes typically load up with 20 grams a day for five days and then keep taking 2 grams daily. Some studies have shown that creatine supplements do enhance sports performance and anaerobic power, but only in activities that require repeated short bursts of high-intensity energy, such as sprints and weight lifting, rather than long-distance running or swimming.[66]

Studies of college football players randomly assigned to placebo or creatine treatment groups have produced inconsistent results.[67] Creatine has not shown any usefulness for lower-intensity, longer-duration exercises, and the water retention and weight gain associated with creatine supplementation may actually hamper performance. Some researchers have observed that only those subjects whose own creatine levels were at the lower end of the normal range benefited from supplementation. It's not known if creatine can benefit the average recreational athlete.

Commercially marketed creatine supplements do not meet the same rigid quality control standards as prescription drugs, so it is difficult to apply efficacy and safety results from published trials to general practice. The dose delivered by a commercially available product may be more or less than that suggested by the labeling. This could influence the effectiveness of the supplement and could lead to unexpected adverse effects.

Muscle cramping, diarrhea, and dehydration have been reported in creatine users, as well as a few cases of kidney dysfunction. Some experts are concerned that creatine may damage internal organs, but there is no evidence of this so

far. In a study of college football players, those taking creatine supplements did not show harmful effects on their kidneys or liver function.[68]

The Food and Drug Administration has warned consumers to consult a physician before taking creatine supplements. The Association of Professional Team Physicians cautions that creatine may cause dehydration and heat-related illnesses, reduced blood volume, and electrolyte imbalances. Some athletes drink large quantities of water hoping to avoid such effects. However, many coaches forbid or discourage creatine use because its long-term effects remain unknown.

Other Ergogenic Aids

Ergogenic aids are substances used to enhance energy and provide athletes with a competitive advantage. By some estimates, more than three of four athletes in some sports use some sort of supplements to enhance their performance and boost energy.[69] These include everyday substances. Caffeine, for instance, may boost alertness in some people but cause jitteriness in others. Baking soda (sodium bicarbonate) is believed to delay fatigue by neutralizing lactic acid in the muscles, but its potential drawbacks include explosive diarrhea, abdominal cramps, bloating, and nausea.[70]

GBL (gamma butyrolactone) is an unapproved drug that is being studied as a treatment for narcolepsy, a disabling sleep disorder. Nevertheless, it is marketed on the Internet and in some professional gyms as a muscle-builder and performance-enhancer. The Food and Drug Administration has warned consumers to avoid any products containing GBL, noting that they have been associated with at least one death and several incidents in which users became comatose or unconscious.

Glycerol is a natural element derived from fats. Some sports-drink manufacturers are testing formulations that include glycerol, which they claim can lower heart rate and stave off exhaustion in marathon events. Glycerol-induced hyperhydration (holding too much water in the blood) can have a negative impact on performance, however, and may be hazardous to health.

❋ Flexibility

Flexibility is the characteristic of body tissues that determines the range of motion achievable without injury at a joint or group of joints. There are two types of flexibility: static and dynamic. **Static flexibility**—the type most people think of as flexibility—refers to the ability to assume and maintain an extended position at one end point in a joint's range of motion. **Dynamic flexibility,** by comparison, involves movement. It is the ability to move a joint quickly and fluidly through its entire range of motion with little resistance. The static flexibility in the hip joint determines whether you can do a split; dynamic flexibility is what would enable you to perform a split leap.

Static flexibility depends on many factors, including the structure of a joint and the tightness of the muscles, tendons, and ligaments attached to it. Dynamic flexibility is influenced by static flexibility, but also depends on additional factors, such as strength, coordination, and resistance to movement.

Genetics, age, gender, and body composition all influence how flexible you are. Girls and women tend to be more flexible than boys and men, to a certain extent because of hormonal and anatomical differences. The way females and males use their muscles and the activities they engage in can also have an effect. Over time, the natural elasticity of muscles, tendons, and joints decreases in both genders, resulting in stiffness.

The Benefits of Flexibility

Just as cardiorespiratory fitness benefits the heart and lungs and muscular fitness builds endurance and strength, a stretching program produces unique benefits, including

enhancement of the ability of the respiratory, circulatory, and neuromuscular systems to cope with the stress and demands of our high-pressure world. Among the other benefits of flexibility are:

:: **Prevention of injuries.** Flexibility training stretches muscles and increases the elasticity of joints. Strong, flexible muscles resist stress better than weak or inflexible ones. Adding flexibility to a training program for sports such as soccer, football, or tennis can reduce the rate of injuries by as much as 75 percent. In one study of competitive runners, weekly stretching sessions significantly reduced the incidence of low back pain.

:: **Relief of muscle strain.** Muscles tighten as a result of stress or prolonged sitting. If you study or work in one position for several hours, you'll often feel stiffness in your back or neck. Stretching helps relieve this tension and enables you to work more effectively.

:: **Relaxation.** Flexibility exercises are great stress-busters that reduce mental strain, slow the rate of breathing, and reduce blood pressure.

:: **Relief of soreness after exercise.** Many people develop delayed-onset muscle soreness (DOMS) one or two days after they work out. This may be the result of damage to the muscle fibers and supporting connective tissue. Some researchers theorize that stretching after exercise can decrease this aftereffect, although others contend that it produces only short-term benefits.[71]

:: **Improved posture.** Bad posture can create tight, stressed muscles. If you slump in your chair, for instance, the muscles in the front of your chest may tighten, causing those in the upper spine to overstretch and become loose.

:: **Better athletic performance.** Good flexibility allows for more efficient movement and exertion of more force through a greater range of motion, a special benefit for any activity, from gymnastics to golf, where positions beyond the normal range of motion are necessary to perform certain skills.

Flexibility can make everyday tasks, like bending over to tie a shoe or reaching up to a high shelf, easier and safer. It can also prevent and relieve the ankle, knee, back, and shoulder pain that many people feel as they get older. If you do other forms of exercise, flexibility lowers your risk of injury and may improve your performance.

Types of Stretching

You should stretch a minimum of two or three times a week. Unlike strength training, flexibility exercises do not require time off between sessions. Ideally you should try to incorporate some stretches into your daily routine. The basic types of stretching include static, passive, active, and ballistic stretching. (See Figure 4-6.)

Static stretching involves a gradual stretch held for a short time (10 to 30 seconds). A shorter stretch provides little benefit; a longer stretch does not provide additional benefits. Since a slow stretch provokes less of a reaction from the stretch receptors, the muscles can safely stretch farther than usual. Fitness experts most often recommend static stretching because it is both safe and effective. An example of such a stretch is letting your hands slowly slide down the front of your legs (keeping your knees in a soft, unlocked position) until you reach your toes and holding this final position for several seconds before slowly straightening up. You should feel a pull, but not pain, during this stretch.

In **passive stretching,** your own body, a partner, gravity, or a weight serves as an external force or resistance to help your joints move through their range of motion. You can achieve a more intense stretch and a greater range of motion with passive stretching. There is a greater risk of injury, however, because the muscles themselves are not controlling the stretch. If working with a partner, it's very important that you communicate clearly so as not to force a joint outside its normal functional range of motion.

Research on stretching demonstrates a 5 to 20 percent increase in static flexibility within four to six weeks of stretching. Much of this long-term increase in range of motion is due to an increased "stretch tolerance," or ability to tolerate the discomfort of a stretched position.

Active stretching involves stretching a muscle by contracting the opposing muscle (the muscle on the opposite side of the limb). In an active seated hamstring stretch, for example, the stretch occurs by actively contracting the muscles on top of the shin, which produces a reflex that relaxes the hamstring. This method allows the muscle to be stretched farther with a low risk of injury.

The disadvantage of active stretching is that a person may not be able to produce enough of a stretch to increase flexibility only by means of contracting opposing muscle groups. Although active stretching is the safest and most convenient approach, an occasional passive assist can be helpful.

Figure 4-6 SOME SIMPLE STRETCHING EXERCISES

(a) *Foot pull for the groin and thigh muscles.* Sit on the ground and bend your legs so that the soles of your feet touch. Pull your feet closer as you press on your knees with your elbows. Hold for 10 seconds; repeat. (b) *Lateral head tilt.* Gently tilt your head to each side. Repeat several times. (c) *Wall stretch for the Achilles tendon.* Stand 3 feet from a wall or post with your feet slightly apart. Keeping your heels on the ground, lean into the wall. Hold for 10 seconds; repeat. (d) *Triceps stretch for the upper arm and shoulder.* Place your right hand behind your neck and grasp it above the elbow with your left hand. Gently pull the elbow back. Repeat with the left elbow. (e) *Knee-chest pull for lower back muscles.* Lying on your back, clasp one knee and pull it toward your chest. Hold for 15–30 seconds; repeat with the other knee.

(a)

(b)

(c)

(d)

(e)

STRATEGIES FOR PREVENTION

How to Avoid Stretching Injuries

■ Never stretch to the point of pain.

■ Don't attempt a ballistic stretch on a weak or injured muscle.

■ Start small. Work the muscles of the smaller joints in the arms and legs first and then work the larger joints like the shoulders and hips.

■ Stretch individual muscles before you stretch a group of muscles, for instance, the ankle, knee, and hip before a stretch that works all three.

■ Don't make any quick, jerky movements while stretching. Even ballistic stretches should be gentle and smooth.

Ballistic stretching is characterized by rapid bouncing movements, such as a series of up-and-down bobs as you try again and again to touch your toes with your hands. These bounces can stretch the muscle fibers too far, causing the muscle to contract rather than stretch. They also can tear ligaments and weaken or rupture tendons, the strong fibrous cords that connect muscles to bones. The heightened activity to stretch receptors caused by the rapid stretches can continue for some time, possibly causing injuries during any physical activities that follow. Because of its potential dangers, fitness experts generally recommend against ballistic stretching.

What Is the Difference Between Stretching and Warming Up?

Warming up means getting the heart beating, breaking a sweat, and readying the body for more vigorous activity. Stretching is a specific activity intended to elongate the muscles and keep joints limber, not simply a prelude to a game of tennis or a three-mile run.

For most sports, light to moderate activity, such as walking at gradually increasing intensity, is a better warm-up than stretching. One of the best times to stretch is after an aerobic workout. Your muscles will be warm, more flexible, and less prone to injury. In addition, stretching after aerobic activity can help a fatigued muscle return to its normal resting length and possibly helps reduce delayed muscle soreness.

✖ Body Composition

A combination of regular exercise and good nutrition is the best way to maintain a healthy body composition. Aerobic exercise helps by burning calories and increasing metabolic rate (the rate at which the body uses calories) for several hours after a workout. Strength training increases the proportion of lean body tissue by building muscle mass, which also increases the metabolic rate.

Body Mass Index (BMI)

Body mass index (BMI), a ratio between weight and height, is a mathematical formula that correlates with body fat. The BMI numbers apply to both men and women. (See Figure 4-7.)

You can also calculate your body mass index by following these three simple steps:

1. Multiply your weight in pounds by 703.
2. Multiply your height in inches by itself.
3. Divide the first number by the second and then round up to the nearest whole number. This is your body mass index.

Doctors use BMI to determine whether a person is at risk for weight-related diseases like diabetes. However, using BMI as an assessment tool has limitations. Muscular individuals, including athletes and body builders, may be miscategorized as overweight or obese because they have greater lean muscle mass. BMI also does not reliably reflect body fat, an independent predictor of health risk, and is not useful for growing children, women who are pregnant or nursing, or the elderly. In addition, BMI, which was developed in Western nations, may not accurately indicate the risk of obesity-related diseases in Asian men and women.[72]

If your BMI is high, you may be at increased risk of developing certain diseases, including hypertension, cardiovascular disease, adult-onset diabetes (type 2), sleep apnea, and osteoarthritis.

Body Composition Assessment

Two simple measures can tell you whether you are at greater risk for disease—your waist size and your waist-to-hip ratio:

:: *Waist size.* Among those with BMIs over 25, men with waists larger than 40 inches and women with waists larger than 35 inches are at greater risk of heart disease. The danger increases along with the waistline. According to one study, women with waists of 30 inches run twice the risk of heart disease as slimmer women. At 38 inches, the risk is three times higher

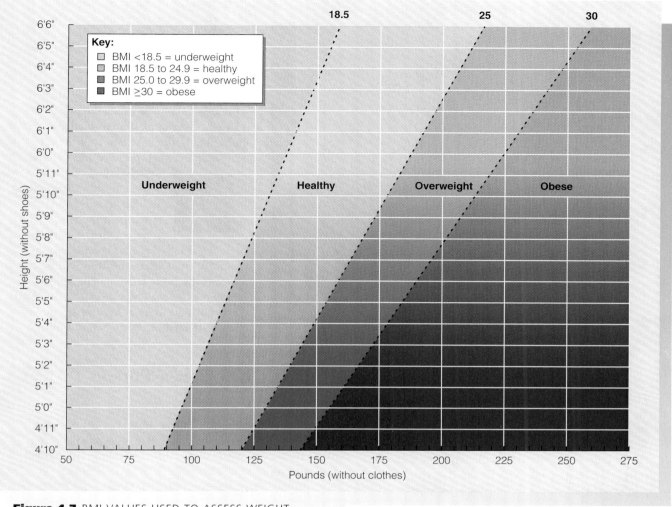

Figure 4-7 BMI VALUES USED TO ASSESS WEIGHT FOR ADULTS

compared to women with waists of 28 inches or less.[73]

:: **Waist-to-hip ratio (WHR).** A WHR greater than 1 for men or .85 for women is considered a signal of high risk for disease; a WHR of .90 to 1 for men or .80 to .85 for women indicates moderately high risk; a WHR less than .90 for men or less than .80 for women indicates lower risk.

Knowing your specific body composition can provide useful information about body fat and health. Ideal body fat percentages for men range from 7 to 25 percent and for women from 16 to 35 percent (see Figure 4-8). Methods of assessing body composition include:

:: **Skinfold fat measurement.** A caliper is used to measure the amount of skinfold. The usual sites include the chest, abdomen, and thigh for men, and the tricep, hip, and thigh for women. Various equations determine body fat percentage, including calculations that take

into account age, gender, race, and other factors. This relatively simple and low-cost method requires considerable technical skill for an accurate reading (see photo on p. 104.)

:: **Bioelectrical Impedance Analysis (BIA).** This noninvasive method is based on the principle that electrical current applied to the body meets greater resistance with different types of tissue (see Figure 4-9). Lean tissue, which contains large amounts of water and electrolytes, is a good electrical conductor; fat, which does not, is a poor conductor. In theory, the easier the electrical conduction, the greater an individual's lean body mass. Although BIA is quick, painless, and safe, some have questioned its accuracy, largely because being overhydrated or underhydrated can throw off the results.

45% muscle

25% organs

15% fat

15% bone

36% muscle

24% organs

27% fat

13% bone

Figure 4-8 AVERAGE BODY COMPOSITION OF MEN AND WOMEN

Source: Data from R. E. C. Wildman and D. M. Medeiros, *Advanced Human Nutrition*. Boca Raton, Fla.: CRC Press, 2000, pp. 321–323.

:: *Home body fat analyzers.* Handheld devices and stand-on monitors sold online and in specialty stores promise to make measuring your body fat percentage as easy as finding your weight. None has been extensively tested.

:: *The Bod Pod®.* This large, egg-shaped fiberglass chamber uses an approach based on air displacement plethysmography, that is, the calculation of the relationship between pressure and volume to derive body volume. Research on undergraduates has shown gender differences in the Bod Pod's accuracy. In comparative studies, skinfold measurements proved more accurate than the Bod Pod in measuring body fat in female athletes.[75] However, in male wrestlers, the Bod Pod proved as accurate as hydrostatic weighing to determine body composition.[76]

:: *Hydrostatic (underwater) weighing.* According to the Archimedes Principle, a body immersed in a fluid is buoyed by a force equal to the weight of the displaced fluid. Since muscle has a higher density than water and fat has a lower density, fat people tend to displace less water than lean people. This method, also known as hydrodensitometry, is expensive and complex.

:: *Dual-energy X-ray absorptiometry (DXA).* X rays are used to quantify the skeletal and soft tissue components of body mass (see Figure 4-9). The test requires just 10 to 20 minutes, and radiation dosage is low (800 to 2,000 times lower than a typical chest X ray). Some researchers believe that DXA will supplant hydrostatic testing as the standard for body composition assessment.[74]

Can a Person Be Fat and Fit?

Most people assume that fitness comes in only one size: small. That's not necessarily so. There is considerable controversy over how to define a healthy weight. But individuals of every size can improve their physical fitness.

In ten years of research on 25,000 men and 8,000 women, scientists led by Steven Blair, director of research at the Cooper Institute for Aerobics Research in Dallas, have found that heavier individuals can be just as healthy and physically fit as their leaner counterparts. In their studies, obese people who exercised moderately (30 minutes of daily walking at three or four miles per hour) had half the death rate of those who were slimmer but more sedentary. Low cardiorespiratory fitness, regardless of an individual's weight, is as great a risk factor for dying of heart disease or other causes such as diabetes, high blood pressure, and other well-recognized threats.

Nonetheless, fitness doesn't completely reverse the increased risks associated with excess weight. In one study of the effects of fitness and fatness on longevity in men and women, both had an impact on mortality from all causes and from cardiovascular disease.[77]

Being overweight also can interfere with physical activities that

Figure 4-9 TWO TYPES OF BODY COMPOSITION ASSESSMENT

Bioelectrical impedance analysis (BIA)   *Dual energy X-ray absorptiometry (DXA)*

enhance fitness. For instance, overweight and obese women find walking difficult because of discomfort and pain.

Nutrition for an Active Life

The food you eat provides the fuel you use to move through life. Nutrition and physical activity are interrelated. Your level of activity influences your calorie needs, and the foods you eat affect your energy and performance.

 Many people assume that individuals with active lifestyles eat more nutritiously, but that's not necessarily so—at least among college students. A study of 109 undergraduates at a Texas state university found no correlation between fitness levels and healthy eating habits. The fittest students were not more likely to eat a nutritious diet, nor were those consuming the most nutrients more likely to rate highly on fitness tests.[78]

In general, active people need the same basic nutrients as others and should follow the recommendations in Chapter 5. However, athletes in competitive sports—amateur as well as professional—may have increased energy requirements.

Not just *what* you eat, but *when* you eat can affect your exercise performance. If you eat immediately prior to a workout, you may feel sluggish or develop nausea, cramping, or diarrhea. If you don't eat, you may feel weak, faint, or tired.

Time your meals so that you exercise three to four hours after a large meal and one to two hours after a small one. Most people can eat a snack right before exercise. After a workout, eat a meal containing both protein and carbohydrates within two hours to help your muscles recover and to replace fuel stores.[79]

How Much Water Should I Drink?

Water, which we need more than any other nutrient, is even more important during exercise and exertion. Thirst, the body's way of telling you to replace lost fluids, is not a good way for athletes to monitor their fluid needs. Rather than waiting until you're already somewhat dehydrated, you should be fully hydrated when you begin your activity or exercise and, depending on the duration and intensity of your workout, continue to replace fluids both during and afterward.

Here are the American Dietetic Association's guidelines for fluid intake for active individuals:

:: Consume at least two cups (16 to 20 ounces) of fluid about two hours before exertion.

Active people need extra fluid, even in cold weather.

:: Drink another two cups of fluid approximately 15 to 20 minutes before endurance exercise.

:: If the climate is hot and humid, take small servings (4 to 6 ounces) every 15 minutes of plain cool water (40 to 50 degrees Fahrenheit) or another rehydration beverage. (Think of an ounce as approximately one "gulp.") Depending on your sport or activity, you may need to drink whenever the opportunity arises (e.g., during breaks or time-outs).

:: After an activity, drink at least two cups (16 ounces) per pound of body weight lost during the activity. Some exercise physiologists recommend an additional 8 ounces (24 ounces total per pound) to compensate for urine losses as you rehydrate.

Loss of more than 2 percent of body weight during an activity indicates that a person is becoming dehydrated. Any degree of dehydration impairs physical performance; extreme dehydration can lead to heat exhaustion or heat stroke, two serious conditions discussed in Chapter 18.

Nutrition and Athletic Performance

Most people, even if physically active, do not require special diets. Contrary to a common misconception, athletes generally do not need more protein; the exception may be those engaged in intense strength training. Like most Americans, athletes typically consume more than the

Recommended Daily Allowance for protein and do not need increased protein. As discussed in Chapter 6, a high-protein diet can be high in fat and low in the nutrients supplied by fruits, vegetables, and grains and can put a strain on the liver and kidneys.

Although complex carbohydrates are essential in an athlete's diet, fat also plays a role. Including the right types of fat in the daily diet can actually improve athletic performance—not just by providing calories, but by replenishing intramuscular fat stores (fat stored within the muscle and used to fuel extended exercise).

Energy Bars

Sold as snacks, meal substitutes, or performance enhancers, energy bars come in different forms. High-carbohydrate bars derive more than 70 percent of their calories from carbohydrates (such as corn syrup, grape and pear juice concentrate, oat bran, and brown rice) and are low in protein and fat. Another type gets 40 percent of its energy from carbohydrate, 30 percent from protein, and 30 percent from fat.

Little scientific research has studied the actual benefits of the various types of energy bars, including their effects on blood glucose levels and athletic performance. According to one nutritional analysis, high-carbohydrate energy bars are similar to candy bars in their impact on glucose—even though sugars composed 31 percent of the high-carbohydrate energy bar and 86 percent of the candy bar. In fact, the high-carbohydrate energy bar caused a more rapid peak in blood glucose followed by a sharper decline than did the candy bar. This effect may be desirable for athletes involved in short-duration events who want a quick increase in blood glucose.

Energy bars with a lower carbohydrate level produce a more moderate, sustained increase in blood glucose level, possibly because the protein and fat in a 40–30–30 bar diminish blood glucose response. These bars would be a better choice for athletes involved in endurance events.

For others, energy bars are of dubious value. Even Americans who eat poorly rarely need additional protein. Despite their marketing claims, energy bars don't build muscle or boost energy more than any other food; they just provide extra and often unneeded calories.

Sport and Protein Drinks

Protein shakes and prepackaged drinks also have become popular. However, many sports nutritionists consider them of dubious value.[80] As explained in Chapter 5, most people obtain adequate protein from their daily diet, and dietary protein is just as beneficial as the "high-quality" proteins advertised as ingredients of sports drinks.

▒ Sports Safety

Whenever you work out, you don't want to risk becoming sore or injured. Starting slowly when you begin any new fitness activity is the smartest strategy. Keep a simple diary to record the time and duration of each workout. Get accustomed to an activity first and then begin to work harder or longer. In this way, you strengthen your musculoskeletal system so you're less likely to be injured, you lower the cardiovascular risk, and you build the exercise habit into your schedule.

Even seasoned athletes should "listen to their bodies." If you develop aches and pains beyond what you might expect from an activity, stop. Never push to the point of fatigue. If you do, you could end up with sprained or torn muscles. Figure 4–10 gives the PRICE prescription for coping with an exercise injury.

Figure 4-10 PRICE: HOW TO COPE WITH AN EXERCISE INJURY

- **P**rotect the area with an elastic wrap, a sling, splint, cane, crutches or an air cast.
- **R**est to promote tissue healing. Avoid activities that cause pain, swelling or discomfort.
- **I**ce the area immediately, even if you're seeking medical help. Repeat every two or three hours while you're awake for the first 48 to 72 hours. Cold reduces pain, swelling and inflammation in injured muscles, joints and connecting tissues and may slow bleeding if a tear has occurred.
- **C**ompress the area with an elastic bandage until the swelling stops. Begin wrapping at the end farthest from your heart. Loosen the wrap if the pain increases, the area becomes numb or swelling is occurring below the wrapped area.
- **E**levate the area above your heart, especially at night. Gravity helps reduce swelling by draining excess fluid.

After 48 hours, if the swelling is gone, you may apply warmth or gentle heat, which improves the blood flow and speed healing. Apply cold to sore areas after a workout to prevent inflammation and swelling.

How Can I Prevent Sports Injuries?

According to the American Physical Therapy Association, the most common exercise-related injury sites are the knees, feet, back, and shoulders, followed by the ankles and hips. **Acute injuries**—sprains, bruises, and pulled muscles—are the result of sudden trauma, such as a fall or collision. **Overuse injuries,** on the other hand, are the result of overdoing a repetitive activity, such as running. When one particular joint is overstressed—such as a tennis player's elbow or a swimmer's shoulder—tendinitis, an inflammation at the point where the tendon meets the bone, can develop. Other overuse injuries include muscle strains and aches and stress fractures, which are hairline breaks in a bone, usually in the leg or foot.

 Men and women may be vulnerable to different types of injuries. Studies of male and female college basketball and soccer players have shown that gender differences in the neuromuscular control of the knee places female athletes at higher risk for knee injuries.[81] Balance training may reduce the risk.[82]

To prevent exercise-related problems before they happen, use common sense and take appropriate precautions, including the following:

:: Get proper instruction and, if necessary, advanced training from knowledgeable instructors.

:: Make sure you have good equipment and keep it in good condition. Know how to check and do at least basic maintenance on the equipment yourself. Always check your equipment prior to each use (especially if you're renting it).

:: Always make sure that stretching and exercises are preventing, not causing, injuries.

:: Use reasonable protective measures, including wearing a helmet when cycling or skating.

:: For some sports, such as boating, always go with a buddy.

:: Take each outing seriously—even if you've dived into this river a hundred times before, even if you know this mountain like you know your own backyard. Avoid the unknown under adverse conditions (for example, hiking unfamiliar terrain during poor weather or kayaking a new river when water levels are unusually high or low) or when accompanied by a beginner whose skills may not be as strong as yours.

:: Never combine alcohol or drugs with any sport.

Beyond the Gym

Many people are trying exhilarating sports that, by their very nature, entail some risk. If you choose these activities, you're responsible for learning how to stay safe as you push to the limit. Here are some sport-specific guidelines:

:: **Inline skating.** The most common injuries are to the wrists. Skaters should always wear protective gear, including a helmet, wrist guards, and knee pads, and should warm up before strapping on their skates. Learn how to fall: Relax, go down to your knees, and roll to one side.

:: **Mountain biking.** Off-road biking requires knowing how to shift your weight to keep a bike stable on rough trails. Know the limits of your endurance and of your equipment. Wear a helmet, bicycle gloves, and glasses or goggles to protect your eyes from dirt and overhanging branches. Carry a bike repair kit and a first aid kit if you head for a remote area.

:: **Rock climbing.** Rock climbing takes strength, balance, and hand-eye coordination. Training with a qualified instructor is essential to learn proper technique. The best place to learn is indoors, with supervised instruction and controlled conditions.

:: **Snowboarding.** Well-fitted snowboarding boots are essential, as is training in how to fall. The most common injuries are to the wrist or thumb, which can fracture if snowboarders put out their palms to break a fall. Sunburn and frostbite are both risks, and snowboarders should wear sunscreen and monitor weather conditions closely.

Thinking of Temperature

Prevention is the wisest approach to heat problems. Always dress appropriately for the weather and be aware of the health risks associated with temperature extremes.

Heeding Heat

Always wear as little as possible when exercising in hot weather. Choose loose-fitting, lightweight, white or light-colored clothes. Cotton is good because it absorbs perspiration. Never wear rubberized or plastic pants and jackets to sweat off pounds. These sauna suits will cause you to lose water only—not fat—and, because they don't allow your body heat to dissipate, they can be dangerous. On humid days, carry a damp washcloth to wipe off perspiration and cool yourself down. Be sure to drink plenty of fluids while exercising (especially water), and watch for the earliest signs of heat problems, including cramps, stress, exhaustion, and heatstroke. (See Chapter 18 for a further discussion of safety precautions.)

Coping with Cold

Protect yourself in cold weather (or cold indoor gyms) by covering as much of your body as possible, but don't overdress. Wear one layer less than you would if you were outside but not exercising. Don't use warm-up clothes made of waterproof material because they tend to trap heat and keep perspiration from evaporating. Make sure your clothes are loose enough to allow movement and exercise of the hands, feet, and other body parts, thereby maintaining proper circulation. Choose dark colors that absorb heat. And because 40 percent or more of your body heat is lost through your head and neck, wear a hat, turtleneck, or scarf. Make sure you cover your hands and feet as well; mittens provide more warmth and protection than gloves.

Toxic Workouts

If you live in a large city, you may have to consider the risks of exercising in polluted air. On smoggy days, avoid a noontime workout. Exposure to ground-level ozone, produced as sunlight reacts with exhaust fumes, can irritate the lungs and constrict bronchial tubes. An ozone level of 0.12 part per million causes, on the average, a 13 percent decline in lung capacity. This level is the maximum considered safe under the Clean Air Act, but it is often surpassed in New York, Los Angeles, and other urban areas.

Overtraining

About half of all people who start an exercise program drop out within six months. One common reason is that they **overtrain,** pushing themselves to work too intensely too frequently. Signs of overdoing it include persistent muscle soreness, frequent injuries, unintended weight loss, nervousness, and an inability to relax. Overtraining for endurance sports like marathon running can damage the lungs and intensify asthma symptoms. If you're pushing too hard, you may find yourself unable to complete a normal workout or to recover after a normal workout.

If you develop any of the symptoms of overtraining, reduce or stop your workout sessions temporarily. Make gradual increases in the intensity of your workouts. Allow 24 to 48 hours for recovery between workouts. Make sure you get adequate rest. Check with a physical education instructor, coach, or trainer to make sure your exercise program fits your individual needs.

Excessive exercise can be a problem, particularly for young men. In a study of 93 male college students, one-third exercised as intensely and often as professional athletes, burning about 1,100 calories at least five days a week. They continued to work out when they were ill or injured; felt annoyed, angry, or agitated if their exercise was interrupted or changed; and said that exercise was of more than average importance to them. Yet none felt they had a problem with overdoing their physical activity.[83]

Evaluating Fitness Products and Programs

As fitness has become a major industry in the United States, consumers have been bombarded with pitches for products that promise to do everything from whittle a waistline to build up biceps. As always, you have to ask questions and do your own research—whether you're buying basic exercise aids (See Savvy Consumer: "Don't Fall for the 'Muscle Hustle.'") or joining a health club. Beware of any promise that sounds too good to be true. And keep in mind that nothing matters more than your own commitment.

How Do I Buy the Right Athletic Shoes?

For many aerobic activities, good shoes are the most important purchase you'll make. Take the time to choose well. Here are some basic guidelines:

:: Shop for shoes in the late afternoon, when your feet are most likely to be somewhat swollen—just as they will be after a workout.

:: For walking shoes, look for a shoe that's lightweight, flexible, and roomy enough for your toes to wiggle, with a well-cushioned, curved sole; one that has good support at the heel; and one with an upper that is made of a material that breathes (allows air in and out).

:: For running shoes, look for good cushioning, support, and stability. You should be able to wiggle your toes easily, but the front of your foot shouldn't slide from side to side, which could cause blisters. Your toes should not touch the end of the shoe because your feet will swell with activity. Allow about half an inch from the longest toe to the tip of the shoe. If you run up to 10 miles a week, replace your shoes every 9 to 12 months.

:: For racquetball shoes, look for reinforcement at the toe for protection during foot drag. The sole should allow minimal slippage. There should be some heel elevation to lessen strain on the back of the leg and Achilles tendon. The shoe should have a long "throat" to ensure greater control by the laces.

:: For tennis shoes, look for reinforcement at the toe. The sole at the ball of the foot should be well padded, because that's where most pressure is exerted. The sides of the shoe should be sturdy, for stability during continuous lateral movements. The toe box should allow ample room and some cushioning at the tips. A long throat ensures greater control by the laces.

Savvy Consumer

DON'T FALL FOR THE "MUSCLE HUSTLE"

Do you want "six-pack abs"? Just wrap an electrical muscle stimulator (EMS) around your middle. Without a single sit-up, you'll end up with washboard-taut abdominal muscles.

Too good to believe? Absolutely. The Federal Trade Commission has filed claims of false advertising against three manufacturers of such devices. Despite what infomercials and advertisements claimed, no device can evaporate fat or build lean muscle mass. EMS devices do have a place—for physical therapy and rehabilitation. Applying electrical current may cause muscles to contract, which leads to some toning and strengthening. However, it will not cause a major change in appearance without the addition of weight loss and regular exercise.

Here are guidelines from the FTC:

- Ignore any claims that an exercise machine or device can provide long-lasting, easy, "no-sweat" results in a short time.
- Don't believe claims about "spot-reducing." While you can tone muscles by exercising, you cannot burn fat off a particular part of the body.
- Be skeptical of dramatic before-and-after photos. The experience pictured may not be typical—and you never know if the photos were doctored or if the results lasted.
- Read the fine print. Often they say that the results are based not just on the device, but on dieting and exercising as well.
- Find out about return policies, warranties, and guarantees.
- If you have questions or complaints, check MedWatch, the FDA's voluntary reporting program at: www.fda.gov/medwatch/how.htm.

Don't wear wet shoes for training. Let wet shoes air-dry, because a heater will cause them to stiffen or shrink. Use powder in your shoes to absorb moisture, lessen friction, and prevent fungal infections. Break in new shoes for several days before wearing them for a long-distance run or during competition.

Exercise Equipment

Always try out equipment before buying it. If you decide to purchase a stationary bicycle, for instance, read all the product information. Ask someone in your physical education department or at a local gym for recommendations. Try out a bicycle at the gym. Make sure any equipment you purchase is safe and durable.

Think about your fitness goals. If you're primarily interested in aerobic fitness, try out stationary bicycles, stair-climbing machines, rowing machines, treadmills, and cross-country skiing machines. Spend 5 to 10 minutes working at moderate intensity. How do your movements on this particular piece of equipment feel to you—awkward or fluid, extremely difficult or surprisingly easy?

If you're considering strength-training equipment, remember that free weights are your least expensive option. The best resistance machines are also the most expensive, with prices over $1,000. Would you use one often enough to justify that cost? Or would an annual health-club membership be more cost-effective?

Your exercise style is also an important consideration. Are you going to find sitting at a stationary bicycle for 30 minutes too boring? Are you motivated enough to hoist free weights on your own several times a week? The best home exercise equipment will do you no good unless you use it.

Not all fitness equipment comes with a big price tag. Here are some affordable ways to expand and enhance a home workout:

:: **Dumbbells.** You can purchase light weights to carry when walking and jogging to build and firm arm muscles. Training with heavier weights increases muscle strength and endurance, improves balance and body composition, and may reverse some bone loss. An adjustable dumbbell set allows you to add more weight as you build strength.

:: **Stretchy bands.** Low in cost, lightweight, and highly portable, elastic exercise bands allow you to create resistance as you exercise. Available in different strengths, they can also provide for progressive overload. Some trainers believe they work best for novice exercisers, since well-conditioned athletes may need more challenge.

:: **Exercise balls.** Popular in group classes, exercise balls come in various sizes. Heavy, weighted balls can be lifted or tossed to tone the upper body. The larger, inflatable balls are mainly used for balance and back workouts. Some trainers think they add fun and variety to a workout; others question their value. Crunches performed on a ball may be somewhat more effective.

Fitness Centers and Trainers

If you decide to join a gym or health club, find out exactly what facilities and programs it offers. The club should be located close to home, campus, or work and should be open at convenient hours. Think about your schedule and when you'll have time to work out. Visit the club at the times you're most likely to use it: During peak hours, you might have to wait half an hour for a turn on the machines.

A club should have facilities for a complete workout, including both aerobic and muscle workouts: exercycles, rowing machines, treadmills, stair-climbing machines, stationary bicycles, a running track, aerobics classes, a swimming pool, strength-training equipment, and, if that's what you're looking for, racquetball and squash courts and a large gym for basketball and volleyball.

Find out whether all facilities are available to all members at all times. Some clubs reserve the pool for families only or kids' lessons at certain times. Ask if you can try out the club before joining. Find out what the membership includes. Will you end up paying extra for lockers, towels, classes, and the like? Are student discounts offered? Beware of long-term memberships; many clubs go out of business or change ownership often. Pay attention to cleanliness and to the atmosphere and people. Do the members seem to be significantly older or younger, or in much better or worse shape, than you are? You're more likely to work out regularly in a place, and with people, you like.

The Bottom Line ▼
Fitness for Life

If you have started to exercise regularly, you know how important physical activity is. You can feel the difference in your energy and vitality. As you've shaped up, you've discovered the daily joys of living in a body that is supple, strong, resilient, and responsive. You can sense the long-term benefits you read about in this chapter, such as a healthier heart, a hardier immune system, and a brighter mental outlook.

Yet about half of people who begin an exercise program drop out within three to six months. Why do some people stick with an exercise program while others quit?

Researchers studied a group of Brown University undergraduates, all of whom had been exercising for at least 20 minutes three times a week. Two months later 87 percent were still exercising, but 13 percent had relapsed. The relapsers had scored lower on measures of self-efficacy, the feelings of competence and control dis-cussed in Chapter 1. They also listed significantly fewer "pros" or advantages of exercising than those who stuck with the program. In time, the "cons" or negatives out-weighed their positive motivators. The researchers con-cluded that one way to prevent relapse might be to reduce the number of "cons" (such as inconvenience, cost, or lack of competence) so that people have less reason to drop out of an exercise program.[84]

In general individuals are most likely to maintain physical activity if they:

:: perceive a net benefit

:: choose an enjoyable activity

:: feel competent doing the activity

:: feel safe doing the activity

:: can easily access the activity on a regular basis

:: can fit the activity into their daily schedule

:: feel the activity does not cost more than they are willing to spend

:: experience minimal negative consequences, such as injury, loss of time, negative peer pressure

:: can handle competing time demands.

What can you do to make sure you remain active? Here are some practical strategies that can help:

:: Aim to do half a workout. Once you get started, you may find you want to keep going.

:: Show up. Once you're at the gym, you're more likely to be in the mood to exercise.

:: If you're embarrassed about your body, remind yourself that you're more concerned about your appearance than anyone else is. Look around: people come in all different shapes and sizes.

:: If you're easily winded, decrease intensity and increase duration. For example, slow your pace as you walk but extend the distance you cover.

:: Vary your routine. Walk one day, bicycle the next. Go dancing. Mow the lawn. Learn how to play tennis.

 After watching the CNN video segment, discuss the following question. What are the behavioral strategies for getting a good nights sleep?

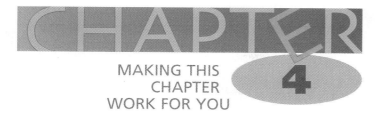

MAKING THIS
CHAPTER
WORK FOR YOU

4

1. Mary Ann takes a step aerobics class three times a week. Which component of physical fitness does her exercise routine emphasize?
   a. muscular strength and endurance
   b. flexibility
   c. cardiorespiratory fitness
   d. body composition

2. The benefits of regular physical activity include:
   a. decreased bone mass.
   b. lowered risk of shin splints.
   c. enhanced immune response.
   d. altered sleep patterns.

3. To motivate yourself to stick to an exercise program:
   a. Watch professional athletic competitions.
   b. Set a long-term goal, then break it down into short-term goals that can be achieved in a few months.
   c. Keep a detailed record of all the times that you avoided working out.
   d. Join an expensive health club so that you feel pressured to get your money's worth.

4. Which of the following best describes the primary benefit of aerobic exercise?
   a. It improves cardiorespiratory endurance.
   b. It helps condition your muscles, enabling them to work efficiently and reliably.
   c. It can enhance weight loss.
   d. It increases the range of motion of your joints.

5. An aerobic workout may consist of
   a. 5 minutes of brisk walking, 30 minutes of flexibility exercises, 5 minutes of brisk walking.
   b. 15 minutes of resistance exercises followed by 10 minutes of stretching.
   c. 10 minutes of sprints, 5 minutes of slow jogging, 5 minutes of stretching, and 10 minutes of sprints.
   d. 5 minutes of stretching, 5 minutes of brisk walking, 45 minutes of jogging, 5 minutes of slow walking, 5 minutes of stretching.

6. Which statement is true about isometric, isotonic, and isokinetic exercises?

   a. Isokinetic exercises usually involves pushing on an object, isotonic exercises involve pulling on an object, and isotonic exercises involve lifting an object.
   b. Isometric and isokinetic exercises can be done with free weights, but isotonic exercises require special resistance machines.
   c. Weight lifting is an isotonic exercise, pushing against the wall is an isometric exercise, and isokinetic exercises require special machines that move muscles through their range of motion.
   d. Isotonic exercises are much more effective at contracting muscles than isometric or isokinetic.

7. A regular flexibility program provides which of the following benefits?
   a. stronger heart and lungs
   b. relief of muscle strain and soreness
   c. increased strength and endurance
   d. increased bone mass and leaner muscles

8. Body composition estimates can be obtained with which of the following methods?
   a. skinfold fat weighing
   b. bioelectrical impedance analysis
   c. biofeedback analysis
   d. basal metabolic rate measurement

9. Which nutrient is the most important during exercise and exertion?
   a. water
   b. carbohydrates
   c. fat
   d. protein

10. Which of the following precautions could help prevent a serious sports injury from occurring?
    a. Wear swimming goggles when doing laps to decrease the irritating effects of chlorine.
    b. Wear knee pads when cycling to prevent knee gashes if you fall off your bicycle.
    c. To eliminate persistent muscle soreness, increase the frequency and/or time period of your workout.
    d. Wear a helmet, wrist guards, and knee pads when inline skating to help prevent fractures and head injuries.

Answers to these questions can be found on page 652.

Critical Thinking

1. Allison knows that exercise is good for her health, but she figures she can keep her weight down by dieting and worry about her heart and health when she gets older. "I look good. I feel okay. Why should I bother exercising?" she asks. What would you reply?

2. When he started working out, Jeff simply wanted to stay in shape. But he felt so pleased with the way his body looked and responded that he kept doing more. Now he runs 10 miles a day (longer on weekends), lifts weights, works out on

Critical Thinking

exercise equipment almost every day, and plays racquetball or squash whenever he gets a chance. Is Jeff getting too much of a good thing? Is there any danger in his fitness program? What would be a more reasonable approach?

3. Your younger brother Andre is hoping to get a starting position on his high school football team. Practices began in July. You are aware that a couple of other players have suffered heat-related incidences, but according to Andre,

Critical Thinking

these players just weren't tough enough. What can you do to help your brother protect his health?

4. Although anabolic steroids have been banned for use by athletes in certain competitions, other performance-enhancing supplements are used routinely to provide a competitive advantage. Do you believe that most athletes use such substances routinely? Do you think that athletes should be able to use these substances without intervention or regulation? Why or why not?

Profile Plus

Assess your current fitness levels and begin planning for a fitter future with these activities on your Profile Plus CD-ROM:

Profile Plus

- Exercise Prescription
- Exercise Log
- Cardiovascular Risk
- Cardiorespiratory Endurance

Profile Plus

- Skill-Related Fitness
- Muscular Strength and Endurance Test
- Heart Rate and Blood Pressure

Sites and Bytes

Just Move.

www.justmove.org

At this website sponsored by the American Heart Association, after a free registration, you can access an interactive exercise diary where you can keep track of your own exercise progress. In addition, an information resource called My Fitness provides recommendations for optimizing your exercise program to match your lifestyle, as well as a list of health and fitness resources.

Sites and Bytes

Georgia State University's Exercise and Physical Fitness Page

www.gsu.edu/~wwwfit

Sponsored by the Department of Kinesiology and Health at Georgia State University, this site features a series of links containing research-based exercise and fitness information, including how to get started on an exercise program and stay with it, aerobic exercises, strength training, flexibility, nutrition, and body composition.

Sites and Bytes

Health A to Z

www.healthatoz.com/healthatoz/ Atoz/hl/fit/demo/excerdemo.html

This website has animated models showing the proper technique for various exercises. The site also has a "Getting Started" section that has tips and short workouts good for the heart.

InfoTrac College Edition

Activity

Suminski, Richard R., et al. "Physical Activity Among Ethnically Diverse College Students" *Journal of American College Health,* Volume 51, No. 2, September 2002, p. 75(6).

1. What is the relationship between ethnicity and gender differences on

InfoTrac College Edition

the rates of physical activity in college students?

2. What factors influence physical activity patterns among college students?

3. Describe some of the explanations for the relatively low levels of physical activity seen in women.

InfoTrac College Edition

You can find additional readings related to fitness with InfoTrac College Edition, an online library of more than 900 journals and publications. Follow the instructions for accessing InfoTrac that were packaged with your textbook; then search for articles using a keyword search.

For addition links, resources, and suggested readings on InfoTrac, visit our Health & Wellness Resource Center at **http://health.wadsworth.com**.

Key Terms

The terms listed are used on the page indicated. Definitions of the terms are in the Glossary at the end of this book.

Key Terms

Key Terms

Key Terms

active stretching 125
acute injuries 130
aerobic exercise 104
anabolic steroids 123
anaerobic exercise 114
ballistic stretching 126
body composition 104
body mass index
    (BMI) 126
cardiorespiratory
    fitness 104
conditioning 104
cross-training 117
dynamic flexibility 124
endorphins 111

endurance 104
ergogenic aids 123
FITT 112
flexibility 104, 124
isokinetic 121
isometric 121
isotonic 121
muscular fitness 104
osteoporosis 111
overload principle 112
overloading 120
overtrain 132
overuse injuries 130
passive stretching 125
physical fitness 104

principle of reversibility
    113
progressive
    overloading 112
Rating of Perceived
    Exertion (RPE) 115
rep (or repetition) 121
resting heart rate 114
sets 122
specificity principle 112
static flexibility 124
static stretching 125
strength 104
target heart rate 114
waist-to-hip ratio 127

References

1. Suminski, Richard, et al. "Physical Activity Among Ethnically Diverse College Students," *Journal of American College Health,* Vol. 51, September 2002, p. 75.
2. Sparling, Phillip, and Teresa Snow. "Physical Activity Patterns in Recent College Alumni." *Research Quarterly for Exercise and Sport,* Vol. 73, No. 2, June 2002, p. 200.
3. "Biology Shows Women and Men Are Different." *Mayo Clinic Women's Healthsource,* September 2002.
4. "Physical Activity and Health: Adults," A Report of the Surgeon General, President's Council on Physical Fitness and Sports, http://www.cdc.gov.
5. "CDC Reports Levels of Physical Activity in the 1990s Remained Unchanged." *Medical Letter on the CDC & FDA,* April 1, 2001.
6. Lindstrom, Martin, et al. "Socioeconomic Differences in Leisure-time Physical Activity." *Social Science & Medicine,* Vol. 52, No. 3, February 2001, p. 441.
7. Hu, Frank, et al. "Television Watching and Other Sedentary Behaviors in Relation to Risk of Obesity and Type 2 Diabetes Mellitus in Women," *Journal of American Medical Association,* Vol. 289, No. 14, April 9, 2003, p. 1785.
8. Suminsky, "Physical Activity Among Ethnically Diverse College Students."
9. Ibid.
10. Kimm, Sue, et al. "Decline in Physical Activity in Black Girls and White Girls During Adolescence," *New England Journal of Medicine,* Vol. 347, September 5, 2002, p. 709.
11. Sparling and Snow, "Physical Activity Patterns in Recent College Alumni."
12. Marcus, Bess, and Beth Lewis. "Physical Activity and the Stages of Motivational Readiness for Change Model," *President's Council on Physical Fitness and Sports Research Digest,* Series 4, No. 1, March 2003, p. 1.
13. Marcus, H. and L. J. Forsyth. *Motivating People to Be Physically Active.* Champaign, IL: Human Kinetics, 2003.
14. Butler, Lawrence, and Steen Anderson. "Inspiring Students for a Lifetime of Physical Activity," *JOPERD—The Journal of Physical Education, Recreation & Dance,* Vol. 73, No. 9, November–December 2002, p. 21.
15. Adams, Daniel, et al. "Body Image and Physical Fitness as a Function of Locus of Control and Gender in College Women and Men." *Research Quarterly for Exercise and Sport,* Vol. 72, No. 1, March 2001, p. A-18.
16. Wallace, Lorraine, et al. "Characteristics of Exercise Behavior Among College Students." *Preventive Medicine,* Vol. 31, No. 5, November 1, 2000.
17. Ibid.
18. DeVoe, Dale, and Cathy Kennedy. "Physical Activity Stages-of-Change and Activity Self-Efficacy of College Students Enrolled in a University-Required Fitness and Wellness Course." *Research Quarterly for Exercise and Sport,* Vol. 72, No. 1, March 2001, p. A-28.
19. "How Fit You Are Determines Your Life Span." *Tufts University Health & Nutrition Letter,* Vol. 20, No. 5, July 2002, p. 6.
20. "Information From Your Family Doctor. Physical Activity For Healthy Weight," *American Family Physician,* Vol. 67, No. 6, March 15, 2003, p. 1266.
21. "How Fit You Are Determines Your Life Span."
22. McInnis, Kyle, et al. "Counseling for Physical Activity in Overweight and Obese Patients," *American Family Physician,* Vol. 67, No. 6, March 15, 2003, p. 1254.
23. Booth, Frank, et al. "Physiologists Claim 'SeDS' Is Second Greatest Threat to U.S. Public Health." *Medical Letter on the CDC & FDA,* June 24, 2001.
24. Booth, Frank, et al. "Waging War on Modern Chronic Diseases: Primary Prevention Through Exercise Biology." *Journal of Applied Physiology,* Vol. 88, No. 2, February 2000.
25. Wallace, Lorraine, et al. "Promoting Physical Activity in the Family Practice Setting," *American Family Physician,* Vol. 67, No. 6, March 15, 2003, p. 1196.
26. MacIntosh, D. "Getting the Facts on Physical Activity," *Canadian Family Physician,* Vol. 49, January 2003, p. 23.
27. College of Family Physicians of Canada, www.cfpc.ca.
28. Gretebeck, K. "Behavioral Counseling in Primary Care to Promote Physical

References

Activity: Recommendation and Rationale," *American Fitness*, Vol. 21, No. 1, January–February 2003, p. 16.

29. Elley, C. Raina, et al. "Effectiveness of Counseling Patients on Physical Activity in General Practice: Cluster Randomised Controlled Trial," *British Medical Journal*, Vol. 326, April 12, 2003, p. 793.

30. Palatini, P., et al. "Exercise Capacity and Mortality," *New England Journal of Medicine*, Vol. 347, No. 4, July 25, 2002, p. 288.

31. Roberts, Shauna. "Why Exercise Matters." *Diabetes Forecast*, Vol. 55, No. 8, August 2002, p. 73.

32. "Heart Beat—Activity Keeps the Blood Flowing." *Harvard Heart Letter*, Vol. 12, No. 11, July 2002.

33. Duncan, Glen. "Exercise and Insulin Resistance Syndrome." *Diabetes Care*, Vol. 26, March 2003, pp. 557–562; Sheard, N. F. "Moderate Changes in Weight and Physical Activity Can Prevent or Delay the Development of Type 2 Diabetes Mellitus in Susceptible Individuals," *Nutrition Review*, Vol. 61, No. 2, February 2003, pp. 76–79.

34. Stevens, J., et al. "Fitness and Fatness as Predictors of Mortality From All Causes and From Cardiovascular Disease in Men and Women in the Lipid Research Clinics Study," *American Journal of Epidemiology*, Vol. 156, No. 9, November 1, 2002, p. 832.

35. "Regular Physical Exertion May Fight Cancer As Well As Heart Disease." *Tufts University Health & Nutrition Letter*, Vol. 18, No. 7, September 2000.

36. Dorn, J., et al. "Lifetime Physical Activity and Breast Cancer Risk in Pre- and Postmenopausal Women," *Medicine and Science in Sports and Exercise*, Vol. 35, No. 2, 2003, pp. 278–285.

37. Hawkins, S. A., et al. "Five-Year Maintenance of Bone Mineral Density in Women Master Runners," *Medicine and Science in Sports and Exercise*, Vol. 35, No. 1, 2003, pp. 137–144.

38. "Mild Aerobic Exercise No Protection From Osteoporosis," *FDA Consumer*, Vol. 37, No. 1, 2003, p. 8.

39. Cussler, E. C., et al. "Weight Lifted in Strength Training Predicts Bone Change in Postmenopausal Women." *Medicine and Science in Sports and Exercise*, Vol. 35, No. 1, 2003, pp. 10–17.

40. "Exercise and Illness." *JOPERD—The Journal of Physical Education, Recreation & Dance*, Vol. 73, No. 6, August 2002, p. 19.

41. Babyak, Michael, et al. "Exercise Treatment for Major Depression: Maintenance of Therapeutic Benefit at 10 Months." *Psychosomatic Medicine*, Vol. 62, No. 5, September–October 2000, pp. 633–638.

42. Abdel-Hamid, T. K. "Exercise and Diet in Obesity Treatment: An Integrative System Dynamics Perspective." *Medicine and Science in Sports and Exercise*, Vol. 35, No. 3, 2003, pp. 400–414."

43. Mayo, M. J., et al. "Exercise-Induced Weight Loss Preferentially Reduces Abdominal Fat," *Medicine and Science in Sports and Exercise*, Vol. 35, No. 2, 2003, pp. 207–213.

44. National Blueprint: Increasing Physical Activity Among Adults Age 50 and Older. National Center for Chronic Disease Prevention and Health Promotion. Washington, DC: May 1, 2001.

45. Grubbs, Laurie, and Jason Carter. "The Relationship of Perceived Benefits and Barriers to Reported Exercise Behaviors in College Undergraduates." *Family and Community Health*, Vol. 25, No. 2, July 2002, p. 76.

46. Plunk, Jamey, et al. "The Relationship Between Fitness Level and Academic Success Among College Students." *Research Quarterly for Exercise and Sport*, Vol. 72, No. 1, March 2001, p. A-34.

47. Hu et al., "Television Watching and Other Sedentary Behaviors."

48. "Exercise and Your Health," *Mayo Clinic Health Letter*, Vol. 21, No. 4, April 2003, p. 1.

49. Haennel, Robert, and Francine Lemire. "Physical Activity to Prevent Cardiovascular Disease," *Canadian Family Physician*, Vol. 48, 2002, p. 65.

50. Panel on Macronutrients; Subcommittees on Upper Reference Levels of Nutrients and Interpretation and Uses of Dietary Reference Intakes, and the Standing Committee on the Scientific Evaluation of Dietary Reference Intakes. *Dietary Reference Intakes for Energy, Carbohydrates, Fiber, Fat, Protein and Amino Acids*. Washington, DC: National Academy of Sciences Press, 2002.

51. Yu, S., et al. "What Level of Physical Activity Protects Against Premature Cardiovascular Death? The Caerphilly Study," *Heart*, Vol. 89, April 2003, p. 502.

52. American College of Sports Medicine, www.acsm.org.

53. Burke, Edmund. "Heart Rate ABCs," *Better Nutrition*, Vol. 64, No. 8, August 2002, p. 48.

54. "Measuring Exercise Intensity," *IDEA Personal Trainer*, Vol. 13, No. 9, October 2002, p. 60.

55. Manson, JoAnn, et al. "Walking Compared with Vigorous Exercise for the Prevention of Cardiovascular Events in Women." *New England Journal of Medicine*, Vol. 347, September 5, 2002, p. 716.

56. Lee, I-Min, et al. "Physical Activity and Coronary Heart Disease in Women: Is

'No Pain, No Gain' Passé?" *Journal of the American Medical Association*, Vol. 285, No. 11, March 21, 2001, p. 1447.

57. "Heart Lines—Walking and Gardening Beneficial for Heart Disease Patients." *Harvard Heart Letter*, Vol. 11, No. 8, April 2001.

58. Yaffe, Kristin, et al. "A Prospective Study of Physical Activity and Cognitive Decline in Elderly Women." *Archives of Internal Medicine*, Vol. 161, No. 14, July 23, 2001, p. 1703.

59. Welch, Gregory. "Learning to Let Go." *American Fitness*, Vol. 19, No. 4, July 2001, p. 61.

60. Hicks, Bernard. "America on the Move: The National Health Campaign for 2003," press release, Aerobics and Fitness Association of America, April 2003.

61. Kofoed, Jennifer, et al. "ACSM Review: Progression Models in Resistance Training," *IDEA Personal Trainer*, Vol. 14, No. 3, March 2003, p. 19; Larew, K., et al. "Muscle Metabolic Function, Exercise Performance, and Weight Gain," *Medicine and Science in Sports and Exercise*, Vol. 35, No. 2, 2003, pp. 230–236.

62. Price, T. B., et al. "Smoking Impairs Muscle Recovery from Exercise," *European Journal of Applied Physiology*, Vol. 89, No. 1, March 2003, p. 85.

63. Mark, Stephen. "Ergogenic Aids: Powders, Pills, and Potions to Enhance Performance." *American Family Physician*, Vol. 63, No. 5, March 1, 2001, p. 842.

64. Broeder, C. E. "Oral Andro-Related Prohormone Supplementation: Do the Potential Risks Outweigh the Benefits?" *Canadian Journal of Applied Physiology*, Vol. 28, No. 1, February 2003, p. 102.

65. Schilling, Brian, et al. "Creatine Supplementation and Health Variables: A Retrospective Study." *Medicine and Science in Sports and Exercise*, Vol. 33, No. 2, February 2001, p. 183.

66. Cho, Hunchul, et al. "The Effect of Creatine Supplementation in Anaerobic Power and Blood Fatigue Factors." *Research Quarterly for Exercise and Sport*, Vol. 72, No. 1, March 2001, p. 19.

67. Wilder, Nathan, et al. "The Effects of Low-Dose Creatine Supplementation Versus Creatine Loading in Collegiate Football Players." *Journal of Athletic Training*, Vol. 36, No. 2, April–June 2001, p. 124.

68. Mayhew, D. L., et al. "Effects of Long-Term Creatine Supplementation on Liver and Kidney Functions in American College Football Players," *International Journal of Sport Nutrition and Exercise Metabolism*, Vol. 12, No. 4, December 2002, pp. 453–460.

References

69. Ahrendt, Dale. "Ergogenic Aids: Counseling the Athlete." *American Family Physician,* Vol. 63, No. 5, March 1, 2001, p. 913.

70. "Performance Boosters: Science vs. Hype." *Berkeley Wellness Letter,* December 2000.

71. Connolly, D. A., et al. "Treatment and Prevention of Delayed Onset Muscle Soreness," *Journal of Strength and Conditioning Research,* Vol. 17, No. 1, February 2003, pp. 187–196.

72. Choo, Vivien. "WHO Reassesses Appropriate Body-Mass Index for Asian Populations." *Lancet,* Vol. 360, No. 9328, July 20, 2002, p. 235.

73. "Use of Body Mass Index and Waist Circumference to Predict Risk of Chronic Disease." *Journal of the American Dietetic Association,* Vol. 101, No. 6, June 2001, p. 708.

74. Tylavsky, F. A., et al. "Comparison of the Effectiveness of 2 Dual-Energy X-Ray Absorptiometers with That of Total Body Water and Computed Tomography in Assessing Changes in Body Composition During Weight Change," *American Journal of Clinical Nutrition,* Vol. 77, No. 2, February 2003, pp. 356–363.

75. Vescovi, J. D., et al. "Evaluation of the BOD POD for Estimating Percent Fat in Female College Athletes," *Journal of Strength Conditioning Research,* Vol. 17, No. 1, February 2003, pp. 197–208.

76. Utter, A. C., et al. "Evaluation of Air Displacement for Assessing Body Composition of Collegiate Wrestlers," *Medicine and Science in Sports and Exercise,* Vol. 35, No. 3, March 2003, p. 500.

77. Stevens et al., "Fitness and Fatness as Predictors of Mortality."

78. Bowden, Rodney, and Jamey Plunk. "The Relationship Between Fitness Level and Nutrition Habits." *Research Quarterly for Exercise and Sport,* Vol. 72, No. 1, March 2001, p. A-25.

79. "Eating and Exercise: When and What to Eat," Mayo Clinic Fitness & Medicine Center, www.mayoclinic.com.

80. Clark, Nancy. "Muscle Mix." *American Fitness,* Vol. 19, No. 3, May 2001, p. 48.

81. White, K., et al. "EMG Power Spectra of Intercollegiate Athletes and Anterior Cruciate Ligament Injury Risk in Females," *Medicine and Science in Sports and Exercise,* Vol. 35, No. 3, 2003, pp. 371–376.

82. Fagenbaum, R., and W. G. Darling, "Jump Landing Strategies in Male and Female College Athletes and the Implications of Such Strategies for Anterior Cruciate Ligament Injury," *American Journal of Sports Medicine,* Vol. 31, No. 2, March–April 2003, p. 233.

83. O'Dea, Jennifer and Suzanne Abraham. "Eating and Exercise Disorders in Young College Men," *Journal of American College Health,* Vol. 50, May 2002, p. 273.

84. Sullum, Julie, et al. "Predictors of Exercise Relapse in a College Population," *Journal of American College Health,* Vol. 48, No. 4, January 2000.

Personal Nutrition

The freshmen on the fifth floor of a university dormitory decided to test a dubious premise: that man—and woman—can live on pizza alone. For a month, they vowed to eat nothing but pizza in all its savory varieties—mushroom, pepperoni, sausage, anchovies, extra cheese, thin crust, double crust. In less than a week, most cringed at the very sight of yet another cardboard delivery box. It wasn't just the boredom of having the same meal that got to them. Some felt bloated. Others had stomachaches. A few complained of headaches and fatigue. One was convinced she had scurvy, a vitamin deficiency disease caused by a lack of fruit and vegetables. None of them managed to stick with pizza for an entire month.

As these students discovered, the foods we choose to eat have an enormous impact on how we feel—and not just in the short term. As demonstrated by the science of **nutrition,** the field that explores the connections between our bodies and the foods we eat, our daily diet affects how long and how well we live. Sensible eating can provide energy for our daily tasks, protect us from many chronic illnesses, and may even extend longevity.

Many foods can serve as the building blocks of a healthy lifestyle. The latest federal guidelines for healthful eating reflect this fact by allowing greater flexibility in putting together a diet tailored to individual activity levels and nutritional needs.[1] However, making good food choices isn't easy. In 1900 people in the United States could choose from about 500 different foods; today we can choose from more than 50,000.[2] Faced with this bewildering array of products in stores and restaurants and a blitz of advertising claims, you may well find it hard to select the foods that not only taste good but also are good for you.

This chapter can help. It translates the latest information on good nutrition into specific advice that you can use to nourish yourself as well as enjoy the pleasure of eating well.

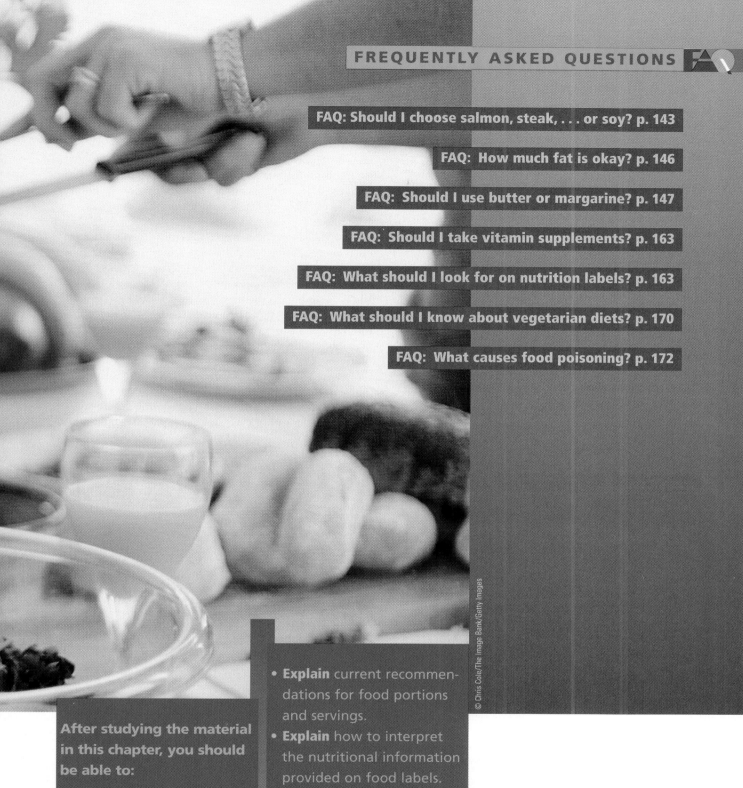

© Chris Cole/The Image Bank/Getty Images

After studying the material in this chapter, you should be able to:

- **List** the basic nutrients necessary for a healthy body and **describe** their functions.
- **Describe** the Food Guide Pyramid and explain its significance.

- **Explain** current recommendations for food portions and servings.
- **Explain** how to interpret the nutritional information provided on food labels.
- **Compare** the advantages and disadvantages of various alternative diets and ethnic foods.
- **List** the food safety hazards and describe prevention measures.

141

☒ What You Need to Know About Nutrients

Every day your body needs certain **essential nutrients** that it cannot manufacture for itself. They provide energy, build and repair body tissues, and regulate body functions. The six classes of essential nutrients, which are discussed in this section, are water, protein, carbohydrates, fats, vitamins, and minerals (see Table 5–1).

Water makes up about 60 percent of the body and is essential for health and survival. Besides water, we also need energy to live, and we receive our energy from the carbohydrates, proteins, and fats in the foods we eat. These three essential nutrients are called **macronutrients,** because they are the nutrients required by the human body in the greatest amounts. The amount of energy that can be derived from the macronutrients is measured in **calories.** There are 9 calories in every gram of fat and 4 calories in every gram of protein or carbohydrate. The other two essential nutrients—the vitamins and minerals—are called **micronutrients** because our bodies need them in only very small amounts.

Digestion is the process that releases nutrients into the body by breaking them down into compounds that are absorbed through the gastrointestinal tract (see Figure 5–1). Most foods provide a combination of nutrients, and a healthy diet contains a variety of foods supplying the entire range of essential nutrients.

In 2002 the federal government, in the latest of a series of reports from the Institute of Medicine, issued its first standards for intakes of macronutrients. These standards are likely to lead to changes in everything from the Food Pyramid to nutrition labels, both discussed later in this chapter.[3]

Individuals' need for macronutrients depends on how much energy they expend. Because fats, carbohydrates, and protein can all serve as sources of energy, they can, to some extent, substitute for one another in providing calories. Adults, according to the new standards, should get 45 to 65 percent of calories from carbohydrates, 20 to 35 percent from fat, and 10 to 35 percent from protein. Children's fat intake should be slightly higher: 25 to 40 percent of their caloric intake.

To eat well without overeating, choose foods that are "nutrient-dense," that is, foods that provide the most nutritional value. For example, both a cup of nonfat milk and an ounce and a half of cheddar cheese provide about 300

TABLE 5-1	The Essential Nutrients	
	Sources	**Functions**
Water	Liquids, fruits, and vegetables	Carries nutrients and removes waste; dissolves amino acids, glucose, and minerals; cleans body by removing toxins; regulates body temperature
Proteins	Meat, poultry, fish, eggs, beans, nuts, cheese, tofu, vegetables, some fruits, pastas, breads, cereal, and rice	Help build new tissue to keep hair, skin, and eyesight healthy; build antibodies, enzymes, hormones, and other compounds; provide fuel for body
Carbohydrates	Grains, cereal, pasta, fruits and vegetables, nuts, milk, and sugars	Provide energy
Fats		
Saturated Fats	Red meat, dairy products, egg yolks, and coconut and palm oils	Provide energy; trigger production of cholesterol (see Chapter 14)
Unsaturated Fats	Some fish; avocados; olive, canola, and peanut oils; shortening; stick margarine; baked goods	Also provide energy, but trigger more "good" cholesterol production and less "bad" cholesterol production (see Chapter 14)
Vitamins	Fruits, vegetables, grains, some meat and dairy products (see Table 5-5)	Facilitate use of other nutrients; involved in regulating growth, maintaining tissue, and manufacturing blood cells, hormones, and other body components
Minerals	Many foods (see Table 5-6)	Help build bones and teeth; aid in muscle function and nervous system activity; assist in various body functions including growth and energy production

This cola and bunch of grapes each provide about 150 calories, but the grapes offer a trace of protein, some vitamins, minerals, and fiber along with the energy; the cola beverage offers only "empty" calories from sugar without any other nutrients.

© Polara Studios Inc.

mg of calcium, but the milk offers the same amount of calcium for half the calories. Foods that are extremely low in nutrient density—such as potato chips, candy, and soft drinks—are "empty," delivering only calories with few, if any, nutrients.[4]

Water

Water, which makes up 85 percent of blood, 70 percent of muscles, and about 75 percent of the brain, performs many essential functions: It carries nutrients, maintains temperature, lubricates joints, helps with digestion, rids the body of waste through urine, and contributes to the production of sweat, which evaporates from the skin to cool the body. Research has correlated high fluid intake with a lower risk of kidney stones, colon cancer, and bladder cancer.

You lose about 64 to 80 ounces of water a day—the equivalent of eight to ten 8-ounce glasses—through perspiration, urination, bowel movements, and normal exhalation. You lose water more rapidly if you exercise, live in a dry climate or at a high altitude, drink a lot of caffeine or alcohol (which increase urination), skip a meal, or become ill. To assure adequate water intake, nutritionists advise drinking a minimum of 64 ounces, enough so that your urine is not dark in color. New research indicates that healthy individuals can get adequate hydration from beverages other than plain water, including juice and soft drinks.[5]

Protein

Critical for growth and repair, **proteins** form the basic framework for our muscles, bones, blood, hair, and fingernails. Supplying 4 calories per gram, they are made of combinations of 20 **amino acids,** 9 of which we must get from our diet because the human body cannot produce them. These are called *essential amino acids.*

Animal proteins—meat, fish, poultry, and dairy products—are **complete proteins** that provide the nine essential amino acids. Grains, dry beans, and nuts are **incomplete proteins** that may have relatively low levels of one or two essential amino acids but fairly high levels of others. Combining incomplete proteins, such as beans and rice, ensures that the body gets sufficient protein.

Based on the latest data, the federal report reaffirms the previously established recommended level of protein intake: 0.8 gram per kilogram of body weight for adults. The panel did not set a tolerable upper intake level because of conflicting or inadequate data on the health risks of high-protein diets, although it did warn about this potential danger. The report also establishes age-based requirements for all nine of the essential amino acids found in dietary protein.

Should I Choose Salmon, Steak, . . . or Soy?

Meat, fish, and soy are high-quality protein sources, and a healthy diet can include all of them. Lean red meat provides important minerals such as zinc and iron and B

FACT OR FICTION?

You shouldn't eat eggs.

Fiction: Eggs, once America's favorite breakfast food, fell out of favor several years ago. The reason: A single egg yolk contains about 200 milligrams of cholesterol, the maximum amount that federal guidelines say you should eat in a day. (Egg whites, rich in protein, have no cholesterol.) There is ongoing debate over the risk of eggs to healthy individuals.

Most people don't have to ban eggs from the breakfast table, but limit how often they are eaten. Avoid high-fat preparations like frying them in butter. If your diet is low in saturated fat, the cholesterol in any eggs you eat will have less impact on your blood cholesterol levels than if you're eating a lot of high-fat foods.

Source: USDA. "Eggs of Evil?" *Better Nutrition,* Vol. 65, No. 3, March 2003, p. 32.

Accessory Organs That Aid Digestion

Salivary Glands
Donate a starch-digesting enzyme
Donate a trace of fat-digesting enzyme (important to infants)

Liver
Manufactures bile, a detergent-like substance that facilitates digestion of fats

Gallbladder
Stores bile until needed

Bile Duct
Conducts bile to small intestine

Pancreatic Duct
Conducts pancreatic juice into small intestine

Pancreas
Manufactures enzymes to digest all energy-yielding nutrients
Releases bicarbonate to neutralize stomach acid that enters small intestine

Digestive Tract Organs That Contain the Food

Mouth
Chews and mixes food with saliva

Esophagus
Passes food to stomach

Stomach
Adds acid, enzymes, and fluid
Churns, mixes, and grinds food to a liquid mass

Small Intestine
Secretes enzymes that digest carbohydrate, fat, and protein
Cells lining intestine absorb nutrients into blood and lymph

Large Intestine (Colon)
Reabsorbs water and minerals
Passes waste (fiber, bacteria, any unabsorbed nutrients) and some water to rectum

Rectum
Stores waste prior to elimination

Anus
Holds rectum closed
Opens to allow elimination

Figure 5-1 THE DIGESTIVE SYSTEM
The organs of the digestive system break down food into nutrients that the body can use.

vitamins, which boost the functioning of the immune and nervous system, as well as amino acids that help build and maintain muscle mass. According to recent research, you can eat 6 ounces of lean red meat five or more days a week and still manage to lower or maintain your cholesterol level.[6]

Fish oils are rich in omega-3 fatty acids, which make molecules such as prostaglandins that enhance cardiovascular health. Fish oils also improve health blood lipids (fats), prevent blood clots, ward off the age-related vision problem called macular degeneration, and may lower blood pressure, especially in people with hypertension or atherosclerosis. The American Heart Association recommends at least two 3-ounce servings of fatty fish, such as salmon, tuna, and sardines, every week.

Unlike other proteins derived from plants, soy is complete, which makes it an important nutrient for vegetarians (vegetarian diets are discussed later in this chapter). But meat-eaters are also trying the vast new array of soy products and supplements on the market because of claims that soy can relieve hot flashes, strengthen bones, lower cholesterol, and reduce the risk of certain cancers. For now, however, no strong scientific proof backs up these promises, especially for soy supplements rather than foods. If you'd like to add soy to your diet, choose whole soy foods rather than isoflavone supplements.[7]

Carbohydrates

Carbohydrates are organic compounds that provide our brains and bodies with *glucose,* their basic fuel. The major sources of carbohydrates are plants—including grains, vegetables, fruits, and beans—and milk. There are two types: *simple carbohydrates* (sugars) and *complex carbohydrates* (starches and fiber). All provide 4 calories per gram. The new federal report recommends that both adults and children consume at least 130 grams of carbohydrates each day, the minimum needed to produce enough glucose for the brain to function.[8]

Forms of Carbohydrates

Simple carbohydrates, include *natural sugars,* such as the lactose in milk and the fructose in fruit, and *added sugars* that are found in candy, soft drinks, fruit drinks, pastries, and other sweets. According to the federal report, added sugars should make up no more than 25 percent of total calories consumed. Those whose diets are higher in added sugars typically have lower intakes of other essential nutrients. Other nutritional advocacy groups, such as the Center for Science in the Public Interest, have challenged this recommendation and suggest a much lower 8 percent of calories, or about 40 grams of added sugar a day, for a person consuming 2,000 calories.

Complex carbohydrates include grains, cereals, vegetables, beans, and nuts. Americans, however, get most of their complex carbohydrates from refined grains, which have been stripped of fiber and many nutrients.

Far more nutritious are whole grains, which are made up of all components of the grain: the *bran* (or fiber-rich outer layer), the *endosperm* (middle layer), and the *germ* (the nutrient-packed inner layer). Increasing whole-grain consumption has become a public health priority, and several national health organizations have joined in recommending that Americans increase their consumption of whole-grain foods to at least three servings every day. Individuals

who eat whole-grain products each day have about a 15 to 25 percent reduction in death from all causes, including heart disease and cancer.[9]

Fiber

Dietary fiber is the nondigestible form of complex carbohydrates occurring naturally in plant foods, such as leaves, stems, skins, seeds, and hulls. **Functional fiber** consists of isolated, nondigestible carbohydrates that may be added to foods and that provide beneficial effects in humans. Total fiber is the sum of both.

The various forms of fiber enhance health in different ways: They slow the emptying of the stomach, which creates a feeling of fullness and aids weight control. They interfere with absorption of dietary fat and cholesterol, which lowers the risk of heart disease and stroke in both middle-aged and elderly individuals.[10] In addition, fiber helps prevent constipation, diverticulosis (a painful inflammation of the bowel), and diabetes.[11] The link between fiber and colon cancer is complex. Some studies have indicated that increased fiber intake reduces risk; a large-scale study of almost 90,000 women found no such correlation.[12]

The federal report on macronutrients set the first-ever recommendations for daily intake levels of total fiber (dietary plus functional fiber): 38 grams of total fiber for men and 25 grams for women. For men and women over 50 years of age, who consume less food, the recommendations are, respectively, 30 and 21 grams. The American Dietetic Association recommends 25 to 35 grams of dietary fiber a day, much more than the amount Americans typically consume.[13]

FACT OR FICTION?

Chocolate is a health food (sort of).

Fact: Researchers at the University of California at Davis who reviewed recent studies on chocolate—particularly dark chocolate—found that it contains minerals and specific antioxidants that help ward off diseases. These phytochemicals, called flavonols, also found in red wine and tea, may enhance heart health by inhibiting blood clotting and widening blood vessels to maintain healthy blood flow.

Source: Shara Aaron. "Chocolate and Cardiovascular Disease," *Journal of the American Dietetic Association,* Vol. 103, No. 2, February 2003, p. 155.

TABLE 5-2	Putting Fiber into Meals and Snacks	

High-Fiber Options for Breakfast

Whole-grain toast		2 g per slice
Bran cereal:		
Bran flakes	1 cup	7 g
All Bran	⅓ cup	10 g
Raisin bran	¾ cup	5 g
Oat bran	⅓ cup	5 g
Bran muffin, with fruit	1 small	3 g
Strawberries	10	2 g
Raspberries	½ cup	3 g
Banana	1 medium	2 g

Lunches That Include Fiber

Whole-grain bread		2 g per slice
Baked beans	½ cup	10 g
Carrot	1 medium	2 g
Raisins	¼ cup	2 g
Peas	½ cup	6 g
Peanut butter	2 tablespoons	2 g

Fiber on the Menu for Supper

Brown rice	½ cup	2 g
Potato	1 medium	3 g
Dried cooked beans	½ cup	8 g
Broccoli	½ cup	3 g
Corn	½ cup	5 g
Tomato	1 medium	2 g
Green beans	½ cup	3 g

Fiber-Filled Snacks

Peanuts	¼ cup	3 g
Apple	1 medium	2 g
Pear	1 medium	4 g
Orange	1 medium	3 g
Prunes*	3	2 g
Sunflower seeds	¼ cup	2 g
Popcorn	2 cups	2 g

*Prunes contain fiber, but their laxative effect is primarily due to a naturally occurring chemical substance that causes an uptake of fluid into the intestines and the contraction of muscles that line the intestines.

Source: Judith E. Brown. *Nutrition Now*. 3rd ed. Belmont, CA: Wadsworth, 2002.

Good fiber sources include wheat and corn bran (the outer layer); leafy greens; the skins of fruits and root vegetables; oats, beans, and barley; and the pulp, skin, and seeds of many fruits and vegetables, such as apples and strawberries. Because sudden increases in fiber can cause symptoms like bloating and gas, experts recommend gradually adding more fiber to your diet with an additional serving or two of vegetables, fruit, or whole wheat bread.[14]

Fats

Fats carry the fat-soluble vitamins A, D, E, and K; aid in their absorption in the intestine; protect organs from injury; regulate body temperature; and play an important role in growth and development. They provide 9 calories per gram—more than twice the amount in carbohydrates or proteins.

Forms of Fat

Saturated fats and **unsaturated fats** are distinguished by the type of fatty acids in their chemical structures. Unsaturated fats can be divided into monounsaturated or polyunsaturated, again depending on their chemical structure. All dietary fats are a mix of saturated and unsaturated fats but are predominantly one or the other (Figure 5-2). Unsaturated fats, like oils, are likely to be liquid at room temperature and saturated fats, like butter, are likely to be solid. In general, vegetable and fish oils are unsaturated, and animal fats are saturated.

Olive, soybean, canola, cottonseed, corn, and other vegetable oils are unsaturated fats. Olive oil is considered a good fat and one of the best vegetable oils for salads and cooking. Used for thousands of years, this staple of the Mediterranean diet, discussed later in this chapter, has been correlated with a lower incidence of heart disease, including strokes and heart attacks. The omega-3 fatty acids in deep-water fish like salmon are unsaturated and may help lower the risk of cardiovascular disease.[15]

In contrast, saturated fats can increase the risk of heart disease and should be avoided as much as possible. In response to consumer and health professionals' demand for less saturated fat in the food supply, many manufacturers switched to partially hydrogenated oils.

The process of hydrogenation creates unsaturated fatty acids called **trans fat.** They are found in some margarine products and most foods made with partially hydrogenated oils, such as baked goods and fried foods. Even though trans fats are unsaturated, they appear similar to saturated fats in terms of raising cholesterol levels. Epidemiological studies have suggested a possible link between cardiovascular disease risk and high intakes of trans fats, and researchers have concluded that they are, gram for gram, twice as damaging as saturated fat. There is no safe level for trans fats, which occur naturally in meats as well as in foods prepared with partially hydrogenated vegetable oils. The federal panel recommends that trans fats be listed on food product labels so people can reduce their intake.

To cut down on both saturated and trans fats, choose soybean, canola, corn, olive, safflower, and sunflower oils, which are naturally free of trans fats and lower in saturated fats. Look for reduced-fat, low-fat, fat-free, and trans fat–free versions of baked goods, snacks, and other processed foods.

How Much Fat Is Okay?

Both high- and low-fat diets can be unhealthy. When people eat very low levels of fat and very high levels of carbohydrates, their levels of high-density lipoprotein, the

☐ Saturated fats ☐ Monounsaturated fats ☐ Polyunsaturated fats

• Animal fats and the tropical oils of coconut and palm are mostly **saturated.**

Coconut oil	
Butter	
Beef tallow	
Palm oil	
Lard	

• Some vegetable oils, such as olive and canola, are rich in **monounsaturated** fatty acids.

Olive oil	
Canola oil	
Peanut oil	

• Many vegetable oils are rich in **polyunsaturated** fatty acids.

Safflower oil	
Sunflower oil	
Corn oil	
Soybean oil	
Cottonseed oil	

Figure 5-2 COMPARISON OF DIETARY FATS

Most fats are a mixture of saturated, monounsaturated, and polyunsaturated fatty acids.

At room temperature, saturated fats (such as those found in butter) are solid, whereas unsaturated fats (such as those found in oil) are usually liquid.

© Polara Studios, Inc.

so-called *good cholesterol,* declines. On the other hand, high-fat diets can lead to obesity and its related health dangers, discussed in Chapter 6.

Ever since the first U.S. food guide was published in 1916, federal dietary guidelines have urged Americans to limit fat intake, but the amounts have varied from "moderate" to "sparingly" to 20–35 percent of calories.[16] The American Heart Association and American Cancer Society suggest no more than 30 percent of calories from fat. Table 5-3 shows the percentage of fat calories in various foods.

High-fat diets are associated with a higher risk of heart disease, but it is not clear whether an extreme reduction in dietary fat invariably lowers this risk. People who eat a high-carbohydrate diet—including excessive hard candies, fat-free cookies, and fat-free frozen yogurt—often have high levels of triglycerides, fats that circulate in the bloodstream.

▣ Should I Use Butter or Margarine?

The debate over what to spread on bread has been raging for years. First, butter was targeted as an unhealthy choice because it is high in saturated fats. (See Table 5-4 on page 149). Then margarines came under fire because they contain harmful trans fats, which can raise bad LDL cholesterol at least as much as saturated fat. Baffled consumers haven't been sure which to choose. Margarine con-

sumption has fallen since 1993, while butter sales have held steady or spiked upward.

Although butter still has its backers, the healthier choice actually is margarine—particularly tub margarine. A tablespoon of butter contains about 7 grams of saturated fat, while the same amount of stick margarine has, at most, 5 grams of saturated fat and trans fats combined. The soft margarines in tubs and tubes have much less because trans fats are formed when the liquid oils used to make margarine are hardened. The harder the margarine, the more trans fats it contains.

When looking for a margarine, try to choose one in which the trans fats and the saturated fat content are the lowest. Trans fat-free margarines are available, but even so, check labels to make sure you're not getting more than 2 grams of saturated fat per serving. If you like the taste of butter, choose a tub margarine that contains whey protein for a close-to-the-real-thing buttery taste.

Some margarines are being marketed as medicines. Benecol, for instance, is a canola-oil based, margarine-like spread that contains phytochemicals from pine trees, soy, corn, and wheat known to inhibit the body's ability to absorb cholesterol—be it cholesterol in foods or cholesterol produced by the liver. Three servings a day may lower LDL by as much as 10 percent.

TABLE 5-3	Percentage of Fat Calories in Foods			
Type of Food	**Less Than 15% of Calories from Fat**	**15%–30% of Calories from Fat**	**30%–50% of Calories from Fat**	**More Than 50% of Calories from Fat**
Fruits and Vegetables	Fruits, plain vegetables, juices, pickles, sauerkraut		French fries, hash browns	Avocados, coconuts, olives
Bread and Cereals	Grains and flours, most breads, most cereals, corn tortillas, pita, matzoh, bagels, noodles, and pasta	Corn bread, flour tortillas, oatmeal, soft rolls and buns, wheat germ	Breakfast bars, biscuits and muffins, granola, pancakes and waffles, donuts, taco shells, pastries, croissants	
Dairy Products	Nonfat milk, dry curd cottage cheese, nonfat cottage cheese, nonfat yogurt	Buttermilk, low-fat yogurt, 1% milk, low-fat cottage cheese	Whole milk, 2% milk, creamed cottage cheese	Butter, cream, sour cream, half & half, most cheeses (including part-skim and lite cheeses)
Meats		Beef round; veal loin, round, and shoulder; pork tenderloin	Beef and veal, lamb, fresh and picnic hams	All ground beef, spareribs, cold cuts, beef, hot dogs, pastrami
Poultry	Egg whites	Chicken and turkey (light meat without skin)	Chicken and turkey (light meat with skin, dark meat without skin), duck and goose (without skin)	Chicken/turkey (dark meat with skin), chicken-turkey hot dogs and bologna, egg yolks, whole eggs
Seafood	Clams, cod, crab, crawfish, flounder, haddock, lobster, perch, sole, scallops, shrimp, tuna (in water)	Bass and sea bass, halibut, mussels, oysters, tuna (fresh)	Anchovies, catfish, salmon, sturgeon, trout, tuna (in oil, drained)	Herring, mackerel, sardines
Beans and Nuts	Dried beans and peas, chestnuts, water chestnuts		Soybeans	Tofu, most nuts and seeds, peanut butter
Fats and Oils	Oil-free and some lite salad dressings			Butter, margarine, all mayonnaise (including reduced-calorie), most salad dressings, all oils
Soups	Bouillons, broths, consommé	Most soups	Cream soups, bean soups, "just add water" noodle soups	Cheddar cheese soup, New England clam chowder
Desserts	Angel food cake, gelatin, some fat-free cakes	Pudding, tapioca	Most cakes, most pies	
Frozen Desserts	Sherbet, low-fat frozen yogurt, sorbet, fruit ices	Ice milk	Frozen yogurt	All ice cream
Snack Foods	Popcorn (air popped), pretzels, rye crackers, rice cakes, fig bars, raisin biscuit cookies, marshmallows, most hard candy, fruit rolls	Lite microwave popcorn, Scandinavian "crisps," plain crackers, caramels, fudge, gingersnaps, graham crackers	Snack crackers, popcorn (popped in oil), cookies, candy bars, granola bars	Most microwave popcorn, corn and potato chips, chocolate, buttery crackers

Sources: American Heart Association and the U.S. Department of Agriculture.

Vitamins and Minerals

Vitamins, which help put proteins, fats, and carbohydrates to use, are essential to regulating growth, maintaining tissue, and releasing energy from foods. Together with the enzymes in the body, they help produce the right chemical reactions at the right times. They're also involved in the manufacture of blood cells, hormones, and other compounds.

The body produces some vitamins, such as vitamin D, which is manufactured in the skin after exposure to sun-

TABLE 5-4	Butter vs. Margarine		
Product (per Tablespoon)	Total Fat (grams)	Saturated Fat (grams)	Trans Fats (grams)
Butter	10.8	7.2	0.3
Margarine, stick (82% fat)	11.4	2.3	2.4
Margarine, tub (80% fat)	11.2	1.9	1.1
Margarine, stick (68% fat)	9.5	1.6	1.8
Margarine, tub (40% fat)	5.6	1.1	0.6

Sources: U.S. Food and Drug Administration and the U.S. Department of Agriculture.

light. Other vitamins must be ingested. Vitamins A, D, E, and K are fat-soluble; they are absorbed through the intestinal membranes and stored in the body. The B vitamins and vitamin C are water-soluble; they are absorbed directly into the blood and then used up or washed out of the body in urine and sweat. They must be replaced daily. Table 5-5 summarizes key information about vitamins.

Carbon, oxygen, hydrogen, and nitrogen make up 96 percent of our body weight. The other 4 percent consists of **minerals** that help build bones and teeth, aid in muscle function, and help our nervous system transmit messages. Every day we need about a tenth of a gram (100 milligrams) or more of the major minerals: sodium, potassium, chloride, calcium, phosphorus, magnesium, and sulfur. We also need about a hundredth of a gram (10 milligrams) or less of each of the trace minerals: iron (although premenopausal women need more), zinc, selenium, molybdenum, iodine, copper, manganese, fluoride, and chromium. See Table 5-6 on page 000 for a summary of mineral information.

How Antioxidants Work

Antioxidants are substances that prevent the harmful effects caused by oxidation within the body. They include vitamins C, E, and beta-carotene (a form of vitamin A) as well as compounds like carotenoids and flavonoids. All share a common enemy: renegade oxygen cells called free radicals released by normal metabolism, as well as by pollution, smoking, radiation, and stress.

Like tiny thugs, free radicals constantly roam through the body and attack cells in the brain, heart, bloodstream, and immune system. Antioxidants rush to the rescue, limit damage, and help repair any harm that's been done. Like bouncers in a nightclub, they wrap up the troublemakers and carry them away.

In the cardiovascular system, free radicals combine with cholesterol and dangerous LDL to damage the inner lining of blood vessels. In clinical studies, vitamin E has generally lowered the risk of heart attacks and strokes by 40 to 60 percent.

Other antioxidants, particularly supplements of vitamin C and beta-carotene, have not proved as helpful in protecting the heart. In epidemiological studies, however, individuals eating lots of dark green, yellow, and orange fruits and vegetables (good sources of vitamin C and beta-carotene) consistently have lower rates of coronary disease.

Diets high in antioxidant-rich fruits and vegetables have been linked with lower rates of esophageal, lung, colon, and stomach cancer. Nevertheless, scientific studies have not proved conclusively that any specific antioxidant, particularly in supplement form, can prevent cancer. In studies of beta-carotene, this carotenoid did not reduce overall cancer rates or mortality. In two studies of smokers, beta-carotene was actually associated with increased mortality from lung cancer.

In theory, though, antioxidants may slow the cumulative effect of free radicals in diseases associated with age, including memory impairment, cataracts, and arthritis. In laboratory and animal studies, vitamin E has shown particular promise in slowing neurological aging and improving cognitive function. Recent research suggests that vitamins C and E may reduce the risk of Alzheimer's Disease[17] and that high doses of vitamin E supplements may provide a modest boost in cognitive performance in the elderly.[18] Certain antioxidants, such as vitamin E, vitamin C, and beta-carotene, may also provide protection against age-related macular degeneration.

© 2000 PhotoDisc, Inc.

Antioxidants are found in vegetables and fruit. By eating an orange at breakfast and half a carrot for lunch, you will have all the antioxidants you need for the day.

TABLE 5-5	Key Information About Vitamins			

Vitamin/ Recommended Intake per Day	Significant Sources	Chief Functions	Signs of Severe, Prolonged Deficiency	Signs of Extreme Excess
Fat-Soluble Vitamins				
Vitamin A Males 19–50: 900 μg Females 19–50: 700 μg	Fortified milk, cheese, cream, butter, fortified margarine, eggs, liver; spinach and other dark, leafy greens, broccoli, deep orange fruits (apricots, cantaloupes) and vegetables (carrots, sweet potatoes, pumpkins)	Antioxidant; needed for vision, health of cornea, epithelial cells, mucous membranes, skin health, bone and tooth growth, reproduction, immunity	Anemia, painful joints, cracks in teeth, tendency toward tooth decay, diarrhea, depression, frequent infections, night blindness, keratinization, corneal degeneration, rashes, kidney stones	Nosebleeds, bone pain, growth retardation, headaches, abdominal cramps and pain, vomiting, diarrhea, weight loss, overreactive immune system, blurred vision, fatigue, irritability, hair loss, dry skin
Vitamin D Males 19–50: 5 μg Females 19–50: 5 μg	Fortified milk or margarine, eggs, liver, sardines; exposure to sunlight	Mineralization of bones (promotes calcium and phosphorus absorption)	Abnormal growth, misshapen bones (bowing of legs), soft bones, joint pain, malformed teeth	Raised blood calcium, excessive thirst, headaches, irritability, loss of appetite, weakness, nausea, kidney stones, stones in arteries
Vitamin E Males 19–50: 15 mg Females 19–50: 15 mg	Polyunsaturated plant oils (margarine, salad dressings, shortenings), green and leafy vegetables, wheat germ, whole-grain products, nuts, seeds	Antioxidant; needed for stabilization of cell membranes, regulation of oxidation reactions	Red blood cell breakage, anemia, muscle degeneration, difficulty walking, leg cramps	Augments the effects of anticlotting medication; general discomfort; blurred vision
Vitamin K Males 19–50: 120 μg Females 19–50: 90 μg	Green leafy vegetables, cabbage-type vegetables, soybeans, vegetable oils	Synthesis of blood-clotting proteins and proteins important in bone mineralization	Hemorrhage	Interference with anticlotting medication; jaundice
Water-Soluble Vitamins				
Vitamin B$_6$ Males 19–50: 1.3 mg Females 19–50: 1.3 mg	Meats, fish, poultry, liver, legumes, fruits, whole grains, potatoes, soy products	Part of a coenzyme used in amino acid and fatty acid metabolism, helps make red blood cells	Anemia, depression, abnormal brain wave pattern, convulsions, skin rashes	Impaired memory, irritability, headaches, numbness, damage to nerves, difficulty walking, loss of reflexes
Vitamin B$_{12}$ Males 19–50: 2.4 μg Females 19–50: 2.4 μg	Animal products (meat, fish, poultry, milk, cheese, eggs)	Part of a coenzyme used in new cell synthesis, helps maintain nerve cells	Anemia, nervous system degeneration progressing to paralysis, hypersensitivity	None known
Vitamin C Males 19–50: 90 mg Females 19–50: 75 mg	Citrus fruits, cabbage-type vegetables, dark green vegetables, cantaloupe, strawberries, peppers, lettuce, tomatoes, potatoes, papayas, mangoes	Antioxidant, collagen synthesis (strengthens blood vessel walls, forms scar tissue, matrix for bone growth), amino acid metabolism, strengthens resistance to infection, aids iron absorption	Anemia, pinpoint hemorrhages, frequent infections, bleeding gums, loosened teeth, muscle degeneration and pain, joint pain, blotchy bruises, failure of wounds to heal	Nausea, abdominal cramps, diarrhea, excessive urination, headache, fatigue, insomnia, rashes; deficiency symptoms may appear at first on withdrawal of high doses

TABLE 5-5	Key Information About Vitamins				
Vitamin/ Recommended Intake per Day	**Significant Sources**	**Chief Functions**	**Signs of Severe, Prolonged Deficiency**	**Signs of Extreme Excess**
Thiamin Males 19–50: 1.2 mg Females 19–50: 1.1 mg	Pork, ham, bacon, liver, whole grains, legumes, nuts; occurs in all nutritious foods in moderate amounts	Part of a coenzyme used in energy metabolism, supports normal appetite and nervous system function	Edema, enlarged heart, nervous/muscular system degeneration, difficulty walking, loss of reflexes, mental confusion	None reported
Riboflavin Males 19–50: 1.3 mg Females 19–50: 1.1 mg	Milk, yogurt, cottage cheese, meat, leafy green vegetables, whole-grain or enriched breads and cereals	Part of a coenzyme used in energy metabolism, supports normal vision and skin health	Cracks at corner of mouth, magenta tongue, hypersensitivity to light, reddening of cornea, skin rash	None reported
Niacin Males 19–50: 16 mg Females 19–50: 14 mg	Milk, eggs, meat, poultry, fish, whole-grain and enriched breads and cereals, nuts, and all protein-containing foods	Part of a coenzyme used in energy metabolism	Diarrhea, black smooth tongue, irritability, loss of appetite, weakness, dizziness, mental confusion, flaky skin rash on areas exposed to sun	Nausea, vomiting, painful flush and rash, sweating, liver damage
Folate Males 19–50: 400 µg Females 19–50: 400 µg	Leafy green vegetables, legumes, seeds, liver, enriched breads, cereal, pasta, and grains	Part of a coenzyme needed for new cell synthesis	Anemia, heartburn, frequent infections, smooth red tongue, depression, mental confusion	Masks vitamin B_{12} deficiency
Panothenic acid Males 19–50: 5 mg Females 19–50: 5 mg	Widespread in foods	Part of a coenzyme used in energy metabolism	Vomiting, intestinal distress, insomnia, fatigue	Water retention (rare)
Biotin Males 19–50: 30 µg Females 19–50: 30 µg	Widespread in foods	Used in energy metabolism, fat synthesis, amino acid metabolism, and glycogen synthesis	Abnormal heart action, loss of appetite, nausea, depression, muscle pain, drying of facial skin	None reported

Source: Adapted from Frances Sizer and Eleanor Whitney. *Nutrition: Concepts and Controversies,* 9th ed. Belmont, CA: Wadsworth, 2003.

Folic Acid

Folate is the generic term used to refer to various chemical forms of a water-soluble B vitamin that can be obtained from a diet high in vegetables and citrus fruit. **Folic acid** is the form used in vitamin supplements and fortified foods. Food manufacturers add folic acid to foods, primarily because insufficient levels increase the risk of neural tube defects (abnormalities of the brain and spinal cord), such as spina bifida, in which a piece of the spinal cord protrudes from the spinal column.[19] Folic acid also reduces blood levels of homocysteine, a chemical associated with increased risk of cardiovascular disease, and reduces the excess risk of breast cancer associated with alcohol consumption.

Calcium

Calcium, the most abundant mineral in the body, builds strong bone tissue throughout life and plays a vital role in heart and brain functioning. Pregnant or nursing women need more calcium to meet the additional needs of their babies' bodies. Calcium may also help control high blood pressure and prevent colon cancer in adults.[20]

Adequate calcium intake during childhood, adolescence, and young adulthood is crucial to prevent **osteoporosis,** the bone-weakening disease that strikes one of every four women over the age of 60. National health organizations are promoting greater calcium consumption among college students, particularly women, to increase bone density and safeguard against osteoporosis.

 In a study of college athletes, the most common food sources of calcium for both European-American and African-American students were mixed dishes and dairy products. There were no racial differences in calcium consumption levels, but male athletes consumed significantly more calcium than females.[21]

In both men and women, bone mass peaks between the ages of 25 and 35. Over the next 10 to 15 years, bone mass remains fairly stable. At about age 40, bone loss

TABLE 5-6	**Key Information About Essential Minerals**			
Mineral	**Significant Sources**	**Chief Functions**	**Signs of Severe, Prolonged Deficiency**	**Signs of Extreme Excess**
Major Minerals				
Sodium	Salt, soy sauce, processed foods	Needed to maintain fluid balance and acid-base balance in body cells; critical to nerve impulse transmission	Mental apathy, poor appetite, muscle cramps	High blood pressure
Potassium	All whole foods: meats, milk, fruits, vegetables, grains, legumes	Needed to maintain fluid balance and acid-base balance in body cells; needed for muscle and nerve activity	Muscle weakness, mental confusion, paralysis	Irregular heartbeat, heart attack; muscular weakness
Chloride	Salt, soy sauce, processed foods	Aids in digestion; needed to maintain fluid balance and acid-base balance in body cells	Muscle cramps, apathy, poor appetite, growth failure in children	Vomiting
Calcium	Milk and milk products, oysters, small fish (with bones), tofu, greens, legumes	Component of bones and teeth, needed for muscle and nerve activity, blood clotting	Stunted growth in children, adult bone loss (osteoporosis)	Constipation, calcium deposits in kidneys, liver, and other tissues, decreased absorption of other minerals
Phosphorus	All animal tissues	Component of bones and teeth, energy formation, needed to maintain cell membranes	Loss of appetite, muscle weakness, impaired growth	Loss of calcium from bones
Magnesium	Nuts, legumes, whole grains, dark green vegetables, seafoods, chocolate, cocoa	Component of bones and teeth, nerve activity, energy and protein formation	Stunted growth in children, weakness, muscle spasms, personality changes	Diarrhea, dehydration, impaired nerve activity
Sulfur	All protein-containing foods	Component of certain amino acids; stabilizes protein shape	None known; protein deficiency would occur first	Depresses growth in animals

Calcium-rich foods such as milk can help prevent bone loss and osteoporosis.

© PhotoDisc, Inc.

STRATEGIES FOR CHANGE

Building Stronger Bones

- Make calcium-rich foods part of your daily diet. These include dairy products, leafy green vegetables, canned fish, and tofu. Also look for products fortified with calcium and vitamin D, which aids in calcium absorption.

- Avoid cigarette smoking, which has been linked with bone loss.

- Drink alcohol only in moderation. Prolonged or heavy use of alcohol may decrease bone metabolism.

- Be wary of high-protein diets. Excess protein intake may increase the rate of calcium loss from the body.

- Do weight-bearing exercises. Activities such as walking, running, doing push-ups and sit-ups, and lifting weights all contribute to the development and maintenance of bone mass.

| TABLE 5-6 | Key Information About Essential Minerals | | | |

Mineral	Significant Sources	Chief Functions	Signs of Severe, Prolonged Deficiency	Signs of Extreme Excess
Trace Minerals				
Iron	Red meats, fish, poultry, shellfish, eggs, legumes, dried fruits	Aids in transport of oxygen, component of myoglobin, energy formation	Anemia, weakness, fatigue, pale appearance, reduced attention span, developmental delays in children	"Iron poisoning," vomiting, abdominal pain, blue coloration of skin, shock, heart failure, diabetes, decreased zinc absorption
Zinc	Protein-containing foods: fish, shellfish, poultry, grains, vegetables	Protein reproduction, component of insulin	Growth failure, delayed sexual maturation, slow wound healing	Nausea, vomiting, weakness, fatigue, susceptibility to infection, copper deficiency, metallic taste in mouth
Selenium	Meats and seafood, eggs, grains	Acts as an antioxidant in conjunction with vitamin E	Anemia, muscle pain and tenderness, Keshar disease, heart failure	Hair and fingernail loss, weakness, liver damage, garlic or metallic breath
Molybdenum	Dried beans, grains, dark green vegetables, liver, milk and milk products	Aids in oxygen transfer from one molecule to another	Rapid heartbeat and breathing, nausea, vomiting, coma	Loss of copper from the body, joint pain, growth failure, anemia, gout
Iodine	Iodized salt, milk and milk products, seaweed, seafood, bread	Component of thyroid hormones that helps regulate energy production and growth	Goiter, cretinism in newborns (mental retardation, hearing loss, growth failure)	Pimples, goiter, decreased thyroid function
Copper	Organ meats, whole grains, nuts and seeds, seafood, drinking water	Component of enzymes involved in the body's utilization of iron and oxygen	Anemia, nerve and bone abnormalities in children, growth retardation	Wilson's disease (excessive accumulation of copper in the liver and kidneys); vomiting, diarrhea, liver disease
Manganese	Whole grains, coffee, tea, dried beans, nuts	Formation of body fat and bone	Weight loss, rash, nausea and vomiting	Infertility in men, disruptions in the nervous system, muscle spasms
Fluoride	Fluoridated water, foods, and beverages; tea; shrimp; crab	Component of bones and teeth (enamel)	Tooth decay and other dental diseases	Fluorosis, brittle bones, mottled teeth, nerve abnormalities
Chromium	Whole grains, liver, meat, beer, wine	Glucose utilization	Poor blood glucose control, weight loss	Kidney and skin damage

Source: Adapted from Judith E. Brown. *Nutrition Now,* 3rd ed. Belmont, CA: Wadsworth, 2002 and Frances Sizer and Eleanor Whitney. *Nutrition: Concepts and Controversies,* 9th ed. Belmont, CA: Wadsworth, 2003.

equivalent to 0.3 to 0.5 percent per year begins in both men and women. Women may experience greater bone loss, at a rate of 3 to 5 percent, at the time of menopause. This decline continues for approximately five to seven years and is the primary factor leading to postmenopausal osteoporosis.

The higher an individual's peak bone mass, the longer it takes for age- and menopause-related bone losses to increase the risk of fractures. Osteoporosis is less common in groups with higher peak bone mass—men versus women, blacks versus whites. A combination of calcium and exercise can boost bone mineral density in teenage girls, which may prevent or delay osteoporosis later in life.[22]

Iron

Iron is an essential ingredient of **hemoglobin,** the protein that makes the blood red and carries oxygen to all our tissues. Because oxygen is needed to convert food into energy, too little iron—and thus too little hemoglobin—can trigger an internal energy crisis. Getting enough iron can be a big problem for women, whose iron stores are drained by menstruation, pregnancy, and nursing. Half of all women of childbearing age get less than the recommended 15 milligrams of iron, and 5 percent suffer from iron-deficiency anemia.

The symptoms of iron deficiency are sensitivity to cold, chronic fatigue, edginess, depression, sleeplessness, and susceptibility to colds and infections. To boost your iron, see the Strategies for Change. Don't take supplements unless you've had a blood test that indicates you should. Excess iron can cause severe constipation and other complications.

Sodium

Sodium helps maintain proper fluid balance, regulates blood pressure, transmits muscle impulses, and relaxes muscles. Excess sodium isn't a problem for most healthy people, but for those who are sodium-sensitive—as many as 30 percent of the population—too much sodium contributes to high blood pressure.

The National Heart, Lung, and Blood Institute recommends less than 2.4 grams (2,400 milligrams) of sodium a day, the equivalent of about one teaspoon of table salt a day. For someone with high blood pressure, a daily intake of less than 1,500 mg of sodium is better for lowering blood pressure.

Phytochemicals

Phytochemicals, compounds that exist naturally in plants, serve many functions, including helping a plant protect itself from bacteria and disease. Some phytochemicals such as solanine, an insect-repelling chemical found in the leaves and stalks of potato plants, are natural toxins, but many are beneficial to humans. Flavonoids, found in apples, strawberries, grapes, onions, green and black tea, and red wine, may decrease atherosclerotic plaque and DNA damage related to cancer developments. Phytochemicals are associated with a reduced risk of heart disease, certain cancers, age-related macular degeneration,

adult-onset diabetes, stroke, and other diseases. However, research has yet to show a cause-and-effect relationship between consumption of phytochemicals and prevention of a specific disease.

✖ Eating for Good Health

No one food can provide all the nutrients we need. To make sure you consume a healthful variety, the federal Dietary Guidelines suggest that you "let the Pyramid guide your food choices." The USDA's Food Guide Pyramid (see Figure 5-5 on page 160), adopted in 1992, has five categories of foods. These categories are not considered nutritional equals. For the sake of good health, you need some food from all the groups every day, but in different amounts.

In 2003 an expert panel commissioned by the World Health Organization (WHO) and the Food and Agriculture Organization recommended a diet low in energy-dense foods that are high in saturated fats and sugars and abundant in fruits and vegetables, coupled with an active lifestyle, as the best measure to combat chronic disease. Based on analysis of the best available scientific evidence, the report called for limited consumption of saturated and trans fats, sugars, and salt and noted that the quality of fats and oils in a diet can influence cardiovascular diseases, such as strokes and heart attacks. Its specific recommendations included limiting fat to between 15 and 30 percent of total calories, with saturated fats less than 10 percent of this total, protein 10 to 15 percent, and the bulk of calories—55 to 75 percent—from carbohydrates. The recommended maximum salt intake is less than 5 grams. In addition, the report recommended one hour a day of moderate intensity activity, such as walking, on most days of the week in order to maintain a healthy body weight.[23]

 College students often change the way they eat. In one recent survey, 59 percent of freshmen said their diet had changed since they began college. Two-thirds reported that they did not eat five fruits or vegetables daily; one-third no longer ate red meat.[24] In other studies, students of different ethnic backgrounds typically ate far less than the recommended amount of fruits and vegetables.[25] (See Student Snapshot: "How Freshmen Change the Way They Eat" on page 157.) Even college athletes, bombarded with nutrition information from coaches, trainers, and popular sports magazines, often do not know the role of various nutrients or which foods or fluids can boost their performance.[26]

Snacking has become more widespread on campuses, as in other places (see Figure 5-3 on page 157). College students snack primarily "to satisfy hunger"; the second most common reason is "no time for meals." Other reasons for munching between meals: "for energy," "to be sociable," and "to relieve stress." One-third snack at 9:00 P.M. or later.[27]

Self Survey
How Healthy Is Your Diet?

Step 1

For a week, write down everything you eat and drink for meals and snacks. Include the approximate amount eaten (for example, ½ cup, 1 large, 12 oz. can, and so on).

	Mon	Tues	Wed	Thurs	Fri	Sat	Sun
Grains							
Vegetables							
Fruits							
Milk, yogurt, cheese							
Meat, poultry, dry beans, eggs, nuts							
Fats, oil, sweets, cheese							

Step 2: Are You Getting Enough Vegetables, Fruits, and Grains?

How often do you eat:	Seldom/never	1–2 times a week	3–5 times a week	Almost daily
At least three servings of vegetables a day?				
Starchy vegetables like potatoes, corn, or peas?				
Foods made with dry beans, lentils, or peas?				
Dark green or deep yellow vegetables (broccoli, spinach, collards, carrots, sweet potatoes, squash)?				
At least two servings of fruit a day?				
Citrus fruits and 100% fruit juices (oranges, grapefruit, tangerines)?				
Whole fruit with skin or seeds (berries, apples, pears)?				
At least six servings of breads, cereals, pasta, or rice a day?				

The best answer for each is "almost daily." Use your food diary to see which foods you should be eating more often.

Step 3: Are You Getting Too Much Fat?

How often do you eat:	Seldom/never	1–2 times a week	3–5 times a week	Almost daily
Fried, deep-fat fried, or breaded food?				
Fatty meats, such as sausages, luncheon meat, fatty steaks or roasts?				
Whole milk, high-fat cheeses, ice cream?				
Pies, pastries, rich cakes?				
Rich cream sauces and gravies?				
Oily salad dressings or mayonnaise?				
Butter or margarine on vegetables, rolls, bread, or toast?				

Ideally, you should be eating these foods no more than one or two times a week. If your food diary indicates that you're eating them more frequently, your fat intake may well be too high.

(continued)

Self Survey **How Healthy Is Your Diet? (continued)**

Step 4: Are You Getting Too Much Sodium?

How often do you eat:	Seldom/never	1–2 times a week	3–5 times a week	Almost daily
Cured or processed meats, such as ham, sausage, frankfurters, or luncheon meats?				
Canned vegetables or frozen vegetables with sauce?				
Frozen TV dinners, entrees, or canned or dehydrated soups?				
Salted nuts, popcorn, pretzels, corn chips, or potato chips?				
Seasoning mixes or sauces containing salt?				
Processed cheese?				
Salt added to table foods before you taste them?				

Ideally, you should be eating these high-sodium items no more than one or two times a week. If your food diary indicates that you're eating them more frequently, your sodium intake may well be too high.

Your Health Change Plan

for Better Nutrition

:: **Eat five servings of fruits and vegetables per day.** For breakfast, have 100 percent juice or add raisins, berries, or sliced fruit to cereal, pancakes, or waffles. For lunch, have vegetable soup or salad with your meal or pile vegetables on your sandwich. For dinner, choose vegetables that are green, orange (such as carrots or squash), and red (such as tomatoes or bell peppers).

:: **Include three servings of whole-grain foods every day.** To identify whole-grain products, check the ingredient list. The first ingredient should be a whole grain, such as "whole-grain oats," "whole-grain wheat," or "whole wheat."

:: **Consume a calcium-rich food at each meal.** Good options include low-fat and nonfat milk, cheese, or yogurt; tofu; broccoli; dried beans; spinach; and fortified soy milk.

:: **Eat less meat.** Rather than making meat the heart of a meal, think of it as a flavoring ingredient.

:: **Avoid high-fat fast foods.** Hot dogs, fried foods, packaged snack foods, and pastries are most likely to be laden with fat.

:: **Check the numbers.** When buying prepared foods, choose items that contain no more than 3 grams of fat per 100 calories.

:: **Think small.** A dinner-size serving of meat should be about the size of a deck of cards; half a cup is the size of a woman's fist; a pancake is the diameter of a CD.

:: **Read labels carefully.** Remember that "cholesterol-free" doesn't necessarily mean fat-free. Avoid products that contain saturated coconut oil, palm oil, lard, or hydrogenated fats.

:: **Switch to low-fat and no-fat dairy products.** Rather than buying whole-fat dairy products, choose skim milk, fat-free sour cream, and low- or nonfat yogurt.

:: **The brighter the better.** When selecting fruits and vegetables, choose the most intense color. A bright orange carrot has more beta-carotene than a pale one. Dark green lettuce leaves have more vitamins than lighter ones. Orange sweet potatoes pack more vitamin A than yellow ones.

Student Snapshot

How Freshmen Change the Way They Eat

33%
Stopped eating red meat

59%
Admit diet has
changed for worse

66%
Don't eat
5 fruits/vegies daily

Source: Data from Tufts University Longitudinal
Health Study, 2002. "Freshman College Student
Dining Habits." *Food Service Director*, Vol. 15,
No. 3, March 15, 2002, p. 1(1).

Portions and Servings

Consumers often are confused by what a *"serving"* actually is, especially since many American restaurants have super-sized the amount of food they put on their customers' plates. The average bagel has doubled in size in the last ten to fifteen years.[28] A standard fast-food serving of french fries is larger in the United States than in the United Kingdom.

According to nutritionists, "marketplace portions"—the actual amounts served to customers—are two to eight times larger than the standard serving sizes defined by the USDA. In fast-food chains, today's portions are two to five times larger than the original size.[29] As studies have shown, people presented with larger portions eat up to 30 percent more than they otherwise would.[30]

In an analysis of quantities of food consumed from the early to the mid-1990s, researchers found that Americans reported drinking more soft drinks, coffee, and tea and eating more ready-to-eat cereal—but less margarine, mayonnaise, macaroni and cheese, and pizza.[31]

Most college students do not calculate portion sizes accurately.[32] One of the best ways to improve such estimates is by using three-dimensional food models. In a study of 380 undergraduates enrolled in an introductory nutrition course, students first estimated the amount of food in three dinners, each with varying portions of five foods (starchy food, cooked vegetables, salad, milk, and meat). After correcting their own estimates, students were asked to estimate portion sizes on a new display with different foods and amounts after one week, and then again after four weeks. Each day between these two tests, different food models were passed around in class. The accuracy of the students' estimates improved significantly afterward.[33]

The Food Guide Pyramid describes the total number of recommended *daily* servings of each of the food groups. It does *not* describe the size of an individual portion. The size of the daily serving is determined by four criteria:

:: The amount of foods from a food group typically reported in surveys as consumed on one eating occasion.

:: The amount of food that provides a comparable amount of key nutrients from that food group; for example, the amount of cheese that provides the same amount of calcium as a cup of milk.

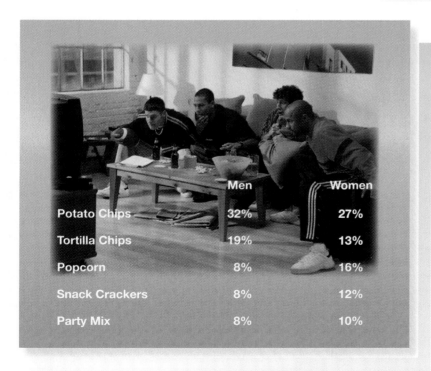

	Men	Women
Potato Chips	32%	27%
Tortilla Chips	19%	13%
Popcorn	8%	16%
Snack Crackers	8%	12%
Party Mix	8%	10%

Figure 5-3 FAVORITE SNACK FOODS ON CAMPUS

Source: Data from "When, Why, and On What Are College Students Snacking,"
The Food Institute Report, February 25, 2002, p. 4.

the X&Y file — Do Men and Women Have Different Nutritional Needs?

Men and women do not need to eat different foods, but their nutritional needs are different. Because most men are bigger and taller than most women, they consume more calories. Eating more means it's easier for them to get the nutrients they need, even though many don't make the wisest food choices.

Women, particularly those who restrict their caloric intake or are chronically dieting, are more likely to develop specific deficiencies. Calcium is one example. Women drink less milk than men, and many do not consume the recommended 800 to 1,200 milligrams of calcium daily. This deficiency increases the risk of bone-weakening osteoporosis.

Many women also get too little iron. Even in adolescence, girls are more prone to iron deficiency than boys; some suffer memory and learning impairments as a result. In adult women, menstrual blood loss and poor eating habits can lead to low iron stores, which puts them at risk for anemia. According to U.S. Department of Agriculture research, most women consume only 60 percent of the recommended 15 milligrams of iron per day. (The recommendation for men is 10 milligrams.) Regular blood tests can monitor a woman's iron status.

Here are some gender-specific strategies for better nutrition:

- Men should cut back on fat and meat in their diets, two things they eat too much.
- Women should increase their iron intake by eating meat (iron from animal sources is absorbed better than that from vegetable sources) or a combination of meat and vegetable iron sources together (for example, a meat and bean burrito). Those with iron deficiencies should consult a physician. Because large doses of iron can be toxic, iron supplements should be taken only with medical supervision.
- Women should consume more calcium-rich foods, including low-fat and nonfat dairy products, leafy greens, and tofu. Women who cannot get adequate amounts of calcium from their daily diet should take calcium supplements. This is not advised for all men because of a possible connection between calcium and prostate cancer.
- Women who could become pregnant should take a multivitamin with 400 micrograms of folic acid, which helps prevent neural tube defects such as spina bifida. Folic acid is also useful to men because it may cut the risk of heart disease, stroke, and colon cancer.
- Both genders should increase their fruit and vegetable intake to ensure that they are getting adequate amounts of vitamins and fiber in their daily diet.

:: The amount of food recognized by most consumers or easily multiplied or divided to describe how much food is actually consumed.

:: The amount traditionally used in previous food guides to describe servings.

A food-label *serving* is a specific amount of food that contains the quantity of nutrients described on the Nutrition Facts label. For many foods, the serving size in the Food Guide Pyramid and on the food label are the same (for example, half a cup of canned fruit or one slice of bread), but in other cases they differ. The Pyramid describes serving units for each food group in ways that consumers find easy to remember (for example, a cup of leafy raw vegetables), while the food label is meant to help consumers compare nutrient information on a number of food products within a category (for example, frozen dinner entrées containing foods from several food groups).

A *portion* is the amount of a specific food that an individual eats at one time. Portions can be bigger or smaller than the servings on food labels or in the Food Guide Pyramid. According to research by the USDA, portion sizes tend to be bigger for men than women, but to decrease for both genders with age. (See The X&Y File: "Do Men and Women Have Different Nutritional Needs?")

If you are trying to balance your diet or control your weight, it's important to keep track of the size of your portions so that you do not exceed the recommended serving. For instance, a 3-ounce serving of meat is about the size of a pack of playing cards—see Figure 5-4. If you eat a larger amount, count it as more than one serving.

The USDA Food Guide Pyramid

Since 1992 the U.S. Department of Agriculture's Food Guide Pyramid (see Figure 5-5 on page 160) has become a familiar icon. Complex carbohydrates (bread, cereal, rice, pasta, etc.) make up the wide base of the pyramid; with vegetables, then fruit and dairy products, then meat and beans on successive tiers. At the very top are fats, oils, and added sugars.

 The USDA has modified the Food Guide Pyramid for children and for the elderly. More than thirty bilingual food pyramids have adapted the guidelines to different cultures and cuisines, including Korean, Puerto

Rican, and Navajo. They vary in the arrangement and types of foods shown in various groups. The Haitian Creole pyramid, for example, contains cabbage rather than spinach; the Korean and Arabic ones feature more root vegetables.[34]

Grains Group (6–11 servings a day)

Breads, cereals, rice, and pasta are the foundation of a healthy diet because they are a good source of complex carbohydrates. Both simple and complex carbohydrates (starches) have 4 calories per gram. The sugars in simple carbohydrates provide little more than a quick spurt of energy, whereas complex carbohydrates are rich in vitamins, minerals, and other nutrients.

A typical serving in this category might be one slice of bread, and 1 ounce of ready-to-eat cereal (or one-half cup of cooked cereal, rice, or pasta). Although many people think of these foods as fattening, it's actually what you put on them, such as butter on a roll or cream sauce on pasta, that adds extra calories.

Here are suggestions for getting more grains in your diet:

:: Add brown rice or barley to soups.

:: Check labels of rolls and bread, and choose those with at least 2 to 3 grams of fiber per slice.

:: Go for pasta power. Pasta has 210 calories per cooked cup and only 9 calories from fat. Like whole-grain breads, whole-grain pastas may provide more nutrients than those made with refined flour.

Eat 6 to 11 servings daily of bread, cereals, and other grain products.

Vegetables Group (3–5 servings a day)

Naturally low in fat and high in fiber, vegetables provide crucial vitamins (such as A and C) and minerals (such as iron and magnesium). A serving in this category consists of one cup of raw leafy vegetables, one-half cup of other vegetables (either cooked or raw), three-quarters cup of vegetable juice, or one potato or ear of corn. Since different types of vegetables provide different nutrients, it's best to eat a variety. Dark green vegetables are especially good sources of vitamins and minerals; certain greens (such as collards, kale, turnip, and mustard) provide calcium and iron. Winter squash, carrots, and the plant family that includes broccoli, cabbage, kohlrabi, and cauliflower (the **crucifers**) are high in fiber, rich in vitamins, and excellent sources of **indoles,** chemicals that help lower cancer risk.

Figure 5-4 QUICK AND EASY ESTIMATES OF PORTION SIZES

| 1 medium fruit is about the size of a baseball. | 1 c cooked vegetables is about the size of your fist. | ½ c ice cream is about the size of a racquet ball. | 3 oz. of meat is about the size of a deck of cards. | 1½ oz. cheese is about the size of six stacked dice. | ¼ c dried fruit is about the size of a golf ball. | 2 tbs peanut butter is about the same size of a marshmallow. | 4 small cookies are about the same size of 4 poker chips. |

Bread, Cereal, Rice, and Pasta Group (Grains Group)—whole grain and refined
- 1 slice of bread
- About 1 cup of ready-to-eat cereal
- 1/2 cup of cooked cereal, rice, or pasta

Vegetable Group
- 1 cup of raw leafy vegetables
- 1/2 cup of other vegetables—cooked or raw
- 3/4 cup of vegetable juice

Fruit Group
- 1 medium apple, banana, orange, pear
- 1/2 cup of chopped, cooked, or canned fruit
- 3/4 cup of fruit juice

Milk, Yogurt, and Cheese Group (Milk Group)[1]
- 1 cup of milk[2] or yogurt[2]
- 1 1/2 ounces of a natural cheese[2] (such as Cheddar)
- 2 ounces of processed cheese[2] (such as American)

Meat, Poultry, Fish, Dry Beans, Eggs, and Nuts Group (Meat and Beans Group)
- 2–3 ounces of cooked lean meat, poultry, or fish
- 1/2 cup of cooked dry beans[3] or 1/2 cup of tofu counts as 1 ounce of lean meat
- 2 1/2-ounce soyburger or 1 egg counts as 1 ounce of lean meat
- 2 tablespoons of peanut butter or 1/3 cup of nuts counts as 1 ounce of meat

NOTE: Many of the serving sizes given above are smaller than those on the Nutritional Facts Label. For example, 1 serving of cooked cereal, rice, or pasta is 1 cup for the label but only 1/2 cup for the Pyramid.
[1] This includes lactose-free and lactose-reduced milk products. One cup of soy-based beverage with added calcium is an option for those who prefer a non-dairy source of calcium.
[2] Choose fat-free or reduced-fat dairy products most often.
[3] Dry beans, peas, and lentils can be counted as servings in either the meat and beans group or the vegetable group. As a vegetable, 1/2 cup of cooked, dry beans counts as 1 serving. As a meat substitute, 1 cup of cooked, dry beans counts as 1 serving (2 ounces of meat).

Figure 5-5 USDA'S FOOD GUIDE PYRAMID
This graphic demonstrates the daily food choices that make up a healthy diet: modest amounts of meat, dairy products, and fats; and a larger number of servings of foods containing grains and cereals.

Source: U.S. Department of Agriculture, *Dietary Guidelines for Americans, 2000.*

Here are ways to increase your vegetable intake:

:: Make or order sandwiches with extra tomatoes or other vegetable toppings.

:: Add extra vegetables whenever you're preparing soups and sauces.

:: If you can't find fresh vegetables, use frozen. They contain less salt than canned veggies.

:: Use raw vegetables for dipping, instead of chips.

Fruits Group (2–4 servings a day)

Like whole grains and vegetables, fruits are excellent sources of vitamins, minerals, and fiber. Along with vegetables, fruits may protect against cancer; those who eat little produce have a cancer rate twice that of people who eat the most fruits and vegetables. A serving consists of a medium apple, banana, or orange; a half-cup of chopped, cooked, or canned fruit; or three-quarters of a cup of fruit juice.

Try the following suggestions to get more fruit into your daily diet:

:: Carry a banana, apple, or package of dried fruit with you as a healthy snack.

© Polara Studios, Inc.

Three to five servings daily of vegetables are recommended.

:: Eat fruit for dessert or a snack. Try poached pears, baked apples, or fresh berries.

:: Start the day with a daily double: a glass of juice and a banana or other fruit on cereal.

:: Add citrus fruits (such as slices of grapefruit or oranges) or apples to green salads, rice, or grains, and to chicken, pork, or fish dishes.

:: Watch out for processed chicken and turkey products; for example, bolognas and salamis made from turkey can contain 45 to 90 percent fat.

:: Select small chickens when you shop: They're leaner than large ones. Broiler-fryers are lowest in fat, followed by roasters. Remove skin before eating poultry.

:: Choose dry-roasted or raw nuts and low-fat peanut butter.

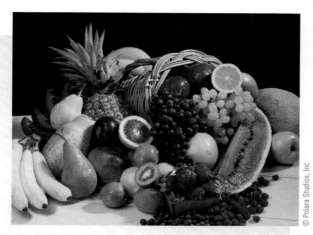

Eat two to four servings daily of fruits to follow the Food Guide Pyramid.

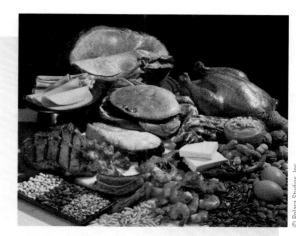

Protein comes in many different forms.

Meat and Beans Group (2–3 servings a day)

Foods in the meat and bean group include meat, poultry, fish, tofu, dry beans (lentils, soy, kidney, black, etc.) and nuts. A serving in this category consists of 2 or 3 ounces of lean, cooked meat, fish, or poultry (roughly the size of an average hamburger or the amount of meat on half a medium chicken breast). An egg or one-half cup of cooked dry beans can substitute for 1 ounce of lean meat. One-third cup of nuts or 2 ounces of peanut butter count as 1 ounce of meat. Thus, one day's total protein intake might include an egg at breakfast; a serving of beans or 2 ounces of sliced chicken in a sandwich or 2 ounces of peanut butter in a sandwich at lunch; and 3 ounces of fish for dinner.

To pick the best protein, follow these recommendations:

:: Choose the leanest meats, such as beef round or sirloin, pork tenderloin, or veal. Broil or roast instead of frying. Trim fat before cooking, which can lower the fat content of the meat you eat by more than 10 percent. Marinate low-fat cuts to increase tenderness.

:: Cook stews, boiled meat, or soup stock ahead of time; refrigerate; and remove the hardened fat before using. Drain fat from ground beef after cooking.

Milk Group (2–3 servings a day)

Most milk products—milk, yogurt, and cheese—are high in calcium, riboflavin, protein, and vitamins A and B_{12}. The Food Guide Pyramid recommends two servings of milk, yogurt, or cheese for most adults and three for women who are pregnant or breast-feeding. In addition, teenagers and young adults up to age 24 should also get three servings of milk products a day. Dairy products, such as milk and yogurt, are the best calcium sources, but be sure you choose products that are low-fat or, preferably, nonfat. A serving in this category consists of an 8-ounce cup of milk, one cup of plain yogurt, 1½ ounces of hard cheese, or 1 tablespoon of cheese spread. An 8-ounce glass of nonfat milk is a more nutritious choice than a tablespoon of a high-fat cheese spread.

As many as 85 percent of adults may be lactose intolerant, especially African Americans, Native Americans, Mexican Americans, and Asian Americans. Beginning in childhood, they gradually lose the ability to digest lactose (the primary sugar in milk) and suffer stomach cramps and diarrhea when they eat dairy products. For them, good alternative sources of calcium include tofu, sardines with bones, dark green leafy vegetables, and calcium-fortified orange juice and cereals.[35] Over-the-counter medicines can also help, and many dairy products are available in special forms for the lactose-intolerant.

To make sure you get more milk with less fat, try the following:

:: Gradually switch from whole milk to 2%-fat (reduced fat) milk, then to 1%-fat (low-fat) milk, then to nonfat (skim) milk.

:: Substitute fat-free sour cream or nonfat plain yogurt for sour cream.

:: Use part-skim or low-fat cheeses whenever possible.

:: Note that cottage cheese is lower in calcium than most cheeses. Thus, one cup of cottage cheese counts as only one-half serving of milk.

Eat fats, oils, and sweets only in small amounts.

Two to three servings of milk products per day are recommended.

Fats, Oils, and Sweets (small amounts each day)

The Food Guide Pyramid places fats, oils, and sweets at the very top so that Americans will realize they should use them only in very small amounts. These foods supply calories but little or no vitamins or minerals.

Added sugars include sweeteners used in processing or at the table (such as jams, jellies, syrups, corn sweetener, molasses, fruit-juice concentrate, and the sugar in candy, cake, and cookies). Sugars often are hidden in favorites—such as soft drinks (9 teaspoons of sugar per can), low-fat fruit yogurt (7 teaspoons per cup), fruit pie (6 teaspoons per serving), and catsup (a teaspoon in every tablespoon).

Try the following:

:: Put a small, child-sized spoon in the sugar bowl.

:: When you crave a sweet, reach for nature's candy: fruit.

:: If you want a daily sweet, have it as dessert, when you'll eat less of it, rather than as a snack.

:: Drink fruit juices and water instead of sugar-laden soft drinks.

Does the Pyramid Need Rebuilding?

The Food Guide Pyramid has won praise, particularly for its emphasis on eating more fruits and vegetables. In long-term studies, women and men who followed the Pyramid's guidelines had a lower mortality rate than those who did not. However, critics have noted that it does not take into account differences in nutrient density. Nonfat milk and ice cream, for instance, are in the same group of milk products but differ greatly in their calorie and fat content. The servings recommended in the Pyramid also are much smaller than real-life portions. Half of a 2-ounce bagel qualifies as a serving of bread, but most bagels today weigh 4 ounces or more.

Compared with the Food Guide Pyramid, the typical American diet is top heavy, with high consumption of the added sugars and fats at the Food Guide's tip, and low in the fruit and leafy vegetables that are at its bottom.[36]

In addition, emerging research has challenged the Pyramid's recommendations for healthy fats like olive oil, fish oil and nuts and for whole grains rather than refined grains.[37] Harvard School of Public Health researchers have proposed an alternative "Healthy Eating" pyramid that incorporates the latest thinking on healthful eating.[38] (See The Cutting Edge: "A New Pyramid?" on page 164.)

Alternative Food Guides

Other nations use different icons—from plates in Mexico to pagodas in China—to provide guidance on healthy eating. In Canada, a brightly colored rainbow illustrates the basic concepts of its food guide (See Fig. 5-7 on page 166):

:: Eat a variety of foods.

:: Choose more grain products.

:: Choose lower fat options such as lowfat milk and trim away excess fat on meat.

:: Maintain a healthy body weight.

:: Participate in regular physical activity.

:: Feel good about yourself.

Nutritional Supplements

More than half of Americans regularly use nutritional supplements—vitamins, minerals, and botanical and biological substances that have not been approved for sale as drugs.[39] There are serious questions about the safety and efficacy of these products.

Marketed as foods, supplements do not have to undergo the same rigorous testing required of drugs. They can carry *structure/function claims*—claims that a product may affect the structure or functioning of the body—but not claims that they can treat, diagnose, cure, or prevent a disease. For example, statements such as "helps maintain a healthy cholesterol level" are acceptable, while statements like "lowers cholesterol levels" are not.

The FDA has issued rules for nutritional supplement labeling. Labels must now include an information panel titled Supplement Facts (similar to the Nutrition Facts panel that appears on processed foods), a clear identity statement, and a complete list of ingredients. Specifically, the "Supplement Facts" panel must show the manufacturer's suggested dose/serving size; information on nutrients when they are present in significant levels (such as vitamins A and C, calcium, iron, and sodium) and the percent Daily Value where a reference has been established; and all other dietary ingredients present in the product, including botanicals and amino acids. Herbal products are identified by the common or usual name and the part of the plant used (such as root, stem, or leaf).

Should I Take Vitamin Supplements?

Many health experts feel that the best way to make sure your body gets the vitamins and minerals it needs is to eat a wide variety of foods. If you rely on vitamin/mineral pills and fortified foods to make up for poor nutrition, you may shortchange yourself. See Table 5-7 for a summary of what we know about different supplements.

As scientists note, most health benefits and dangers stem from more than one source, so it's unlikely that changing any one nutrient will in itself produce great benefits—and may, by interfering with the complex balance of nutrients, do harm. In particular, the fat-soluble vitamins, primarily A and D, can build up in our bodies and cause serious complications, such as damage to the kidneys, liver, or bones. Large doses of water-soluble vitamins, including

the B vitamins, may also be harmful. Excessive intake of vitamin B_6 (pyridoxine), often used to relieve premenstrual bloating, can cause neurological damage, such as numbness in the mouth and tingling in the hands. (An excessive amount in this case is 250 to 300 times the recommended dose.) High doses of vitamin C can produce stomachaches and diarrhea. Niacin, often taken in high doses to lower cholesterol, can cause jaundice, liver damage, and irregular heartbeats as well as severe, uncomfortable flushing of the skin. Table 5-5 provides more information about the effects of vitamin excess.

Knowing What You Eat

Because of the Nutrition Labeling and Education Act, food manufacturers must provide information about fat, calories, and ingredients in large type on packaged food labels, and they must show how a food item fits into a daily diet of 2,000 calories. The law also restricts nutritional claims for terms such as *healthy, low-fat,* and *high-fiber.*

In evaluating food labels and product claims, keep in mind that while individual foods vary in their nutritional value, what matters is your total diet. If you eat too much of any one food—regardless of what its label states—you may not be getting the variety and balance of nutrients that you need.

What Should I Look For on Nutrition Labels?

As Figure 5-8 on page 167 shows, the Nutrition Facts on food labels present a wealth of information—if you know what to look for. The label focuses on those nutrients most clearly associated with disease risk and health: total fat, saturated fat, cholesterol, sodium, total carbohydrate, dietary fiber, sugar, and protein.

:: **Calories.** Calories are the measure of the amount of energy that can be derived from food. Science defines a *calorie* as the amount of energy required to raise the temperature of 1 gram of water by one degree Celsius. In the laboratory, the caloric content of food is measured in 1,000-calorie units called *kilocalories.* The calorie referred to in everyday usage is actually the equivalent of the laboratory kilocalorie.

The Nutrition Facts label lists two numbers for calories: calories per serving and calories from fat per serving. This allows consumers to calculate how many calories they'll consume and to determine the percentage of fat in an item.

:: **Serving size.** Rather than the tiny portions manufacturers sometimes used in the past to keep down the number of calories per serving, the new labels reflect more realistic portions. Serving sizes, which have been defined for approximately 150 food categories, must

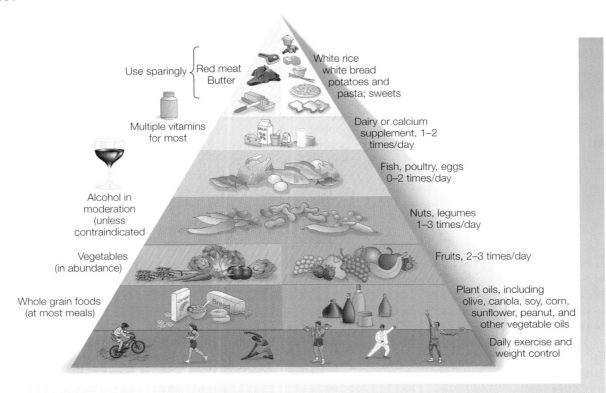

Figure 5-6 THE "HEALTHY EATING" PYRAMID

Source: Based on Walter C. Willett. *Eat, Drink, and Be Healthy,* NY: Simon & Schuster, 2001.

THE CUTTING EDGE

A New Pyramid?

Is the USDA Food Guide Pyramid in need of an update? Yes, say Harvard School of Public Health researchers, who have proposed an alternative "Healthy Eating" pyramid (see Figure 5-6). With daily exercise and weight control at its base, it calls for whole grain foods and plant oils at most meals; vegetables in abundance; two to three servings of fruit; one to three servings of nuts and legumes; zero to two servings of fish, poultry, and eggs; and one to two servings of dairy foods (or calcium supplements). At the tip of the pyramid—to be used sparingly—are red meat, butter, white rice, white bread, potatoes, pasta, and sweets. The Healthy Eating Pyramid also suggests alternate protein sources such as nuts and soy, multivitamins, and moderate alcohol intake for disease prevention.

Which pyramid is better for you? In an analysis of almost 105,000 health professionals, the Harvard scientists compared the rates of chronic diseases in those who followed the USDA pyramid guidelines and those whose diets were more in line with their proposed "Healthy Eating" pyramid. Men who adhered to the Harvard pyramid lowered their risk of heart disease by 39 percent, compared with 28 percent for the USDA diet. Women following the Harvard plan lowered their risk by 28 percent, compared with a 14 percent reduction for those on the USDA guidelines.

Sources: Walter Willett and Meir Stampfer. "Rebuilding the Food Pyramid," *Scientific American,* January 2003. "Food Pyramid in Need of Renovation," *Harvard Women's Health Watch,* February 2003.

TABLE 5-7	Do Nutritional Supplements Work?	
Supplement	**Claims**	**What We Know**
Amino acids	Increase muscle mass.	No solid evidence that amino acid supplements promote muscle building. Little is known about the side effects of high doses of single or combination amino acid supplements.
Beta-carotene	Reduces your risk of cancer.	Converts into vitamin A in the body. No evidence that beta-carotene supplements reduce cancer risk.
B complex vitamins	Provide energy; help relieve stress and may help reduce heart disease risk.	No evidence that B vitamins relieve stress. Long thought to be nontoxic, but some B vitamins, such as B_6 and niacin, may have serious side effects when taken in very high doses.
Vitamin C	Prevents colds, certain cancers, and heart disease.	Vitamin C supplements can lessen the severity of colds but not prevent them. Observational studies have shown that vitamin C may help prevent cancer and heart disease, but too few clinical trials have been conducted to substantiate those results.
Calcium	Prevents osteoporosis and colon cancer; reduces high blood pressure.	Calcium plays a critical role in preventing osteoporosis if taken with vitamin D. Results of research on calcium's role in preventing colon cancer are still preliminary. It may help regulate blood pressure in some people, but there is no way of knowing who might benefit.
Chromium picolinate	Reduces body fat, builds muscle, and improves overall fitness.	Scientists have found that this popular nutritional and dietary supplement causes DNA breakage and may be a cancer risk.
Vitamin E	Reduces the risk of heart disease and cancer.	Supplements of 400–800 IU may protect against heart disease. Very few side effects have been reported, but high doses of vitamin E supplements should not be used by anyone taking anticoagulation medication.
Niacin	Helps lower cholesterol.	Niacin, in the form of nicotinic acid, is an inexpensive alternative to cholesterol-lowering drugs but should be prescribed by a doctor. Side effects include flushing, itching, and gastrointestinal distress. Time-released niacin can be toxic to the liver.
Zinc	Boosts immunity, wards off colds, and improves sex drive.	Zinc taken at the onset of a cold can lessen its severity. High doses of zinc, however, may *suppress* immune function. No evidence that zinc supplements affect sexual performance.

be the same for similar products (for example, different brands of potato chips) and for similar products within a category (for example, snack foods such as pretzels, potato chips, and popcorn). This makes it easier to compare the nutritional content of foods.

:: **Daily Values (DVs).** DVs refer to the total amount of a nutrient that the average adult should aim to get or not exceed on a daily basis. The DVs for cholesterol, sodium, vitamins, and minerals are the same for all adults. The DVs for total fat, saturated fat, carbohydrate, fiber, and protein are based on a 2,000-calorie daily diet—the amount of food ingested by many American men and active women.

:: *Percent Daily Values (%DVs).* The goal for a full day's diet is to select foods that together add up to 100 percent of the DVs. The %DVs show how a particular food's nutrient content fits into a 2,000-calorie diet.

Individuals who consume (or should consume) fewer than 2,000 total calories a day have to lower their DVs for total fat, saturated fat, and carbohydrates. For example, if their caloric intake is 10 percent less than 2,000 calories, they would lower the DV by 10 percent. Similarly, those who consume more than 2,000 calories should adjust the DVs upward.

:: *Calories per gram.* The bottom of the food label lists the number of calories per gram for fat, carbohydrates, and protein.

People zero in on different figures on the food label—for example, calories if they're watching their weight, specific ingredients if they have food allergies. Among the useful items to check are the following:

:: *Calories from fat.* Get into the habit of calculating the percentage of fat calories in a food before buying or eating it.

Figure 5-7 FOOD GUIDES FROM OTHER COUNTRIES

The United States uses a pyramid to convey the message of proportionality. Canada's unique rainbow design also illustrates proportionality. Puerto Rico (and the Philippines) adopted and modified the pyramid design. Puerto Rico adds a blue shadow to illustrate water, and the Philippines combines the milk and meat groups into one group of animal foods. China (and Korea) use a pagoda to depict their food guides. Germany (and most European countries, as well as Australia) illustrate their food guides with a circle. Mexico (and Great Britain) transform a circular food guide into a sectioned plate of foods.

Source: Journal of THE AMERICAN DIETETIC ASSOCIATION. April 2002, pp. 484–485.

:: **Total fat.** Since the average person munches on 15 to 20 food items a day, it's easy to overload on fat. Saturated fat is a figure worthy of special attention because of its reported link to several diseases.

:: **Cholesterol.** Cholesterol is made by and contained in products of animal origin only. Many high-fat products, such as potato chips, contain 0 percent choles-

terol because they're made from plants and are cooked in vegetable fats. However, the vegetable fats they contain can be processed and made into saturated fats that are more harmful to the heart than cholesterol.

:: **Sugars.** There is no Daily Value for sugars because health experts have yet to agree on a daily limit. The

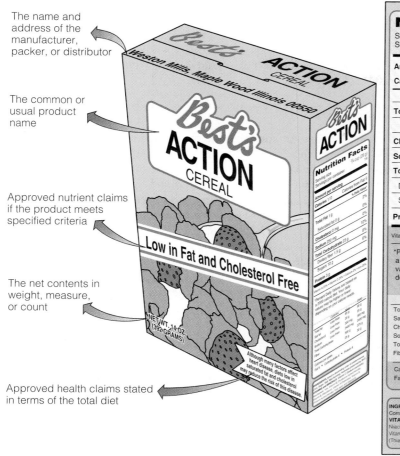

The name and address of the manufacturer, packer, or distributor

The common or usual product name

Approved nutrient claims if the product meets specified criteria

The net contents in weight, measure, or count

Approved health claims stated in terms of the total diet

The serving size and number of servings per container

Calorie information and quantities of nutrients per serving, in actual amounts

Quantities of nutrients as "% Daily Values" based on a 2000-calorie energy intake

Daily Values reminder for selected nutrients for a 2000- and a 2500-calorie diet

Calorie per gram reminder

The ingredients in descending order of predominance by weight

A container with fewer than 40 square inches of surface area can present fewer facts in this format.

Packages with fewer than 12 square inches of surface area need not carry nutrition information, but they must provide an address or telephone number for obtaining information.

Figure 5-8 UNDERSTANDING NUTRITION LABELS
The Nutrition Facts label lists the essential nutrient content of packaged food as well as the amount of potentially harmful substances such as fat and sodium.

figure on the label includes naturally present sugars, such as lactose in milk and fructose in fruit, as well as those added to the food, such as table sugar, corn syrup, or dextrose.

:: *Fiber.* A "high–fiber" food has 5 or more grams of fiber per serving. A "good" source of fiber provides at least 2.5 grams. "More" or "added" fiber means at least

2.5 grams more per serving than similar foods—10 percent more of the DV for fiber.

:: **Calcium.** "High" equals 200 milligrams (mg) or more per serving. "Good" means at least 100 mg, while "more" indicates that the food contains at least 100 mg more calcium—10 percent more of the DV—than the item usually would have.

:: **Sodium.** Since many foods contain sodium, most of us routinely get more than we need. Read labels carefully to avoid excess sodium, which can be a health threat.

:: **Vitamins.** A Daily Value of 10 percent of any vitamin makes a food a "good" source; 20 percent qualifies it as "high" in a certain vitamin.

Nutrition labeling for fresh produce, fish, meat, and poultry remains voluntary. Packages too small for a full-sized label must provide an address or phone number so consumers can obtain information from the manufacturer.

Functional Foods

As the American Dietetic Association has noted, all foods are functional at some physiological level. However, the term *functional* generally applies to a food specifically created to have health-promoting benefits. The International Food Information Council defines functional foods as those "that provide health benefits beyond basic nutrition."

Some manufacturers are adding herbs, such as the cold-fighter echinacea, to food products and promoting them as functional foods. However, the amounts added are often too low to have any effect, and many herb-sprinkled foods are high-sugared drinks and snack foods. These products have other dangers, including the use of low-quality or contaminated herbs and adverse drug and food interactions.[40]

◾ The Way We Eat

For centuries, Native Americans ate a diet of corn, beans, fish, game, wild greens, wild fruits, squash, and tomatoes. Over time the United States, a nation of immigrants, has imported a wide variety of ethnic cuisines. Although many people think of foods such as hamburgers, steak, potatoes, cheesecake, and ice cream as all-American favorites, in most cities across the country, all-American also includes dozens of different cultural cuisines.

Dietary Diversity

Whatever your cultural heritage, you have probably sampled Chinese, Mexican, Indian, Italian, and Japanese foods. If you belong to any of these ethnic groups, you may eat these cuisines regularly. Each type of ethnic cooking has its own nutritional benefits and potential drawbacks, yet all recommend eating more carbohydrate-rich grains, vegetables, and fruits, and less high-protein meat and dairy. None of these "all-American" cuisines endorses a high-protein diet as a healthy eating pattern.[41]

African-American Diet

African-American cuisine traces some of its roots to food preferences from west Africa (for example, peanuts, okra, and black-eyed peas), as well as to traditional American foods, such as fish, game, greens, and sweet potatoes. Cajun cuisine, most closely associated with New Orleans, blends both African and French traditions in dishes such as gumbo (thick spicy soup), sausage, red beans, and seafood. African-American cooking uses many nutritious vegetables, such as collard greens and sweet potatoes, as well as legumes. However, some dishes include high-fat food products such as peanuts and pecans or involve frying, sometimes in saturated fat.

Chinese Diet

The mainland Chinese diet, which is plant-based, high in carbohydrates, and low in fats and animal protein, is considered one of the healthiest in the world. The Food Guide Pagoda recommends plenty of cereals, vegetables, fruits, and beans, with physical activity balancing food intake.[42] However, Chinese food is prepared differently in America. Chinese restaurants here serve more meat and sauces than are generally eaten in China. According to laboratory tests of typical take-out dishes from Chinese restaurants, many have more fats and cholesterol than hamburger or egg dishes from fast-food outlets.

To eat healthfully when you choose Chinese cuisine, select boiled, steamed, or stir-fried dishes; mix entrées with steamed rice; and lift food out of a container with chopsticks or a fork and transfer it to serving bowls to leave excess sauce behind. Order wonton soup rather than egg rolls or pork spareribs. To avoid the cholesterol in egg yolks, steer away from egg foo yung and items made with lobster sauce. If you are prone to high blood pressure, watch out for the high sodium content of soy and other sauces, and of a seasoner called MSG (monosodium glutamate).

French Diet

Traditional French cuisine, which includes rich, high-fat sauces and dishes, has never been considered healthful. Yet nutritionists have been stumped to explain the so-called French paradox. Despite a diet high in saturated fats, the French have had one of the lowest rates of coronary artery disease in the world.

In today's ethnically diverse United States, all-American food ranges from Indian to Japanese. The vegetables and legumes in the Indian diet are healthy and high in protein, but too much saturated fat can cancel some of the benefits. The Japanese diet is high in seafood and rice and low in fats, cheese, and meat.

Recent reports indicate that the French diet is changing. Until 1990 the French ate much less animal fat and had significantly lower blood cholesterol levels than Americans and Britons. Fat consumption in France has since risen as the French have begun eating more meat and fast foods, snacking more, eating fewer relaxed meals, exercising less, and drinking less wine. They've also been getting fatter, and some researchers contend that their rates of heart disease will inevitably rise in the coming decades. The French diet increasingly resembles the American diet, but French portions tend to be one-third to one-half the size of American portions.

Indian Diet

Many Indian dishes highlight healthful ingredients such as vegetables and legumes (beans and peas). However, many also use *ghee* (a form of butter) or coconut oil; both are rich in harmful saturated fats. The best advice in an Indian restaurant is to ask how each dish is prepared. Good choices include *daal* or *dal* (lentils), *karbi* or *karni* (chickpea soup), and *chapati* (tortilla-like bread). Hold back on *bhatura* or *naan* (fried bread), coconut milk, and *samosas* (fried meat or vegetables in dough).

Japanese Diet

The traditional Japanese diet is very low in fat, which may account for the low incidence of heart disease in Japan. Dietary staples include soybean products, fish, vegetables,

noodles, and rice. A variety of fruits and vegetables are also included in many dishes. However, Japanese cuisine is high in salted, smoked, and pickled foods. Watch out for deep-fried dishes such as tempura, and salty soups and sauces (which you can ask for on the side). In a restaurant, ask for broiled entrées or nonfried dishes made with tofu, which has no cholesterol.

Mediterranean Diet

Several years ago epidemiologists noticed something unexpected in the residents of regions along the Mediterranean Sea: a lower incidence of deaths from heart disease. Scientists have identified antioxidants in red wine and olive oil that may account for the beneficial effects on the heart of the Mediterranean diet.[43]

As illustrated by the Mediterranean Food Pyramid (see Figure 5-9), the region's diet features lots of fruits and vegetables, legumes, nuts, and grains. Meat is used mainly as a condiment rather than as a main course, and fish, yogurt, and low-fat feta cheese are the predominant animal foods. The diet is relatively high in fat, but the main source is olive oil, an unsaturated fat.

Mexican Diet

The cuisine served in Mexico features rice, corn, and beans, which are low in fat and high in nutrients. However, the dishes Americans think of as Mexican are far

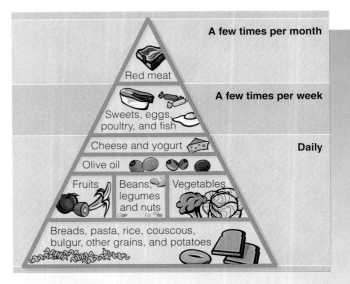

Figure 5-9 MEDITERRANEAN FOOD PYRAMID

The Mediterranean diet relies heavily on fruits, vegetables, grain, and potatoes and includes considerable olive oil.

Source: Oldways Preservation & Exchange Trust. Reprinted by permission of the *New York Times.*

less healthful. Burritos, especially when topped with cheese and sour cream, are very high in fat. Although guacamole has a high fat content, it contains mostly monounsaturated fatty acids, a better form of fat.

When eating at Mexican restaurants, ask that cheese and sour cream be served on the side. Avoid refried beans, which are usually cooked in lard. Hold back on guacamole, quesadillas, and enchiladas. Nutritious choices include rice, beans, and shrimp or chicken tostadas on unfried cornmeal tortillas.

Southeast Asian Diet

A rich variety of fruits and vegetables—bamboo shoots, bok choy, cabbage, mangoes, papayas, cucumbers—provides a sound nutritional basis for this diet. In addition, most foods are broiled or stir-fried, which keeps fat low. However, coconut oil and milk, used in many sauces, are high in fat.

The use of MSG and pickled foods means the sodium content is high. At Thai or Vietnamese restaurants, choose salads (*larb* is a chicken salad with mint) or seafood soup (*po tak*).

❓ What Should I Know About Vegetarian Diets?

Not all vegetarians avoid all meats. Some, who call themselves *lacto-ovo-pesco-vegetarians,* eat dairy products, eggs, chicken, and fish, but not red meat. **Lacto–vegetarians** eat dairy products as well as grains, fruits, and vegetables; **ovo-lacto-vegetarians** also eat eggs. Pure vegetarians, called **vegans,** eat only plant foods; often they take vitamin B_{12} supplements because that vitamin is normally found only in animal products. If they select their food with care, vegetarians can get sufficient amounts of protein, vitamin B_{12}, iron, and calcium without supplements (see Figure 5-10).

The key to getting sufficient protein from a vegetarian diet is understanding the concept of **complementary proteins.** Meat, poultry, fish, eggs, and dairy products are *complete proteins* that provide the nine essential amino acids—substances that the human body cannot produce itself. *Incomplete proteins,* such as legumes or nuts, may have relatively low levels of one or two essential amino acids,

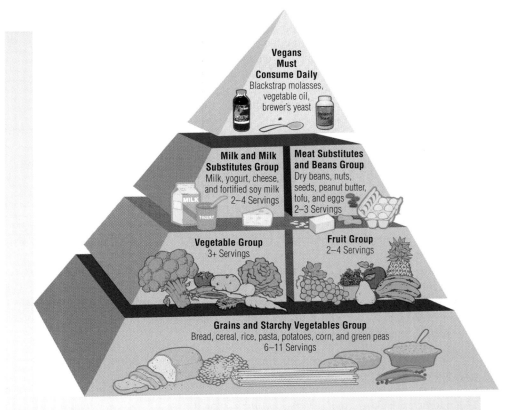

Figure 5-10 NEW YORK MEDICAL COLLEGE VEGETARIAN PYRAMID

This version of the Food Guide Pyramid has been modified for use by vegetarians. Compare it to the Pyramid shown in Figure 5-5 on page 160.

but fairly high levels of others. By combining complementary protein sources, you can make sure that your body makes the most of the nonanimal proteins you eat. Many cultures rely heavily on complementary foods for protein. In Middle Eastern cooking, sesame seeds and chickpeas are a popular combination; in Latin American dishes, beans and rice, or beans and tortillas; in Chinese cuisine, soy and rice.

Vegetarian diets have proven health benefits. Studies show that vegetarians' cholesterol levels are low, and vegetarians are seldom overweight. As a result, they're less apt to be candidates for heart disease than those who consume large quantities of meat. Vegetarians also have lower incidences of breast, colon, and prostate cancer; high blood pressure; and osteoporosis. When combined with exercise and stress reduction, vegetarian diets have helped reverse the buildup of harmful plaque within the blood vessels of the heart. (See Chapter 14 for further discussion of the connections between diet and heart disease.)

Fast Food: Nutrition on the Run

On any given day, about 25 percent of adults in the United States go to a fast-food restaurant. The typical American consumes three hamburgers and four orders of french fries every week.[44] Not all fast foods are junk foods—that is, high in calories, sugar, salt, and fat, and low in beneficial nutrients. But while it's not all bad, fast food has definite disadvantages. A meal in a fast-food restaurant may cost twice as much as the same meal prepared at home and may provide half your daily calorie needs. The fat content of many items is extremely high. A Burger King Whopper with cheese contains 723 calories and 48 grams of fat, 18 grams from saturated fat. A McDonald's Sausage McMuffin with egg has 517 calories and 33 grams of fat, 13 grams from saturated fat. Many fast-food chains have switched from beef tallow or lard to unsaturated vegetable oils for frying, but the total fat content of the foods remains the same. Some consumer advocacy groups have sued fast-food restaurant changes, asserting that because of their aggressive marketing, particularly to children, they should bear responsibility for the costs of the nation's obesity epidemic.[45]

At regular restaurants or cafeterias, you can usually get a better nutritional value for the calories you consume. For example, you can request that your entrée be baked or broiled without fat. You can also ask that fresh vegetables be steamed without salt or butter. When possible, ask for luncheon rather than dinner-sized portions.

◼ Food Safety

Increasingly, Americans are concerned not just with whether the food they eat is nutritious, but whether it's safe. Many unsuspected safety hazards have been identified by **food toxicologists,** specialists who detect toxins (potentially harmful substances) in food and treat the conditions they produce.

Pesticides, Irradiation, and Genetic Engineering

Plants and animals naturally produce compounds that act as pesticides to aid in their survival. The vast majority of the pesticides we consume are therefore natural, not added by farmers or food processors. *Commercial pesticides* save billions of dollars of valuable crops from pests, but they also may endanger human health and life.

Fearful of potential risks in pesticides, many consumers are purchasing **organic** foods. The term *organic* refers to foods produced without the use of commercial chemicals at any stage. Independent groups now certify foods before they can be labeled organic. Foods that are truly organic are cleaner and have much lower levels of residues than standard commercial produce. There's no guarantee that the organic produce you buy at a grocery or health-food store is more nutritious than other produce.

STRATEGIES FOR PREVENTION

A Guide to Fast Foods

▪ For breakfast, avoid croissants or muffins stuffed with eggs or meat; they pack as many as 700 calories. Better options include plain scrambled eggs (150–180 calories), pancakes without butter or syrup (400 calories), and English muffins (185 calories each).

▪ For lunch or dinner, if you want meat, go for plain hamburgers (no cheese), which average 275 to 350 calories. An even better choice is roast beef, which is lower in fat and calories.

▪ Be wary of fast-food fish. With frying oil trapped in the breading and creamy tartar sauce on top, fried-fish sandwiches supply more calories (425–500) and fat than regular hamburgers.

▪ Avoid fried chicken; the coatings tend to retain grease. If you want bite-sized chicken, select bites made of chicken breast, not processed chicken (which contains fatty, ground-up skin).

▪ Ask for unsalted items; they are available. (Many chains have also reduced the amount of sodium used in cooking.)

▪ If you sample the salad bar, steer clear of mayonnaise, bacon bits, oily vegetable salads, and rich dressings.

Wash produce thoroughly in fresh water to remove dirt and any pesticide residue, scrubbing when necessary to clean off soil.

However, buying organic foods is one way in which you can work toward a healthier environment.

Irradiation is the use of radiation, either from radioactive substances or from devices that produce X rays, on food. It doesn't make the food radioactive. Its primary benefit is to prolong the shelf life of food. Like the heat in canning, irradiation can kill all the microorganisms that might grow in a food, and the sterilized food can then be stored for years in sealed containers at room temperature without spoiling. Are irradiated foods safe to eat? The best available answer is a qualified yes, because we don't have complete data yet.

Genetically engineered foods—custom built to improve quality or remove unwanted traits—may become an important part of our diets in the future. By modifying the genetic makeup of plants, engineers will be able to produce apples that resist insects, raspberries that last longer, and potatoes that absorb less fat in cooking. Will these items be as tasty and healthful as foods grown the old-fashioned way? And will they have unforeseen health hazards? That's yet to be seen.

Additives: Risks Versus Benefits

Additives are substances added to foods to lengthen storage time, change taste in a way the manufacturer thinks is better, alter color, or otherwise modify them to make them more appealing. The average American takes in approximately 160 pounds of food additives per year: more than 140 pounds of sweeteners, 15 pounds of table salt, and 5 to 10 pounds of all others.

Additives provide numerous benefits. Sodium and calcium propionate, sodium benzoate, potassium sorbate, and sulfur dioxide prevent the growth of bacteria, yeast, and mold in baked goods. BHA (butylated hydroxyanisole), BHT (butylated hydroxytoluene), propyl gallate, and vitamin E protect against the oxidation of fats (rancidity). Other additives include leavening agents, emulsifiers, stabilizers, thickeners, dough conditioners, and bleaching agents.

Some additives can pose a risk to eaters. For example, nitrites—used in bacon, sausages, and lunch meats to inhibit spoilage, prevent botulism, and add color—can react with other substances in your body or in food to form potentially cancer-causing agents called *nitrosamines*. In the last decade, the food industry has reduced the amount of nitrite used to cure foods, so there should be less danger than in the past. Sulfites, used to prevent browning, can produce severe, even fatal, allergic reactions in sensitive individuals. The FDA has required the labeling of sulfites in packaged foods and has banned the use of sulfites on fresh fruits and vegetables, including those in salad bars.

What Causes Food Poisoning?

Salmonella is a bacterium that contaminates many foods, particularly undercooked chicken, eggs, and sometimes processed meat. Eating contaminated food can result in salmonella poisoning, which causes diarrhea and vomiting. The Centers for Disease Control and Prevention (CDC) estimates 40,000 reported cases of salmonella poisoning a year; the actual number of cases could be anywhere from 400,000 to 4 million. The FDA has warned consumers about the dangers of unpasteurized orange juice because of the risk of salmonella contamination.

Another bacterium, *Campylobacter jejuni,* may cause even more stomach infections than salmonella. Found in water, milk, and some foods, Campylobacter poisoning causes severe diarrhea and has been implicated in the growth of stomach ulcers.

Bacteria can also cause illness by producing toxins in food. *Staphylococcus aureus* is the most common culprit. When cooked foods are cross-contaminated with the bacteria from raw foods and not stored properly, staph infections can result, causing nausea and abdominal pain anywhere from thirty minutes to eight hours after ingestion.

Even many healthy foods can pose dangers. The FDA has urged consumers to avoid eating raw sprouts because of the risk of getting sick. Sprouts, particularly alfalfa and clover, can be contaminated by salmonella or *E. coli* bacteria, which can cause nausea, diarrhea, and cramping in healthy adults. Children and senior citizens can experience serious symptoms that lead to kidney failure and compromised immune systems. The FDA advises people to either cook sprouts before eating them or request that they be and by washing everything that may come into contact with raw meat.

 College students who often begin preparing their own meals for the first time as undergraduates, are more likely to engage in risky food handling behaviors than the general public. As shown in Figure 5-11, a higher percentage of students eat pink hamburger meat, while fewer read or remember the labels on raw meat or poultry and change food preparation because of the information on the label.[46]

"Hamburger Disease"/Barbecue Syndrome

Barbecue syndrome is the common name for a type of food poisoning caused by the bacteria *verotoxigenic E. coli*, or VTEC. People who develop this syndrome frequently report that they ate ground beef hamburgers prior to getting sick. Other kinds of undercooked meat and poultry, drinking unpasteurized milk or unchlorinated water also are culprits.

Symptoms, which can range from mild to life-threatening, usually develop within two to ten days and include severe stomach cramps, vomiting, and a mild fever. Most people recover within seven to ten days. Proper handling and cooking of food can practically eliminate hamburger disease.[47]

Foodborne Illnesses

Americans may be more likely to get sick from what they eat today than they were half a century ago. According to the CDC, the frequency of serious gastrointestinal illness—one indicator of food poisoning—is significantly higher

STRATEGIES FOR PREVENTION

Protecting Yourself from Food Poisoning

- Clean food thoroughly. Wash produce thoroughly. Wash utensils, plates, cutting boards, knives, blenders, and other cooking equipment with very hot water and soap after preparing raw meat, poultry, or fish to avoid contaminating other foods or the cooked meat.

- Drink only pasteurized milk. Raw or unpasteurized milk increases the danger of microbial infections.

- Don't eat raw eggs. Since raw eggs can be contaminated with salmonella, don't use them in salad dressings, eggnog, or other dishes.

- Cook chicken thoroughly. About a third of all poultry sold contains harmful organisms. Thorough cooking eliminates any danger.

- Cook pork thoroughly. An internal temperature of 170° Fahrenheit must be reached to kill a parasite called *trichina* occasionally found in the muscles of pigs.

- Know how to store foods. Bacteria cannot survive in temperatures hotter than 140° Fahrenheit or colder than 40° Fahrenheit. The temperatures in between are a danger zone. If you must leave foods out—perhaps at a buffet or picnic—don't let them stay in the temperature danger zone for more than two hours. After that time, throw the food away.

- Stored food doesn't last forever. Refrigerate leftovers as soon as possible and use them within three days. If frozen, use leftovers within two to three months.

left off sandwiches and other food ordered in restaurants. Homegrown sprouts can also present a risk if they come from contaminated seeds.

An uncommon but sometimes fatal form of food poisoning is **botulism,** caused by the *Clostridium botulinum* organism. Improper home-canning procedures are the most common cause of this potentially fatal problem.

There have been several outbreaks of listeriosis, caused by the bacteria **listeria,** commonly found in deli meats, hot dogs, soft cheeses, raw meat, and unpasteurized milk. At greatest risk are pregnant women, infants, and those with weakened immune systems. You can reduce your risk by cooking meats and leftovers thoroughly

	20	40	60	80	100

Ate hamburgers... 86.3% / 90.4%

Ate pink hamburgers... 19.7% / 43.5%

Ate runny eggs... 50.2% / 50.8%

☐ General public
■ Student sample

Figure 5-11 COMPARING THE FOOD SAFETY BEHAVIOR OF STUDENTS TO THE GENERAL PUBLIC

Source: Data from Michele Morrone and Ann Rathbun. "Health Education and Food Safety Behavior in the University Setting." *Journal of Environmental Health,* March 2003, Vol. 65, No. 7, p. 9.

Savvy Consumer

SPOTTING NUTRITION MISINFORMATION

- Don't believe everything you read. A quick way to spot a bad nutrition self-help book is to look in the index for a diet to prevent or treat rheumatoid arthritis (none exists). If you find one, don't buy the book.

- Before you try any new nutritional approach, check with your doctor or a registered dietitian or call the American Dietetic Association's consumer hot line, (800)366-1655.

- Don't believe ads or advisers basing their nutritional recommendations on hair analysis, which is not accurate in detecting nutritional deficiencies.

- Be wary of anyone who recommends megadoses of vitamins or nutritional supplements, which can be dangerous. High doses of vitamin A, which some people take to clear up acne, can be toxic.

- Question personal testimonies about the powers of some magical-seeming pill or powder, and be wary of "scientific articles" in journals that aren't reviewed by health professionals.

- Be wary of any nutritional supplements sold in health stores or through health and body-building magazines. These products may contain ingredients that have not been tested and proven safe.

Quick and easy fixes
Even proven treatments take time to be effective.

One product does it all
No one product can possibly treat such a diverse array of conditions.

Phony terms hide the lack of scientific proof.

Personal testimonials
Hearsay is the weakest form of evidence.

Time-tested
Such findings would be widely publicized and accepted by health professionals.

Meaningless medical jargon

Paranoid accusations
And this product's company doesn't want money? At least the drug company has scientific research proving the safety and effectiveness of its products.

Satisfaction guaranteed
Marketers may make generous promises, but consumers won't be able to collect on them.

Natural
Natural is not necessarily better or safer; any product that is strong enough to be effective is strong enough to cause side effects.

than it was in 1948. Every year food poisoning causes 5,000 deaths, 325,000 hospitalizations, and 76 million illnesses. Cases of potentially deadly *E. coli* infection more than doubled in the last five years of the twentieth century.

According to the Government Accounting Office, 85 percent of food poisoning comes from fruits, vegetables, cheeses, and seafood. People aren't washing fruits thoroughly or cooking vegetables before eating, increasing the chance of infection with viruses or bacteria. They're also eating more precooked foods rather than sit-down meals served right out of the oven. And the sheer number and types of products on the market far exceed the government's ability to monitor them.

Foodborne infections generally produce nausea, vomiting, and diarrhea from twelve hours to five days after infection. The symptoms and severity depend on the specific microorganism and the victim's overall health. Although the illnesses tend to be short-term and not usually severe, they can be fatal to those whose immune systems are impaired or whose general health is poor.

A foodborne illness that generated international alarm several years ago is **mad cow disease,** the popular term for deadly bovine spongiform encephalopathy (BSE). After attacking British cattle in 2001, BSE crossed species to kill dozens of people in the United Kingdom, Ireland, and France. Caused by eating beef containing brain or spinal tissue from infected cows, BSE seems to be transmitted by a misshapen protein called a prion that cannot be detected by testing blood or tissue. In humans, BSE causes mood swings, hallucinations, uncontrollable body movements, progressive dementia, and eventual death.[48]

The U.S. Department of Agriculture confirmed the first case of mad cow disease in the United States in December, 2003. In January, 2004, the government issued new rules to enhance safeguards against the disease.

Food Allergies

An estimated 12 to 20 percent of adults have some form of food hypersensitivity, an adverse reaction to a particular food. Women are more prone to report hypersensitivity or food allergies than men.[49]

Physicians disagree as to which foods are the most common triggers of food allergies. Cow's milk, eggs, seafood, wheat, soybeans, nuts, seeds, and chocolate have all been identified as culprits. The symptoms they provoke vary. One person might sneeze if exposed to an irritating food; another might vomit or develop diarrhea; others might suffer headaches, dizziness, hives, or a rapid heartbeat. Symptoms may not develop for up to 72 hours, making it hard to pinpoint which food was responsible.

If you suspect that you have a food allergy, see a physician with specialized training in allergy diagnosis. Medical opinion about the merits of many treatments for food allergies is divided. Once you've identified the culprit, the wisest and sometimes simplest course is to avoid it.

Nutritional Quackery

The American Dietetic Association describes nutritional quackery as a growing problem for unsuspecting consumers. Because so much nutritional nonsense is garbed in scientific-sounding terms, it can be hard to recognize bad advice when you get it. One basic rule: If the promises of a nutritional claim sound too good to be true—they probably are. (See Savvy Consumer: "Spotting Nutrition Misinformation.")

If you seek the advice of a nutrition consultant, carefully check his or her credentials and professional associations. Because licensing isn't required in all states, almost anyone can use the label "nutritionist," regardless of qualifications. Be wary of diplomas from obscure schools and organizations that allow anyone who pays dues to join. (One physician obtained a membership for his dog!) A registered dietitian (R.D.), who has a bachelor's degree and specialized training (including an internship), and who passed a certification examination, is usually a member of the American Dietetic Association (ADA), which sets the standard for quality in diets. A nutrition expert with an M.D. or Ph.D. generally belongs to the ADA, the American

Institute of Nutrition, or the American Society of Clinical Nutrition; all have stringent membership requirements.

The Bottom Line ▼
A Lifetime of Healthy Eating

As nutritional knowledge expands and evolves, it's easy to be confused by changing advice on which foods to avoid and which to eat. But even though research may challenge or change thinking on a specific food, some basic principles always apply. At the very least, keep in mind the American Dietetic Association's ABCs.

:: **Aim for fitness.** In order to maintain a healthy weight, build physical activity into your daily routine.

:: **Build a healthy base.** Select a variety of foods to help you get all the nutrients and fiber you need.

:: **Choose sensibly.** Put together a diet that is low in saturated fat and cholesterol and moderate in total fat.

Here are some other guidelines that never go out of style:

:: **Eat breakfast.** Easy to prepare breakfasts include: cold cereal with fruit and lowfat milk, whole-wheat toast with peanut butter, yogurt with fruit, or whole-grain waffles.

:: **Snack smart.** Choose snacks from different food groups—a glass of lowfat milk and a few graham crackers, an apple or celery sticks with peanut butter and raisins, or some dry cereal.

:: **Don't eat too much of one thing.** Your body needs protein, carbohydrates, fat, and many different vitamins and minerals such as vitamins C and A, iron, and calcium from a variety of foods.

:: **Eat more grains, fruits, and vegetables.** These foods give you carbohydrates for energy, plus vitamins, minerals, and fiber. Try breads such as whole-wheat, bagels, and pita. Spaghetti and oatmeal are also in the grain group.

:: **Don't ban any food.** Fit in a higher-fat food, like pepperoni pizza, at dinner by choosing lower-fat foods at other meals. And don't forget about moderation. If two pieces of pizza fill you up, don't eat a third.

:: **Make every calorie count.** Load up on nutrients, not on big portions. Choosing foods that are nutrient dense will help protect against disease and keep you healthy.

 After watching the CNN video segment, discuss the following question. How can eating fish twice a week help reduce cardiovascular disease?

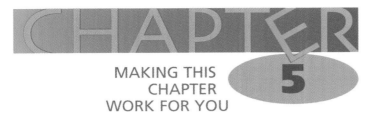

MAKING THIS CHAPTER WORK FOR YOU

5

1. The classes of essential nutrients include which of the following?
   a. amino acids, antioxidants, fiber and cholesterol
   b. proteins, calcium, calories, and folic acid
   c. carbohydrates, minerals, fat, and water
   d. iron, whole grains, fruits, and vegetables

2. Which type of fat is *not* considered a threat to heart health?
   a. omega-3 fatty acids
   b. trans fat
   c. triglycerides
   d. saturated fats

3. Antioxidants
   a. are nutrients important in the production of hemoglobin.
   b. are substances added to foods to make them more flavorful or physically appealing.
   c. are suspected triggers of food allergies.
   d. are substances that prevent the harmful effects of free radicals.

4. Which of the following is true about the Food Guide Pyramid?
   a. It advises that, on a daily basis, you eat the same amounts of food from each of the food groups represented in the Pyramid.
   b. The foods at the top of the pyramid are considered to be the most nutritionally essential.
   c. According to the Pyramid, one should eat six to eleven servings of bread, cereals, rice, and pasta every week
   d. The Pyramid advises no more than two to three servings daily of both dairy foods and meat and other high-protein foods.

5. Which statement about essential nutrients is *false*?
   a. Carbohydrates provide body cells with glucose.
   b. Fats are necessary for the growth and repair of body cells.
   c. Water is an essential nutrient but doesn't provide any energy.
   d. Vitamins are necessary for the body to manufacture blood cells and hormones.

6. Food labels on packaged food include all of the following *except*
   a. total weight of the package.
   b. total amount of nutrients contained in the food.
   c. the percent of nutrient Daily Values provided in the food.
   d. serving size.

7. Which of the following statements is true?
   a. The Chinese diet, which is high in fats and low in carbohydrates, leads to high incidence of obesity and heart disease.
   b. The French diet is considered to be healthful because the food is high in saturated fats.
   c. The Mediterranean diet is rich in fruits, vegetables, wine, and olive oil and may help prevent heart disease.
   d. Mexican and African-American recipes often include MSG, which is unhealthy for people with high blood pressure.

8. Some vegetarians may
   a. include chicken and fish in their diets.
   b. avoid vitamin B_{12} supplements if they eat only plant foods.
   c. eat only legumes or nuts because these provide complete proteins.
   d. have high cholesterol levels because of the saturated fats in fruits and vegetables.

9. Food hazards include all the following *except*
   a. nitrites
   b. raw eggs
   c. pesticides
   d. refrigerated leftovers used within 3 days.

10. Common causes of foodborne infections include which of the following?
    a. the influenza virus
    b. salmonella and *E. coli* bacteria
    c. additives
    d. irradiation

Answers to these questions can be found on page 652.

Critical Thinking

1. Joel's grandparents seem to eat a fairly balanced diet, but he knows that elderly adults are more susceptible to disease. What recommendations could he make to them to ensure that they are getting all the nutrients they need to enhance their health?

Critical Thinking

2. Scientists are using genetic engineering to develop foods, such as tomatoes that won't bruise easily, cows that will produce more milk, or corn that will grow larger ears. Some consumer advocates argue that these items shouldn't be put on the market because they

Critical Thinking

haven't been studied carefully enough. What do you think of these foods? Would you eat them?

3. Which alternative or ethnic diet do you think has the best-tasting food? Which is the most healthy? Why?

Critical Thinking

4. Is it possible to meet nutritional requirements on a limited budget? Have you ever been in this situation? What would you recommend

Critical Thinking

to someone who wanted to eat healthfully on $30 a week?

5. Consider the number of times a week you eat fast food. How much

Critical Thinking

money would you have saved if you had eaten home-prepared meals? Which fast foods could you have selected that would have provided more nutritional value?

Profile Plus

Find the nutrient values of the food you are eating and plan a diet that supports a healthy lifestyle with this activity on your Profile Plus CD-ROM:

Profile Plus

• Nutrient Analysis and Diet Planning

Profile Plus

Sites and Bytes

USDA Center for Nutrition Policy and Promotion
www.usda.gov/cnpp

This interactive site sponsored by the United States Center for Nutrition Policy and Promotion features the Interactive Health Eating Index, an online dietary assessment that enables you to receive a personalized score on the overall quality of your diet, on a daily basis, based on the recommendations of the Food Guide Pyramid. This tool provides you with information on total fat, cholesterol, sodium, and other nutrients. You can also download a series of brochures featuring dietary guidelines as well as healthy recipes.

Sites and Bytes

Health Canada
www.hc-sc.gc.ca

Select *Healthy Living*, then *Food & Nutrition* to find information on Canadian nutrition guidelines and food labels.

Nutrient Analysis Tool
www.nat.uiuc.edu

This site, provided as a public service by the Food Science and Human Nutrition Department at the University of Illinois, features a free nutrient analysis interactive program that calculates the amount of calories, carbohydrates, protein, fat, vitamins, minerals, and fiber in the foods that make up your daily diet.

Sites and Bytes

Mayo Clinic Food and Nutrition
www.mayoclinic.com

Select *Food and Nutrition* on the Home page. This site features a wealth of reliable information, including current news, feature articles, interactive tools, nutrition basics, diet planning, nutrition and disease management, dietary supplements, as well as a virtual cookbook featuring healthy recipes, serving sizes, and shopping lists.

InfoTrac College Edition

Activity

Dundas, Mary L. and Jay R. Keller. "Herbal, Vitamin, and Mineral Supplement Use and Beliefs of University Students." *Topics in Clinical Nutrition*, Vol. 18, No. 1, January–March 2003, p. 49(5).

1. According to the study, what are the three most frequently used herbs by college students? What are the most frequently used vitamins and minerals?

InfoTrac College Edition

2. According to the college and university students surveyed, what is the most common reason for using vitamins and herbal supplements? Name three perceived benefits of using vitamins and herbal supplements.

3. What were the limitations of this study?

You can find additional readings related to nutrition with InfoTrac College Edition, an online library of

InfoTrac College Edition

more than 900 journals and publications. Follow the instructions for accessing InfoTrac College Edition that were packaged with your textbook; then search for articles using a key word search.

For additional links, resources, and suggested readings on InfoTrac College Edition, visit our Health & Wellness Resource Center at **http://health.wadsworth.com**.

Key Terms

The terms listed are used on the page indicated. Definitions of the terms are in the Glossary at the end of this book.

additives 172
amino acids 143
antioxidants 149
botulism 173
calories 142
carbohydrates 145
complementary
   proteins 170
complete proteins 143
complex
   carbohydrates 145
crucifers 159
Daily Values (DV) 165
dietary fiber 145
essential nutrients 142

folate 151
folic acid 151
food toxicologists 171
functional fiber 145
hemoglobin 153
incomplete proteins 143
indoles 159
irradiation 172
lacto-vegetarians 170
listeria 173
macronutrients 142
mad cow disease 174
micronutrients 142
minerals 149
nutrition 140

organic 171
osteoporosis 151
ovo-lacto-vegetarians
   170
phytochemicals 154
proteins 143
saturated fats 146
simple
   carbohydrates 145
trans fat 146
unsaturated fats 146
vegans 170
vitamins 148

References

1. Panel on Micronutrients, Subcommittees on Upper Reference Levels of Nutrients and Interpretation and Uses of Dietary Reference Intakes, and the Standing Committee on the Scientific Evaluation of Dietary Reference Intakes. *Dietary Reference Intakes for Energy, Carbohydrates, Fiber, Fat, Protein and Amino Acids.* Washington, DC: National Academy of Sciences Press, 2002.
2. Sizer, Frances, and Eleanor Whitney. *Nutrition: Concepts and Controversies,* 9th ed. Belmont, CA: Wadsworth, 2003.
3. Panel on Micronutrients.
4. Sizer and Whitney, *Nutrition: Concepts and Controversies.*
5. Grandjean, Ann, et al. "The Effect on Hydration of Two Diets, One with and One without Plain Water." *Journal of the American College of Nutrition.* Vol. 22, April 2003, p. 165.
6. "Beef: Nutrients That Work As Hard As You Do." American Dietetic Association, www.eatright.org.
7. Fitzpatrick, L. A. "Soy Isoflavones: Hope or Hype?" *Maturitas,* Vol. 44, No. 1, March 14, 2003, p. S21-29.
8. Panel on Micronutrients.
9. Harder, B. "Wholesome Grains: Insulin Effects May Explain Healthful Diet." *Science News,* Vol. 161, No. 20, May 18, 2002, p. 308.
10. Mozaffarian, Dariush, et al. "Cereal, Fruit, and Vegetable Fiber Intake and the Risk of Cardiovascular Disease in Elderly Individuals." *Journal of the American Medical Association,* Vol. 289, No. 13, April 2, 2003, p. 1659.
11. Liu, Simin. "Whole-Grain Foods, Dietary Fiber, and Type 2 Diabetes: Searching for a Kernel of Truth." *American Journal of Clinical Nutrition,* Vol. 77, 2003, pp. 527–529.
12. Panel on Micronutrients.
13. "Position of the American Dietetic Association: Health Implications of Dietary Fiber." *Journal of the American Dietetic Association,* Vol. 102, No. 7, July 2002, p. 993.
14. "Eating More Fiber Doesn't Have to Be Uncomfortable." *Tufts University Health & Nutrition Letter,* Vol. 20, No. 5, July 2002, p. 7.
15. "Evidence for Fish/Heart Health Connection Strengthens Even More." *Tufts University Health & Nutrition Letter,* Vol. 20, No. 4, June 2002, p. 3.
16. Gifford, K. D. "Dietary Fats, Eating Guides, and Public Policy: History, Critique, and Recommendations." *American Journal of Medicine,* Vol. 113, No. 9B, December 30, 2002, pp. 89S–106S.
17. Martin, A., et al. "Antioxidant Vitamins E and C and Risk of Alzheimer's Disease." *Nutrition Review,* Vol. 61, No. 2, February 2003, p. 69.
18. Grodstein, F., et al. "High-Dose Antioxidant Supplements and Cognitive Function in Community-Dwelling Elderly Women." *American Journal of Clinical Nutrition,* Vol. 77, No. 4, April 2003, p. 975.
19. Moyers, Susan, and Lynn Bailey. "Fetal Malformations and Folate Metabolism: Review of Recent Evidence." *Nutrition Reviews,* Vol. 59, No. 7, July 2001, p. 215.
20. "What You Need to Know About Calcium." *Harvard Health Letter,* Vol. 28, No. 6, April 2003, p. 1.
21. Slawson, Deborah, et al. "Food Sources of Calcium in a Sample of African-American and Euro-American Collegiate Athletes." *International Journal of Sport Nutrition and Exercise Metabolism,* Vol. 11, No. 2, June 2001.
22. Stear, Samantha, et al. "Effect of a Calcium and Exercise Intervention on the Bone Mineral Status of 16–18 Year-Old Adolescent Girls." *American Journal of Clinical Nutrition,* Vol. 77, No. 4, April 2003, p. 985.
23. "Independent Expert Report on Diet and Chronic Disease." World Health Organization news release, March 3, 2003.
24. "Freshman College Student Dining Habits." *Food Service Director,* Vol. 15, No. 3, March 15, 2002, p. 1.
25. Evans, Alexandra, et al. "Fruit and Vegetable Consumption Among Mexican-American College Students." *Journal of the American Dietetic Association.* Vol. 100, No. 11, November 2000, p. 1399.
26. "Nutrition Knowledge of Collegiate Athletes." *Nutrition Research Newsletter,* Vol. 21, No. 4, April 2002, p. 3.
27. "When, Why, and On What Are College Students Snacking." *The Food Institute Report,* February 25, 2002, p. 4.
28. Glanz, Karen. "Reducing Chronic Diseases Risk Through Nutrition." *Facts of Life: Issue Briefing for Health Reporters,* Vol. 5, No. 9, November 2000, p. 2.
29. Smiciklas-Wright, H., et al. "Foods Commonly Eaten in the United States, 1989–1991 and 1994–1996: Are Portion Sizes Changing?" *Journal of the American Dietetic Association,* Vol. 103, No. 1, January 2003, p. 39.

References

30. Critser, Greg. *Fat Land: How Americans Became the Fattest People in the World.* Boston: Houghton-Mifflin, 2003.
31. Smiciklas-Wright et al. "Food Commonly Eaten in the United States."
32. Knaust, Gretchen, and Irene Foster. "Estimation of Food Guide Pyramid Serving Sizes by College Students." *Family and Consumer Sciences Research Journal,* Vol. 29, No. 2, December 2000, p. 101.
33. Brown, C. Hsing-Kuan. "A Food Display Assignment and Handling Food Models Improves Accuracy of College Students' Estimates of Food Portions." *Journal of The American Dietetic Association,* Vol. 100, No. 9, September 2000, pp. 1063–1064.
34. Fly, Alyce, et al. "Keeping the Culture with Food Guide Pyramids." *Physical Educator,* Vol. 59, No. 4, Winter 2002, p. 193.
35. Ibid.
36. Frazao, E. and J. Allshouse. "Strategies for Intervention: Commentary and Debate." *Journal of Nutrition,* Vol. 33, No. 3, March 2003, pp. 844S–847S.

References

37. "Food Pyramid in Need of Renovation." *Harvard Women's Health Watch,* February 2003.
38. Willett, Walter, and Meir Stampfer. "Rebuilding the Food Pyramid." *Scientific American,* January 2003, www.sciam.com/
39. Halsted, C. H. "Dietary Supplements and Functional Foods: Two Sides of a Coin?" *American Journal of Clinical Nutrition,* Vol. 77, No. 4, April 2003, p. 1001.
40. Ibid.
41. "Whether Pyramid, Plate, or Pagoda, All Countries Recommend Less Protein and More Carbohydrate." *Tufts University Health & Nutrition Letter,* Vol. 20, No. 4, June 2002, p. 6.
42. "Dietary Guidelines and the Food Guide Pagoda." *Journal of the American Dietetic Association,* Vol. 100, No. 8, August 2000.
43. Carluccio, M. A., et al. "Olive Oil and Red Wine Antioxidant Polyphenols Inhibit Endothelial Activation, Antiatherogenic Properties of Mediterranean Diet Phytochemicals." *Arteriosclerosis, Thrombosis, Vascular Biology,* February 20, 2003. Available at www.ahajaurals.org.

References

44. Schlosser, Eric. *Fast Food Nation.* New York: Simon & Schuster, 2001.
45. Elliott, Victoria. "Fast-Food Sellers Under Fire for Helping Supersize People." American Medical News, April 21, 2003.
46. Morrone, M. and A. Rathbun. "Health Education and Food Safety Behavior in the University Setting." *Journal of Environmental Health,* Vol. 65, No. 7, March 2003, p. 9.
47. "Hamburger Disease/Barbecue Syndrome." *Health Canada,* www.hcsc.gc. ca/english/feature/summer/food_drink/ bbq.html
48. Bovine spongiform encephalopathy, www.fda.gov/oc/opacom/hottopics/bse. html
49. Crespo, J. F .and J. Rodriguez. "Food Allergy in Adulthood." *Allergy,* Vol. 58, March 2003, p. 98.

CHAPTER 6

Eating Patterns and Problems

By the time she went away to college, Gia had lost and gained 10 pounds again and again. During her frantic first semester, Gia never seemed to stop eating. Come spring, she was 12 pounds heavier—and determined to slim down by summer. Gia tried every diet she heard of. For a while, she ate no fat, although she couldn't resist wolfing down entire boxes of no-fat cookies. She started counting carbohydrates and wouldn't eat a single slice of bread or strand of spaghetti. Her favorite was the high-protein diet that allowed her to load up on eggs, bacon, hamburgers, and steak.

Even though Gia began every diet with enthusiasm, she invariably fell off each one. Sooner or later, she started craving the foods she'd been forcing herself to live without.

And once she went back to her old eating habits, she felt out of control. When she stepped onto the scale, she weighed more than she did before she went on the diet.

Like Gia, many Americans struggle with their weight. An estimated 64.5 percent of adult Americans—almost two of every three men and women—and 15 percent of children ages 6 to 19 are overweight or obese.[1] Each year obesity costs approximately $100 billion in health care expenses and causes at least 300,000 excess deaths.[2]

Ironically, as average weights have increased, the quest for thinness has become a national obsession. In a society where slimmer is

seen as better, anyone who is less than lean may feel like a failure. Individuals who are overweight or embarrassed by their appearance often assume that they would be happier, sexier, or more successful in thinner bodies. And so they diet. Each year, 15 to 35 percent of Americans go on diets, but no matter how much they lose, 90 to 95 percent regain extra pounds within five years.

This chapter explores our national preoccupation with slimness; examines unhealthy eating patterns and eating disorders; tells what obesity is and why excess pounds are dangerous; shows why fad diets don't work; and offers guidelines for how to control weight safely, sensibly, and permanently.

FREQUENTLY ASKED QUESTIONS FAQ

FAQ: How many calories do I need? p. 184

FAQ: Who develops eating disorders? p. 188

FAQ: How did we get so fat? p. 193

FAQ: Which diets are safe and effective? p. 199

• **Identify** and **describe** the symptoms and dangers associated with eating disorders.

• **Define** obesity and **describe** its relationship to genetics, lifestyle, and major health problems.

• **Assess** various approaches to weight loss.

• **Design** a personal plan for sensible weight management.

After studying the material in this chapter, you should be able to:

• **Identify** factors that influence hunger, appetite, and food consumption.

• **Discuss** types of unhealthy eating behavior.

© David Oliver/Taxi/Getty Images

181

Body Image

Throughout most of history, bigger was better. The great beauties of centuries past, as painted by such artistic masters as Rubens and Renoir, were soft and fleshy, with rounded bellies and dimpled thighs. Culture often shapes views of beauty and health.

Many developing countries still regard a full figure, rather than a thin one, as the ideal. Fattening huts, in which brides-to-be eat extra food to plump up before marriage, still exist in some African cultures. Among certain Native American tribes of the Southwest, if a girl is thin at puberty, a fat woman places her foot on the girl's back so she will magically gain weight and become more attractive.

Influenced by the media, many Americans are paying more attention to their body images than ever before—and at a younger age. In a study of high school girls, those who regularly read women's health and fitness magazines, which may present unrealistic physical ideals, were more likely to go on low-calorie diets, take pills to suppress their appetites, use laxatives, or force themselves to vomit after eating. In other research, girls who watched a lot of television and expressed concern about slimness and popularity were more dissatisfied with their bodies than girls involved in sports.[3] Boys' body images also are influenced by media images depicting superstrong, highly muscular males.

"Thinner is better" is not the global standard, and in past centuries, the fuller figure was considered healthy and beautiful. This painting by Renoir from the late 1880s shows the feminine ideal of the time.

African-American women often have more positive attitudes toward their bodies, feeling more satisfied with their weight and seeing themselves as more attractive. However, there are no significant differences between African-American women who diet and white women who diet in terms of self-esteem and body dissatisfaction.

Being overweight for a long period of time has a cumulative negative impact on body image. In a study of 266 college women, those who described themselves as "always overweight" ranked much lower in current body self-esteem than those with more recent weight problems.[4]

College students of different ethnic and racial backgrounds, including Asians, express as much—and sometimes more—concern about their body shape and weight as whites.[5] Men and women are prone to different distortions in body image. Women tend to see themselves as overweight, whether or not they are; men perceive themselves as underweight, even when their weights are normal or above normal. In a study of university students, African-American and Caucasian men were similar in their ideals for body size and in their perceptions of their own shapes. As shown in Student Snapshot: "Body Dissatisfaction in African-American and White Students," both African-American and white women perceived themselves as smaller than they actually were and desired an even smaller body size. (BMI, or body mass index, is defined in Chapter 4.) However, the African-American women were more accepting of larger size.[6]

As men and women age, their attitudes about their bodies change. In a study comparing college students, parents, and grandparents, older men and women were more dissatisfied with their appearance than younger people. Women were more concerned with aging than men, but there were no gender differences in overall body dissatisfaction.

Weight Assessment

As discussed in Chapter 4, health experts have shifted from body weight to Body Mass Index (BMI) as the primary tool for evaluating body composition and health risks. A BMI equal to or greater than 25 defines **overweight** and marks the point at which excess weight increases the risk of disease. (See Figure 4-7 on page 127.) A BMI equal to or greater than 30 defines **obesity** and marks the point at which excess weight increases the risk of death. Among Asians the relative risk of obesity-related diseases increases above a BMI of 23.4.[7]

Student Snapshot

Body Dissatisfaction in African-American and White Students

In a study of 630 undergraduates, both African-American and white women perceived themselves to be smaller than they actually were—and wished to be even smaller. However, the white students saw themselves and desired to be considerably smaller than the African-American women. Both African-American and white men rated the silhouette depicting a BMI of 20 as the most desirable.

Source: "Body Dissatisfaction Among College Students," *Nutrition Research Newsletter*, Vol. 21, No. 3, March 2002, p. 9.

BMI 17   18   20   22.5   24   32   35

Desired · Desired · Perceived · Current · Perceived · Current

☐ White women
■ African-American women

The degree of an individual's risk from excess weight also depends on waist circumference, waist–hip ratio, and lifestyle habits related to diet and exercise. A waist circumference of 40 inches or more in men and 35 or more inches in women indicates central obesity, which is characterized by fat deposited deep within the central abdominal area of the body. (See Figure 6-1.) Such "visceral" fat is more dangerous than "subcutaneous" fat just below the skin because it moves more readily into the bloodstream and directly raises levels of harmful cholesterol.

The **waist-to-hip ratio,** which considers the distribution of weight and the location of excess fat, also is important. Excess weight around the abdominal area, creating an apple-shaped silhouette, is associated with increased cardiovascular risk for both men and women. (See Figure 6–2.) Men of all ages are more prone to develop the "apple" shape characteristic of central obesity; women in their reproductive years are more likely to accumulate fat around the hips and thighs and acquire a pear shape.

When men and women diet, men lose more visceral fat located around the abdominal area. This weight loss produces more cardiovascular benefits for men, including a decrease in triglycerides (fats circulating in the blood) and an increase in the "good" form of cholesterol, high–density lipoprotein (HDL).

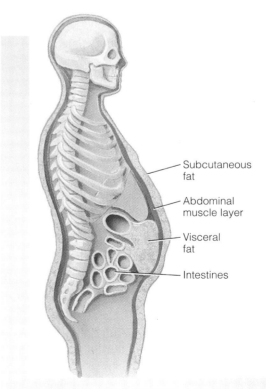

Subcutaneous fat

Abdominal muscle layer

Visceral fat

Intestines

Figure 6-1 VISCERAL FAT AND SUBCUTANEOUS FAT
The fat deep within the body's abdominal cavity may pose an especially high risk to health.

PEAR
Fat stores around hips predominate

APPLE
Fat stores around waist predominate

Figure 6-2 PEAR-SHAPED VERSUS APPLE-SHAPED BODIES

How Many Calories Do I Need?

Calories, as noted in Chapter 5, are the measure of the amount of energy that can be derived from food. How many calories you need depends on your gender, age, body-frame size, weight, percentage of body fat, and your **basal metabolic rate (BMR)**—the number of calories needed to sustain your body at rest. Your activity level also affects your calorie requirements. (See Table 6-1.) Regardless of whether you consume fat, protein, or carbohydrates, if you take in more calories than required to maintain your size and don't work them off in some sort of physical activity, your body will convert the excess to fat.

The Anatomy of Appetite

Why do you wake up starving? Why does your stomach rumble during a late afternoon lecture? The simple answer is **hunger:** the physiological drive to consume food. **Appetite** is the psychological desire to eat. More than a dozen different signals may influence and control our desire for food. Researchers at the National Institutes of Health have discovered appetite receptors within the hypothalamus region of the brain that specifically respond to hunger messages carried by chemicals (Figure 6-3).

Appetite usually begins with the fear of the unpleasant sensation of hunger. We learn to avoid hunger by eating a certain amount of food at certain times of the day, just as dogs in the laboratory learn to avoid electric shocks by jumping at the sound of a warning bell. But appetite is easily led into temptation. In one famous experiment, psy-

chologists bought bags of high-calorie goodies—peanut butter, marshmallows, chocolate-chip cookies, and salami—for their test rats. The animals ate so much on this "supermarket diet" that they gained more weight than any laboratory rats ever had before. The snack-food diet that fattened up these rats was particularly high in fats. Biologists speculate that creamy, buttery, or greasy foods may cause internal changes that increase appetite and, consequently, weight.

A hormone called leptin, produced by fat cells, sends signals to the brain that affect appetite. When leptin levels are normal, people eat just enough to maintain weight. When leptin is low, the brain responds as if fat stores had been depleted and slows down metabolism. This may be one reason why it is so difficult to lose weight by dieting alone.

Other hormones made in the stomach also influence how hungry we feel. One is ghrelin, a natural appetite stimulant. When given shots of ghrelin, people become very hungry and eat 30 percent more than they normally would. Ghrelin typically rises before meals and falls afterward. Dieters tend to have high levels of ghrelin, as if their bodies were trying to stimulate appetite so they regain lost fat.

We stop eating when we feel satisfied; this is called **satiety,** a feeling of fullness and relief from hunger, which also is influenced by hormones. PYY, another hormone made in the gut, travels to the brain after a meal and

TABLE 6-1	**Daily Energy Requirements (in Calories) for People of Various Sizes and Levels of Activity**	
Sedentary	**Active**	
5'1", 98 to 132 pounds		
Women	1,688 to 1,834	2,104 to 2,290
Men	1,919 to 2,167	2,104 to 2,290
5'5", up to 150 pounds		
Women	1,816 to 1,982	2,267 to 2,477
Men	2,068 to 2,349	2,490 to 2,842
5'9", 125 to 169 pounds		
Women	1,948 to 2,134	2,434 to 2,670
Men	2,222 to 2,538	2,683 to 3,078
6'1", 139 to 188 pounds		
Women	2,083 to 2,290	2,605 to 2,869
Men	2,382 to 2,736	2,883 to 3,325

Source: Panel on Micronutrients, Subcommittees on Upper Reference Levels of Nutrients and Interpretation and Uses of Dietary Reference Intakes, and the Standing Committee on the Scientific Evaluation of Dietary Reference Intakes. *Dietary Reference Intakes for Energy, Carbohydrates, Fiber, Fat, Protein and Amino Acids (Macronutrients):* Washington, DC: National Academy of Sciences Press, 2002.

Appetite receptors in hypothalamus respond to hormonal messages

Ghrelin stimulates appetite before meals

Leptin regulates appetite to maintain weight

PPY depresses appetite after meals

Figure 6-3 HOW HORMONES HELP REGULATE OUR APPETITE

switches off the urge to eat more. In experiments, people given PYY and then offered a buffet two hours later ate a third fewer calories than when they did not get the hormone. Scientists are experimenting with PYY and other chemicals as potential agents to help treat obesity.[8]

From this perspective, diets are doomed to fail because they pit the dieter against tireless internal enemies: the set point and its enforcer, appetite. The only effective alternative is lowering, or resetting, the set point. And the safest, most effective way to do so is through physical activity, which dampens appetite in the short run and lowers the set point for the long term. As discussed later in this chapter, moderate activity not only works up an appetite but also helps work it off.

Unhealthy Eating Behavior

Unhealthy eating behavior takes many forms, ranging from not eating enough to eating too much too quickly. Its roots are complex. In addition to media and external pressures, a family history can play a role. Researchers have linked specific genes to some cases of anorexia nervosa and binge eating, but most believe that a variety of factors, including stress and culture, combine to cause disordered eating.[9]

About a third of female athletes in every sport show symptoms of disordered eating or eating disorders. Girls and adolescent females who participate regularly in sports are at risk for disordered eating, menstrual dysfunction, and decreased bone mineral density, according to the American Academy of Pediatrics. The combination of these three disorders is known as the *female athlete triad*.

Sooner or later many people don't eat the way they should. They may skip meals, thereby increasing the likelihood that they'll end up with more body fat, a higher weight, and a higher blood cholesterol level. They may live on diet foods, but consume so much of them that they gain weight anyway. Some even engage in more extreme eating behavior: Dissatisfied with almost all aspects of their appearance, they continuously go on and off diets, eat compulsively, or binge on high-fat treats. Such behaviors can be warning signs of potentially serious eating disorders that should not be ignored.

Disordered Eating in College Students

College students—particularly women, including varsity athletes—are at risk for unhealthy eating behaviors. The prevalence of disordered eating symptoms and eating disorders has increased dramatically in the last 20 years.

In a recent survey at a large, public, rural university in the mid-Atlantic states, 17 percent of the women were struggling with disordered eating. Younger women (ages 18 to 21) were more likely than older students to have an eating disorder. In this study, eating disorders did not discriminate, equally affecting women of different races (white, Asian, African-American, Native American, and Hispanic), religions, athletic involvement, and living arrangements (on or off campus, with roommates, boyfriends, or family). Although the students viewed eating disorders as both mental and physical problems, and felt that individual therapy would be most helpful, all said that they would first turn to a friend for help.[10] In another study of 1,620 students, almost 11 percent of the women and 4 percent of the men were at risk for eating disorders. About 17 percent of the women and 10 percent of the men said concerns about weight interfered with their academic work. Women in sororities were at slightly increased risk of an eating disorder compared with those in dormitories.[11]

In a study of Australian male undergraduates, one in four men worried about shape and weight; one in five displayed attitudes and behaviors characteristic of disordered eating and eating disorders. (See Table 6-2.) None ever sought treatment, even if the students recognized they had

a problem. The reason, the researchers theorized, may be that the young men hesitated to seek treatment for an illness stigmatized as a problem that affects only women. Some men exercised extremely intensively almost every day, even if ill or injured. None felt they had a problem with excessive exercise.[12]

The unique demands and stressors of the transition to college do not increase the likelihood of disordered eating for all freshmen. One study that followed more than 100 undergraduate women through their freshman year found that those who reported the most body dissatisfaction and unhealthy eating patterns at the beginning of the first semester were most likely to experience more eating problems, such as losing control of their eating when feeling strong emotions. The strongest predictor that eating symp-

TABLE 6-2	Eating Behavior and Concerns About Body Weight and Exercise of Australian Male College Students	
Behavior or Concern	**Percentage Reporting "a lot" or "a great deal"**	
Eating behavior		
Follow rules about eating for any reason	23	
Follow rules about eating for weight/shape	20	
Limit what eat for weight/shape	20	
Eat only 1 or 2 meals each day	19	
Try to avoid eating liked foods for weight/shape	18	
Body weight/shape concern		
Worry about shape and weight	25	
Shape important for self-esteem	16	
Feel fat	12	
Unhappy about shape	10	
Seriously want to lose weight	9	
Feel inhibited about my weight	9	
Afraid of gaining weight and becoming fat	8	
Unhappy about weight	8	
Feel distressed if had to be weighed regularly	7	
Thinking of food affects concentration on other things	3	
Exercise concerns		
Exercise important for self-esteem	48	
Distressed if not exercising as much as wanted	34	
Exercise to feel good	33	
Exercise for weight and shape	33	
Follow rules about exercising	27	
Worry about exercise	14	

Source: Jennifer O'Dea and Suzanne Abraham. "Eating and Exercise Disorders in Young College Men." *Journal of American College Health*, Vol. 50, No. 4, May 2002, p. 273. Reprinted with permission of the Helen Dwight Reid Educational Foundation. Published by Heldref Publications, 1319 Eighteenth Street, NW, Washington, DC 20036-1802. Copyright © 2002.

toms would get worse over the freshman year was not BMI or weight, but body dissatisfaction.

The most common weight-related problem on campuses may be gaining weight, particularly in the first year away from home. As many students discover, it's easy to gain weight on campuses, which are typically crammed with vending machines, fast-food counters, and cafeterias serving up hearty meals. But the infamous *freshman 15,* the extra pounds acquired in the first year at college, seems to be a myth. Several studies have documented much lower weight gains, ranging from 2.45 to 7 pounds. In one recent study of changes in both weight and body fat, freshman estimated that they had gained an average of 4.1 pounds. In fact, their weights fluctuated from a gain of 15 pounds to a loss of 15 pounds (Figure 6-4). Among the 60 percent of freshmen who did put on weight, the average gain was 4.6 pounds.[13]

 Even international students may gain weight and body fat after arriving on American campuses. Ohio University researchers found that after 20 weeks, foreign students, who had incorporated foods high in fat, salt, and sugar into their diets, gained about 3 pounds on average and their percentage of body fat rose by about 5 percent.

Extreme Dieting

About half of girls attempt to control their weight by dieting. In a year-long study of teenagers, both parents and the media had the most influence on the development of weight concerns and weight control practices, including dieting, among adolescents and preadolescents.

Extreme dieters go beyond cutting back on calories or increasing physical activity. They become preoccupied with what they eat and weigh. Although their weight never falls below 85 percent of normal, their weight loss is severe enough to cause uncomfortable physical consequences, such as weakness and sensitivity to cold. Technically, these dieters do not have anorexia nervosa (discussed later in the chapter), but they are at increased risk for it.

Extreme dieters may think they know a great deal about nutrition, yet many of their beliefs about food and weight are misconceptions or myths. For instance, they may eat only protein because they believe complex carbohydrates, including fruits and breads, are fattening. When they're anxious, angry, or bored, they focus on food and their fear of fatness. Dieting and exercise become ways of coping with any stress in their lives.

Sometimes nutritional education alone can help change this eating pattern. However, many avid dieters who deny that they have a problem with food may need counseling (which they usually agree to only at their family's insistence) to correct dangerous eating behavior and prevent further complications.

Figure 6-4 THE MYTH OF THE FRESHMAN 15: CHANGES IN WEIGHT AND BODY FAT DURING FRESHMAN YEAR

In this study of 44 freshmen at a small Midwestern liberal arts college, weight change ranged from a loss of 15 pounds to a gain of 15 pounds.

Source: Melody Graham and Amy Jones. "Freshman 15: Valid Theory or Harmful Myth?" *Journal of American College Health*, Vol. 50, No. 4, January 2002, p. 171.

Compulsive Overeating

People who eat compulsively cannot stop putting food in their mouths. They eat fast and they eat a lot. They eat even when they're full. They may eat around the clock rather than at set meal times, often in private because of embarrassment over how much they consume.

Some mental health professionals describe compulsive eating as a food addiction that is much more likely to develop in women. According to Overeaters Anonymous (OA), an international 12-step program, many women who eat compulsively view food as a source of comfort against feelings of inner emptiness, low self-esteem, and fear of abandonment.

The following behaviors may signal a potential problem with compulsive overeating:

:: Turning to food when depressed or lonely, when feeling rejected, or as a reward.

:: A history of failed diets and anxiety when dieting.

:: Thinking about food throughout the day.

:: Eating quickly and without pleasure.

:: Continuing to eat even when you're no longer hungry.

:: Frequent talking about food, or refusing to talk about food.

:: Fear of not being able to stop eating once you start.

Recovery from compulsive eating can be challenging because people with this problem cannot give up entirely the substance they abuse. Like everyone else, they must eat. However, they can learn new eating habits and ways of dealing with underlying emotional problems. An OA survey found that most of its members joined to lose weight but later felt the most important effect was their improved emotional, mental, and physical health. As one woman put it, "I came for vanity but stayed for sanity."

Binge Eating

Binge eating—the rapid consumption of an abnormally large amount of food in a relatively short time—often occurs in compulsive eaters. Individuals with a binge-eating disorder typically eat a larger-than-ordinary amount of food during a relatively brief period, feel a lack of control over eating, and binge at least twice a week for at least a six-month period. During most of these episodes, binge eaters experience at least three of the following:

:: Eating much more rapidly than usual.

:: Eating until they feel uncomfortably full.

:: Eating large amounts of food when not feeling physically hungry.

:: Eating large amounts of food throughout the day with no planned mealtimes.

:: Eating alone because they are embarrassed by how much they eat and by their eating habits.

Binge eaters may spend up to several hours eating, and consume 2,000 or more calories worth of food in a single binge—more than many people eat in a day. After such binges, they usually do not induce vomiting, use laxatives, or rely on other means (such as exercise) to control weight. They simply get fatter. As their weight climbs, they become depressed, anxious, or troubled by other psychological symptoms to a much greater extent than others of comparable weight.

Probably the most common eating disorder, binge-eating strikes up to 4 million Americans, according to the National Institutes of Health. Binge-eaters are usually overweight or obese. An estimated 8 to 19 percent of obese patients in weight loss programs are binge eaters.

A recent study suggests that a weak gene, not feeble willpower, may be the cause of binge eating for some people.[14] There is no established ideal treatment, and psychological and cognitive behavior approaches generally lead to only modest weight loss. New research indicates that medication may help at least as a short-term treatment.[15]

Eating Disorders

According to the American Psychiatric Association, patients with **eating disorders** display a broad range of symptoms that occur along a continuum between those of anorexia nervosa and those of bulimia nervosa.

As many as 10 percent of teenage girls develop symptoms of or full-blown eating disorders.[16] Among the factors that increase the risk are: Preoccupation with a thin body, social pressure, and childhood traits such as perfectionism and excessive cautiousness, which reflect an obsessive-compulsive personality.[17]

The best known eating disorders are anorexia nervosa, which affects fewer than 1 percent of adolescent women, and bulimia nervosa, which strikes 2 to 3 percent. Many more young women do not have the characteristic symptoms of these disorders but are preoccupied with their weight or experiment with unhealthy forms of dieting.

The American Psychiatric Association has developed practice guidelines for the treatment of patients with eating disorders, which include medical, psychological, and behavioral approaches. One of the most scientifically supported is cognitive-behavior therapy, described in Chapter 2.[18]

Who Develops Eating Disorders?

Eating disorders affect an estimated 5 to 10 million women and 1 million men. Despite past evidence that eating disorders were primarily problems for white women, they are increasing among men and members of different ethnic and racial groups. (See The X&Y File: "Men, Women, and Weight" on page 190.)

In the few studies of eating disorders in minority college students that have been completed, African-American female undergraduates had a slightly lower prevalence of eating disorders than whites. Asian Americans reported fewer symptoms of eating disorders but more body dissatisfaction, concerns about shape, and more intense efforts to lose weight.

STRATEGIES FOR PREVENTION

Do You Have an Eating Disorder?

Physicians have developed a simple screening test for eating disorders, consisting of the following questions:

- Do you make yourself sick because you feel uncomfortably full?

- Do you worry you have lost control over how much you eat?

- Have you recently lost more than 14 pounds in a three-month period?

- Do you believe yourself to be fat when others say you are too thin?

- Would you say that food dominates your life?

Score one point for every "yes." A score of two or more is a likely indication of anorexia nervosa or bulimia nervosa.

Source: Karl Miller. "Treatment Guideline for Eating Disorders." *American Family Physician,* Vol. 62, No. 1, July 1, 2000.

Researchers in one study analyzed the importance of BMI in evaluating eating disorders in different ethnic groups. The BMIs of Hispanics are generally higher than those of whites, and more Hispanics are categorized as overweight. Asians, as a group, weigh less than whites. In the study, college women with higher BMIs were most concerned about their weights and shapes—regardless of their ethnic backgrounds. Data on Hispanics, Asians, and whites of similar weights show equivalent concern about their weight.[19]

In a study of Iranian-born young women living in Teheran (Iran) and Los Angeles, those in Teheran were more concerned about their weight than the California women, even though most had little access to images from the Western media and were obliged to wear clothes that hid the shape of their body. They also were as dissatisfied with their body and as likely to have symptoms of disordered eating as those in the United States.[20]

In a survey of health care professionals at the country's largest colleges and universities, 70 percent said that eating disorders are common among their undergraduates; 11 percent said they were widespread; 19 percent described them as rare. While 99 percent of the schools surveyed provide general mental health services, 69 percent have professionals on staff who specialize in diagnosing and treating eating disorders. Of all the hurdles to helping students with eating disorders, 39 percent said denial is the biggest, while 24 percent felt it was unwillingness to seek treatment, and 20 percent blamed pressure from peers and the media to stay thin.

Eating disorders affect every aspect of college students' lives, including dating. Both men and women tend to avoid dating individuals with eating disorders, but men are far less accepting of obesity than women.

Male and female athletes are vulnerable to eating disorders, either because of the pressure to maintain ideal body weight or to achieve a weight that might enhance their performance. Many female athletes, particularly those participating in sports or activities that emphasize leanness (such as gymnastics, distance running, diving, figure skating, and classical ballet) have "subclinical" eating disorders that could undermine their nutritional status and energy levels. However, there is often little awareness or recognition of their disordered eating.

If someone you know has an eating disorder, let your friend know you're concerned and that you care. Don't criticize or make fun of his or her eating habits. Encourage your friend to talk about other problems and feelings, and suggest that he or she talk to the school counselor or someone at the mental health center, the family doctor, or another trusted adult. Offer to go along if you think that will make a difference.

Anorexia Nervosa

Although *anorexia* means "loss of appetite," most individuals with **anorexia nervosa** are, in fact, hungry all the time. For them, food is an enemy—a threat to their sense of self, identity, and autonomy. In the distorted mirror of their mind's eye, they see themselves as fat or flabby even at a normal or below-normal body weight. Some simply feel fat; others think that they are thin in some places and too fat in others, such as the abdomen, buttocks, or thighs.

The characteristics of anorexia nervosa include:

:: A refusal to maintain normal body weight (weight loss leading to body weight of less than 85 percent of that expected for age and height).

:: An intense fear of gaining weight or becoming fat, even though underweight.

:: A distorted body image, so that the person feels fat even when emaciated.

:: In women, the absence of at least three menstrual cycles.

The incidence of anorexia nervosa has increased in the last three decades in most developed countries. The peak ages for its onset are 14½ and 18 years.[21] According to the American Psychiatric Association's Work Group on Eating Disorders, cases are increasing among males, minorities, women of all ages, and possibly preteens.

the X & Y file   *Men, Women, and Weight*

Women have long been bombarded by the media with idealized images of female bodies that bear little resemblance to the way most women look. Increasingly, more advertisements and men's magazines are featuring idealized male bodies. Sleek, strong, and sculpted, they too do not resemble the bodies most men inhabit. The gap between reality and ideal is getting bigger for both genders.

In the last decade, numerous studies have shown that women in *Playboy* centerfolds and Miss America pageants weigh less than they did in the 1970s. In one analysis, 29 percent of *Playboy* centerfolds and 17 percent of Miss America pageant winners had BMIs below 17.5, one of the criteria for anorexia nervosa and a definite indication of being severely underweight.

As beauty pageant queens and female models have been shrinking, the men featured in *Playgirl* centerfolds have been bulking up. Their BMIs are higher than in the past, as are the BMIs of a sample of Canadian and American men between the ages of 18 and 24. Researchers do not know if the higher BMIs are the result of an increase in lean body mass or body fat. Their theory: The models have become more muscular over time,

accounting for their high BMIs, while real guys may simply have gotten fatter.

When college men and women step on a scale or look in a mirror, they react in different ways. In a study of 525 undergraduates, the women failed to see themselves as underweight, even when they were, and perceived themselves as overweight, even when they were not. Many of the women who considered themselves normal weight nonetheless desired to be thinner. Men in the study generally saw themselves as underweight, even when they were not. Most desired to be heavier, though not obese. Women yearning to be thinner and men wanting to be heavier were equally likely to experience what the researchers dubbed *social physique anxiety*.

Women are more prone to unhealthy eating and eating disorders than men, but the incidence among men is increasing. Men and women with these problems share many psychological similarities and experience similar symptoms. However, men are more likely to have other psychiatric disorders and are less likely to seek professional treatment. Some feel that eating disorders fall under the category of "women's diseases." Others may not recognize the symptoms because eating disorders have long been assumed to plague only women.

In the *restricting* type of anorexia, individuals lose weight by avoiding any fatty foods, and by dieting, fasting, and exercising. Some start smoking as a way of controlling their weight. In the *binge-eating/purging* type, they engage in binge eating, purging (through self-induced vomiting, laxatives, diuretics, or enemas), or both. Obsessed with an intense fear of fatness, they may weigh themselves several times a day, measure various parts of their body, check mirrors to see if they look fat, and try on different items of clothing to see if they feel tight.

What Causes Anorexia Nervosa?

Many complex factors interact and contribute to this disorder, including biological, psychological, and social ones. Anorexia is more common among close relatives, particularly sisters, than it is in the general population. The relatives of anorexics also have a higher than expected frequency of depressive disorders.

Anorexia is associated with changes within the brain, including abnormalities in the stress-hormone cortisol, the neurotransmitters dopamine, serotonin, and norepinephrine—all of which influence appetite and satiety—and the peptide cholecystokinin, which affects feelings of fullness. It is not clear whether these changes are a cause or a consequence of this disorder.

Anorexia also may be a response to a personal loss or a sign of a driven, perfectionist personality. Often young anorexics have above-average grades and an unwarranted fear of failure. Some theorists speculate that young teenage girls may starve themselves because of fear of their budding sexuality. By drastically reducing their weight, they can prevent or stop menstruation and breast development.

Girls who develop anorexia often have little insight or awareness of their feelings, needs, and wants. After years of reacting to the expectations of others, they may feel inadequate as they approach the age of independence. In some ways, starvation may serve as a way of creating an identity and asserting independence.

In one study that followed 21 college women with eating disorders for six years, 11 got better during their post-college years, while 10 continued to struggle with disordered eating. The major difference between the two groups revolved around issues of autonomy and relation. Those who could better negotiate the tension between being independent and relating to others had higher self-esteem, a more positive self-concept, and a healthier relationship with food.

About one-third of those with anorexia initially were mildly overweight and cut back on food just to lose a few pounds. Others had normal weights but began to diet to look more attractive or, in the case of male and female athletes and dancers, to gain a performance advantage.

Sometimes, illness, stress, or surgery triggers weight loss. Often the initial response to their weight loss—from parents, coaches, or friends—is positive. However, starvation seems to take on a life of its own, and anorexics cannot return to a healthy eating pattern. In time, they may place so much value on thinness that they cannot recognize the dangers to their health.

Health Dangers and Treatment

The medical consequences of anorexia nervosa are serious (see Figure 6-5). Menstrual periods stop in women; testosterone levels decline in men. Adolescents with this disorder do not undergo normal sexual maturation, such as breast development, and may not reach their anticipated height. Even individuals who look and feel reasonably healthy may have subtle or hidden abnormalities, including heart irregularities and arrhythmias that can increase their risk of sudden death. Women who do not menstruate for six months or more may develop osteoporosis and suffer irreversible weakening and thinning of their bones as a result.

Even when they realize that they are jeopardizing their health, people with anorexia tend to fear that treatment will make them worse—that is, fatter. They need repeated reassurance that they will not become overweight and that they can and will find healthier ways of coping with life.

According to current practice guidelines, treatment of anorexia nervosa includes medical therapy (such as "refeeding" to overcome malnutrition) and behavioral, cognitive, psychodynamic, and family therapy. Antidepressant medication sometimes can help, particularly when there is a personal or family history of depression. Most people who get help do return to normal weight, but it can take a long time for their eating behaviors to become normal and for them to deal with troubling body image issues. In a study that followed 95 patients with anorexia, about half—56 percent—had no symptoms of an eating disorder after five years; three had died.[22]

Bulimia Nervosa

Individuals with **bulimia nervosa** go on repeated eating binges and rapidly consume large amounts of food, usually sweets, stopping only because of severe abdominal pain or sleep, or because they are interrupted. Those with *purging* bulimia induce vomiting or take large doses of laxatives to relieve guilt and control their weight. In *nonpurging* bulimia, individuals use other means, such as fasting or excessive exercise, to compensate for binges.

The characteristics of bulimia nervosa include:

:: Repeated binge eating.

:: A feeling of lack of control over eating behavior.

:: Regular reliance on self-induced vomiting, laxatives, or diuretics.

:: Strict dieting or fasting, or vigorous exercise, to prevent weight gain.

:: A minimum average of two bingeing episodes a week for at least three months.

:: A preoccupation with body shape and weight.

An estimated 1 to 3 percent of adolescent and young American women develop bulimia.[23] Some experiment with bingeing and purging for a few months and then stop when they change their social or living situation. Others develop longer-term bulimia. Among males, this disorder is about one-tenth as common. The average age for developing bulimia is 18.

What Causes Bulimia Nervosa?

Bulimia usually begins after a rigid diet that lasted from several weeks

Loss of fat and muscle mass, including heart muscle

Increased sensitivity to cold

Irregular heartbeats

Bloating, constipation, abdominal pain

Amenorrhea (absence of menstruation)

Growth of fine babylike hair over body

Abnormal taste sensations

Osteoporosis

Depression

Sudden death

© William Thompson/Index Stock Imagery

Figure 6-5 MEDICAL COMPLICATIONS OF WEIGHT LOSS FROM ANOREXIA NERVOSA to a year or more. Strict dieting may affect brain chemistry in such a way as to disrupt the normal mechanisms for appetite and satiety. Semi-starvation eventually sets off a binge; bingeing leads to purging. Once dieters realize that vomiting reduces the anxiety triggered by gorging, they no longer fear overeating. When this happens, bingeing may become more frequent and severe until, in time, it becomes an all-purpose way of coping with stress. However, the driving force in this disorder may not be the overeating but the vomiting or laxative use. If individuals felt they couldn't get rid of food, they might not overeat.

Obesity in adolescence may increase the likelihood of bulimia in adulthood. Extremely obese individuals may lose weight by vomiting and not want to stop because they fear regaining it. Sometimes bulimia develops after recovery from anorexia. Purging becomes an alternative way of staying thin.

As with anorexia, bulimia is associated with changes in brain chemistry, particularly low levels of the peptide cholescystokinin, which produces feelings of satiety. The cycle of bingeing and purging seems to wreak havoc on the biological controls that keep weight at a certain level.

Family conflicts, life stresses such as going away to school, and struggles with the transition to independent adulthood also may play a role. Bulimia also may be a symptom of depression. About 20 to 30 percent of those with this problem are chronically depressed; others have a history of depressive episodes. Bulimic individuals also are more likely to experience other problems, including anxiety disorders, substance abuse, and impulse disorders, such as shoplifting (kleptomania) and cutting themselves. A significant percentage of bulimics—from a quarter to a half, by some estimates—may have been victims of incest, sexual molestation, or rape, but this correlation is controversial.

Bulimia may continue for many years, with binges alternating with periods of normal eating. Physiological consequences are cumulative (see Figure 6-6). Often dentists are the first to detect bulimia because they notice damage to teeth and gums, including erosion of the enamel from the stomach acids in vomit. Repeated vomiting can lead to other complications as it robs the body of essential nutrients and fluids, causes dehydration and electrolyte imbalances, and impairs the ability of the heart and other muscles to function. Bulimia can trigger cardiac arrhythmias and, occasionally, sudden death.

Most mental health professionals treat bulimia with a combination of nutritional counseling, psychodynamic, cognitive-behavior therapy, individual or group psychotherapy, and medication. The drug most often prescribed is an antidepressant medication such as fluoxetine (Prozac), which increases levels of the neurotransmitter serotonin. About 70 percent of those who complete treatment programs reduce their bingeing and purging, although flareups are common in times of stress.

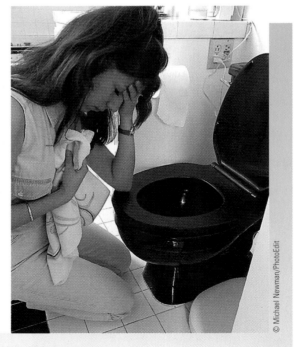

Abnormal levels of crucial chemicals

Inflammation of the salivary glands

Erosion of the esophagus and stomach

Severe abdominal pain

Erosion and decay of dental enamel, particularly of front teeth

Fatigue and weekness

Seizures

© Michael Newman/PhotoEdit

Figure 6-6 MEDICAL COMPLICATIONS RELATED TO PURGING

⬤ The Silent Epidemic: "Globesity"

The weight problem some have dubbed "globesity" has emerged as the major preventable health threat of the twenty-first century.[24] An estimated 1.1 billion people around the world—seven in ten of the Dutch and Spanish, two in three Americans and Canadians, and one in two Britons, Germans, and Italians—are overweight or obese. In Europe excess weight ranks as the most common childhood disorder. Obesity rates have quadrupled in Japan and are soaring in South America.

The obesity epidemic is not restricted to industrialized societies. According to the International Obesity Task Force, more than 115 million people in developing countries suffer from obesity-related problems. In many poor countries obesity is common among city dwellers, while people in rural areas remain underweight and malnourished.

In the United States, obesity rates have skyrocketed in recent decades (see Figure 6-7). Nine million American children aged 6 to 19 are overweight, triple the number of 20 years ago, according to the Centers for Disease Control and Prevention.[25] Young adults are becoming obese 28 percent faster than those born in the early 1960s.[26] By

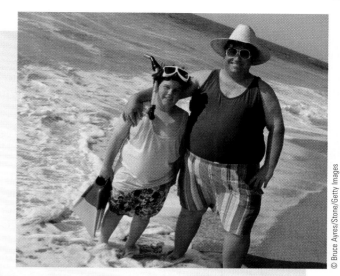

Heredity plays a role in the tendency toward obesity, but so do environment and behavior.

middle age, 70 percent of American adults are overweight or obese.[27]

Although more men than women are overweight, more adult women (38 percent) are obese than men (28 percent). Non-Hispanic black women have the highest obesity rate (50 percent), compared with 40 percent of Hispanic women and 30 percent of white women.[28] In some Native American communities, up to 70 percent of all adults are dangerously overweight. Differences in metabolic rates may be one factor.

⬤ How Did We Get So Fat?

As one obesity expert puts it, we are all "swimming against the tide of a fattening American lifestyle."[29] Bombarded by nonstop commercials for taste treats, tempted by foods in every form to munch and crunch, Americans are eating more—some 200 to 400 calories more a day than they did several decades ago. Many of these extra calories come from refined carbohydrates, which can raise heart-damaging blood fats called triglycerides and increase the risk of diabetes as well as obesity.

Our plates literally are running over. Both in restaurants and at home, portions have ballooned. (See Table 6-3.) The portions at many popular restaurant and in packaged foods has increased two to five times during the past twenty years. Some foods, like chocolate bars, have grown more than 10 times since they were first introduced.[30] Popular 64-ounce sodas can pack a whopping 800 calories—half of the total amount of calories a child needs in a day.[31] According to studies in satiety, people presented with larger portions eat up to 30 percent more than they otherwise would.[32]

Overweight (prevalence)

Black — Men 60.1%, Women 78%
Mexican-American — Men 74.4%, Women 71.8%
White — Men 67.5%, Women 57.5%

Obesity

Black — Men 28.8%, Women 50.8%
Mexican-American — Men 29.4%, Women 40.1%
White — Men 27.7%, Women 30.6%

Men / Women

Figure 6-7 WEIGHT PROBLEMS BY RACE/ETHNIC GROUP AND GENDER

Source: American Obesity Association, "Obesity in Minority Populations," www.obesity.org.

As Americans eat more, they exercise less. Experts estimate that most adults expend 200 to 300 fewer calories than people did 25 years ago. One reason is the couch potato lifestyle. The rise in obesity in recent decades has paralleled a steady increase in the number of homes with multiple TVsets, cable TV, and remote controls as well as in the number of hours spent watching TV.[33]

Scientists now realize that obesity is a complex and serious disorder with multiple causes, including:

:: **Genetics.** Scientists have identified a gene for a protein that signals the brain to halt food intake or to step up metabolic rate to make use of extra calories. If this gene is defective or malfunctions, it could contribute to weight problems. The discovery of a genetic predisposition to excess weight could explain, at least in part, why having one obese parent doubles the likelihood that a child under age ten will be obese.

A child's age also affects the likelihood that fatness will persist. The earlier the weight gain, the greater the danger. A child who is chubby at age ten is six times more likely to remain heavy into adulthood than a thinner youngster.

:: **Developmental factors.** Some obese people have a high number of fat cells, others have large fat cells, and the most severely obese have both a high number and large fat cells. Whereas the size of fat cells can increase at any time in life, the number is set during childhood, possibly the result of genetics or overfeeding at a young age.

:: **Social determinants.** In affluent countries, people in lower socioeconomic classes tend to be more obese. For reasons unknown, those in the upper classes, who can afford as much food as they want, tend to be leaner. Education may be a factor.

:: **Physical activity.** Obesity tends to go with a sedentary lifestyle. In countries where many people tend to work at physically demanding jobs, obesity is rare. Physical activity prevents obesity by increasing caloric expenditure, decreasing food intake, and increasing metabolic rate.

:: **Emotional influences.** Obese people are neither more nor less psychologically troubled than others. Psychological problems, such as irritability, depression, and anxiety, are more likely to be the result of obesity than the cause. As discussed later in this chapter, emotions do play a role in weight problems. Just as some people reach for a drink or a drug when they're upset, others cope by overeating, bingeing, or purging.

:: **Lifestyle.** Television is a culprit in an estimated 30 percent of new cases of obesity. TV viewing may increase weight in several ways: It takes up time that otherwise might be spent in physical activities. It increases food intake since people tend to eat more while watching TV. And compared with sewing, reading, driving, or other sedentary pursuits, television watching lowers metabolic rate so viewers burn fewer calories.[34] The combination of watching television (at least 2½ hours a day) and eating fast food more than twice a week triples the risk of obesity, according to a 15-year study of more than 3,700 white and black young adults.[35]

Health Dangers of Being Overweight or Obese

Excess weight has become the single greatest preventable threat to health and well-being. It weakens hearts, raises blood pressure, clogs arteries, strains backs and joints, and increases the risk of diabetes, stroke, and certain cancers (Figure 6-8). The annual cost

TABLE 6-3	**Supersized Portions**	
Food/Beverage	**Original Size (Year Introduced)**	**Today (Largest Available)**
Budweiser (bottle)	7 oz (1976)	40 oz
Nestle's Crunch	1.6 oz (1938)	5 oz
French Fries (Burger King)	2.6 oz (1954)	6.9 oz
Hamburger (McDonald's) (Beef only)	1.6 oz (1955)	8 oz
Soda (Coca Cola)	6.5 oz (1916)	34 oz

© Tony Freeman/PhotoEdit (both)

Source: "Are Growing Portion Sizes Leading to Expanding Waistlines?" American Dietetic Association, www.eatright.org.

Cancer:

Breast, ovary, cervix, endometrium (women)

esophagus

kidney

gall bladder

nonHodgkins disease

stomach and prostate (men)

colorectal

Type 2 Diabetes

High blood cholesterol

High blood pressure

Stroke

Daytime sleepiness/sleep apnea

Impaired breathing

Heart disease

Pancreatitis

Kidney disease

Liver disease

Gall bladder disease

Carpal tunnel syndrome

Low back pain

Pain

Urinary stress incontinence

Surgical complications

Infections following wounds

Infertility

Impaired immunity

Osteoarthritis

Gout

Figure 6-8 HEALTH DANGERS OF EXCESS WEIGHT

of weight-related health problems totals more than $117 billion.

A recent study of 900,000 people, the largest ever of its kind, found that excess weight may account for 14 percent of all cancer deaths in men and 20 percent of those in women. Losing weight, the researchers estimated, could prevent as many as one of every six cancer deaths.[36]

While earlier research had linked excess weight to cancers of the breast and uterus, colon and rectum, kidney, esophagus, and gallbladder, this study also linked weight to other cancers, including non-Hodgkins lymphoma, multiple myeloma, cancers of the pancreas and liver, the cervix and ovary (in women), and the stomach and prostate (in men). Those with BMIs over 40 had death rates from cancer that were 52 percent higher for men and 62 percent higher for women than those of normal-weight individuals.[37]

Too much body fat can influence cancer in several ways: It increases the amount of estrogen in the blood, rais-

ing the risk of cancers of the female reproductive system. It raises the levels of insulin, which prompts the body to create a hormone that causes cells to multiply. Acid reflux, which can cause cancer of the esophagus, occurs more frequently in heavy men and women. Obesity also makes cancer harder to diagnose and treat.

The incidence of diabetes, gallstones, hypertension, heart disease, and colon cancer increases with the degree of overweight in both sexes. Those with BMIs of 35 or more are approximately 20 times more likely to develop diabetes. Individuals who are overweight but not obese, with BMIs between 25 and 29.9, are significantly more likely than leaner women to develop gallstones, high blood pressure, high cholesterol, and heart disease. Overweight men are also more likely to suffer strokes.

Even relatively small amounts of excess fat—as little as 5 pounds—can add to the dangers in those already at risk for hypertension and diabetes. According to the National Heart, Lung, and Blood Institute, being overweight, even if not obese, increases the risk of heart failure. Obesity also causes alterations in various measures of immune function.

Obesity now is considered a greater threat to a healthy heart than smoking. People who both smoke and are obese are at especially high risk of cardiovascular disease. Although some smokers have felt that they couldn't lose weight until they stopped smoking, researchers have found that weight loss among smokers is possible and beneficial, leading to a reduction in other risk factors, such as lower blood pressure and lower cholesterol.[38] Health educators also are targeting teenage dieters, who are more likely to begin smoking, often to help control their weight.

Researchers estimate that the effects of obesity on health are the equivalent of twenty years of aging. However, as discussed in Chapter 4, activity levels are critically important. Fat-and-fit people who exercise regularly are at less risk of dying prematurely than leaner sedentary men and women. Unfortunately, many heavy Americans are inactive and in increased danger of dying of all causes, particularly heart disease and cancer.

In our calorie-conscious and thinness-obsessed society, obesity also affects quality of life, including sense of vitality and physical pain. Many see it as a heavy psychological burden, a sign of failure, laziness, or inadequate willpower. Overweight men and women often blame themselves for becoming heavy, and feel guilty and depressed as a result. In fact, the psychological problems once considered the cause of obesity may be its consequence.

The earlier that obesity begins, the greater the long-term health dangers. The greatest immediate consequences may be psychosocial. "Obesity is one of the most stigmatizing and least socially acceptable conditions of childhood," conclude a research team that found that obese youngsters rate significantly lower than others on various measurements of quality of life. Only children and teens with cancers scored as low.[39]

Years of Life Lost (YLL)

Obesity affects not just how our bodies look, feel, and function, but how long they survive. According to recent research taking race and gender into account, obesity can subtract years from a person's life.[40] The earlier the age at which a person becomes obese, the greater the number of years of life lost (YLL). This means that an obese twenty year old can die twenty years prematurely. Being even moderately overweight at age 40 can steal three to seven years of life expectancy.[41]

African-American men who become obese (with BMIs over 45), while young stand to lose two decades of potential life; young white men, 13 years. A woman's YLL is lower, but still significant. Young obese white women can expect to lose eight years of life; African American women, five years.

Physicians are using the YLL as a powerful incentive to convince patients to undertake a diet and exercise program to shed unhealthy pounds.[42]

The following recommendations from the American Dietetic Association's "Complete Food and Nutrition Guide" may help:

STRATEGIES FOR CHANGE

Getting Ready for Weight Loss

- **Make health,** not appearance, your weight-management priority. Strive for your best weight for health. That's not necessarily the lowest weight you could be—or what you consider your "ideal" number.

- **For weight loss gains,** follow these tactics for weight management: (1) healthful eating, (2) regular physical activity, and (3) acceptance of the weight you can achieve through a healthy lifestyle.

- **Set realistic, attainable goals**—for you! Start with your current weight or your lifestyle, not where you want to be. The challenge of trimming 5 pounds at a time may seem more doable than losing 25 or more pounds.

- **Focus on a healthy lifestyle**—for a lifetime—not on "dieting." Dieting alone is often a short-term tactic without long-term results. The concept of "dieting" carries a lot of negative baggage: guilt, "shoulds," and "can't haves." For most people, "dieting" results in failure.

- **Focus your strategies:** action-oriented and specific. Perhaps you'll walk for 15 minutes each day during your lunch break, or you'll drink milk rather than a milk shake with your fast-food lunch.

- **Tailor your strategies** to your schedule, your budget, your family situation, and your personal needs, to name a few. Experts have found that two out of three people who were successful at weight control personalized their efforts to fit their lifestyles.

- **Think long-term** and act gradually. It's true that fasting and starvation-type diets can peel off pounds, but most of the weight that's lost quickly is only water loss! Grueling exercise regimens may tone the body, but for most people, these tactics aren't realistic ways to live—and they may not be healthful, either.

✖ Overcoming Weight Problems

The best approach to a weight problem depends on how overweight a person is. For extreme obesity, medical treatments, including surgery, may be necessary to overcome the danger to a person's health and life. People who are

Self Survey

Are You Ready to Lose Weight?

Take this readiness quiz to see if you're mentally ready before you begin a weight loss program. Mark each statement "true" or "false." Be honest with yourself! The answers should reflect the way you really think—not how you'd like to be!

1. I have thought a lot about my eating habits and physical activities, and I know what I might change.
2. I know that I need to make permanent, not temporary, changes in my eating and activity patterns.
3. I will feel successful only if I lose a lot of weight.
4. I know that it's best if I lose weight slowly.
5. I'm thinking about losing weight now because I really want to, not because someone else thinks I should.
6. I think losing weight would solve other problems in my life.
7. I am willing and able to increase my regular physical activity.
8. I can lose weight successfully only if I have no slip-ups.
9. I am willing to commit time and effort each week to organize and plan my food and activity choices.
10. Once I lose a few pounds but reach a plateau (I can't seem to lose more), I usually lose the motivation to keep going toward my weight goal.

11. I want to start a weight-loss program, even though my life is unusually stressful right now.

Now Score Yourself

Look at your answers for items 1, 2, 4, 5, 7, and 9. Score "1" if you answered "true" and "0" if you answered "false." For items 3, 6, 8, 10, and 11, score "0" for each "true" answer and "1" for each false answer.

No one score indicates if you're ready to start losing weight. But the higher your total score, the more likely you'll be successful.

If you scored 8 or higher, you probably have good reasons to lose weight now. And you know some of the steps that can help you succeed.

If you scored 5 to 7 points, you may need to reevaluate your reasons for losing weight and the strategies you'd follow.

If you scored 4 or less, now may not be the right time for you to lose weight. You may be successful initially, but you may not be able to sustain the effort to reach or maintain your weight goal. Reconsider your reasons and approach.

From America Dietetic Association's *Complete Food & Nutrition Guide*, 2/e by Rebecca Duyff. Copyright © 2002. Used by permission of John Wiley & Sons, Inc.

Your Health Change Plan

for Weight Loss

Any item you scored as "0" suggests a misconception about weight loss, or a problem area for you. So let's look at each item a bit more closely.

:: You can't change what you don't understand, and that includes your eating habits and activity pattern. Keep records for a week to pinpoint when, what, why, and how much you eat—as well as patterns and obstacles to regular physical activity.

:: You may be able to lose weight in the short run with drastic or highly restrictive changes in your eating habits or activity pattern. But they may be hard to live with permanently. Your food and activity plans should be healthful ones you can enjoy and sustain.

:: Many people fantasize about reaching a weight goal that's unrealistically low. If that sounds like you, rethink your meaning of success. A reasonable goal takes body type into consideration—and sets smaller, achievable "mile markers" along the way.

:: If you equate success with fast weight loss, you'll have problems keeping weight off. This "quick fix" attitude can backfire when you face the challenges of weight maintenance. The best and healthiest approach is to lose weight slowly while learning strategies to keep weight off permanently.

:: To be successful, the desire for and commitment to weight loss must come from you—not your best friend or a family member. People who lose weight, then keep it off, take responsibility for their weight goals and choose their own approach.

:: Being overweight may contribute to some social problems, but it's rarely the single cause. While body image and self-esteem are strongly linked, thinking you can solve all your problems by losing weight isn't realistic. And it may set you up for disappointment.

:: A habit of regular, moderate physical activity is a key factor to successfully losing weight—and keeping it off. For weight control, physical activity doesn't need to be strenuous to be effective. Any moderate physical activity that you enjoy and do regularly counts.

:: Most people don't expect perfection in their daily lives, yet they often feel they must stick to a weight-loss program perfectly. Perfection at weight loss isn't realistic. Rather than viewing lapses as catastrophes, see them as opportunities to find what triggers your problems and develop strategies for the future.

(Continued)

moderately or mildly obese can lose weight through different approaches, including

:: behavioral modification (monitoring food intake, altering eating style, avoiding eating "triggers," and similar strategies)

:: cognitive therapy (changing thoughts or beliefs that lead to overeating)

:: social support (participating in groups such as Overeaters Anonymous).

The keys to overcoming obesity are acknowledging biological limits, addressing individual differences, altering unrealistic expectations, setting limits, and learning coping skills to provide self-nurturing without relying on food.

Severe Obesity

An estimated 3 percent of adults in the United States—some six million people—are "morbidly" obese, with BMIs of 40 or greater. Another 10 million have BMIs between 35 and 40.[43] Because of the medical dangers they face, some severely obese men and women, as a last resort, may undergo surgery. According to the American Society for Bariatric Surgery, some 63,100 individuals undergo weight-reduction operations, including bypassing or stapling the stomach, each year. Gastric bypass surgery has a long-term success rate of nearly 90 percent and patients maintain a weight loss of 50 percent or more for more than ten years. About 15 percent experience complications, which are fatal in 0.5 to 1 percent of cases.[44]

Mild to Moderate Obesity

For individuals with a BMI of 30 to 39, doctors recommend a six-month trial of lifestyle therapy, including a supervised diet and exercise. The initial goal should be a 10 percent reduction in weight, an amount that reduces obesity-related risks.[45] With success and if warranted, individuals can attempt to lose more weight.

Overweight

Rather than going on a low-calorie diet, people with BMIs of 25 to 29 should cut back moderately on their food intake and concentrate on developing healthy eating and exercise habits. Many moderately to mildly overweight people turn to national organizations such as Weight Watchers or to other commercial weight-loss groups. Most of these programs offer behavior-modification techniques, inspirational lectures, and carefully designed nutritional programs, but dropout rates are high. As many as half the members drop out in six weeks.

▣ A Practical Guide to Weight Loss

Never before have so many had so much to lose. At any given time about 40 percent of women and 25 percent of men are attempting to lose weight. Every year approximately 45 million Americans diet, while 55 percent of Americans are trying to maintain current weight.[46]

Weight loss has become a national obsession, with treatments falling into two categories: cognitive (including diet, lifestyle change, and exercise) and noncognitive (such as drugs and surgery).[47] Increasingly, physicians view overweight and obesity as chronic conditions requiring long-term care.[48]

An estimated 13 percent of obese women and 5 percent of obese men turn to formal diet and exercise programs. Although drop-out rates are high, they generally produce a "modest" weight loss.[49] Behavioral counseling from a health professional also helps, both in person and with e-mail follow up and support.[50] However, most people who shed excess pounds and keep them off do so on their own by making a lifelong commitment to healthy weight management. (See Fact or Fiction? "It is possible to lose weight . . .")

Realistic goals are crucial. Doctors recommend starting with a modest goal of 10 percent of initial weight over a six-month period. Such a weight loss produces significant

It is possible to lose weight and keep it off without weight-loss pills or programs.

Fact: In surveys of successful dieters who lost significant amounts of weight and kept it for several years, most did so on their own, without medication, meal substitutes, or membership in an organized weight loss group. According to the National Weight Control Registry, most men and women who maintain a significant weight loss for five years assume personal responsibility for changing their eating and exercise habits. The secrets of their success include a psychological commitment to change, a low-fat diet, frequent monitoring of weight, and an hour of moderate physical activity almost every day.

Source: Mary Serdula, et al. "Weight Loss Counseling Revisited," *Journal of the American Medical Association,* Vol. 289, No. 14, April 9, 2003, p. 1747; National Weight Control Registry.

health benefits, including lowering the risks of diabetes and heart disease.[51]

College students tend to have more realistic weight loss goals than others. When 379 undergraduates reported their "goal," "dream," "happy," "acceptable," and "disappointed" weights, most had realistic weight goals, particularly if they were not overweight. The nonoverweight women chose a "dream" weight about 10 percent less than their current weights but said a loss of just about 1 percent would be acceptable. Overweight women dreamed of weighing 22 percent less than they currently did but would consider a loss of about 8 percent acceptable. Nonoverweight men dreamed of weighing about 10 percent more, probably from increased muscle mass, but considered a gain of 1 percent acceptable. Overweight men had dream weights about 4 percent lower than their current weights, but said a loss of 1 percent would be acceptable.[52]

FAQ Which Diets Are Safe and Effective?

High protein? Low carbohydrate? No fat? Low calorie? The ongoing debate over popular diets has left many weight-conscious Americans more confused than ever about what they should or shouldn't put on their plates. (See Table 6-4.)

Most controversial is the diet popularized by the late Dr. Robert Atkins, which is high in protein and extremely low in carbohydrates. Followers of the Atkins diet eat unlimited amounts of meat, eggs, and cheese and cut back on bread, pasta, crackers, cakes, cookies, and other carbohydrates.

Because they avoid many high-calorie foods and fill up on proteins, which take longer to digest, these dieters typically lose weight without feeling hungry. Particularly in

TABLE 6-4	Dueling Diets	
Low Carbohydrate	**Low Fat**	**Low Calorie**
Dieters limit carbohydrates to varying degrees and eat more protein	Dieters eat lots of complex carbohydrates, such as fruits, vegetables, and whole grains and cut down on saturated fats	Dieters focus on total intake, not particular types of food
Pros: Quick weight loss without hunger	Pros: Very low fat diets can reverse heart disease	Pros: Balanced, flexible eating plan
Cons: Vitamin and mineral deficiencies, risk of kidney stones. Unknown if saturated fats in some protein sources might increase cardiovascular risk in the long term	Cons: Difficult to maintain a very low fat diet over time; critics charge that more "good" fats should be allowed	Cons: Have to keep track of calories or points
Best Known: The Atkins Diet, The Zone, Carb Addicts	Best Known: The Ornish Diet	Best Known: Weight Watchers

the initial stages, followers of the Atkins diet may consume 40 percent of their calories in fat, much of it saturated, which may increase the long-term risk of heart disease.[53] (See Fact or Fiction? "High-protein, low-carb . . .")

Other low-carbohydrate diets, such as The Zone, which advises a daily diet made up of protein (30 percent of calories), carbohydrates (40 percent), and fat (30 percent), also have come under fire.[54] A high protein intake may strain the liver and kidneys and leach some calcium from bones. A lack of complex carbohydrates may lead to vitamin deficiencies and digestive problems, such as constipation. It also triggers an abnormal body process called ketosis, which occurs during starvation and can cause fatigue, constipation, nausea, and vomiting. Potential long-term side effects of ketosis include heart problems, bone loss, and kidney damage.

The very-low-fat diet developed by Dr. Dean Ornish, which limits fat to 10 percent of daily calories, has proven effective in reversing atherosclerotic buildup. Low-fat diets also may enhance the immune response. However, although experts support a decrease in trans and saturated fats for the sake of cardiovascular health, they have challenged the scientific evidence for reducing fat below 30 to 35 percent for the sake of preventing heart disease in healthy individuals.[55] Epidemiological studies have not shown that dietary fat directly increases body fat.[56] "Healthy" fats such as olive oil and fatty acids in fish oils may help control appetite and maintain long-term weight loss.

Which diet is best? A systematic review of 107 studies published from 1966 to 2003 found "insufficient" evidence to recommend or advise against low-carbohydrate diets. Individuals on these diets did lose weight, not because they ate fewer carbohydrates, but because they consumed fewer calories. Their initial weight loss mainly resulted from a loss of fluids over a 7 to 14 day period.[57]

Medical experts advise cutting back 500 to 100 calories a day. Very low calorie diets produce faster weight loss, but because of weight regain, follow-up studies show no benefit a year later. As confirmed by current research, all low-calorie diets produce weight loss, regardless of their composition. The inclusion or exclusion of macronutrients like protein or fat does not seem to play a major role.[58]

FACT OR FICTION? ??????????????

High-protein, low-carbohydrate diets are hazardous to health

The jury is still out: For years professional groups such as the American Dietetic Association and the American Heart Association warned that low-carbohydrate weight loss plans like the Atkins diet pose serious health dangers, primarily because the high fat content may increase the risk of heart disease, diabetes, stroke, and kidney and liver disease. Some recent research has challenged this view.

In a six-month study of 53 obese women, a diet very low in carbohydrate led to a greater loss of weight and body fat than a low-fat diet (30 percent of calories)—and produced no harmful effects on blood pressure, blood fats (including triglycerides and good forms of cholesterol), or other cardiovascular risk factors. Other studies have confirmed greater weight loss after six to twelve months on a low-carbohydrate diet compared with a conventional low-fat, calorie-restricted diet. However, dropout rates were high for all the dieters, with no significant differences in weight loss a year after starting a diet. The long-term health impact of a high-protein, low-carbohydrate diet has not yet been studied.

Source: D. K. Layman, et al. "Increased Dietary Protein Modifies Glucose and Insulin Homeostasis in Adult Women During Weight Loss," *International Journal of Nutrition*, Vol. 133, No. 2, February 2003, p. 405. Joan Stephenson. "Low-Carb, Low-Fat Diet Gurus Face Off," *Journal of the American Medical Association*, Vol. 289, No. 14, April 9, 2003, p. 1767. F. F. Samaha, et al. "A low carbohydrate as compared with a low-fat diet in severe obesity," *New England Journal of Medicine*, Vol. 348, May 22, 2003, p. 2074. G. D. Foster, et al. "A randomized trial of a low-carbohydrate diet for obesity," *New England Journal of Medicine*, Vol. 348, May 22, 2003, p. 2082.

Avoiding Diet Traps

Whatever your eating style, there are only two effective strategies for losing weight: eating less and exercising more. Unfortunately, most people search for easier alternatives that almost invariably turn into dietary dead ends or unexpected dangers. (See Savvy Consumer: "How to Spot Diet Dangers.") Four common traps to avoid are diet foods, the yo-yo diet, the very low-calorie diet, and diet pills.

Diet Foods

According to the Calorie Control Council, 90 percent of Americans choose some foods labeled "light." But even though these foods keep growing in popularity, Americans' weight keeps rising. There are several reasons: Many people think choosing a food that's lower in calories, fat-free, or light gives them a license to eat as much as they want. What they don't realize is that many foods that are low in fat are still high in sugar and calories. Refined carbohydrates, rapidly absorbed into the bloodstream, raise blood glucose levels. As they fall, appetite increases.

What about the artificial sweeteners and fake fats that appear in many diet products? Nutritionists caution to use them in moderation, and not to substitute them for basic foods, such as grains, fruits, and vegetables. Foods made with fat substitutes may have fewer grams of fat, but they don't necessarily have significantly fewer calories. Many

Savvy Consumer

HOW TO SPOT DIET DANGERS

The National Council Against Health Fraud cautions dieters to watch for these warnings of dangerous or fraudulent programs.

- Promises of very rapid weight loss.
- Claims that the diet can eliminate "cellulite" (a term used to describe dimply fatty tissue on the arms and legs).
- "Counselors" who are really salespersons pushing a product or program.
- No mention of any risks associated with the diet.
- Unproven gimmicks, such as body wraps, starch blockers, hormones, diuretics, or "unique" pills or potions.
- No maintenance program.

If you hear about a new diet that promises to melt away fat, don't try it until you get answers to the following questions:

- Does it include a wide variety of nutritious foods?
- Does it provide at least 1,200 calories a day?
- Is it designed to reduce your weight by one-half to two pounds per week?
- Does it emphasize moderate portions?
- Does it use foods that are easy to find and prepare?
- Can you follow it wherever you eat—at home, work, restaurants, or parties?
- Is its cost reasonable?

If the answer to any of these questions is no, don't try the diet; then ask yourself one more question: Is losing weight worth losing your well-being?

---

people who consume reduced-fat, fat-free, or sugar-free sodas, cookies, chips, and other snacks often cut back on more nutritious foods, such as fruits and vegetables. They also tend to eat more of the low- or no-fat foods so that their daily calorie intake either stays the same or actually increases.

The Yo-Yo Syndrome

On-and-off-again dieting, especially by means of very low-calorie diets (under 800 calories a day), can be self-defeating and dangerous. Some studies have shown that weight cycling may make it more difficult to lose weight or keep it off. (See Figure 6-9.) Repeated cycles of rapid weight loss followed by weight gain may even change food preferences. Chronic crash dieters often come to prefer foods that combine sugar and fat, such as cake frosting.

To avoid the yo-yo syndrome and overcome its negative effects: Exercise. Researchers at the University of Pennsylvania found that when overweight women who also exercised went off a very low-calorie diet, their metabolism did not stay slow but bounced back to the appropriate level for their new, lower body weight. The reason may be exercise's ability to preserve muscle tissue. The more muscle tissue you have, the higher your metabolic rate.

Very Low-Calorie Diets

Any diet that promises to take pounds off fast can be dangerous. For reasons that scientists don't fully understand,

Figure 6-9 WEIGHT-CYCLING EFFECT OF REPEATED DIETING

Each round of dieting is typically followed by a rebound leading to a greater weight gain.

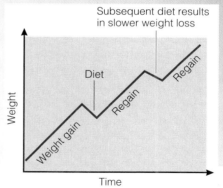

rapid weight loss is linked with increased mortality. Most risky are very low-calorie diets that provide fewer than 800 calories a day. Whenever people cut back drastically on calories, they immediately lose several pounds because of a loss of fluid. As soon as they return to a more normal way of eating, they regain this weight.

On a very low-calorie diet, as much as 50 percent of the weight you lose may be muscle (so you'll actually look flabbier). Because your heart is a muscle, it may become so weak that it no longer can pump blood through your body. In addition, your blood pressure may plummet, causing dizziness, light-headedness, and fatigue. You may develop nausea and abdominal pain. You may lose hair. If you're a woman, your menstrual cycle may become irregular, or you may stop menstruating altogether. As you lose more water, you also lose essential vitamins, and your metabolism slows down. Even reaction time slows, and crash dieters may not be able to respond as quickly as usual.

Once you go off an extreme diet—as you inevitably must—your metabolism remains slow, even though you're no longer restricting your food intake. The human body appears to alter its energy use to compensate for weight loss. These metabolic changes may make it harder for people to maintain a reduced body weight after dieting.

Diet Pills and Products

In their search for a quick fix to weight problems, millions of people have tried often-risky remedies. In the 1920s, some women swallowed patented weight-loss capsules that turned out to be tapeworm eggs. In the 1960s and 1970s, addictive amphetamines were common diet aids. In the 1990s, appetite suppressants known as fen-phen became popular. They were taken off the market after being linked to heart valve problems.

In 2003 the Food and Drug Administration proposed labels warning of heart attacks, strokes, and even death for users of the popular herb ephedra (also identified as ephedrine and ma huang and often combined with caffeine).[59] This action came shortly after the heat stroke death of a Baltimore Orioles pitcher was linked to his use of ephedra. The FDA, which has reports of at least 100 deaths linked to ephedra supplements, had been under pressure from doctors for years to ban the herb after more than 1,000 reports of adverse effects.[60]

In a meta-analysis of studies conducted on ephedra products for weight loss, researchers concluded that use of high doses of ephedra or ephedra and caffeine for six months or less does promote weight loss—but also takes a toll on physical and mental well-being. Ephedra products are associated with two to three times the normal risk of psychiatric symptoms, upper gastrointestinal symptoms, and heart palpitations.[61]

Obesity medications are recommended only for patients with BMIs equal to or greater than 30 or those with a BMI equal to or greater than 27 with risk factors (like high blood pressure) that increase their risk of disease.[62] Researchers are experimenting with other medications, such as the epilepsy drug zonisamide, to enhance weight loss.[63] Currently, only two weight loss drugs are approved.

Xenical (Orlistat) blocks fat absorption by the gut but also inhibits absorption of water and vitamins in some patients and may cause cramping and diarrhea. It produces a weight loss of 2 to 3 percent of initial weight beyond the weight lost by dieting over the course of a year. Meridia (sibutramine) is in the same chemical class as amphetamines and works by suppressing appetite. It also may increase blood pressure, heart rate, or both. Health officials in the United States and other countries are investigating reports of adverse effects. Health Canada considered a ban but decided that the potential benefits outweighed the risks. Both drugs cause rebound weight gain when patients stop taking them.[64]

Other diet products, including diet sodas and low-fat foods, also are a very big business. Many people rely on meal replacements, usually shakes or snack bars, to lose or keep off weight. If used appropriately—as actual replacements rather than supplements to regular meals and snacks—they can be a useful strategy for weight loss. Yet people who use these products aren't necessarily sure to slim down. In fact, people who consume such products often gain weight because they think that they can afford to add high-calorie treats to their diet.

◼ The Psychology of Weight Loss

Diets focus on the symptoms of weight gain rather than its underlying causes. The key to lasting weight loss is changing the attitudes, beliefs, feelings, choices, and habits that determine what, when, why, how often, and how much we eat.

One common challenge is learning to control "emotional eating," using food as a way of coping with anger, frustration, stress, boredom, or fatigue. Whatever its motivation, emotional eating always involves eating for reasons other than physiological hunger. The first step to overcoming it is being able to distinguish between emotional and physical hunger (see Table 6-5).

"Train yourself to take a step back," says Kathy McManus, Ph.D., director of nutrition at the Brigham and Women's Hospital in Boston. She suggests asking yourself a series of questions before you take a bite: Am I hungry? If not, what am I feeling—stressed, tired, bored, anxious, sad, happy? Once you identify your true feelings, push deeper and ask why you feel this way. Writing down your answers is even more effective in making sure that every bite you take is a conscious one.

To avoid temptation, keep favorite foods out of sight. "Availability makes a big difference," says McManus. "If carrots are competing with chocolate chip cookies, they'll lose. If they're your only option, you probably aren't going to run out and buy something else."[65]

You don't have to "stuff" your feelings inside or deny they exist. "Let yourself feel how you're feeling without eating," the College of Family Physicians of Canada advises. "After you let yourself feel your emotions without eating, you may discover that eating doesn't really help you feel better. In fact, it may make you feel worse."[66]

TABLE 6-5	Is It Physical Hunger or Emotional Hunger?	
Physical Hunger	**Emotional Hunger**	
• Builds gradually	• Develops suddenly	
• Strikes below the neck (e.g., growling stomach)	• Above the neck (e.g., a "taste" for ice cream)	
• No sense of compulsion	• An urgent need to eat	
• Occurs several hours after a meal	• Unrelated to time since last meal	
• General	• Specific, often for a particular food or brand	
• Goes away when full	• Persists despite fullness	
• Eating leads to feeling of satisfaction	• Eating leads to guilt and shame	

The most effective and healthful way to manage your weight is to combine dietary changes with regular physical exercise.

When you're feeling emotionally overwhelmed, try a physical form of release. Roll up a towel and tug with all your might. Pound a pillow with your fist. Stomp, growl, throw punches into the air. Put your palms together and press as hard as you can. Grunting at the same time intensifies the feeling of relief. For additional motivation, write the name of the person who's triggered your rage or frustration on the bottom of your athletic shoes before you work out.

✖ The 60-Minute Solution

You may think that exercise will make you want to eat more. Actually, it has the opposite effect. The combination of exercise and cutting back on calories may be the most effective way of taking weight off and keeping it off. According to the National Weight Control Registry, a database of people who have kept off a minimum of 30 pounds for more than five years, most successful weight losers both restrict how much they eat and increase their physical activity.

Exercise has other benefits: It increases energy expenditure, builds up muscle tissue, burns off fat stores, and stimulates the immune system. Exercise also may reprogram metabolism so that more calories are burned during and after a workout.

As discussed in Chapter 4, the latest national guidelines recommend 60 minutes of moderate physical activity a day to maintain a healthy weight. Even though briefer, less intense workouts provide health benefits, researchers

have found that healthy people with a BMI of less than 25 need an hour's worth of exercise to avoid excess weight.

An exercise program designed for both health benefits and weight loss should include both aerobic activity and resistance training. (See Chapter 4 for an in-depth description.) Once you start an exercise program, keep it up. People who've started an exercise program during or after a weight-loss program are consistently more successful in keeping off most of the pounds they've shed.

The Bottom Line ▼ Healthy Weight Management for Life

No diet—high protein, low-fat, or high-carbohydrate—can produce permanent weight loss. Successful weight management, the American Dietetic Association has concluded, "requires a lifelong commitment to healthful lifestyle behaviors emphasizing sustainable and enjoyable eating practices and daily physical activity."[67] Studies have shown that successful dieters were highly motivated, monitored their food intake, increased their activity, set realistic goals, and received social support from others. Another key to long-term success is tailoring any weight-loss program to an individual's gender, lifestyle, and cultural, racial, and ethnic values.

Here are some practical guidelines.

:: ***Establish your goals.*** Subtract your target weight from your actual weight and calculate how long it will take you to lose the difference, based on a weekly loss of 1½ pounds.

:: ***Never say diet.*** Going on a diet implies going off a diet sooner or later.

:: ***Be realistic.*** Trying to shrink to an impossibly low weight dooms you to defeat. Start off slowly and make steady progress. If your weight creeps up 5 pounds, go back to the basics of your program. Take into account normal fluctuations, but watch out for an upward trend. If you let your weight continue to creep up, it may not stop until you have a serious weight problem—again.

:: ***Recognize that there are no quick fixes.*** Ultimately, quick-loss diets are very damaging physically and psychologically because when you stop dieting and put the pounds back on you feel like a failure.

:: ***Note your progress.*** Make a graph, with your initial weight as the base, to indicate your progress. View plateaus or occasional gains as temporary setbacks rather than disasters.

:: ***Adopt the 90 percent rule.*** If you practice good eating habits 90 percent of the time, a few indiscretions won't make a difference. In effect, you should allow for occasional cheating, so that you don't have to feel guilty about it.

:: ***Try, try again.*** Remember, dieters don't usually keep weight off on their first attempt. The people who eventually succeed try various methods until they find the plan that works for them.

 After watching the CNN video segment, discuss the following question. How do nutrients fuel the bodies of active teens?

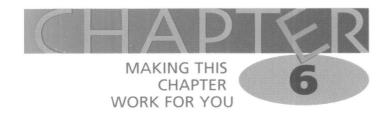

MAKING THIS CHAPTER WORK FOR YOU **6**

1. Excess weight
   a. is not a problem until you reach 50 years of age.
   b. increases your metabolism.

   c. is caused by fast food.
   d. increases the risk of type 2 diabetes, heart disease, and colorectal cancer.

2. Which of the following statements about body weight is *not* true?
   a. Visceral fat is more of a health risk than subcutaneous fat.
   b. Only women have body weight shapes and concerns.
   c. Daily energy requirements depend on your activity level.
   d. The infamous "freshman 15"—the 15 pounds that first-year students gain—turns out to be a myth.

3. Research on hunger and appetite has shown that
   a. the hormones ghrelin, leptin, and PYY stimulate the appetite.
   b. appetite receptors in the cerebellum of the brain respond to hormonal signals.
   c. people presented with larger portions of food eat more than they otherwise would.
   d. eating fast food and watching TV do not increase the risk of obesity.

4. Which of the following eating behaviors may be a warning sign of a serious eating disorder?
   a. vegetarianism
   b. compulsive food washing
   c. binge eating
   d. weight gain during the first year of college

5. Individuals with anorexia nervosa
   a. believe they are overweight even if they are extremely thin.
   b. typically feel full all the time, which limits their food intake.
   c. usually look overweight even though their body mass index is normal.
   d. have a reduced risk for heart-related abnormalities.

6. Bulimia nervosa is
   a. characterized by excessive sleeping followed by periods of insomnia.
   b. found primarily in older women who are concerned with the aging process.
   c. associated with the use of laxatives or excessive exercise to control weight.
   d. does not have serious health consequences.

7. Which of the following statements is *not* true?
   a. Obesity is a greater threat to heart health than smoking.
   b. Men who accumulate fat around their waist are at increased risk for cardiovascular risk.

c. Individuals who are obese are neither more nor less psychologically troubled than people of normal weight.

d. Children with an obese parent are more likely to be thin because of their embarrassment about the parent's appearance.

8. Weight management strategies that work include which of the following?

a. Increase your activity level and eat less, aiming for a weekly weight loss of about 1½ pounds.

b. Ask friends for recommendations for methods that helped them lose weight quickly.

c. Practice good eating habits about 50 percent of the time so that you can balance your cravings with healthy food.

d. Try a number of weight-loss diets to find the one that works best for you.

9. Which of the following statements is true?

a. Very low-calorie diets increase metabolism, which helps burn calories more quickly.

b. An individual eating low-calorie or fat-free foods can increase the serving sizes.

c. High-protein, low-carbohydrate diets may increase the risk of heart disease.

d. Yo-yo dieting works best for long-term weight loss.

10. Which of the following nonprescription diet products has been shown to have dangerous health effects?

a. Meridia and Xenical

b. ephedra

c. liquid meal replacements

d. diet snack bars

Answers to these questions can be found on page 652.

Critical Thinking

1. Do you think you have a weight problem? If so, what makes you think so? Is your perception based on your actual BMI measurement or on how you believe you look? If you found out that your BMI is within the ideal range, would that change your opinion about your body? Why or why not?

Critical Thinking

2. Different cultures have different standards for body weight and attractiveness. Within our society, men and women often seem to follow different standards. What influences have shaped your personal feelings about desired weight?

Critical Thinking

3. Suppose one of your roommates appears to have symptoms of an eating disorder. You have told him or her of your concerns, but your roommate has denied having a problem and brushed off your fears. What can you do to help this individual? Should you contact his or her parent? Why or why not?

Profile Plus

Discover the health risks associated with where you store fat, by participating in the following activity on your Profile Plus CD-ROM:

Profile Plus

• Weight and Health: Disease Risk

Profile Plus

Sites and Bytes

Count Your Calories Because Your Calories Count
www.wfubmc.edu/nutrition/in.html

This interactive site sponsored by Wake Forest University Baptist Medical Center features a four-step assessment of your diet, including "How's Your Diet," "Fit or Not Quiz," "Calorie Counter," and "Drive Through Diet." There is also an "Eating Disorders" quiz.

Sites and Bytes

Something Fishy Website on Eating Disorders
www.something-fishy.org

This comprehensive site features a wealth of information on all aspects of eating disorders, including facts, prevention, causes, symptoms, information on helping others, resources, treatment, cultural issues, recovery, chat rooms, and an online support center featuring bulletin boards and an e-mail newsletter.

Sites and Bytes

NHLBI Obesity Education Initiative
www.nhlbi.nih.gov/about/oei/index.htm

This site by the Obesity Education Initiative is sponsored by the National Heart, Lung, and Blood Institute (NHLBI) of the National Institutes of Health. The overall purpose of the initiative is to help reduce the prevalence of overweight and physical inactivity, thereby reducing the risk, morbidity, and mortality of coronary heart disease. The site features information on weight management and obesity for the general public and for health professionals. Interactive features include a BMI calculator, a menu planner, and treatment guidelines.

InfoTrac College Edition

Activity

"Childhood Overweight—A Public Health Issue. (Case Studies)" *Journal of the American Dietetic Association,* Vol. 102, No. 11, November 2002, p. S4(2).

1. What are the goals and objectives of the New York program "The Dutchess County Eat Well Play Hard" initiative?

InfoTrac College Edition

2. How did this program meet its objectives?

3. What is the most important factor regarding the ability of this initiative to be replicable?

You can find additional readings relating to eating patterns and problems with InfoTrac College Edition, an online library of more than 900 journals and publications. Follow the

InfoTrac College Edition

instructions for accessing InfoTrac that were packaged with your textbook; then search for articles using a keyword search.

For additional links, resources, and suggested readings on InfoTrac College Edition, visit our Health & Wellness Resource Center at **http://health.wadsworth.com**.

Key Terms

The terms listed are used on the page indicated. Definitions of the terms are in the Glossary at the end of this book.

Key Terms

anorexia nervosa 189
appetite 184
basal metabolic rate (BMR) 184
binge eating 188

Key Terms

bulimia nervosa 191
calories 184
eating disorders 188
hunger 184
obesity 182

Key Terms

overweight 182
satiety 184
waist-to-hip ratio (WHR) 183

References

1. Manson, JoAnn. "Obesity in the United States: A Fresh Look at Its High Toll." *Journal of the American Medical Association*, Vol. 289, No. 2, January 8, 2003, p. 229.

2. "What Is Obesity?" AOA Fact Sheet, American Obesity Association, www.obesity.org.

3. Tiggeman, Marika. "The Impact of Adolescent Girls' Life Concerns and Leisure Activities on Body Dissatisfaction, Disordered Eating, and Self-Esteem."

References

Journal of Genetic Psychology, Vol. 162, No. 2, June 2001, p. 133.

4. McLaren, L. and L. Gauvin. "The Cumulative Impact of Being Overweight on Women's Body Esteem: A Preliminary Study." *Eating and Weight Disorders,* Vol. 7, No. 4, December 2002, p. 324.

5. Arriaza, Ceceilia, and Traci Mann. "Ethnic Differences in Eating Disorders Among College Students: The Confounding Role of Body Mass Index." *Journal of American College Health,* Vol. 49, No. 6, May 2001, p. 309.

6. DiGioacchino, Rita, et al. "Body Dissatisfaction Among White and African American Male and Female College Students." *Eating Behaviors,* Vol. 2, December 2001, p. 39.

7. "Controlling the Global Obesity Epidemic." International Obesity Task Force (IOTF), www.iotf.org.

8. Vastag, Brian. "Experimental Drugs Take Aim at Obesity." *Journal of the American Medical Association,* Vol. 289, No. 14, April 9, 2003, p. 1763.

9. Branson, Ruth, et al. "Binge Eating as a Major Phenotype of Melanocortin 4 Receptor Gene Mutations." *New England Journal of Medicine,* Vol. 348, No. 12, March 20, 2003, pp. 1096–1103.

10. Prouty, Ann, et al. "College Women: Eating Behaviors and Help-Seeking Preferences." *Adolescence,* Vol. 37, No. 146, Summer 2002, p. 353.

11. Roerr, Sharon, et al. "Eating Disorder a Risk in Sorority and Dorm Students." *Journal of the American College of Nutrition,* Vol. 21, August 2002, p. 307.

12. O'Dea, Jennifer, and Suzanne Abraham. "Eating and Exercise Disorders in Young College Men." Journal of American College Health, Vol. 50, No. 4, May 2002, p. 273.

13. Graham, Melody, and Amy Jones. "Freshman 15: Valid Theory or Harmful Myth?" *Journal of American College Health,* Vol. 50, No. 4, January 2002, p. 171.

14. Branson, "Binge Eating as a Major Phenotype."

15. McElroy, Susan, et al. "Topiramate in the Treatment of Binge Eating Disorder Associated with Obesity." *American Journal of Psychiatry,* Vol. 160, No. 2, February 2003, p. 255.

16. The McKnight Investigators. "Risk Factors for the Onset of Eating Disorders in Adolescent Girls." *American Journal of Psychiatry,* Vol. 160, No. 2, February 2003, p. 248.

17. Anderluh, Marija, et al. "Childhood Obsessive-Compulsive Personality Traits in Adult Women with Eating Disorders." *American Journal of Psychiatry,* Vol. 160, No. 2, February 2003, p. 242.

18. Hales, Robert, and Stuart Yudofsky (editors). *Textbook of Clinical Psychiatry* (4th edition). Washington, DC: American Psychiatric Publishing, Inc., 2003, p. 975.

19. Arriaza and Mann, "Ethnic Differences in Eating Disorders Among College Students."

20. "Eating Disorders and Culture." *Harvard Mental Health Letter,* Vol. 18, No. 12, June 2002.

21. Halmi, Katherine. "From Giacometti to Botero: Images of Eating Disorders under Investigation." *American Journal of Psychiatry,* Vol. 160, No. 2, February 2003, p. 205.

22. Ben-Tovim, David I. "Outcomes in Patients with Eating Disorders: A 5-Year Study." *Journal of the American Medical Association,* Vol. 286, No. 1, July 4, 2001, p. 21.

23. Hales and Yudofsky, *Textbook of Clinical Psychiatry* (4th edition).

24. International Obesity Task Force (IOTF), www.iotf.org.

25. Willi, Denise. "Couch Potato Crisis: Diabetes, Obesity, Little Physical Exercise." *Instructor,* Vol. 112, No. 6, March 2003, p. 20(2).

26. Berkowitz, Robert, et al. "Behavior Therapy and Sibutramine for the Treatment of Adolescent Obesity." *Journal of the American Medical Association,* Vol. 289, No. 14, April 9, 2003, p. 1833.

27. "Obesity in the U.S." AOA Fact Sheet, American Obesity Association, www.obesity.org.

28. National Center for Health Statistics, www.hhs.gov.

29. Stephenson, Joan. "Low-Carb, Low-Fat Diet Gurus Face Off." *Journal of the American Medical Association,* Vol. 289, No. 14, April 9, 2003, p. 1767.

30. Smiciklas-Wright, H., et al. "Foods Commonly Eaten in the United States, 1989–1991 and 1994–1996: Are Portion Sizes Changing?" *Journal of the American Dietetic Association,* Vol. 103, No. 1, January 2003, p. 39.

31. Moore, Barbara. "Supersized America," *Cleveland Clinic Journal of Medicine,* Vol. 70, No. 3, March 2003, p. 237.

32. Critser, Greg. *Fat Land: How Americans Became the Fattest People in the World.* Boston: Houghton-Mifflin, 2003.

33. Hu, Frank, et al. "Television Watching and Other Sedentary Behaviors in Relation to Risk of Obesity and Type 2 Diabetes Mellitus in Women." *Journal of American Medical Association,* Vol. 289, No. 14, April 9, 2003, p. 1785.

34. Hu et al., "Television Watching and Other Sedentary Behaviors."

35. Pereira, Mark. Presentation, American Heart Association, Miami Beach, FL, February 2003.

36. Calle, Eugenia, et al. "Overweight, Obesity, and Mortality from Cancer in a Prospectively Studied Cohort of U.S. Adults." *New England Journal of Medicine,* Vol. 348, No. 17, April 24, 2003, p. 1625.

37. Ibid.

38. "Dangers Are Overlooked." *Medical Letter on the CDC & FDA,* August 12, 2001.

39. Schwimmer, Jeffrey, et al. "Health-Related Quality of Life of Severely Obese Children and Adolescents." *Journal of the American Medical Association,* Vol. 289, No. 14, April 9, 2003, p. 1813.

40. Peeters, Anna, et al. "Obesity in Adulthood and Its Consequences for Life Expectancy: A Life-Table Analysis." *Annals of Internal Medicine,* Vol. 138, No. 1, January 7, 2003, p. 24.

41. Fontaine, K. R., et al. "Years of Life Lost Due to Obesity." *Journal of the American Medical Association,* Vol. 289, No. 2, April 9, 2003, p. 183.

42. "Your Message to Patients: Supersize, Shorter Life." *American Medical News,* February 17, 2003.

43. Mitka, Mike. "Surgery for Obesity." *Journal of the American Medical Association,* Vol. 289, No. 14, April 9, 2003, p. 1761.

44. Rasheid, S. "Gastric Bypass is an Effective Treatment for Obstructive Sleep Apnea in Patients with Clinically Significant Obesity." *Obesity Surgery,* Vol. 13, No. 1, February 2003, pp. 58–61.

45. Torpy, Janet. "Obesity." *Journal of the American Medical Association,* Vol. 289, No. 14, April 9, 2003, p. 1880.

46. "Consumer Protection." American Obesity Association, www.obesity.org.

47. Bray, George. "Low-Carbohydrate Diets and Realities of Weight Loss." *Journal of the American Medical Association,* Vol. 289, No. 14, April 9, 2003, p. 1853.

48. Serdula, Mary, et al. "Weight Loss Counseling Revisited." *Journal of the American Medical Association,* Vol. 289, No. 14, April 9, 2003, p. 1747.

49. Heshka, Stanley, et al. "Weight Loss with Self-Help Compared with a Structured Commercial Program." *Journal of the American Medical Association,* Vol. 289, No. 14, April 9, 2003, p. 1792.

50. Tate, Deborah, et al. "Effects of Internet Behavioral Counseling on Weight Loss in Adults at Risk for Type 2 Diabetes." *Journal of the American Medical Association,* Vol. 289, No. 14, April 9, 2003, p. 1833.

51. Torpy, "Obesity."

References

52. Anderson, Drew A., et al. "Weight Goals in a College-age Population." *Obesity Research,* Vol. 11, 2003, pp. 274–278.

53. Stephenson, J. "Low-Carb, Low-Fat Diet Gurus Face Off."

54. Cheuvront, S. N. "The Zone Diet Phenomenon: A Closer Look at the Science Behind the Claims." *Journal of the American College of Nutrition,* Vol. 22, No. 1, February 2003, p. 9–17.

55. Sanders, T. A. "High- Versus Low-Fat Diets in Human Diseases." *Current Opinion of Clinical Nutrition and Metabolic Care,* Vol. 6, No. 2, March 2003, p. 151.

56. Willett W. C., and R. L. Leibel. "Dietary Fat is Not a Major Determinant of Body Fat." *American Journal of Medicine,* Vol. 113, No. 9B, December 30, 2002, pp. 47S–59S.

References

57. Bravata, Dena, et al. "Efficacy and Safety of Low-Carbohydrate Diets: A Systematic Review." *Journal of the American Medical Association,* Vol. 289, No. 14, April 9, 2003, p. 1837.

58. Serdula, et al. "Weight Loss Counseling Revisited."

59. Torpy, Janet. "Ephedra and Ephedrine." *Journal of the American Medical Association,* Vol. 289, No. 12, March 26, 2003, p. 1590.

60. Fontanarosa, Phil, et al. "The Need for Regulation of Dietary Supplements: Lessons from Ephedra." *Journal of the American Medical Association,* Vol. 289, No. 12, March 26, 2003, p. 1568.

61. Shekelle, Paul, et al. "Efficacy and Safety of Ephedra and Ephedrine for Weight Loss and Athletic Performance: A Meta-Analysis." *Journal of the American Medical*

References

Association, Vol. 289, No. 12, March 26, 2003, p. 1537.

62. Serdula et al. "Weight Loss Counseling Revisited."

63. Gadde, Kishore, et al. "Zonisamide for Weight Loss in Obese Adults." *Journal of the American Medical Association,* Vol. 289, No. 14, April 9, 2003, p. 1820.

64. Vastag, "Experimental Drugs Take Aim at Obesity."

65. McManus, Kathy. Personal Interview.

66. "Weight Control." Ontario, Canada: College of Family Physicians of Canada, 2003.

67. Cummings, Sue, et al. "Position of the American Dietetic Association: Weight Management." *Journal of the American Dietetic Association,* Vol. 102, No. 8, August 2002, pp. 11, 1145.

RESPONSIBLE SEXUALITY

OUR most special relationships are those that bring us closer to others—our friends, partners, spouses, parents, and children. Such intimacy is the most rewarding and often the most demanding of human involvements. The giving of ourselves to another—sharing thoughts, feelings, experiences, and sexual pleasure—touches the essence of what it means to be human. This section provides a comprehensive philosophical and practical view of relating to others. Each of the chapters focuses on the unique form of personal responsibility involved in every close relationship: a responsibility that looks beyond the self to those we care for and love.

Communication and Relationships

Oona compares the people in her life to threads in a magnificent tapestry. Each brings different tones and textures that complement and contrast with others. Her earliest childhood memories are of loving circles of family and friends that she once thought revolved around only her. Now she sees that she is part of these concentric rings and that the friendship and support she offers others enrich all of their lives.

When she left for a college thousands of miles from her home, Oona worried about the people she was leaving behind and the strangers she would be living among. She wondered if she'd be welcomed or shunned, judged by her looks or her race, invited to join social groups or excluded from them. What she discovered was that the choice was largely hers. She could reach out to others, smile and hope that others would smile in return, communicate clearly and honestly, strive to forge connections. Within months of her arrival, Oona was sure she had made friends she would keep forever.

Whether we are shy or outgoing, reserved or exuberant, we all crave human connection. As individuals and as part of society, we need to care about others and to know that others care about us, to feel for others and have others feel for us, to share what we know and to learn from what others know.

Sending clear messages through words, gestures, expressions, and behaviors is the essence of good communication. The more effectively we communicate, the more likely we are to create good relationships built on honesty, understanding, and mutual trust. Such relationships can infuse our lives with a richness no solitary pleasure can match.

This chapter discusses the social needs we all share, the ways some of us respond to those needs, and the possibilities that exist for coming together from our solitude to warm ourselves in each other's glow.

© JFB/Stone/Getty Images.

After studying the material in this chapter, you should be able to:

- **Describe** the role verbal and nonverbal communication plays in forming and maintaining relationships and **discuss** gender differences in communication.
- **Define** friendship and **explain** how friendship grows.
- **Discuss** the behavior and emotional expectations for friendship, dating, and intimate relationships.

- **Compare** and **contrast** romantic love and mature love.
- **List** and **describe** the various living arrangements today's adults might choose.
- **Identify** the problems likely to affect long-term relationships and **explain** how they can be prevented.
- **Describe** the different types of families and **discuss** some of the major issues facing them.
- **Identify** the behaviors that may result in dysfunctional relationships.

◼ Personal Communication

Getting to know someone is one of life's greatest challenges and pleasures. When you find another person intriguing—as a friend, as a teacher, as a colleague, as a possible partner—you want to find out as much as you can about him or her and to share more and more information about yourself. Roommates may talk for endless hours. Friends may spend years getting to know each other. Partners in committed relationships may delight in learning new things about each other.

Communication stems from a desire to know and a decision to tell. Each of us chooses what information about ourselves we want to disclose and what we want to conceal or keep private. But in opening up to others, we increase our own self-knowledge and understanding.

Communicating Feelings

A great deal of daily communication focuses on facts: on the who, what, where, when, and how. Information is easy to convey and comprehend. Emotions are not. Some people have great difficulty saying "I appreciate you" or "I care about you," even though they are genuinely appreciative and caring. Others find it hard to know what to say in response and how to accept such expressions of affection. Men and women vary in their communication styles. (See the X&Y File: "How Men and Women Communicate.")

Some people feel that relationships shouldn't require any effort, that there's no need to talk of responsibility between people who care about each other. Yet responsibility is implicit in our dealings with anyone or anything we value—and what can be more valuable than those with whom we share our lives? Friendships and other intimate relationships always demand an emotional investment, but the rewards they yield are great.

Sometimes people convey strong emotions with a kiss or a hug, a pat or a punch, but such actions aren't precise enough to communicate exact thoughts. Stalking out of a room and slamming the door may be clear signs of anger, but they don't explain what caused the anger or suggest what to do about it. You must learn how to communicate all feelings clearly and appropriately if you hope to become truly close to another person.

As two people build a relationship, they must sharpen their communication skills so that they can discuss all the issues they may confront. They must learn how to communicate anger as well as affection, hurt as well as joy—and they must listen as carefully as they speak.

Listening involves more than waiting for the other person to stop talking. Listening is an active process of trying to understand the other person's feelings and motivation. Effective listeners ask questions when they're not sure they understand the other person and prompt the other person to continue.

Nonverbal Communication

More than 90 percent of communication may be nonverbal. While we speak with our vocal cords, we communicate with our facial expressions, tone of voice, hands,

Good communication is essential to a healthy and successful relationship.

© 2000 David Roth/Stone/Getty Images

Body language can send powerful nonverbal messages about your true state of mind and feelings.

© 2000 PhotoDisc, Inc.

the X&Y file *How Men and Women Communicate*

In the past decade scientists have begun to explore gender differences in the way women and men use language. In ongoing research, psychologist James Pennebaker of the University of Texas developed a computer program to analyze four 450-word essays by more than 900 university students. The preliminary findings suggest that sex differences in written language are huge—larger, in fact, than many other psychological and personality characteristics.

In writing, women use more words overall, more words related to emotion (positive and negative), more idea words, more hearing, feeling, and sensing words, more causal words, such as *because,* and more modal words (*would, should, could*). Men use more numbers, more prepositions, and more articles, such as *an* and *the,* that, Pennebaker notes, "make language more concrete." Women use more question marks, more pronouns (especially *I*), and more references to other people. Men use more body words and, even in an academic assignment, twice as many swear words.[1]

Gender differences also appear online. In general, women tend to write e-mails in much the same way that they talk, using words to build a connection with people. Men's e-mails are briefer and more utilitarian. In chat rooms and online groups, men are more likely to make strong assertions, disagree with others, and to use profanities and sarcasm. Women are more prone to posing questions, making suggestions, and including polite expressions. Communication researchers studying the differences between "he-mails" and "she-mails" have also found that people who are not generally verbally expressive—mainly men—often convey more feelings in e-mails than they do in face-to-face conversations.

When men and women speak, other gender differences emerge. In her insightful studies of language, linguist Deborah Tannen has noted that men speak more often and for longer periods in public, often as a way of putting themselves in a "one-up" situation; women speak more in private, usually to build better connections to oth-ers. In a male's hierarchical social order, she explains, conversations "are negotiations in which people try to achieve and maintain the upper hand if they can and protect themselves from others' attempts to put them down and push them around." To women, who see the world as a network of connectedness, conversations are something else entirely: "negotiations for closeness in which people try to seek and give confirmation and support, and to reach consensus." While men use words to preserve independence, women talk to draw others closer.

Perhaps this is why, in public and private, women generally are better listeners, facilitating conversation by nodding, asking questions, and signaling interest by saying "uh-huh," or "yes." Men interrupt more, breaking in on another's monologue if they aren't getting the information they need. Women are more likely to wait for the speaker to finish. "There's more than one interpretation for why a woman is less likely to interrupt," says psychologist Judith Hall. "It could show that she's being submissive and not playing the aggressive role. But it also could mean that she is less of a social blunderer and is more adept at reading the other person's signals."[2]

Beginning in their preteen and teen years, women consistently outsmile men in all sorts of situations—with children, other women, or men—when they're in positions of authority or power. They even manage to grin under stress. "If you put a man and a woman in an equally nerve-wracking situation, the woman will laugh and smile," notes Hall. In hospitals, women physicians smile considerably more than their male colleagues.

 In social interactions, two white women talking together look into each other's eyes far more often than two men; African-American women are less likely to do so. When a man and a woman are together, the man gazes into the woman's eyes more often than he would a man's, while a woman makes eye contact less often than she would if she were with another woman—a nice exercise in reciprocity. "A man talking with a woman will act more like a woman, and a woman will act more like a man," observes Hall. "It's as if they're adjusting to accommodate each other's cultural norm."

shoulders, legs, torsos, posture. "Body language is a very elementary level of communication that people react to without realizing why," observes Albert Mehrabian, a professor of psychology at the University of California, Los Angeles (UCLA) and author of *Silent Messages.* "It's the building block upon which more advanced verbal forms of communication rest."[3]

Learning to interpret what people *don't* say can reveal more than what they *do* say. "Understanding nonverbal communication is probably the best tool there is for a good life of communicating, be it personally or profession-ally," says Marilyn Maple, an educator at the University of Florida. "It's one of the most practical skills you can develop. When you can consciously read what others are saying unconsciously, you can deal with issues before they become problems."[4]

 In a survey of 233 undergraduates at a large southeastern university, those who saw themselves as "involved" daters were more concerned about nonverbal communication than "casual" daters. These individuals were more likely to "work hard" to ensure that their nonverbal behavior backed up the words they said—and to say their partners did the same. Regardless of their dating status, the female students valued nonverbal behavior more than men. They also engaged in more forms of nonverbal communication, such as looking their partners straight in the eye and nodding their heads as their partners spoke.[5]

Culture has a great deal of influence over body language. In some cultures, for example, establishing eye contact is considered hostile or challenging; in others, it conveys friendliness. A person's sense of personal space—the distance he or she feels most comfortable in keeping from others—varies in different societies.

⚙ Forming Relationships

We first learn how to relate in our families, as children. Our relationships with parents and siblings change dramatically as we grow toward independence. Relationships between friends also change as they move or develop different interests; between lovers, as they come to know more about each other; between spouses, as they pass through life together; and between parents and children, as youngsters develop and mature. But throughout life, close relationships, tested and strengthened by time, allow us to explore the depths of our souls and the heights of our emotions. (See Self-Survey: "How Strong Are the Communication and Affection in Your Relationship?")

I, Myself, and Me

The way each of us perceives himself or herself affects all the ways we reach out and relate to others. If we feel unworthy of love, others may share that opinion. Self-esteem (discussed in Chapter 2) provides a positive foundation for our relationships with others. Self-esteem doesn't mean vanity or preoccupation with our own needs; rather, it is a genuine concern and respect for ourselves so that we remain true to our own feelings and beliefs. We can't know or love or accept others until we know and love and accept ourselves, however imperfect we may be.

Partners with low self-esteem may feel responsible for a partner's unhappiness. In studies of college students, those who scored low on measures of self-esteem were far more likely to feel rejected or hostile if their partners seemed distraught. Regardless of the reason for the distress, insecure, self-doubting individuals may "read nonexistent meaning into their partners' ambiguous cues." As a result, they may unwittingly sabotage their relationships. This misreading of cues occurs not just in dating couples, but among long-married partners who still fear that their spouses love them less than they actually do.[6]

Friendship

Friendship has been described as "the most holy bond of society." Every culture has prized the ties of respect, tolerance, and loyalty that friendship builds and nurtures. An anonymous writer put it well:

> A friend is one who knows you as you are,
> Understands where you've been,
> Accepts who you've become,
> And still gently invites you to grow.

Friends can be a basic source of happiness, a connection to a larger world, a source of solace in times of trouble. Although we have different friends throughout life, often the friendships of adolescence and young adulthood are the closest we ever form. They ease the normal break from parents and the transition from childhood to independence.

In the past, many people believed that men and women couldn't become close friends without getting romantically involved. But as the genders have worked together and come to share more interests, this belief has changed. Yet unique obstacles arise in male-female friendships, such as distinguishing between friendship and romantic attraction and dealing with sexual tension. However, men and women who overcome such barriers and become friends benefit from their relationship—but in different ways. For men, a friendship with a woman offers support and nurturance. What they report liking most is talking and relating to women, something they don't do

STRATEGIES FOR CHANGE

Being a Good Friend

- **Be willing to open up.** The more you share, the deeper the bond between you and your friend will become.

- **Be sensitive to your friend's feelings.** Keep in mind that, like you, your friend has unique needs, desires, and dreams.

- **Express appreciation.** Be generous with your compliments. Let your friends know you recognize their kindnesses.

- **Know that friends will disappoint you from time to time.** They, too, are only human. Accept them as they are. Admitting their faults need not reduce your respect for them.

- **Talk about your friendship.** Evaluate the relationship periodically. If you have any gripes or frustrations, air them.

Self Survey | How Strong Are the Communication and Affection in Your Relationship?

Effective, caring communication and loving affection markedly enhance a couple's relationship. The following self-test may help you to assess the degree of good communication, love, and respect in your intimate relationship. If you agree or mostly agree with a statement, answer yes. If you disagree or mostly disagree, answer no. You may wish to have your partner respond to this assessment as well. If so, mark your answers on a separate sheet.

1.	My partner seeks out my opinion.	Yes	No
2.	My partner cares about my feelings.	Yes	No
3.	I don't feel ignored very often.	Yes	No
4.	We touch each other a lot.	Yes	No
5.	We listen to each other.	Yes	No
6.	We respect each other's ideas.	Yes	No
7.	We are affectionate toward one another.	Yes	No
8.	I feel my partner takes good care of me.	Yes	No
9.	What I say counts.	Yes	No
10.	I am important in our decisions.	Yes	No
11.	There's lots of love in our relationship.	Yes	No
12.	We are genuinely interested in one another.	Yes	No
13.	I love spending time with my partner.	Yes	No
14.	We are very good friends.	Yes	No
15.	Even during rough times, we can be empathetic.	Yes	No
16.	My partner is considerate of my viewpoint.	Yes	No
17.	My partner finds me physically attractive.	Yes	No
18.	My partner expresses warmth toward me.	Yes	No
19.	I feel included in my partner's life.	Yes	No
20.	My partner admires me.	Yes	No

Scoring:

A preponderance of yes answers indicates that you enjoy a strong relationship characterized by good communication and loving affection. If you answered yes to fewer than seven items, it is likely that you are not feeling loved and respected and that the communication in your relationship is decidedly lacking.

Source: John Gottman, *Why Marriages Succeed or Fail*. New York: Simon & Schuster, 1994.

Your Health Change Plan

for Better Communication

Like other skills, communication improves with practice. Here are some suggestions that can enhance your ability to express yourself more precisely and to understand spoken and unspoken messages from others.

:: **Tune into your body talk.** Notice details about the way you speak, gesture, and move. If possible, watch yourself on videotape. Analyze the emotions you're feeling at the time and think of how they may be influencing your body language.

:: **Learn to establish good eye contact, but don't glare or stare.** If you sense that someone feels uncomfortable with an intense eye grip, shift your focus so that your gaze hits somewhere between the eyes and the chin, rather than pupil-to-pupil.

:: **Avoid putting up barriers.** If you fold your arms across your chest, you'll look defensive or uninterested in contact. Crossing your legs or ankles also can seem like a way of keeping your distance.

:: **Identify the little things you characteristically do when you're tense.** Some people pat their hair or pick at their ears; others rub their necks, twist a ring or watch, twirl a lock of hair, or play with a pen. Train yourself to become aware of what you're doing (have a friend give your a signal, if necessary) and to control your mannerisms.

:: **Use "I" statements.** Describe what's going on with you. Say, "I worry about being liked" or "I get frustrated when I can't put my feelings into words." Avoid generalities such as "You never think about my feelings," or "Nobody understands me."

:: **Gently ask how the other person feels.** If your friend or partner describes thoughts rather than feelings, ask for more adjectives. Was he or she sad, excited, angry, hurt?

:: **Become a very good listener.** When another person talks, don't interrupt, ask why, judge, or challenge. Nod your head. Use your body language and facial expression to show you're eager to hear more.

:: **Respect confidences.** Treat a friend's or partner's secrets with the discretion they deserve. Consider them a special gift entrusted to your care.

with their male buddies. Women view their friendships with men as more light-hearted and casual, with more joking and less fear of hurt feelings. They especially like getting insight into what guys really think.

Friendship transcends all boundaries of distance and differences and enhances feelings of warmth, trust, love, and affection between two people. It is a common denominator of human existence that cuts across major social categories: In every country, culture, and language, human beings make friends. Friendship is both a universal and a deeply satisfying experience.

"Wishing to be friends," Aristotle wrote, "is quick work, but friendship is a slowly opening fruit." The qualities that make a good friend include honesty, acceptance, dependability, empathy, and loyalty. To sustain a close friendship, both people must be able to see the other's perspective, anticipate each other's needs, and take each other's viewpoint into account. More than anything else, good friends are there when we need them. They see us at our worst but never lose sight of our best. They share our laughter and tears, our triumphs and tragedies.

Can Relationships Be Bad for You?

Although they enrich and fulfill us in many ways, our relationships with friends, siblings, parents, or colleagues can also sabotage our health. Mental health professionals define a "toxic" relationship as one in which either person is made to feel worthless or incompetent. Dysfunctional relationships are so common and troubling that mental health professionals are debating whether they constitute a psychiatric disorder.

"Physical symptoms, such as headaches, digestive troubles, tics, and inability to sleep well, can be signs of a destructive relationship," says sociologist Robert Billingham, professor of human development and family

studies at Indiana University.[7] Yet, although one person may repeatedly attack, abandon, betray, badger, bully, criticize, deceive, dominate, or demean the other, the responsibility for changing the unhealthy dynamic belongs to both.

"The big question is, 'Do I want or have to keep this relationship going?'" says sociologist Jan Yager, author of *When Friendship Hurts.* "If yes, are you willing to invest time and energy to turn it around?"[8]

Dating

A date is any occasion during which two people share their time. It can be a Friday night dance, a bicycle ride, a dinner for two, or a walk in the park. Friends and lovers go on dates; so do complete strangers. Some men date other men; some women date other women. We don't expect to love, or even like, everyone we date. Yet the people you date reveal something about the sort of person you are.

 Dating peaks among young adults. Nearly 50 percent of 18-year-olds go out at least once a week. By age 32, only about 25 percent date that often.[9] While in school, you may go out with people you meet in class or on campus. Some students form such close relationships that they are practically "joined at the hip." Others "hook up," connecting only for a one-time sexual encounter that might involve anything from kissing to intercourse.

With more people remaining single longer, the search for a good date has become more complex. Singles bars have become less popular because of the dangers of excessive drinking and casual sex. Cafés, laundromats, health clubs, and bookstores have become more acceptable as places to meet new people. Personal ads and cyberspace are alternative ways to meet potential dates. (See Savvy Consumer: "Do's and Don'ts of Online Dating.")

Dating can do more than help you meet people. By dating, you can learn how to make conversation, get to know more about others as well as yourself, and share feelings, opinions, and interests. In adolescence and young adulthood, dating also provides an opportunity for exploring your sexual identity. Some people date for months and never share more than a good-night kiss. Others may fall into bed together before they fall in love or even "like."

Separating your emotional feelings about someone you're dating from your sexual desire is often difficult. The first step to making responsible sexual decisions is respecting your sexual values and those of your partner. If you care about the other person—not just his or her body—and the relationship you're creating, sex will be an important, but not the all-important, factor while you're dating.

Dating has potential dangers. As discussed in Chapter 18, approximately one in five female teens is physically and/or sexually abused by a dating partner,[10] though in some cases girls are the aggressors.[11]

STRATEGIES FOR CHANGE

Coping with an Unhealthy Relationship

■ **Start a dialogue.** Focus on communication, not confrontation. Start with a positive statement, for instance, saying what you really value in the relationship. Volunteer what you might do to make it better, and state what you need from the other person.

■ **Distance yourself.** Take a vacation from a toxic friendship. Skip the family reunion or Thanksgiving dinner. When forced into proximity, be polite. If you refuse to engage—not arguing, not getting angry, not trying to make things better—toxic people give up trying to get under your skin.

■ **Consult a professional.** A therapist or minister can help people recognize and change toxic behavior patterns. Changes you make in how you act and react can trigger changes in others.

■ **Save yourself.** If you can never get what you need in a relationship, you may need to let it go. Nothing is worth compromising your mental or physical health.

Savvy Consumer

DO'S AND DON'TS OF ONLINE DATING

Forget personal ads or single bars. If you're looking for love in the new millennium, the place more people are turning is cyberspace. Some estimate that thousands, perhaps millions of people, are using the Internet to find a companion.

E-mail flirtations can be fun, but they also entail some risks, particularly if you decide to go off-line and meet in person. Here are some guidelines:

- Be careful of what you type. Anything you put on the Internet can end up almost anywhere. To avoid embarrassment, don't say anything you wouldn't want to see in newspaper print.

- Don't give out your address, telephone number, or any other identifying information. The people you meet online are strangers, and you should keep your guard up.

- Don't "date" on an office or university computer. You could end up supplying your professors, classmates, or coworkers with unintentional entertainment. Also, many organizations and institutions consider e-mail messages company property.

- Remember that you have no way of verifying if a correspondent is telling the truth about anything—sex, age, occupation, marital status. If your online partner seems insincere or strange in any way, stop corresponding.

- If you do decide to meet, make your first face-to-face encounter a double or group date, and make it somewhere public, like a cafe or museum. Don't plan a full-day outing. Coffee or a drink in a crowded place makes the best transition from e-mails.

- Make sure you tell a friend or family member your plans and have your own way of getting home. It's also a good idea to schedule the first meeting in the afternoon or early in the evening rather than later at night.

- Don't let your expectations run wild. Finding Mr. or Ms. Right is no easier in cyberspace than anywhere else, so be realistic about where your relationship might lead.

- Don't rely on the Internet as your only method of meeting people. Continue to get out in the real world and meet potential dates the old-fashioned ways.

Most longitudinal studies on dating relationships have shown little change in love over time, although love has been found to increase for individuals who advance to a deeper, more long-lasting commitment. Romantic partners in enduring relationships generally perceive their love, commitment, and satisfaction as increasing over time. A four-year study of romantic couples, all dating as the study began, found that those who remained together perceived that their love, satisfaction, and commitment had grown.[12]

:: Intimate Relationships

The term **intimacy**—the open, trusting sharing of close, confidential thoughts and feelings—comes from the Latin word for *within*. Intimacy doesn't happen at first sight, or in a day or a week or a number of weeks. Intimacy requires time and nurturing; it is a process of revealing rather than hiding, of wanting to know another and to be known by that other. (See Figure 7-1 for the elements of love.) Although intimacy doesn't require sex, an intimate relationship often includes a sexual relationship, heterosexual or homosexual.

All of our close relationships, whether they're with parents or friends, have a great deal in common. We feel we can count on these people in times of need. We feel that they understand us and we understand them. We give and receive loving emotional support. We care about their happiness and welfare. However, when we choose one person above all others, there is something even deeper and richer—something we call romantic love.

Figure 7-1 STERNBERG'S LOVE TRIANGLE
The three components of love are intimacy, passion, and commitment. The various kinds of love are composed of different combinations of the three components.

Liking
(intimacy alone)

Intimacy

Romantic love
(intimacy + passion)

Companionate
love
(intimacy +
commitment)

Consummate
love
(intimacy +
passion +
commitment)

Passion   Commitment

Infatuation
(passion alone)

Empty love
(commitment alone)

Fatuous love
(passion + commitment)

What Causes Romantic Attraction?

What draws two people to each other and keeps them together: chemistry or fate, survival instincts or sexual longings? "Probably it's a host of different things," reports sociologist Edward Laumann, coauthor of *Sex in America,* a landmark survey of 3,432 men and women conducted by the National Opinion Research Center at the University of Chicago.[13] "But what's remarkable is that most of us end up with partners much like ourselves—in age, race, ethnicity, socioeconomic class, education."

Why? "You've got to get close for sexual chemistry to occur," says Laumann. "Sparks may fly when you see someone across a crowded room, but you only see a pre-selected group of people—people enough like you to be in the same room in the first place. This makes sense because initiating a sexual relationship is very uncertain. We all have such trepidations about being too fat, too ugly, too undesirable. We try to lower the risk of rejection by looking for people more or less like us."

Scientists have tried to analyze the combination of factors that attracts two people to each other. In several studies of college students, four predictors ranked as the most important reasons for attraction: warmth and kindness, desirable personality, something specific about the person, and reciprocal liking.[14]

Romantic attraction is characterized by a high-level of emotional arousal, reciprocal liking, and mutual sexual desire.

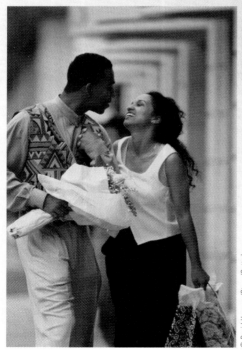

© David Hanover/Stone/Getty Images

In his cross-cultural research, psychologist David Buss, author of *The Evolution of Desire,* found that men in 37 sample groups drawn from Africa, Asia, Europe, North and South America, Australia, and New Zealand rated youth and attractiveness as more important in a possible mate than did women. Women placed greater value on potential mates who were somewhat older, had good financial prospects, and were dependable and hardworking.[15]

The reason for this gender difference could be evolutionary. Throughout time, men have sought fertile females of "high reproductive value." Two outward signs of female fertility are youth and a more subtle factor: waist-to-hip ratio. When researchers analyzed the physical dimensions of the women considered most attractive by men, those with the slimmest waists and roundest hips were consistently rated as most desirable. Women have had to look for mates who could provide greater security for their offspring. For them, a man's power, wealth, and status—which require more time to assess—mattered more than appearance.

In a national survey of more than 13,000 adults in the United States, researchers asked how willing they would be to marry an individual, based on education, income, age, and other factors. Figure 7-2 shows that the women were significantly more willing than men to marry someone who was older, better educated, would earn more, and was not good-looking. The men were more willing than women to marry someone who had less education, was younger, wasn't likely to hold a steady job, and who would earn less. There were minor differences on items related to prior marriages, religion, and already having children.

The Science of Romantic Love

Falling in love is an intense, dizzying experience. A person not only enters our life but takes possession of it as well. We are intrigued, flattered, delighted—but is this love, or a love of loving? At the time you're experiencing it, you may not care. You're in such a state of giddy elation that it doesn't matter, at least for the moment, whether it stems from a strong sexual attraction, a fear of loneliness, loneliness itself, or a hunger for approval.

We like to think of this powerful force, this source of both danger and delight, as something that defies analysis. However, in recent years, as scientists have attempted to study love objectively, they have provided new perspectives on its nature. (See Fact or Fiction? "Two people . . .")

An Anthropological View

When you first fall in love, you may be sure that no one else has ever known the same dizzying, wonderful feelings. Yet, while every romance may be unique, romantic love is anything but. Anthropologists have found evidence of romantic love in most of the cultures they studied. Intense attraction between individuals seems to be a human universal, or at the least, a near-universal.

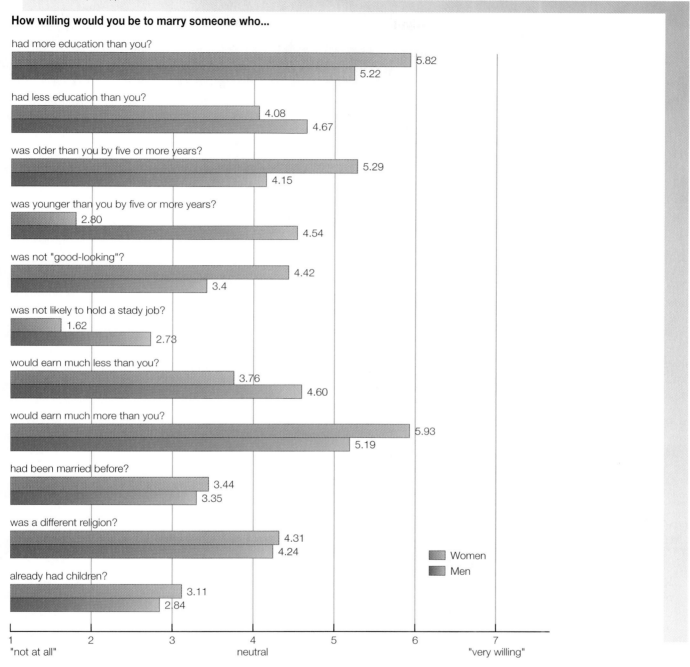

Figure 7-2 MEN, WOMEN, AND MARITAL PREFERENCES

Source: Data from Robert Crooks and Karla Baur. *Our Sexuality*, 8th ed. Pacific Grove, CA: Wadsworth, 2002, p. 190.

How willing would you be to marry someone who...

had more education than you?
5.82
5.22

had less education than you?
4.08
4.67

was older than you by five or more years?
5.29
4.15

was younger than you by five or more years?
2.80
4.54

was not "good-looking"?
4.42
3.4

was not likely to hold a stady job?
1.62
2.73

would earn much less than you?
3.76
4.60

would earn much more than you?
5.93
5.19

had been married before?
3.44
3.35

was a different religion?
4.31
4.24

Women
Men

already had children?
3.11
2.84

1 "not at all"   2   3   4 neutral   5   6   7 "very willing"

Another anthropologist, Helen Fisher, author of *Anatomy of Love: The Natural History of Monogamy, Adultery and Divorce,* describes romantic love "as a very primitive, basic human emotion, as basic as fear, anger or joy." As she explains, it pulled men and women of prehistoric times into the sort of partnerships that were essential to child rearing. But after about four years—just "long enough to rear one child through infancy," says Fisher—romantic love seemed to wane, and primitive couples tended to break up and find new partners. This "four-year itch" may well have endured through the centuries, contends Fisher, who notes that divorce statistics from most of the 62 cultures she has

Standards of physical attractiveness vary widely around the world.

studied still show a pattern of restlessness four years into a marriage.[16]

A Biochemical View

The heart is the organ we associate with love, but the brain may be where the action really is. According to research on **neurotransmitters** (messenger chemicals within the brain), love sets off a chemical chain reaction that causes our skin to flush, our palms to sweat, and our lungs to breathe more deeply and rapidly. The "love chemicals" within the brain—dopamine, norepinephrine, and phenylethylamine (PEA)—have effects similar to those of amphetamines, stimulant drugs that intensify physiological reactions (see Chapter 12).

Infatuation may indeed be a natural high, but like other highs, this rush doesn't last—possibly because the body develops tolerance for love-induced chemicals, just as it does with amphetamines. However, as the initial lovers' high fades, other brain chemicals may come into play: the endorphins, morphinelike chemicals that can help produce feelings of well-being, security, and tranquility. These feel-good molecules may increase in partners who develop a deep attachment.

The hormone **oxytocin,** best known for its role in inducing labor during childbirth, seems particularly important in our ability to bond with others. By measuring blood levels of women as they recalled positive and negative relationships, researchers have found that women whose oxytocin levels rose when remembering a positive relationship reported having little difficulty setting appropriate boundaries, being alone, or trying too hard to please others. Women whose oxytocin levels fell in response to remembering a negative emotional relationship reported greater anxiety in close relationships.

Mature Love

Social scientists have distinguished between *passionate love* (characterized by intense feelings of elation, sexual desire, and ecstasy) and *companionate love* (characterized by friendly affection and deep attachment). Often relationships begin with passionate love and evolve into a more companionate love. Sometimes the opposite happens and two people who know each other well discover that their friendship has "caught fire" and the sparks have flamed an unexpected passion.

A romantic relationship shows definite promise if:

:: You feel at ease with your new partner.

:: You feel good about your new partner both when you're together and when you're not.

FACT OR FICTION????????????????

Two people can deliberately fall in love.

Fact: "Yes, you can make yourself deliberately fall in love with someone you presently like but do not really love," says noted therapist Albert Ellis, Ph.D., of the Albert Ellis Institute, "but not easily." Other experts agree, despite the popular notion that love either finds two people or not. "Romantic falsehoods tend to obscure the actual work involved in creating love between two people," says James Morris, Ph.D., president of the American Association for Marriage and Family Therapy. "When we say that people 'fall' in love, we would do well to think more in terms of 'choosing' and 'creating' love together."

Source: "Heads Up: Can Two People Deliberately Fall in Love?" *Psychology Today,* Vol. 36, No. 1, February 2003, p. 46.

:: Your partner is open with you about his or her life—past, present, and future.

:: You can say no to each other without feeling guilty.

:: You feel cared for, appreciated, and accepted as you are.

:: Your partner really listens to what you have to say.

Mature love is a complex combination of sexual excitement, tenderness, commitment, and—most of all—an overriding passion that sets it apart from all other love relationships in one's life. This passion isn't simply a matter of orgasm, but also entails a crossing of the psychological boundaries between oneself and one's lover. You feel as if you're becoming one with your partner while simultaneously retaining a sense of yourself.

When Love Ends

Breaking up is indeed hard to do. Sometimes two people grow apart gradually, and both of them realize that they must go their separate ways. More often, one person falls out of love first. It hurts to be rejected; it also hurts to inflict pain on someone who once meant a great deal to you.

In a survey of 259 undergraduates, about eight in ten said they knew how to end a relationship, but three in ten reported feeling ambivalent about breaking up. (See Student Snapshot: "Is Breaking Up Hard to Do?") Most students supported getting out of an unsatisfactory dating relationship. About three in four felt that breaking up an unhappy relationship while dating would make for happier marriages in the long term. Non-whites were more likely to end relationships with no future than whites.[17]

In surveys, college students say it's more difficult to initiate a breakup than to be rejected. Those who decided to end a relationship reported greater feelings of guilt, uncertainty, discomfort, and awkwardness than those with whom they broke up. However, students with high levels of jealousy are likely to feel a desire for vengeance that can lead to aggressive behavior.[18]

Research suggests that people do not end their relationships because of the disappearance of love. Rather a sense of dissatisfaction or unhappiness develops, which may then cause love to stop growing. The fact that love does not dissipate completely may be one of the reasons why breakups are so painful. While the pain does ease over time, it can help both parties if they end their relationship in a way that shows kindness and respect. Your basic guideline should be to think of how you would like to be treated if someone were breaking up with you. Would it

hurt more to find out from someone else? Would it be more painful if the person you cared for lied to you or deceived you, rather than admitted the truth? Saying, "I don't feel the way I once did about you; I don't want to continue our relationship," is hard, but it's also honest and direct.

◼ Living Arrangements

Today's adults have many choices to explore regarding how and with whom they might live: returning to one's primary family, staying single, living with one or more friends, living in a long-term relationship with a lover of the same or opposite sex, or getting married. Increasingly, men and women in their twenties are spending more time considering all their options before committing themselves to an exclusive relationship.

Living with Parents

According to the Census Bureau, young adults between the ages of 18 and 24 are more likely to be living in their parents' homes than young people were in the 1970s. Some 18 million Americans between the ages of 18 and 34 are still living with their parents. Of those between ages 19 and 24, 66 percent (including college students) are living at home, compared to 50 percent in 1980.[19] Their

Student Snapshot   **Is Breaking Up Hard to Do?**

Students who...

Know how to end a relationship
77.9%

Seldom or never stay in a relationship they think they should end
59.9%

Seldom or never stay in relationships that become unhappy
58.6%

Sometimes remain in relationships they think they should end
31%

Sometimes remain in relationships that become unhappy
32.3%

Have felt ambivalent about ending a relationship
30%

Source: Data from a sample of 259 undergraduates at a large southeastern university: David Knox et al. "College Students' Attitudes and Behaviors Toward Ending an Unsatisfactory Relationship," *College Student Journal,* Vol. 36, No. 4, December 2002, p. 630.

reasons include the high cost of housing and the low incomes most men and women earn in their early twenties.

Single Life

In young adulthood, single men outnumber single women; after age 40, however, there are more single women than single men. Perhaps because there are so many singles, more and more Americans are living alone. The number of women living alone has doubled since 1970 and has nearly tripled for men.[20] Approximately one-quarter of the households in the nation are one-person homes. (See Figure 7-3).

Among Americans between 25 and 34 years old, about 35 percent (14 million) have never been married. Of African Americans in this age group, 53 percent have never been married. Being single no longer marks a transition phase between living with parents and living with a spouse, but is an accepted, appealing lifestyle for millions of men and women.

The number-one reason people remain single is not being able to find the right person, according to psychologist Florence Kaslow, director of the Florida Couples and Family Institute. For women, the next two reasons for staying single are their careers and independence. For men, independence and resolving personal issues are the second

1960   2000

13%   26%

87%   74%

Figure 7-3 PERCENT OF ALL HOUSEHOLDS OCCUPIED BY ONE PERSON

Between 1960 and 2000, the number of single households doubled.

Source: U.S. Census Bureau.

and third reasons for not marrying. Most of the women and all of the men in her study said that they would like to get married—someday. Yet only 5 percent of bachelors over age 40 ever marry.

STRATEGIES FOR CHANGE

How to Stay Single and Satisfied

- Fill your life with meaningful work, experiences, and people.

- Build a network of supportive friends who care for and about you.

- Be open to new experiences that can expand your feelings about yourself and your world.

- Don't miss out on a special event because you don't have someone to accompany you: Go alone.

- Volunteer to help others less fortunate, or become involved in church and social organizations.

Cohabitation

Although couples have always shared homes in informal relationships without any official ties, "living together," or **cohabitation,** has become more common. Some 55 million couples are cohabiting in the United States, a tenfold increase since 1960. The vast majority are heterosexual.[21]

 As shown in Figure 7-4, Asians and non-Hispanic white couples are the least likely to cohabit. A higher percentage of Native American, black, and Hispanic couples are unmarried. "Cohabiters" tend to have lower income and education levels. They also are younger—on average, some twelve years younger than married men and women.[22]

According to the Census Bureau, unmarried couples tend to cluster in several zones in the United States, including the western states and the Northeast. In these regions, married couples flock to the suburbs, while unmarried couples, especially same-sex ones, are most likely to live in central cities.[23]

Unmarried couples are much like those joined in wedlock.[24] The great majority—an estimated 95 percent—expect to remain faithful to each other.[25] But women who do not wed seem to have more clout. According to the Census Bureau, women are identified as the head of the household in 46 percent of unmarried couples, compared to only 13 percent of married couples.

Cohabitation doesn't necessarily lead to marriage.[26] (See Fact or Fiction?: "Couples who live together . . .") In a study of 700 women living with boyfriends, one in four said she did not expect to marry the man whose address she shared. Among white and Hispanic women with both high levels of education and income and who were living with men of equal socioeconomic standing, about 80 percent expected to marry their partners. This fell to 50 percent when the women were living with men with less education and income than their own. Women who have been married or cohabited before are less likely to expect to walk down the aisle and wed.[27]

Unmarried couples are gaining legal recognition. Some cities in the United States have domestic partnership laws that grant a variety of spousal rights—such as insurance benefits and bereavement leave—to partners, heterosexual or homosexual, who live together. Canada has recognized marriages between homosexual partners as legitimate unions.

Figure 7-4 TO WED OR NOT TO WED?

Source: From American Demographics Forecast (April 2003). Copyright © 2003, PRIMEDIA Business Magazines & Media, Inc. All Rights Reserved.

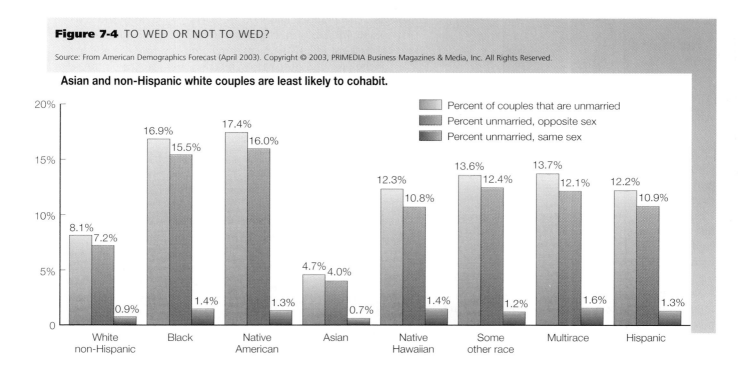

Asian and non-Hispanic white couples are least likely to cohabit.

FACT OR FICTION??????????????

Couples who live together usually get married.

Fiction: According to recent research, couples who live together are much less likely to wed than in the past. In the 1970s two-thirds of cohabiting couples married within three years. Today about half of men and women living together get married within five years; 40 percent break up; 10 percent continue to cohabit for a longer period. Among women cohabiting with a man, one in four says she doesn't ever expect to marry him.

Source: Alternatives to Marriage Project, www.unmarried.org.

◖ Committed Relationships

Even though men and women today may have more sexual partners than in the past, most still yearn for an intense, supportive, exclusive relationship, based on mutual commitment and enduring over time. In our society, most such relationships take the form of heterosexual marriages, but partners of the same sex or heterosexual partners who never marry also may sustain long-lasting, deeply committed relationships. These couples are much like married people: They make a home, handle daily chores, cope with problems, celebrate special occasions, plan for the future—all the while knowing that they are not alone, that they are part of a pair that adds up to far more than just the sum of two individual souls.

Marriage

> *Like everything which is not the involuntary result of fleeting emotion but the creation of time and will, any marriage, happy or unhappy, is infinitely more interesting and significant than any romance, however passionate.*

W. H. Auden

Contemporary marriage has been described as an institution that everyone on the outside wants to enter and everyone on the inside wants to leave. According to the Census Bureau, nine in ten people marry, but about half of first marriages end in divorce after an average of seven or eight years. The median age of first marriage is 26.8 for men and 25.1 for women.[28]

Not too long ago, marriage was often a business deal, a contract made by parents for economic or political reasons when the spouses-to-be were still very young. Today, in some countries, it is still culturally acceptable to arrange marriages in this manner. Even in America, certain ethnic groups, such as Asians who have recently immigrated to the United States, plan marriages for their children. In such arrangements, the marriage partners are likely to have similar values and expectations. However, the newlyweds also start out as strangers who may not even know whether they like—let alone love—each other. Sometimes arranged marriages do lead to loving unions; sometimes they trap both partners in loneliness and longing.

Most of today's marriages aren't arranged, but even in this day and age, partners often marry because they have to: One of every six brides is pregnant on her wedding day. Other young couples marry as a way to escape from their parents' homes and authority. But most people say they marry for one far-from-simple reason: love.

Preparing for Marriage

With more than half of all marriages ending in divorce, there's little doubt that modern marriages aren't made in heaven. Are some couples doomed to divorce even before they swap "I do's"? Could counseling before a marriage increase its odds of success? According to recent research findings, the answer to both questions is yes.

There have been government attempts to set requirements for couples who want to marry. Some states, such as Arizona and Louisiana, have established "covenant" marriages in which engaged couples are required to get premarital counseling. Utah allows counties to require counseling before issuing marriage licenses to minors and people who have been divorced. Florida requires high school students to take marriage education classes.[29]

Finding Mr. or Ms. Right

Generally, men and women marry people from the geographical area they grew up in and from the same social background. Differences in religion and race can add to the pressures of marriage, but they also can enrich the relationship if they aren't viewed as obstacles. In our culturally diverse society, interracial and crosscultural marriages are becoming more common and widely accepted, although the odds are much greater for partners of the same race to live together or marry.

 In a study of 75,000 couples who lived together and 480,000 married couples in the United States, researchers found that African Americans were 365 times more likely to marry a black than a nonblack spouse and 110 times more likely to live with, or cohabit with, a black partner than someone of another racial group. Asians were 55 times more likely to marry another Asian and 17 times more likely to cohabit with another Asian. Hispanics were 12 times more likely to select a Hispanic spouse and nine times more likely to live with a Hispanic partner. Whites were about eight times more likely to marry another white person and five times more likely to cohabit with someone who is white rather than nonwhite.[30]

Some of the traits that appeal to us in a date become less important when we select a mate; others become key ingredients in the emotional cement holding two people together. According to psychologist Robert Sternberg of Yale University, the crucial ingredients for commitment are the following:

:: Shared values.

:: A willingness to change in response to each other.

:: A willingness to tolerate flaws.

:: A match in religious beliefs.

:: The ability to communicate effectively.

The single best predictor of how satisfied one will be in a relationship, according to Sternberg, is not how one feels toward a lover, but the difference between how one would like the lover to feel and how the lover actually feels. Feeling that the partner you've chosen loves too little or too much is, as he puts it, "the best predictor of failure."[31]

Premarital Assessments

There are scientific ways of predicting marital happiness. Some premarital assessment inventories identify strengths and weaknesses in many aspects of a relationship: realistic expectations, personality issues, communication, conflict resolution, financial management, leisure activities, sex, children, family and friends, egalitarian roles, and religious orientation. Couples who become aware of potential conflicts by means of such inventories may be able to resolve

STRATEGIES FOR PREVENTION

Think Twice About Getting Married If:

■ You or your partner is constantly asking the other such questions as "Are you sure you love me?"

■ You spend most of your time together disagreeing and quarreling.

■ You're both still very young (under the age of 20).

■ Your boyfriend or girlfriend has behaviors (such as non-stop talking), traits (such as bossiness), or problems (such as drinking too much) that really bother you and that you're hoping will change after you're married.

■ Your partner wants you to stop seeing your friends, quit a job you enjoy, or change your life in some other way that diminishes your overall satisfaction.

them through professional counseling. In some cases, they may want to reconsider or postpone their wedding.

Other common predictors of marital discord, unhappiness, and separation are:

:: A high level of arousal during a discussion.

:: Defensive behaviors such as making excuses and denying responsibility for disagreements.

:: A wife's expressions of contempt.

:: A husband's stonewalling (showing no response when a wife expresses her concerns).

By looking for such behaviors, researchers have been able to predict with better than 90 percent accuracy whether a couple will separate within the first few years of marriage.

Types of Marriage

Sociologists have categorized marriages as traditional or companion-oriented. In **traditional marriages,** the couples assume prescribed societal roles. In **companion-oriented marriages,** the partnership and its rewards—rather than the roles of fathering, mothering, and breadwinning—are primary. In addition, there are **romantic marriages,** in which sexual passion never seems to die, and **rescue marriages,** in which one partner suffered a traumatic childhood and sees marriage as a way of healing. About a fifth of all marriages belong to another category that has grown significantly in recent years: marriages of equally dependent spouses. Each partner in these unions earns between 40 and 59 percent of the total family income. According to research on these marriages, divorces are more common and occur more often at the wife's initiative. Researchers theorize that wives who are not economically dependent on their spouses may be more likely to leave an emotionally unfulfilling relationship.[32] Regardless of type, a marriage can succeed if it fulfills basic tasks, such as providing a sense of intimacy and autonomy and providing a safe haven that is strong enough to absorb inevitable conflicts.

Issues Couples Confront

No two people can live together in perfect harmony all the time. Some of the issues that crop up in any long-term relationship include expectations, how to disagree, money, sex, and careers.

Unrealistic Expectations

Partners may think that their significant others should always be as attractive, charming, and tolerant as they were when they were dating. They may assume that their

A relationship is just as alive as the individuals who create it. It grows if there is caring; it can blossom if there is emotional nourishment; and it endures if there is commitment.

partners will always agree with them or will automatically see their point of view; or they may believe that their one true love will always be able to meet all their needs. Because no one could ever live up to such expectations, the partners are doomed to disappointment.

Togetherness does not necessarily guarantee happiness. According to one study of more than 2,000 couples, too much time together—particularly doing shopping and chores—may be bad for a marriage.[33]

Settling Differences

Contrary to what you may assume, arguments can be good for the health of a relationship. According to the National Institute of Mental Health, couples who learn how to fight fairly and effectively have a 50 percent lower divorce rate than those who haven't mastered the art of disagreeing. Results of a study of 150 couples from premarriage through the first ten years of marriage (the highest risk period for divorce) led researchers to conclude that "nondestructive" arguing lowers the likelihood for physical violence, helps couples stay together longer, and benefits children by preparing them to build good intimate relationships as adults.

Money

Money may make the business world go around, but it has the opposite effect on relationships: It knocks them off their tracks, brings them to a halt, twists them upside down. However, even though almost all couples quarrel about money, they rarely fight over how much they have. What matters more—whether they make $10,000 or $100,000 a year—is what money means to both partners. How does each person use money to meet emotional needs? Who decides how the money is spent? Who keeps track? Until they resolve these issues, couples may quarrel over money as long as they're together.

To avoid fighting over money, understand that having different money values or expectations doesn't make one of you right and the other wrong. Recognize the value of unpaid work. A partner who's finishing school or taking care of the children is making an important contribution to the family and its future. It also helps to go over your finances together, so you have a firm basis in reality for what you can and can't afford. Talk about the financial goals you hope to attain five years from now. Set priorities to meet them. Also, set aside money for each of you to spend without asking or answering to the other. Even a small amount can make each partner feel more independent.

STRATEGIES FOR PREVENTION

Making the Most of a Committed Relationship

■ Focus on what's right with your partner. Be kinder to your partner. Don't take for granted the nice things your spouse does.

■ Learn to negotiate for what you want. One effective approach is offering your mate what he or she wants in return.

■ Look for the problem behind the problem. Often an affair or a lack of sexual interest is merely a symptom; the real question is why this problem has developed.

■ Keep your perspective. Uncapped toothpaste tubes or food not prepared exactly to your taste may be annoying, but are they worth a fight?

■ Rather than thinking of all the things your partner is or isn't doing, look for things you can do to make your marriage better.

Fight fair. You can learn to argue effectively, without attacking others or damaging relationships.

Sex

Like every other aspect of a relationship, sex evolves and changes over the course of marriage. The redhot sexual chemistry of the early stages of intimacy invariably cools down. Even so, the happiest couples have sex more often than unhappily married pairs do.

What matters most isn't quantity alone, but the quality of sexual activity and intimacy (discussed in Chapter 8). Are both partners satisfied with their sexual relationship? Does one partner always initiate sex? Do the partners talk about their preferences and pleasures? Sexuality, like personality, is dynamic and changes throughout life. Do the partners acknowledge and adapt to these changes? Do they feel sufficiently at ease with each other to discuss anxieties about sex? The answers to these questions can determine how sexually gratifying a marriage is for both spouses.

Extramarital Affairs

How faithful are American mates? The answer depends on the questions researchers ask and whom they ask. In face-to-face interviews, University of Chicago researchers found that 25 percent of men and 15 percent of women had had affairs, and that 94 percent of the married subjects had been monogamous in the last year. Another survey of Americans found that one out of six Americans had had an extramarital relationship—19 percent of the men and 15 percent of the women.[34]

High or low, numbers are little comfort when affairs do occur. A husband or wife who learns about a spouse's affair typically feels a devastating sense of betrayal as well as deep feelings of shame, fear of abandonment, depression, and anger. Two crucial questions determine whether a marriage can survive: Do the spouses still feel a serious commitment to each other? And do they love each other and want to grow old together?

Two-Career Couples

More than 75 percent of women with children work—a dramatic increase from the 1960s, when only 30 percent of mothers worked outside the home. Two careers can bring pressure to a relationship: Both individuals may come home tired and irritable; both may have to spend a great deal of time on their jobs; both may have to travel or work on weekends. Two-career couples must be able to discuss their problems openly to resolve these pressures.

Couples pursuing individual careers sometimes face difficult choices. What happens, for example, if one of them is offered a promising job in another city? Does the spouse quit his or her job, pack up, and move? Some couples resolve such dilemmas by working in different cities and spending weekends together. Others try to alternate career and home priorities. However imperfect these arrangements may be, they work for some couples.

Do dual careers affect a couple's sex lives? The answers are complex. Some researchers have theorized that long hours and multiple roles would dampen sexual expression in working couples. But that's not necessarily the case. Except for spouses working unusually demanding jobs (more than 54 hours a week), work per se does not cause psychological distress (in women, it actually promotes better mental health) nor does it affect sexual frequency.

In studies comparing homemakers and women working part or full time, there have been no significant differences in frequency of intercourse, sexual satisfaction, or decreased sexual desire. Fatigue does dampen a woman's sex life—but is just as common in homemakers without paid jobs as in employed women.

Breadwinner Wives

According to the Bureau of Labor Statistics, 29 percent of wives—an estimated 10.5 million women—outearn their spouses, double the percent with heftier incomes thirty years ago. With more women studying for advanced degrees and charging up corporate ladders, the number of "breadwinner" wives is expected to soar.

How will their marriages fare? Experts once predicted that as a wife's paycheck grew, her marriage would be doomed to discord and divorce. But the few academic studies that have focused on such couples have found not more challenges, but different ones. As they make more money, wives generally report greater marital happiness and well-being.

Yet both partners face issues. "Even though we've progressed beyond Ozzie and Harriet, the idea that a wife cannot outearn a husband is still deeply embedded in our society," says Pam Klainer, author of *How Much Is Enough?* "The wife has to admit that she consciously or unconsciously chose someone less ambitious. The husband has to acknowledge that he's not living up to expectations. It can

Two-career couples cope with balancing family and work in various and sometimes imperfect ways.

be painful, but if couples are open and support each other, they come to see the benefits to both of them."[35]

Why Do People Still Get Married?

Despite its problems, marriage endures because it is a fulfilling way for two people to live. As researchers have proven, good marriages make people happy and healthy. For years researchers thought that marriage was especially beneficial to men. Married men have lower rates of alcohol and drug abuse, depression, and risk-taking behavior than divorced men. They also earn more money—possibly because they have more incentive to do so.

However, more recent research indicates that marriage boosts mental health and well-being in both spouses. Married men and women have lower rates of most mental disorders than single or divorced individuals.[36] Both husbands and wives live longer than single or divorced individuals. In one national survey, about 90 percent of husbands and wives survived until at least age 65, compared with only about 60 to 70 percent of divorced and never-married men and women. Although there has not been much research on same-sex committed relationships, most experts believe that gay couples are likely to enjoy similar benefits, as long as they remain together and receive social support for doing so.

Spouses undeniably influence each other's behavior—for better or for worse. While married individuals report generally better health habits, they can emulate and acquire each other's bad behaviors, including substance use and abuse and antisocial behaviors.[37]

Couples Therapy

According to the Association of Family and Marital Therapists, at least one of every five couples in this country needs professional counseling—and increasing numbers are seeking help. An estimated five million couples—married or not—now turn to the 50,000 licensed family therapists in the United States, a dramatic increase since 1980. The relationships of about two-thirds of those who get counseling do improve, according to both the couples' own judgments and objective measures of satisfaction.

A well-trained counselor can spot destructive behavior patterns and help couples see their situations in a new light. Therapy often helps stop spouses from hurting each other so badly that they can't stay together. If nothing else, it can help both partners decide whether to continue or end the relationship.[38]

What Is the Current Divorce Rate?

About half of all marriages end in divorce, but the odds of a first marriage lasting are slightly better. According to a CDC analysis of the most recent census data, about 43 percent of first marriages end in separation or divorce within 15 years. The older the bride, the better the chance the marriage will last. Nearly 60 percent of brides under age 18 eventually separate or divorce, compared with 36 percent of those age 20 or older. Women who marry and divorce young are more apt to wed again: 81 percent of those divorced before age 25 remarry within ten years, compared with 68 percent of those divorced at age 25 or older.

Race also influences marriage and divorce rates. African-American couples are more likely to break up than white couples, and black divorcées are less likely to marry again. Researchers have found that African Americans place an equally high value on marriage. However, there is a smaller "marriageable pool" of black men for a variety of reasons, including a higher mortality rate.[39]

Even after their hopes for happiness with one spouse end, men and women still yearn to mesh two personalities, two life histories, and two persons' dreams into a marriage. Eighty percent of divorced men and women remarry, and the remarriage rate increases with the number of times an individual has been divorced. The remarriage rate after a second divorce is 90 percent; after a third divorce, it's even higher. However, more second, third, and fourth marriages fail than original unions.

⬤ Family Ties

America's families are growing—and changing. According to the Census Bureau, the number of households in the United States increased 15 percent from 1990 to 2000, with nonfamily households increasing about twice as much (23 percent) as family households (11 percent). Married couples make up the majority of households, though by a smaller number than in 1990 (see Figure 7-5). Family households headed by women with no husbands outnumber by almost three times households headed by men without wives. The average family numbers 3.16 people.

Diversity Within Families

The all-American **family**—as portrayed on television and in movies—is typically white and middle-class. But families of different cultures—Italian to Indian to Indonesian—reflect different traditions, beliefs, and values. Within African-American families, for instance, traditional gender roles are often reversed, with women serving as head of the household, a kinship bond uniting several households, and a strong religious commitment or orientation. In Chinese-American families, both spouses may work and see themselves as breadwinners, but the wife may not have an equal role in decision making. In Hispanic families, wives and mothers are acknowledged and respected as healers and dispensers of wisdom. At the same time, they are expected to defer to their husbands, who see themselves as the strong, protective, dominant head of the family. As time passes and families from different cultures become more integrated into American life, traditional gender roles and decision-making patterns often change, particularly among the youngest family members.

American families are diverse in other ways. *Multigenerational families,* with children, parents, and grand-

parents, make up 3.7 percent of households. They occur most often in areas where new immigrants live with relatives, where housing shortages or high costs force families to double up their living arrangements, or where high rates of out-of-wedlock childbearing force unwed mothers to live with their children in their parents' home.

Three of every ten households consist of **blended families,** formed when one or both of the partners bring children from a previous union. In the future, social scientists predict, American families will become even more diverse, or pluralistic. But as norms or expectations about the configurations of families have changed, values or ideas about the intents and purposes of families have not. American families of every type still support each other and strive toward values such as commitment and caring.

Figure 7-5 A COMPARISON OF HOUSEHOLDS BY TYPE: 1990 AND 2000

The percent of married-couple households has decreased while the number of other types of households have increased.

Source: U.S. Census Bureau.

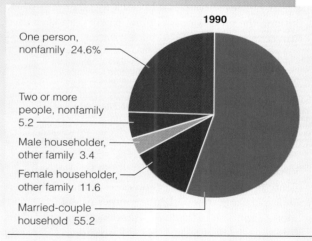

1990

- One person, nonfamily 24.6%
- Two or more people, nonfamily 5.2
- Male householder, other family 3.4
- Female householder, other family 11.6
- Married-couple household 55.2

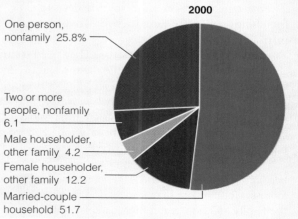

2000

- One person, nonfamily 25.8%
- Two or more people, nonfamily 6.1
- Male householder, other family 4.2
- Female householder, other family 12.2
- Married-couple household 51.7

Becoming Parents

Parenting is a 24-hour-a-day, 7-day-a-week, 52-week-a-year job, with no sabbaticals or sick leaves and no opportunity to renegotiate the contract. Having a child is an experience that deeply affects, involves, and changes a man and a woman.

When Baby Makes Three

New parents are likely to feel proud one moment and anxious the next. The infant may fascinate them both, but the adjustment to a baby-centered life can cause resentment. The husband who feels that his wife is more concerned with the baby than with him often feels jealous, which in turn makes him feel guilty. The mother, still recovering from childbirth, may feel overwhelmed by new responsibilities and the daunting physical demands of caring for a newborn.

Experts in family development, who have been studying the changes a baby brings to a marriage, note that marital satisfaction invariably declines, if only slightly, while the number of separations and divorces rises after a baby's arrival. However, couples who stick together as partners through the process of becoming parents can keep their marriages strong.

As Children Grow

A child's greatest need is for love—the feeling of being wanted and cared for, of being special, and of realizing that the parents like the child for him- or herself. According to a study that followed 379 kindergarten-aged children for 36 years, warm, loving parenting—the kind that supplies plenty of hugs, kisses, and cuddles—has more influence on adult social adjustment than any other parental or childhood factor. The individuals whose mothers and fathers were openly affectionate were able to sustain long and relatively happy marriages, raise children, develop close friendships, and enjoy varied activities outside their marriage.

Children have other needs, too. They need security—assurance that their parents will be there when needed most; protection; confidence; and a feeling of belonging. They need role models to learn behavior from and a sense of clear limits and controls. Parents are responsible for establishing values of what is right or wrong and for guiding by example as well as with words.

With each year that passes in a child's life, the conflict between independence and dependence becomes more intense. Children are drawn into the larger world outside the family and home, and their parents are torn between clinging to them and pushing them out of the nest. It's not enough to set rules; parents must also advise a child on how to make decisions within those rules.

The teen years—the transition from childhood to adulthood—are, for parents and children, the best and worst of times. Children becoming teenagers develop more responsibility, a greater sense of self, and more independence. Simultaneously, they may rebel, challenging and testing their parents. Setting limits—such as curfews and dating guidelines—may set off a confrontation instead of being a simple matter of stating policy. A teen's emerging sexuality may be difficult for the parents to acknowledge and accept. (Chapter 8 discusses adolescent sexuality.)

Siblings

The ways in which siblings relate as children often affect their interactions with each other—and with others, including their mates—when they grow up. Sibling rivalry, for instance, though normal, can lead to unhealthy ways of relating to others. For example, siblings who had to compete fiercely for parental attention or affection may remain competitive throughout life, doing anything necessary in order to come out on top. And youngsters who feel that their parents clearly prefer another child in the family may come to think that they're inadequate or somehow unworthy of love.

Siblings typically grow more distant during adolescence, as they focus on developing their own identities. This separation continues during early adulthood. However, in middle age, most adults report positive relationships with siblings. Some are bound by loyalty, even if they don't feel friendly toward a brother or sister. Others socialize with siblings but are closer to friends. In old age, sisters and brother-sister pairs have more positive relationships than brothers; elderly African Americans tend to have more positive relationships with their siblings than do elderly whites.

Working Parents

The traditional family with a breadwinner and a homemaker has been replaced by what some call "the juggler family." Two working parents or an unmarried working parent head 70 percent of American families with children. As a result, American parents have 22 fewer hours to spend with their children than parents did in 1969.[40] Women, balancing multiple roles as parents, spouses, caregivers, and employees often give their own personal needs the lowest priority.[41]

The Family and Work Institute of New York calculates that American husbands put in 75 percent as much time as wives on workday chores—a dramatic rise from 30 percent in 1977. In actual clocktime, the gender difference in domestic "scutwork" amounts to just 45 minutes a day.

Plenty of sociologists—and lots of weary women still doing the lioness share of chores—doubt whether all men in all income groups are doing as much. However, the trend toward greater husbandly involvement is real—and likely to continue.

Single Parents

About 28 percent of all children under age 18 live with just one parent, the majority with their mothers. The number of families headed by single mothers has increased 25 percent since 1990, to more than 7.5 million households. About a third of all babies are born to unmarried women, compared to just 3.8 percent in 1940.

The new breed of single mother doesn't fit the old stereotype of an unwed minority teenager. The median age for unmarried mothers is the late 20s; the fastest growing group is white women. She may be divorced or, like celebrities Calista Flockhart and Rosie O'Donnell, unmarried. Forty percent live with men who may be the fathers of one or more of their children. There has been a 72 percent increase in the number of cohabiting couples, many of whom bring along children from other relationships. This change represents a dramatic transition in the demographic makeup of the United States, although it is not yet clear whether having children outside of marriage will become as widespread as it is in other nations, such as Sweden.[42]

Single fathers head over two millions households. Men now comprise 1 in 6 of the nation's 11.9 million single parents, up from 1 in 7 in 1995 and 1 in 10 in 1980.

The typical single father is 38 years old. One in 9 is under age 25; and 1 in 70 is 60 or older. About 5 of every 6 (83 percent) of the nation's single fathers are white. African Americans and Hispanics together constitute about 13 percent.

Median family income for one-parent families is significantly lower than the median for two-parent families. Twenty percent are poor, compared with 9 percent of two-parent families. Half live in rental housing, compared with one-quarter of two-parent families.

How Does Divorce Affect Children?

Each year divorce separates more than a million children from their parents. The breakup of a marriage has an enormous impact on many aspects of a child's life, including his or her standard of living. While there are no good times for divorce, long-term studies have found that children are especially vulnerable at two stages: infancy and puberty. Babies need continuity of care and the opportunity to bond with both parents. At age 12 or 13, youngsters need a strong, stable family as strong biological drives of sexuality and aggression emerge.[43]

Children whose parents divorced are less likely to marry and to stay married. However, their adult relationships aren't doomed to fail. "Divorce isn't in the genes," says child psychologist, Judith Wallerstein, who has studied divorced families for thirty years. "Divorce is an avoidable human error."

Blended Families

Each year about half a million children become part of new, blended families when their parents remarry. Over the years many studies have found significant differences in family and relationship processes in these families. However, improved communication and problem solving can help blended families work through their problems.

Children can also be encouraged to spend time with members of the extended family or friends to experience other role models.

Bill Bachmann/Stock, Boston/Picture Quest

Although the majority of single parents are women, about 17 percent of single-parent families are headed by fathers.

✺ Dysfunctional Relationships

Relationships that don't promote healthy communication, honesty, and intimacy are sometimes called **dysfunctional.** Individuals with addictive behaviors or dependence on drugs or alcohol (see Chapters 12 and 10), and the children or partners of such people, are especially likely to find themselves in such relationships.

Often partners have magical, unrealistic expectations (e.g., they expect that a relationship with the right person will make their life okay), and one person uses the other almost as if he or she were a mood-altering drug. The partners may compulsively try to get the other to act the way they want. Both persons may not trust or may deceive each other. Often they isolate themselves from others, thus trapping themselves in a recurring cycle of pain.

Dysfunctional families exist in every economic, social, educational, religious, and racial group. They inflict emotional pain on children through destructive behaviors, such as physical, emotional, verbal, or sexual abuse; physical or emotional neglect; and alcoholism or drug use. Although alcohol or drugs do not in themselves create dysfunctional families, they can push parents over a psychological brink. The results can be emotionally devastating. The children of alcoholics, drug users, and parents with other addictive behaviors are prone to learning disabilities, eating disorders, compulsive achievement, and addiction.

✺ What Is Codependence?

Contemporary therapists use the term **codependence** (or coaddiction) for the tendency of the spouses, partners, parents, and friends of individuals with addictive behaviors to allow or *enable* their loved ones to continue their self-destructive habits. Codependent individuals focus on their loved ones, even to the extent of giving up their own lives. They change who they are and what they feel in order to please others, feel responsible for meeting others' needs, have low self-esteem, and frequently have compulsions of their own. However, codependent behaviors need to be evaluated in the context of an individual's culture. For example, the emphasis on family values and support that is part of the value system of many Latinos would not be considered codependent behavior.

Codependents Anonymous, founded in 1986 for men and women whose common problem is an inability to maintain functional relationships, is one of the fastest-growing support programs in the country. Other self-help groups for codependents include Al-Anon (for adult family members of alcoholics), Alateen (for the teenaged children of addicts), Nar-Anon (for people in relationships with individuals who abuse drugs), O-Anon (for those whose family members have eating disorders), and Gam-Anon (for those living with people who have gambling problems). Local chapters of these groups can be found in the white pages of the telephone book. Through such groups, codependent individuals can learn how to leave behind guilt feelings, how to become less judgmental and moralistic, how to understand their powerlessness over their loved one's problem, and how to do what needs to be done for themselves as well as the addict.

If you wonder if you may be codependent, read through the following list of characteristics of codependence and check any that apply to you:

:: I find myself covering for another person's alcohol or drug use, eating or work habits, gambling, sexual escapades, or general behavior.

:: I spend a great deal of time talking about and worrying about other people's behavior/problems/future instead of living my own life.

:: I have marked or counted bottles, searched for a hidden stash, or in other ways monitored someone else's behavior.

:: I find myself taking on more responsibility at home or in a relationship, even though I resent it.

:: I ignore my own needs in favor of meeting someone else's.

:: I'm afraid that if I get angry, the other person will leave or not love me.

:: I worry that if I leave a relationship or stop controlling the other person, that person will fall apart.

:: I spend less time with friends and more with my partner/parent/child in activities that I wouldn't normally choose.

:: My self-esteem depends on what others say and think of me, or on my possessions or job.

:: I grew up in a family in which there was little communication, in which expressing feelings wasn't acceptable, and in which there were either rigid rules or none at all.

If you identify with more than three of these statements, you may be codependent. There are many useful books on codependence at libraries and bookstores. You may also wish to visit a support group on campus or in your area or talk with a counselor.

Enabling

Experts on the subject of addiction first identified traits of codependence in spouses of alcoholics, who followed a predictable pattern of behavior: While intensely trying to control the drinkers, the codependent mates would act in ways that allowed the drinkers to keep drinking. For example, if an alcoholic found it hard to get up in the morning, his wife would wake him up, pull him out of bed and into the shower, and drop him off at work. If he was late, she made excuses to his boss. The husband was the one with the substance-abuse problem, but without realizing it, his wife was enabling him to continue drinking. In fact, he might not have been able to keep up his habit without her unintentional cooperation.

The different styles or components of **enabling** include the following:

:: *Shielding.* Codependents may cover up for abusers, preventing them from experiencing the full impact of the harmful consequences of their behavior—for example, by dropping off a paper or report so that the addicted person can avoid a missed deadline.

:: *Controlling.* A codependent may try to control the significant other—for instance, by withholding sex or using sex as a reward for cutting down on an addictive behavior.

:: *Taking over responsibilities.* The codependent may take over such household chores as shopping or running errands.

:: *Rationalizing.* Codependents try to rationalize their partners' addiction by telling themselves that a compulsive behavior pattern, like workaholism, is making the person more successful, or that drinking helps him or her relax.

:: *Cooperating.* Sometimes codependents become involved in the person's compulsion, perhaps placing bets for a gambler or buying alcohol for a drinker.

:: *Rescuing.* The codependent may become overprotective—for example, by allowing the user to use drugs at home to avoid the risk of an accident or arrest.

Codependence progresses just as an addiction does, and codependents excuse their own behavior with many of the same defense mechanisms used by addicts, such as rationalization ("I cut class so I could catch up on my reading, not to keep an eye on my partner") and denial ("He likes to gamble, but he never loses more than he can afford"). In time, just as an addict's world becomes smaller and smaller, codependents lose sight of everything but their loved one. They feel that if they can only "fix" this person, everything will be fine.

The Bottom Line ▼
Building Better
Relationships

We are born social. From our first days of life, we reach out to others, struggle to express ourselves, strive to forge connections. The fabric of our lives becomes richer as family and friends weave through it the threads of their experiences. No solitary pleasure can match the gifts that we gain by reaching out and connecting with others.

As with other significant endeavors, good relationships require work—through hard times, despite conflicts, over months and years and decades. As you strive to improve the ties that bind you to others, keep in mind the characteristics of a good relationship. They can serve as the goals you strive to attain:

:: *Trust.* Partners are able to confide in each other openly, knowing their confidences will be respected.

:: *Togetherness.* In a healthy relationship, two people create a sense of both intimacy and autonomy. They enjoy each other's company but also pursue solitary interests.

:: *Expressiveness.* Partners in healthy relationships say what they feel, need, and desire.

:: *Staying power.* People in committed relationships keep their bond strong through tough times by proving that they will be there for each other.

:: *Security.* Because a good relationship is strong enough to absorb conflict and anger, partners know they can express their feelings honestly. They also are willing to risk vulnerability for the sake of becoming closer.

:: *Laughter.* Humor keeps things in perspective—always crucial in any sort of ongoing relationship or enterprise.

:: *Support.* Partners in good relationships continually offer each other encouragement, comfort, and acceptance.

:: *Physical affection.* Sexual desire may fluctuate or diminish over the years, but partners in loving, long-term relationships usually retain some physical connection.

:: *Personal growth.* In the best relationships, partners are committed to bringing out the best in each other and have the other's best interests at heart.

:: *Respect.* Caring partners are aware of each other's boundaries, need for personal space, and vulnerabilities. They do not take each other or their relationship for granted.

 After watching the CNN video segment, discuss the following question. What important factors should parents consider when blending stepfamilies?

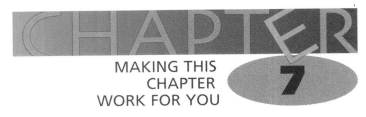

MAKING THIS
CHAPTER
WORK FOR YOU

7

1. In friendships and other intimate relationships, which of the following is *not* true?
   a. Friends can communicate feelings as well as facts.
   b. Listening is just as important as talking.
   c. Emotional investment is required but the rewards are great.
   d. There is no need to pay attention to nonverbal communication.

2. Which of the following scenarios demonstrates what might be considered gender differences in verbal and nonverbal communication styles?
   a. While Alyssa and Peter are discussing their vacation plans, Alyssa is gazing at the television and Peter is looking at Alyssa.
   b. Good friends Eva and Julia see each other for the first time after Christmas break and greet each other with a nod and a quick "Hi."
   c. New bank manager Alejandro tells the staff that they should consider him "the team coach and the keeper of the playbook."
   d. During an argument, Tony complains to Nicki, "I don't appreciate your crude jokes and constant swearing."

3. Romantic love
   a. is associated with the depletion of the hormone oxytocin.
   b. is an emotional phenomenon between humans that has its roots in prehistoric times and occurs in almost all cultures.
   c. can only occur between people who share interests and goals.
   d. always results in a committed long-term relationship.

4. The characteristics of a good relationship include which of the following?
   a. trust
   b. financial stability
   c. identical interests
   d. physical attractiveness

5. Which of the following statements is true?
   a. About 25 percent of bachelors over age 40 usually marry by the time they are 50.
   b. Research strongly supports the belief that living with a person before marrying is a good idea.
   c. The number-one reason women remain single is to focus on their career.
   d. Approximately 10 percent of today's young adults will never marry.

6. Partners in successful marital relationships
   a. are generally from the same social and ethnic background.
   b. usually lived together before marrying.
   c. were usually very young at the time of their marriage.
   d. have premarital agreements.

7. Married people
   a. have sex less frequently than unmarried partners.
   b. are more likely to become alcoholics and drug users.
   c. typically have at least one extramarital affair during their marriage.
   d. live longer than single or divorced individuals.

8. When couples have a child,
   a. their marital satisfaction typically increases.
   b. they should resist being openly affectionate to each other to avoid embarrassing situations.
   c. they have a slightly higher risk of divorce.
   d. they are less likely to get divorced for the sake of the child.

9. Which of the following statements about divorce is *false?*
   a. The older the bride, the more likely the chance that the marriage will endure.
   b. African-American couples are more likely to divorce than white couples.
   c. Infants are less likely to be affected by the divorce of their parents than teenagers.
   d. The majority of divorced men and women remarry, even after multiple divorces.

10. Which of the following is more likely a sign of a dysfunctional relationship?
    a. The partners have frequent disagreements about money.
    b. One partner makes all the decisions for the couple and the other partner.
    c. Each partner has a demanding career.
    d. One partner is much older than the other partner.

Answers to these questions can be found on page 652.

Critical Thinking

1. Reread the section on Personal Communication in this chapter, and think about your own communication skills. How does your communication style compare to the patterns Pennebaker and Tannen have revealed for your gender? Do your personal experiences support or contradict the research results?

Critical Thinking

2. While our society has become more tolerant, marriages between people of different religious and racial groups still face special pressures. What issues might arise if a Christian marries a Jew or Muslim? What about the issues facing partners of different races? How could these issues be resolved? What are your own feelings about mixed marriages? Would you date someone of a different religion or race? Why or why not?

Critical Thinking

3. What are your personal criteria for a successful relationship? Develop a brief list of factors you consider important, and support your choices with examples or experiences from your own life.

Profile Plus

Caring communication is the key to most healthy relationships. Assess the degree of good communication in your intimate relationship with this activity on your Profile Plus CD-ROM:

Profile Plus

• How Strong is the Communication and Affection in Your Relationship?

Profile Plus

Sites and Bytes

Family and Relationships Information from the American Psychological Association
http://helping.apa.org/family/index.html

This site features information on a variety of parenting topics, including how to handle stress, stepfamilies, marriage, and raising children to resist violence.

Sites and Bytes

Communicating About Sex
http://healthydevil.studentaffairs.duke.edu/info/sex/com.html

Information written specifically for college students, sponsored by the Duke University Student Health Service.

Sites and Bytes

Youth.org
www.youth.org

This website provides information on gay, lesbian, bisexual, and questioning youth and provides young people with a safe space online to be themselves, to know they are not alone, and to interact with others who have already accepted their sexuality.

InfoTrac College Edition

Activity

Wolak, Janis, et al. "Close Online Relationships in a National Sample of Adolescents." *Adolescence,* Vol. 37, No. 147, Fall 2002, p. 441(15).

1. What are some of the factors that increase the likelihood that adolescents who establish online relationships will actually meet face-to-face?

InfoTrac College Edition

2. What is the relationship between gender and age on the likelihood of forming a close or romantic online relationship?

3. Based on the results of the study, in what ways were the close online relationships that resulted in face-to-face meetings different from other close online friendships?

InfoTrac College Edition

You can find additional readings related to communication and relationships with InfoTrac College Edition, an online library of more than 900 journals and publications. Follow the instructions for accessing InfoTrac that were packaged with your textbook; then search for articles using a key word search.

For additional links, resources, and suggested readings on InfoTrac College Edition, visit our Health & Wellness Resource Center at **http://health.wadsworth.com**.

Key Terms

The terms listed are used on the page indicated. Definitions of the terms are in the Glossary at the end of this book.

blended families 229
codependence 232
cohabitation 223
companion-oriented marriages 225

dysfunctional 232
enabling 233
family 229
intimacy 217
neurotransmitters 220

oxytocin 220
rescue marriages 225
romantic marriages 225
traditional marriages 225

References

1. Pennebaker, James. Personal interview.
2. Hall, Judith. Personal interview.
3. Mehrabian, Albert. Personal interview.
4. Maple, Marilyn. Personal interview.
5. McGinty, Kristen, et al. "Nonverbal and Verbal Communication in 'Involved' and 'Casual' Relationships Among College Students." *College Student Journal*, Vol. 37, No. 1, March 2003, p. 68.
6. Perina, Kaja. "Taking the Blame for a Partner's Bad Mood." *Psychology Today*, Vol. 36, No. 3, May–June 2003, p. 16.
7. Billingham, Robert. Personal interview.
8. Yager, Jan. Personal interview.
9. Anderson, David, and Rosemary Clandos. "Dating After Divorce." *Psychology Today*, Vol. 36, No. 1, February 2003, p. 46.
10. Silverman, Jay, et al. "Dating Violence Against Adolescent Girls and Associated Substance Use, Unhealthy Weight Control, Sexual Risk Behavior, Pregnancy, and Suicidality." *Journal of the American Medical Association*, Vol. 286, No. 5, August 1, 2001, p. 572.
11. Lewis, S. F., et al. "Characteristics of Female Perpetrators and Victims of Dating Violence." *Violence and Victims*, Vol. 17, No. 5, October 2002, p. 593.
12. Sprecher, Susan. "Insiders' Perspectives on Reasons for Attraction to a Close Other." *Social Psychology Quarterly*, Vol. 61, No. 4, December 1998.
13. Laumann, Edward. Personal interview.

14. Sprecher. "Insiders' Perspectives on Reasons for Attraction to a Close Other."
15. Buss, David. *The Evolution of Desire*. New York: Basic Books, 1994.
16. Fisher, Helen. Personal interview.
17. Knox, David, et al. "College Students Attitudes and Behaviors Toward Ending an Unsatisfactory Relationship." *College Student Journal*, Vol. 36, No. 4, December 2002, p. 630.
18. Sommers, Jennifer, and Stephen Vodanovich. "Vengeance Scores Among College Students: Examining the Role of Jealously and Forgiveness." *Education*, Vol. 121, No. 1, Fall 2000.
19. U.S. Census Bureau.
20. Anderson and Clandos, "Dating After Divorce."
21. "What Happened to the Wedding Bells?" *Forecast*, Vol. 23, No. 4, April 2003, p. 1.
22. "Cohabitation, Marriage, Divorce, and Remarriage in the United States." Series Report 23, No. 22. Hyattsville, MD: National Center for Health Statistics, 2002.
23. Wellner, Alison. "Mapping the Unmarried: Cohabiting Couples are Found in Clusters Around the Country." *Forecast*, Vol. 23, No. 4, April 2003, p. 5.
24. Alternatives to Marriage Project, www.unmarried.org.
25. Solott, Dorian, and Marshall Miller. *Unmarried to Each Other*. New York:

Marlowe & Co; November 2002.
26. Hymowitz, Kay. "The Cohabitation Blues." *Commentary*, Vol. 115, No. 3, March 2003, p. 56.
27. Schulman, Dan. "No Finance? No Romance." *Psychology Today*, Vol. 36, No. 3, April 2003, p. 16.
28. "Stats & Facts." *Psychology Today*, Vol. 36, No. 3, April 2003, p. 16.
29. Kantrowitz, Barbara, and Pat Wingert. "Unmarried, with Children." *Newsweek*, May 28, 2001, p. 46.
30. Crooks, Robert, and Karla Baur. *Our Sexuality*, 8th ed. Pacific Grove, CA: Wadsworth, 2002.
31. Sternberg, Robert. Personal interview.
32. Nock, Steven. "Marriages of Equally Dependent Spouses." *Journal of Family Issues*, Vol. 22, No. 6, September 2001, p. 755.
33. "Does Togetherness Equal Happiness?" *Marriage Partnership*, Vol. 20, No. 1, Spring 2003, p. 13.
34. Crooks and Baur. *Our Sexuality*.
35. Klainer, Pamela. Personal interview.
36. de Vaus, David. "Marriage and Mental Health: Does Marriage Improve the Mental Health of Men at the Expense of Women?" *Family Matters*, No. 62, Winter 2002, p. 26.
37. Arehart-Treichel, Joan. "Antisocial Behavior Contagious for Some Married Couples." *Psychiatric News*, Vol. 38, No. 3, February 7, 2003, p. 26.

References

38. Johnson, Susan, and Aviva Patz. "Save Your Relationship." *Psychology Today,* Vol. 36, No. 3, April 2003, p. 51.
39. Bramlett, Matthew, and William Mosher. "Love and Marriage." *Forecast,* Vol. 21, No. 10, July 2, 2001, p. 11. Also available at www.cdc.gov/nchs/data/ad/ad323.pdf.
40. Kornbluh, Karen. "The Parent Trap." *Atlantic Monthly,* Vol. 291, No. 1, January–February 2003, p. 111.

References

41. Wyn, Roberta, and Victoria Ojeda. *Women, Work, and Family Health: A Balancing Act.* Menlo Park, CA: Kaiser Family Foundation, April 2003.
42. Raley, R. Kelly. "Increasing Fertility in Cohabiting Unions: Evidence for the Second Demographic Transition in the United States?" *Demography,* Vol. 38, No. 1, February 2001, p. 59.

References

43. Wallerstein, Judith, and Sandra Blakeslee. *What About the Kids? Raising Your Children Before, During, and After Divorce.* New York: Hyperion, 2003.

Personal Sexuality

Charles, several years older than the typical college freshman, usually doesn't think much about the age difference—until the conversation turns to sex. He understands his younger classmates' seemingly endless fascination with sex, but his perspective is different. As a teenager, he had plunged recklessly into dangerous territory of every type. Sex—casual and sometimes unprotected—was one of them. Looking back, he feels lucky that he didn't, as he puts it, "end up a statistic." But he still regrets the irresponsible ways he acted.

At 25, Charles is a veteran of military service, a married man, and an expectant father. His enjoyment of sex hasn't faded—in many ways, it's deepened and become more gratifying. He now realizes that there is no such thing as casual sex, that sexual choices have consequences and effects on one's own life and on other people. These are the lessons he hopes someday to pass on to his own children.

As Charles learned with time and experience, you are ultimately responsible for your sexual health and behavior. You make decisions that affect how you express your **sexuality,** how you respond sexually, and how you give and get sexual pleasure. Yet most sexual activity involves another person. Therefore, your decisions about sex—more so than those you make about nutrition, drugs, or exercise—have important effects on other people. Recognizing this fact is the key to responsible sexuality.

Human sexuality—the quality of being sexual—is as rich, varied, and complex as life itself. Along with our **sex,** or biological maleness or femaleness, it is an integral part of who we are, how we see ourselves, and how we relate to others. Of all of our involvements with others, sexual **intimacy,** or physical closeness, can be the most rewarding. But while sexual expression and experience can provide intense joy, they also can involve great emotional turmoil.

Sexual responsibility means learning about your body, your partner's body, your sexual development and preferences, and the health risks associated with sexual activity. This chapter is an introduction to your sexual self and an exploration of sexual issues in today's world. It provides the information and insight you can use in making decisions and choosing behaviors that are responsible for all concerned.

© Michael Jang/Stone/Getty Images

After studying the material in this chapter, you should be able to:

- **Explain** the roles of hormones in sexual development.
- **Describe** the male and female reproductive systems and the functions of the individual structures of each system.
- **Describe** conditions or issues unique to women's and men's sexual health.

- **Define** sexual health and **list** behaviors that can contribute to sexually healthy relationships.
- **Define** sexual orientation and **give examples** of sexual diversity.
- **List** the range of sexual behaviors practiced by adults.
- **Describe** the phases of sexual response.
- **List** the common sexual concerns of men and women.

◼ Becoming Male or Female

Physiological maleness or femaleness, or biological sex, is indicated by the sex chromosomes, hormonal balance, and genital anatomy. **Gender** refers to the psychological and sociological, as well as the physical, aspects of being male or female. You are born with a certain *sexual identity* based on your sexual anatomy and appearance; you, your parents, and society mold your *gender identity.*

Are You an X or a Y?

Biologically, few absolute differences separate the sexes: Males alone can make sperm and contribute the chromosome that causes embryos to develop as males; females alone are born with sex cells (eggs or ova), menstruate, give birth, and breast-feed babies. But the process of becoming male or female is a long and complex one.

In the beginning, all human embryos have undifferentiated sex organs. Only after several weeks do the sex organs differentiate, becoming either male or female **gonads** (testes or ovaries), the structures that produce the future reproductive cells of an individual. This initial differentiation process depends on genetic instructions in the form of the sex chromosomes, referred to as X and Y. (See Figure 8-1.) If a Y (or male) chromosome is present in the embryo, about seven weeks after conception, it signals the sex organs to develop into testes. If a Y chromosome isn't present, an embryo begins developing ovaries in the eighth week. From this point on, the sex hormones produced by the gonads, not the chromosomes, play the crucial role in making a male or female.

Figure 8-1 GENETIC SEXUAL DIFFERENTIATION
Human cells contain 23 pairs of chromosomes. One of these pairs is the sex chromosomes. A normal female has two X chromosomes and a normal male has an X and a Y chromosome.

© Custom Medical Stock

◼ How Do Hormones Work?

In Greek, *hormone* means "set into motion"—and that's exactly what our **hormones** do. These chemical messengers, produced by various organs in the body, including the sex organs, and carried to target structures by the bloodstream, arouse cells and organs to specific activities and influence the way we look, feel, develop, and behave.

The group of organs that produce hormones is referred to as the **endocrine system.** Except for the sex organs, males and females have identical endocrine systems. Directing the endocrine system is the *hypothalamus,* a pea-sized section of the brain. The pituitary gland, directly beneath the hypothalamus, turns the various glands on and off in response to messages from it.

The ovaries produce the sex hormones most crucial to women, **estrogen** and **progesterone.** The primary sex hormone in men is **testosterone,** which is produced by the testes and the adrenal glands. However, both men and women have small amounts of the hormones of the opposite sex. Estrogen, in fact, is crucial to male fertility and gives sperm what researchers describe as their "reproductive punch."

The sex hormones begin their work early in an embryo's development. As soon as the testes are formed, they start releasing testosterone, which stimulates the development of other structures, such as the penis. The absence of testosterone in an embryo causes female genitals to form. (If the testes of a genetic male don't produce testosterone, the fetus will develop female genitals. Similarly, if a genetic female is exposed to excessive testosterone, the fetus will have ovaries but will also develop male genitals.)

As puberty begins, the pituitary gland initiates the changes that transform boys into men and girls into women. When a boy is about 14 years old and a girl about 12, their brains stimulate the hypothalamus to secrete a hormone called *gonadotropin-releasing hormone (GnRH).* This substance causes the pituitary gland to release hormones called **gonadotropins.** These, in turn, stimulate the gonads to make sex hormones. (See Figure 8-2.)

The gonadotropins are *follicle-stimulating hormone (FSH)* and *luteinizing hormone (LH).* In girls, these hormones travel to the ovary and stimulate the production of estrogen. As estrogen increases, a girl's **secondary sex characteristics** develop. Her breasts become fuller, her external genitals enlarge, and fat is deposited on her hips and buttocks. Estrogen keeps her hair thick and skin smooth. She begins menstruating because she has begun ovulating, the process that prepares her body to conceive and carry a baby.

This process seems to be beginning earlier than in the past. "By eight, 15 per-

Figure 8-2 PUBERTY

The body's endocrine system produces hormones that trigger body changes in males and females. Additional body changes include growth spurts and changes to the skeleton.

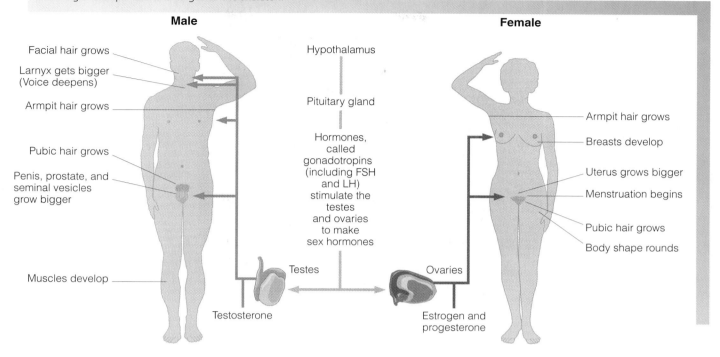

cent of white girls and 48 percent of African-American girls show signs of sexual development," says Marcia Herman-Giddens, Ph.D., of the University of North Carolina at Chapel Hill, who analyzed 17,077 growth charts from pediatricians around the country. In her study, the mean ages for breast development were 8.87 years for African-American girls and 9.96 years for white girls. African-American girls reach **menarche**—the term for first menstruation—at a mean age of 12.16 years; white girls, at 12.88 years. By comparison, a hundred years ago girls didn't reach menarche until the relatively ripe age of fifteen.[1]

"We don't know precisely why development is starting sooner or why there's a racial discrepancy," notes Herman-Giddens. Improved nutrition and good health seem to be the primary factors. Girls today are bigger, taller, better fed, more sedentary, and have a higher percentage of body fat (one of the triggers of sexual maturation). They also grow up amid a host of environmental influences that may further speed development.

Cultural influences affect a girl's response to menarche. In a cross-cultural study of college students, the most common emotions expressed by American women at menarche were embarrassment, pride, and anxiety. Malaysian women cited fear, embarrassment, and worry. Lithuanian women described themselves as happy or scared, while Sudanese women cited fear, anxiety, embar-

rassment, and anger. On the positive side, the Lithuanian women reported feeling more valuable and believing they had entered the world of women. American girls worried about whether they could still play sports, but felt superior to friends who had not reached menarche, and became eager to learn about sex. Malaysians described feeling wise, respected, and mature. Sudanese women felt more beautiful and aware that they could now have children.

In boys, the gonadotropins stimulate the testes to produce testosterone, which triggers the development of male secondary sex characteristics. Their voices deepen, hair grows on their faces and bodies, their penises become thicker and longer, and their muscles become stronger.

The sex hormones released during puberty change the growth pattern of childhood, so that a boy or girl may now spurt up 4 to 6 inches in a single year. The skeleton matures very rapidly until, at the end of puberty (usually around age 18), the growth centers at the ends of the bones close off. Estrogen causes girls' bones to stop growing at an earlier age than boys' bones.

Sexual Stereotypes

Being male is not the same as being masculine, and being female is not the same as being feminine. Today more men and women are breaking out of traditional stereotypes.

In today's world, traditional sexual stereotypes do not hinder the career aspirations or personal desires of men and women.

AP/Wide World Photos

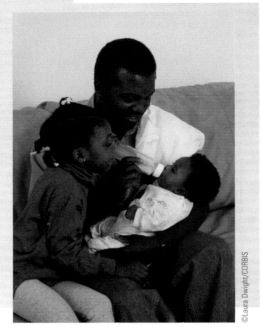

©Laura Dwight/CORBIS

Men are acknowledging their feelings and fears and taking on what were formerly women's jobs—becoming nurses and secretaries at work, and doing the grocery shopping and laundry at home. Although there still aren't any female linebackers in the National Football League (and no one expects that there will be), women have become astronauts, truck drivers, engineers, pilots, coal miners, physicians, and executives.

An alternative to both male and female sexual typecasting is the concept of **androgyny,** a word that literally translates (from the Greek) as "man woman." Androgynous individuals combine aspects of both masculinity and femininity into their personalities and lifestyles. They act in ways that seem appropriate to a given relationship or situation—instead of in ways that seem appropriately masculine or feminine. Such behaviors can enhance compatibility and satisfaction in a relationship.

◼ Women's Sexual Health

Only recently has medical research devoted major scientific investigations to issues in women's health. Until about a decade ago the National Institutes of Health routinely excluded women from experimental studies because of concerns about menstrual cycles and pregnancy. In clinical settings, women are more likely to have their symptoms dismissed as psychological and not to be referred to a specialist than are men with identical complaints. Some physicians are suggesting the creation of a new medical specialty

(distinct from obstetrics and gynecology) that would be devoted to women's health to provide more comprehensive care and overcome the current gender gap in health services. A lack of health insurance, a topic discussed in Chapter 16, is another barrier to adequate health care, particularly for low-income women.

Female Sexual Anatomy

As illustrated in Figure 8-3A, the **mons pubis** is the rounded, fleshy area over the junction of the pubic bones. The folds of skin that form the outer lips of a woman's genital area are called the **labia majora.** They cover soft flaps of skin (inner lips) called the **labia minora.** The inner lips join at the top to form a hood over the **clitoris,** a small elongated erectile organ, and the most sensitive spot in the entire female genital area. Below the clitoris is the **urethral opening,** the outer opening of the thin tube that carries urine from the bladder. Below that is a larger opening, the mouth of the **vagina,** the canal that leads to the primary internal organs of reproduction. The **perineum** is the area between the vagina and the anus (the opening to the rectum and large intestine).

At the back of the vagina is the **cervix,** the opening to the womb, or **uterus** (see Figure 8-3B). The uterine walls are lined by a layer of tissue called the **endometrium.** The **ovaries,** about the size and shape of almonds, are located on either side of the uterus, and con-

Figure 8-3 THE FEMALE SEX ORGANS AND REPRODUCTIVE STRUCTURES

A. External structure

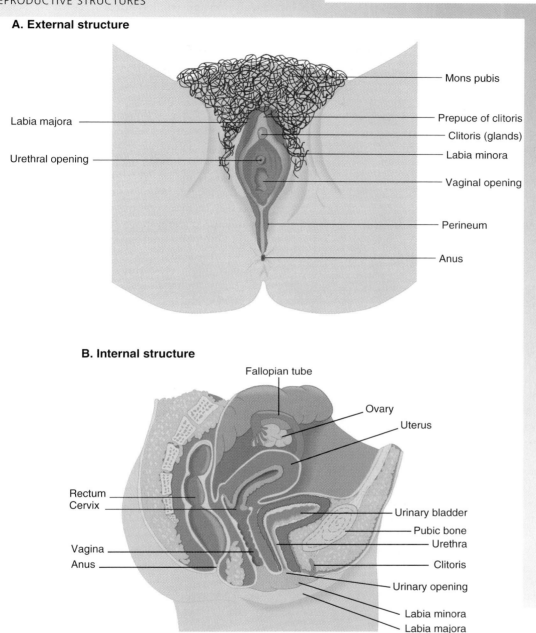

Mons pubis

Prepuce of clitoris

Clitoris (glands)

Labia minora

Vaginal opening

Perineum

Anus

Labia majora

Urethral opening

B. Internal structure

Fallopian tube

Ovary

Uterus

Rectum

Cervix

Urinary bladder

Pubic bone

Urethra

Vagina

Anus

Clitoris

Urinary opening

Labia minora

Labia majora

tain egg cells called **ova** (singular, **ovum**). Extending outward and back from the upper uterus are the **fallopian tubes,** the canals that transport ova from the ovaries to the uterus. When an egg is released from an ovary, the finger-like ends of the adjacent fallopian tube "catch" the egg and direct it into the tube.

Discharge and changes in odor normally occur in a healthy vagina. They typically fluctuate through the menstrual cycle, depending on hormone level. In the past, many women practiced douching, the introduction of a liq-

uid into the vagina, to cleanse the vagina. However, particularly if done frequently, douching may increase the risk of pelvic inflammatory disease (discussed in Chapter 13) and ectopic or out-of-uterus pregnancy. Despite the potential dangers, according to data from a southern university, four in ten female students had douched in the past; half currently douche. African-American women were encouraged to douche by their mothers; white women were more influenced by television advertisements. When advised to stop douching by a doctor or nurse, most students do so.[2]

What Is The Menstrual Cycle?

Scientists have discovered that the menstrual cycle actually begins in the brain with the production of gonadotropin-releasing hormone (GnRH). Each month a surge of GnRH sets into motion the sequence of steps that lead to ovulation, the potential for conception, and, if conception doesn't occur, menstruation. As shown in Figure 8-4, the hypothalamus monitors hormone levels in the blood and sends messages to the pituitary gland to release follicle-stimulating hormone (FSH) and luteinizing hormone (LH).

In the ovaries, these hormones stimulate the growth of a few of the immature eggs, or ova, stored in follicles in every woman's body. Usually, only one ovum matures completely during each monthly cycle. As it does, it increases its production of the female sex hormone estrogen, which in turn triggers the release of a larger surge of LH.

At midcycle, the increased LH hormone levels trigger **ovulation,** the release of the egg cell, or ovum from the follicle. Estrogen levels drop, and the remaining cells of the follicle then enlarge, change character, and form the **corpus luteum,** or yellow body. In the second half of the menstrual cycle, the corpus luteum secretes estrogen and larger amounts of progesterone. The endometrium (uterine lining) is stimulated by progesterone to thicken and become more engorged with blood in preparation for nourishing an implanted, fertilized ovum.

If the ovum is not fertilized, the corpus luteum disintegrates. As the level of progesterone drops, **menstruation** occurs; the uterine lining is shed during the course of a menstrual period. If the egg is fertilized and pregnancy occurs, the cells that eventually develop into the placenta secrete *human chorionic gonadotropin (HCG),* a messenger hormone that signals the pituitary not to start a new cycle. The corpus luteum then steps up its production of progesterone.

A woman's attitudes toward menstruation can affect her sexual attitudes and behaviors. In a Canadian study of 114 romantically involved women, those who had engaged in sex during their periods were significantly more comfortable with menstruation, less sensitive to disgust in general, and more aroused by romantic and unconventional sexual activities.[3]

Many women experience physical or psychological changes, or both, during their monthly cycles. Usually the changes are minor, but more serious problems can occur.

Premenstrual Syndrome

Women with **premenstrual syndrome (PMS)** experience bodily discomfort and emotional distress for up to two weeks, from ovulation until the onset of menstruation. Up to 85 percent of menstruating women report one or more premenstrual symptoms; 2 to 10 percent experience disabling, incapacitating symptoms.[4]

Once dismissed as a psychological problem, PMS has been recognized as a very real physiological disorder that may be caused by a hormonal deficiency; abnormal levels of thyroid hormone; an imbalance of estrogen and progesterone; or social and environmental factors, particularly stress. Recent studies indicate that PMS may originate in the brain. Women with too little of the messenger chemical serotonin may be more sensitive to progesterone and develop premenstrual symptoms.[5]

The most common symptoms of PMS are mood changes, anxiety, irritability, difficulty concentrating, forgetfulness, impaired judgment, tearfulness, digestive symptoms (diarrhea, bloating, constipation), hot flashes, palpitations, dizziness, headache, fatigue, changes in appetite, cravings (usually for sweets or salt), water retention, breast tenderness, and insomnia. For a diagnosis to be made, women—using a self-rating symptom scale or calendar—must report troubling premenstrual symptoms in the period before menstruation in at least two successive menstrual cycles.

Treatments for PMS depend on specific symptoms. Diuretics (drugs that speed up fluid elimination) can relieve water retention and bloating. Relaxation techniques have led to a 60 percent reduction in anxiety symptoms. Sleep deprivation, or the use of bright light to adjust a woman's circadian or daily rhythm, also has proven beneficial. Behavioral approaches, such as exercise or charting cycles, help by letting women know when they're vulnerable.

Low doses of medications known as *selective serotonin-reuptake inhibitors* (SSRIs), such as fluoxetine (marketed as Prozac, Sarafem, and in generic forms) provide relief for symptoms such as tension, depression, irritability, and mood swings, even when taken only during the premenstrual phase rather than daily throughout the month. SSRIs are not effective in all women with PMS, and other factors, including a genetic susceptibility, may play a role.

Oral contraceptives, though widely prescribed for PMS, have not been shown to be consistently effective. One particular brand, Yasmin, which has a diuretic effect, has been associated with relief of premenstrual symptoms such as bloating and breast tenderness.[6] One of the most controversial treatments is the use of progesterone during the second half of the menstrual cycle. However, its efficacy has not been demonstrated, and doctors currently advise against its use.[7]

Calcium supplements may be beneficial. Other treatments with some reported success include vitamins; exercise; less caffeine, alcohol, salt and sugar; acupuncture; and

Figure 8-4 MENSTRUAL CYCLE

A. In response to the hypothalamus, the pituitary gland releases the gonadotropins FSH and LH.
B. Levels of FSH and LH stimulate the cycle (and in turn are affected by production of estrogen and progesterone).
C. FSH does what its name says—it stimulates follicle development in the ovary. The follicle matures and ruptures, releasing an ovum (egg) into the fallopian tube.
D. The follicle produces estrogen, and the corpus luteum produces estrogen and progesterone. The high level

of estrogen at the middle of the cycle produces a surge of LH, which triggers ovulation.
E. Estrogen and progesterone stimulate the endometrium, which becomes thicker and prepares to receive an implanted, fertilized egg.

If a fertilized egg is deposited in the uterus, pregnancy begins. If the egg is not fertilized, progesterone production decreases, and the endometrium is shed (menstruation). At this point, both estrogen and progesterone levels have dropped, so the pituitary responds by producing FSH, and the cycle begins again.

stress management techniques such as meditation or relaxation training.

Premenstrual Dysphoric Disorder

Premenstrual dysphoric disorder (PMDD), which is not related to PMS, occurs in an estimated 3 to 5 percent of all menstruating women. It is characterized by regular symptoms of depression (depressed mood, anxiety, mood swings, diminished interest or pleasure) during the last week of the menstrual cycle. Women with PMDD cannot function as usual at work, school, or home. They feel better a few days after menstruation begins. SSRIs, which are used to treat PMS, also are effective in relieving symptoms of PMDD.

PMDD remains controversial, primarily for political reasons. Some women's advocacy groups oppose labeling women with menstruation-linked symptoms as mentally ill. Others contend that a diagnosis of PMDD simply recognizes the distress some women experience and may make it easier for them to obtain needed help.

Menstrual Cramps

Dysmenorrhea is the medical name for the discomforts—abdominal cramps and pain, back and leg pain, diarrhea, tension, water retention, fatigue, and depression—that can occur during menstruation. About half of all menstruating women suffer from dysmenorrhea. The cause seems to be an overproduction of bodily substances called *prostaglandins,* which typically rise during menstruation.

Women who produce excessive prostaglandins have more severe menstrual cramps. During a cramp, the uterine muscles may contract too strongly or frequently, and temporarily deprive the uterus of oxygen, causing pain. Medications that inhibit prostaglandins can reduce menstrual pain, and exercise can also relieve cramps.

Amenorrhea

Women may stop menstruating—a condition called **amenorrhea**—for a variety of reasons, including a hormonal disorder, drastic weight loss, strenuous exercise, or change in the environment. "Boarding-school amenorrhea" is common among young women who leave home for school. Distance running and strenuous exercise also can lead to amenorrhea. The reason may be a drop in body fat from the normal range of 18 to 22 percent to a range of 9 to 12 percent. To be considered amenorrheic, a woman's menstrual cycle is typically absent for three or more consecutive months. Prolonged amenorrhea can have serious health consequences, including a loss of bone density that may lead to stress fractures or osteoporosis.

Scientists have developed chemical mimics, or analogues, of GnRH—usually administered by nasal spray—that trigger ovulation in women who don't ovulate or menstruate normally.

Toxic Shock Syndrome

This rare, potentially deadly bacterial infection primarily strikes menstruating women under the age of 30 who use tampons. Both *Staphylococcus aureus* and group A *Streptococcus pyogenes* can produce **toxic shock syndrome (TSS).** Symptoms include a high fever; a rash that leads to peeling of the skin on the fingers, toes, palms, and soles; dizziness; dangerously low blood pressure; and abnormalities in several organ systems (the digestive tract and the kidneys) and in the muscles and blood. Treatment usually consists of antibiotics and intense supportive care; intravenous administration of immunoglobulins that attack the toxins produced by these bacteria also may be beneficial.

Menstruating women should follow these guidelines to reduce their risk of TSS:

:: Use sanitary napkins instead of tampons.

:: If you do use tampons, check the box label for information on absorbency (required by the FDA) and avoid superabsorbent brands.

:: Change tampons every four to eight hours.

:: Use napkins during the night or for some time during each day of menstrual flow.

STRATEGIES FOR PREVENTION

Reducing Premenstrual Problems

■ Get plenty of exercise. Physically fit women usually have fewer problems both before and during their periods.

■ Eat frequently and nutritiously. In the week before your period, your body doesn't regulate the levels of sugar, or glucose, in your blood as well as it usually does.

■ Swear off salt. If you stop using salt at the table and while cooking, you may gain less weight premenstrually, feel less bloated, and suffer less from headaches and irritability.

■ Cut back on caffeine. Coffee, colas, diet colas, chocolate, and tea can increase breast tenderness and other symptoms.

■ Don't drink or smoke. Some women become so sensitive to alcohol's effects before their periods that a glass of wine hits with the impact of several stiff drinks. Nicotine worsens low blood sugar problems.

■ Watch out for sweets. Premenstrual cravings for sweets are common, but try to resist. Sugar may pick you up, but later you'll feel worse than before.

:: As menstrual flow decreases, switch to less-absorbent tampons, which are less likely to cause problems.

◼ Men's Sexual Health

Because the male reproductive system is simpler in many ways than the female, it's often ignored—especially by healthy young men. However, men should make regular self-exams (including checking their penises and testes, as described in Chapter 15) part of their routine.

Male Sexual Anatomy

The visible parts of the male sexual anatomy are the **penis** and the **scrotum**, the pouch that contains the **testes** (see Figure 8-5). The testes manufacture testosterone, the hormone that stimulates the development of a male's secondary characteristics, and **sperm**, the male reproductive cells. Immature sperm are stored in the **epididymis**, a collection of coiled tubes adjacent to each testis.

The penis contains three hollow cylinders loosely covered with skin. The two major cylinders, the *corpora cavernosa*, extend side by side through the length of the penis.

Figure 8-5 MALE SEX ORGANS AND REPRODUCTIVE STRUCTURES

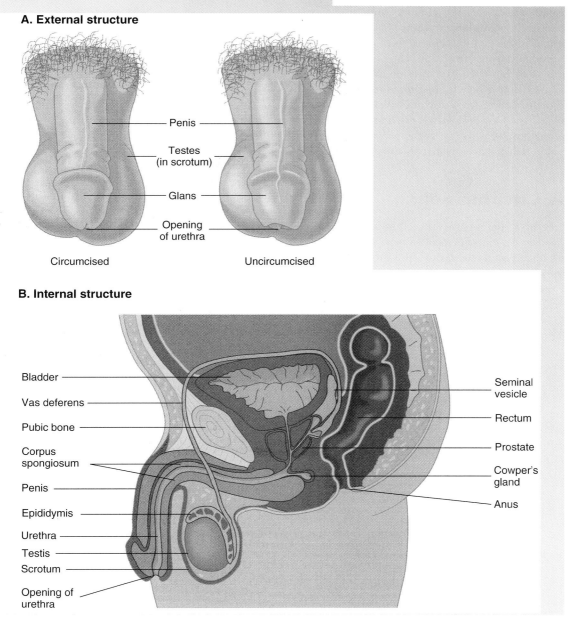

A. External structure

Penis

Testes (in scrotum)

Glans

Opening of urethra

Circumcised

Uncircumcised

B. Internal structure

Bladder

Vas deferens

Pubic bone

Corpus spongiosum

Penis

Epididymis

Urethra

Testis

Scrotum

Opening of urethra

Seminal vesicle

Rectum

Prostate

Cowper's gland

Anus

The third cylinder, the *corpus spongiosum,* surrounds the **urethra,** the channel for both seminal fluid and urine (see Figure 8-5).

When hanging down loosely, the average penis is about 3¾ inches long. During erection, its internal cylinders fill with so much blood that they become rigid, and the penis stretches to an average length of 6¼ inches. About 90 percent of all men have erect penises measuring between 5 and 7 inches in length. There is no relation, however, between penis size and female sexual satisfaction: A woman's vagina naturally adjusts during intercourse to the size of her partner's penis.

Inside the body are several structures involved in the production of seminal fluid, or **semen,** the liquid in which sperm cells are carried out of the body during ejaculation. The **vas deferens** are two tubes that carry sperm from the epididymis into the urethra. The **seminal vesicles,** which make some of the seminal fluid, join with the vas deferens to form the **ejaculatory ducts.** The **prostate gland** produces some of the seminal fluid, which it secretes into the urethra during ejaculation. The **Cowper's glands** are two pea-sized structures on either side of the urethra (just below where it emerges from the prostate gland) and connected to it via tiny ducts. When a man is sexually aroused, the Cowper's glands often secrete a fluid that appears as a droplet at the tip of the penis. This fluid is not semen, although it occasionally contains sperm.

What Is Circumcision?

In its natural state, the tip of the penis is covered by a fold of skin called the *foreskin.* About 60 percent of baby boys in the United States undergo **circumcision,** the surgical removal of the foreskin. However, increasingly more parents are opting for the natural look.

An estimated 1.2 million newborn males are circumcised in the United States annually for reasons that vary from religious traditions to preventive health measures. Until the last half century, scientific evidence to support or repudiate routine circumcision was limited. The American Academy of Pediatrics (AAP) reviewed 40 years of data and concluded that although there are potential medical benefits, the data are not strong enough to recommend routine neonatal circumcision.[8] However, other experts, challenging this controversial view, argue that lack of circumcision increases the risk of sexually transmitted diseases, including HIV and syphilis.[9]

Boys who are not circumcised are four times as likely to develop urinary tract infections in their first year; however, such infections develop in only 1 percent of circumcised boys. Uncircumcised men are three times as likely to develop penile cancer, but the absolute risk is low. (Only about nine in every million American men ever gets cancer of the penis.) The drawbacks of circumcision include the risk of complications (which tend to be uncommon and minor) and pain. The AAP recommends that when circumcision is performed, analgesic creams or anesthetic shots be used to minimize discomfort.

Parents who choose not to have their sons circumcised should not attempt to retract the foreskin. This could lead to infection, bleeding, or scarring. As a boy gets older, gradual retraction of the foreskin during bath time helps it dilate, with full retraction possible by age two to four. There is little consensus on what impact the presence or absence of a foreskin has on sexual functioning or satisfaction.

Parents have mixed feelings about the decisions they make. In one study, families who did not have their sons circumcised were less satisfied with their decision. They were more likely to feel that they had not been adequately informed and to reconsider their decision.[10]

Responsible Sexuality

The World Health Organization defines **sexual health** as "the integration of the physical, emotional, intellectual, and social aspects of sexual being in ways that are positively enriching, and that enhance personality, communication, and love. . . . Every person has a right to receive sexual information and to consider sexual relationships for pleasure as well as for procreation."

Sexuality education is a lifelong process. Your own knowledge about sex may not be as extensive as you might assume. Most people grow up with a lot of myths and misconceptions about sex. (See Self-Survey: "How Much Do You Know About Sex?") Rather than relying on what peers say or what you've always thought was true, find out the facts. This textbook is a good place to start. The student health center and the library can provide additional materials on sexual identity, orientation, behavior, and health, as well as on options for reducing your risk of acquiring sexually transmitted infections (discussed in Chapter 13) or becoming pregnant.

Sexually Healthy Relationships

A sexually healthy relationship, as defined by the Sexuality Information and Education Council of the United States (SIECUS), is based on shared values and has five characteristics: It is consensual, nonexploitative, honest, mutually pleasurable, and protected against unintended pregnancy and sexuality transmitted infections (STIs), including HIV/AIDS. All individuals also have sexual rights, which include the right to the information, education, skills, support, and services they need to make responsible decisions about their sexuality consistent with their own values, as well as the right to express their sexual orientation without violence or discrimination.

Self Survey | How Much Do You Know About Sex?

Mark each of the following statements True or False:

1. Men and women have completely different sex hormones.
2. Premenstrual syndrome (PMS) is primarily a psychological problem.
3. Circumcision diminishes a man's sexual pleasure.
4. Sexual orientation may have a biological basis.
5. Masturbation is a sign of emotional immaturity.
6. Only homosexual men engage in anal intercourse.
7. Despite their awareness of AIDS, many college students do not practice safe sex.
8. After age 60, lovemaking is mainly a fond memory, not a regular pleasure of daily living.
9. Doctors advise against having intercourse during a woman's menstrual period.
10. Only men ejaculate.
11. It is possible to be infected with HIV during a single sexual encounter.
12. Impotence is always a sign of emotional or sexual problems in a relationship.

Answers:

1. False. Men and women have the same hormones, but in different amounts.
2. False. PMS has been recognized as a physiological disorder that may be caused by a hormonal deficiency, abnormal levels of thyroid hormone, or social and environmental factors, such as stress.
3. False. Sex therapists have not been able to document differences in sensitivity to stimulation between circumcised and uncircumcised men.
4. True. Researchers documented structural differences in the brains of homosexual men and women.
5. False. Throughout a person's life, masturbation can be a form of sexual release and pleasure.
6. False. As many as one in every four married couples under age 35 have reported that they occasionally engage in anal intercourse.
7. True. In one recent study, more than a third of college students had engaged in vaginal or anal intercourse at least once in the previous year without using effective protection from conception or sexually transmitted infections (STIs).
8. False. More than a third of American married men and women older than 60 make love at least once a week as do 10% of those older than 70.
9. False. There's no medical reason to avoid intercourse during a woman's menstrual period.
10. False. Stimulation of the Grafenberg spot in a woman's vagina may lead to a release of fluid from her urethra during orgasm.
11. True. Although the risk increases with repeated sexual contact with an infected partner, an individual can contract HIV during a single sexual encounter.
12. False. Many erection difficulties have physical causes.

Your Health Change Plan

for Responsible Sexuality

Your score on this self-survey may indicate that you know a lot more—or less—about sex than you thought you did. Part of sexual responsibility is being informed about sexuality, including reproductive anatomy, sexual orientation, the range of sexual behaviors, and ways of protecting yourself from sexually transmitted diseases.

The Sexuality Information and Education Council of the United States (SIECUS) has worked with nongovernmental organizations around the world to develop a consensus about the life behaviors of a sexually healthy and responsible adult. These include:

:: Appreciating one's own body.
:: Seeking information about reproduction as needed.
:: Affirming that sexual development may or may not include reproduction or genital sexual experience.
:: Interacting with both genders in respectful and appropriate ways.
:: Affirming one's own sexual orientation and respecting the sexual orientation of others.

:: Expressing love and intimacy in appropriate ways.
:: Developing and maintaining meaningful relationships.
:: Avoiding exploitative or manipulative relationships.
:: Making informed choices about family options and lifestyles.
:: Enjoying and expressing one's sexuality throughout life.
:: Expressing one's sexuality in ways congruent with one's values.
:: Discriminating between life-enhancing sexual behaviors and those that are harmful to self and/or others.
:: Expressing one's sexuality while respecting the rights of others.
:: Seeking new information to enhance one's sexuality.
:: Using contraception effectively to avoid unintended pregnancy.
:: Preventing sexual abuse.
:: Seeking early prenatal care.
:: Avoiding contracting or transmitting a sexually transmitted infection, including HIV.

(Continued)

:: Practicing health-promoting behaviors, such as regular checkups, breast and testicular self-exam, and early identification of potential problems.

:: Demonstrating tolerance for people with different sexual values and lifestyles.

:: Exercising democratic responsibility to influence legislation dealing with sexual issues.

:: Assessing the impact of family, cultural, religious, media, and societal messages on one's thoughts, feelings, values, and behaviors related to sexuality.

:: Promoting the rights of all people to accurate sexuality information.

:: Avoiding behaviors that exhibit prejudice and bigotry.

:: Rejecting stereotypes about the sexuality of diverse populations.

Sexual Decision Making

Sexual decision making always takes place within the context of an individual's values and perceptions of right and wrong behavior. Making sexually responsible decisions means considering all the possible consequences of sexual behavior for both yourself and your partner. It must always take into account, not just personal preferences and desires, but the very real risks of unwanted pregnancy, sexually transmitted infections (STIs), and long-term medical consequences (such as impaired fertility). You also must consider the emotional consequences of a sexual relationship—not just for yourself but also for your partner.

:: What role do we want relationships and sex to have in our life at this time?

:: What are my values and my potential partner's values as they pertain to sexual relationships? Does each of us believe that intercourse should be reserved for a permanent partnership or committed relationship?

:: Will a decision to engage in sex enhance my positive feelings about myself or my partner? Does either of us have questions about sexual orientation or the kinds of people we are attracted to?

:: Do I and my partner both want to have sex? Is my partner pressuring me in any way? Am I pressuring

Talking About Sex

Prior to any sexual activity that involves a risk of sexually transmitted infection or pregnancy, both partners should talk about their prior sexual histories (including number of partners and exposure to STIs) and other high-risk behavior, such as the use of injection drugs. They should also discuss the issue of birth control and which methods might be best for them to use. If you know someone well enough to consider having sex with that person, you should be able to talk about such sensitive subjects. If a potential partner is unwilling to talk or hedges on crucial questions, you shouldn't be engaging in sex.

Styles of communicating vary among white Americans, African Americans, Hispanic Americans, and Asian Americans. While white and African Americans may openly discuss sex with partners, Hispanic-American couples generally do not discuss their sexual relationship. Asian Americans also are less inclined to discuss sex and to value nonverbal, indirect, and intuitive communication over explicit verbal interaction.[11]

Here are some questions to consider as you think and talk about the significance of becoming sexually intimate with a partner:

STRATEGIES FOR CHANGE

Improving a Sexual Relationship

■ Use "I" statements, such as "I really enjoy making love, but I'm so tired right now that I won't be a responsive partner. Why don't we get the kids to bed early tomorrow so we can enjoy ourselves a little earlier?"

■ Speak up if something hurts during sex. Be specific.

■ If you would like to try something different, say so. Practice saying the words first if they embarrass you. If your partner feels uncomfortable, don't force the issue, but do try talking it through.

■ If you want to request changes or tackle a touchy topic, start with positive statements. Let your partner know how much you enjoy having sex, and then express your desire to enjoy lovemaking more often or in different ways.

■ Encourage small changes. If you want your partner to be less inhibited, start slowly, perhaps by suggesting sex in a different room or place.

my partner? Am I making this decision for myself or my partner?

:: Have my partner and I discussed our sexual histories and risk factors? Have I spoken honestly about any STIs I've had in the past? Am I sure that neither my partner nor I have a sexually transmitted infection?

:: Have we taken precautions against unwanted pregnancy and STIs?

Whether couples are on a first date or have been married for years, each partner always has the right not to have sex. Unfortunately, "no" sometimes seems to mean different things to men and women.

 At some campuses, such as Antioch College in Ohio, freshmen must attend workshops on sexual consent and adhere to a campus policy that requires "willing and verbal consent" for each sexual act. (Chapter 18 also discusses sexual coercion.)

✸ Sexual Behavior

From birth to death, we are sexual beings. Our sexual identities, needs, likes, and dislikes emerge in adolescence and become clearer as we enter adulthood, but we continue to change and evolve throughout our lives. In men, sexual interest is most intense at age 18; in women, it reaches a peak in the 30s. Although age brings changes in sexual responsiveness, we never outgrow our sexuality.

Adolescent Sexuality

Early in adolescence, sexual curiosity explodes, and sexual exploration—both alone and with a partner—takes on new meaning and intensity. Sexual education programs can make a difference by helping young people become sexually responsible, enabling them to form satisfying relationships, helping them assess their own attitudes toward sex, and giving them information on sexuality. Good programs can clarify values and enhance communication.

It's not unusual for teenage boys to experience frequent erections during the day and night, including **nocturnal emissions,** or wet dreams, during which ejaculation occurs. **Masturbation** (discussed later in this chapter) is the primary form of sexual expression for many teenagers, especially boys. Self-stimulation helps teens learn about their bodies and their sexual potential and serves as an outlet for sexual tension. By the end of adolescence, the majority of teens have masturbated to orgasm.

Other common sexual activities during adolescence include kissing and petting—erotic physical contact that may include holding, touching, manual stimulation of the genitals, and oral sex. As many as 25 percent of teens experience some same-sex attractions. Although many experi-

ment with heterosexual and homosexual sexual experiences, adolescent sexual behavior does not always foretell sexual orientation. Young people, who often feel confused about their sexual identity, may engage in sexual activity with members of the same or the other sex as a way of testing how they really feel.

For the first time since the federal government started keeping statistics in the early 1970s, fewer American teenagers are becoming sexually active. According to the CDC, the percentage of high school students who had intercourse dropped from 54.1 to 45.6 percent.[12]

The popular media have reported an increase in oral sex among teenagers. In a study of 212 tenth-graders, adolescents were more likely to report engagement in oral sex than intercourse and more oral sex partners than intercourse partners. Teens were less likely to use any form of protection against sexually transmitted infection during oral sex than during intercourse.[13]

About nine in ten teenagers have been educated about HIV/AIDS. About 25 percent more students say they used a condom during their last sexual encounter than those surveyed a decade ago. Every year, an estimated one in four sexually active adolescents—approximately 3 million—acquires an STI.

Teenagers say they'd like their parents to provide more information about sexuality, but parents often do not initiate or engage in such discussions, particularly with boys. In a recent survey of older teens and their parents, more than a third of boys said no one spoke to them prior to or during puberty about sexual development or sexuality issues. Parents were more likely to talk with girls and to do so at an earlier age: 13 rather than 15.[14]

According to a national survey of 1,800 teenagers and young adults sponsored by the Kaiser Family Foundation, young people are more concerned about sex and sexual health than any other health issue in their lives. Most—but especially males—report peer pressure to have sex. Three in five respondents described putting off sex as a "nice idea," but something nobody does (Figure 8-6). One in five reported initial sexual intercourse by age 15. Sexually experienced young teens were far more likely than virgins to engage in other risky behaviors, such as smoking, drinking, and using drugs. Almost a third said they had "done more sexually" because of alcohol or drug use.[15]

A third of adolescents say they have engaged in oral sex, but one in five did not know that STIs can be transmitted via oral sex. One in six young adults and adolescents regard unprotected sex as "not that big a deal." Males are twice as likely as females to feel this way. Pregnancy remains a real concern among young people. Seven in ten college age young adults have or have had a partner who had a pregnancy test. Nearly two in five reported that they or a partner has been pregnant.[16]

Figure 8-6 WHAT STUDENTS SAY ABOUT RELATIONSHIPS AND SEX

These percentages of adolescents and young adults (ages 15–24) say they "strongly" or "somewhat" agree with each of these statements.

Source: "National Survey of Adolescents and Young Adults: Sexual Health Knowledge, Attitudes, and Experiences." Menlo Park, CA: Kaiser Family Foundation, 2003.

Waiting to have sex is a nice idea but nobody really does
61%

There is pressure to have sex by a certain age
58%

Once you have had sex it is harder to say no the next time
55%

If you have been seeing someone for a while it is expected that you will have sex
47%

Oral sex is not as big of a deal as sexual intercourse
42%

0   10   20   30   40   50   60   70   80   90   100

How Sexually Active Are College Students?

According to various reports, 74 to 90 percent of American college students are sexually active.[17] (See Student Snapshot: "Behind Closed Doors . . .") Most are not engaging in frequent casual sex and take sex and monogamy seriously.[18] (See Fact or Fiction? "Most college students . . .")

College students see sexual activity as normal behavior for their peer group. When researchers at Pennsylvania State University conducted focus groups with undergraduates, most agreed that the majority of college students (80 to 90 percent, in their estimate) are sexually active and that alcohol and drug use make sexual activity more likely.[19]

Yet students' assumptions about their peers' behaviors may be grossly inaccurate. In one study, undergraduates believed that the "average" college student engaged in significantly more frequent HIV-risky sexual activity (such as intercourse without a condom) far more frequently than they did themselves. According to their self-reports, 14 percent of the students engaged in unprotected intercourse, 19 percent in oral sex, and 2 percent had sexual relations with someone they had just met. Yet they believed that much higher percentages of students—more than half in some cases—engaged in these behaviors, particularly if drunk or high.[20]

Memory is not a reliable source of information about college students' sexual experiences. In one experiment, researchers compared the e-mail diaries of 37 sexually active heterosexual students with their recollections six to twelve months later. The students underreported the number of partners they'd had, but overreported both their sexual encounters and their use of condoms.[21]

College students who first got drunk before age 13 are twice as likely to have unplanned and unprotected sex because of drinking than those who did not drink until age 19 or older—regardless of age, race or ethnicity, marital status, parents' drinking history, and age of first smoking or marijuana use.[22]

Annual spring breaks provide what researchers describe as "ideal conditions for the potentially lethal interaction between alcohol, drugs, and sexual risk-taking."[23] Students typically engage in binge drinking, illicit drug use, and unsafe sexual practices. The likelihood of casual sex depends on several factors, including peer influences, prior experiences with casual sex, alcohol consumption prior to sex, and impulsivity.

A substantial proportion of college students—male and female—report that they engage in unwanted sexual activity. Sometimes this is the result of sexual coercion (a problem discussed in Chapter 18) or alcohol use. However, some students admit to feigning desire and consenting to an unwanted sexual activity for various reasons, including satisfying a partner's needs, promoting intimacy, and avoiding relationship tension.

FACT OR FICTION? ???????????????

Most college students are not engaging in frequent, casual sex.

Fact: In a recent national survey of 1,051 students ages 18 to 24, about 25 percent said they had never engaged in sexual intercourse: 34 percent of men and 18 percent of women. One in four said they had passed on an opportunity to have sex during the previous year. Three in four agreed that sex and contraception should be discussed in advance. The average number of sex partners reported by the students during the previous year was 1.2. Two in three women and one in three men described themselves as being in committed relationships.

Source: "Smarter Sex Survey," results available at www.SmarterSex.org.

Student Snapshot — Behind Closed Doors on Campus

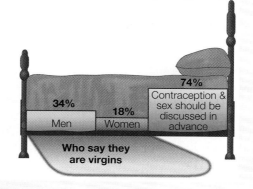

74% Students who are sexually active

34% Men

24% Women

Who said their first sexual experience was unplanned

34% Men

18% Women

74% Contraception & sex should be discussed in advance

Who say they are virgins

Source: Data from 1,051 students (526 men and 525 women) ages 18–24 who participated in the online Smarter Sex Survey. www.smartersex.org/resources/behind.asp.

Men also report nonconsensual sexual activity. In studies of college-age men, one in four reported at least one incident in which a woman (often a friend or ex-partner) attempted to engage them in unwanted kissing, petting, oral sex, or intercourse.[24]

During adolescence, sexuality develops rapidly. Teens explore different social and intimate relationships as they begin to develop a sexual identity.

Why Don't College Students Practice Safer Sex?

Decades of education about sexual risks has had an impact. More students today are aware of and use safer sex practices—but not consistently. In a survey of 119 American colleges, condom use varied from 32 to 52 percent among unmarried sexually active students.[25] Heterosexual students—male and female—were more likely to say they always used condoms than gay men. Of those engaging in heterosexual sex, 52 percent of men and 43 percent of women reported consistent condom use, compared with 32 percent of men with only male partners.

Researchers explain that the college environment "provides students with a sense of new independence, self-determination, and strong peer pressure to experiment with a variety of sexual behaviors." Yet by engaging in sex with multiple partners and not regularly using condoms, college students in general—and African-American students in particular—put themselves at high risk of contracting HIV and other sexual infections.

In a recent study of African-American undergraduates, male and female students identified barriers to their use of safer sex practices. Negative views of condoms rank first. But the reason men and women don't like condoms is not reduced sensitivity or pleasure, but a sense that not wearing a condom provides a sense of greater intimacy.[26]

Trust is another issue. Men trust a women as safe and healthy on the basis of the way she looks. Women trust a man because they believe they are in a monogamous relationship after a period of time (one month on average) or number of encounters (twelve). Neither men nor women base their feelings of trust on a discussion with a partner. They simply assume that a partner can be trusted and that condoms are not necessary.

Another reason not to practice safer sex is the sense of invincibility that is common among college students, who are in the healthiest years of their lives and filled with the optimism of youth. Students also cite a desire to live for and in the moment. Peer pressure and lack of self-control also influence student behavior. Particularly for women, alcohol and drugs present another major barrier to safer sex.

The Sex Life of American Adults

The scientific study of Americans' sexual behavior began in 1938, when Alfred Kinsey, Ph.D., a professor of biology at the University of Indiana, and his colleagues asked 5,300 white men and 5,940 white women about their sexual practices. In his landmark studies—*Sexual Behavior in the Human Male,* published in 1948, and *Sexual Behavior in the Human Female* published in 1953—Kinsey reported that 73 percent of men and 20 percent of women had premarital intercourse by age 20, and 37 percent of men and 17 percent of women had some homosexual experience in their lifetime.

The Janus Report on Sexual Behavior, published in 1993, was based on a survey of 2,765 individuals across the United States. A larger survey, conducted by researchers at the University of Chicago, was based on face-to-face interviews with 3,432 Americans, aged 18 to 59. It became the basis for two books published in 1994: *Sex in America,* aimed at a lay audience, and *The Social Organization of Sexuality,* a more scholarly work. Since then, the researcher's General Social Survey (GSS) database on sexual activity has grown to nearly 10,000 respondents.

The GSS data indicate that overall sexual activity in America is relatively infrequent, with an average of 58 episodes per year, or slightly more than one a week. Yet sexual activity increased compared with earlier decades— even though the population is aging, works longer hours, and can choose among a growing number of distractions. About 15 percent of adults engage in half of all sexual activity; 42 percent of adults engage in 85 percent of all sex.[27]

The average adult reports having sex about once a week. However, 1 in 5 Americans has been celibate for at least a year, and 1 in 20 engages in sex at least every other day. Men report more sexual frequency than women—not because men are more boastful about their prowess, the researchers contend, but because the sample of women includes many widows and older women without partners. Among married people, the frequency reports of hus- bands and wives (not in the same couples) are within one episode per year—58.6 for married men and 57.9 for married women. And if other differences between men and women are statistically controlled (such as sexual preference, age, and educational attainment), married women actually report a slightly higher frequency than men.

Sexual frequency peaks among those with some college education, then decreases among four-year college graduates, and declines even further among those with professional degrees. Americans who have attended graduate school are the least sexually active educational group in the population. These respondents may be more honest than others in reporting sexual activity, or they may be more precise in their definition of what counts as sex.

Does sex make people happier or healthier? Based on their analysis, the researchers concluded that the more sex a person has, the more likely he or she is to report having a happy life and a happy marriage. This connection is stronger among women than men. A second and more important predictor of sexual frequency is the feeling that one's life is exciting rather than routine or dull. "Being excited by life is most strongly associated with being happier," the researchers noted. "It seems that increased sexual activity is one of the many benefits of having a positive attitude."

✖ Sexual Diversity

Human beings are diverse in all ways—including sexual preferences and practices. Physiological, psychological, and social factors determine whether we are attracted to members of the same sex or the other sex. This attraction is our **sexual orientation.** Sigmund Freud argued that we all start off **bisexual,** or attracted to both sexes. But by the time we reach adulthood, most males prefer female sexual partners, and most females prefer male partners. **Heterosexual** is the term used for individuals whose primary orientation is toward members of the other sex. In virtually all cultures, some men and women are **homosexuals,** preferring partners of their own sex.

In our society, we tend to view heterosexuality and homosexuality as very different. In reality, these orientations are opposite ends of a spectrum. Sex researcher Alfred Kinsey devised a seven-point continuum representing sexual orientation in American society. At one end of the continuum are those exclusively attracted to members of the other sex; at the opposite end are people exclusively attracted to members of the same sex. In between are varying degrees of homosexual, bisexual, and heterosexual orientation.

According to Kinsey's original data, 4 percent of men and 2 percent of women are exclusively homosexual. More recent studies have found lower numbers. For instance, in the University of Chicago's national survey, 2.8 percent of men and 1.4 percent of women defined themselves as homosexual. However, when asked if they'd had sex with a person of the same gender since age 18, about 5 percent of men and 4 percent of women said yes. When asked if they found members of the same gender sexually attractive, 6 percent of men and 5.5 percent of women said yes.

In a recent survey of lesbian and bisexual women, most reported that their first sexual experience occurred with a man (at the median age of 18) and that sex with a women followed a few years later (at median age 21). Their most frequently reported sexual activities with men were mutual masturbation and vaginal penetration with penis or fingers. Their most common sex practices with women were oral sex, vaginal penetration with fingers, and mutual masturbation.[28]

Bisexuality

Bisexuality—sexual attraction to both males and females—can develop at any point in one's life. In some cultures, bisexual activity is considered part of normal sexual experimentation. Among the Sabmia Highlanders in Papua New Guinea, for instance, boys perform oral sex on one another as part of the rites of passage into manhood.[29]

Some people identify themselves as bisexual even if they don't behave bisexually. Some are *serial* bisexuals— that is, they are sexually involved with same-sex partners for a while and then with partners of the other sex, or vice versa. An estimated 7 to 9 million men, about twice the number thought to be exclusively homosexual, could be described as bisexual during some extended period of their lives. The largest group are married, rarely have sexual relations with women other than their wives, and have secret sexual involvements with men.

Fear of HIV infection has sparked great concern about bisexuality, particularly among heterosexual women who worry about becoming involved with a bisexual man. About 20 to 30 percent of women with AIDS were infected by bisexual partners, and health officials fear that bisexual men who hide their homosexual affairs could transmit HIV to many more women.

Homosexuality

Homosexuality—social, emotional, and sexual attraction to members of the same sex—exists in almost all cultures. Men and women homosexuals are commonly referred to as *gay;* women homosexuals are also called *lesbians.*

Homosexuality threatens and upsets many people, perhaps because homosexuals are viewed as different, or perhaps because no one understands why some people are heterosexual and others homosexual. *Homophobia* has led to an increase in *gay bashing* (attacking homosexuals) in

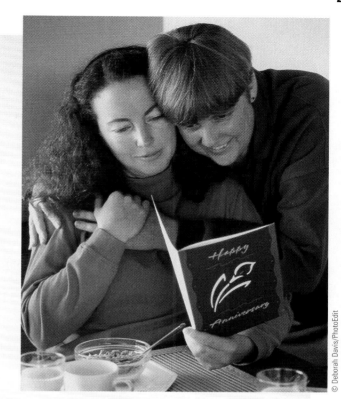

Close-couple homosexual relationships are similar to stable heterosexual relationships.

many communities, including college campuses. Some blame the emergence of AIDS as a societal danger. However, researchers have found that fear of AIDS has not created new hostility but has simply given bigots an excuse to act out their hatred.

Violations of basic human rights for homosexuals remain common around the globe. Amnesty International has documented abuses ranging from exile to labor camps in China to social cleansing death squads in Colombia to the death penalty in Iran.

Roots of Homosexuality

Most mental health experts agree that nobody knows what causes a person's sexual orientation. Research has discredited theories tracing homosexuality to troubled childhoods or abnormal psychological development. Sexual orientation probably emerges from a complex interaction that includes biological and environmental factors.

For decades, behavioral and medical specialists have debated whether homosexuality is biologically or socially determined. Some say that sexual orientation is genetically determined. However, new research has cast doubt on the existence of a homosexuality gene. Others contend that prenatal hormones influence sexual preference. Today, questions and controversies persist about the roots and nature of sexual orientation.

Homosexuality on Campus

In a study of almost 700 heterosexual students at six small liberal arts colleges, attitudes toward homosexuals and homosexuality varied, depending on students' membership in fraternities or sororities, sex role attitudes, religion and religiosity, and contact with and knowledge of gays, lesbians, and bisexuals. The students most likely to be accepting were those who were women, had less traditional sex-role attitudes, were less religious, attended colleges that did not have Greek social clubs, and had gay lesbian, and/or bisexual friends.[30]

A survey of 119 colleges and universities found great variation in the resources available to gay, lesbian, and bisexual students. Most (71 percent) have a student organization; 32 percent provide a paid staff member to deal with the students' needs and issues; 40 percent provide a support identification program; 36 percent offered at least one course on gay, lesbian, and bisexual issues.[31]

Homosexual Relationships

Extensive studies of male and female homosexuals have shown that only a minority have problems coping with their homosexuality. The happiest and best adjusted tend to be those in close-couple relationships, the equivalent of stable heterosexual partnerships. An estimated 3 to 5 million gays and lesbians have conceived children in heterosexual relationships; others have become parents through adoption or artificial insemination. These men and women describe their families as much like any other, and studies of lesbian mothers have found that their children are essentially no different from children of heterosexual couples in self-esteem, gender-related issues and roles, sexual orientation, and general development.

Different ethnic groups respond to homosexuality in different ways. To a greater extent than white homosexuals, gays and lesbians from ethnic groups tend to stay in the closet longer rather than risk alienation from their families and communities. Often they feel forced to choose between their gay and their ethnic identities.

In general, the African-American community has stronger negative views of homosexuals than whites, possibly because of the influence of strong fundamentalist Christian beliefs. Hispanic culture, with its emphasis on machismo, also has a very negative view of male homosexuality. Asian cultures, which tend to view an individual as a representative of his or her family, tend to view open declarations of sexual orientation as shaming the family and challenging their reputation and future.

⚙ Sexual Activity

Part of learning about your own sexuality is having a clear understanding of human sexual behaviors. Understanding frees us from fear and anxiety, so that we can accept ourselves and others as the natural sexual beings we all are.

Celibacy

A celibate person does not engage in sexual activity. Complete **celibacy** means that the person doesn't masturbate (stimulate himself or herself sexually) or engage in sexual activity with a partner. In partial celibacy, the person masturbates but doesn't have sexual contact with others. Many people decide to be celibate at certain times of their lives. Some don't have sex because of concerns about pregnancy or STIs; others haven't found a partner for a permanent, monogamous relationship. Many simply have other priorities, such as finishing school or starting a career and realize that sex outside of a committed relationship is a threat to their physical and psychological well-being.

STRATEGIES FOR CHANGE

How to Say No to Sex

- First of all, recognize your own values and feelings. If you believe that sex is something to be shared only by people who've already become close in other ways, be true to that belief.

- If you're at a loss for words, try these responses: "I like you a lot, but I'm not ready to have sex." "You're a great person, but sex isn't something I do to prove I like someone." "I'd like to wait until I'm married to have sex."

- If you're feeling pressured, let your date know that you're uncomfortable. Be simple and direct. Watch out for emotional blackmail. If your date says, "If you really like me, you'd want to make love," point out that if he or she really likes you, he or she wouldn't try to force you to do something you don't want to do.

- If you're a woman, monitor your sexual signals. Men impute more sexual meaning to gestures (such as casual touching) that women perceive as friendly and innocent.

- Communicate your feelings to your date sooner rather than later. It's far easier to say, "I don't want to go to your apartment," than to fight off unwelcome advances once you're there.

- Remember that if saying no to sex puts an end to a relationship, it wasn't much of a relationship in the first place.

the X&Y file *The Other Sex*

While differences in sexual anatomy between men and women are obvious, the differences and similarities in sexual response and behavior can be more subtle:

- **A woman's sexual response varies more.** As researchers have demonstrated, women may respond quickly to stimulation and reach orgasm. Women may become excited and remain so for some time but not experience orgasm. Or women may have multiple orgasms. The most typical male response is a steady buildup from excitement to ejaculation, although a man may have several mild orgasmic peaks prior to ejaculation or may have prolonged pelvic contractions following ejaculation.

- **Only men have a refractory period.** After ejaculation, a man is incapable of another climax for a certain minimum time, which lengthens with age. This occurs not just in humans but in other species, including rats, dogs, and chimpanzees.

- **Women are much more likely to experience multiple orgasms.** According to sex researchers, a minority of women—an estimated 14 to 16 percent—may have more than one orgasm within a short time interval. Although men may actually be capable of a series of orgasms in a short time period, this seems rare.

- **Both men and women have sexual fantasies.** The brain plays a key role in the sex lives of men and women. Both are about equally likely to fantasize during sexual intercourse. Men's fantasies tend to be more active and focus on the female body, explicit sexual acts, and physical gratification. Women's, with more romance and emotional context, often focus on men's interest in their bodies.

- **Most men and women have engaged in oral sex.** According to national data, 81 percent of men report performing and receiving oral sex. Among women, 75 percent have performed oral sex; 78 percent have received it.

Fantasy

The mind is the most powerful sex organ in the body, and erotic mental images can be sexually stimulating. Sexual fantasies can accompany sexual activity or be pleasurable in themselves. Fantasies generally enhance sexual arousal, reduce anxiety, and boost sexual desire. They're also a way to anticipate and rehearse new sexual experiences, as well as to bolster a person's self-image and feelings of desirability. Part of what makes fantasies exciting is that they provide an opportunity for expressing forbidden desires, such as sex with a different partner or with a past lover.

In the University of Chicago survey, more than half the men (54 percent)—but only 19 percent of the women—said they thought about sex every day or several times a day. Men and women also have different types of sexy thoughts, with men's fantasies containing more explicit genital images and culminating in sexual acts more quickly than women's. In women's fantasies, emotional feelings play a greater role, and there is more kissing and caressing rather than genital contact. For many women, fantasy helps in reaching orgasm during intercourse; a loss of fantasy often is a sign of low sexual desire.

What Does It Mean to Abstain?

The CDC defines **abstinence** as "refraining from sexual activities which involve vaginal, anal, and oral intercourse." The definition of abstinence remains a subject of debate and controversy, with some emphasizing positive choices and others avoidance of specific behaviors.[32] In reality abstinence means different things to different people, cultures, and religious groups.

Increasing numbers of adolescents and young adults are choosing to remain virgins and abstain from sexual intercourse until they enter a permanent, committed, monogamous relationship. About 2.5 million teens have taken pledges to abstain from sex. According to a major study, teens who do so are 34 percent less likely to have premarital sex than others, and are far older when they finally engage in intercourse.[33] The federal government, which has promoted abstinence as a means of preventing pregnancy and sexually transmitted infections, funded abstinence education programs for two decades. Research on abstinence-only sex education training has found a significant impact at the three-month follow-up, but this disappeared after one year. A program emphasizing safer sex was consistently effective throughout the one-year period.[34]

Many people who were sexually active in the past also are choosing abstinence because the risk of medical complications associated with STIs increases with the number of sexual partners a person has. Abstinence is the safest, healthiest option for many. However, there is confusion about what it means to abstain, and individuals who think they are abstaining may still be engaging in behaviors that put them at risk for HIV and STIs. (See Chapter 9 for more on abstinence as a form of birth control.)

Sex in Cyberspace

The Internet has become a new medium for relationships, including those that might be described as sexual. In certain chat rooms, individuals can share explicit sexual fantasies or engage in the cyberspace equivalent of mutual fantasizing. In some ways, the Internet is the perfect venue for a safe form of sexual risk-taking. Individuals can assume any name, gender, race, or personality, and can pretend to lead lives entirely different from their actual existences. However, studies of individuals who had sexual intercourse with partners they met through the Internet found a greater risk for sexually transmitted infections.[35]

Many see cybersex as a harmless way of adding an extra erotic charge to their daily lives. In some cases, individuals who meet in cybersex chat rooms develop what they come to think of as a meaningful relationship and arrange to meet in person. Sometimes these meetings are awkward; sometimes they do lead to a real-life romance. However, they rarely survive the intrusive reality of everyday existence and sometimes they end disastrously in disappointment or danger.

In a study of 506 undergraduates at a public university in Texas, 43 percent had logged on to sexually explicit materials through the Internet, although only 2.9 percent said they did so frequently. About one in ten campus computer users logged on to sexually explicit websites from university computers; one in four home computer users searched for sexually explicit material. Male students were much more likely to have done so; curiosity about sex was their motivation for this behavior. Women were significantly more likely to have experienced sexual harassment while online. Asked about specific behaviors while online, 15 percent of the students reported masturbating online.[36] (See Figure 8-7.)

For some individuals, particularly gays and lesbians, the Internet provides the opportunity to join a virtual community. In addition to sexual exchanges, they can find access to information and resources that may not be available elsewhere. For adolescents struggling with gender identity or for closeted homosexuals, going online can be their only opportunity to be open about their sexuality. But they do face an increased risk of syphilis and HIV if they pursue a relationship off-line.[37]

Among college-age young adults who seek sex partners on the Internet, the majority are white males. They report significantly different patterns of sexual behavior, both on- and off-line, than young adults who do not seek sex on the Internet and are at much greater risk of sexually transmitted infections.[38]

Because young people go online so often, the Internet may emerge as an effective tool for improving sexual health awareness, particularly if messages were incorporated into websites they enjoy.[39] Among patients treated for sexually transmitted infections, those who used the Internet to find sexual partners also went online for information about STIs.[40] While some worry that blocking pornographic sites would also restrict sexual health availability online, this is likely to occur only with the most restrictive blocking configurations.[41]

Masturbation

Not everybody masturbates, but most people do. Kinsey estimated that 7 out of 10 women and 19 out of 20 men masturbate (and admit they do). Their reason is simple: It feels good. Masturbation produces the same physical responses as sexual activity with a partner and can be an enjoyable form of sexual release.

Masturbation has been described as immature; unsocial; tiring; frustrating; and a cause of hairy palms, warts, blemishes, and blindness. None of these myths is true. Even Freud felt that masturbation was normal for children. Sex educators recommend masturbation to adolescents as a means of releasing tension and becoming familiar with their sexual organs. Throughout adulthood, masturbation often is the primary sexual activity of individuals not involved in a sexual relationship and can be particularly useful when illness, absence, divorce, or death deprives a person of a partner. In the University of Chicago survey, about 25 percent of men and 9 percent of women said they masturbate at least once a week.

White men and women have a higher incidence of masturbation than African-American men and women. Latino women have the lowest rate of masturbation, compared with Latino men, white men and women, and black men and women. Individuals with a higher level of education are more likely to masturbate than those with less schooling, and people living with sexual partners masturbate more than those who live alone.

Masturbation helps some people make better decisions about getting sexually involved with others. Self-stimula-

What do students do?	Percentage
Access sexual material on the Internet	43.5%
Search for sex online	56.5% of men 35.2% of women
Access these materials frequently	2.9%
Click on sex sites to become aroused	19%
Go online to enhance their sex lives with their real-life boyfriend or girlfriend	13%
Masturbate while online	15% of men 12% of women
Had cybersex with an online partner	3.1% of men 5.3% of women

Figure 8-7 CYBERSEX ON CAMPUS
A study of more than 500 undergraduates found that many students use the Internet as a resource for a variety of sexual activities.

Source: Patricia Goodson et al "Searching for Sexually Explicit Materials on the Internet: An Exploratory Study of College Students' Behavior and Attitudes." *Archives of Sexual Behavior*, Vol. 30, No. 3, April 2001, p. 101.

Savvy Consumer

X-RATED ONLINE SITES

Sex is the number-one word searched for online. About 15 percent of Americans logging onto the Internet visit sexually oriented sites. Men are the largest consumers of sexually explicit material and outnumber women by a ratio of six to one. However, while men look for visual erotica, women are more likely to visit chat rooms, which offer more interactions. Most people who check out sex sites on the Internet do not suffer any negative impact, but psychologists warn of some potential risks, including the following:

- *Dependence.* Individuals who spend eleven hours or more a week online in sexual pursuits show signs of psychologi-

cal distress and admit that their behavior interferes with some areas of their lives.

- *Interference with work and study.* While most individuals use their home computers when surfing the Internet for sex-related sites, one in ten has used a school computer. Some universities have strict policies barring such practices and may take punitive actions against employees who violate the rules.

- *Sexual compulsivity.* A small but significant number of users are at risk of a serious problem as a result of their heavy Internet use.

- *Dishonesty.* Most Internet surfers admit that they occasionally "pretend" about their age on the Internet. Most keep secret how much time they spend on sexual pursuits in cyberspace.

tion also can aid women learning to experience orgasms or men experimenting with ways of delaying ejaculation. Some people find that masturbation enables them to relax and fall asleep more easily at night.

Kissing and Touching

A kiss is a universal sign of affection. A kiss can be just a kiss—a quick press of the lips—or it can lead to much more. Usually kissing is the first sexual activity that couples engage in, and even after years of sexual experimentation and sharing, it remains an enduring pleasure for partners.

Touching is a silent form of communication between friends and lovers. Although a touch to any part of the body can be thrilling, some areas, such as the breasts and

Rob Lewine/CORBIS

The magic of touch. Thrilling, soothing, stimulating— touch is a powerful way to communicate affection and sexual pleasure.

genitals, are especially sensitive. Stimulating these **erogenous** regions can lead to orgasm in both men and women. Though such forms of stimulation often accompany intercourse, more couples are gaining an appreciation of these activities as primary sources of sexual fulfillment— and as safer alternatives to intercourse.

Intercourse

Vaginal **intercourse,** or coitus, refers to the penetration of the vagina by the penis (see Figure 8-8). This is the preferred form of sexual intimacy for most heterosexual couples, who may use a wide variety of positions. The most familiar position for intercourse in our society is the so-called missionary position, with the man on top, facing the woman. An alternative is the woman on top, either lying down or sitting upright. Other positions include lying side by side (either face to face or with the man behind the woman, his penis entering her vagina from the rear); lying with the man on top of the woman in a rear-entry position; and kneeling or standing (again, in either a face-to-face or rear-entry position). Many couples move into several different positions for intercourse during a single episode of lovemaking; others may have a personal favorite or may choose different positions at different times.

Sexual activity, including intercourse, is possible throughout a woman's menstrual cycle. However, some women prefer to avoid sex while menstruating because of uncomfortable physical symptoms, such as cramps, or concern about bleeding or messiness. Others use a diaphragm or cervical cap (see Chapter 9) to hold back menstrual flow. Since different cultures have different views on intercourse during a woman's period, partners should discuss their own feelings and try to respect each other's views. If

Fallopian tube
Uterus
Cervix
Bladder
Grafenberg spot (G spot)
Penis
Urethra
Clitoris
Rectum
Anus

Vas deferens
Seminal vesicle
Prostate gland
Rectum
Cowper's gland
Anus
Testis

Figure 8-8 A CROSS-SECTIONAL VIEW OF SEXUAL INTERCOURSE

Sperm are formed in each of the testes and stored in the epididymis. When a man ejaculates, sperm traveling in semen travel up the vas deferens. (The prostate gland and seminal vesicles contribute components of the semen.) The semen is expelled from the penis through the urethra and deposited in the vagina, near the cervix. During sexual excitement and orgasm in a woman, the upper end of the vagina enlarges and the uterus elevates. After orgasm, these organs return to their normal states, and the cervix descends into the pool of semen.

they choose not to have intercourse, there are other gratifying forms of sexual activity.

Vaginal intercourse, like other forms of sexual activity involving an exchange of bodily fluids, carries a risk of sexually transmitted infections, including HIV infection. In many other parts of the world, in fact, heterosexual intercourse is the most common means of HIV transmission. (See Chapter 13.)

Oral-Genital Sex

Our mouths and genitals give us some of our most intense pleasures. Though it might seem logical to combine the two, some people are very uncomfortable with it. Some people consider oral-genital sex a perversion; it is against the law in some states and a sin in some religions. However, others find it normal and acceptable. (The same comments apply to anal sex as well—see the next section.)

The formal terms for oral sex are **cunnilingus,** which refers to oral stimulation of the woman's genitals, and **fellatio,** oral stimulation of the man's genitals. For many couples, oral-genital sex is a regular part of their lovemaking. For others, it's an occasional experiment. Oral sex with a partner carrying a sexually transmitted infection, such as herpes or HIV infection, can lead to infection, so a condom should be used (with cunnilingus, a condom cut in half to lay flat can be used).

 Different groups of the population have diverse views of oral sex. In one survey, more African-American than white men reported never having performed or received oral sex.[42]

Anal Stimulation and Intercourse

Because the anus has many nerve endings, it can produce intense erotic responses. Stimulation of the anus by the fingers or mouth can be a source of sexual arousal; anal intercourse involves penile penetration of the anus. An estimated 25 percent of adults have experienced anal intercourse at least once. However, anal sex involves important health risks, such as damage to sensitive rectal tissues and the transmission of various intestinal infections, hepatitis, and STIs, including HIV.

 ## Cultural Variations

While the biological mechanisms underlying human sexual arousal and response are essentially universal, the particular sexual stimuli or behaviors that people find arousing are greatly influenced by cultural conditioning. For example, in Western societies, where the emphasis during sexual activity tends to be heavily weighted toward achieving orgasm, genitally focused activities are frequently defined as optimally arousing. In contrast, devotees to Eastern Tantric traditions (where spirituality is interwoven with sexuality) often achieve optimal pleasure by emphasizing the sensual and spiritual aspects of shared intimacy rather than orgasmic release.

Kissing on the mouth, a universal source of sexual arousal in Western society, may be rare or absent in many other parts of the world. Certain North American Eskimo people and inhabitants of the Trobriand Islands would rather rub noses than lips, and among the Thonga of South Africa, kissing is viewed as odious behavior. The Hindu people of India are also disinclined to kiss because they believe such contact symbolically contaminates the act of sexual intercourse. One survey of 190 societies found that mouth kissing was acknowledged in only 21 societies and practiced as a prelude or accompaniment to coitus in only 13.

Oral sex (both cunnilingus and fellatio) is a common source of sexual arousal among island societies of the South Pacific, in industrialized nations of Asia, and in much of the Western world. In contrast, in Africa (with the exception of northern regions), such practices are likely to be viewed as unnatural or disgusting behavior.

Foreplay in general, whether it be oral sex, sensual touching, or passionate kissing, is subject to wide cultural variation. In some societies, most notably those with Eastern traditions, couples may strive to prolong intense states of sexual arousal for several hours. While varied patterns of foreplay are common in Western cultures, these activities often are of short duration as lovers move rapidly toward the "main event" of coitus. In still other societies, foreplay is either sharply curtailed or absent altogether. For example, the Lepcha farmers of the southeastern Himalayas limit foreplay to men briefly caressing their partners' breasts, and among the Irish inhabitants of Inis Beag, pre-coital sexual activity is reported to be limited to mouth kissing and rough fondling of the woman's lower body by her partner.

Sexual Response

Sexuality involves every part of you: mind and body, muscles and skin, glands and genitals. The pioneers in finding out exactly how human beings respond to sex were William Masters and Virginia Johnson, who first studied more than 800 individuals in their laboratory in the 1950s. They discovered that sexual response is a well-ordered sequence of events, so predictable it could be divided into four phases: excitement, plateau, orgasm, and resolution (see Figure 8-9). In real life, individuals don't necessarily follow this well-ordered pattern. But the responses for both sexes are remarkably similar. And sexual response always follows the same sequence, whatever the means of stimulation.

Males

Excitement

Testes enlarge and elevate, penis becomes partially erect

Plateau

Testes are fully elevated; penis reaches full erection, glans swell, drops of fluid are released

Orgasm

Contractions release semen into urethra; urethral sphincter relaxes, penile contractions occur, semen is ejaculated

Resolution

Erection disappears, testes descend

Females

Excitement

Inner vagina expands, clitoris swells, and labia swell

Plateau

Inner vagina becomes fully expanded, outer vagina swells, and clitoris retracts under hood

Orgasm

Anal sphincter contracts, uterus contracts, and outer vagina contracts

Resolution

Uterus lowers, vagina returns to normal

Figure 8-9 HUMAN SEXUAL RESPONSE

The four stages of sexual response are excitement, plateau, orgasm, and resolution.

Excitement

Stimulation is the first step: a touch, a look, a fantasy. In men, sexual stimuli set off a rush of blood to the genitals, filling the blood vessels in the penis. Because these vessels are wrapped in a thick sheath of tissue, the penis becomes erect. The testes lift.

Women respond to stimulation with vaginal lubrication within 10 to 20 seconds of exposure to sexual stimuli. The clitoris becomes larger, as do the vaginal lips (the labia), the nipples, and later the breasts. The vagina lengthens, and its inner two-thirds increase in size. The uterus lifts, further increasing the free space in the vagina.

Plateau

During this stage, the changes begun in the excitement stage continue and intensify. The penis further increases in both length and diameter. The outer one-third of the vagina swells. During intercourse, the vaginal muscles grasp the penis to increase stimulation for both partners. The upper two-thirds of the vagina become wider as the uterus moves up; eventually its diameter is 2½ to 3 inches.

Orgasm

Men and women have remarkably similar **orgasm** experiences. Both men and women typically have 3 to 12 pelvic muscle contractions approximately four-fifths of a second apart and lasting up to 60 seconds. Both undergo contractions and spasms of other muscles, as well as increases in breathing and pulse rates, and blood pressure. Both can sometimes have orgasms simply from kisses, stimulation of the breasts or other parts of the body, or fantasy alone.

The process of **ejaculation** (the discharge of semen by a male) requires two separate events. First, the vas deferens, the seminal vesicles, the prostate, and the upper portion of the urethra contract. The man perceives these subtle contractions deep in his pelvis just before the point of no return—which therapists refer to as the point of "ejaculatory inevitability." Then, seconds later, muscle contractions force semen out of the penis via the urethra.

Female orgasms follow several patterns. Some women experience a series of mini-orgasms—a response sometimes described as "skimming." Another pattern consists of rapid excitement and plateau stages, followed by a prolonged orgasm. This is the most frequent response to stimulation by a vibrator.

Female orgasms are primarily triggered by stimulating the clitoris. When stimulation reaches an adequate level, the vagina responds by contracting. Although it sometimes seems that vaginal stimulation alone can set off an orgasm, the clitoris is usually involved—at least indirectly during full penile penetration.

Some researchers have identified what they call the *Grafenberg* (or *G*) *spot* (or *area*) just behind the front wall of the vagina, between the cervix and the back of the pubic bone (see Figure 8-8). When this region is stimulated, women report various sensations, including slight discomfort, a brief feeling that they need to urinate, and increasing pleasure. Continued stimulation may result in an orgasm of great intensity, accompanied by ejaculation of fluid from the urethra. However, other researchers have failed to confirm the existence and importance of the G spot, and sex therapists disagree about its significance for a woman's sexual satisfaction.

Resolution

The sexual organs of men and women return to their normal, nonexcited state during this final phase of sexual response. Heightened skin color quickly fades after orgasm, and the heart rate, blood pressure, and breathing rate soon return to normal. The clitoris also resumes its normal position and appearance very shortly thereafter, whereas the penis may remain somewhat erect for up to 30 minutes.

After orgasm, men typically enter a **refractory period,** during which they are incapable of another orgasm. The duration of this period varies from minutes to days, depending on age and the frequency of previous sexual activity. If either partner doesn't have an orgasm after becoming highly aroused, resolution may be much slower and may be accompanied by a sense of discomfort.

▪ Sexual Concerns

Many sexual concerns stem from myths and misinformation. There is no truth, for instance, behind these misconceptions: men are always capable of erection, sex always involves intercourse, partners should experience simultaneous orgasms, or people who truly love each other always have satisfying sex lives.

Cultural and childhood influences can affect our attitudes toward sex. Even though America's traditionally puritanical values have eased, our society continues to convey mixed messages about sex. Some children, repeatedly warned of the evils of sex, never accept the sexual dimensions of their identity. Others—especially young boys—may be exposed to macho attitudes toward sex and feel a need to prove their virility. Young girls may feel confused by media messages that encourage them to look and act provocatively and a double standard that blames them for leading boys on. In addition, virtually everyone has individual worries. A woman may feel self-conscious about the shape of her breasts; a man may worry about the size of his penis; both partners may fear not pleasing the other.

The concept of sexual normalcy differs greatly in different times, cultures, or racial and ethnic groups. In certain times and places, only sex between a husband and wife has been deemed normal. In other circumstances, "normal" has been applied to any sexual behavior—alone or with others—that does not harm others or produce great anxiety and guilt. The following are some of the most common contemporary sexual concerns.

Safer Sex

Having sex is never completely safe; the only 100 percent risk-free sexual choice is abstinence. If you choose to be sexually active, you can greatly reduce your risk by restricting sexual activity to the context of a mutually exclusive, monogamous relationship in which both partners know, on the basis of laboratory testing, that neither has HIV antibodies or a sexually transmitted infection (STI). Sober sex, in which both partners are not under the influence of drugs or alcohol, is more likely to be safer sex.

For centuries, sexually transmitted infections, such as gonorrhea and syphilis, caused great suffering and many deaths. Modern medicine has developed effective treatments for these health threats, but other STIs, such as herpes and chlamydia, have become serious health problems. The incidence of STIs has been rising, particularly among the young. A quarter of all STIs in the United States occur among adolescents, and a quarter of sexually active adolescents acquire an STI each year. The United States has the highest rate of STIs among all developed countries, yet there is no effective national system of STI prevention. (Chapter 13 provides a complete discussion of the symptoms, diagnosis, and treatment of sexually transmitted infections, including HIV infection and AIDS.)

Sex with a person who has never been exposed to HIV or to other STIs is safe (for you), regardless of what type of sexual activity you engage in. The only way of knowing for certain that a prospective partner doesn't have an STI or is not infected with HIV is through laboratory testing (see Chapter 13). Sex educators and health professionals strongly encourage couples to abstain from any sexual activity that puts them at risk for STIs until they both undergo medical examinations and testing for STIs. This process greatly reduces the danger of disease transmission and can also help foster a deep sense of mutual trust and commitment. Many campus and public health clinics provide exams or laboratory testing either free of charge or on a sliding scale determined by your income.

 In a study of college students, information on how many couples practice safer sex had unexpected effects. On the one hand, when students learn that the prevalence of safer sex is high, they see this as "normative" or typical, acceptable behavior. On the other hand, they conclude that because of this, their perceived risk is lower—so they are less likely to say they intend to use condoms the next time they engage in sex.[43]

Talking to a potential partner is the first step toward safer sex. Professionals offer advice on how to discuss a topic that makes many people uncomfortable: Choose a time and place that is relaxed and comfortable. Arm yourself with facts so you can answer any questions or objections your partner raises. Start on a positive note—for instance, by saying how much you care for your partner and saying that this is the reason you want to discuss something important. This is the time for you to be honest about any STIs you might have had or still carry. Give your partner time to take in what you've said. If you find out about a partner's STI, you may feel a range of emotions. You also will need to acquire information about symptoms, treatment, and how the disease is spread.[44]

Sex educators also are urging greater use of the media to promote responsible sexual behavior, as occurs in other countries. Several international studies have shown that exposure to family planning messages through television, radio, and print increases condom use. In the United States, safe sex media campaigns are linked with a decrease in sexual activity by teens and an increase in condom use with casual partners.[45]

What Are the Most Common Sexual Problems?

A sexual difficulty may occur anywhere in the sexual response sequence. A man's penis may not become erect; a woman's vagina may not become moist. A man may lose

Sexual problems can be difficult for partners to talk about, but lack of communication can create tension and anxiety.

his erection while attempting intercourse; the woman's vagina may become dry after penetration. Some men and women become excited, enjoy the plateau stage, but then don't achieve an orgasm; or their sexual cycle may be too long or too short for one of the partners. Sometimes the cause of the problem is alcohol or drugs, disease, injury, stress, or chronic pain. Often, however, it's fear or ignorance.

One of the most common feelings associated with sex—along with curiosity, desire, and love—is anxiety. No one is born knowing about sex. Most of us learn from our experiences, and—as with most activities, from skiing to speaking French—our first attempts tend to be awkward. A caring, loving relationship can make all the difference.

Sexual Dysfunction

SIECUS defines **sexual dysfunction** as the inability to react emotionally and/or physically to sexual stimulation in a way expected of the average healthy person or according to one's own standards. Sexual dysfunctions, which have a wide range of psychological and physiological origins, can affect different stages in the sexual response cycle. They are not all-or-nothing problems but vary considerably in how severe they are and how frequently they occur. In as many as one-third of people with sexual problems, the partner also has a sexual dysfunction.

Most men and women at one time or another experience some sort of sexual difficulty, but they tend to develop different types. Men are more likely to seek and receive treatment for sexual problems. Nevertheless, they find them very difficult to talk about and may delay or avoid seeking help. In women, the most common sexual dysfunction is loss of desire for sexual activity.

Problems with Arousal

Perfectly healthy couples with no physical impairment sometimes simply become bored with sex, even though they love each other and find each other attractive and enjoyable. Men and women may lose interest in sex, and often neither partner has had previous arousal or orgasm problems. Physical disorders, including neurological and endocrine diseases, can affect sexual desire, as can psychological conditions such as depression and fatigue. Many medications and drugs of abuse also can inhibit desire.

Often stress—perhaps caused by a recent move, a new baby, or a high-pressure job—is the real culprit. Severe stress can short-circuit normal sexual response. Couples who try to unwind by drinking or using tranquilizers usu-

ally make the problem worse by further dampening their sexual responses.

Erectile Dysfunction

An NIH consensus conference has defined **erectile dysfunction** (ED, also referred to as **impotence**) as the consistent inability to maintain a penile erection sufficient for adequate sexual relations.[46] Virtually all men are occasionally unable to achieve or maintain an erection because of fatigue, stress, alcohol, or drug use.

Psychological factors, such as anxiety about performance, may cause erectile dysfunction. But in as many as 80 percent of cases, the problem has physical origins. Diabetes and reactions to drugs—including an estimated 200 prescription medications—are the most frequent organic causes. Even cigarettes can create erection problems for men sensitive to nicotine. Erectile dysfunction increases with advancing age. An estimated 45 percent of men ages 65 to 69 have moderate or complete ED.[47]

Viagra

A little blue pill called Viagra (sildenafil), which delays the breakdown of an enzyme involved in deflating the penis after ejaculation, revolutionized therapy for ED. However, urologists estimate that less than 15 percent of the 150 million men with erectile dysfunction have used Viagra.

FACT OR FICTION?

Viagra is a permanent cure for erectile dysfunction.

Fiction: The effects of Viagra are temporary, lasting no longer than four hours. Although scientists had theorized that regular use of Viagra might bolster a man's erectile function over time, this has not proven to be the case. Men who need Viagra continue to require the medication for intercourse despite frequent long-term use. In a study of 200 men who had used Viagra for at least two years, 20 percent of men had to increase the dose to get the same benefits as they did initially. Another 17 percent stopped using the drug because it no longer had any impact, even at higher doses.

Source: "Viagra and Erections: Do the Benefits Persist?" *Harvard Men's Health Watch*, January 2003. www.health.harvard.edu/medline/Men/N0103b.html.

About half of men don't refill their prescriptions within a year, usually because of side effects or lack of efficacy. Contrary to early assumptions, Viagra does not lead to permanent improvement in sexual functioning.[48] (See Fact or Fiction? "Viagra is a permanent cure . . .")

There are medical risks associated with Viagra use, and more than 130 deaths have been associated with the drug.[49] The FDA requires health labels on bottles of Viagra that warn doctors and patients that men with heart problems and very high or very low blood pressure should be carefully examined before getting a prescription. Interactions with certain drugs, such as heart medications containing nitrate, have proven fatal. Other medications, including antifungal medications and the antibiotic erythromycin, also can affect Viagra's metabolism and excretion. Some users experience visual side effects, but these are temporary and are not considered serious. However, despite the warnings and risks, many men have bought Viagra online after filling out an application reviewed by a medical doctor—a practice condemned by medical societies and by the drug's manufacturer.

Alternatives to Viagra, recently released in the U.S., claim to work faster and last longer than the original. Women have tried Viagra to increase their sexual responsiveness. Generally it has not proven beneficial, but researchers are testing other products, such as a prostaglandin cream, that may improve female sexual satisfaction.

Orgasm Problems in Men

About 20 percent of men complain of **premature ejaculation,** which is defined as ejaculating within 30 to 90 seconds of inserting the penis into the vagina, or after 10 to 15 thrusts. Another definition is that a premature ejaculator cannot control or delay his ejaculation long enough to satisfy a responsive partner at least half the time. By this definition, a man may be premature with some women but not with others.[50]

To delay orgasm, men may try to think of baseball or other sports, but this just makes sex boring. Others may masturbate before intercourse, hoping to take advantage of the refractory period, during which they cannot ejaculate again. Others may bite their lips or dig their nails into their palms—although usually this just results in premature ejaculators with bloody lips and scarred palms. Topical anesthetics used to prevent climax dull pleasurable sensations for the woman as well as for the man.

Researchers are studying several medications, including clomipramine, SSRIs, and Viagra in the treatment of premature ejaculation. The combination of medication and psychological and behavioral counseling seems most effective.[51]

Men can learn to control their ejaculation by concentrating on their sexual responses, rather than by trying to distract themselves or ignore their reactions. Some men find that they have greater control by lying on their backs with their partner on top, by relaxing during intercourse, and by communicating with their partner about when to stop or slow down movements.

Other techniques for delaying ejaculation include *stop-start,* in which a man learns to sense the feelings that precede ejaculation and stop his movements before the point of ejaculatory inevitability, allowing his arousal to subside slightly before restarting sexual activity. In the *squeeze technique,* a man's partner applies strong pressure with her thumb on the frenum (the thin strip of skin that connects the glans to the shaft on the underside of the penis) and her second and third fingers on the top side of the penis, one above and one below the corona (rim of penile glans), until the man loses the urge to ejaculate.

Female Sexual Dysfunction

The American Foundation for Urological Disease classifies female sexual dysfunction into four categories: sexual desire disorders, arousal disorders, orgasmic disorders, and sexual pain disorders.[52] How common are these problems? That's hard to estimate. In a recent online survey, 40 percent of women reported that they did not seek help from a physician for sexual complaints, even though 5 percent said that they would like to.[53] Some sex therapists have speculated that as many as 43 percent of American women may have some form of sexual dysfunction.[54]

Many health professionals remain dubious about the "medicalization" of various patterns of female sexual response.[55] Scientists at the Kinsey Institute for Research in Sex, Gender, and Reproduction, for instance, caution that a pill, whatever its nature, may not be the solution to many women's sexual concerns. In women, psychology often is as or even more important than physiology, and effective therapy must address psychological problems in a sexual relationship as well as social constraints and inhibitions.[56]

Some forms of female sexual dysfunction do respond to various therapies. These include **dyspareunia,** or pain during intercourse, and **vaginismus,** an extreme form of painful intercourse in which involuntary contractions of the muscles of the outer third of the vagina are so intense that they totally or partially close the vaginal opening. This problem often derives from a fear of being penetrated. Relaxation techniques, such as *Kegel exercises* (alternately tightening and relaxing the muscles of the pelvic floor), or the use of fingers or dilators to gradually open the vagina, can make penetration easier.

The female orgasm has long been a controversial sexual topic. According to recent estimates, about 90 percent of sexually active women have experienced orgasm, but only a much smaller percentage achieve orgasm through intercourse alone. Even fewer reach orgasm if intercourse isn't accompanied by direct stimulation of the clitoris. Is intercourse without orgasm a sexual problem? The best answer is that it is a problem if a woman wants to experience orgasm during intercourse but doesn't.

Many counseling programs urge women who have never had orgasms to masturbate. They are then encouraged to share with their partners what they've learned, communicating with words or gestures what is most pleasing to them. Some women want more than a single orgasm during intercourse. Partners can help by varying positions and experimenting with sexual techniques. However, in sexual response, more is not necessarily better, and the couple should keep in mind that no one else is counting.

Sex Therapy

Modern sex therapy, pioneered by Masters and Johnson in the 1960s, views sex as a natural, healthy behavior that enhances a couple's relationship. Their approach emphasizes education, communication, reduction of performance anxiety, and sexual exercises that enhance sexual intimacy.

Today most sex therapists, working either alone or with a partner, have modified Masters and Johnson's approach. Most see couples once a week for eight to ten weeks; the focus of therapy is on correcting dysfunctional behavior, not exploring underlying psychodynamics.

Contrary to common misconceptions, sex therapy does not involve conducting sexual activity in front of therapists. The therapist may review psychological and physiological aspects of sexual functioning and evaluate the couple's sexual attitudes and ability to communicate. The core of the program is the couple's "homework"—a series of exercises, carried out in private, that enhances their sensory awareness and improves nonverbal communication. These techniques have proven effective for couples regardless of their age or general health.

You and your partner should consider consulting a sex therapist if any of the following is true for you:

:: Sex is painful or physically uncomfortable.

:: You're having sex less and less frequently.

:: You have a general fear of, or revulsion toward, sex.

:: Your sexual pleasure is declining.

:: Your sexual desire is diminishing.

:: Your sexual problems are increasing in frequency or persisting for longer periods.

Drugs and Sex

Many recreational drugs, such as alcohol and marijuana, are believed to enhance sexual performance. However, none of the popular drugs touted as *aphrodisiac*—including amphetamines, barbiturates, cantharides ("Spanish fly"), cocaine, LSD and other psychedelics, marijuana, amyl nitrite ("poppers"), and L-dopa (a medication used to treat Parkinson's disease)—is truly a sexual stimulant. In fact, these drugs often interfere with normal sexual response. Researchers are studying one drug that may truly enhance sexual performance: yohimbine hydrochloride, which is derived from the sap of the tropical yohimbe tree that grows in West Africa.

Because many psychiatric problems can lower sexual desire and affect sexual functioning, medications appropriate to the specific disorders can help. In addition, psychiatric drugs may be used as part of therapy. Drugs such as certain antidepressants may be used to prolong sexual response in conditions such as premature ejaculation.

Medications can also cause sexual difficulty. In men, drugs that are used to treat high blood pressure, anxiety, allergies, depression, muscle spasms, obesity, ulcers, irritable colon, and prostate cancer can cause impotence, breast enlargement, testicular swelling, priapism (persistent erection), loss of sexual desire, inability to ejaculate, and reduced sperm count. In women, they can diminish sexual desire, inhibit or delay orgasm, and cause breast swelling or secretions.

Atypical Behavior

Although sexual desire and response are universal, some individuals develop sexual appetites or engage in activities that are not typical sexual behaviors.

Sexual Addiction

Some men and women can get relief from their feelings of restlessness and worthlessness only through sex (either masturbation or with a partner). Once the sexual high ends, however, they're overwhelmed by the same negative feelings and driven, once more, to have sex.

Some therapists describe this problem as **sexual addiction;** others, as **sexual compulsion.** Professionals continue to debate exactly what this controversial condition is, how to diagnose it, and how to overcome it. However, most agree that for some people, sex is more than a normal pleasure: It is an overwhelming need that must be met, even at the cost of their careers and marriages.

Sex addicts can be heterosexual or homosexual, male or female. Their behaviors include masturbation, phone sex, reading or viewing pornography, attending strip shows, having affairs, engaging in anonymous sex with strangers or prostitutes, exhibitionism, voyeurism, child molestation, incest, and rape. Many were physically and emotionally abused as children or have family members who abuse drugs or alcohol. They typically feel a loss of control and a compulsion for sexual activity, and they continue their unhealthy (and sometimes illegal) sexual behavior despite the dangers, including the risk of contracting STIs. Characteristics exhibited by sex addicts include:

:: A preoccupation with sex so intense and chronic that it interferes with a normal sexual relationship with a spouse or lover.

:: A compulsion to have sex again and again within a short period of time, and to engage in sexual behavior that results in feelings of anxiety, depression, guilt, or shame.

:: A great deal of time spent away from family or work, in order to look for sex partners or engage in sex.

:: Use of sex to hide from troubles.

With help, sex addicts can deal with the shame that both triggers and follows sexual activity. Professional therapy may begin with a month of complete sexual abstinence, to break the cycle of compulsive sexual behavior. Several organizations, such as Sexaholics Anonymous and Sexual Addicts Anonymous, offer support from people who share the same problem.

Sexual Deviations

Sexual deviations listed by the American Psychiatric Association include the following:

:: **Fetishism:** Obtaining sexual pleasure from an inanimate object or an asexual part of the body, such as the foot.

:: **Transvestitism:** Becoming sexually aroused by wearing the clothing of the opposite sex.

:: **Exhibitionism:** Exposing one's genitals to an unwilling observer.

:: **Voyeurism:** Obtaining sexual gratification by observing people undressing or involved in sexual activity.

:: **Sadism:** Becoming sexually aroused by inflicting physical or psychological pain.

:: **Masochism:** Obtaining sexual gratification by suffering physical or psychological pain.

Another, increasingly common sexual variation, hypoxyphilia, involves attempts to enhance the pleasure of orgasm by reducing oxygen intake. Individuals who do so by tying a noose around the neck have accidentally killed themselves.

Psychiatrists distinguish between passive sexual deviancy, which doesn't involve actual contact with another, and aggressive deviancy. Most voyeurs and obscene phone callers don't seek physical contact with the objects of their sexual desire. These behaviors are performed predominantly, but not exclusively, by males.

Transgenderism

Transgendered individuals, formerly called *transsexuals,* have gender identities opposite their biological sex. Most are males who feel deeply that they are more truly females. More than 3,000 Americans have undergone complex medical procedures to change their genital and secondary sex characteristics. Those who desire *sex-change operations* should be carefully screened and counseled to determine whether such extreme measures would be appropriate and beneficial.

Sex sells. Topless bars and strip clubs are among the businesses that cater to those who enjoy sexual stimulation outside a loving relationship.

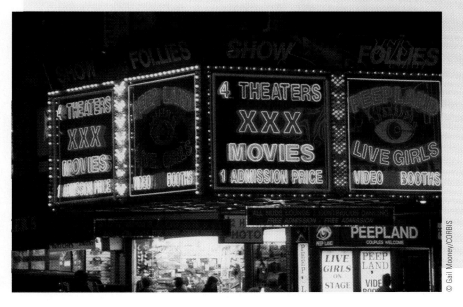

© Gail Mooney/CORBIS

The Business of Sex

Sex, without affection and individuality, becomes a product to be packaged, marketed, traded, bought, and sold. Two of the billion-dollar industries that treat sex as a commodity are prostitution and pornography.

Prostitution, described as the world's oldest profession, is a nationwide industry grossing more than $1 billion annually. In every state except Nevada (and in all but a few counties there), prostitution is illegal. Besides the threat of jail and fines, prostitutes and their clients face another danger: sexually transmitted infections, including HIV infection and hepatitis B.

Pornography is a multimedia industry—books, magazines, movies, the Internet, phone lines, and computer games are available to those who find sexually explicit material entertaining or exciting. Most laws against pornography are based on the assumption that such materials can set off uncontrollable, dangerous sexual urges, ranging from promiscuity to sexual violence. Research indicates that exposure to scenes of rape or other forms of sexual violence against women, or to scenes of degradation of women, does lead to tolerance of these hostile and brutal acts.

Bottom Line ▼
Smarter Sex

We remain sexual beings throughout life. At different ages and stages, sexuality can take on different meanings. As you forge relationships and explore your sexuality, you may encounter difficult situations and unfamiliar feelings. But sex is never just about hormones and body parts. People describe the brain as the sexiest of our organs. Using your brain to make responsible sexual decisions leads to both a smarter and a more fulfilling sex life.

:: *Be sure sexual activity is consensual.* Coercion can take many forms: physical, emotional, and verbal. All cause psychological damage and undermine trust and respect.

:: *No means no.* At any point in a relationship, whether the couple is dating or married, either individual has the right to say no.

:: *In sexual situations, always think ahead.* For the sake of safety, think about potential dangers—parking in an isolated area, going into a bedroom with someone you hardly know, and the like—and options to protect yourself.

:: *Be aware of your own and your partner's alcohol and drug intake.* The use of such substances impairs judgment and reduces the ability to say no. While under

their influence, you may engage in sexual behavior you'll later regret.

:: *Be prepared.* If there's any possibility that you may be engaging in sex, be sure you have the means to protect yourself against unwanted pregnancy and sexually transmitted infections.

:: *Communicate openly.* If you or your partner cannot talk openly and honestly about your sexual histories and contraception, you should avoid having sex. For the sake of protecting your sexual health, you have to be willing to ask—and answer—questions that may seem embarrassing.

:: *Share responsibility in a sexual relationship.* Both partners should be involved in protecting themselves and each other from STIs and, if heterosexual, unwanted pregnancy.

:: *Respect sexual privacy.* Revealing sexual activities violates the trust between two partners. Bragging about a sexual conquest demeans everyone involved.

:: *Do not sexually harass others.* Pinches, pats, sexual comments or jokes, and suggestive gestures are offensive and disrespectful. (See Chapter 18 for more on harassment.)

:: *Be considerate.* A public display of sexual affection can be extremely embarrassing to others. Roommates, in particular, should be sensitive and discrete in their sexual behavior.

Source: Adapted from: Robert Hatcher et al. *Sexual Etiquette 101.* Atlanta, GA: Emory University School of Medicine.

 After watching the CNN video segment, discuss the following question. What does research say about the connection between chat rooms and STDs?

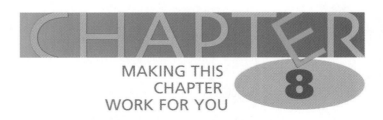

MAKING THIS CHAPTER WORK FOR YOU **8**

1. The hormones that influence the early development of sexual organs
   a. are released by the ovaries in the female and the testes in the male.
   b. begin to work soon after conception during the embryo's development.

c. begin to work during puberty, when they stimulate the development of secondary male and female sex characteristics.

d. determine one's biological sex.

2. Which of the following statements about the menstrual cycle is true?

a. The pituitary gland releases estrogen and progesterone.

b. Ovulation occurs at the end of the menstrual cycle.

c. Premenstrual syndrome is a physiological disorder that usually results in amenorrhea.

d. The endometrium becomes thicker during the cycle and is shed during menstruation.

3. Which statement about male anatomy is *incorrect*?

a. The testes manufacture testosterone and sperm.

b. Sperm cells are carried in the liquid semen.

c. Cowper's glands secrete semen.

d. Circumcision is the surgical removal of the foreskin of the penis.

4. Which of the following behaviors is most likely to be a characteristic of sexually healthy and responsible adults?

a. engages in frequent sexual encounters with many partners

b. avoids the use of condoms in order to heighten sexual enjoyment for both partners

c. uses alcohol sparingly and only to help loosen the inhibitions of a resistant partner

d. engages in sex that is unquestionably consensual

5. Which of the following statements is true about sexual orientation?

a. Most individuals who identify themselves as bisexual are really homosexual.

b. Homosexuality is caused by a poor family environment.

c. Homosexual behavior is found only in affluent and well-educated cultures.

d. The African-American, Hispanic, and Asian cultures tend to be less accepting of homosexuality than the white community.

6. According to the Centers for Disease Control, abstinence is defined as

a. refraining from all sexual behaviors that result in arousal.

b. refraining from all sexual activities that involve vaginal, anal, and oral intercourse.

c. having sexual intercourse with only one partner exclusively.

d. refraining from drinking alcohol before sexual activity.

7. Which statement about college students is *not* true?

a. They consider sexual activity as normal for their peer group.

b. Most take sex and monogamy seriously.

c. More than 40 percent do not use condoms.

d. Women trust a man as safe and healthy on the basis of the way he looks.

8. Which of the following statements about erectile dysfunction is false?

a. ED is usually caused by physical factors.

b. A popular treatment for ED is Viagra.

c. ED is usually caused by psychological factors.

d. Men who are heavy smokers are at risk for developing ED.

9. Women may experience which of the following problems during intercourse?

a. vaginismus

b. excitement

c. vaginal expansion

d. amenorrhea

10. Atypical sexual behaviors include which of the following?

a. masochism

b. sexual desire

c. masturbation

d. celibacy

Answers to these questions can be found on page 652.

Critical Thinking

1. Bill has told his girlfriend, Anita, that he has never taken any sexual risks. But when she suggested that they get tested for STIs, he became furious and refused. Now Anita says she doesn't know what to believe. Could Bill be telling the truth, or is he hiding something? If he is telling the truth, why is Bill so upset? Anita doesn't want to take any risks, but she doesn't want to lose him either. What would you advise her to say or do? What would you advise Bill to say or do?

Critical Thinking

2. Do you think it is okay to read or look at pornographic books, magazines, websites, and videos? Why or why not?

Critical Thinking

3. What do you think about the legalization of homosexual marriages? Many gay people feel that they will never be fully accepted in society unless they can legally marry. In

Critical Thinking

addition, without the sanction of marriage, homosexual partners may not be recognized as the legal "next of kin" in medical emergencies or in inheritance situations.

Critical Thinking

Some heterosexuals think that gay marriages would violate the sanctity of marriage. Do you think homosexual marriages should be accepted? Why or why not?

Profile Plus

What is your sex IQ? Discover how accurate your knowledge is about sexual issues with this activity on your Profile Plus CD-ROM.

Profile Plus

• How Much Do You Know About Sex?

Profile Plus

Sites and Bytes

The Sexuality Information and Education Council of the U.S. (SIECUS)

www.siecus.org

This website is sponsored by SIECUS, a national, nonprofit organization that promotes comprehensive education about sexuality and advocates the right of all individuals of all sexual orientations to make responsible sexual choices. The site features a library of facts sheets and articles on a variety of sexuality topics and STIs, designed for educators, adults, teens, parents, media, international audiences, and religious organizations.

Sites and Bytes

Sexually Transmitted Disease Risk Profiler

www.unspeakable.com/truth.jsp

The Naked Truth, a public health outreach project sponsored as an educational service by Pfizer Inc. pharmaceuticals, sponsors this informative website featuring two interactive sections. First, the Risk Profiler can help you determine your risk of acquiring an STI with thirteen questions about your age, gender, sexual history, and behavior, and shows you how these factors play a part in creating your own personal risk profile. The second interactive site is a ten-question STI Quiz that will give you an opportunity to test your knowledge of STIs, and learn more about their symptoms, prevention, and treatment.

Sites and Bytes

National Center for HIV, STD, and TB Prevention

www.cdc.gov/hiv/dhap.htm

This site, sponsored by the Centers for Disease Control and Prevention (CDC) features current information, fact sheets, conferences, media campaigns, publications, the 20-year history of HIV/AIDS, information on prevention and treatment, FAQ section, as well as the most current HIV/AIDS statistics.

InfoTrac College Edition

Activity

Synovitz, Linda, et al. "Sexual Knowledge of College Students in a Southern State: Relationship to Sexuality Education," *American Journal of Health Studies,* Vol. 17, No. 4, Fall 2002, p. 163(10).

1. According to the study results, what is the relationship between the college students' perceptions about the quality of their previous HIV/AIDS and STI sexuality educa-

InfoTrac College Edition

tion to their HIV/AIDS and STI knowledge scores?

2. Based on a number of scientific studies, what are the benefits of sexuality education? Does sexuality education increase or decrease sexual activity? Why or why not?

3. What were the results of this study and the implications for colleges and universities?

You can find additional readings related to sexuality with InfoTrac

InfoTrac College Edition

College Edition, an online library of more than 900 journals and publications. Follow the instructions for accessing InfoTrac College Edition that were packaged with your textbook; then search for articles using a key word search.

For additional links, resources, and suggested readings on InfoTrac College Edition, visit our Health & Wellness Resource Center at **http://health.wadsworth.com**.

Key Terms

The terms listed are used on the page indicated. Definitions of the terms are in the Glossary at the end of this book.

Key Terms

Key Terms

Key Terms

References

1. Herman-Giddens, Marcia. Personal interview.
2. Funkhouser, Ellen, et al. "Vaginal Douching Practices Among Women Attending a University in the Southern United States." *Journal of American College Health,* Vol. 50, No. 4, p. 177.
3. Rempel, J. K., and B. Baumgartner. "The Relationship Between Attitudes Towards Menstruation and Sexual Attitudes, Desires, and Behavior in Women," *Archives of Sexual Behavior,* Vol. 32, No. 2, April 2003, p. 155.
4. Dickerson, Lori, et al. "Premenstrual Syndrome." *American Family Physician,* Vol. 67, No. 8, April 15, 2003, p. 1743.
5. Ibid.
6. Freeman, E. W. "Evaluation of a Unique Oral Contraceptive (Yasmin) in the Management of Premenstrual Dysphoric Disorder." *European Journal of Contraception and Reproductive Health Care,* Vol. 7, No. 3, December 2002, p. 27.
7. Dickerson et al., "Premenstrual Syndrome."
8. "Just the Facts . . . Circumcision." American Academy of Pediatrics, www.aap.org/mrt/factscir.htm.
9. Schoen, Edgar, et al. "New Policy on Circumcision—Cause for Concern." *Pediatrics,* Vol. 105, No. 3, March 2000.
10. Adler, Robert, et al. "Circumcision: We Have Heard from the Experts; Now Let's Hear from the Parents." *Pediatrics,* Vol. 107, No. 2, February 2001, p. 395.
11. Crooks, Robert, and Karla Baur. *Our Sexuality,* 8th ed. Pacific Grove, CA: Wadsworth, 2002.
12. www.cdc.gov.
13. Prinstein, M. J., et al. "Adolescent Oral Sex, Peer Popularity, and Perceptions of Best Friends' Sexual Behavior." *Journal of Pediatric Psychology,* Vol. 28, No. 4, June 2003, p. 243.
14. Omar, H., et al. "Educating Adolescents About Puberty: What Are We Missing?" *International Journal of Adolescent Medicine and Health,* Vol. 15, No. 1, January–March 2003, p. 79.
15. "National Survey of Adolescents and Young Adults: Sexual Health Knowledge, Attitudes, and Experiences." Menlo Park, CA: Kaiser Family Foundation, 2003.
16. Ibid.
17. Eisenberg, M. E. "The Association of Campus Resources for Gay, Lesbian, and Bisexual Students with College Students' Condom Use." *Journal of American College Health,* Vol. 51, No. 3, November 2002, p. 109.
18. www.smartersex.org/resources/behind.asp.
19. Luquis, R., et al. "College Students' Perceptions of Substance Use and Sexual Behaviors." *Research Quarterly for Exercise and Sport,* Vol. 72, No. 1, March 2001, p. A-33.
20. Bon, Rebecca, et al. "Normative Perceptions in Relation to Substance Use and HIV-Risky Sexual Behaviors of College Students." *Journal of Psychology,* Vol. 135, No. 2, March 2001, p. 165.
21. Sharman, Garry. "Examining Memory for Heterosexual College Students' Sexual Experiences Using an Electronic Mail Diary." *Health Psychology,* Vol. 21, No. 6, November 2002, p. 629.
22. Hingson, R., et al. "Early Age of First Drunkenness as a Factor in College Students' Unplanned and Unprotected Sex Attributable to Drinking." *Pediatrics,* Vol. 111, No. 1, January 2003, p. 34.
23. Apostolopoulos, Y., et al. "HIV-Risk Behaviours of American Spring Break Vacationers: A Case of Situational Disinhibition?" *International Journal of STDs and AIDS,* Vol. 13, No. 11, November 2002, p. 733.
24. Krahe, B. "Men's Reports of Nonconsensual Sexual Interactions with Women: Prevalence and Impact." *Archives of Sexual Behavior,* Vol. 32, No. 2, April 2003, p. 165.
25. Eisenberg, "The Association of Campus Resources."
26. Duncan, C., et al. "Barriers to Safer Sex Practices Among African American College Students." *Journal of National Medical Association,* Vol. 94, No. 11, November 2002, p. 944.
27. Robinson, John, and Geoffrey Godbey. "No Sex, Please . . . We're College Graduates." *American Demographics,* February 1998.
28. Bailey, J. V., et al. "Sexual Behavior of Lesbians and Bisexual Women." *Sexually Transmitted Infections,* Vol. 79, No. 2, April 2003, p. 147.
29. Crooks and Baur, *Our Sexuality.*
30. Hinrichs D. W., and P. J. Rosenberg. "Attitudes Toward Gay, Lesbian, and Bisexual Persons Among Heterosexual Liberal Arts College Students." *Journal of Homosexuality,* Vol. 43, No. 1, 2002, p. 61.
31. Eisenberg, "The Association of Campus Resources."
32. Goodson, P., et al. "Defining Abstinence: Views of Directors, Instructors, and Participants in Abstinence-Only-Until-Marriage Programs in Texas." *Journal of School Health,* Vol. 73, No. 3, March 2003, p. 91.
33. "Better than Condoms in a Cookie Jar." *American Enterprise,* Vol. 12, No. 3, April 2001, p. 10.
34. Witkin, A., et al. "Comprehensive Versus Abstinence-Only Sex Education: What Works?" *Focus,* Vol. 18, No. 2, January 2003, p. 1.
35. Toomey, Kathleen, and Richard Rothenberg, "Sex and Cyberspace— Virtual Networks Leading to High-Risk Sex." *Journal of the American Medical Association,* Vol. 284, No. 4, July 26, 2000.
36. Goodson, Patricia, et al. "Searching for Sexually Explicit Materials on the Internet: An Exploratory Study of College Students' Behavior and Attitudes." *Archives of Sexual Behavior,* Vol. 30, No. 2, April 2001, p. 101.
37. McFarlane, M., et al. "The Internet as a Newly Emerging Risk Environment for Sexually Transmitted Diseases." *Journal of the American Medical Association,* Vol. 384, No. 4, July 26, 2000.
38. McFarlane, M. "Young Adults on the Internet: Risk Behaviors for Sexually Transmitted Diseases and HIV." *Journal of Adolescent Health,* Vol. 31, No. 1, 2002, p. 11.
39. Goold, P. C., et al. "Can the Internet Be Used to Improve Sexual Health Awareness in Web-Wise Young People?" *Journal of Family Planning and Reproductive Health Care,* Vol. 29, No. 1, January 2003, p. 28.
40. Rietmeijer C. A., et al. "Risks and Benefits of the Internet for Populations at Risk for Sexually Transmitted Infections (STIs): Results of an STI Clinic Survey." *Sexually Transmitted Diseases,* Vol. 30, No. 1, January 2003, p. 15.
41. Richardson, C. R., et al. "Does Pornography-Blocking Software Block Access to Health Information on the Internet?" *Journal of the American Medical Association,* Vol. 288, No. 22, December 11, 2002, p. 2887.
42. Crooks and Baur, *Our Sexuality.*

References

43. Buunk, Bram, et al. "The Double-Edged Sword of Providing Information About the Prevalence of Safer Sex." *Journal of Applied Social Psychology,* Vol. 32, No. 4, 2002, p. 684.

44. "It's Your (Sex) Life." Menlo Park, CA: Henry J. Kaiser Family Foundation, 2002.

45. Keller, S. N., and J. D. Brown. "Media Interventions to Promote Responsible Sexual Behavior." *Journal of Sex Research,* Vol. 39, No. 1, February 2002, p. 67.

46. Gaile, G., and H. Trummer. "The Etiology of Erectile Dysfunction and Mechanisms by Which Drugs Improve Erection." *Drugs Today,* Vol. 39, No. 3, March 2003, p. 193.

47. "Erectile Dysfunction." *Advanced Nurse Practitioner,* Vol. 11, No. 4, April 2003, p. 72.

48. "Viagra and Erections: Do the Benefits Persist?" *Harvard Men's Health Watch,* January 2003. www.health.harvard. ed/medline/Men/N0103b.html.

49. Jackson, G. "Sildenafil (Viagra) and Cardiac Patients: An Open Outpatient Study." *Heart,* Vol. 85, No. 5, May 2001, p. 42.

50. Jannini, E. A., et al. "Disorders of Ejaculation." *Journal of Endocrinology Investigation,* Vol. 25, No. 11, December 2002, p. 1006.

51. Chen, J., et al. "Efficacy of Sildenafil as Adjuvant Therapy to Selective Serotonin Reuptake Inhibitor in Alleviating Premature Ejaculation." *Urology,* Vol. 61, No. 1, January 2003, p. 197.

52. Ragucci, K. R., and N. S. Culhane. "Treatment of Female Sexual Dysfunction." *Annals of Pharmacotherapy,* Vol. 37, No. 4, April 2003, p. 546.

53. Berman, L., et al. "Seeking Help for Sexual Function Complaints: What Gynecologists Need to Know About the Female Patient's Experience." *Fertility and Sterility,* Vol. 79, No. 3, March 2003, p. 57.

54. Moynihan, R. "The Making of a Disease: Female Sexual Dysfunction." *British Medical Journal,* Vol. 326, No. 7379, p. 45.

55. Doogan, D. P. "The Making of a Disease: Female Sexual Dysfunction. Inaccuracies Are Not Helpful." *British Medical Journal,* Vol. 326, No. 7390, March 22, 2003, p. 658.

56. Bancroft, J. "Distress About Sex: A National Survey of Women in Heterosexual Relationships." *Archives of Sexual Behavior,* Vol. 32, No. 3, June 2003, p. 193.

Reproductive Choices

Jess and Sara, juniors at the same community college, can't remember a time when abortion was illegal, when AIDS wasn't a deadly threat, and when safe sex wasn't a concern of every sexually active individual. Yet even though they were aware of the risks and the realities involved, neither used contraception during every single sexual encounter. Then one of Jess's partners had a pregnancy scare. He decided never again to engage in unprotected sex. Sara had a different reality check: At her regular physical, she learned that she had contracted chlamydia, the most common sexually transmitted infection in the United States (see Chapter 13).

When Jess and Sara started dating, both of them felt that something was special about their relationship. Despite their mutual attraction, they decided to take every step toward intimacy slow. Both considered and talked about their personal priorities and concerns. Even though it was awkward, they also discussed their own sexual histories and underwent tests for STIs. Looking toward a continuing committed relationship, they decided on, not one, but two forms of contraception: the birth control pill and a condom. In the future, they realized that they might switch to other forms of birth control—and might well consider different options, including both marriage and parenthood.

As human beings, we have a unique power: the ability to choose to conceive or not to conceive. No other species on Earth can separate sexual activity and pleasure from reproduction. However, simply not wanting to get pregnant is never enough to prevent conception, nor is wanting to have a child always enough to get pregnant. Both desires require individual decisions and actions.

Anyone who engages in vaginal intercourse must be willing to accept the consequences of that activity—the possibility of pregnancy and responsibility for the child who might be conceived—or take action to avoid those consequences. Although many people are concerned about the risks associated with contraception, using birth control is safer and healthier than not using it. According to the Population Reference Bureau, the use of contraceptives, including oral contraceptives, saves millions of lives each year. Some forms of contraception also reduce the risk of sexually transmitted infections.

This chapter provides information on conception, birth control, abortion, infertility, adoption, and the processes by which a new human life develops and enters the world.

© Stephen Simpson/Taxi/Getty Images

After studying the material in this chapter, you should be able to:

• **Describe** the process of human conception.
• **List** the major options available for contraception, and **identify** the advantages and risks of each.
• **Describe** the commonly used abortion methods.

• **Discuss** the physiological effects of pregnancy on a woman and **describe** fetal development.
• **Give examples** of prenatal care measures.
• **Describe** the three stages of labor and the birth process.
• **Identify** the options available to infertile couples wanting children.

275

Conception

The equation for making a baby is quite simple: One sperm plus one egg equals one fertilized egg, which can develop into an infant. But the processes that affect or permit **conception** are quite complicated. The creation of sperm, or **spermatogenesis,** starts in the male at puberty, and the production of sperm is regulated by hormones. Sperm cells form in the seminiferous tubules of the testes and are passed into the epididymis, where they are stored until ejaculation (see Figure 9-1); a single male ejaculation may contain 500 million sperm. Each sperm released into the vagina during intercourse moves on its own, propelling itself toward its target, an ovum.

To reach its goal, the sperm must move through the acidic secretions of the vagina, enter the uterus, travel up the fallopian tube containing the ovum, then fuse with the nucleus of the egg (**fertilization**). Just about every sperm produced by a man in his lifetime fails to accomplish its mission.

There are far fewer human egg cells than there are sperm cells. Each woman is born with her lifetime supply of ova, and between 300 and 500 eggs eventually mature and leave her ovaries during ovulation. As discussed in Chapter 8, every month, one or the other of the woman's ovaries releases an ovum to the nearby fallopian tube. It travels through the fallopian tube until it reaches the uterus, a journey that takes three to four days. An unfertilized egg lives for about 24 to 36 hours, disintegrates, and, during menstruation, is expelled along with the uterine lining.

Even if a sperm, which can survive in the female reproductive tract for two to five days, meets a ripe egg in a fallopian tube, its success is not assured. It must penetrate the layer of cells and a jellylike substance that surround each egg. Every sperm that touches the egg deposits an enzyme that dissolves part of this barrier. When a sperm bumps into a bare spot, it can penetrate the egg membrane and merge with the egg. (See Figure 9-2.) The fertilized egg travels down the fallopian tube, dividing to form a tiny clump of cells called a **zygote.** When it reaches the uterus, about a week after fertilization, it burrows into the endometrium, the lining of the uterus. This process is called **implantation.**

Conception can be prevented by **contraception.** Some contraceptive methods prevent ovulation or implantation, and others block the sperm from reaching the egg. Some methods are temporary; others permanently alter one's fertility.

Figure 9-1 THE TESTES

Spermatogenesis takes place in the testes. Sperm cells form in the seminiferous tubules and are stored in the coils of the epididymis. Eventually, the sperm drain into the vas deferens, ready for ejaculation.

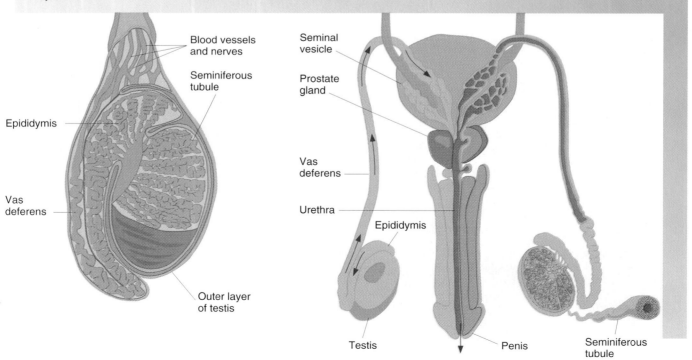

Figure 9-2 FERTILIZATION

(a) The efforts of hundreds of sperm may allow one to penetrate the ovum's corona radiata, an outer layer of cells, and then the zona pellucida, a thick inner membrane. (b)The nuclei of the sperm and the egg cells merge, and the male and female chromosomes in the nuclei come together, forming a zygote. (c)The zygote divides into two cells, then four cells, and so on. (d) As fluid enters the ball, cells form a ball of cells called a blastocyst. (e)The blastocyst implants itself in the endometrium.

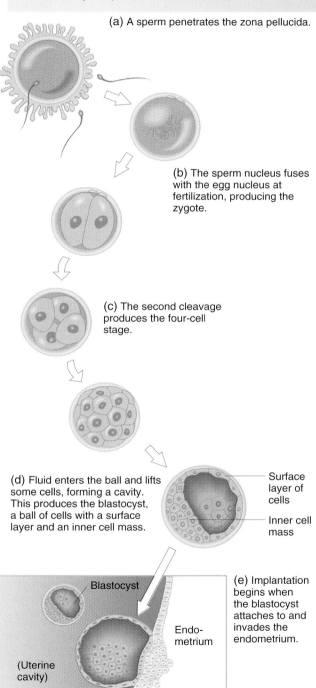

(a) A sperm penetrates the zona pellucida.

(b) The sperm nucleus fuses with the egg nucleus at fertilization, producing the zygote.

(c) The second cleavage produces the four-cell stage.

(d) Fluid enters the ball and lifts some cells, forming a cavity. This produces the blastocyst, a ball of cells with a surface layer and an inner cell mass.

Surface layer of cells

Inner cell mass

Blastocyst

(Uterine cavity)

Endo-metrium

(e) Implantation begins when the blastocyst attaches to and invades the endometrium.

Birth Control Basics

A heterosexual woman in Western countries spends 90 percent of her reproductive years trying to prevent pregnancy and 10 percent of these years trying to become or being pregnant. Today birth control is safer, more effective, and more convenient than in the past—yet none of today's contraceptives are 100 percent safe, 100 percent effective, or 100 percent convenient. And even protection that is effective 95 percent of the time (which, some contend, is the best available in real-life use) isn't as good as it may sound. With just a 5 percent failure rate, statistically speaking, seven in ten women who want no more than two children would have to undergo one or more abortions in order to achieve their desired family size.

Ideally, two partners should decide together which form of birth control to use. However, female methods account for 63 percent of all contraceptive methods reported by women between ages 15 and 44.[1] Lack of male involvement may account for 40 percent of each year's unwanted pregnancies.

If you are engaging in sexual activity that could lead to conception, you have to be realistic about your situation. This may mean assuming full responsibility for your reproductive ability, whether you're a man or a woman. The more you know about contraception, the more likely you are to use birth control. (See Fact or Fiction? "You can't get pregnant . . .") You also have to recognize the risks associated with various methods of contraception. If you're

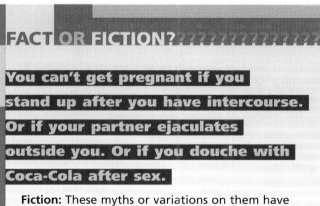

FACT OR FICTION? ????????????????????

You can't get pregnant if you stand up after you have intercourse. Or if your partner ejaculates outside you. Or if you douche with Coca-Cola after sex.

Fiction: These myths or variations on them have spread among young people for years. None prevents pregnancy. If you don't want to get pregnant, you must use some form of birth control every single time you engage in sexual intercourse. A couple that engages in unprotected intercourse around the time of ovulation faces about a 10 percent risk of pregnancy. Immediately after a woman's period, the chance of pregnancy is lower—about 2 to 3 percent, but is not zero.

Source: Mary Jane Minkin and Carol Wright. *The Yale Guide to Women's Reproductive Health.* New Haven: Yale University Press, 2003.

a woman, the risks are chiefly yours. Although most women never experience any serious complications, it's important to be aware of the potential for long-term risks. Risks that are acceptable to others may not be acceptable to you.

In one recent study at a Western college, undergraduates were more likely to report "almost always" using a reliable, proven method of birth control after completing an introductory health course.[2]

🔲 🔳 How Do I Choose a Birth Control Method?

When it comes to deciding which form of birth control to use, there's no one "right" decision. In a study of contraceptive decisionmaking among African-American, Hispanic, and European-American women ages 18 to 50, those who made contraceptive decisions alone were older, single, African American, used pregnancy prevention, or had histories of sexually transmitted infections and unintended pregnancies. Older African-American women were more likely to choose no contraception. Among contraceptive users, African Americans used effective methods of pregnancy prevention, but not disease prevention. Women who had a history of sexually transmitted infections and younger, more educated women were more likely to use methods that prevent both pregnancy and infections.

Regardless of pregnancy history, about half of adolescents do not use effective contraception. Adolescents who have had previous abortions are three times more likely than never-pregnant adolescents to use hormonal contraception. However, although more likely to use contraceptive injections or implants, adolescent mothers are not more likely than never-pregnant adolescents to use oral contraceptives.[3]

In an online survey of undergraduates, 6 percent of female students said they have had an unintended pregnancy during the last year. One-third said they have been afraid of getting pregnant in the past year.[4]

Good decisions are based on sound information. You should consult a physician or family-planning counselor if you have questions or want to know how certain methods might affect existing or familial medical conditions, such as high blood pressure or diabetes. Table 9-1 presents your contraceptive choices. As the table indicates, contraception doesn't always work. When you evaluate any contraceptive, always consider its *effectiveness* (the likelihood that it will indeed prevent pregnancy). The **failure rate** refers to the number of pregnancies that occur per year for every 100 women using a particular method of birth control.[5]

The reliability of contraceptives in actual, real-life use is much lower than those reported in national surveys or clinical trials. In general, failure rates are highest among cohabiting and other unmarried women, very poor families, black and Hispanic women, adolescents, and women in their twenties.

Some couples use withdrawal or **coitus interruptus,** removal of the penis from the vagina before ejaculation, to prevent pregnancy, even though this is not a reliable form of birth control. About half the men who have tried coitus interruptus find it unsatisfactory, either because they don't know when they're going to ejaculate or because they can't withdraw quickly enough. Also, the Cowper's glands, two pea-sized structures located on each side of the urethra, often produce a fluid that appears as drops at the tip of the penis any time from arousal and erection to orgasm. This fluid can contain active sperm and, in infected men, human immunodeficiency virus (HIV).

As many as 3 million unintentional pregnancies each year in the United States are the result of contraceptive failure, either from problems with the drug or device itself or from improper use. Partners can lower the risk of unwanted pregnancy by using backup methods—that is, more than one form of contraception simultaneously. Emergency or after-intercourse contraception (discussed later in this chapter) could prevent as many as 2.3 million unwanted pregnancies each year.[6]

Even college students aware of the risks associated with unprotected sexual intercourse often do not practice safe-sex behaviors. There are many reasons, ranging from the influence of sex and alcohol to embarrassment about buying condoms. Generally, the ability to talk

STRATEGIES FOR PREVENTION

Choosing a Contraceptive

Your contraceptive needs may change throughout your life. To decide which method to use now, you need to know:

- How well will it fit into your lifestyle?
- How convenient will it be?
- How effective will it be?
- How safe will it be?
- How affordable will it be?
- How reversible will it be?
- Will it protect against sexually transmitted infections?

Source: "Facts About Birth Control." www.plannedparenthood.org.

TABLE 9-1	Your Contraceptive Choices				
Type of Contraceptive	**Failure Rate** (number of pregnancies expected per 100 women per year)	**Some Risks** (serious medical risks from contraceptives are rare)	**Protection from Sexually Transmitted Infections (STIs)**	**Convenience**	**Availability**
Oral Contraceptives—combined pill	1	Dizziness; nausea; changes in menstruation, mood, and weight; rarely cardiovascular disease, including high blood pressure, blood clots, heart attack, and strokes	None, except some protection against pelvic inflammatory disease.	Must be taken on daily schedule, regardless of frequency of intercourse	Prescription
Oral Contraceptives—progestin-only minipill	2	Irregular bleeding, weight gain, breast tenderness, less protection against ectopic pregnancy	None	Must be taken on daily schedule, regardless of frequency of intercourse	Prescription
Patch (Ortho Evra)	1 Appears to be less effective in women weighing more than 198 pounds	Similar to oral contraceptives—combined pill	None	New patch is applied once a week for 3 weeks. Patch is not worn during the fourth week, and woman has a menstrual period	Prescription
Vaginal Contraceptive Ring (NuvaRing)	1	Vaginal discharge, vaginitis, irritation. Similar to oral contraceptives—combined pill	None	Inserted by the woman; remains in the vagina for 3 weeks, then is removed for 1 week. If ring is expelled and remains out for more than 3 hours, another birth control method must be used until ring as been used continuously for 7 days	Prescription
Emergency Contraceptives (Preven and Plan B)	Almost 80 percent reduction in risk of pregnancy for a single act of unprotected sex	Nausea, vomiting, abdominal pain, fatigue, headache	None	Must be taken within 72 hours of having unprotected intercourse	Prescription
Injection (Depo-Provera)	less than 1	Irregular bleeding, weight gain, breast tenderness, headaches	None	One injection every 3 months	Prescription
Injection (Lunelle)	less than 1	Changes in menstrual cycle, weight gain. Similar to oral contraceptives—combined	None	Injection given once a month	Prescription
IUD (Intrauterine Device)	less than 1	Cramps, bleeding, pelvic inflammatory disease, infertility, perforation of uterus	None	After insertion by physician, can remain in place for up to one or 10 years, depending on type	Prescription

(continued)

TABLE 9-1	**Your Contraceptive Choices (continued)**				
Type of Contraceptive	**Failure Rate (number of pregnancies expected per 100 women per year)**	**Some Risks (serious medical risks from contraceptives are rare)**	**Protection from Sexually Transmitted Infections (STIs)**	**Convenience**	**Availability**
Diaphragm with Spermicide	17	Irritation and allergic reactions, urinary tract infection Risk of Toxic Shock Syndrome when kept in place longer than recommended	None	Inserted before intercourse and left in place at least 6 hours after; can be left in place for 24 hours, with additional spermicide for repeated intercourse	Prescription
Cervical Cap with Spermicide	17	Irritation and allergic reactions, abnormal Pap test. Risk of Toxic Shock Syndrome when kept in place longer than recommended	None	May be difficult to insert; can remain in place for 48 hours without reapplying spermicide for repeated intercourse	Prescription
Male Condom Latex/Polyurethane	11	Irritation and allergic reactions (less likely with polyurethane)	Except for abstinence, latex condoms are the best protection against STIs, including herpes and AIDS	Applied immediately before intercourse; used only once and discarded. Polyurethane condoms are available for those with latex sensitivity	Nonprescription
Female Condom	21	Irritation and allergic reactions	May give some STI protection; not as effective as latex condom	Applied immediately before intercourse; used only once and discarded	Nonprescription
Sponge with Spermicide	14–28	Irritation and allergic reactions, difficulty in removal Risk of Toxic Shock Syndrome when kept in place longer than recommended	None	Inserted before intercourse and protects for repeated acts of intercourse for 24 hours without additional spermicide; must be left in place for at least 6 hours after intercourse; must be removed within 30 hours of insertion. Is discarded after use	Nonprescription
Spermicide Alone	20–50 (studies have shown varying failure rates)	Irritation and allergic reactions, urinary tract infections	None	Instructions vary; check labeling. Inserted between 5 and 90 minutes before intercourse and usually left in place at least 6 to 8 hours after	Nonprescription
Periodic Abstinence	20	None	None	Requires frequent monitoring of body functions (for example, body temperature for one method)	Instructions from health-care provider

TABLE 9-1	Your Contraceptive Choices (continued)				
Type of Contraceptive	**Failure Rate** (number of pregnancies expected per 100 women per year)	**Some Risks** (serious medical risks from contraceptives are rare)	**Protection from Sexually Transmitted Infections (STIs)**	**Convenience**	**Availability**
Surgical Sterilization—female	less than 1	Pain, bleeding, infection, other post-surgical complications	None	One-time surgical procedure	Surgery
Surgical Sterilization—male	less than 1	Pain, bleeding, infection, other minor postsurgical complications	None	One-time surgical procedure	Surgery

Source: FDA

about a desire to use condoms has been found to be associated with a greater use of condoms. However, a recent survey of college students found that a significant percentage of both men and women either tried to dissuade a potential partner from condom use or had a sexual partner who'd tried to discourage condom use. Both men and women generally used the same arguments against condoms: that sex felt better without them, that the woman wouldn't get pregnant, and that neither would get a sexually transmitted infection.[7]

The bottom line is that it takes two people to conceive a baby, and two people should be involved in deciding not to conceive a baby. In the process, they can also enhance their skills in communication, critical thinking, and negotiating.

❖ Abstinence and Outercourse

The contraceptive methods discussed in this chapter are designed to prevent pregnancy as a consequence of vaginal intercourse. Couples who choose abstinence make a very different decision—to abstain from vaginal intercourse and other forms of sexual activity (any in which ejaculation occurs near the vaginal opening) that could result in conception.

For many individuals, abstinence represents a deliberate choice regarding their bodies, minds, spirits, and sexuality. People choose abstinence for various reasons, including waiting until they are ready for a sexual relationship or until they find the "right" partner, respecting religious or moral values, enjoying friendships without sexual involvement, recovering from a breakup, or preventing pregnancy and sexually transmitted infection.

Abstinence is the only form of birth control that is 100 percent effective and risk-free. It is also an important, increasingly valued lifestyle choice. A growing number of

© Michael Dwyer/Stock, Boston

Some couples refrain from intercourse but engage in "outercourse," or intimacy that includes kissing, hugging, and sensual touching.

individuals, including some who have been sexually active in the past, are choosing abstinence until they establish a relationship with a long-term partner.

Abstinence offers special health benefits for women. Those who abstain until their twenties and engage in sex with fewer partners during their lifetime are less likely to get sexually transmitted infections, to suffer infertility, or to develop cervical cancer. However, some people find it difficult to abstain for long periods of time. There also is a risk that people will abruptly end their abstinence without being prepared to protect themselves against pregnancy or infection.

Individuals who choose abstinence from vaginal intercourse often engage in activities sometimes called *outercourse*, such as kissing, hugging, sensual touching, and

STRATEGIES FOR PREVENTION

Is Abstinence the Right Choice for You?

■ Think about your values, goals, and priorities. Would abstinence support them?

■ Realize that drugs and alcohol could affect your ability to make sexual decisions. Are you prepared to avoid their use to be sure to maintain your abstinence?

■ Talk about your feelings before a relationship gets sexual. Can you put your thoughts and feelings about abstinence into words?

■ Abstinence does not mean an end to all sexual experiences. What behaviors would you consider? What limits would you set?

mutual masturbation. Outercourse is nearly 100 percent effective as a contraceptive measure, but pregnancy is possible if there is genital contact. If the man ejaculates near the vaginal opening, sperm can swim up into the vagina and fallopian tubes to fertilize an egg. Except for oral-genital and anal sex, outercourse also may lower the risk of contracting sexually transmitted infections. It is an effective form of safe sex as long as no body fluids are exchanged.

Some couples routinely restrict themselves to outercourse; others temporarily choose such sexual activities when it is inadvisable for them to have vaginal intercourse—for example, after childbirth. Other benefits: Outercourse has no medical or hormonal side effects; it may prolong sex play and enhance orgasm, and it can be used when no other methods are available.

✴ Hormonal Contraceptives

In recent years birth control methods made with synthetic hormones have become available in a variety of forms. Oral contraceptives have been available for decades, and the birth control pill is one of the most well-researched medications. Other options for hormonal birth control include a skin patch, a vaginal ring, and a monthly or quarterly injection. All are extremely effective when used consistently and conscientiously.[8]

Hormonal contraceptives do not protect against HIV infection and other STIs, so condoms and spermicides should also be used if you need protection against infections.

Oral Contraceptives

The pill—the popular term for **oral contraceptives**—is the method of birth control preferred by unmarried women and by those under age 30, including college students. Women 18 to 24 years old are most likely to choose oral contraceptives. In use for 40 years, the pill is one of the most researched, tested, and carefully followed medications in medical history—and one of the most controversial.[9] The impact of the pill has been enormous. By virtually eliminating the risk of pregnancy, the pill encouraged women's careers. It also altered the marriage market by enabling young men and women to delay marriage while not having to delay sex.[10]

Although many women incorrectly think that the risks of the pill are greater than those of pregnancy and childbirth, long-term studies show that oral contraceptive use does not increase mortality rates. Combination oral contraceptives significantly reduce the risk of ovarian and endometrial cancer and produce no increase in serious disease, including breast cancer, diabetes, multiple sclerosis, rheumatoid arthritis, and liver disease.[11]

Combination Pills

These pills consist of two hormones, synthetic estrogen and progestin, which play important roles in controlling ovulation and the menstrual cycle. The doses in today's oral contraceptives are much lower—less than one-fourth the amount of estrogen and one-twentieth the progestin in the original pill. This means fewer side effects and lower risk of heart disease and stroke.[12]

Monophasic pills release a constant dose of estrogen and progestin throughout a woman's menstrual cycle. **Multiphasic pills** mimic normal hormonal fluctuations of the natural menstrual cycle by providing different levels of estrogen and progesterone at different times of the month. Multiphasic pills reduce total hormonal dose and side effects. Both constant-dose combination and multiphasic pills block the release of hormones that would stimulate the process leading to ovulation. They also thicken and alter the cervical mucus, making it more hostile to sperm, and they make implantation of a fertilized egg in the uterine lining more difficult.

One combination pill, Yasmin, contains a unique progestin that works like a mild diuretic and prevents fluid retention. Researchers have found that it lessens symptoms of premenstrual problems.[13] Women who are taking potassium supplements, daily anti-inflammatory drugs, or heparin, a blood-thinner, should not take Yasmin because of potentially dangerous drug interactions.[14] Other pills offer different benefits, such as clearer skin and reduced facial hair.

Self Survey | Which Contraceptive Method Is Best for You?

Answer yes or no to each statement as it applies to you and, if appropriate, your partner.

1. You have high blood pressure or cardiovascular disease.
2. You smoke cigarettes.
3. You have a new sexual partner.
4. An unwanted pregnancy would be devastating to you.
5. You have a good memory.
6. You or your partner have multiple sexual partners.
7. You prefer a method with little or no bother.
8. You have heavy, crampy periods.
9. You need protection against STIs.
10. You are concerned about endometrial and ovarian cancer.
11. You are forgetful.
12. You need a method right away.
13. You're comfortable touching your own and your partner's genitals.
14. You have a cooperative partner.
15. You like a little extra vaginal lubrication.
16. You have sex at unpredictable times and places.
17. You are in a monogamous relationship and have at least one child.

Scoring:

Recommendations are based on Yes answers to the following numbered statements:

The combination pill: 4, 5, 6, 8, 10, 16
The progestin-only pill: 1, 2, 5, 7, 16
The patch: 4, 7, 8, 11, 16
The NuvaRing: 4, 7, 8, 11, 13, 16
Condoms: 1, 2, 3, 6, 9, 12, 13, 14
Depo-Provera: 1, 2, 4, 7, 11, 16
Lunelle: 4, 7, 11, 16
Diaphragm, cervical cap, or FemCap: 1, 2, 13, 14
Mirena IUD: 1, 2, 7, 8, 11, 13, 16, 17
Copper T IUD: 1, 2, 7, 11, 13, 16, 17
Spermicides: 1, 2, 12, 13, 14, 15
Sponge: 1, 2, 12, 13

Your Health Change Plan
for Choosing a Contraceptive

Your responses may indicate that there's more than one appropriate method of birth control for you. Remember that you may choose different types of birth control at different stages of your life, or switch contraceptives for various reasons. You and your partner should always consider and discuss these factors:

:: **Effectiveness.** Keep in mind that your own conscientiousness will play an important role. If you forget to take your daily pill, or if you decide not to use a condom "just this once," you'll increase the odds of pregnancy by interfering with effective birth control.

:: **Suitability.** If you don't have sex very often, a contraceptive with many risks and side effects, such as the pill, may be wrong for you. If you have many sexual partners and are at risk of contracting a sexually transmitted infection, a condom may provide protection against pregnancy and infection, especially if used with a diaphragm or cervical cap.

:: **Side effects.** Some complications related to contraceptives are serious health threats. Be sure to ask questions and gather as much information as possible about what side effects to expect.

:: **Safety.** The risks of certain contraceptives, such as the pill, may be too great to allow their use, if, for example, you have high blood pressure. Be honest in describing your medical history to your physician.

:: **Future fertility.** Some women don't return to regular menstrual cycles for six months to a year after discontinuing oral contraceptives. This possibility may or may not be important to you now, but you should try to look ahead.

:: **Cost.** The only free contraceptive methods are abstinence and rhythm methods. If you're on a tight budget, you might consider the relative costs of a year's prescription of oral contraceptives compared to a year's supply of condoms or spermicidal foam or jelly. You should also think about the long-term costs and consequences.

:: **Reduced risk of sexually transmitted infections.** Some forms of contraception, in particular barrier contraceptives and spermicides, help reduce the risk of transmission of some STIs. However, none provides complete protection.

Progestin-Only Pills

Progestin-only **"minipills"** contain only a small amount of progestin and no estrogen. They work somewhat differently than combination pills. Women taking **progestin-only pills** probably ovulate, at least occasionally. In those cycles, the pills prevent pregnancy by thickening cervical mucus, making it hard for sperm to penetrate, and by interfering with implantation of a fertilized egg.

The risk of heart disease and stroke is lower with progestin-only pills than with any combination pill. For this reason, they are a good choice for women over age 35 and others who cannot take estrogen-containing pills because of high blood pressure, diabetes, or clotting disorders. Because they do not affect the quality or quantity of breast milk, progestin-only pills often are recommended for nursing mothers, and they are recommended for smokers. Because progestin can affect mood and worsen the symptoms of depression, progestin-only pills are not recommended for women with a history of depression. Antiseizure medications, such as Dilantin, which accelerate liver metabolism, may make the minipill less effective.[15]

Users of progestin-only pills have to be conscientious about taking these pills, not just every day, but at the same time every day. If you take a progestin-only pill three or more hours later than usual, use a back-up method of contraception, such as a condom, for two days after you resume taking the pill.

Advantages Birth control pills have several advantages: They are extremely effective. Among women who miss no pills, only 1 in 1,000 becomes pregnant in the first year of use. They are reversible, so a woman can easily stop using them. They do not interrupt sexual activity. Women on the pill have more regular periods, less cramping, and fewer tubal, or ectopic, pregnancies (discussed later in this chapter). After five years of use, the pill halves the risk of endometrial and ovarian cancer.

In a major study in 2002, scientists at the Centers for Disease Control and Prevention and the National Institutes of Health looked at more than 9,200 women ages 35 to 64 and found that the pill does not raise the risk of breast cancer, even among women who started taking it early or who have close relatives with the disease.[16] This held true regardless of a woman's race, weight, whether she had started taking contraceptives before age 20, took the early

higher-dose oral contraceptives, or had a family history of breast cancer.[17] The pill also reduces the risk of benign breast lumps, ovarian cysts, iron-deficiency anemia, and pelvic inflammatory disease (PID). In actual use, the failure rate is 1 to 5 percent for estrogen/progesterone pills and 3 to 10 percent for minipills.

Disadvantages The hormones in oral contraceptives may cause various side effects, including spotting between periods, weight gain or loss, nausea and vomiting, breast tenderness, and decreased sex drive. Most lessen after the first three months of use. Combination pills with the lowest amount of estrogen (20 mcg) are more likely to cause spotting between periods.[18]

Oral contraceptives can interact with other medications and diminish their effectiveness; women should inform any physician providing medical treatment that they are taking the pill. Herbal medicines, like St. John's Wort, as well as commonly used prescription drugs, such as certain antibiotics, may affect the efficacy of all oral contraceptives. However, the risk of pregnancy may be greatest with progestin-only pills because their effectiveness rate is lower.

The pill increases the risk of cardiovascular problems, primarily for women over 35 who smoke and those with other health problems, such as high blood pressure. Heart attacks strike an estimated 1 in 14,000 pill users between the ages of 30 and 39, and 1 in 1,500 between the ages of 40 and 44. Strokes occur five times more frequently among women taking oral contraceptives, and clots in the veins develop in 1 of every 500 previously healthy women. Combination pills have somewhat different effects on a woman's circulatory system, which may affect her risk of blood clotting.[19] (See Savvy Consumer: "Evaluating the Risks of Contraceptives.")

Before Using Oral Contraceptives Before starting on the pill, you should undergo a thorough physical examination that includes the following tests:

> Routine blood pressure test.
> Pelvic exam, including a Pap smear.
> Breast exam.
> Blood test.
> Urine sample.

Let your doctor know about any personal or family incidence of high blood pressure or heart disease, diabetes, liver dysfunction, hepatitis, unusual menstrual history, severe depression, sickle-cell anemia, cancer of the breast, ovaries, or uterus, high cholesterol levels, or migraine headaches.

How to Use Oral Contraceptives An estimated 2 million women worldwide become unintentionally pregnant every year because they do not use the pill as directed. The pill usually comes in 28-day packets: 21 of the pills contain the hormones, and 7 are "blanks," included so that the woman can take a pill every day, even during her men-

Various types of birth control pills contain different hormones and combinations of hormones.

© Joel Gordon Photography

Savvy Consumer

EVALUATING THE RISKS OF CONTRACEPTIVES

For individuals with certain medical conditions, specific types of birth control can pose a health risk. To be safe, follow these guidelines:

- **High blood pressure** (180/110 mmHg or higher): Avoid birth control pills or injectables containing estrogen, which may increase your risk of a heart attack or stroke.

- **Episodes of depression:** Avoid products that contain progestin, such as Depo-Provera, contraceptive implants, and the minipill. In some women with depression, pro-

gestin may worsen depressive symptoms. Also, check with your doctor if you are taking an antidepressant medication; it may affect or be affected by oral contraceptives and you may require a different dose.

- **Seizure disorder:** Avoid low-dose birth control pills. Some antiseizure medications, such as Dilantin, accelerate liver metabolism of all substances, including oral contraceptives, and make them less effective.

- **Ectopic pregnancy:** Avoid IUDs. Although IUDs do not cause ectopic pregnancies, if your fallopian tubes have been scarred by a previous ectopic gestation, you're more likely to have another ectopic if you use an IUD.

- **Hepatitis** (discussed in Chapter 13): Avoid birth control pills or injectables containing estrogen, which is metabolized in the liver—an organ damaged by hepatitis.

---

strual period. If a woman forgets to take one pill, she should take it as soon as she remembers. However, if she forgets during the first week of her cycle or misses more than one pill, she should rely on another form of birth control until her next menstrual period.

Even if you experience no discomfort or side effects while on the pill, see a physician at least once a year for an examination, which should include a blood pressure test, a pelvic, and a breast exam. Notify your doctor at once if you develop severe abdominal pain, chest pain, coughing, shortness of breath, pain or tenderness in the calf or thigh, severe headaches, dizziness, faintness, muscle weakness or numbness, speech disturbance, blurred vision, a sensation of flashing lights, a breast lump, severe depression, or yellowing of your skin.

Generally, when a woman stops taking the pill, her menstrual cycle resumes the next month, but it may be irregular for the next couple of months. However, 2 to 4 percent of pill users experience prolonged delays. Women who become pregnant during the first or second cycle after discontinuing use of the pill may be at greater risk of miscarriage; they also are more likely to conceive twins. Most physicians advise women who want to conceive to change to another method of contraception for three months after they stop taking the pill.

Extended Use Oral Contraceptives

For years physicians have prescribed prolonged use of birth control pills to lessen the number of menstrual cycles for women with asthma, migraines, rashes or other conditions that flare up during their periods. Eliminating periods eliminates symptoms, and having fewer cycles also may lower a woman's long-term risk of ovarian cancer. A new package of standard combination birth control pills, called

Seasonale, provides pills for 84 days of continuous use so women have four periods a year rather than twelve.

The Patch (Ortho Evra)

The Ortho Evra birth control patch, the first transdermal (through the skin) contraceptive, works like a combination pill but looks like a bandaid. Embedded in its adhesive layer are two hormones, a low-dose estrogen and a progestin. It prevents pregnancy by delivering continuous levels of estrogen and progestin through the skin into the bloodstream. The patch is waterproof and stays on in the shower, swimming pools, or hot tubs.[20]

Advantages The patch is a good option for women who can't remember, don't like, or have problems swallowing pills. Because the patch bypasses the digestive tract, nausea is less likely to be a problem for patch wearers. Its steady release of contraceptive hormones also reduces breakthrough bleeding, mood swings, and other symptoms that occur with pill use. A woman can become pregnant quickly once she stops its use.

Disadvantages Users have an increased risk of blood clots, heart attack, and stroke. Cigarette smoking increases the risk of serious cardiovascular side effects. The patch may be less effective in women who weigh more than 198 pounds.[21] Wearers of contact lenses may experience a change in vision or be unable to continue to wear lenses.

In clinical studies, about 5 percent of women reported that at least one patch had slipped off, and skin irritation occurred in 2 percent of women. Side effects include breast tenderness, headache, and upper respiratory infections. Some women may feel self-conscious wearing a matchbook-sized bandaid on their skin.

The hormones in Ortho Evra are slowly released when the patch is applied to the skin.

Ortho-McNeil Pharmaceutical

How to Use the Patch

A woman applies that 1¾-inch square to her back, upper arm, lower abdomen, or buttocks and changes it every seven days for three weeks. During the patch-free week, she experiences menstrual bleeding. A user should check every day to make sure the patch is still in place. If you don't replace a detached patch within 24 hours, use a back-up method of contraception until your next period.

The NuvaRing

The silver-dollar-sized NuvaRing, a 2-inch ring made of flexible, transparent plastic, slowly emits the same hormones as oral contraceptives through the vaginal tissues. Smaller than the smallest diaphragm, it contains less estrogen than any pill. As effective as the pill, it provides a steady dose of hormones and causes fewer side effects.[22]

Advantages Under medical supervision, the ring may be a safer alternative than the pill for women with conditions such as mild hypertension or diabetes. There is less likelihood of pill-related side-effects, like nausea or mood swings; less spotting, menstrual bleeding and cramping.

Women have no need for a daily pill, a fitting by a doctor, or the use of a spermicide. A woman's ability to become pregnant returns quickly once she stops using the ring. In European studies, overall acceptance of the contraceptive ring was high. The primary reasons for liking the ring were not having to remember anything and ease of use.[23]

Disadvantages In clinical trials, a small percentage of women reported vaginal discharge, irritation, and infection. Some women don't feel comfortable placing something inside their vaginas and then trying to retrieve it.

Women cannot use oil-based vaginal medicine to treat yeast infections while the ring is in place, or a diaphragm or cervical cap for a backup method of birth control.

How to use the ring Unlike a diaphragm, the NuvaRing does not have to be exactly positioned within the vagina or used with a spermicide.

The flexible plastic 2-inch ring compresses so a woman can easily insert it. Each ring stays in place for three weeks, then is removed for the fourth week of the menstrual cycle. Like the pill and the patch, the ring works by preventing ovulation. The ring remains in place for 21 days, then is removed for a week of withdrawal bleeding.

Figure 9-3 NUVARING (ACTUAL SIZE)
The NuvaRing releases estrogen and progestin, preventing ovulation. The exact position of NuvaRing in the vagina is not important for it to work.

If a NuvaRing pops out (uncommon but possible), it should be washed, dried and replaced within three hours. If a longer time passes, users should rely on a back-up form of birth control until the ring has been reinserted for a week and the protective medications have risen to protective levels again.

Contraceptive Injectables

Two different hormonal contraceptives are available in the form of "shots" or injections. Lunelle, which consists of the same hormones as combination birth control pills, is administered monthly. Depo-Provera, which contains only progestin, must be given every 12 weeks. Injectable contraceptives provide no protection against HIV and other STIs.

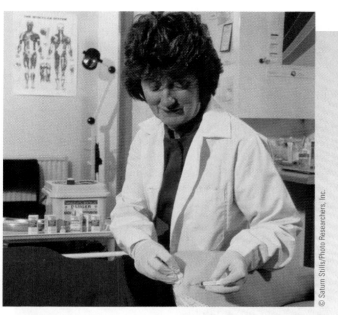

Women must go to a doctor's office or clinic for contraceptive injectables—once a month for Lunelle and every

Lunelle

Lunelle is a contraceptive injection of estrogen and progestin, given by a health professional (doctor, nurse or, in some places, pharmacist) into the arm, thigh, or buttocks during the first five days of a woman's menstrual cycle. It is considered 99.5 percent effective in preventing pregnancy.[24]

Advantages Lunelle eliminates any risk of user error and eliminates worry about buying, storing, using, or remembering contraceptives. It is a popular choice among travelers, college students, or athletes, who prefer not to tote and store contraceptives or who do not want to bother with contraception for four weeks at a time.

Disadvantages A woman must visit a doctor's office or clinic every month for an injection. The most troublesome side effect for many Lunelle users is weight gain. The average is 4 pounds, but some women gain 10 or 20 pounds. Other side effects include nausea, breakthrough bleeding, acne, headache, change in sexual desire, depression, and breast tenderness, particularly during the first few months of use.

How to Use Lunelle You must receive injections within 28 to 30 days of the last one to protect against pregnancy. The maximum safe period between injections is 33 days.

Depo-Provera

One injection of Depo-Provera, a synthetic version of the natural hormone progesterone, provides three months of contraceptive protection. This long-acting hormonal contraceptive raises levels of progesterone, thereby simulating pregnancy. The pituitary gland doesn't produce FSH and LH, which normally cause egg ripening and release. The endometrial lining of the uterus thins, preventing implantation of a fertilized egg.

Advantages The main advantage is that women do not need to take a daily pill. Because Depo-Provera contains only progestin, it can be used by women who cannot take oral contraceptives containing estrogen (such as those who've had breast cancer). Depo-Provera also may have some protective action against endometrial and ovarian cancer.

Disadvantages Depo-Provera causes menstrual irregularities in most users, and in a small percentage of users it causes a delayed return of fertility, excessive endometrial bleeding, and other side effects, including decreased libido, depression, headaches, dizziness, weight gain, frequent urination, and allergic reactions. Long-term use may lead to significantly reduced bone density.

How to Use Depo-Provera Women must receive an injection of Depo-Provera once every 12 weeks, ideally within five days of the beginning of menstruation.

Contraceptive Implants

Hormonal implants, placed under the skin, deliver a constant low dose of progestin. They work primarily by suppressing ovulation, but they also thicken the cervical mucus (which inhibits sperm migration), inhibit the development and growth of the uterine lining, and limit secretion of progesterone during the second or luteal half of the menstrual cycle. The best candidates for implants are women who desire reversible long-term contraception, those who don't want to insert or ingest a contraceptive, those who cannot take estrogen-containing oral contraceptives, those who would face high medical risks if they did become pregnant, and those who are undecided about sterilization.

Norplant, consisting of six thin silicone rubber capsules containing a synthetic form of progestin, was the first such implant available in the United States. Approximately 9 million women used this method before it was taken off the market for reasons unrelated to its efficacy. Women with Norplant implants, who include many adolescents and young adults, should consult their doctors. They can safely leave the rods in place for the entire five-year period of contraceptive protection. However, they should discuss all options, including removal of the Norplant rods and switching to an alternative form of contraception.

A newer generation of implants may provide the benefits of long-term pregnancy protection with fewer complications. Implanon, a single silastic rod, that is simpler to insert and remove than Norplant, provides at least three years of contraception. Available in Europe and Canada, it uses a different type of progestin than Norplant and may cause fewer side effects like weight gain or acne. It should be available in the United States soon.[25]

⠿ Intrauterine Contraceptives

Centuries ago women inserted objects, such as small pebbles, into the uterus to prevent pregnancy. Today women have far more sophisticated options: Mirena, a hormonal "intrauterine system," and a highly effective intrauterine device (IUD). An **intrauterine device (IUD)** is a small piece of molded plastic, with a nylon string attached, that is inserted into the uterus through the cervix. It prevents pregnancy by interfering with implantation. Once widely used, IUDs became less popular after most brands were removed from the market because of serious complications such as pelvic infection and infertility.

Intrauterine contraceptives do not protect against HIV infection and other STIs, so condoms and spermicides should also be used if you need protection against disease.

Mirena

The Mirena Intrauterine System consists of a T-shaped device, inserted in the uterus by a physician, that releases a continuous low dose of progestin and provides five years of protection from pregnancy. Used in Europe, Asia, and Latin America for years, it is 99 percent effective.

Mirena is increasingly being used, not just for contraception, but as an alternative to hysterectomy for extremely heavy menstrual bleeding and as a treatment for problems such as iron-deficiency anemia.

Advantages With Mirena, a woman does not need to think about contraception for five years after insertion. Her periods are likely to become shorter and lighter, with less cramping. About 20 percent of Mirena users stop menstruating altogether, a plus for women with conditions like migraines that flare up during their periods.[26] Perimenopausal women report that Mirena eases their symptoms.

Mirena is a small, flexible plastic T-frame about the size of a quarter.

Courtesy © Berlex Laboratories, Inc.

Disadvantages Side effects include breakthrough bleeding during the first three to six months, acne, headaches, nausea, breast tenderness, mood changes. Mirena users have an increased risk of benign ovarian cysts, and it may take longer (sometimes up to a year) for fertility to return with Mirena than other methods.

Mirena is not recommended for women who have not had children, primarily because of the difficulty of insertion through the cervix of a woman who has never given birth. The system is not advised for women with more than one sexual partner, who face a greater risk of pelvic infections that could impair their fertility. Women who have had an ectopic pregnancy should not use Mirena because of the danger of another misplaced pregnancy.

How to Use the Mirena System A physician must insert the Mirena in a woman's uterus. In a five-year clinical trial, about 5 in every 100 women reported that the Mirena had slipped out of the uterus. Users should check for the string that extends from the device through the vagina at least once a month.

Copper T (ParaGard)

The Copper T (ParaGard) contains copper, which reduces the sperm's ability to reach the egg and interferes with the growth of a fertilized egg by causing biochemical reactions with the uterine lining. The Copper T remains effective for ten years, making it the longest-acting reversible contraceptive available to women in the United States. Its cumulative failure rate is 2.6.

Advantages According to recent analyses, the Copper T is the cheapest and most cost-effective form of birth control. It causes fewer complications than the pill and does not interrupt sexual activity.

© Joel Gordon Photography

The Copper T is made of flexible plastic, with copper bands around the arms and copper thread around the stem.

Disadvantages Many gynecologists recommend other forms of birth control for childless women who someday may want to start a family. Women who have never given birth and have used an IUD for an extended period of time may find it more difficult to conceive after discontinuing its use. In addition, women with many sexual partners, who are at highest risk of pelvic inflammatory disease, are not good candidates for this method.

During insertion of an IUD, women may experience discomfort, cramping, bleeding, or pain, which may continue for a few days or longer. An estimated 2 to 20 percent of users expel an IUD within a year of insertion.

If a woman using an IUD does become pregnant, the IUD is removed to reduce the risk of miscarriage (which can be as high as 50 percent). In addition, physicians generally offer a therapeutic abortion to the pregnant patient because of the serious risks (including infection, premature delivery, and possibly a higher rate of birth defects) of continuing the pregnancy.

How to Use an IUD A physician inserts an IUD during a woman's period, when the cervix is slightly softened and dilated. Antibiotics may be prescribed to lower any risk of infection. An IUD can be removed at any time during her cycle. A woman should check regularly, particularly after each menstrual period, for the nylon string attached to the IUD, because she may not otherwise notice if an IUD has been expelled.

▌ Barrier Contraceptives

As their name implies, **barrier contraceptives** block the meeting of egg and sperm by means of a physical barrier (a diaphragm, cervical cap, FemCap, or condom) or a chemical one (vaginal spermicide in jellies, foams, creams, suppositories, or film). These forms of birth control can do more than prevent conception—they can also help reduce the risk of STIs.

Prescription Barriers

The prescription barrier contraceptives are used by women: the diaphragm, cervical cap, and FemCap. They are placed in the vagina with a spermicide. They do not protect against HIV infection and most STIs.

Diaphragm

The **diaphragm** is a bowl-like rubber cup with a flexible rim that is inserted into the vagina to cover the cervix and prevent the passage of sperm into the uterus during sexual intercourse. (See Figure 9-4.) When used with a spermicide, the diaphragm is both a physical and a chemical barrier to sperm. The effectiveness of the diaphragm in preventing pregnancy depends on strong motivation (to use it faithfully) and a precise understanding of its use. If diaphragms with spermicide are used consistently and carefully, they can be 95 to 98 percent effective. Without a spermicide, the diaphragm is not effective.

Advantages Diaphragms have become increasingly popular, most likely because of concern about the side effects of hormonal contraceptives. Many women feel that using a diaphragm makes them more knowledgeable and comfortable about their bodies.

Disadvantages Some people find that the diaphragm is inconvenient and interferes with sexual spontaneity. The spermicidal cream or jelly is messy, detracts from oral-genital sex, and can cause irritation. A poorly fitted diaphragm may cause discomfort during sex; some women report bladder discomfort, urethral irritation, or recurrent cystitis as a result of diaphragm use.

How to Use a Diaphragm Diaphragms are fitted and prescribed by a qualified health-care professional in diameter sizes ranging from 2 to 4 inches (50 to 105 millimeters). The diaphragm's main function is to serve as a container for a spermicidal (sperm-killing) foam or jelly, which is available at pharmacies without a prescription. A diaphragm should remain in the vagina for at least six hours after intercourse to ensure that all sperm

Figure 9-4 DIAPHRAGM

When used correctly and consistently and with a spermicide, the diaphragm is effective in preventing pregnancy. It must be fitted by a health-care professional.

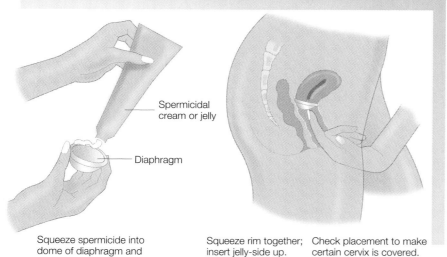

Squeeze spermicide into dome of diaphragm and around the rim.

Spermicidal cream or jelly

Diaphragm

Squeeze rim together; insert jelly-side up.

Check placement to make certain cervix is covered.

are killed. If intercourse occurs again during this period, additional spermicide must be inserted with an applicator tube.

The key to proper use of the diaphragm is having it available. A sexually active woman should keep it in the most accessible place—her purse, bedroom, bathroom. Before every use, a diaphragm should be checked for tiny leaks (hold up to the light or place water in the dome). A health-care provider should check its fit and condition every year when the woman has her annual Pap smear. Oil-based lubricants will deteriorate the latex of the diaphragm and should not be used with one.

Cervical Cap

Like the diaphragm, the **cervical cap,** combined with spermicide, serves as both a chemical and physical barrier blocking the path of the sperm to the uterus. The rubber or plastic cap is smaller and thicker than a diaphragm and resembles a large thimble that fits snugly around the cervix. It is about as effective as a diaphragm (95 to 98 percent).

Advantages Women who cannot use a diaphragm because of pelvic-structure problems or loss of vaginal muscle tone can often use the cap. Also, the cervical cap is less messy and does not require additional applications of spermicide if intercourse occurs more than once within several hours.

Disadvantages A cervical cap is more difficult to insert and remove, and may damage the cervix. Some women find it uncomfortable to wear. In the past, only four sizes of conventional cervical caps were available, and about 25 percent of women had difficulty getting a proper fit. Newer products, such as Lea's Shield, come in one size and are designed to fit all women.

The cervical cap is very similar to the diaphragm and may work better for some women. It is smaller than the diaphragm and covers only the cervix.

© Joel Gordon Photography

Some cap users have developed abnormal Pap smears within three months of beginning this birth control method. Doctors recommend a Pap smear before beginning and after three months of cervical cap use.

How to Use a Cervical Cap Like the diaphragm, the cervical cap is fitted by a qualified health-care professional. For use, the woman fills it one-third to two-thirds full with spermicide and inserts it by holding its edges together and sliding it into the vagina. The cup is then pressed onto the cervix. (Most women find it easiest to do so while squatting or in an upright sitting position.) The cap can be inserted up to 6 hours prior to intercourse and should not be removed for at least 6 hours afterward. It can be left in place up to 24 hours. Pulling on one side of the rim breaks the suction and allows easy removal. Oil-based lubricants should not be used with the cap because they can deteriorate the latex.

The FemCap

Approved by the FDA in 2003, the FemCap is a nonhormonal latex-free barrier contraceptive that works with a spermicide. (See Figure 9-5.) The FemCap, designed to conform to the anatomy of the cervix and vagina, comes in three sizes. The smallest usually best suits women who have never been pregnant; the medium size, for women who have been pregnant but have not had a vaginal delivery; the largest, for those who have delivered a full-term baby vaginally.

Advantages The FemCap can be inserted several hours prior to sexual intimacy. Each FemCap can be used for two years. There is no impact on fertility.

Disadvantages Less effective than hormonal contraception, the FemCap requires planning and insertion prior to sex. A woman may forget about the FemCap and leave it in longer than 48 hours. Because it is new, data on efficacy and problems with use are limited.

How to Use FemCap A prescription is required to purchase FemCap, and the woman selects the appropriate size. Apply spermicide to the bowl of the FemCap (which goes over the cervix), to the outer brim, and to the groove that will face into the vagina. Insert the squeezed, flattened cap into the vagina with the bowl facing upward. The FemCap must be pushed all the way in to cover the cervix completely and left in place at least six hours after intercourse.

Nonprescription Barriers

The nonprescription barrier contraceptives include the male and female condom, vaginal spermicides, the contraceptive sponge, and vaginal contraceptive film. Both condoms provide protection against HIV infection and other STIs; spermicides, sponges, and films do not.

Figure 9-5 FEMCAP

The FemCap must be used with spermicide and must be correctly positioned to cover the cervix completely.

Reproduced with permission from FemCap, Inc. and Alfred Shihata, MD.

Male Condom

The male **condom** covers the erect penis and catches the ejaculate, thus preventing sperm from entering the woman's reproductive tract. (See Figure 9-6.) Most are made of thin surgical latex or sheep membrane; a new type is made of polyurethane, which is thinner, stronger, more heat-sensitive, and more comfortable than latex. In a study of 901 couples over six months, the polyurethane condom was not as effective as the latex condom for pregnancy prevention.[27] Condoms with a spermicidal lubricant (nonoxynol-9) kill most sperm on contact and are thus more effective than other brands.

Although the theoretical effectiveness rate for condoms is 97 percent, the actual rate is only 80 to 85 per-cent. The condom can be torn during the manufacturing process or during its use; testing by the manufacturer may not be as strenuous as it could or should be. Careless removal can also decrease the effectiveness of condoms. However, the major reason that condoms have such a low actual effectiveness rate is that couples don't use them each and every time they have sex. Users who have little experience with condoms—who are young, single, or childless, or who engage in risky behaviors—are more likely to have condoms break.

Condoms are second only to the pill in popularity among college-age adults. [See Student Snapshot: "Condoms on Campus"] Condom use has increased in the last decade. Approximately one in five women ages 15

Figure 9-6 MALE CONDOM

Condoms effectively reduce the risk of pregnancy as well as STIs if used consistently and correctly.

Pinch or twist the tip of the condom, leaving one-half inch at the tip to catch the semen.

Holding the tip, unroll the condom.

Unroll the condom until it reaches the pubic hairs.

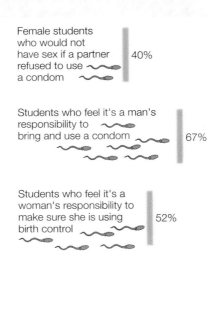

Student Snapshot **Condoms on Campus**

Male students who know how to use a condom correctly — 87%

Female students who know how use a condom correctly — 60%

Male students who believe men should carry condoms "just in case" — 70%

Female students who would not have sex if a partner refused to use a condom — 40%

Students who feel it's a man's responsibility to bring and use a condom — 67%

Students who feel it's a woman's responsibility to make sure she is using birth control — 52%

Source: 1,051 students (526 men and 525 women) ages 18–24 participated in the online Smarter Sex Survey. www.smartersex.org/resources/behind.asp.

to 44 who used contraception rely on their partner's use of condoms as their primary method of birth control.[28]

More teens also are using condoms but not consistently. (See the X&Y File: "Sex, Lies, and Condom Use"). From one-third to one-half of sexually active teens report using condoms for every act of intercourse. However, condom use decreases as teens get older, with fewer males ages 18 and 19 using condoms than those 15 to 17 years old. Teenage girls report less frequent use of condoms than males.[29]

According to the National Longitudinal Study of Adolescent Health, one-fifth to one-half of sexually active adolescents share common misconceptions about condoms.[30] Many believe that there is no space at the tip of a condom or think that Vaseline can be used with condoms; some say that lambskin protects against HIV better than latex. None of these is true.[31] Television advertising of condoms, which has been controversial in the past, may help correct such misinformation. According to a recent study, nine in ten Americans surveyed endorsed condom advertising on TV, either freely, like any other product, or at restricted times.

Advantages Condoms made of latex or polyurethane, especially when used with spermicides containing nonoxynol-9, can help reduce the risk of certain STIs, including syphilis, gonorrhea, chlamydia, and herpes. They appear to lower a woman's risk of pelvic inflammatory disease (PID) and may protect against some parasites that cause urinary tract and genital infections. Public health officials view condoms as the best available defense against HIV infection. They are available without a prescription or medical appointment, and their use does not cause harmful side effects. Some men appreciate the slight blunting of sensation they experience when using a condom because it helps prolong the duration of intercourse before ejaculation.

Disadvantages Condoms are not 100 percent effective in preventing pregnancy or STIs, including infection with HIV or HPV (human papilloma virus, discussed in Chapter 13). For anyone, heterosexual or homosexual, not in a monogamous relationship with a mutually exclusive, healthy partner, condoms can reduce the risks of sexual involvement, but they cannot eliminate them. Condoms

the XY file *Sex, Lies, and Condom Use*

In a series of focus groups with 92 sexually active, young, ethnically and racially diverse individuals, ages 15 to 20, in five American cities, researchers focused on their views and motivations for sex and for condom use. Most found it difficult to believe that people their age used condoms every single time they had sex. Although they acknowledged that everyone is at risk for sexually transmitted infections, the young people saw their own risk as minimal.

The genders had very different motives both for engaging in sex and for using condoms. In the interviews, young women said they engaged in sexual relations because of a desire for physical intimacy and a committed relationship. They generally reported having sex only with men they cared for and deeply trusted, and expected that these men would be honest and forthright about their sexual history. This trust played a significant role in their decision whether to insist on condom use.

In contrast, few of the young men said relationships were an important dimension of their sexual involvements. Their primary motivation was a desire for physical and sexual satisfaction. Most said they were not interested in commitment and viewed emotional expectations as a complication of becoming sexually involved with a woman. The young men also admitted to making judgments about types of girls. To them, young women they didn't care about were "sluts" with whom they used a condom for their own protection.

Which partner determined whether a couple would use a condom? In these interviews, the answer was the women—if they chose to do so. Regardless of race or ethnicity, many of the young women were adamant in demanding that their partners use condoms—and many young men said they would not challenge such a demand out of fear of losing the opportunity for sex. Men often expected potential partners to want to use condoms and described themselves as "suspicious" of women who did not.

Both sexes named two primary reasons for using condoms: preventing pregnancy and protecting against sexually transmitted infections. Young women saw an unwanted pregnancy as an occurrence that would be disruptive, expensive, and could "ruin" their lives and their parents' lives. Young men saw condom use as a way of protecting themselves against emotional entanglements and paternity issues.

The young people were most strongly motivated to use condoms when they did not know a potential sexual partner well or were at the earliest stages of sexual involvement with others. Nearly all said they solicited information about a potential partner's sexual history from this person or from friends. Rather than directly asking about the number of past partners, they more often relied on feelings and visual observations. Some admitted to lying when asked about their own sexual experience in order to avoid being seen as promiscuous. Once a couple had sex without a condom, both partners—but especially women—found it awkward to resume condom use because doing so would imply a lack of trust.

---

may have manufacturing defects, such as pin-size holes, or they may break or slip off during intercourse.

The main objections to condoms include odor, lubrication (too much or too little), rips or breaks, access, disposal, feel, taste, and difficulty opening the packages. Some couples feel that putting on a condom interferes with sexual spontaneity; others incorporate it into their sex play. Some men dislike the reduced penile sensitivity or will not use them because they believe they interfere with sexual pleasure. Others cannot sustain an erection while putting on a condom. A small number are allergic to latex condoms.

How to Use a Condom Most physicians recommend prelubricated, spermicide-treated American-made latex or polyurethane condoms, not membrane condoms ("natural" or "sheepskin"). Before using a condom, check the expiration date, and make sure it's soft and pliable. If it's yellow or sticky, throw it out. Don't check for leaks by blowing up a condom before using it; you may weaken or tear it.

The condom should be put on at the beginning of sexual activity, before genital contact occurs. (See Figure 9-6.) There should be a little space at the top of the condom to catch the semen. Wait until just before intercourse to apply spermicide. Any vaginal lubricant should be water-based. Petroleum-based creams or jellies (such as Vaseline, baby oil, massage oil, vegetable oils, or oil-based hand lotions) can deteriorate the latex. After ejaculation, the condom should be held firmly against the penis so that it doesn't slip off or leak during withdrawal. Couples engaging in anal intercourse should use a water-based lubricant as well as a condom, but should never assume the condom will protect them from HIV infection or other STIs.

Female Condom

The female condom, made of polyurethane, consists of two rings and a polyurethane sheath, and is inserted into the vagina with a tampon-like applicator. (See Figure 9-7.) Once in place, the device loosely lines the walls of the vagina. Internally, a thickened rubber ring keeps it anchored near the cervix. Externally, another rubber ring, 2 inches in diameter, rests on the labia and resists slippage.

Figure 9-7 FEMALE CONDOM
This device is less effective than the male condom for preventing pregnancy and STIs (since no spermicide is used). Like the male condom, this method does not require a prescription.

Although not widely used in the West, the female condom is gaining acceptance in Africa, Asia, and Latin America. Properly used, it is believed to be as good or better than the male condom for preventing infections, including HIV, because it is stronger and covers a slightly larger area. However, it is slightly less effective at preventing pregnancy. The efficacy of female condoms does increase with a woman's experience in using it.[32]

Advantages The female condom gives women more control in reducing their risk of pregnancy and STIs. It does not require a prescription or medical appointment. One size fits all.

Disadvantages The failure rate for the female condom is higher than for other contraceptives. The statistical failure rate is 12.2 percent, which means that 12 of every 100 women using the device could expect to get pregnant during a six-month period. In clinical trials, the actual failure rate was even higher—20.6 percent. Since it does not have spermicide on it, the female condom does not provide as much risk-reduction against STIs as male condoms with spermicide. Women complained that the condom, which retails for $2 to $3, was too expensive, difficult to use, squeaked, and looked odd.

How to Use a Female Condom As illustrated in Figure 9-7, a woman removes the condom and applicator from the wrapper and inserts the condom slowly by gently pushing the applicator toward the small of the back. When properly inserted, the outer ring should rest on the folds of skin around the vaginal opening, and the inner ring (the closed end) should fit against the cervix. The condom should be used with a spermicide and a water-based lubricant.

The female condom can be washed and reused several times and still meet the standards set by the Food and Drug Administration (FDA), according to the study con-

ducted in South Africa in which a sample of women washed, dried and relubricated female condoms up to seven times.

Vaginal Spermicide

The various forms of **vaginal spermicide** include chemical foams, creams, jellies, vaginal suppositories, and gels. (See Figure 9-8.) Some creams and jellies are made for use

---

STRATEGIES FOR PREVENTION

Seven Steps of Correct Condom Use

- Use a new condom at each act of intercourse.

- Handle the condom carefully to avoid damage from fingernails, teeth, or other sharp objects.

- Put on condom after penis is erect and before any genital contact with a partner.

- Make sure that air is trapped in the tip of the condom.

- Ensure adequate lubrication during intercourse.

- Use only water-based lubricants with latex condoms.

- Withdraw the penis while it is still erect to prevent slippage. Hold the condom firmly against the base of the penis during withdrawal.

with a diaphragm; others can be used alone. Several vaginal suppositories claim high effectiveness, but no American studies have confirmed these claims. In general, failure rates for vaginal suppositories are as high as 10 to 25 percent.

Advantages Conscientious use of a spermicide together with another method of contraception, such as a condom, can provide safe and effective birth control and reduce the risk of some vaginal infections, pelvic inflammatory disease, and STIs. The side effects of vaginal spermicides are minimal.

Disadvantages Even though spermicides can be applied in less than a minute, couples may feel that they interfere with sexual spontaneity. Some people are irritated by the chemicals in spermicides, but often a change of brand solves this problem. Others find foam spermicides messy or feel they interfere with oral-genital contact. Spermicidal suppositories that do not dissolve completely can feel gritty.

How to Use a Vaginal Spermicide The various types of spermicide come with instructions that should be followed carefully for maximum protection. Contraceptive vaginal suppositories take about 20 minutes to dissolve and cover the vaginal walls. Foam, inserted with an applicator, goes into place much more rapidly. You must apply additional spermicide before each additional intercourse. After sex, women should shower rather than bathe to prevent the spermicide from being rinsed out of the vagina, and they should not douche for at least six hours.

Contraceptive Sponge

The Today Sponge, a soft, disposable polyurethane sponge permeated with a spermicide, returned to the U.S. market in 2003. The Sponge was withdrawn in 1995 because of

The contraceptive sponge, which contains spermicide, fits over the cervix to block and absorb semen and kill sperm. The string loop helps with removal.

problems at the manufacturing plant, including bacterial contamination of water and sanitizing equipment. With processing problems corrected and a new manufacturer, the Sponge can be purchased online and in pharmacies.

The sponge, which works by releasing a protective spermicidal gel that kills or immobilizes sperm, can be inserted several hours prior to intercourse and left in place for twelve hours later. If used consistently and conscientiously, the effectiveness rate is 84 to 87 percent. Some research has indicated that the sponge is much less effective in women who have had children, possibly because of changes in the vagina and cervix following childbirth. However, a review of studies both in the United States and abroad found little significant difference between women who have never given birth and those who have. Side effects include vaginal irritation and allergic reactions.[33] Vaginal sponges do not protect against HIV infection and other STIs.

Uterus — Spermicidal foam — Applicator — Vagina

Figure 9-8 VAGINAL SPERMICIDES
These various creams, foams, and jellies are available without a prescription and have minimal side effects. They are most effective in preventing pregnancy and STIs when used together with a condom.

Figure 9-9 HOW TO USE VAGINAL CONTRACEPTIVE FILM (VCF)
This thin film is laced with spermicide. Its effectiveness is similar to other spermicides, and is most effective with a condom.

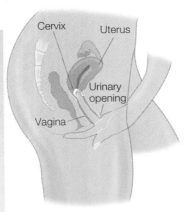

With one swift movement, place VCF high in your vagina against the cervix. VCF is effective for one hour. One film should be used for each act of intercourse. Follow the instructions in the product leaflet.

Vaginal Contraceptive Film

Available from pharmacies without a prescription, the 2-inch-by-2-inch thin film known as **vaginal contraceptive film (VCF)** is laced with spermicide. (See Figure 9-9.) Once folded and inserted into the vagina, it dissolves into a stay-in-place gel. Its theoretical effectiveness is similar to that of other forms of spermicide; paired with a condom, it is almost 100 percent effective.

Advantages VCF film can be used by people allergic to foams and jellies. Unlike foams and jellies, it dissolves gradually and almost unnoticeably.

Disadvantages Some people feel that insertion, even though it takes only seconds, interrupts sexual spontaneity.

How to Use Vaginal Contraceptive Film Fold one square of VCF in half, place it on your second or third finger, then insert high into the vagina, near the cervix. VCF is effective for one hour. One film should be used for each act of intercourse.

:: Periodic Abstinence and Fertility Awareness Methods

Awareness of a woman's cyclic fertility can help in both conception and contraception. The different methods of birth control based on a woman's menstrual cycle are sometimes referred to as *natural family planning* or *fertility awareness methods*. They include the calendar method, the basal-body-temperature method, and the cervical mucus

method (all described below). New fertility monitors that use saliva to determine time of ovulation can improve the accuracy of these methods.

Women's menstrual cycles vary greatly. To use one of the fertility awareness methods, a woman must know and understand her cycle. She should track her cycle for at least eight months—marking day one (the day bleeding begins) on a calendar, and counting the length of each cycle. Figure 9-10 shows the days in a 28-day cycle when abstinence or other contraceptive methods would be necessary.

Calendar Method

In this approach, often called the **rhythm method,** a woman counts forward eight days from day 1 of her period. This is the first day she is likely to be fertile, and she and her partner should abstain or use back-up contraception.

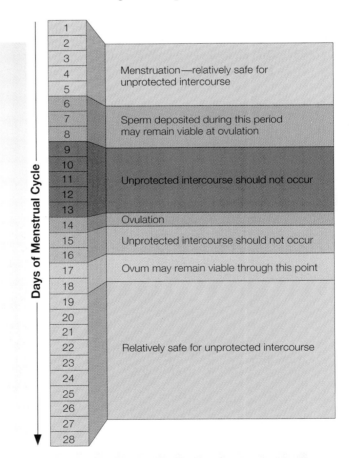

Figure 9-10 SAFE AND UNSAFE DAYS
Events in the menstrual cycle determine the relatively safe days for unprotected intercourse.

CycleBeads are an easy way for a woman to track her cycle and clearly identify the days she could become pregnant and the days when pregnancy is most unlikely.

Cycle Technologies and Institute for Reproductive Health, Georgetown University

The Standard Days Method

The Standard Days Method (SDM) is a sophisticated version of the calendar method for women with regular cycles. This new option is based on computerized analysis of reproductive physiology data. SDM identifies the 12-day "fertile window" of a woman's menstrual cycle: cycle days 8 through 19, during which the couple can protect against the risk of pregnancy through contraception or abstinence. The SDM formula is based on information on more than 7,500 menstrual cycles from women in five countries.[35]

To help women identify and keep track of days on which they are likely to get pregnant, the Institute for Reproductive Health at Georgetown University developed Cycle Beads™, a string of 32 color-coded beads with each bead representing a day of the menstrual cycle. A woman moves a small rubber ring one bead each day. Brown beads designate the days when pregnancy is very unlikely; glow-in-the-dark white beads represent fertile days. The method is 88 to 95 percent effective in preventing pregnancy when used correctly by women with regular menstrual cycles between 26 and 32 days long.[36]

There are different ways of calculating a woman's fertile days, but the longer the time of abstinence, the lower the risk of pregnancy. To determine unsafe days, she can subtract 18 from the total number of days in her shortest cycle. Some doctors recommend subtracting 21 rather than 18, but again, the longer the time of abstinence, the more likely you are to prevent pregnancy.

To find her last fertile day, a woman subtracts 11 days from her longest cycle. This is the last day she and her partner must abstain or use backup contraception.[34]

Basal–Body-Temperature Method

In this method the woman measures her **basal body temperature,** the body temperature upon waking in the morning, using a specially calibrated rectal thermometer, which is more precise than an oral one. She records her temperature on a chart. (See Figure 9-11.) The basal body temperature remains relatively constant from the beginning of the menstrual cycle to ovulation. After ovulation, however, the basal body temperature rises by more than 0.5 degree Fahrenheit. The woman knows that her safe period has begun when her temperature has been elevated for three consecutive days. After eight to ten months, she should have a sense of her ovulatory pattern, in addition to knowing her daily readings.

Cervical Mucus Method

This method, also called the **ovulation method,** is based on the observation of changes in the consistency of the mucus in the vagina. In the first days after menstruation, the vagina feels dry

Figure 9-11 BASAL-BODY TEMPERATURE METHOD
When her temperature has been elevated for three consecutive days, a woman knows that a relatively safe period for unprotected intercourse has begun.

because of a decline in hormone production, indicating a safe period for unprotected intercourse. Within a few days, estrogen levels rise, and the mucus begins to thin out and becomes less cloudy: The fertile period begins. At peak estrogen levels, the mucus is smooth, stretchable, and slippery (like raw egg white), and very clear. Mucus with these characteristics is usually observed within 24 hours of ovulation and lasts one to two days, signaling maximum fertility. The mucus becomes sticky and cloudy again three days thereafter, and the second safe period begins. Most women using this method have to refrain from unprotected intercourse for about 9 days of each 28-day menstrual cycle.

Advantages of Fertility Awareness Methods Birth control methods based on the menstrual cycle involve no expense, no side effects, and no need for prescriptions or fittings. On the days when the couple can have intercourse, there is nothing to insert, swallow, or check. In addition, abstinence during fertile periods complies with the teachings of the Roman Catholic Church.

Disadvantages of Fertility Awareness Methods
During times of possible fertility (usually eight to eleven days a month), couples must abstain from vaginal intercourse or use some form of contraception. Conscientious planning and scheduling are essential. Women with irregular cycles may not be able to rely on the calendar method. Others may find the mucus or temperature methods difficult to use. For all these reasons, this approach to birth control is less reliable than many others. In theory, the overall effectiveness rate for the various fertility awareness methods is 80 percent. In practice, of every 100 women using one of these methods for a year, 24 become pregnant. However, using a combination of the basal-body-temperature method and the cervical mucus method may be 90 to 95 percent effective in preventing pregnancy.

What Is Emergency Contraception?

Emergency contraception (EC) is the use of a method of contraception to prevent unintended pregnancy after unprotected intercourse or the failure of another form of contraception, such as a condom breaking or slipping off. Medical researchers do not fully understand how EC works. Emergency contraception pills (ECPs) may inhibit or delay ovulation, prevent union of sperm and ovum, or alter the endometrium so a fertilized ovum cannot implant itself. (See Fact or Fiction? "Emergency Contraception . . .") The copper-bearing intrauterine device (IUD) is also an EC option.[37]

There are two types of emergency contraceptive pills. Combined ECPs use estrogen and progestin, the same hormones used in ordinary birth control pills. A brand

FACT OR FICTION? ??????????????

Emergency contraception is not a form of abortion.

Fact: Emergency contraception consists of the same hormones found in ordinary birth control pills. When taken in a concentrated dose shortly after unprotected sex, these hormones reduce the risk of a pregnancy by about 75 percent. They do so in the same way as other hormonal contraceptives: they delay or inhibit ovulation, inhibit fertilization, or block implantation of a fertilized egg, depending on a woman's phase of the menstrual cycle. They have no effect once a pregnancy has been established.

Source: "Emergency Contraception: Increasing Public Awareness," *Issues Brief* (Alan Guttmacher Institute), Vol. 2, February 2003, p. 1.

called Preven is specifically packaged for emergency use, but several other brands can be used as well. Combined ECPs reduce the risk of unintended pregnancy by 75 to 88 percent. The second type of ECP contains only the hormone progestin and is packaged under the brand name Plan B. It has proven more effective than the first type, reducing the risk of pregnancy by 89 percent, with a lower risk of nausea and vomiting.[38]

Although ECPs are sometimes called *morning-after pills,* it is not necessary to wait until the morning after. A woman can start the pills right away or up to three days after unprotected sex. Therapy is more effective the earlier it is initiated, ideally within 24 hours. The second dose is generally taken 12 hours after the first dose. Each dose may consist of 1, 2, 4, or 5 pills, depending on the brand. Most women can safely use them, even if they cannot use birth control pills as their regular method of birth control. (Although ECPs use the same hormones as birth control pills, not all brands of birth control pills can be used for emergency contraception.) Some women may experience spotting or a full menstrual period a few days after taking ECPs, depending on where they were in their cycle when they began therapy. Most women have their next period at the expected time.

Another alternative is the copper IUD, which can be inserted by a physician up to five days after ovulation to prevent pregnancy. IUDs are more effective at preventing pregnancy than hormonal ECPs and reduce the risk of pregnancy by 99 percent. However, they are not used as commonly as hormonal methods for EC. Once inserted, the IUD can provide highly effective continuous contraceptive protection for 10 years.

The American College of Obstetricians and Gynecologists (ACOG) estimates that emergency contraception has the potential to reduce by half the 3 million unintended pregnancies each year in the United States.[39]

Along with other women's health groups, ACOG supports over-the-counter availability for ECP and has recommended that physicians offer women of reproductive age an advance prescription for use in any future emergency.

Despite its safety and effectiveness, many physicians do not regularly discuss it with patients, and many Americans are unaware of this option.[40] This is especially true of minority women.[41] As emergency contraception has become more well known, women increasingly turn to the Internet for answers to frequent questions, such as the occurrence of spotting and menstrual bleeding following EC use.[42]

In a recent national survey of colleges and universities, slightly more than half—52.2 percent—of student health centers offer emergency contraception. Private institutions, as well as those with a high proportion of commuter students, were less likely to do so than large public schools. Half of the schools that offered ECP had begun doing so within the previous five years. The primary benefit they cited was pregnancy prevention. Student health centers in the Midwest and South are less likely to offer ECP than those in the Northeast.[43]

Sterilization

The most popular method of birth control among married couples in the United States is **sterilization** (surgery to end a person's reproductive capability). Each year an estimated 1 million men and women in the United States undergo sterilization procedures. Fewer than 25 percent ever seek reversal.

Advantages Sterilization has no effect on sex drive in either men or women. Many couples report that their sexual activity increases after sterilization because they're free from the fear of pregnancy or the need to deal with contraceptives.

Disadvantages Sterilization should be considered permanent and should be used only if both individuals are sure they want no more children. Although sterilization doesn't usually create psychological or sexual problems, it can worsen existing problems, particularly marital ones. Couples should discuss sterilization, with each other and with a physician, to understand fully the possible physical and emotional consequences. Although a link between vasectomy and an increased risk of prostate cancer was reported, the most recent research did not find a correlation.

Male Sterilization

In men, the cutting of the vas deferens, the tube that carries sperm from one of the testes into the urethra for ejac-

ulation, is called **vasectomy.** During the 15- or 20-minute office procedure, done under a local anesthetic, the doctor makes small incisions in the scrotum, lifts up each vas deferens, cuts them, and ties off the ends to block the flow of sperm. (See Figure 9-12.) Sperm continue to form, but they are broken down and absorbed by the body.

The man usually experiences some local pain, swelling, and discoloration for about a week after the procedure. More serious complications, including the formation of a blood clot in the scrotum (which usually disappears without treatment), infection, and an inflammatory reaction, occur in a small percentage of cases. The National Institute of Child Health and Human Development, in a 15-year follow-up study of nearly 5,000 men, found that sterilization poses no increased danger of heart disease, even decades after the procedure. The pregnancy rate among the wives of men who've had vasec-

THE CUTTING EDGE

Future Contraceptives

What's the next best thing in birth control? Here are some of the birth control options currently under development:

- **Extended use hormonal contraceptives.** Manufacturers are testing once-a-week and once-a-month birth control pills as well as pills, patches, and vaginal rings that could provide pregnancy protection for three months or longer.

- **Invisible condoms.** A new generation of chemicals called microbicides kill sperm as well as sexually transmitted bacteria or viruses, including HIV. One, currently in clinical trials, is applied to the vagina in liquid form but turns into a gel when activated by body heat.

- **Contraceptive nasal spray.** In experiments with mice, Japanese researchers have been developing a nasal vaccine that changes female vaginal secretions to block sperm penetration.

- **Male pill.** In animal studies in England, a hormone-free contraceptive pill rendered male mice completely but reversibly infertile for up to six months but had no effect on testosterone levels or sexual behaviors. The mice regained fertility within four weeks of stopping the drug.

- **Male implants and patches.** Researchers are combining testosterone with a progestin in various forms, including pellets and patches, to block sperm production.

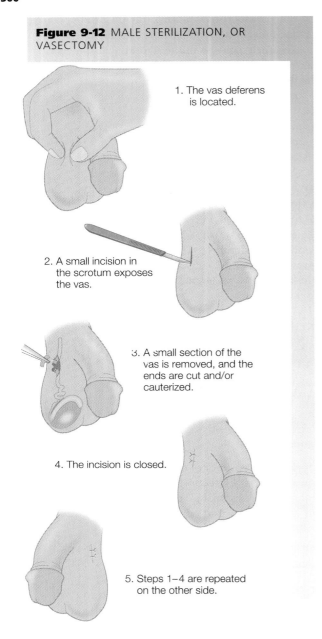

Figure 9-12 MALE STERILIZATION, OR VASECTOMY

1. The vas deferens is located.

2. A small incision in the scrotum exposes the vas.

3. A small section of the vas is removed, and the ends are cut and/or cauterized.

4. The incision is closed.

5. Steps 1–4 are repeated on the other side.

Female Sterilization

Female sterilization is the most commonly used "modern" contraceptive in the United States. About 27 percent of women who have chosen to use contraception have opted for tubal sterilization. Women are three times more likely to undergo sterilization than are men.[44] Female sterilization procedures modify the fallopian tubes, which each month normally carry an egg from the ovaries to the uterus. The two terms used to describe female sterilization are **tubal ligation** (the cutting or tying of the fallopian tubes) and **tubal occlusion** (the blocking of the tubes). The tubes may be cut or sealed with thread, a clamp, or a clip, or by coagulation (burning) to prevent the passage of eggs from the ovaries. (See Figure 9-13.) They can also be blocked with bands of silicone.

The procedures used for sterilization are laparotomy, laparoscopy, and colpotomy. **Laparotomy** involves making an abdominal incision about 2 inches long and cutting the tubes. A laparotomy usually requires a hospital stay and up to several weeks of recovery. It leaves a scar and carries the same risks as all major surgical procedures: the side effects of anesthesia, potential infection, and internal scars. In a **minilaparotomy,** an incision about an inch long is made just above the pubic hairline. The tubes may be tied, cut, plugged, or sealed by electrical coagulation. The operation can be performed by a skilled physician in 10 to 30 minutes, usually under local anesthesia, and the woman can generally go home the same day. The failure (pregnancy) rate is only 1 in 1,000.

Tubal ligation or occlusion can also be performed with the use of **laparoscopy,** commonly called *belly-button* or *band-aid surgery.* This procedure is done on an outpatient basis and takes 15 to 30 minutes. A lighted tube called a *laparoscope* is inserted through a half-inch incision made

tomies is about 15 in 10,000 women per year. Most result from a couple's failure to wait several weeks after the operation, until all sperm stored in each vas deferens have been ejaculated, before having unprotected coitus.

Sometimes men want to reverse their vasectomies, usually because they want to have children with a new spouse. Although anyone who chooses to have a vasectomy should consider it permanent, surgical reversal (*vasovasostomy*) is sometimes successful. New microsurgical techniques have led to annual pregnancy rates for the wives of men undergoing vasovasostomies of about 50 percent, depending on such factors as the doctor's expertise and the time elapsed since the vasectomy.

Figure 9-13 FEMALE STERILIZATION, OR TUBAL LIGATION

Fallopian tube

Cauterized

Tied and cut

Ovary

Uterus

right below the navel, giving the doctor a view of the fallopian tubes. Using surgical instruments that may be inserted through the laparoscope or through other tiny incisions, the doctor then cuts or seals the tubes, most commonly by electrical coagulation. The cumulative failure rate of the procedures is reported to be about 1.85 percent during a 10-year period. Complications include problems with anesthesia, hemorrhage, organ damage, and mortality.[45]

In a **colpotomy,** the fallopian tubes are reached through the vagina and cervix. This procedure leaves no external scar, but is somewhat more hazardous and less effective. A **hysterectomy** (removal of the uterus) is a major surgical procedure that is too dangerous to be used as a method of sterilization, unless there are other medically urgent reasons for removing the uterus.

Essure

This new method for permanent sterilization involves placement of small, flexible micro-coils into the fallopian tubes via the vagina by a physician. Unlike other methods it does not require the risks of general anesthesia and surgery. The procedure itself does not require incisions and takes an average of about 35 minutes. Recovery occurs quickly. In clinical trials, about 90 percent of women returned to work within 24 hours. For the first three months after insertion, women should use another form of contraception. An X ray called a hysterosalpingogram must confirm that the inserts are correctly placed and the fallopian tubes are completely blocked.

Like traditional forms of tubal ligation, Essure cannot be reversed. It is recommended only for women who definitely do not want more children and especially for those with medical and health problems (such as diabetes or obesity) that make surgery and anesthesia more dangerous. There is a risk that the microinserts may not be placed correctly at the first attempt (this occurred in 14 percent of women in one study). Because the procedure is new, long-term data on the effectiveness of Essure are not yet available.[46]

❖ Abortion

More than half of unintended pregnancies end in induced abortions. Abortion rates vary greatly around the world. The U.S. abortion rate, which has declined, still remains higher than that of many Western countries, including Canada, Great Britain, the Netherlands, and Sweden. Although there is no one single or simple explanation for this difference, researchers focus on America's high rate of unintended pregnancies. In many nations with fewer unwanted pregnancies and lower abortion rates, contraceptives are generally easier and cheaper to obtain, and early sex education strongly emphasizes their importance.[47]

No woman in any country ever elects to be in a situation where she has to consider abortion. But if faced with an unwanted pregnancy, many women consider *elective abortion* as an option.

After rising steadily through the 1970s, the number of legal abortions leveled off in the 1980s and declined in the 1990s (Figure 9-14).[48] According to the most recent data, the U.S. abortion rate is at its lowest in thirty years. The decline is greatest among young women. The reasons include decreased sexual activity among adolescents and increased use of effective contraceptives.[49] Although women of all backgrounds have abortions, abortion in the United States is increasingly likely to occur among single women, racial or ethnic minorities, low-income women, and women who have had at least one child.[50]

Thinking Through the Options

A woman faced with an unwanted pregnancy—often alone, unwed, and desperate—can find it extremely difficult to decide what to do. The political debate over the

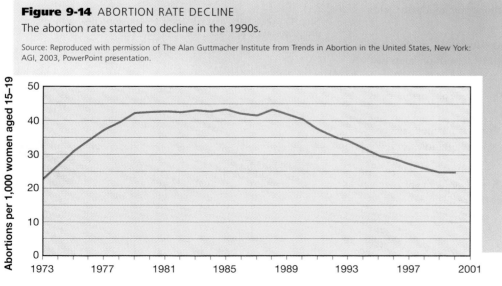

Figure 9-14 ABORTION RATE DECLINE
The abortion rate started to decline in the 1990s.

Source: Reproduced with permission of The Alan Guttmacher Institute from Trends in Abortion in the United States, New York: AGI, 2003, PowerPoint presentation.

right to life almost always is secondary to practical and emotional matters, such as the quality of her relationship with the baby's father, their capacity to provide for the child, the impact on any children she already has, and other important life issues.

Giving up her child for adoption is an option for women who do not feel abortion is right for them. Because the number of would-be adoptive parents greatly exceeds the number of available newborns, some women considering adoption may feel pressured by offers of money from couples eager to adopt. Others, particularly minority women, may feel cultural pressures to keep a child—regardless of their age, economic situation, or ability to care for an infant. Advocates of adoption reform are pressing for mandatory counseling for all pregnant women considering adoption (available now in agency-arranged, but not private, adoptions) and for extending the period of time during which a new mother can change her mind about giving up her child for adoption.

In deciding whether or not to have an abortion, women report asking themselves many questions, including the following:

:: How do I feel about the man with whom I conceived this baby? Do I love him? Does he love me? Is this man committed to staying with me?

:: What sort of relationship, if any, have we had or might we have in the future?

:: If I continue the pregnancy and give birth, could I love the baby?

:: Who can help me gain perspective on this problem?

:: Have I thought about adoption? Do I think I could surrender custody of my baby? Would it make a difference if the adoption process were open and I could know the adoptive parents?

:: If I keep my child, can I properly care for him or her?

:: How would the birth of another baby affect my other children?

:: Do I have marketable skills, an education, an adequate income? Would I be able to go to school or keep my job if I have a child? Who would help me?

:: Would this child be born with serious abnormalities? Would it suffer or thrive?

:: How does each option fit with what I believe is morally correct? Could I emotionally handle each option?

Answering these questions honestly and objectively may help women as they think through the realities of their situation.

Medical Abortion

The term **medical abortion** describes the use of drugs, also called *abortifacients,* to terminate a pregnancy. In 2000 the abortion pill mifepristone (Mifeprex), formerly known

as RU-486, became available for use in the United States. Mifepristone, which is 97 percent effective in inducing abortion, blocks progesterone, the hormone that prepares the uterine lining for pregnancy. Two days after taking this compound, a woman takes a prostaglandin to increase uterine contractions. The uterine lining is expelled along with the fertilized egg. (See Figure 9-15.) Women have

Figure 9-15 MEDICAL ABORTION
Mifepristone works by blocking the action of progesterone.

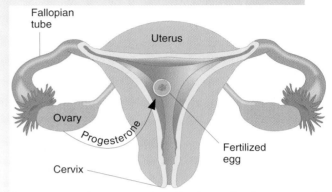

Progesterone, a hormone produced by the ovaries, is necessary for the implantation and development of a fertilized egg.

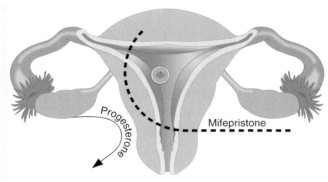

Step 1. Taken early in pregnancy, mifepristone blocks the action of progesterone and makes the body react as if it isn't pregnant.

Step 2. Prostaglandins, taken two days later, cause the uterus to contract and the cervix to soften and dilate. As a result, the fertilized egg is expelled in 97 percent of the cases.

compared the discomfort of this experience to severe menstrual cramps. Common side effects include excessive bleeding, nausea, fatigue, abdominal pain, and dizziness. About 1 woman in 100 requires a blood transfusion.

Within months of FDA approval of mifepristone, medical abortions accounted for 6 percent of all abortions. In European countries, where medical abortion was legalized a decade or more ago, the method has accounted for a growing share of early abortions each year without increasing the overall abortion rate.[51]

Other agents used in medical abortion are methotrexate, widely used to treat certain cancers and arthritis, and misoprostol (Cytotec), primarily prescribed in the United States to prevent gastrointestinal ulcers. Methotrexate interferes with the ability of cells to multiply and divide, which halts development of an embryo or placenta. Misoprostol causes the uterus to contract, which helps expel a fertilized egg. Although misoprostol has been used in combination with mifespristone, researchers are investigating whether it can be used alone to terminate pregnancy.

Although condemned by right-to-life advocates, abortion medications may in time lower the public profile of pregnancy termination. They are not painless, cheap, or equally available to all, but they do offer women a chance to carry through on their personal choice in greater privacy and safety. In a recent study, women who had a medical abortion reported a significantly higher level of satisfaction than those undergoing a surgical abortion.

Medical abortion does not require anesthesia, can be performed very early in pregnancy, and may feel more private. However, women experience more cramping and bleeding during medical abortion than during surgical abortion, and bleeding lasts for a longer period.

Other Abortion Methods

More than nine in ten abortions are performed in clinics, which account for 46 percent of all abortion providers. The number of providers is declining; one-third of American women now live in counties with no source of abortion services.[52] About half of all abortions (54 percent) are performed within the first 8 weeks of pregnancy. Only about 1 percent of abortions occur after 20 weeks. Medically, first-trimester abortion is less risky than childbirth. However, the likelihood of complications increases when abortions are performed in the second trimester (the second three-month period) of pregnancy.

The vast majority of abortions performed in the United States today are surgical. **Suction curettage,** usually done from 7 to 13 weeks after the last menstrual period, involves the gradual dilation (opening) of the cervix, often by inserting into the cervix one or more sticks of *laminaria* (a sterilized seaweed that absorbs moisture and expands, thus gradually stretching the cervix). Some women feel pressure or cramping with the laminaria

in place. Occasionally, the laminaria itself starts to bring on a miscarriage.

At the time of abortion, the laminaria is removed, and dilators are used to further enlarge the cervical opening, if needed. The physician inserts a suction tip into the cervix, and the uterine contents are drawn out via a vacuum system. (See Figure 9-16.) A *curette* (a spoon-shaped surgical instrument used for scraping) is used to check for complete removal of the contents of the uterus. With suction curettage, the risks of complication are low. Major complications, such as perforation of the uterus, occur in fewer than 1 in 100 cases.

For early second-trimester abortions, physicians generally use a technique called **dilation and evacuation (D and E),** in which they open the cervix and use medical instruments to remove the fetus from the uterus. D and E procedures are performed under local or general anesthesia.

To induce abortion from week 16 to week 20, prostaglandins (natural substances found in most body tissues) are administered as vaginal suppositories or injected into the amniotic sac by inserting a needle through the abdominal wall. They induce uterine contractions, and the fetus and placenta are expelled within 24 hours. Injecting saline or urea solutions into the amniotic sac can also terminate the pregnancy by triggering contractions that expel the fetus and placenta. Sometimes vaginal suppositories or drugs that help the uterus contract are used. Complications from abortion techniques that induce labor include nausea, vomiting, diarrhea, tearing of the cervix, excessive bleeding, and possible shock and death.

Hysterotomy involves surgically opening the uterus and removing the fetus. This is generally done from week

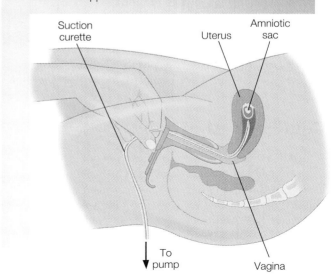

Figure 9-16 SUCTION CURETTAGE
The contents of the uterus are extracted through the cervix with a vacuum apparatus.

Suction curette

Amniotic sac

Uterus

To pump

Vagina

16 to week 24 of the pregnancy, primarily in emergency situations when the woman's life is in danger, or when other methods of abortion are considered too risky. However, late pregnancy abortions increase the risk of spontaneous abortion or premature labor in subsequent pregnancies and should be avoided if possible.

What Is the Psychological Impact of Abortion?

Many assume that abortion must be psychologically devastating, that women who abort a fetus sooner or later develop what some have termed *post-abortion trauma syndrome*. In her studies at the University of Chicago, psychiatrist Nada Stotland found that there is no such thing. The primary emotion of women who have just had an abortion, she discovered, is relief. Although many women also express feelings of sadness or guilt, their anxiety levels eventually drop until they are lower than they were immediately before the abortion.

Nonetheless, although psychologists consider the mental-health risks minimal compared to those of bearing an unwanted child, this does not mean women who have abortions never have regrets. In one recent study, nearly one in five women reported sadness, dissatisfaction, and regret about her abortion two years later.[53] But a feeling—even one as painful as loss, sadness, or guilt—is not a syndrome, and a woman's responses to abortion often change with passing days, weeks, months, or years. Anniversaries—of conception, of the date a woman found out she was pregnant, of the abortion, of the delivery date—can trigger memories and a sense of loss, but most women deal with these and move on with their lives.

The best predictor of psychological well-being after abortion is a woman's emotional well-being prior to pregnancy. At highest risk are women who have had a psychiatric illness, such as an anxiety disorder or clinical depression, prior to an abortion, and those whose abortions occurred among complicated circumstances (such as a rape, or coercion by parents or a partner). The vast majority of women manage to put the abortion into perspective as one of many life events.

Politics of Abortion

Abortion is one of the most controversial political, religious, and ethical issues of our time. The issues of when life begins, a woman's right to choose, and an unborn child's right to survival are among the most divisive Americans face. Abortions were legal in the United States until the 1860s. For decades after that, women who decided to terminate unwanted pregnancies did so by attempting to abort themselves or by obtaining illegal abortions—often performed by untrained individuals using

unsanitary and unsafe procedures. In the late 1960s, some states changed their laws to make abortions legal. In 1973, the U.S. Supreme Court, following a 1970 ruling on the case of *Roe v. Wade* by the New York Supreme Court, said that an abortion in the first trimester of pregnancy was a decision between a woman and her physician, and was protected by privacy laws. The Court further ruled that abortion during the second trimester could be performed on the basis of health risks and that abortion during the final trimester could be performed only for the sake of the mother's health.

Since then, several laws have restricted the availability of legal abortions for low-income women. In 1989, the U.S. Supreme Court narrowed the interpretation of *Roe v. Wade* by upholding a law that sharply restricted publicly funded abortions and required doctors to test if a fetus more than 20 weeks old could survive. In 1992, in *Planned Parenthood v. Casey*, the Court upheld the right to legalized abortion but gave states the right to restrict abortion as long as they did not place an "undue burden" on a woman. This limited the availability of abortion to young, rural, and low-income women. In 2000, in *Sternberg v. Carhart*, the U.S. Supreme Court struck down Nebraska's ban on "partial birth abortions," a term abortion opponents use for dilation and extraction, a second-trimester surgical procedure.

The debate over abortion continues to stir passionate emotions, with pro-life supporters arguing that life begins

The controversy over abortion has resulted in countless demonstrations and encounters between pro-choice and pro-life supporters.

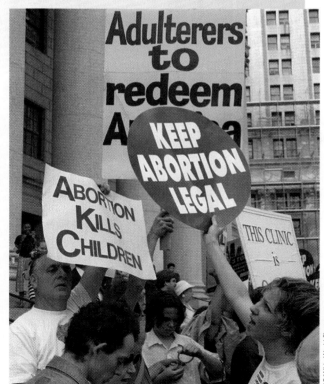

AP/Wide World Photos

at conception and that abortion is therefore immoral, and pro-choice advocates countering that an individual woman should have the right to make decisions about her body and health. The controversy over abortion has at times become violent: Physicians who performed abortions have been shot and killed; abortion clinics have been bombed, wounding and killing patients and staff members.[54]

Although the majority of Americans continue to support abortion, many feel that it should be more restricted and difficult to obtain. While 61 percent of Americans say abortion should be permitted during the first three months of pregnancy, only 15 percent support second-trimester abortions and 7 percent feel that abortions in the last trimester should be legal.

A Cross-Cultural Perspective

Throughout the world an estimated 10 to 20 million illegal abortions are performed each year. About 1 in 100 women dies as a result. Women who survive illegal abortions may suffer chronic health problems related to the lack of adequate medical care.

In other countries, abortion laws vary greatly. In Eastern Europe, where abortions were once legal and common, the collapse of communism has led to new restrictions on abortion. By contrast, Spain's supreme court has relaxed legal restrictions on abortions performed on social grounds. In Pakistan, new, more liberal rules on abortion state that abortion is no longer a crime if carried out to provide "necessary treatment." In Latin America, where anti-abortion laws are very strict, Cuba is the only country in which abortion on request is legal in early pregnancy. In other nations of Central and South America, women obtaining abortions and those performing them face criminal penalties, including imprisonment.

Childfree by Choice

In Europe, fertility rates in many nations are at an all-time low. In the United States, one in five women in the baby boom generation has not given birth—many because of a decision not to. More women and men are deliberately choosing to remain "childfree."

According to the limited data available, single childfree women tend to be better educated, more cosmopolitan, less religious, and more professional than those in the general population. In general, childfree women are high achievers, often in demanding careers, who describe their work as exciting and satisfying. Childless couples are predominantly urban, well-educated, and upper middle class, with egalitarian and long-running marriages.

Their reasons for not having children are diverse: a desire to maintain their freedom, more time with their

partners, career ambitions, concern about overpopulation and the fate of the Earth. Some women cite the hostile work environment for mothers and the inadequacy of day care. Others say they're disillusioned with the have-it-all hopes of baby boomers and believe in a have-most-of-it philosophy.

Some observers theorize that childfree women will regret their choice after it's too late to do anything about it. However, this doesn't seem to be the case. In a study of 90 childless women over age 60, a Philadelphia anthropologist found that, while the women who believed that a woman's primary duty is to have children did express some regret, most women had come up with satisfying alternative ways of living. In another study of nearly 700 Canadian women and men over age 55, those who chose childlessness were just as happy as parents who had good relationships with their children—and happier than parents who described their relationships with their children as distant.[55] "Not everybody needs children to have a full life," says Leslie Lafayette, who founded the ChildFree Network (CFN) to create a sense of belonging among people without children.[56]

Pregnancy

In the last half century, pregnancy rates have generally declined, although the absolute number of births has risen.[57] The average age of mothers in the United States has risen, but about 70 percent of babies are still born to women in their twenties. Mothers are now averaging slightly fewer than two children each. Not every married couple is opting for parenthood.

Of course, you don't have to be part of a couple to want or to conceive a child. The number of never-married, college-educated, career women who are becoming single parents has risen dramatically. They want children—with or without an ongoing relationship with a man—and may feel that, because of their age, they can't delay getting pregnant any longer.

Preconception Care: A Preventive Approach

The time *before* a child is conceived can be crucial in assuring that an infant is born healthy, full-size, and full-term. Women who smoke, drink alcohol, take drugs, eat poorly, are too thin or too heavy, suffer from unrecognized infections or illnesses, or are exposed to toxins at work or home may start pregnancy with one or more strikes against them and their unborn babies. The best chance for lowering the infant mortality rate and preventing birth defects is before pregnancy. **Preconception care**—the enhancement of a woman's health and well-being prior to conception in order to ensure a healthy pregnancy and baby—includes risk assessment (evaluation of medical, genetic, and lifestyle risks), health promotion (such as teaching good nutrition), and interventions to reduce risk (such as treatment of infections and other diseases, and assistance in quitting smoking or drug use).

How a Woman's Body Changes During Pregnancy

The 40 weeks of pregnancy transform a woman's body. At the beginning of pregnancy, the woman's uterus becomes slightly larger, and the cervix becomes softer and bluish due to increased blood flow. Progesterone and estrogen trigger changes in the milk glands and ducts in the breasts, which increase in size and feel somewhat tender. The pressure of the growing uterus against the bladder causes a more frequent need to urinate. As the pregnancy progresses, the woman's skin stretches as her body shape changes, her center of gravity changes as her abdomen protrudes, and her internal organs shift as the baby grows. (See Figure 9-17.) Pregnancy is typically divided into three-month periods called trimesters.

How a Baby Grows

Silently and invisibly, over a nine-month period, a fertilized egg develops into a human being. When the zygote reaches the uterus, it's still smaller than the head of a pin. Once nestled into the spongy uterine lining, it becomes an **embryo.** The embryo takes on an elongated shape, rounded at one end. A sac called the **amnion** envelops it (see photo, Figure 9-17). As water and other small molecules cross the amniotic membrane, the embryo floats freely in the absorbed fluid, cushioned from shocks and bumps. At nine weeks the embryo is called a **fetus.**

A special organ, the **placenta,** forms. Attached to the embryo by the umbilical cord, it supplies the growing baby with fluid and nutrients from the maternal bloodstream and carries waste back to the mother's body for disposal. (See Figure 9-18.)

🔲🎧 Why Is Prenatal Care Important?

A pregnant woman has to take good care of herself to provide good care for her unborn child. This means regular medical and dental checkups. A woman should have her first prenatal visit as soon as she discovers that she's pregnant. A study group of the American College of Obstetricians and Gynecologists (ACOG) has recommended seven or eight prenatal visits for women with low-risk pregnancies; women at higher risk require more frequent checkups. Many teenage and unmarried pregnant women don't get adequate prenatal care, and some don't

see a health-care professional until late in their pregnancy, because they can't afford or don't have access to medical services. Even women who begin prenatal care in the second and third trimester lower their risk of having a low-birthweight baby.[58]

Age

Risks to the fetus are greater when mothers are older than 35, primarily an increase in fetal birth defects due to chromosomal abnormalities, such as Down syndrome. At age 30, the estimated risk of 2.6 per thousand; the incidence rises to 5.6 per thousand at age 35; 15.8 at age 40; and 53.7 at age 45. However, pregnancy itself for healthy women over age 35 is safe. As discussed later in this chapter, assisted reproductive technologies have enabled women in their forties, fifties, and even sixties to have successful pregnancies.

Nutrition

A well-balanced diet throughout pregnancy is critical for a mother and her fetus both before and at birth. If a woman—regardless of her prepregnancy weight—gains too little weight, the risk to the growing fetus is high. ACOG recommends a weight gain of 22 to 27 pounds during pregnancy. The National Academy of Sciences' Food and Nutrition Board advises a maximum weight gain of 35 pounds, based on findings that weight gain aids fetal growth and lowers the risk of infant mortality and mental retardation.

Substance Use

Smoking endangers two lives: the mother's and the fetus's. The sooner a mother-to-be stops smoking, the better the chances that the fetus will develop normally. Smoking increases the risk of miscarriage, stillbirth, low birthweight, heart defects, and premature birth, and also impairs growth. The fetus's oxygen supply is impaired by the increased levels of carbon monoxide in the smoking mother's bloodstream. Passive smoking (inhaling other people's smoke) can be hazardous for the mother and fetus as well. (See Chapter 11.)

Approximately 16 percent of pregnant women report drinking in the previous month. According to the CDC, more than 8,000 alcohol-damaged babies are born every year. One of every 750 newborns has a cluster of physical and mental defects called **fetal alcohol syndrome (FAS):** low birthweight, smaller-than-normal head circumference, smaller and shorter size, irritability as newborns, and permanent mental impairment as a result of

First Trimester

Increased urination because of hormonal changes and the pressure of the enlarging uterus on the bladder.

Enlarged breasts as milk glands develop.

Darkening of the nipples and the area around them.

Nausea or vomiting, particularly in the morning.

Fatigue.

Increased vaginal secretions.

Pinching of the sciatic nerve, which runs from the buttocks down through the back of the legs, as the pelvic bones widen and begin to separate.

Irregular bowel movements.

Before conception   At 4 months

Second Trimester

Thickening of the waist as the uterus grows.

Weight gain.

Increase in total blood volume.

Slight increase in size and change in position of the heart.

Darkening of the pigment around the nipple and from the navel to the pubic region.

Darkening of the face.

Increased salivation and perspiration.

Secretion of colostrum from the breasts.

Indigestion, constipation, and hemorrhoids.

Varicose veins.

At 7 months

At 9 months

Third Trimester

Increased urination because of pressure from the uterus.

Tightening of the uterine muscles (called Braxton-Hicks contractions).

Shortness of breath because of increased pressure by the uterus on the lungs and diaphragm.

Heartburn and indigestion.

Trouble sleeping because of the baby's movements or the need to urinate.

Descending ("dropping") of the baby's head into the pelvis about two to four weeks before birth.

Navel pushed out.

© Petit Format/Nestle/ScienceSource/Photo Researchers, Inc.

Figure 9-17 PHYSIOLOGICAL CHANGES OF PREGNANCY

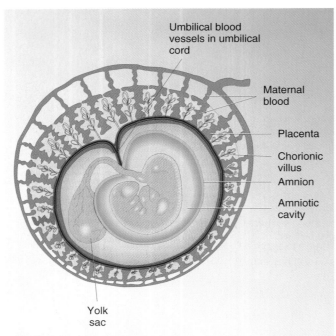

Figure 9-18 THE PLACENTA

The placenta supplies the growing embryo with fluid and nutrients from the maternal bloodstream and carries waste back for disposal.

Most pregnant women benefit from regular, moderate exercise. For women who were very active before their pregnancies, a higher level of activity is probably fine, but they should consult with their physician first.

their mothers' alcohol consumption. The milder forms of these problems, particularly impaired intellectual ability and school performance, are called fetal alcohol effects (FAE). (See Chapter 10.)

The risk of fetal alcohol syndrome is greatest if a mother drinks 3 ounces or more of pure alcohol (the equivalent of six or seven cocktails) a day. However, moderate drinking—one or two cocktails daily—may also have an effect. Even one drink a day has been associated with birth defects; binge drinking (five or more drinks on one occasion) is most toxic. The National Institute on Alcohol Abuse and Alcoholism and the Surgeon General advise pregnant women—and those trying to become pregnant—to abstain from drinking alcohol.[59]

Prenatal Testing

All parents worry that their unborn baby might not be normal and healthy. Sophisticated new tests can answer some, but not all, of their questions and can identify more than 250 diseases and defects. Prenatal tests are being performed earlier and with less risk to a fetus than ever before. The most common prenatal tests include the following:

:: *Ultrasonography* uses high-frequency sound waves to produce an image of the fetus on a video screen and as a photographic picture. Ultrasound can check fetal age and spot certain birth defects.

:: *Alpha-fetoprotein (AFP) screening,* performed from the 13th to 20th week of pregnancy, measures a substance produced by the baby's kidneys in the mother's blood. Levels that are too high could indicate a neural tube defect; levels that are too low may signal Down syndrome.

:: *Chorionic villi sampling (CVS),* performed from the eighth to tenth week of pregnancy, involves suctioning a small sample of the chorionic villi, the tissue surrounding the fetus, for laboratory analysis (see Figure 9-19). Results are generally available within a week.

:: *Amniocentesis,* performed from the 14th to 16th week of pregnancy, consists of removing a small amount of the amniotic fluid surrounding the fetus. This fluid contains cells shed by the fetus, which can be grown in tissue culture and then checked for any chromosomal or genetic defects (see Figure 9-19).

There are no known risks for ultrasonography and AFP screening. For both amniocentesis and CVS, there is about a 1 percent risk of miscarriage. Some testing centers have reported a higher incidence of both limb defects and miscarriage following CVS than others using this technique. Before choosing a facility for testing, pregnant women should inquire about that facility's experience and complication rate. Prenatal tests are usually recommended only if the mother is over age 35, has had a child with a genetic

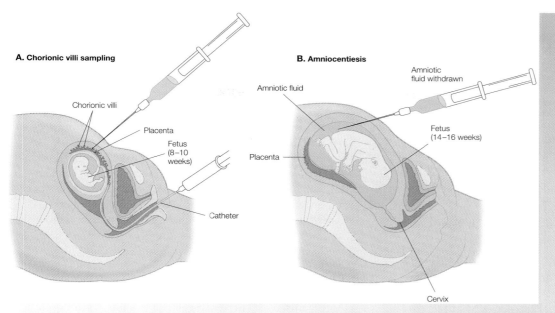

A. Chorionic villi sampling

Chorionic villi

Placenta

Fetus
(8–10
weeks)

Catheter

B. Amniocentiesis

Amniotic fluid

Amniotic
fluid withdrawn

Fetus
(14–16 weeks)

Placenta

Cervix

Figure 9-19 PRENATAL TESTING

(A) In chorionic villi sampling (CVS), a tissue sample of the villi is removed from the uterus through either a catheter into the uterus or a needle through the abdominal wall. The tissue sample is then analyzed for chromosomal defects. (B) In amniocentesis, a sample of the amniotic fluid is withdrawn; fetal cells found in that fluid can then be grown in tissue culture and checked for chromosomal defects.

disorder, or is a known carrier of a detectable genetic disorder.

Complications of Pregnancy

In about 10 to 15 percent of all pregnancies, there is increased risk of some problem, such as a baby's failure to grow normally. **Perinatology,** or maternal-fetal medicine, focuses on the special needs of high-risk mothers and their unborn babies. Perinatal centers, with state-of-the-art equipment and 24-hour staffs of specialists in this field, have been set up around the country. Several of the most frequent potential complications of pregnancy are discussed below.

Ectopic Pregnancy

Any woman who is of childbearing age, has had intercourse, and feels abdominal pain with no reasonable cause may have an **ectopic pregnancy.** In this type of pregnancy, the fertilized egg remains in the fallopian tube instead of traveling to the uterus. Ectopic, or tubal, pregnancies have increased dramatically in recent years, now accounting for 2 percent of all reported pregnancies. STIs, particularly chlamydia infections (discussed in Chapter 13), have become a major cause of ectopic pregnancy. Other risk factors include previous pelvic surgery, particularly

involving the fallopian tubes; pelvic inflammatory disease; infertility; and use of an IUD.

In an ectopic pregnancy, a misplaced egg develops normally, producing the usual signs of pregnancy, until the cramped amniotic sac bursts, damaging the fallopian tube. The women will bleed internally and feel lower abdominal pains, or she may feel an aching in her shoulders, as the blood flows upward toward the diaphragm. If the bleeding is substantial, the women can go into shock, with low blood pressure and a high pulse rate. Symptoms are hot and cold flashes, nausea, dizziness, fainting, pelvic pain, and irregular bleeding.

Treatment for the damaged fallopian tube is usually removal, but microsurgery can often repair the damage. About 50 percent of the women who have had an ectopic pregnancy conceive again; 10 percent have another ectopic pregnancy. Ectopic pregnancies can lead to permanent infertility.

Miscarriage

About 10 to 20 percent of pregnancies end in **miscarriage,** or spontaneous abortion, before the 20th week of gestation. Major genetic disorders may be responsible for 33 to 50 percent of pregnancy losses. The most common cause is an abnormal number of chromosomes. About 0.5 to 1 percent of women suffer three or more miscarriages, possibly because of genetic, anatomic, hormonal, infectious, or autoimmune factors. An estimated 70 to 90 percent of women who miscarry eventually become pregnant again.

Physicians typically recommend bed rest if a woman begins bleeding or cramping early in pregnancy. In some cases, the cramping stops, and the pregnancy continues normally. In others, the bleeding becomes intense, the cervix widens, and the embryo is expelled. If the miscar-

STRATEGIES FOR PREVENTION

A Mother-to-Be's Guide to a Healthy Pregnancy

■ ACOG recommends consuming about 300 more calories a day than before pregnancy and concentrating on eating the right foods, not on watching your weight. Never diet during pregnancy. Don't restrict salt intake either, unless specifically directed to by your doctor.

■ Drink six to eight glasses of liquids each day, including water, fruit and vegetable juices, and milk.

■ Don't exercise strenuously for more than 15 minutes, ACOG advises. Avoid vigorous exercise in hot, humid weather. Never let your body temperature rise above 100°F or your heart rate climb above 140 beats per minute.

■ Stretch and flex carefully because the joints and connective tissue soften and loosen during pregnancy. After the fourth month of pregnancy, don't do any exercises while lying on your back, as this could impair blood flow to the placenta.

■ Walk, swim, and jog in moderation; play tennis only if you played before pregnancy. Ski only if you're experienced, and stick to low altitudes and safe slopes. Do not water-ski, surf, or ride a horse.

riage is complete, the bleeding stops and the uterus returns to its normal state and shape. If it is incomplete, a physician has to remove any bits of tissue remaining in the uterus.

Few medical events are more emotionally devastating than a pregnancy loss. Women often feel the loss in an extremely intense, almost physical way. Many who miscarry had not reached the point in pregnancy where the fetus seems separate from them. Typically, women feel both vulnerable and responsible, as if they did something to cause the loss or should have, could have, done something to prevent it. They try to identify what they did wrong: exercising or not exercising, working or not working; eating too much or not enough. Some women interpret a loss as a punishment for past sins, imagined or real. Such self-inflicted guilt, allowed to fester, can lead to major depression.

Infections

The infectious disease most clearly linked to birth defects is **rubella** (German measles). All women should be vaccinated against this disease at least three months prior to conception, to protect themselves and any children they

may bear. (See Chapter 13 for more on immunization.) The most common prenatal infection today is *cytomegalovirus*. This infection produces mild flulike symptoms in adults but can cause brain damage, retardation, liver disease, cerebral palsy, hearing problems, and other malformations in unborn babies.

STIs, such as syphilis, gonorrhea, and genital herpes, can be particularly dangerous during pregnancy if not recognized and treated. If a woman has a herpes outbreak around the date her baby is due, her physician will deliver the baby by caesarean section to prevent infecting the baby. HIV infection endangers both a pregnant woman and her unborn baby, and all pregnant women and new mothers should be aware of the HIV epidemic, the risks to them and their babies, and the availability of anonymous testing.

Premature Labor

Approximately 10 percent of all babies are born too soon (before the 37th week of pregnancy). According to researchers, prematurity is the main underlying cause of stillbirth and infant deaths within the first few weeks after birth. Bed rest, close monitoring, and, if necessary, medications for at-risk women can buy more time in the womb for their babies. But women must recognize the warning signs of **premature labor**—dull, low backache; a feeling of tightness or pressure on the lower abdomen; and intestinal cramps, sometimes with diarrhea. Low-birthweight premature babies face the highest risks, but comprehensive, enriched programs can reduce developmental and health problems.

Childbirth

A generation ago, delivering a baby was something a doctor did in a hospital. Today parents can choose from an almost bewildering array of birthing options. The first decision parents-to-be face is choosing a birth attendant, who can be a physician or a nurse-midwife. Certified nurse-midwives in the United States deliver more than 90,000 babies a year, mostly in hospitals and birth centers. Their approach is based on the belief that the typical pregnant woman can deliver her baby naturally without technological intervention. Lay midwives have a similar orientation but less formal training; only a handful of states permit lay midwives to deliver babies.

Preparing for Childbirth

The most widespread method of childbirth preparation is **psychoprophylaxis,** or the **Lamaze method.** Fernand Lamaze, a French doctor, instructed women to respond to

Today's fathers are routinely present at the birth of their children and often act as birth coaches after both parents participate in childbirth preparation classes.

labor contractions with prelearned, controlled breathing techniques. As the intensity of each contraction increases, the laboring woman concentrates on increasing her breathing rate in a prescribed way. Her partner coaches her during each contraction and helps her cope with discomfort.

Women who attend prenatal classes are less likely to undergo Cesarean deliveries and more likely to breast feed.[60] They also tend to have fewer complications and require fewer medications. However, painkillers or anesthesia are always an option if labor is longer or more painful than expected. The lower body can be numbed with an **epidural block,** which involves injecting an anesthetic into the membrane around the spinal cord, or a **spinal block,** in which the injection goes directly into the spinal canal. General anesthesia is usually used only for emergency caesarean births.

What Is Childbirth Like?

There are three stages of **labor.** The first starts with *effacement* (thinning) and *dilation* (opening up) of the cervix. Effacement is measured in percentages, and dilation in centimeters or finger-widths. Around this time, the amniotic sac of fluids usually breaks, a sign that the woman should call her doctor or midwife.

The first contractions of the early, or *latent,* phase of labor are usually not uncomfortable; they last 15 to 30 seconds, occur every 15 to 30 minutes, and gradually increase in intensity and frequency. The most difficult contractions come after the cervix is dilated to about 8 centimeters, as the woman feels greater pressure from the fetus. The first stage ends when the cervix is completely dilated to a diameter of 10 centimeters (or five finger-widths) and the baby is ready to come down the birth canal. (See Figure

9-20.) For women having their first baby, this first stage of labor averages 12 to 13 hours. Women having another child often experience shorter first-stage labor.

When the cervix is completely dilated, the second stage of labor occurs, during which the baby moves into the vagina, or birth canal, and out of the mother's body. As this stage begins, women who have gone through childbirth preparation training often feel a sense of relief from the acute pain of the transition phase and at the prospect of giving birth.

This second stage can take up to an hour or more. Strong contractions may last 60 to 90 seconds and occur every two to three minutes. As the baby's head descends, the mother feels an urge to push. By bearing down, she helps the baby complete its passage to the outside.

As the baby's head appears, or *crowns,* the doctor may perform an *episiotomy*—an incision from the lower end of the vagina toward the anus to enlarge the vaginal opening. The purpose of the episiotomy is to prevent the baby's head from causing an irregular tear in the vagina, but routine episiotomies have been criticized as unnecessary. Women may be able to avoid this procedure by trying different birthing positions or having an attendant massage the perineal tissue.

Usually the baby's head emerges first, then its shoulders, then its body. With each contraction, a new part is born. However, the baby can be in a more difficult position, facing up rather than down, or with the feet or buttocks first (a **breech birth**), and a caesarean birth may then be necessary.

In the third stage of labor, the uterus contracts firmly after the birth of the baby and, usually within five minutes, the placenta separates from the uterine wall. The woman may bear down to help expel the placenta, or the doctor may exert gentle external pressure. If an episiotomy has been performed, the doctor sews up the incision. To help the uterus contract and return to its normal size, it may be massaged manually, or the baby may be put to the mother's breast to stimulate contraction of the uterus.

Caesarean Birth

In a **caesarean delivery** (also referred to as a *caesarean section*), the doctor lifts the baby out of the woman's body through an incision made in the lower abdomen and uterus. The most common reason for caesarean birth is *failure to progress,* a vague term indicating that labor has gone on too long and may put the baby or mother at risk. Other reasons include the baby's position (if feet or buttocks are first) and signs that the fetus is in danger.

Thirty years ago, only 5 percent of babies born in America were delivered by caesarean birth; the current rate is 22.6 percent, substantially higher than in most other industrialized countries. About 36 percent of caesarean sections are performed because the woman has had a previous caesarean birth. However, four of every five women who

Figure 9-20 BIRTH

(a)

Umbilical cord
Uterus
Placenta
Vagina
Cervix

(b)

Sacrum

(c)

Perineum

(d)

Uterus
Placenta (detaching)
Umbilical cord

have had caesarean births can have successful vaginal deliveries in subsequent pregnancies.

Caesarean birth involves abdominal surgery, so many women feel more physical discomfort after a caesarean than a vaginal birth, including nausea, pain, and abdominal gas. Women who have had a caesarean section must refrain from strenuous activity, such as heavy lifting, for several weeks.

After the Birth

Hospital stays for new mothers are shorter than in the past. The average length of stay is now only 2.6 days for a vaginal delivery and 4.1 days after a caesarean birth. A primary reason has been pressure to reduce medical costs. Obstetricians have voiced concern that the rush to release new mothers may jeopardize their well-being and the health of their babies, who are more likely to require emergency care for problems such as jaundice. The American College of Obstetricians and Gynecologists and the American Academy of Pediatrics recommend that women remain in the hospital two days after a vaginal delivery and four days after a caesarean birth.

Breast-Feeding Versus Bottle-Feeding

A generation ago, most middle- and upper-class women bottle-fed their babies. Today, an increasing number of medical professionals state that breast milk is best. Breast-fed babies have fewer illnesses, a much lower hospitalization rate, and a lower mortality rate. Breast milk seems not only to prevent disease, but also to help bring infection under control. When breast-fed babies do get sick, they recover more quickly. Breastfeeding women are generally advised not to use contraceptives containing estrogen.

Despite the benefits of breast-feeding, there are valid reasons to choose bottle-feeding. According to the American Council on Science and Health, at least 20 percent of women are unable to breast-feed after their first deliveries, and 50 percent of new mothers encounter significant difficulties nursing. Sometimes the woman's breasts become inflamed, or she must take medications that would endanger her infant; sometimes the infant is unable to suckle vigorously enough to get an adequate milk supply. Another problem is that in certain areas of the country, the levels of pesticides and other chemical contaminants in mother's milk can be high.

 ## Babies at Risk

According to the National Center for Health Statistics, a record percentage of U.S. newborns are surviving to their first birthday. The infant mortality rate is a record low of 6.9 deaths per 1,000 live births. However, African-American babies are not faring as well. They face a much greater risk of dying, primarily because of prematurity and dangerously low birthweight, before their first birthday. Babies of Chinese and Japanese descent have the lowest mortality rates.

In all, more than 1.3 million newborns each year require special care after birth because of prematurity, low birthweight, birth defects, jaundice, respiratory difficulties, or other problems. About 6 percent of newborns—more than 200,000 babies a year—require immediate intensive care for potentially life-threatening problems that developed before, during, or after birth.

Genetic Disorders

In some sense, each of us is a carrier of a genetic problem. Every individual has an estimated four to six defective genes, but the chances of passing them on to a child are slim. Almost all are recessive, which means they are "masked" by a more influential dominant gene. The likelihood of a child inheriting the same faulty recessive gene from both parents is remote—unless the parents are so closely related that they have very similar genetic makeup.

The child of a parent with an abnormal dominant gene has a 50 percent likelihood of inheriting it. The most common of such defects are minor, such as the growth of an extra finger or toe. However, some single-gene defects can be fatal. Huntington's chorea, for example, is a degenerative disease that in the past was usually not diagnosed until midlife.

Genetic tests can identify "carriers" of abnormal recessive genes for diseases such as sickle-cell anemia (the most common genetic disorder among African Americans), beta-thalassemia (found in families of Mediterranean origin), and Tay-Sachs (found in Jews of Eastern European origin). Two carriers of the same abnormal recessive genes can pass such problems on to their children.

The most common genetic disorders are not fatal. They include:

:: *Cystic fibrosis.* The most common genetic problem among white Americans, this is a disabling abnormality of the respiratory system and sweat and mucous glands.

:: *Down syndrome.* This disorder is caused by an extra number 21 chromosome and occurs in one of every 600 to 1,000 births. Infants are born with varying degrees of physical and mental retardation. The chances of a woman delivering an infant with Down syndrome increase with her age. At age 25, the chances are 1 in 1,200; at age 35, they rise to 1 in 365; and at age 40, they are 1 in 100.

:: *Sickle-cell anemia.* About 8 to 10 percent of North America's 25 million African Americans carry a gene for sickle-cell anemia, a blood disorder that occurs when hemoglobin, the oxygen-carrying protein of red blood cells, is abnormal and causes red blood cells to assume a crescent (sickle) shape. Unable to provide adequate oxygen to vital organs of the body, sickled cells cause fatigue, loss of interest and appetite, pain, and a host of other symptoms.

:: *Phenylketonuria (PKU).* This disease occurs when the liver enzyme needed by the body for the metabolism of the amino acid phenylalanine is absent. If both parents are carriers, there's a one-in-four chance that the child will develop phenylketonuria (PKU). In most states, the law requires testing newborns for PKU. If PKU is detected, an immediate, long-term phenylalanine-free diet can reduce the effects of the disorder. If untreated, the victim becomes severely mentally retarded.

:: *Tay-Sachs disease.* Occurring almost exclusively among young children of Eastern European Jewish ancestry, Tay-Sachs disease is caused by an enzyme deficiency. Infants with this disorder appear normal for perhaps nine months, but then gradually deteriorate physically and mentally. Death usually occurs before the fifth birthday. Carriers can be identified by a blood test.

Sudden Infant Death Syndrome (SIDS)

SIDS, or **crib death**—the unexplained death of an apparently healthy baby under one year of age—is the second-leading cause of infant mortality in the United States. About 900 infants die of crib death each year, a significant decrease from the past. Typically, a seemingly healthy infant, usually 1 to 7 months old, is put to bed according to the daily routine. The baby may have some signs of a cold or cough. When the parents return to the crib, they find the child dead. There is no sign of a struggle, nor does the baby suffocate in the blankets. Determining the cause of death often proves impossible. Premature and very small babies are the most vulnerable. A recognized risk factor, based on studies of 20,000 infants during the first week of life, is the "resonance frequency" of each cry—an acoustic measure of a child's cry that cannot be easily determined by listening. Computer analysis found that infants with a high-resonance frequency were more likely to die of SIDS. A screening test based on this factor may be developed to detect newborns at risk.

Based on a review of studies on SIDS from around the world, health professionals have found that sleeping on its stomach increases a baby's risk of SIDS. As a result, pediatricians now recommend that normal, full-term infants be placed on their backs for the first six months. Parents should remove pillows, quilts, comforters, stuffed toys, and other soft products from the crib.

✖ Infertility

The World Health Organization defines **infertility** as the failure to conceive after one year of unprotected intercourse. Infertility affects one in seven couples. Women between ages 35 and 44 are about twice as likely to have fertility problems as women ages 30 to 34.[61]

Infertility is a problem of the couple, not of the individual man or woman. In 40 percent of cases, infertility is caused by female problems, in 40 percent by male problems, in 10 percent by a combination of male and female problems, and in 10 percent by unexplained causes. A thorough diagnostic workup can reveal a cause for infertility in 90 percent of cases.

In women, the most common causes of subfertility or infertility are age, abnormal menstrual patterns, suppression of ovulation, and blocked fallopian tubes. A woman's fertility peaks between ages 20 and 30 and then drops quickly: by 20 percent after 30, by 50 percent after 35, and by 95 percent after 40. In a survey of 1,168 professional women in the United States, 42 percent of those over 40 were childless—only 14 percent by choice.[62]

Male subfertility or infertility is usually linked to either the quantity or the quality of sperm, which may be inactive, misshapen, or insufficient (less than 20 million sperm per milliliter of semen in an ejaculation of 3 to 5 milliliters). Sometimes the problem is hormonal or a blockage of a sperm duct. Some men suffer from the inability to ejaculate normally, or from retrograde ejaculation, in which some of the semen travels in the wrong direction, back into the body of the male.

Fertility drugs can increase the chances of multiple births.

© Dana Fineman/CORBIS-Sygma

Infertility can have an enormous emotional impact.[63] Many women long to experience pregnancy and childbirth and feel great loss if they cannot conceive. Women in their thirties and forties fear that their biological clock is running out of time. Men may be confused and surprised by the intensity of their partner's emotions.

▣ What Are the Options for Infertile Couples?

The treatment of infertility has become a $2 billion a year enterprise in the United States. The odds of successful pregnancy range from 30 to 70 percent, depending on the specific cause of infertility. One result of successful infertility treatments has been a boom in multiple births, including quintuplets and sextuplets. Multiple births are associated with greater risk, both to the babies—including prematurity, low birthweight, neonatal death, and lifelong disability—and to the mothers, including caesarean section and hemorrhage.[64]

Artificial Insemination

Since the 1960s, **artificial insemination**—the introduction of viable sperm into the vagina by artificial means—has led to an estimated 250,000 births in the United States, primarily in couples in which the husband was infertile. However, some states do not recognize such children as legitimate; others do, but only if the woman's husband gave his consent for the insemination.

Assisted Reproductive Technology

New approaches to infertility include microsurgery, sometimes with lasers, to open destroyed or blocked egg and sperm ducts; new hormone preparations to induce ovulation; and the use of balloons, inserted through the cervix and inflated, to open blocked fallopian tubes (a procedure called *balloon tuboplasty*). More than 35,000 babies are born each year as a result of assisted reproductive technology (ART).[65]

The most common ART procedure is *in vitro fertilization (IVF)*, which involves removing the ova from a woman's ovary and placing the woman's egg and her mate's sperm in a laboratory dish for fertilization. If the fertilized egg cell shows signs of development, within several days it is returned to the woman's uterus, the egg cell implants itself in the lining of the uterus, and the pregnancy continues as normal. The success rate varies but is generally about 25 percent, and the costs are high.

Less time-consuming and less expensive than IVF, *gamete intrafallopian transfer (GIFT)* involves placing sperm and eggs into the fallopian tubes. GIFT mimics nature by allowing fertilized eggs to develop in the fallopian tubes according to a normal timetable. The success rate is about 20 percent. In *zygote intrafallopian transfer (ZIFT),* eggs are collected from the mother-to-be and combined with the father's sperm in a laboratory dish. One day after fertilization occurs, the single-celled zygote that forms is placed in the fallopian tube. In a variation called *intracytoplasmic sperm injection (ICSI),* several eggs are harvested, and each is injected with a single sperm by means of a fine hollow needle. (This overcomes problems related to the inability of sperm to penetrate the egg.) The fertilized eggs are then placed in the fallopian tube. Fertilization rates are comparable to in vitro fertilization with sperm from normal ejaculation.

In *gestational surrogacy,* an embryo is conceived in a laboratory dish using a woman's egg and her partner's sperm and then implanted into another woman's (the surrogate's) uterus. Alternatively, the fertilized donor egg can later be transferred to the uterus of the infertile woman, who carries and delivers the developing embryo.

Embryos can be frozen for later implantation in a process (called *cryopreservation*) that is highly controversial because of legal issues concerning the "ownership" of the unborn. Nearly 400,000 embryos are stored in the United States; the majority (88.2%) are targeted for patient use.[66] Some women are considering an experimental technique to freeze some of their eggs at a young age for later use.

Older women are just as likely as younger women to have a successful pregnancy after implantation of a donor embryo. In some experimental and controversial cases, donor eggs and embryos have been successfully implanted in women in their forties, fifties, and (in at least two cases) sixties. The use of a donor egg from a younger woman eliminates the risk of increased genetic problems. There are ethical questions about using expensive assisted reproductive technologies for the sake of enabling older women to become mothers or of allowing creation of "designer" babies of a certain racial or ethnic identity or with certain attributes, such as sex, height, or intelligence.

▌ Adoption

Men and women who cannot conceive children biologically can still become parents. **Adoption** matches would-be parents yearning for youngsters to love with infants or children who need loving. Couples interested in adoption can work with either public agencies or private counselors who contact obstetricians directly. Or they can contact organizations that arrange adoptions of children in need from other countries.

Although there are no reliable statistics on the annual number of adoptions in the United States, census records indicate there are currently 1.5 million adopted children in the U.S.[67] Each year some 50,000 U.S. children become available for adoption—far fewer than the number of would-be parents looking for youngsters to adopt. By some estimates, only 1 in 30 couples receive a child—and they spend an average of two years and as much as $100,000 on the adoption process.

Not only are the stakes high, but adoption arrangements often are chaotic. Private adoptions are legal in some states, banned in others. In some places, birth mothers sign over all claims to a child within 72 hours of giving birth; in others they have up to a year to change their minds. Sometimes foster parents are encouraged to adopt—particularly if they're African Americans caring for an African-American child. In others, they face a daunting series of bureaucratic barriers. What's needed most, say experts on every side of the issue, are uniform adoption laws in all fifty states.

An increasing number of people support *open adoptions,* which allow for visiting and communication with the biological parents even though the adoptive parents retain legal custody. Even after a *closed adoption,* the biological (or birth) parents may at some point search for their children, if only to explain why they chose to give them up for adoption.

Although fewer than 2 percent of each year's 50,000 adoptions of American children are contested, adoptive parents are nervous and confused.

The best advice for prospective adoptive parents is to learn as much as they can about their state's adoption laws and to prepare for the reality that their plans might not work out.

Adoption matches would-be parents yearning for youngsters to love with infants or children who need loving.

Mike Greenlar/The Image Works

The Bottom Line ▼
Reproductive Health

The decisions and choices you make about birth control can affect your current and future reproductive health—and your partner's. Here are some guidelines that can help both prevent pregnancy and protect your reproductive well-being.

:: *Abstain.* The only 100 percent safe and effective way to avoid unwanted pregnancy is not to engage in heterosexual intercourse.

:: *Limit sexual activity to "outercourse."* You can engage in many sexual activities—kissing, hugging, touching, massage, oral-genital sex—without risking pregnancy.

:: *Talk about birth control with any potential sex partner.* If you are considering sexual intimacy with a person, you should feel comfortable enough to talk about contraception.

:: *Know what doesn't work—and don't rely on it.* There are many misconceptions about ways to avoid getting pregnant, such as having sex in a standing position or during menstruation. Only the methods described in this chapter are reliable forms of birth control.

:: *Talk with a health-care professional.* A great deal of information and advice is available—in writing, from family planning counselors, from physicians on the Internet. Check it out.

:: *Choose a contraceptive method that matches your personal habits and preferences.* If you can't remember to take a pill every day, oral contraceptives aren't for you. If you're constantly forgetting where you put things, a diaphragm might not be a good choice.

:: *Consider long-term implications.* Since you may well wish to have children in the future, find out about the reversibility of various methods and possible effects on future fertility.

:: *Resist having sex without contraceptive protection "just this once."* It only takes once—even the very first time—to get pregnant. Be wary of drugs and alcohol. They can impair your judgment and make you less conscientious about using birth control—or using it properly.

:: *Use backup methods.* If there's a possibility that a contraceptive method might not offer adequate protection (for instance, if it's been almost three months since your last injection of Depo-Provera), use an additional form of birth control.

:: *Inform yourself about emergency contraception.* Just in case a condom breaks or a diaphragm slips, find out about the availability of forms of after-intercourse contraception.

 After watching the CNN video segment, discuss the following questions. Are emergency contraceptives like the morning-after pill safe? Should they be made available over the counter?

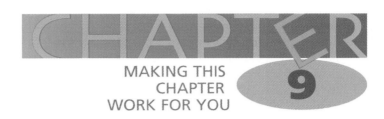

MAKING THIS
CHAPTER
WORK FOR YOU

9

1. Conception occurs
   a. when a fertilized egg implants in the lining of the uterus.
   b. when sperm is blocked from reaching the egg.
   c. when a sperm fertilizes the egg.
   d. after the uterine lining is discharged during the menstrual cycle.

2. Factors to consider when choosing a contraceptive method include all of the following *except*
   a. cost.
   b. failure rate.
   c. effectiveness in preventing sexually transmitted diseases.
   d. preferred sexual position.

3. When used correctly, which is the most effective non-hormonal contraceptive method?
   a. Copper T intrauterine device
   b. condom
   c. spermicide
   d. diaphragm

4. Which of the following contraceptive choices offers the best protection against STIs?
   a. condom alone
   b. condom plus spermicide
   c. abstinence
   d. withdrawal plus spermicide

5. Which statement about prescription contraceptives is *not* true?
   a. Prescription contraceptives do not offer protection against STIs.
   b. Some prescription contraceptives contain estrogen and progestin, and some contain only progestin.
   c. The contraceptive ring must be changed every week.
   d. IUDs prevent pregnancy by preventing or interfering with implantation.

6. Which of the following statements is true about sterilization?
   a. In women, the most frequently performed sterilization technique is hysterectomy.

b. Many couples experience an increase in sexual encounters after sterilization.

c. Vasectomies are easily reversed with surgery.

d. Sterilization is recommended for single men and women who are unsure about whether they want children.

7. The incidence of abortion is
   a. highest in women older than 30 and who have several children.
   b. lower in the United States than in countries where birth control education begins early and contraceptives are easier and cheaper to obtain.
   c. higher in affluent women, who can afford the procedure, than in poor women.
   d. higher in Catholic women than in Protestant women.

8. In the third trimester of pregnancy,
   a. the woman experiences shortness of breath as the enlarged uterus presses on the lungs and diaphragm.
   b. the embryo is now called a fetus.
   c. the woman should begin regular prenatal checkups.

d. the woman should increase her activity level to ensure that she is fit for childbirth.

9. During childbirth,
   a. breech birth can be prevented by practicing the Lamaze method.
   b. the cervix thins and dilates so that the baby can exit the uterus.
   c. the intensity of contractions decreases during the second stage of labor.
   d. the placenta is expelled immediately before the baby's head appears.

10. Which of the following statements is true about infertility?
    a. Infertility is most often caused by female problems.
    b. In men, infertility is usually caused by a combination of excess sperm production and an ejaculation problem.
    c. In vitro fertilization involves introducing sperm into the vagina with a long needle.
    d. In some cases of infertility no cause can be demonstrated.

Answers to these questions can be found on page 652.

Critical Thinking

1. After reading about the various methods of contraception, which do you think would be most effective for you? What factors enter into your decision (convenience, risks, effectiveness, etc.)?

Critical Thinking

2. In Wyoming, a pregnant woman went to the police station to report that her husband had beaten her. Instead of charges being brought against him, she was arrested for intoxication and charged with abusing her fetus by drinking. Across the country, other women who use hard drugs or alcohol while pregnant or whose newborns test positive for drugs have been arrested and put on trial for abusing their unborn children. Prosecutors argue that they are defending the innocent victims of substance abuse. Some health officials, on the other hand, argue that addicted women need help, not punishment. What do you think? Why?

Critical Thinking

3. Suppose that you and your partner were told that your only chance of having a child is by using fertility drugs. After taking the drugs, you and your partner are informed that there are seven fetuses. Would you carry them all to term? What if you knew that the chances of them all surviving were very slim and that eliminating some of them would improve the odds for the others? What ethical issues do cases like these raise?

Profile Plus

Make informed choices about your method of birth control. Discover which method is best for you with this activity on your Profile Plus CD-ROM.

Profile Plus

• Which Contraceptive Method is Best for You?

Profile Plus

Sites and Bytes

American Society for Reproductive Medicine
www.asrm.org

This professional site features information for patients, health professionals, and the media on a variety of topics, including contraception and infertility. The site contains fact sheets, annual meeting information, and information about current clinical trials.

Sites and Bytes

National Women's Health Information Center
www.4woman.gov

This site, by the U.S. Public Health Office on Women's Health, features current women's health topics and press releases, as well as information on screening and immunization schedules, violence, smoking cessation, prevention, pregnancy, disabilities, and body image. Also, there is information for health professionals and an online newsletter.

Sites and Bytes

Planned Parenthood
www.plannedparenthood.org

This site features current health information pertaining to family planning, including emergency contraception, as well as pregnancy, sexually transmitted infections, safer sex, and political action.

InfoTrac College Edition

Activity

Frey, Keith A. "Preconception care." *Primary Care Reports,* Vol. 8, No. 25, December 9, 2002, p. 222(5).

1. What are the benefits of preconception care?
2. List the seven health categories that should be addressed by a woman's primary care physician as part of her medical history.

InfoTrac College Edition

3. What are some of the concerns about pregnancy in women who are over the age of 35, who consume alcohol, who smoke, and who are obese?

You can find additional readings related to contraception and reproduction with InfoTrac College Edition, an online library of more than 900 journals and publications. Follow the

InfoTrac College Edition

instructions for accessing InfoTrac College Edition that were packaged with your textbook; then search for articles using a keyword search.

For additional links, resources, and suggested readings on InfoTrac College Edition, visit our Health & Wellness Resource Center at **http://health.wadsworth.com**.

Key Terms

The terms listed are used on the page indicated. Definitions of the terms are in the Glossary at the end of this book.

Key Terms

Key Terms

Key Terms

Key Terms

rubella 310
spermatogenesis 276
spinal block 311

Key Terms

sterilization 299
suction curettage 303
sudden infant death
    syndrome (SIDS) 313

Key Terms

tubal ligation 300
tubal occlusion 300
vaginal contraceptive
    film (VCF) 296

Key Terms

vaginal spermicide 294
vasectomy 299
zygote 276

References

1. Darroch, Jacqueline. "The Pill and Men's Involvement in Contraception." *Family Planning Perspective,* Vol. 32, No. 2, March 2000.
2. Murray, Steven, and Jessica L. Miller. "Birth Control and Condom Usage Among College Students." *Research Quarterly for Exercise and Sport,* Vol. 71, No. 1, March 2000.
3. Paukku, M., et al. "Adolescents' Contraceptive Use and Pregnancy History: Is There a Pattern?" *Obstetrics and Gynecology,* Vol. 101, No. 3, March 2003, p. 534.
4. www.smartersex.com.
5. "Birth Control: Comparing the Choices." Association of Reproductive Health Professionals, www.arhp.org/patienteducation.
6. Pennachio, Dorothy. "New Approaches to Emergency Contraception." *Patient Care,* Vol. 35, No. 5, March 15, 2001, p. 19.
7. Oncale, Renee, and Bruce King. "Comparisons of Men's and Women's Attempts to Dissuade Sexual Partners from the Couple Using Condoms." *Archives of Sexual Behavior,* Vol. 30, No. 4, August 2001, p. 379.
8. Murphy, P. A. "New Methods of Hormonal Contraception." *Nurse Practitioner,* Vol. 28, No. 2, February 2003, p. 11.
9. "Hormonal Contraception Forty Years after Approval of 'The Pill.'" *Kaiser Family Foundation Issue Update,* June 2002, p. 1.
10. Goldin, Claudia, and Lawrence Katz. "The Power of the Pill: Oral Contraceptives and Women's Career and Marriage Decisions." *Journal of Political Economy,* Vol. 110, No. 4, August 2002, p. 730.
11. Kemmeren, Jeanet, et al. "Third Generation Oral Contraceptives and Risk of Venous Thrombosis: Meta-Analysis." *British Medical Journal,* Vol. 323, No. 7305, July 21, 2001.
12. Akert, Jacqueline. "A New Generation of Contraceptives." *RN,* Vol. 66, No. 2, February 2003, p. 54.
13. Freeman, E. W. "Evaluation of a Unique Oral Contraceptive (Yasmin) in the Management of Premenstrual Dysphoric Disorder." *European Journal of Contraception and Reproductive Health Care,* Vol. 7, No. 3, December 2002, p. 27.

14. Apter, D., et al. "Effect of an Oral Contraceptive Containing Drospirenone and Ethinylestradiol on General Well-Being and Fluid-Related Symptoms." *European Journal of Contraception and Reproductive Health Care,* Vol. 8, No. 1, March 2003, p. 37.
15. "You and the Pill." www.plannedparenthood.org.
16. Davidson, N., and K. Helzsouer. "Good News About Oral Contraceptives." *New England Journal of Medicine,* Vol. 346, June 27, 2002, p. 2078.
17. Marchbanks, P., et al. "Oral Contraceptives and the Risk of Breast Cancer." *New England Journal of Medicine,* Vol. 346, June 27, 2002, p. 2025.
18. Minkin, Mary Jane, and Carol Wright. *The Yale University Guide to Women's Reproductive Health.* New Haven: Yale University Press, 2003.
19. Oral Contraceptive and Hemostasis Study Group. "The Effects of Seven Monophasic Oral Contraceptive Regimens on Hemostatic Variables." *Contraception,* Vol. 67, No. 3, March 2003, p. 173.
20. "Is Ortho Evra Right for You?" www.plannedparenthood.org.
21. "Does Weight Play a Role in Effectiveness?" *Contraceptive Technology Update,* Vol. 23, No. 7, July 2002, p. 81.
22. "Is NuvaRing Right for You?" www.plannedparenthood.org.
23. Novak, A., et al. "The Combined Contraceptive Vaginal Ring, NuvaRing®: An International Study of User Acceptability." *Contraception,* March 2003, Vol. 67, No. 3, March 2003, p. 173.
24. "Is Lunelle Right for You?" www.plannedparenthood.org.
25. Sivin, I. "Risks and Benefits, Advantages and Disadvantages of Levonorgestrel-Releasing Contraceptive Implants." *Drug Safety,* Vol. 26, No. 5, 2003, p. 303.
26. Baldaszi, E., et al. "Acceptability of the Long-Term Contraceptive Levonorgestrel-Releasing Intrauterine System (Mirena): A 3-Year Follow-Up Study." *Contraception,* Vol. 67, No. 2, February 2003, p. 87.
27. Steiner, M. J. "Contraceptive Effectiveness of a Polyurethane Condom and a Latex

Condom: A Randomized Controlled Trial." *Obstetrics and Gynecology,* Vol. 101, No. 3, March 2003, p. 539.
28. Michaels Opinion Research. "In the Heat of the Moment." Menlo Park, CA: Henry J. Kaiser Family Foundation, June 2001.
29. "Condom Use by Adolescents." *Pediatrics,* Vol. 107, No. 6, June 2001, p. 463.
30. Rimsza, M. E. "Counseling the Adolescent About Contraception," *Pediatric Reviews,* Vol. 24, No. 5, May 2003, p. 162.
31. "Perceived Versus Actual Knowledge About Correct Condom Use Among U.S. Adolescents: Results from a National Study." *Journal of Adolescent Health,* Vol. 28, No. 5, May 2001, p. 415.
32. Macaluso, M., et al. "Efficacy of the Female Condom as a Barrier to Semen During Intercourse." *American Journal of Epidemiology,* Vol. 157, No. 4, February 15, 2003, p. 289.
33. "Contraceptive Sponge: The Right Form of Birth Control for You?" www.mayoclinic.com.
34. Minkin and Wright, *The Yale University Guide to Women's Reproductive Health.*
35. "Standard Days Method: Family Planning Option." *Contraceptive Technology Update,* Vol. 23, No. 10, October 2002, p. 114.
36. www.cyclebeads.com.
37. "Questions for Recommendations for Clinical Practice Emergency Contraception." *Journal of Family Planning and Reproductive Health Care,* Vol. 29, No. 2, April 2003, p. 16.
38. Gainer, E., et al. "Progestogen-Only Emergency Contraception." *Journal of Family Planning and Reproductive Health Care,* Vol. 29, No. 2, April 2003, p. 58.
39. Haggai, D. N. "Emergency Contraception: The Journey So Far." *British Journal of Obstetrics and Gynaecology,* Vol. 110, No. 4, April 2003, p. 339.
40. "Emergency Contraception: Increasing Public Awareness," *Issues Brief* (Alan Guttmacher Institute) Vol. 2, February 2003, p. 1. www.guttmacher.org.
41. Shaban, Danny. "Emergency Contraception." Presentation, meeting of American College of Obstetricians and Gynecologists, April 2003.

References

42. Gainer, E., et al. "Surfing on the Morning After: Analysis of an Emergency Contraception Website." *Contraception,* Vol. 67, No. 3, March 2003, p. 18.

43. McCarthy, Susan. "Availability of Emergency Contraceptive Pills at University and College Student Health Centers." *Journal of American College Health,* Vol. 51, No. 1, July 2002, p. 15.

44. Baill, Cori, et al. "Counseling Issues in Tubal Sterilization." *American Family Physician,* Vol. 67, April 15, 2003, p. 1287.

45. Ibid.

46. "Essure FDA Approval." *American Family Physician,* Vol. 67, No. 1, January 1, 2003, p. 205.

47. Marston, C., et al. "Relationships Between Contraception and Abortion: A Review of the Evidence." *International Family Planning Perspectives,* Vol. 29, No. 1, March 2003, p. 6.

48. "Trends in Abortion in the United States, 1973–2000." New York, NY: Alan Guttmacher Institute, January 2003.

49. Henshaw, Stanley. "U.S. Teenage Pregnancy Statistics with Comparative Statistics for Women Aged 20–24." New York, NY: Alan Guttmacher Institute, May 2003.

50. Finer, Lawrence, and Stanley Henshaw. "Abortion Incidence and Services in the United States in 2000." *Perspectives on Sexual and Reproductive Health,* Vol. 35, No. 1, January/February 2003, p. 6.

References

51. Beson, J., et al. "Early Abortion Services in the United States." *Contraception,* Vol. 67, No. 4, April 2003, p. 287.

52. Finer, Lawrence, and Stanley Henshaw. "The Accessibility of Abortion Services in the United States, 2001." *Perspectives on Sexual and Reproductive Health,* Vol. 35, No. 1, January/February 2003, p. 16.

53. Bower, B. "Study Explores Abortion's Mental Aftermath." *Science News,* Vol. 158, No. 8, August 19, 2000.

54. Elliott, Victoria. "30 Years After Roe v. Wade, Doctors Reflect on its Impact." *American Medical News,* January 27, 2003.

55. Stotland, Nada. *Abortion: Facts and Feelings.* Washington, DC: American Psychiatric Press, 1998.

56. Lafayette, Leslie. Personal interview.

57. "Births, Marriages, Divorces, and Deaths." *National Vital Statistics Reports,* Vol. 50, No. 15, September 16, 2002, p. 100.

58. Hueston, W. J. "Delayed Prenatal Care and the Risk of Low Birth Weight Delivery." *Journal of Community Health,* Vol. 28, No. 3, June 2003, p. 199.

59. Ingersoll, K., et al. "Reducing the Risk of Alcohol-Exposed Pregnancies: A Study of a Motivational Intervention in Community Settings." *Pediatrics,* Vol. 111, No. 5, May 2003, p. 1131.

References

60. Spinelli A., et al. "Do Antenatal Classes Benefit the Mother and Her Baby?" *Journal of Maternal and Fetal Neonatal Medicine,* Vol. 13, No. 2, February 2003, p. 94.

61. Minkin and Wright, *The Yale University Guide to Women's Reproductive Health.*

62. Hewlett, Sylvia. *Creating a Life: Professional Women and the Quest for Children.* New York: Miramax Books, 2002.

63. Devine, K. S. "Caring for the Infertile Woman." *American Journal of Maternal and Child Nursing,* Vol. 28, No. 2, March–April 2003, p. 100.

64. Reynolds, M. A. "Trends in Multiple Births Conceived Using Assisted Reproductive Technology, United States, 1997–2000." *Pediatrics,* Vol. 111, No. 5, May 2003, p. 1159.

65. *Assisted Reproductive Technology Success Rates.* Atlanta, GA: Centers for Disease Control and Prevention, 2002. www.cdc.gov/nccdphp/drh/art.htm.

66. Hoffman, D. I. "Cryopreserved Embryos in the United States and Their Availability for Research." *Fertility & Sterility,* Vol. 79, No. 5, May 2003, p. 1063.

67. "Adoption Guide." *Health & Medicine Week,* March 24, 2003, p. 40.

SECTION IV

AVOIDING HEALTH RISKS

© Network Productions/Index Stock Imagery

WE constantly hear messages encouraging us to take risks with our health, to try drugs, to have a drink, to smoke cigarettes. We also live with the consequences of others' drug abuse, alcoholism, and smoking. That's why it's important to know about potentially harmful habits—even if you never rely on drugs to pick you up or bring you down, never smoke, and never drink to excess. This section provides information you can use to avoid or overcome habits that could destroy your health, happiness, and life.

Drug Use, Misuse, and Abuse

Amelia doesn't do drugs. That's what she says to anyone who asks. Sure, she and her friends occasionally pass a joint around while listening to music. She's tried a tab of ecstasy at a couple of raves. And when she was stressed out after finals, she took some of her roommate's Vicodin. But she thinks of drug users as desperate addicts craving a fix. She's not like that. That's what she tells herself.

Although she doesn't realize it, Amelia is at risk of drug-related problems—physical, psychological, and legal—and of developing a substance abuse disorder. Like Amelia, the people who try illegal drugs don't think they'll ever lose control. Even regular drug users are convinced that they are smart enough, strong enough, lucky enough not to get caught and not to get hooked. But with continued use, drugs produce changes in an individual's body, mind, and behavior. In time, a person's need for a drug can outweigh everything else, including the values, people, and relationships he or she once held dearest.

Drug use patterns are changing around the world. According to the United Nations Office on Drugs and Crime, heroin and cocaine use have stabilized and even declined in some countries, while the use of marijuana and illicit synthetic or designer drugs is rising.[1] The majority of teenagers in the United States (about 55 percent) have tried an illicit drug by the time they leave high school. In a recent survey of substance use on college campuses, 56 percent of undergraduates reported that they had smoked marijuana at least once; approximately one-fifth had used pot within the previous month.[2]

This chapter provides information on the nature and effects of drugs, the impact of drugs on individuals and society, and the drugs Americans most commonly use, misuse, and abuse.

© Gary S. and Vivian Chapman/The Image Bank/Getty Images

After studying the material in this chapter, you should be able to:

- **Describe** the different types of drug actions and factors affecting individuals' response to drugs.
- **Give examples** of appropriate and inappropriate use of over-the-counter and prescription medications.

- **Identify** the types of drug dependence, and **discuss** the factors affecting drug dependence.
- **Describe** the methods of use and the effects of common drugs of abuse.
- **Describe** the treatment methods available for individuals seeking help for drug dependence.
- **Explain** codependency and some ways that a codependent person can enable another to continue an addictive behavior.

✶ Understanding Drugs and Their Effects

A **drug** is a chemical substance that affects the way you feel and function. In some circumstances, taking a drug can help the body heal or relieve physical and mental distress. In other circumstances, taking a drug can distort reality, undermine well-being, and threaten survival. No drug is completely safe; all drugs have multiple effects that vary greatly in different people at different times. Knowing how drugs affect the brain, body, and behavior is crucial to understanding their impact and making responsible decisions about their use.

Drug misuse is the taking of a drug for a purpose or by a person other than that for which it was medically intended. Borrowing a friend's prescription for penicillin when your throat feels scratchy is an example of drug misuse. The World Health Organization defines **drug abuse** as excessive drug use that's inconsistent with accepted medical practice. Taking prescription painkillers to get high is an example of drug abuse.

Risks are involved with all forms of drug use. Even medications that help cure illnesses or soothe symptoms have side effects and can be misused. Some substances that millions of people use every day, such as caffeine, pose some health risks. Others—like the most commonly used drugs in our society, alcohol and tobacco—can lead to potentially life-threatening problems. With some illicit drugs, any form of use can be dangerous.

Many factors determine the effects a drug has on an individual. These include how the drug enters the body, the dosage, the drug action, and the presence of other drugs in the body—as well as the physical and psychological make-up of the person taking the drug and the setting in which the drug is used.

Routes of Administration

Drugs can enter the body in a number of ways (see Figure 10-1). The most common way of taking a drug is by swallowing a tablet, capsule, or liquid. However, drugs taken orally don't reach the bloodstream as quickly as drugs introduced into the body by other means. A drug taken orally may not have any effect for 30 minutes or more.

Drugs can enter the body through the lungs either by inhaling smoke, for example, from marijuana, or by inhaling gases, aerosol sprays, or fumes from solvents or other compounds that evaporate quickly. Young users of such inhalants, discussed later in this chapter, often soak a rag with fluid and press it over their nose. Or they may place inhalants in a plastic bag, put the bag over their nose and mouth, and take deep breaths—a practice called *huffing* and one that can produce serious, even fatal consequences.

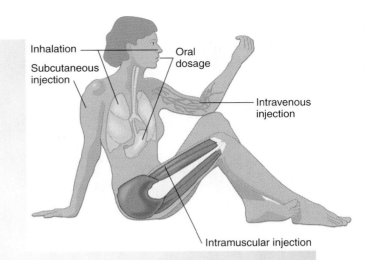

Figure 10-1 ROUTES OF ADMINISTRATION OF DRUGS

Drugs can also be injected with a syringe subcutaneously (beneath the skin), intramuscularly (into muscle tissue, which is richly supplied with blood vessels), or intravenously (directly into a vein). **Intravenous** (IV) injection gets the drug into the bloodstream immediately (within seconds in most cases); **intramuscular** injection, moderately fast (within a few minutes); and **subcutaneous** injection, more slowly (within ten minutes).

Approximately 1.5 million Americans use illegal injected drugs. This practice is extremely dangerous because many diseases, including hepatitis and infection with human immune deficiency virus (HIV), can be transmitted by sharing contaminated needles. Injection-drug users who are HIV-positive are the chief source of transmission of HIV among heterosexuals. (See Chapter 13 for more on HIV infection and AIDS.)

Dosage and Toxicity

The effects of any drug depend on the amount an individual takes. Increasing the dose usually intensifies the effects produced by smaller doses. Also, the kind of effect may change at different dose levels. For example, low doses of barbiturates may relieve anxiety, while higher doses can induce sleep, loss of sensation, even coma and death.

The dosage level at which a drug becomes poisonous to the body, causing either temporary or permanent damage, is called its **toxicity.** In most cases, drugs are eventually broken down in the liver by special body chemicals called *detoxification enzymes.*

Individual Differences

Each person responds differently to different drugs, depending on circumstances or setting. The enzymes in the body reduce the levels of drugs in the bloodstream;

CHAPTER 10 • DRUG USE, MISUSE, AND ABUSE

325

because there can be 80 variants of each enzyme, every person's body may react differently.

Often drugs intensify the emotional state a person is in. If you're feeling depressed, a drug may make you feel more depressed. A generalized physical problem, such as having the flu, may make your body more vulnerable to the effects of a drug. Genetic differences among individuals also may account for varying reactions.

Personality and psychological attitude also play a role in drug effects, so that one person may have a frighteningly bad trip on the same LSD dosage on which another person has a positive experience. To a certain extent, this depends on each user's *mind-set*—his or her expectations or preconceptions about using the drug. Someone who snorts cocaine to enhance sexual pleasure may feel more stimulated simply because that's what he or she expects.

Setting

The setting for drug use also influences its effects. Passing around a joint of marijuana at a friend's is not a healthy or safe behavior, but the experience of going to a crack house is very different—and entails greater dangers.

Types of Action

A drug can act *locally,* as novocaine does to deaden pain in a tooth; *generally,* throughout a body system, as barbiturates do on the central nervous system; or *selectively,* as a drug does when it has a greater effect on one specific organ or system than on others, such as a spinal anesthetic. A drug that accumulates in the body because it's taken in faster than it can be metabolized and excreted is called *cumulative;* alcohol is such a drug.

Interaction with Other Drugs or Alcohol

A drug can interact with other drugs in four different ways:

:: An **additive** interaction is one in which the resulting effect is equal to the sum of the effects of the different drugs used.

:: A **synergistic** interaction is one in which the total effect of the two drugs taken together is greater than the sum of the effects the two drugs would have had if taken by themselves on separate occasions. Mixing barbiturates and alcohol, for example, has up to four times the depressant effect than either drug has alone.

:: A drug can be **potentiating**—that is, one drug can increase the effect of another. Alcohol, for instance, can increase the drowsiness caused by antihistamines (antiallergy medications).

:: Drugs can interact in an **antagonistic** fashion—that is, one drug can neutralize or block another drug with opposite effects. Tranquilizers, for example, may counter some of the nervousness and anxiety produced by cocaine.

The danger of mixing alcohol with other drugs cannot be emphasized too strongly. Alcohol and marijuana intensify each other's effects, making driving and many other activities extremely dangerous. Some people have mixed sedatives or tranquilizers with alcohol and never regained consciousness.

Medications

Many of the medications and pharmaceutical products available in this country do indeed relieve symptoms and help cure various illnesses. However, improper use of medications leads to more than 170,000 hospitalizations and costs of about $750 million every year. Because drugs are powerful and increasingly marketed directly to consumers, it's important to know how to evaluate and use them appropriately.[3]

What Should I Know About Buying Over-the-Counter Drugs?

More than half a million health products—remedies for everything from bad breath to bunions—are readily available without a doctor's prescription. This doesn't mean that they're necessarily safe or effective. Indeed, many widely used **over-the-counter (OTC) drugs** pose unsuspected hazards.

Among the most potentially dangerous is aspirin, the "wonder drug" in practically everyone's home pharmacy. When taken by someone who's been drinking (often to prevent or relieve hangover symptoms), for instance, aspirin increases blood-alcohol concentrations (see Chapter 11). Along with other nonsteroidal anti-inflammatory drugs, such as ibuprofen (brand names include Advil and Nuprin), aspirin can damage the lining of the stomach and lead to ulcers in those who take large daily doses for arthritis or other problems. Kidney problems have also been traced to some pain relievers including acetaminophen (Tylenol).

Some health products that aren't even considered true drugs can also cause problems. Many Americans take food supplements, even though the Food and Drug Administration (FDA) has never approved their use for any medical disorder.

A growing number of drugs that once were available only with a doctor's prescription can now be bought over the counter. These include Gyne-Lotrimin and Monistat, which combat vaginal yeast infections, and famotidine (sold as Pepcid AC) and cimetidine (sold as Tagamet),

OTC drugs. Practically all of these packages have warnings on the back. Read them before you use the drug.

which offer an alternative to antacids for people suffering from heartburn and acid indigestion. For consumers, the advantages of this greater availability include lower prices and fewer visits to the doctor. The disadvantages, however, are the risks of misdiagnosing a problem and misusing or overusing medications.

Like other drugs, OTC medications can be used improperly, often simply because of a lack of education about proper use. Among those most often misused are the following:

:: **Nasal sprays.** Nasal sprays relieve congestion by shrinking blood vessels in the nose. If they are used too often or for too many days in a row, the blood vessels widen instead of contracting, and the surrounding tissues become swollen, causing more congestion. To make the vessels shrink again, many people use more spray more often. The result can be permanent damage to nasal membranes, bleeding, infection, and partial or complete loss of smell.

:: **Laxatives.** Believing that they must have one bowel movement a day (a common misconception), many people rely on laxatives. Brands that contain phenolphthalein irritate the lining of the intestines and cause muscles to contract or tighten, often making constipation worse rather than better. Bulk laxatives are less dangerous, but regular use is not advised. A high-fiber diet and more exercise are safer and more effective remedies for constipation.

:: **Eye drops.** Eye drops make the blood vessels of the eye contract. However, as in the case of nasal sprays, with overuse (several times a day for several weeks), the blood vessels expand, making the eye look redder than before.

:: **Sleep aids.** Although over-the-counter sleeping pills are widely used, there has been little research on their use and possible risks.

:: **Cough syrup.** Chugging cough syrup (also called roboing, after the over-the-counter medication Robitussin) is a growing problem, in part because young people think of dextromethorphan (DXM), a common ingredient in cough medicine, as a "poor man's version" of the popular drug ecstasy.

Prescription Drugs

Medications are a big business in this country. However, the latest, most expensive drugs aren't necessarily the best. Each year the FDA approves about 20 new drugs, yet no more than 4 are rated as truly meaningful advances. The others often are no better or worse than what's already on the market. (For tips on using prescription drugs, see Savvy Consumer: "Getting the Most Out of Medications.")

College students, like other consumers, often take medicines, particularly nonprescription pain pills, without discussing them with their physician. Both doctors and patients make mistakes when it comes to prescription drugs. The most frequent mistakes doctors make are over- or under-dosing, omitting information from prescriptions, ordering the wrong dosage form (a pill instead of a liquid, for example), and not recognizing a patient's allergy to a drug.

Nonadherence

Many prescribed medications aren't taken the way they should be; millions simply aren't taken at all. As many as 70 percent of adults have trouble understanding dosage information and 30 percent can't read standard labels, according to the FDA, which has called for larger, clearer drug labeling. The dangers of nonadherence (not properly taking prescription drugs) include recurrent infections, serious medical complications, and emergency hospital treatment. The drugs most likely to be taken incorrectly are those that treat problems with no obvious symptoms (such as high blood pressure), that require complex dosage schedules, that treat psychiatric disorders, or that have unpleasant side effects.

Some people skip prescribed doses or stop taking medications because they fear that any drug can cause tolerance and eventual dependence. Others fail to let doctors know about side effects. For instance, patients may stop taking anti-inflammatory drugs because they irritate their stomach. However, taking the drugs with food can eliminate this problem. The side effects of other drugs may disappear as the person's body becomes accustomed to the drug.

Savvy Consumer

GETTING THE MOST OUT OF MEDICATIONS

Before you leave with a prescription, be sure to ask the following questions:

- What is the name of the drug?
- What's it supposed to do?
- How and when do I take it? For how long?
- What foods, drinks, other medications, or activities should I avoid while taking this drug?
- Are there any side effects? What do I do if they occur?
- What written information is available on this drug?
- How should I store my prescriptions? (A hot, damp bathroom medicine chest is often the worst place.)

- Are there other, possibly cheaper alternatives?
- Are there nondrug alternatives, such as using a vaporizer, gargling with salt water, and drinking plenty of liquids for a viral infection; or losing weight and exercising to lower blood pressure?

If you're taking a medication, tell your doctor if you plan to change your diet significantly—cutting calories or fat, stopping or starting vitamin supplements, or changing the amount of fiber you consume.

Don't keep old medications (discard after the expiration date). Don't take drugs prescribed for someone else unless your doctor tells you to. Keep medications out of the reach of small children.

Have all prescriptions filled at the same pharmacy, and ask your pharmacist to keep a record of your medications to avoid hazardous interactions.

Physical Side Effects

Most medications, taken correctly, cause only minor complications. However, no drug is entirely without side effects for all individuals taking it. Serious complications that may occur include heart failure, heart attack, seizures, kidney and liver failure, severe blood disorders, birth defects, blindness, memory problems, and allergic reactions.

Allergic reactions to drugs are common. The drugs that most often provoke allergic responses are penicillin and other antibiotics (drugs used to treat infection). Aspirin, sulfa drugs, barbiturates, anticonvulsants, insulin, and local anesthetics can also provoke allergic responses. Allergic reactions range from mild rashes or hives to anaphylaxis—a life-threatening constriction of the airways and sudden drop of blood pressure that causes rapid pulse, weakness, paleness, confusion, nausea, vomiting, unconsciousness, and collapse. This extreme response, which is rare, requires immediate treatment with an injection of epinephrine (adrenaline) to open the airways and blood vessels.

Psychological Side Effects

Dozens of drugs—both over-the-counter and prescription—can cause changes in the way people think, feel, and behave. Unfortunately, neither patients nor their physicians usually connect such symptoms with medications. Doctors may not even mention potential mental and emotional problems because they don't want to scare patients away from what otherwise may be a very effective treatment.

What you don't know about a drug's effects on your mind *can* hurt you.

Among the medications most likely to cause psychiatric side effects are drugs for high blood pressure, heart disease, asthma, epilepsy, arthritis, Parkinson's disease, anxiety, insomnia, and depression. Some drugs—such as the powerful hormones called *corticosteroids,* used for asthma, autoimmune diseases, and cancer—can cause different psychiatric symptoms, depending on dosage and other factors. Other drugs, such as ulcer medications, can cause delirium and disorientation, especially when given in high doses or to elderly patients. More subtle problems, such as forgetfulness or irritability, are common reactions to many drugs that are likely to be ignored or dismissed. The older you are, the sicker you are, and the more medications you're taking, the greater your risk of developing some psychiatric side effects. Even medications that don't usually cause problems, such as antibiotics, can cause psychiatric side effects in some individuals.

Any medication that slows down bodily systems, as many high blood pressure and cardiac drugs do, can cause depressive symptoms. Estrogen in birth control pills can cause mood changes. As many as 15 percent of women using oral contraceptives have reported feeling depressed or moody. For many people, switching to another medication quickly lifts a drug-induced depression.

All drugs that stimulate or speed up the central nervous system can cause agitation and anxiety—including the almost 200 allergy, cold, and congestion remedies containing pseudoephedrine hydrochloride (Sudafed). Other common culprits in inducing anxiety are caffeine and theophylline, a chemical relative of caffeine found in many medications for asthma and other respiratory problems.

These drugs act like mild amphetamines in the body, making people feel hyper and restless.

Drug Interactions

OTC and prescription drugs can interact in a variety of ways. For example, mixing some cold medications with tranquilizers can cause drowsiness and coordination problems, thus making driving dangerous. Moreover, what you eat or drink can impair or completely wipe out the effectiveness of drugs or lead to unexpected effects on the body. For instance, aspirin takes five to ten times as long to be absorbed when taken with food or shortly after a meal than when taken on an empty stomach. If tetracyclines encounter calcium in the stomach, they bind together and cancel each other out.

To avoid potentially dangerous interactions, check the label(s) for any instructions on how or when to take a medication, such as "with a meal." (See Figure 10-2.) If the directions say that you should take a drug on an empty stomach, take it at least one hour before eating or two or three hours after eating. Don't drink a hot beverage with a medication; the temperature may interfere with the effectiveness of the drug. Don't open, crush, or dissolve tablets or capsules without checking first with your physician or pharmacist.

Whenever you take a drug, be especially careful of your intake of alcohol, which can change the rate of metabolism and the effects of many different drugs. Because it dilates the blood vessels, alcohol can add to the dizziness sometimes caused by drugs for high blood pressure, angina, or depression. Also, its irritating effects on the stomach can worsen stomach upset from aspirin, ibuprofen, and other anti-inflammatory drugs.

Generic Drugs

The **generic** name is the chemical name for a drug. A specific drug may appear on the pharmacist's shelf under a variety of brand names, which may cost more than twice the generic equivalent. About 75 percent of all prescriptions specify a brand name, but pharmacists may—and in some states must—switch to a generic drug unless the doctor specifically tells them not to. Prescriptions filled with generic drugs cost 20 to 85 percent less than their brand-name counterparts.

Generic drugs have the same active ingredients as brand-name prescriptions, but their fillers and binders, which can affect the absorption of a drug, may be different. For some serious illnesses, the generics may not be as effective; some experts recommend sticking with brand names for heart medications, psychiatric drugs, and anticonvulsant drugs (for epilepsy and other seizure disorders).

To determine whether you should buy the generic version of a drug, ask your physician whether it matters if you get a brand-name or generic drug. If it does, ask which brand name is best. Also, find out if switching to a generic or from one generic to another might harm your condition in any way.

What Should I Know About Buying Drugs Online?

Millions of people in the United States purchase prescription medications online. Although some websites fill only faxed prescriptions from medical doctors, others ignore or sidestep traditional regulations and safeguards. Cyberspace distributors often ship pills across state lines without requiring a physical examination by a medical doctor. Instead, a "cyberdoc," who may or may not be qualified or up-to-date in a given specialty, reviews information submitted by a "patient." International pharmacies sometimes sell drugs that are not available or approved in the United States. And patients themselves use bulletin boards and other web areas to sell unused or unwanted medications to each other.

Many individuals turn to the Internet for "lifestyle" drugs such as

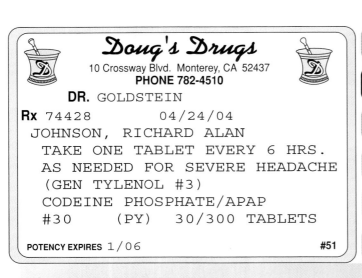

Figure 10-2 DRUG INTERACTIONS
When you take a prescription medication, be sure to read warning labels about interactions, possible side effects, and whether the medication interacts with certain foods.

Viagra for erectile dysfunction and Propecia, a baldness treatment. Other medications commonly bought online include Xenical, a diet pill; Zyban, an antismoking treatment; Celebrex, for arthritis; and Claritin, for allergies. Customers like the convenience and anonymity of buying drugs online. Although many assume drugs cost less on the Internet, shipping costs tend to drive prices up to the same amount or more than the price at a pharmacy.

The dangers of unregulated distribution of medications have alarmed government agencies and medical groups. The American Medical Association has declared it unethical for physicians to write prescriptions for people they've never met. The National Association of Boards of Pharmacy has developed a seal of approval to help customers determine which sites are legitimate. The FDA and other federal agencies, such as the Federal Trade Commission, which regulates advertising, are trying to find ways to impose some controls.

Consumers have to be wary. Ordering a drug like Accutane, an acne treatment, online may seem harmless. However, without close monitoring by a physician, you could develop complications, such as a bad reaction that aggravates hepatitis or inflames the pancreas. Quality control is another concern. Cyberspace pharmacies provide no information on how the drug was stored or whether its expiration date has passed. In addition, since importing medications without a prescription is against the law, you could find yourself in legal trouble.

Abuse of Prescription Painkillers

Almost 7 million young adults between ages 18 and 25 report using prescription drugs nonmedically at least once. Narcotic painkillers, such as Vicodin and OxyContin, are the most commonly abused.[4] OxyContin, the most widely prescribed narcotic in the United States, is particularly deadly. In a recent two-year period, OxyContin was linked to 464 deaths.[5] Most of those who died swallowed the pills whole or crushed them into powder, which had been considered less dangerous forms of administration than injecting or snorting crushed pills.

Many prescription painkillers work by blocking the pathway that pain signals travel to the brain and by triggering production of the chemical dopamine in the brain. Users can become accustomed to the changes dopamine causes in the brain. When they stop taking the medications, they develop a craving for the dopamine-induced feelings. Individuals who've had prior problems with drug dependence may be especially prone to addiction to prescription painkillers.

◆ Caffeine Use and Misuse

Caffeine, which has been drunk, chewed, and swallowed since the Stone Age, is the most widely used **psychotropic** (mind-affecting) drug in the world. Eighty percent of

Americans drink coffee, our principal caffeine source—an average of 3.5 cups a day. Coffee contains 100 to 150 milligrams of caffeine per cup; tea, 40 to 100 milligrams; cola, about 45 milligrams. Most medications that contain caffeine are one-third to one-half the strength of a cup of coffee. However, some, such as Excedrin, are very high in caffeine. (See Table 10-1.)

The effects of caffeine vary. As a **stimulant,** it relieves drowsiness, helps in the performance of repetitive tasks, and improves the capacity for work. Caffeine improves performance and endurance during prolonged, exhaustive exercise and, to a lesser degree, enhances short-term, high-intensity athletic performance. Additional benefits include improved concentration, reduced fatigue, and sharpened alertness. Major sport organizations ban excessive use of caffeine, but these policies remain controversial.[6]

Consumption of high doses of caffeine can lead to dependence, anxiety, insomnia, rapid breathing, upset stom- ach and bowels, and dizziness. In a study of college men and women who normally consumed fewer than three caffeinated beverages per day, caffeine boosted anxiety but did not significantly affect performance on various low-intensity tasks, except for hand-eye coordination, which improved.[7]

Although there is no conclusive proof that caffeine causes birth defects, it does cross the placenta into the tissues of a growing fetus. Because of an increased risk of miscarriage, the U.S. surgeon general has recommended that pregnant women avoid or restrict their caffeine intake. Some fertility specialists also have urged couples trying to conceive to reduce caffeine to increase their chance of success. Women who are heavy caffeine users tend to have shorter menstrual cycles than nonusers. A recent analysis drawing upon data from the ongoing Nurses Health Study

TABLE 10-1	Caffeine Counts
Substance (typical serving)	**Caffeine (milligrams)**
No Doz, one pill	200
Coffee (drip), one 5-ounce cup	130
Excedrin, two pills	130
Espresso, one 2-ounce cup	100
Instant coffee, one 5-ounce cup	74
Coca-Cola, 12 ounces	46
Tea, one 5-ounce cup	40
Dark chocolate, 1 ounce	20
Milk chocolate, 1 ounce	6
Cocoa, 5 ounces	4
Decaffeinated coffee, one 5-ounce cup	3

Coffee and work often go hand in hand, but too much caffeine can lead to dependence, anxiety, and other physical and psychological symptoms.

found that moderate amounts of coffee may protect women from Parkinson's disease.[8]

Is It Possible to Overdose on Caffeine?

Yes, you can overdose on caffeine. The characteristic symptoms of caffeine intoxication are restlessness, nervousness, excitement, insomnia, flushed face, increased urination, digestive complaints, muscle twitching, rambling thoughts and speech, rapid heart rate or arrhythmias, periods of inexhaustibility, and physical restlessness. Some people develop these symptoms after as little as 250 milligrams of caffeine a day; others, only with much larger doses. Higher doses may produce ringing in the ears or flashes of light, grand mal seizures, and potentially fatal respiratory failure.

Caffeine withdrawal for those dependent on this substance can cause headaches and other neurological symptoms. Those who must cut back should taper off gradually. One approach is to mix regular and decaffeinated coffee, gradually decreasing the quantity of the former.

Substance Use Disorders

People have been using mind-altering, or **psychoactive,** chemicals for centuries. Citizens of ancient Mesopotamia and Egypt used opium. More than 3,000 years ago Hindus included cannabis products in religious ceremonies. For centuries the Inca in South America have chewed the leaves of the coca bush. Yet while drugs existed in most societies, their use was usually limited to small groups. Today millions of people regularly turn to drugs to pick them up, bring them down, alter perceptions, or ease psychological pain.

Both men and women are vulnerable to substance use disorders, although they tend to have different patterns of drug use. (See X & Y File: "Men, Women, and Drugs.") The 1960s ushered in an explosive increase in drug use and in the number of drug users in our society. Marijuana use soared in the 1960s and 1970s; cocaine, in the 1980s. In 1986, crack—a cheap, smokeable form of cocaine—hit the streets and cities of the United States, and the number of regular cocaine users zoomed. By the twenty-first century, overall drug use was down, but club or designer drugs, such as ecstasy (MDMA), were growing in popularity.

The United Nations Office on Drugs and Crime has warned that these illicit synthetic drugs could become the world's most severe drug problem in the next five years. Drug use in Eastern Europe, Russia, and Central Asia has spread blood-borne infections, including HIV/AIDS and hepatitis C. Increasingly, as terrorist groups have become involved in the drug trade, the battle against drugs overlaps with the war on terrorism.[9]

Understanding Substance Use Disorders

In early Roman law, *addictus* referred to someone who, because he could not pay his debts, was sentenced into slavery. Indeed, one of the meanings of addiction given by the *Oxford Latin Dictionary* is "enslavement." For much of the twentieth century, addiction to drugs was viewed as a social or criminal problem, and the only people called addicts were "drug-crazed junkies" desperate for a fix. In the 1960s, however, when scientists switched to the *medical model* for understanding addictions, they began to view addictions to chemicals—such as alcohol and psychoactive drugs—as lifelong chronic diseases that affect a person's mind and body.

Today the word **addiction** has moved out of the realm of scientific terminology and into the cultural mainstream. Among laypeople, addiction refers to the habitual use of substances, such as alcohol, psychoactive drugs, and nicotine, and also to compulsive behaviors, such as overeating (discussed in Chapter 6). Like drugs, these activities can be used repeatedly to numb pain or enhance pleasure; some may alter a person's brain chemistry or create cravings; all can lead to a loss of internal control.

Chemical addiction is now viewed as a lifelong, chronic illness that affects mind, body, and spirit. Its key characteristics are repeated drug use, loss of control over how much or how often a person takes a drug, and continued use despite harmful consequences.

Because addiction is considered too broad and judgmental a term for scientific use, mental health professionals describe drug-related problems in terms of *dependence* and *abuse.* However, they agree that addiction has four characteristic symptoms: compulsion to use the substance, loss of

the XY file *Men, Women, and Drugs*

Beginning at a very early age, males and females show different patterns in drug use. Among 12-year-olds who have been offered drugs, boys are more likely to have received those offers from other males or their parents. Girls are most likely to have been offered drugs by a female friend or family member. The social setting and nature of drug offers also differ by gender. Boys are more likely to receive offers in a public setting, such as on the street or in a park, and the offers typically emphasize "benefits," such as improved status or self-image. Girls are more likely to receive a straightforward "do you want some?" offer or one that minimizes the risks of drug use. For girls, these offers are usually made in a private setting such as a friend's home.

Later in life men generally encounter more opportunities to use drugs than women, but given an opportunity to use drugs for the first time, both genders are equally likely to do so and to progress from initial use to dependence. Vulnerability to some drugs varies with gender. Both are equally likely to become addicted to or dependent on cocaine, heroin, hallucinogens, tobacco, and inhalants. Women are more likely than men to become addicted to or dependent on sedatives and drugs designed to treat anxiety or sleeplessness, and less likely than men to abuse alcohol and marijuana.

Males and females may differ in their biological responses to drugs. In studies of animals given the opportunity to self-administer intravenous doses of cocaine or heroin, females began self-administration sooner than males and administered larger amounts of the drugs. Women may be more sensitive than men to the cardiovas-

cular effects of cocaine. In human studies, women and men given equal doses of cocaine experienced the same cardiovascular response despite the fact that blood concentrations of cocaine did not rise as high in women as in men. Male and female long-term cocaine users showed similar impairment in tests of concentration, memory, and academic achievement following sustained abstinence, even though women in the study had substantially greater exposure to cocaine. Women cocaine users also were less likely than men to exhibit abnormalities of blood flow in the brain's frontal lobes. These findings suggest a gender-related mechanism that may protect women from some of the damage cocaine inflicts on the brain. However, women are more vulnerable to poor nutrition and below-average weight, depression, physical abuse, and if pregnant, preterm labor or early delivery.

Substance abuse compounds the risk of AIDS for women, who may become infected with HIV by sharing needles with other injection-drug users and by engaging in unprotected sex. In all, drug abuse is nearly twice as likely to be directly or indirectly associated with AIDS in women as in men.

There are also differences between men and women who seek treatment for drug abuse. Women in treatment programs are less likely than men to have graduated from high school and to be employed, and are more likely than men to have other health problems, to have sought previous drug treatment, to have attempted suicide, and to have suffered sexual abuse or other physical abuse. Traditional drug treatment programs, created for men, have proven to be less effective for women than programs that provide more comprehensive services, including child care, assertiveness training, and parenting training.

---

control, negative consequences, and denial. (See Self-Survey:"Is It a Substance Use Disorder?")

Dependence

Individuals may develop **psychological dependence** and feel a strong craving for a drug because it produces pleasurable feelings or relieves stress and anxiety. **Physical dependence** occurs when a person develops *tolerance* to the effects of a drug and needs larger and larger doses to achieve intoxication or another desired effect. Individuals who are physically dependent and have a high tolerance to a drug may take amounts many times those that would produce intoxication or an overdose in someone who was not a regular user.

Men and women with a substance dependence disorder may use a drug to avoid or relieve withdrawal symptoms, or they may consume larger amounts of a drug or

use it over a longer period than they'd originally intended. They may repeatedly try to cut down or control drug use without success; spend a great deal of time obtaining or using drugs or recovering from their effects; give up or reduce important social, occupational, or recreational activities because of their drug use; or continue to use a drug despite knowledge that the drug is likely to cause or worsen a persistent or recurring physical or psychological problem.

Specific symptoms of dependence vary with particular drugs. Some drugs, such as marijuana, hallucinogens, and phencyclidine, do not cause withdrawal symptoms. The degree of dependence also varies. In mild cases, a person may function normally most of the time. In severe cases, the person's entire life may revolve around obtaining, using, and recuperating from the effects of a drug.

Self Survey **Is It a Substance Use Disorder?**

Individuals with a substance dependence or abuse disorder may

:: Use more of an illegal drug or a prescription medication or use a drug for a longer period of time than they desire or intend. _____

:: Try, repeatedly and unsuccessfully, to cut down or control their drug use. _____

:: Spend a great deal of time doing whatever is necessary in order to get drugs, taking them, or recovering from their use. _____

:: Be so high or feel so bad after drug use that they often cannot do their job or fulfill other responsibilities. _____

:: Give up or cut back on important social, work, or recreational activities because of drug use. _____

:: Continue to use drugs even though they realize that they are causing or worsening physical or mental problems. _____

:: Use a lot more of a drug in order to achieve a "high" or desired effect or feel fewer such effects than in the past. _____

:: Use drugs in dangerous ways or situations. _____

:: Have repeated drug-related legal problems, such as arrests for possession. _____

:: Continue to use drugs, even though the drug causes or worsens social or personal problems, such as arguments with a spouse. _____

:: Develop hand tremors or other withdrawal symptoms if they cut down or stop drug use. _____

:: Take drugs to relieve or avoid withdrawal symptoms. _____

The more blanks that you or someone close to you checks, the more reason you have to be concerned about drug use. The most difficult step for anyone with a substance use disorder is to admit that he or she has a problem. Sometimes a drug-related crisis, such as being arrested or fired, forces individuals to acknowledge the impact of drugs. If not, those who care—family, friends, boss, physician—may have to confront them and insist that they do something about it. This confrontation, planned beforehand, is called an *intervention* and can be the turning point for drug users and their families.

Your Health Change Plan

for Recognizing Substance Abuse

How can you tell if a friend or loved one has a substance use disorder? Look for the following warning signs:

:: **An abrupt change in attitude.** Individuals may lose interest in activities they once enjoyed or in being with friends they once valued.

:: **Mood swings.** Drug users may often seem withdrawn or "out of it," or they may display unusual temper flareups.

:: **A decline in performance.** Students may start skipping classes, stop studying, or not complete assignments; their grades may plummet.

:: **Increased sensitivity.** Individuals may react intensely to any criticism or become easily frustrated or angered.

:: **Secrecy.** Drug users may make furtive telephone calls or demand greater privacy concerning their personal possessions or their whereabouts.

:: **Physical changes.** Individuals using drugs may change their pattern of sleep, spending more time in bed or sleeping at odd hours. They also may change their eating habits and lose weight.

:: **Money problems.** Drug users may constantly borrow money, seem short of cash, or begin stealing.

:: **Changes in appearance.** As they become more involved with drugs, users often lose regard for their personal appearance and look disheveled.

:: **Defiance of restrictions.** Individuals may ignore or deliberately refuse to comply with deadlines, curfews, or other regulations.

:: **Changes in relationships.** Drug users may quarrel more frequently with family members or old friends and develop new, strong allegiances with new acquaintances, including other drug users.

Individuals with drug dependence become intoxicated or high on a regular basis—whether every day, every weekend, or several binges a year. They may try repeatedly to stop using a drug and yet fail, even though they realize their drug use is interfering with their health, family life, relationships, and work.

Abuse

Some drug users do not develop the symptoms of tolerance and withdrawal that characterize dependence, yet they use drugs in ways that clearly have a harmful effect on them. These individuals are diagnosed as having a *psychoactive substance abuse disorder*. They continue to use drugs despite their awareness of persistent or repeated social, occupational, psychological, or physical problems related to drug use, or they use drugs in dangerous ways or situations (before driving, for instance).

Intoxication and Withdrawal

Intoxication refers to maladaptive behavioral, psychological, and physiologic changes that occur as a result of substance use. **Withdrawal** is the development of symptoms that cause significant psychological and physical distress when an individual reduces or stops drug use. (Intoxication and withdrawal from specific drugs are discussed later in this chapter.)

Polyabuse

Most users prefer a certain type of drug but also use several others; this behavior is called **polyabuse.** The average user who enters treatment is on five different drugs. The more drugs anyone uses, the greater the chance of side effects, complications, and possibly life-threatening interactions.

Coexisting Conditions

Mental disorders and substance abuse disorders have a great deal of overlap. "A little more than a third of those with a psychiatric disorder also have a chemical dependency problem, and a little more than a third of those with a chemical dependency problem have a psychiatric disorder," notes psychiatrist Richard Frances, M.D., founding president of the American Association of Addiction Psychiatry.[10] Individuals with such *dual diagnoses* require careful evaluation and appropriate treatment for the complete range of complex and chronic difficulties they face.

What Causes Drug Dependence and Abuse?

No one fully understands why some people develop drug dependence or abuse disorders, whereas others, who may experiment briefly with drugs, do not. Inherited body chemistry, genetic factors, and sensitivity to drugs may make some individuals more susceptible. These disorders may stem from many complex causes.

The Biology of Dependence

Scientists now view drug dependence as a brain disease triggered by frequent use of drugs that change the biochemistry and anatomy of neurons and alter the way they

---

STRATEGIES FOR PREVENTION

Saying No to Drugs

If people offer you a drug, here are some ways to say no:

- Let them know you're not interested. Change the subject. If the pressure seems threatening, just walk away.

- Have something else to do: "No, I'm going for a walk now."

- Be prepared for different types of pressure. If your friends tease you, tease them back.

- Keep it simple. "No, thanks," "No," or "No way" all get the point across.

- Hang out with people who won't offer you drugs.

---

work. A major breakthrough in understanding dependence has been the discovery that certain mood-altering substances and experiences—a puff of marijuana, a slug of whiskey, a snort of cocaine, a big win at blackjack—trigger a rise in a brain chemical called *dopamine,* which is associated with feelings of satisfaction and euphoria. This brain chemical or neurotransmitter is one of the crucial messengers that links nerve cells in the brain (see Figure 2-5), and its level rises during any pleasurable experience, whether it be a loving hug or a taste of chocolate.

The mechanism governing the rise in dopamine levels is not the same for all drugs. Figure 10-3 shows the one for cocaine. Normally, after dopamine is released from the axon terminal of a neuron and activates dopamine receptors on the adjacent neuron, the dopamine is then transported back to its original neuron by "uptake pumps." Cocaine binds to the uptake pumps and prevents them from transporting dopamine back into the neuron terminal. So more dopamine builds up in the synapse and is free to activate more dopamine receptors.

Addictive drugs have such a powerful impact on dopamine and its receptors that they change the pathways within the brain's pleasure centers. Various psychoactive chemicals create a craving for more of the same. According to this hypothesis, addicts do not specifically yearn for heroin, cocaine, or nicotine but for the rush of dopamine that these drugs produce. Other brain chemicals, including glutamate, GABA (gamma-aminobutyric acid) and possibly norepinephrine, may also be involved. Some individuals, born with low levels of dopamine, may be particularly susceptible to addiction.

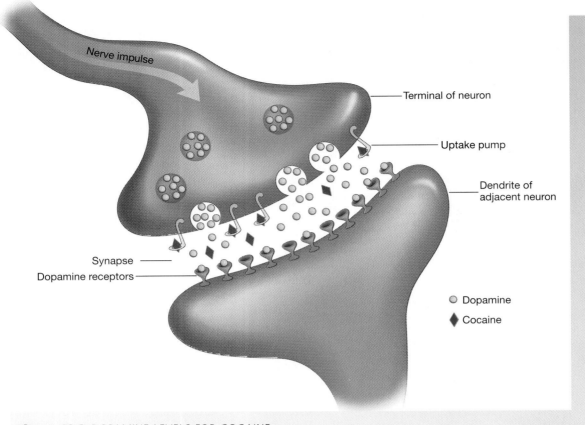

Figure 10-3 DOPAMINE LEVELS FOR COCAINE
Within the synapses between adjacent neurons, cocaine binds to the dopamine uptake pumps and thus allows the neurotransmitter dopamine to build up in the synapse and bind to more dopamine receptors.

The Psychology of Vulnerability

Although scientists do not believe there is an addictive personality, certain individuals are at greater risk of drug dependence because of psychological factors, including difficulty controlling impulses, a lack of values that might constrain drug use (whether based in religion, family, or society), low self-esteem, feelings of powerlessness, and depression. The one psychological trait most often linked with drug use is denial. Young people in particular are absolutely convinced that they will never lose control or suffer in any way as a result of drug use.

Many diagnosed drug users have at least one mental disorder, particularly depression or anxiety. Disorders that emerge in adolescence, such as bipolar disorder, may increase the risk of substance abuse. Many people with psychiatric disorders abuse drugs. Individuals may self-administer drugs to treat psychiatric symptoms; for example, they may take sedating drugs to suppress a panic attack. Contrary to past concerns, treatment of attention-deficit/hyperactivity disorder (ADHD) with stimulant medication does not increase the risk of substance abuse disorders later in life but may in fact decrease their likelihood.[11] (See Fact of Fiction? "Children treated . . .")

Early Influences

Young people from lower socioeconomic backgrounds are more likely to use drugs than their more affluent peers, possibly because of economic disadvantage; family instability; a lack of realistic, rewarding alternatives and role models; and increased hopelessness.

Those whose companions are substance abusers are far more likely to use drugs. Peer pressure to use drugs can be a powerful factor for adolescents and young adults. The likelihood of drug abuse is also related to family instability, parental rejection, and divorce.

Parents' own attitudes and drug-use history affect their children's likelihood of using marijuana, according to the Substance Abuse and Mental Health Services Administration. Parents who perceived little risk associated with marijuana use had children with similar attitudes, and the children of parents who had used marijuana were about three times more likely to try the drug than children whose parents had never used the drug.[12]

Teen Drug Use

Most individuals who use drugs first try them as adolescents. Teens are likely to begin experimenting with tobacco, beer, wine, or hard liquor, then smoke marijuana or sniff inhalants.

New research sponsored by the National Institute on Drug Abuse (NIDA) has confirmed earlier studies linking early use of tobacco and alcohol with a greater likelihood of marijuana use, which in turn increases the likelihood of other illegal drug use.[13] Overall, alcohol or tobacco users are seven times more likely to start using marijuana than individuals who use neither alcohol nor tobacco. Prior marijuana use is closely associated with the opportunity to try cocaine and the likelihood of starting to use cocaine.

Other investigators, analyzing data from individuals aged 12 to 25, focused on "drug exposure opportunities." According to this concept, some young people actively seek out opportunities to try marijuana or cocaine, whereas others are more passive recipients of drug exposure opportunities.

A much smaller percentage of teens try opioids. Over time some individuals give up certain drugs, such as hallucinogens, and return to old favorites, such as alcohol and marijuana. A smaller number continues using several drugs.

The Toll of Drugs

Drugs affect a person's physical, psychological, and social health. The effects of drugs can be *acute* (resulting from a single dose or series of doses) or *chronic* (resulting from long-term use). Acute effects vary with different drugs. Stimulants may trigger unpredictable rage; an overdose of heroin may lead to respiratory depression, a breathing impairment that can be fatal.

Over time, chronic drug users may feel fatigued, cough constantly, lose weight, become malnourished, and ache from head to toe. They may suffer blackouts, flashbacks, and episodes of increasingly bizarre behavior, often triggered by escalating paranoia. Their risk of overdose rises steadily, and they must live with constant stress: the fear of getting busted for possession or of losing a job if they test positive for drugs, the worry of getting enough money for their next fix, the dangers of associating with dealers and other users.

The toll of drug use can be especially great on the young because it disrupts many critical developmental tasks of adolescence and young adulthood. Early use of drugs can lead to drug-related crime (including stealing), poor achievement in high school or college, and job instability.

◾ Drugs in Society

Drug abuse remains a major problem even though drug use among teenagers has declined in recent years. The estimated medical and social costs of drug abuse are believed to exceed $276 billion. Addiction to drugs, alcohol, or tobacco accounts for a third of all hospital admissions and a quarter of all deaths. Heroin, cocaine, and alcohol are the deadliest drugs of abuse.[14]

A growing percentage of teenagers are choosing not to smoke, drink, or experiment with drugs and are voicing disapproval of drug use. According to the most recent data

More teenagers are saying no to drugs.

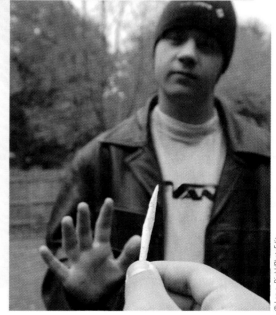

© Lon c. Diehl/PhotoEdit

from the annual Monitoring the Future Study, the percentage of adolescents smoking marijuana has fallen to its lowest level in eight years. Use of MDMA (ecstasy) dropped for the first time since it was added to the annual survey in 1996. More teens now view drugs like ecstasy as harmful and disapprove of their use.[15]

For the first time, the survey asked students about nonmedical use of the prescription painkillers OxyContin and Vicodin. The highest rates of use were reported by high school seniors: 4 percent said they had used OxyContin without a doctor's order in the last year; 9.6 percent had taken Vicodin.[16]

How Common Is Drug Use on Campus?

Alcohol is the number-one drug of abuse on college campuses. Marijuana remains the most commonly used illegal drug. Although the use of alcohol and most other drugs has remained steady in recent years, ecstasy use more than doubled on campus. The Harvard College Alcohol Study revealed an increase of almost 70 percent in ecstasy use by undergraduates over a two-year period.[17] In another study of the drug-using behaviors of 14,520 college students, 3 percent reported use of ecstasy within the past 12 months.[18]

There is a large gap between actual drug use on campus and how prevalent students believe drug use to be. When researchers have compared students' self-reports of frequency of drug use with what students perceived to be the frequency of drug use by "the average student," they greatly overestimate the use of a variety of drugs.[19]

Various factors influence which students use drugs, including the following:

:: **Race/ethnicity.** In general, white students have higher levels of alcohol and drug use than do African-American students. In a comparison of African-American students at predominantly white and predominantly black colleges, those at historically black colleges had lower rates of alcohol and drug use than did either white or African-American students at white schools. The reason, according to the researchers, may be that these colleges provide a greater sense of self-esteem, which helps prevent alcohol and drug use.

:: **Perception of risk.** Students seem most likely to try substances they perceive as being "safe," or low risk. Of these, the top three are caffeine, alcohol, and tobacco; marijuana is listed fourth in terms of perceived safety. Other agents—barbiturates, heroin, cocaine, PCP, speed, LSD, crack, and inhalants—are viewed as more risky and are used much less often.

:: **Alcohol use.** Often individuals engage in more than one "risk behavior," and researchers have documented correlations among smoking, drinking, and drug use. Among college students, researchers have found that those who report binge drinking (discussed in depth in Chapter 11) are much more likely than other students to report current or past use of marijuana, cocaine, or other illegal drugs.[20]

:: **Environment.** As with alcohol use, students are influenced by their friends, their residence, the general public's attitude toward drug use, and even the Internet. College health officials are realizing that, rather than simply trying to change students' substance abuse, they also must change the environment to promote healthier lifestyle choices. One successful innovation is substance-free dorms.

:: **Sexual identity.** In a recent survey of 3,607 undergraduate students, self-identified lesbian women were significantly more likely than heterosexual women to use marijuana, ecstasy, and other drugs.[21] Gay and bisexual men were significantly less likely than heterosexual men to drink heavily but were more likely to use some drugs.[22] In another survey, college women with both male and female sex partners were up to three times more likely to smoke cigarettes, binge drink, and use marijuana than exclusively heterosexual women.[23]

Drugs and Driving

One important impact of drugs is their effect on driving ability (see Chapter 18). Alcohol and drug use are equally common in drivers injured in traffic accidents. Often drivers using alcohol also test positive for other drugs. Different drugs affect driving ability in different ways. Here are the facts from the National Institute on Drug Abuse:

:: Alcohol affects perception, coordination, and judgment, and increases the sedative effects of tranquilizers and barbiturates.

:: Marijuana affects a wide range of driving skills—including the ability to track (stay in the lane) through curves, brake quickly, and maintain speed and a safe distance between cars—and slows thinking and reflexes. Normal driving skills remain impaired for four to six hours after smoking a single joint.

:: Sedatives, hypnotics, and antianxiety agents slow reaction time, and interfere with hand–eye coordination and judgment; the greatest impairment is in the first hour after taking the drug. The effects depend on the particular drug: some build up in the body and can impair driving skills the morning after use; others make drivers very sleepy and, therefore, incapable of driving safely.

:: Amphetamines, after repeated use, impair coordination. They can also make a driver more edgy and less coordinated, and thus more likely to be involved in an accident.

:: Hallucinogens distort judgment and reality, and cause confusion and panic, thus making driving extremely dangerous.

Drugs on the Job

According to the National Household Survey on Drug Abuse, seven in ten illegal drug users have full-time jobs. Workers of every variety—from truck drivers to stockbrokers—use drugs. However, young adults, men, whites, and those with less than a high school education are more likely to use drugs than other workers. At the very least, drug-abusing employees may affect their workplace by being unproductive, making poor decisions, and having strained relationships with coworkers. Even more frightening, however, is the threat to themselves and others from accidents due to their drug use.

Along with alcohol and nicotine, cocaine and marijuana are the primary drugs of abuse on or off the job. As a result of widespread drug use, the military and a growing number of companies are requiring drug tests of job applicants and employees. However, drug testing is not 100 percent precise. For example, individuals who have recently eaten poppy seeds (as in a muffin or bagel) can test positive for opiates. Increasingly, employers are shifting from policing employees to setting up programs to help those with drug problems overcome their drug dependence. (See Fact or Fiction? "Drug testing of students . . .")

Drug use is also common among the unemployed. In particular, unemployed young adults are much more likely to use cocaine and marijuana than those who are working full-time.

◼ Common Drugs of Abuse

Table 10-2 describes the common drugs of abuse within these categories: cannabis, club drugs, stimulants, depressants, hallucinogens, and inhalants. Alcohol, a depressant, is

FACT OR FICTION?

Drug testing of students is not effective in reducing drug use.

Fact: According to a large, multiyear study, the use of school drug tests does not deter adolescents from using drugs. At every grade level tested, beginning in middle school, investigators found virtually identical rates of drug use among students in schools that had drug testing and those that did not.

Source: Patti Meyer. "Student Drug Testing Not Effective in Reducing Drug Use," University of Michigan, May 19, 2003. www.umich.edu/news

discussed in Chapter 11, and tobacco, a stimulant, is covered in Chapter 12.

Cannabis

Marijuana (pot) and **hashish** (hash)—the most widely used illegal drugs—are derived from the cannabis plant. The major psychoactive ingredient in both is *THC (delta-9-tetrahydrocannabinol)*. Nearly half of Americans have smoked marijuana at least once.[24] Some 12 million Americans use cannabis; more than 1 million cannot control this use.

THC triggers a series of reactions in the brain that ultimately lead to the high that users experience when they smoke marijuana. Heredity influences an individual's response to marijuana. Identical male twins, who share all their genes, are more likely than fraternal male twins, who share only about half their genes, to report similar responses to marijuana use, indicating a genetic basis for their response.

Different types of marijuana have different percentages of THC. Because of careful cultivation, the strength of today's marijuana is much greater than that used in the 1970s. Today a marijuana joint contains 150 mg of THC, compared to 10 mg in the 1960s.

Usually, marijuana is smoked in a joint (hand-rolled cigarette) or pipe; it may also be eaten as an ingredient in other foods (as when baked in brownies), though with a less predictable effect. The drug high is enhanced by holding the marijuana smoke in the lungs, and experienced smokers learn to hold the smoke for longer periods to increase the amount of drug diffused into the bloodstream. The circumstances in which marijuana is smoked, the communal aspects of its use, and the user's experience all can affect the way a marijuana-induced high feels.

Marijuana has shown some medical benefits, including boosting appetite in patients who are HIV-positive or undergoing chemotherapy, alleviating cancer and neck pain, helping reduce pressure on the eyeball in glaucoma patients, and helping people with spasticity (extreme muscle tension) due to multiple sclerosis or injuries.

Support for the legalization of marijuana for medicinal purposes has grown in recent years, although the majority of Americans still oppose such legislation.[25] (See Student Snapshot: "Do Students Want Marijuana Legalized?" on page 340) Several states, including California, Alaska, Arizona, Colorado, Hawaii, Maine, Nevada, Oregon, and Washington, allow marijuana to be grown and distributed to people with a doctor's recommendation. In 2003 the Canadian government, responding to a court order, begin selling marijuana to people with severe arthritis, cancer, HIV/AIDS and multiple sclerosis.[26]

TABLE 10-2 **Common Drugs of Abuse**

Type of Drug	Drug Name	Street Name	Description	How It's Used	Related Paraphernalia	Signs and Symptoms of Use
Cannabis	Marijuana	Pot, grass, reefer, weed, Colombian hash, sinsemilla, joint, blunts, Acapulco gold, Thai sticks	Like dried oregano leaves, dark green or brown	Usually smoked in hand-rolled cigarettes, pipes, or thin cigars, or eaten	Rolling papers, pipes, bongs, baggies, roach clips	Sweet burnt odor, neglect of appearance, loss of motivation, slow reactions, red eyes, memory lapses
Club Drugs/ Designer Drugs (Stimulants, depressants, and/or hallucinogens)	MDMA, MDA, MDEA	Ecstasy, XTC, X, Adam, Clarity	Tablet or capsule; colorless, tasteless, and odorless	Swallowed, can be added to beverages by individuals who want to intoxicate others	Pacifiers, glow sticks (used at all-night dance parties, raves, or trances)	Agitated state, confusion, sleep problems, paranoia
	Date-rape drug Rohypnol	Roofies, roche, love drug, forget-me pill	Tasteless, odorless, dissolves easily in all beverages	Swallowed, can be added to beverages by individuals who want to sedate others	Drinks, soda cans	1 milligram can impair a victim for 8 to 12 hours, can cause amnesia, decreased blood pressure, urinary retention
	GHB	Liquid Ecstasy, Grievous Bodily Harm, G	Clear liquid, tablet, capsule	Swallowed, dissolved in drinks	Drinks, soda cans	Can relax or sedate
Stimulants (Stimulate the nervous system)	Amphetamines amphetamine, dextroamphetamine methamphetamine	Speed, uppers, pep pill, bennies, dexies, meth, crank, crystal, black beauties, white crosses	Variety of tablets, capsules, and crystal-like rock salt	Swallowed in pill or capsule form, or injected	Syringe, needles	Excess activity, irritability, nervousness, mood swings, needle marks, dilated pupils, talkativeness then depression
	Cocaine	Coke, snow, toot, white lady	White odorless powder	Usually inhaled; can be injected, swallowed, or smoked	Razor blade, straws, glass surfaces	Restlessness, dilated pupils, oily skin, talkativeness; euphoric short-term high, followed by depression
	Tobacco/ Nicotine	Smokes, butts, cigs, cancer sticks, snuff, dip, chew, plug	Dried brown organic material, bidis flavored with mint or chocolate; smokeless is moist	Burned and inhaled as cigarettes, pipes, cigars, cigarillos; chewed; or inhaled through the nose as snuff.	Rolling papers, pipes, spit cups, cigar cutters, lighters, matches	Shortness of breath, respiratory illnesses; oral, lung, and other cancers

How Users Feel

In low to moderate doses, marijuana typically creates a mild sense of euphoria, a sense of slowed time (five minutes may feel like an hour), a dreamy sort of self-absorption, and some impairment in thinking and communicating. Users report heightened sensations of color, sound, and other stimuli, relaxation, and increased confidence. The sense of being stoned peaks within half an hour and usually lasts about three hours. Even when alterations in perception seem slight, as noted earlier, it is not safe to drive a car for as long as four to six hours after smoking a single joint.

TABLE 10-2	Common Drugs of Abuse—continued

Type of Drug	Drug Name	Street Name	Description	How It's Used	Related Paraphernalia	Signs and Symptoms of Use
Depressants (Depress the nervous system)	**Alcohol**	Booze, hooch, juice, brew, alcopops (hard lemonade or fruit juices)	Clear or amber-colored liquid; sweet, fruit-flavored malt-based drinks	Swallowed in liquid form	Flask, bottles, cans, use of food color to disguise it; colorful and innocent-looking labels	Impaired judgment, poor muscle coordination, lowered inhibitions
	Barbiturates Amyl, Seconal, Nembutal, Butisol, Tuinal	Barbs, downers, yellow jackets, red devils, blue devils	Variety of tablets, capsules, powder	Swallowed in pill form or injected into the veins	Syringe, needles	Drowsiness, confusion, impaired judgment, slurred speech, needle marks, staggering gait
	Tranquilizers/ Benzodiazepines Valium, Librium, Miltown, Xanax	V's, blues, downers, candy	Variety of tablets	Swallowed in pill form or injected	Syringe, pill bottles, needles	Drowsiness, faulty judgment, disorientation
	Narcotics/ Opioids heroin, morphine	Dreamer, junk, smack, horse	White or brown powders, tablets, capsules, liquid	Injected, smoked, may be blended with marijuana	Syringes, spoon, lighter, needles, medicine dropper	Lethargy, loss of skin color, needle marks, constricted pupils, decreased coordination
Hallucinogens (Alter perceptions of reality)	**PCP** (Phencyclidine)	Angel dust, killer weed, supergrass, hog, peace pill	White powder or tablet	Usually smoked, can be inhaled (snorted), injected, or swallowed in tablets	Tinfoil	Slurred speech, blurred vision, lack of coordination, confusion, agitation, violence, unpredictability, "bad trips"
	LSD (Lysergic Acid Diethylamide)	Acid, cubes, purple haze, white lightning	Odorless, colorless, tasteless powder	Injected, or swallowed in tablets or capsules	Blotter papers, tinfoil	Dilated pupils, illusions, hallucinations, disorientation, mood swings, nausea, flashbacks
	Mescaline caps, psilocybin, psilocin, mushrooms	Mesc, cactus, caps, magic mushroom, shrooms	Capsules, tablets, mushrooms	Ingested in its natural form, smoked, or brewed as tea	Dried mushrooms	Same as LSD above
Inhalants (Substances abused by sniffing)	**Solvents, aerosols** airplane glue, gasoline, dry cleaning solution, correction fluid		Chemicals that produce mind-altering vapors	Inhaled or sniffed, often with the use of paper or plastic bags	Cleaning rags, empty spray cans, tubes of glue, baggies	Poor motor coordination; bad breath; impaired vision, memory and thoughts; violent behavior
	Nitrates Amyl & Butyl	Poppers, locker room, rush, snappers	Clear yellowish liquid	Inhaled or sniffed from gauze or single-dose glass vials	Cloth-covered bulb that pops when broken, small bottles	Slowed thought, headache
	Nitrous oxide	Laughing gas, whippets	Colorless gas with sweet taste and smell	Inhaled or sniffed by mask or cone	Aerosol cans such as whipped cream, small canisters	Light-headed, loss of motor control

Source: "A Parent's Guide for the Prevention of Alcohol, Tobacco and Other Drug Use." Copyright © 2000 Lowe Family Foundation, Inc., Revised 2001. (Lowe Family Foundation, 3339 Stuyvesant Pl. NW, Washington DC, 20015, 202-362-4883.) Used with permission.

Some users—particularly those smoking marijuana for the first time or taking a high dose in an unpleasant or unfamiliar setting—experience acute anxiety, which may be accompanied by a panicky fear of losing control. They may believe that their companions are ridiculing or threatening them and experience a panic attack, a state of intense terror.

Student Snapshot **Do Students Want Marijuana Legalized?**

The percentage of students who say marijuana should be legal has risen from the record low of 1989 but remains below the high of 1977. Significantly more men in the Class of 2006 (45.8 percent) favor legalization than women (34.7 percent).

Source: Linda Sax et al. *The American Freshman: National Norms for Fall 2002.* Los Angeles: Higher Education Research Institute, UCLA, 2002.

1977   51.3%

1989   16.7%

2002   39.7%

The immediate physical effects of marijuana include increased pulse rate, bloodshot eyes, dry mouth and throat, slowed reaction times, impaired motor skills, increased appetite, and diminished short-term memory. (See Figure 10-4.) High doses reduce the ability to perceive and to react; all the reactions experienced with low doses are intensified, leading to sensory distortion and, in the case of hashish, vivid hallucinations and LSD-like psychedelic reactions. The drug remains in the body's fat cells 50 hours or more after use, so people may experience psychoactive effects for several days after use. Drug tests may produce positive results for days or weeks after last use.

Risks

Marijuana produces a range of effects in different bodily systems, such as diminished immune responses and impaired fertility in men. Other risks include damage to the brain, lungs, and heart, and to babies born to mothers who use marijuana during pregnancy or while nursing. (See Figure 10-4.)

Brain. THC produces changes in the brain that affect learning, memory, and the way the brain integrates sensory experiences with emotions and motivations. Short-term effects include problems with memory and learning; distorted perceptions; difficulty thinking and problem-solving; loss of coordination; increased anxiety; and panic attacks.

Long-term use produces changes in the brain similar to those seen with other major drugs of abuse.

 According to a study of college students, heavy marijuana use impairs critical skills related to attention, memory, and learning, even 24 hours after its use. Heavy users who smoked marijuana almost every day showed significant difficulty sustaining attention, shifting attention to meet the demands of changes in the environment, and registering, processing, and using information.[27]

Teenagers below college age who use marijuana have lower achievement than nonusers, more acceptance of illegal or socially deviant behavior, more aggression, greater rebelliousness, poorer relationships with parents, and more delinquent and drug-using friends. Those who regularly smoke marijuana often lose interest in school and do not remember what they learned when they were high. Some long-term regular users may experience *burnout,* a dulling of their senses and responses termed *amotivational syndrome.*

Over time, continued heavy marijuana use can interfere with students' ability to learn and perform well in school and in challenging careers. Marijuana contributes significantly to accidental death and injury among adolescents, especially through motor vehicle crashes.

Lungs. Smoking cannabis may cause similar effects to smoking tobacco, with many of them appearing at a younger age. They include chronic bronchitis, emphysema, and other lung disorders and increased risk of heart attacks and sudden death.[28] The amount of tar inhaled by marijuana smokers and the level of carbon monoxide absorbed

Negative Long-Term Effects

Brain and central nervous system
- Dulls sensory and cognitive skills
- Impairs short-term memory
- Alters motor coordination
- Causes changes in brain chemistry
- Leads to difficulty in concentration, attention to detail, and learning new, complex information

Cardiovascular system
- Increases heart rate
- Increases blood pressure
- Decreases blood flow to the limbs, which in extreme cases could require an amputation

Respiratory system
- Damages the lungs (50% more tar than tobacco)
- May cause lung cancer
- May damage throat from inhalation

Reproductive system
- In women, may impair ovulation and cause fetal abnormalities if used during pregnancy
- In men, may suppress sexual functioning and may reduce the number, quality and mobility of sperm, possibly affecting fertility

Positive Short-Term Therapeutic Effects for Patients

Brain and central nervous system
- May help minimize pain from the spread of cancer

Vision
- Reduces intraocular pressure, helping those afflicted with glaucoma

Digestive system
- Combats nausea from chemotherapy and helps minimize vomiting
- Helps restore appetite in people who have lost weight from cancer or AIDS

Muscular system
- May help calm spasms from spinal-cord injury, multiple sclerosis, and possibly epilepsy

Figure 10–4 SOME EFFECTS OF MARIJUANA ON THE BODY
Some negative long-term effects and positive short-term therapeutic effects of marijuana use.

Source: *Time,* November 4, 2002.

are three to five times greater than among tobacco smokers. The reasons may be that marijuana users inhale more deeply, hold the smoke in the lungs longer, and do not use filters. Smoking a single joint can be as damaging to the lungs as smoking five tobacco cigarettes. Someone who smokes five joints a week may take in as many cancer-causing chemicals as a person who smokes a pack of cigarettes a day.[29]

Heart. Otherwise healthy people have suffered heart attacks shortly after smoking marijuana. Experiments have also linked marijuana use to elevated blood pressure and decreased oxygen supply to the heart muscle. According to recent estimates, the risk of heart attack triples within an hour of smoking pot.[30] Smoking marijuana while shooting cocaine can potentially cause deadly increases in heart rate and blood pressure.[31]

Pregnancy. Babies born to mothers who use marijuana during pregnancy are smaller than those born to mothers who did not use the drug, and the babies are more likely to develop health problems.[32] A nursing mother who uses marijuana passes some of the THC to the baby in her breast milk. This may impair the infant's motor development (control of muscle movement).

Withdrawal

Marijuana users can develop a compulsive, often uncontrollable craving for the drug. More than 120,000 people enter treatment every year for marijuana addiction. In addition, animal studies suggest that marijuana causes physical dependence. Stopping after long-term marijuana use can produce *marijuana withdrawal syndrome,* which is characterized by insomnia, restlessness, loss of appetite, and irritability. People who smoked marijuana daily for many years may become aggressive after they stop using it and may relapse to prevent aggression and other symptoms.

Club Drugs (Designer Drugs)

The National Institute on Drug Abuse identifies a variety of drugs—alcohol, LSD (acid), MDMA(ecstasy), GHB, GBL, Ketamine (Special-K), Fentanyl, Rohypnol, amphetamines and methamphetamine—as **"club drugs,"** popular among teens and young adults at nightclubs, bars, or raves and trances—night-long dances often held in warehouses or other unusual settings.

Although many who attend raves do not generally use drugs, they may be told that club drugs are cheap, energizing, and safe. As scientists are demonstrating, this is not true. Brain scans reveal changes in critical parts of the brain from use of club drugs. (See Figure 10-5.) In high doses most of these drugs can cause a sharp increase in body temperature (a condition called malignant hyperthermia), leading to muscle breakdown, kidney and cardiovascular system failure, and possible death.

Ecstasy

Ecstasy (Adam, XTC, X, hug, beans, love drug) is the most common street name for methylene-dioxymethamphetamine (MDMA), a synthetic compound with both stimulant and mildly hallucinogenic properties. MDMA is spreading beyond the young white populations frequenting raves to mainstream dance clubs

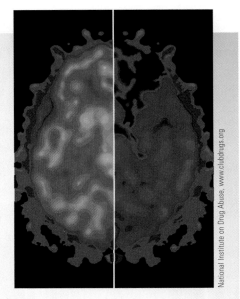

National Institute on Drug Abuse, www.clubdrugs.org

Figure 10-5 EFFECTS OF ECSTASY ON THE BRAIN

These brain scans show the sharp difference in human brain function for an individual who has never used drugs (left) and one who used the club drug ecstasy many times but had not used any drugs for at least three weeks before the scan (right). In the left scan, the bright reddish color shows active serotonin sites in the brain. Serotonin is a critical neurochemical that regulates mood, emotion, learning, memory, sleep, and pain. In the right scan, the dark sections indicate areas where serotonin is not present even after three weeks without any drugs.

and house parties, with use increasing among African-Americans, Hispanics, and people in their thirties.[33]

As noted, ecstasy use has greatly increased on campus. Students who use ecstasy do not differ from others in terms of academic achievement (as measured by GPA) or commitment to community service. In one study, they are significantly more likely to be white, to belong to a fraternity/sorority, and to have used other drugs of abuse during the previous year.[34] Ecstasy users are more likely to use marijuana, binge drink, spend more time socializing and less time studying, have more sexual partners, smoke cigarettes, rate parties as more important than academics, and view religion as less important.[35]

How It Feels. Although it can be smoked, inhaled (snorted), or injected, ecstasy is almost always taken as a pill or tablet. Its effects begin in 45 minutes and last for two to four hours.

MDMA belongs to a family of drugs called *enactogens,* which literally means "touching within." As a mood elevator, it produces a relaxed, euphoric state but does not produce hallucinations. Users of ecstasy often say they feel at peace with themselves and at ease and empathic with oth-

Club drugs are often used at raves, even those that are alcohol-free.

© Scott Houston/CORBIS

ers. In some settings, they reveal intimate details of their lives (which they may later regret); in other settings, they join in collective rejoicing. Like hallucinogenic drugs, MDMA can enhance sensory experience, but it rarely causes visual distortions, sudden mood changes, or psychotic reactions. Regular users may experience depression and anxiety the week after taking MDMA.

Psychologists have experimented with MDMA as a way to enhance self-revelation, self-criticism, and self-exploration, and to boost trust between a patient and a therapist. Most clinicians are highly skeptical of its benefits, and there has been no officially sanctioned research on its therapeutic benefits.

Risks. Ecstasy poses risks similar to those of cocaine and amphetamines. These include psychological difficulties (confusion, depression, sleep problems, drug craving, severe anxiety, and paranoia) and physical symptoms (muscle tension, involuntary teeth clenching, nausea, blurred vision, rapid eye movement, faintness, chills, sweating, and increases in heart rate and blood pressure that pose a special risk for people with circulatory or heart disease).[36]

Continued use of ecstasy can lead to psychological dependence because users seek to recreate the exhilarating high and avoid the plunge into unhappiness and emptiness that comes after use. Because ecstasy is *neurotoxic* (damaging to brain cells), it depletes the brain of serotonin, a messenger chemical involved with mood, sleep, and appetite, and can lead to depression, anxiety, and impaired thinking and memory.[37]

According to brain-imaging studies, users, although as mentally alert as nonusers, fared far worse on measures of memory, learning, and general intelligence. The more frequently they took ecstasy, the worse they did, probably because ecstasy alters neuronal function in a brain structure called the hippocampus, which helps create short-term memory.[38] (See Figure 10-5.) Other experiments have shown increased impulsiveness and attention deficits in MDMA users.

MDMA can produce nausea, vomiting, and dizziness. When combined with extended physical exertion like dancing, club drugs can lead to hyperthermia (severe overheating), severe dehydration, serious increases in blood pressure, stroke, and heart attack. Without sufficient water, dancers at raves may suffer dehydration and heat stroke, which can be fatal. Individuals with high blood pressure, heart trouble, or liver or kidney disease are in the greatest danger. Several deaths have occurred in teens who suffered brain damage by drinking large amounts of water to counteract the raised body temperature induced by the drug.

MDMA has been implicated in some cases of acute hepatitis, which can lead to liver failure. Even after liver transplantation, the mortality rate for individuals with this condition is 50 percent. Another danger comes from the practice of taking Prozac, a drug that modulates the mood-altering brain chemical serotonin, before ecstasy. This can

cause jaw clenching, nausea, tremors, and, in extreme cases, potentially fatal elevations in body temperature.

Although not a sexual stimulant (if anything, MDMA has the opposite effect), ecstasy fosters strong feelings of intimacy that may lead to risky sexual behavior. The psychological effects of ecstasy become less intriguing with repeated use, and the physical side effects become more uncomfortable. Ecstasy poses risks to a developing fetus, including a greater likelihood of heart and skeletal abnormalities and long-term learning and memory impairments in children born to women who used MDMA during pregnancy.[39]

MDMA pills may contain caffeine, dextromethorphan, heroin, and mescaline. The MDMA-like substance para-methoxyamphetamine (PMA) has been implicated in the deaths of people who mistakenly thought they were taking true MDMA. The deaths were due to complications from hyperthermia.[40]

GHB and GBL

The brain messenger chemical called **GHB (gammahydroxybutyrate)** stimulates the release of human growth hormone but has no known effects on muscle growth. Although this central nervous system depressant is banned by the FDA, users obtain it illegally either for its high, which is similar to that caused by alcohol or marijuana, or for its alleged ability to trim fat and build muscles.

The main ingredient is **GBL (gamma butyrolactone),** an industrial solvent often used to strip floors. Once ingested, GBL converts into GHB, an odorless, colorless sedative that can be slipped into a beverage to knock an individual out.

In small doses, GHB and GBL are believed to induce euphoria and enhance sex by increasing dopamine in the brain. However, a larger dose can cause someone to pass

Club drugs, made in a laboratory and sold on the street, aren't subject to quality controls and don't always contain what the buyer expects.

out in 15 minutes and fall into a coma within half an hour. Other side effects include nausea, amnesia, hallucinations, decreased heart rate, convulsions, and sometimes blackouts. Long-term use at high doses can lead to a withdrawal reaction: rapid heartbeat, tremor, insomnia, anxiety, and occasionally hallucinations that last a few days to a week. According to the Drug Enforcement Administration, the use of GHB has been associated with more than 5,700 reported overdoses and at least 66 deaths, mainly from respiratory depression. The danger is greatest when mixed with alcohol or opiates.

Ketamine

"K," or ketamine, is an anesthetic used by veterinarians. When cooked, dried, and ground into a powder for snorting, K blocks chemical messengers in the brain that carry sensory input. As a result, the brain fills the void with hallucinations.

Ketamine has become common in club and rave scenes and has been used as a date rape drug. At high doses, it can cause delirium, amnesia, impaired motor function, high blood pressure, depression, and potentially fatal respiratory problems.

Herbal Ecstasy

Herbal ecstasy, also known as Herbal Bliss, Cloud 9, and Herbal X, is a mixture of stimulants such as ephedrine, pseudoephedrine, and caffeine. Sold in tablet or capsule form as a "natural" and safe alternative to ecstasy, its ingredients vary greatly.

Herbal pills can have dangerous and unpleasant side effects, including stroke, heart attack, and a disfiguring skin condition. They are sold at head shops, night clubs, and raves. The FDA has received hundreds of complaints of strokes, seizures, and possibly even some deaths.

Other Designer Drugs

Methcathinone, or "cat," is a powerful synthetic stimulant that can produce a high that lasts up to six days. Cat usually contains a mix of chemicals along with small doses of Drano or battery acid, which act as a catalyst.

College and street chemists have also produced synthetic opiates that are particularly dangerous because they're far more potent than those derived from natural substances. Derivatives of *fentanyl,* an anesthetic widely used for surgery in the United States, are 20 to 2,000 times as powerful as heroin, and the risk of a fatal overdose or brain damage is much greater.

Stimulants

Central nervous system stimulants are drugs that increase activity in some portion of the brain or spinal cord. Some stimulants increase motor activity and enhance mental alertness, and some combat mental fatigue. Amphetamine, methamphetamine, caffeine, cocaine, and khat are stimulants.

Amphetamine and Methamphetamine

Amphetamines trigger the release of epinephrine (adrenaline), which stimulates the central nervous system. They were once widely prescribed for weight control because they suppress appetite, but they have emerged as a global danger. Amphetamines are sold under a variety of names: amphetamine (brand name Benzedrine, streetname bennies), dextroamphetamine (Dexedrine, dex), methamphetamine (Methedrine, meth, speed), and Desoxyn (copilots). Related *uppers* include the prescription drugs methylphenidate (Ritalin), pemoline (Cylert), and phenmetrazine (Preludin). Amphetamines are available in tablet or capsule form.

Methamphetamine (meth, crank, crystal, fast, glass, speed, beanies, black beauties, blade, christmas tree meth, cinnamon, sugar, crys, shabu, tic, wash) is a powerful addictive stimulant that comes in three forms—powder, crystal, and pills—and can be ingested by mouth, injected, or snorted. "Ice," the slang name for crystallized methamphetamine hydrochloride, is smokeable methamphetamine, highly addictive and toxic.

A new form of methamphetamine called Ya-ba/Thai Tabs, which tastes sweet like candy, may seem less dangerous but is actually more powerful and dangerous than other forms of methamphetamine. It has hallucinogenic effects and may cause increased heart rate, dehydration, paranoia and depression.[41]

Unlike cocaine, which is quickly removed from the brain, methamphetamine remains in the central nervous system and the body, producing prolonged stimulant

**Methamphetamine Pills
Ya-ba/Thai Tabs**

effects. Chronic abuse produces a psychosis similar to schizophrenia, characterized by paranoia, picking at the skin, preoccupation with one's thoughts, and auditory and visual hallucinations. Symptoms can persist for months or even years after discontinuing use.[42]

Methamphetamine "laboratories," created to meet the black-market demand for stimulants, have spread across the country. Using a relatively simple process, meth "cooks" in kitchens, basements, and garages make powder amphetamines in makeshift laboratories, especially in the Midwest. Fires and explosions are common because of the volatile chemicals involved. Large amounts of methamphetamines are also smuggled into the United States from Mexico.[43]

How Users Feel. Amphetamines produce a state of hyper-alertness and energy. Users feel confident in their ability to think clearly and to perform any task exceptionally well—although amphetamines do not, in fact, significantly boost performance or thinking. Higher doses make users feel *wired:* talkative, excited, restless, irritable, anxious, moody.

If taken intravenously, amphetamines produce a characteristic rush of elation and confidence, as well as adverse effects, including confusion, rambling or incoherent speech, anxiety, headache, and palpitations. Individuals may become paranoid; be convinced they are having profound thoughts; feel increased sexual interest; and experience unusual perceptions, such as ringing in the ears, a sensation of insects crawling on their skin, or hearing their name called. Crank users may feel high and sleepy or may hallucinate and lose contact with reality. Methamphetamine, which produces a rapid high when inhaled, produces exceptionally long-lasting toxic effects, including psychosis, violence, seizures, and cardiovascular abnormalities. Brain-imaging studies show changes in heavy users' brains that may affect learning and memory for as long as a year.[44]

Risks. Dependence on amphetamines can develop with episodic or daily use. Users typically take amphetamines in large doses to prevent crashing. Bingeing—taking high doses over a period of several days—can lead to an extremely intense and unpleasant crash characterized by a craving for the drug, shakiness, irritability, anxiety, and depression. Two or more days are required for recuperation.

Amphetamine intoxication may cause the following symptoms:

:: Feelings of grandiosity, anxiety, tension, hypervigilance, anger, social hypersensitivity, fighting, jitteriness or agitation, paranoia, and impaired judgment in social or occupational functioning.

:: Increased heart rate, dilated pupils, elevated blood pressure, perspiration or chills, and nausea or vomiting.

:: Less frequent effects such as speeding up or slowing down of physical movement; muscular weakness; impaired breathing, chest pain, heart arrhythmia; con-

fusion, seizures, impaired movements or muscle tone; or even coma.

:: In high doses, a rapid or irregular heartbeat, tremors, loss of coordination, and collapse.

Smokeable methamphetamine, or ice, also increases heart rate and blood pressure; high doses can cause permanent damage to blood vessels in the brain. Other physical effects of methamphetamine include dilated pupils, blurred vision, dry mouth, and increased breathing rate. Prolonged use can cause fatal lung and kidney disorders. Injecting propylexedrine can lead to convulsions, strokes, and respiratory and kidney failure. Abusers also may develop infected veins, and if they share needles, they risk HIV infection.

The long-term effects of amphetamine abuse include malnutrition, skin disorders, ulcers, insomnia, depression, vitamin deficiencies, and, in some cases, brain damage that results in speech and thought disturbances. Sexual dysfunction and impaired concentration or memory also may occur.

Withdrawal. When the immediate effects of amphetamines wear off, users experience a *crash*—they crave the drug and become shaky, irritable, anxious, and depressed. Amphetamine withdrawal usually persists for more than 24 hours after cessation of prolonged, heavy use. Its characteristic features include fatigue, disturbing dreams, much more or less than usual sleep, increased appetite, and speeding up or slowing down of physical movements. Those who are unable to sleep despite their exhaustion often take sedative-hypnotics (discussed later in this chapter) to help them rest, and may then become dependent on them as well as amphetamines. Symptoms usually reach a peak in two to four days, although depression and irritability may persist for months. Suicide is a major risk.

Cocaine

Cocaine (coke, snow, lady) is a white crystalline powder extracted from the leaves of the South American coca plant. Usually mixed with various sugars and local anesthetics like lidocaine and procaine, cocaine powder is generally inhaled. When sniffed or snorted, cocaine anesthetizes the nerve endings in the nose and relaxes the lung's bronchial muscles.

Cocaine can be dissolved in water and injected intravenously. The drug is rapidly metabolized by the liver, so the high is relatively brief, typically lasting only about 20 minutes. This means that users will commonly inject the drug repeatedly, increasing the risk of infection and damage to their veins. Many intravenous cocaine users prefer the practice of *speedballing,* the intravenous administration of a combination of cocaine and heroin.

Cocaine alkaloid, or *freebase,* is obtained by removing the hydrochloride salt from cocaine powder. *Freebasing* is smoking the fumes of the alkaloid form of cocaine. *Crack,* pharmacologically identical to freebase, is a cheap, easy-to-use, widely available, smokeable, and potent form of cocaine named for the popping sound it makes when burned. Because it is absorbed rapidly into the bloodstream and large doses reach the brain very quickly, it is particularly dangerous. However, its low price and easy availability have made it a common drug of abuse in poor urban areas. An estimated 5 million people in the United States use cocaine.[45]

How Users Feel. A powerful stimulant to the central nervous system, cocaine targets several chemical sites in the brain, producing feelings of soaring well-being and boundless energy. Users feel they have enormous physical and mental ability, yet are also restless and anxious. After a brief period of euphoria, users slump into a depression. They often go on cocaine binges, lasting from a few hours to several days, and consume large quantities of cocaine.

With crack, dependence develops quickly. As soon as crack users come down from one high, they want more crack. Whereas heroin addicts may shoot up several times a day, crack addicts need another hit within minutes. Thus, a crack habit can quickly become more expensive than heroin addiction.

Cocaine may cause changes in the brain that affect a user's ability to sense pleasure and may contribute to depression.[46] With continuing use, cocaine users experience less pleasure and more unpleasant effects. Eventually they may reach a point at which they no longer experience euphoric effects and crave the drug simply to alleviate their persistent hunger for it. They constantly think about it, dream about it, spend all their money on it, and borrow, steal, or deal to pay for it. They cannot concentrate on work; they become increasingly irritable and confused. They may also become dependent on alcohol, sedatives, or opioids, which they use to calm down from cocaine's aftereffects.

Risks. Cocaine dependence is an easy habit to acquire. With repeated use, the brain becomes tolerant of the drug's stimulant effects, and users must take more of it to get high. Those who smoke or inject cocaine can develop dependence within weeks. Those who sniff cocaine may not become dependent on the drug for months or years. It is thought that 5 to 20 percent of all coke users—a group as large as the estimated total number of heroin addicts—are dependent on the drug.

The physical effects of acute cocaine intoxication include dilated pupils, elevated or lowered blood pressure, perspiration or chills, nausea or vomiting, speeding up or slowing down of physical activity, muscular weakness, impaired breathing, chest pain, and impaired movements or muscle tone. Prolonged cocaine snorting can result in ulceration of the mucous membrane of the nose and damage to the nasal septum (the membrane between the nostrils) severe enough to cause it to collapse.

Although some users initially try cocaine as a sexual stimulant, it does not enhance sexual performance. At low doses, it may delay orgasm and cause heightened sensory awareness, but men who use cocaine regularly have problems maintaining erections and ejaculating. They also tend to have low sperm counts, less active sperm, and more abnormal sperm than nonusers. Both male and female chronic cocaine users tend to lose interest in sex and have difficulty reaching orgasm.

Cocaine use can cause blood vessels in the brain to clamp shut and can trigger a stroke, bleeding in the brain, and potentially fatal brain seizures. Cocaine users can also develop psychiatric or neurological complications. (See Figure 10-6.) Repeated or high doses of cocaine can lead to impaired judgment, hyperactivity, nonstop babbling, feelings of suspicion and paranoia, and violent behavior. The brain never learns to tolerate cocaine's negative effects; users may become incoherent and paranoid, and may experience unusual sensations, such as ringing in their ears, feeling insects crawling on the skin, or hearing their name called.

Cocaine can damage the liver and cause lung damage in freebasers. Smoking crack causes bronchitis as well as lung damage, and may promote the transmission of HIV through burned and bleeding lips. Some smokers have died of respiratory complications, such as pulmonary edema (the buildup of fluid in the lungs).

Cocaine causes the heart rate to speed up and blood pressure to rise suddenly. Its use is associated with many cardiac complications, including arrhythmia (disruption of heart rhythm), angina (chest pain), and acute myocardial infarction (heart attack). These cardiac complications can lead to sudden death. The most common ways of dying from cocaine use are persistent seizures that result in respiratory collapse, cardiac arrest from arrhythmias, myocardial infarction, and intracranial hemorrhage or stroke. Cocaine-induced elevations in blood pressure can lead to kidney failure. Cocaine may reduce the immune system's ability to fight infections.[47]

Cocaine users who inject the drug and share needles put themselves at risk for another potentially lethal problem: HIV infection. Other complications of injecting cocaine include skin infections, hepatitis, inflammation of the arteries, and infection of the lining of the heart.

The combination of alcohol and cocaine is particularly lethal. Alcohol and cocaine together are second only to the combination of heroin and alcohol in causing deaths related to substance abuse. When people mix cocaine and alcohol, they compound the danger each drug poses. The liver combines the two agents and manufactures cocaethylene, which intensifies cocaine's euphoric effects, while possibly increasing the risk of sudden death.

Cocaine is dangerous for pregnant women and their babies, causing miscarriages, developmental disorders, and life-threatening complications during birth. Women who use the drug while pregnant are more likely to miscarry in the first three months of pregnancy than women who do not use drugs or who use heroin and other opioids. Cocaine can reduce the fetal oxygen supply, possibly inter-

Central nervous system
- Repeated use or high dosages may cause severe psychological problems
- Suppresses desire for food, sex, and sleep
- Can cause strokes, seizures, and neurological damage

Nose
- Damages mucous membrane

Cardiovascular system
- Increases blood pressure by constricting blood vessels
- Causes irregular heartbeat
- Damages heart tissue

Respiratory system
- Freebasing causes lung damage
- Overdose can lead to respiratory arrest

Reproductive system
- In men, affects ability to maintain erections and ejaculate; also causes sperm abnormalities
- In women, may affect ability to carry pregnancy to term

Figure 10-6 SOME EFFECTS OF COCAINE ON THE BODY

fering with the development of the fetus's nervous system. Infants born to cocaine and crack users can suffer withdrawal and may have major complications or permanent disabilities. Cocaine babies have higher-than-normal rates of respiratory and kidney troubles, visual problems, and developmental retardation, and they may be at greater risk of sudden infant death syndrome.

Withdrawal. When addicted individuals stop using cocaine, they often become depressed. This may lead to further cocaine use to alleviate depression. Other symptoms of cocaine withdrawal include fatigue, vivid and disturbing dreams, excessive or too little sleep, irritability, increased appetite, and physical slowing down or speeding up. This initial crash may last one to three days after cutting down or stopping the heavy use of cocaine. Some individuals become violent, paranoid, and suicidal.

Symptoms usually reach a peak in two to four days, although depression, anxiety, irritability, lack of pleasure in usual activities, and low-level cravings may continue for weeks. As memories of the crash fade, the desire for

cocaine intensifies. For many weeks after stopping, individuals may feel an intense craving for the drug. Experimental medical approaches for treating cocaine dependence include antidepressant drugs, anticonvulsant drugs, and the naturally occurring amino acids tryptophan and tyrosine. However, these have only limited benefit, and much more research into medical treatments is needed. Recent research has found that, depending on personal characteristics such as abstract reasoning ability and religious motivation, some cocaine abusers fare better with cognitive-behavioral therapy (discussed in Chapter 2); others, with 12-step programs (discussed later in this chapter).

The drug's effects seem to be long-lasting. Former users who have been drug-free for at least a year have lower test scores than people who never used stimulants like cocaine.[48]

Khat (kat, catha, chat, Abyssinian tea)

For centuries people in East Africa and the Arabian peninsula consumed the fresh young leaves of the *Catha edulis* shrub in ways similar to our drinking coffee. Its active ingredients are two controlled substances, cathinone and cathine.

Chewing alleviates fatigue and reduces appetite. Compulsive use may result in manic behavior, grandiose illusions, paranoia, and hallucinations.[49]

Depressants

Depressants depress the central nervous system, reduce activity, and induce relaxation, drowsiness, or sleep. They include the benzodiazepines and the barbiturates, the opioids, and alcohol.

Benzodiazepines and Barbiturates

These depressants are the sedative-hypnotics, also known as anxiolytic or antianxiety drugs. The **benzodiazepines**—the most widely used drugs in this category—are commonly prescribed for tension, muscular strain, sleep problems, anxiety, panic attacks, anesthesia, and in the treatment of alcohol withdrawal. They include such drugs as *chlordiazepoxide* (Librium), *diazepam* (Valium), *oxazepam* (Serax), *lorazepam* (Ativan), *flurazepam* (Dalmane), and *alprazolam* (Xanax). They differ widely in their mechanism of action, absorption rate, and metabolism, but all produce similar intoxication and withdrawal symptoms.

Rohypnol, a trade name for flunitrazepam, is one of the benzodiazepines, and it has been of particular concern for the last few years because of its abuse in date rape.

When mixed with alcohol, Rohypnol can incapacitate victims and prevent them from resisting sexual assault. It produces "anterograde amnesia," which means individuals may not remember events they experienced while under the effects of the drug. Rohypnol may be lethal when mixed with alcohol or other depressants.

Benzodiazepine sleeping pills have largely replaced the **barbiturates,** which were used medically in the past for inducing relaxation and sleep, relieving tension, and treating epileptic seizures. These drugs are usually taken by mouth in tablet, capsule, or liquid form. When used as a general anesthetic, they are administered intravenously. Barbiturates such as *pentobarbital* (Nembutal, yellow jackets), *secobarbital* (Seconal, reds), and *thiopental* (Pentothal) are short-acting and rapidly absorbed into the brain. The longer-acting barbiturates, such as *amobarbital* (Amytal, blues, downers) and *phenobarbital* (Luminal, phennies), are usually taken orally and absorbed slowly into the bloodstream, taking a while to reach the brain and having an effect for several days.

How Users Feel. Low doses of these drugs may reduce or relieve tension, but increasing doses can cause a loosening of sexual or aggressive inhibitions. Individuals using this class of drugs may experience rapid mood changes, impaired judgment, and impaired social or occupational functioning. High doses produce slurred speech, drowsiness, and stupor.

Young people in their teens or early twenties who have used many illegal substances typically take sedative-hypnotics to obtain a high or a state of euphoria. Some use them in combination with other drugs. Less commonly, individuals may first obtain sedatives, hypnotics, or antianxiety medications by prescription from a physician for insomnia or anxiety, and then gradually increase the dose or frequency of use on their own, often by seeking prescriptions from several physicians. While they justify this

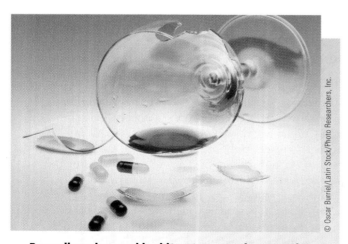

Benzodiazepines and barbiturates react dangerously with alcohol.

© Oscar Burriel/Latin Stock/Photo Researchers, Inc.

continued use because of their symptoms, the fact is that they reach a state in which they cannot function normally without the drug.

Risks. All sedative-hypnotic drugs can produce physical and psychological dependence within two to four weeks. A complication specific to sedatives is *cross-tolerance* (cross-addiction), which occurs when users develop tolerance for one sedative or become dependent on it and develop tolerance for other sedatives as well.

Intoxication with these drugs can produce changes in mood or behavior, such as inappropriate sexual or aggressive acts, mood swings, and impaired judgment. Physical signs include slurred speech, poor coordination, unsteady gait, involuntary eye movements, impaired attention or memory, and stupor or coma.

Taken in combination with alcohol, these drugs have a synergistic effect that can be dangerous or even lethal. For example, an individual's driving ability, already impaired by alcohol, will be made even worse, increasing the risk of an accident. Alcohol in combination with sedative-hypnotics leads to respiratory depression and may result in respiratory arrest and death. Regular users of any of these drugs who become physically dependent should not try to cut down or quit on their own. If they try to quit suddenly, they run the risk of seizures, coma, and death.

Withdrawal. Withdrawal from sedative-hypnotic drugs may range from relatively mild discomfort to a severe syndrome with grand mal seizures, depending on the degree of dependence. Withdrawal symptoms include malaise or weakness, sweating, rapid pulse, coarse tremors (of the hands, tongue, or eyelids), insomnia, nausea or vomiting, temporary hallucinations or illusions, physical restlessness, anxiety or irritability, and grand mal seizures. Withdrawal may begin within two to three days after stopping drug use, and symptoms may persist for many weeks.

Opioids

The **opioids** include *opium* and its derivatives (*morphine, codeine,* and *heroin*) and nonopioid synthetic drugs that have similar sleep-inducing and pain-relieving properties. The opioids come from a resin taken from the seedpod of the Asian poppy. **Nonopioids,** such as *meperidine* (Demerol), *methadone,* and *propoxyphene* (Darvon), are chemically synthesized. Whether natural or synthetic, these drugs are powerful *narcotics,* or painkillers.

Heroin (also known as horse, junk, smack, or downtown), the most widely abused opioid, is illegal in this country. In other nations it is used as a potent painkiller for conditions such as terminal cancer. There are an estimated 600,000 heroin addicts in the United States, with men outnumbering women addicts by three to one. Among people aged 18 to 25, the percentage of heroin users who inject the drug has doubled in the last decade. While the number of young heroin users in major cities has dropped by 50 percent, their numbers almost tripled in suburban and rural areas.[50]

Heroin users typically inject the drug into their veins. However, individuals who experiment with recreational drugs often prefer *skin-popping* (subcutaneous injection) rather than *mainlining* (intravenous injection); they also may snort heroin as a powder, or dissolve it and inhale the vapors. To try to avoid addiction, some users begin by *chipping*, taking small or intermittent doses. Regardless of the method of administration, tolerance can develop rapidly.

Morphine, used as a painkiller and anesthetic, acts primarily on the central nervous system, eyes, and digestive tract. By producing mental clouding, drowsiness, and euphoria, it does not decrease the physical sensation of pain as much as it alters a person's awareness of the pain; in effect, he or she no longer cares about it.

Two semisynthetic derivatives of morphine are *hydromorphone* (trade name Dilaudid, little D), with two to eight times the painkilling effect of morphine, and *oxycodone* (OxyContin, Percocet, Percodan, perkies), similar to codeine but more potent. The synthetic narcotic *meperidine* (Demerol, demies) is now probably second only to morphine for use in relieving pain. It is also used by addicts as a substitute for morphine or heroin.

Codeine, a weaker painkiller than morphine, is an ingredient in liquid products prescribed for relieving coughs and in tablet and injectable form for relieving pain. The synthetic narcotic *propoxyphene* (Darvon), a somewhat less potent painkiller than codeine, is no more effective than aspirin in usual doses. It has been one of the most widely prescribed drugs for headaches, dental pain, and menstrual cramps. At higher doses, Darvon produces a euphoric high, which may lead to misuse.

Prescription opioids are taken orally in pill form but can also be injected intravenously. Some individuals first take a medically prescribed opioid for pain relief or cough suppression, then gradually increase the dose and frequency of use on their own, often justifying this because of their symptoms rather than for the sensations the drug induces. They expend increasing efforts to obtain the drug, frequently seeking out several doctors to write prescriptions.

How Users Feel. All opioids relax the user. When injected, they can produce an immediate *rush* (high) that lasts 10 to 30 minutes. For two to six hours thereafter, users may feel indifferent, lethargic, and drowsy; they may slur their words and have problems paying attention, remembering, and going about their normal routine. The primary attractions of heroin are the euphoria and pain relief it produces. However, some people experience very unpleasant feelings, such as anxiety and fear. Other effects include a sensation of warmth or heaviness, dry mouth, facial flushing, and nausea and vomiting (particularly in first-time users).

Some addicts report a rush when heroin is injected directly into their veins. Since the effects of heroin do not last long—usually only two to four hours—addicts have to "shoot up" two to five times a day. With large doses, the pupils become smaller; and the skin becomes cold, moist, and bluish. Breathing slows down; the user cannot be awakened and may stop breathing completely.

Risks. Addiction is common. Almost all regular users of opioids rapidly develop drug dependence, which can lead to lethargy, weight loss, loss of sex drive, and the continual effort to avoid withdrawal symptoms through repeated drug administration. In addition, they experience anxiety, insomnia, restlessness, and craving for the drug. Users continue taking opioids as much to avoid the discomfort of withdrawal, a classic sign of opioid addiction, as to experience pleasure.

Opioid intoxication is characterized by changes in mood and behavior, such as initial euphoria followed by apathy or discontent and impaired judgment. Physical symptoms include constricted pupils (although pupils may dilate from a severe overdose), drowsiness, slurred speech, and impaired attention or memory. Morphine affects blood pressure, heart rate, and blood circulation in the brain. Both morphine and heroin slow down the respiratory system; overdoses can cause fatal respiratory arrest.

Opioid poisoning or overdose causes shock, coma, and depressed respiration and can be fatal. Emergency medical treatment is critical, often with drugs called *narcotic antagonists* that rapidly reverse the effects of opioids when administered intravenously.

Over time, users who inject opioids may develop infections of the heart lining and valves, skin abscesses, and lung congestion. Infections from unsterile solutions, syringes, and shared needles can lead to hepatitis, tetanus, liver disease, and HIV transmission. Depression is common, and may be both an antecedent and a risk factor for needle-sharing.

© Roy Marsch/CORBIS

Opioid drugs, made from the Asian poppy, come in both legal and illegal forms. In any form, it can readily become addictive.

Withdrawal. If a regular user stops taking an opioid, withdrawal begins within 6 to 12 hours. The intensity of the symptoms depends on the degree of the addiction; they may grow stronger for 24 to 72 hours and gradually subside over a period of 7 to 14 days, though some symptoms, such as insomnia, may persist for several months. Individuals may develop craving for an opioid, irritability, nausea or vomiting, muscle aches, runny nose or eyes, dilated pupils, sweating, diarrhea, yawning, fever, and insomnia. Desperately craving the drug, users may plead, demand, or manipulate others to obtain more. Opioid withdrawal usually is not life-threatening.

Methadone Maintenance

Opioid dependence is a very difficult addiction to overcome. Studies demonstrate that only 10 to 30 percent of heroin users are able to maintain abstinence. This fact contributed to the development of a unique, yet still controversial, treatment for opioid dependence: the use of methadone, a long-acting opioid that users can substitute for heroin or other opioids.

Methadone is used in two basic ways to treat opioid dependence: as an opioid substitute for detoxification, usually with a gradual tapering of methadone over a period of 21 to 180 days, and as a maintenance treatment. Methadone maintenance has been criticized by some as nothing more than the substitution of a legal opioid, methadone, for an illegal opioid, heroin.

Methadone maintenance may be the most thoroughly studied drug treatment. Research has clearly documented several important positive benefits, including decreased use of illicit opioids; decreased criminal behavior; decreased

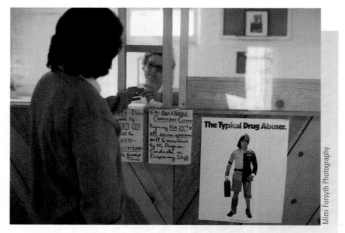

Methadone has been criticized as a treatment for opioid addiction, but research clearly demonstrates positive benefits. Those who participate in long-term methadone maintenance programs usually move out of the drug culture and are candidates for eventually leaving methadone dependence behind them.

risk of contracting HIV infection (through sharing of infected needles); and improvements in physical health, employment, and other lifestyle factors. Individuals who have been on methadone maintenance for a long time (often years), have stable relationships and employment, have assimilated themselves into the nondrug culture, and are highly motivated to get off methadone have the best chance for successful detoxification from methadone.

Other medications are used to treat narcotics dependence. Orlam (LAAM, levo alphacetylmethadol), has a longer duration of action than methadone, but also has a high abuse potential. Buprenorphine, recently approved and available in sublingual (under the tongue) and injectable forms, may be safer in overdose than the other treatment medications.

Hallucinogens

The drugs known as **hallucinogens** produce vivid and unusual changes in thought, feeling, and perception. Hallucinogens do not produce dependence in the same way as cocaine or heroin. Individuals who have an unpleasant experience after trying a hallucinogen may stop using the drug completely without suffering withdrawal symptoms. Others continue regular or occasional use because they enjoy the effects.

LSD and Mescaline

LSD (*lysergic acid diethylamide,* acid) was initially developed as a tool to explore mental illness. It became popular in the 1960s and resurfaced among teenagers in the 1990s. LSD is taken orally, either blotted onto pieces of paper that are held in the mouth or chewed along with another substance, such as a sugar cube. *Peyote* (whose active ingredient is *mescaline*) is another hallucinogen, but it is much less commonly used in this country.

How Users Feel. LSD produces hallucinations, including bright colors and altered perceptions of reality. Effects from a single dose begin within 30 to 60 minutes and last 10 to 12 hours. During this time, there are slight increases in body temperature, heart rate, and blood pressure. Sweating, chills, and goose pimples may appear. Some users develop headache and nausea. Mescaline produces vivid hallucinations—including brightly colored lights, animals, and geometric designs—within 30 to 90 minutes of consumption. These effects may persist for 12 hours.

The effects of hallucinogens depend greatly on the dose, the individual's expectations and personality, and the setting for drug use. Many users report religious or mystical imagery and thoughts; some feel they are experiencing profound insights. Usually the user realizes that perceptual changes are caused by the hallucinogen, but some become convinced that they have lost their minds. Drugs sold as hallucinogens are frequently mixed with other drugs, such as PCP and amphetamines, combinations that can produce unexpected and frightening effects.

Risks. Physical symptoms include dilated pupils, rapid heart rate, sweating, heart palpitations, blurring of vision, tremors, and poor coordination. These effects may last 8 to 12 hours. Hallucinogen intoxication also produces changes in emotions and mood, such as anxiety, depression, fear of losing one's mind, and impaired judgment.

LSD can trigger irrational acts. LSD users have injured or killed themselves by jumping out of windows, swimming out to sea, or throwing themselves in front of cars. Some individuals develop a delusional disorder in which they become convinced that their distorted perceptions and thoughts are real. They may experience *flashbacks* (re-experiencing symptoms felt while intoxicated), which include geometric hallucinations, flashes of color, halos around objects, and other perceptual changes.

Individuals having a *bad trip* may blame themselves and feel excessively guilty, tense, and so agitated that they cannot stop talking and have trouble sleeping. They may fear that they have destroyed their brains and will never return to normal. Someone who already is depressed may take a hallucinogen to lift his or her spirits, only to become more depressed. Suicide is a real danger.

Phencyclidine (PCP)

PCP (phencyclidine, brand name Sernyl; street names angel dust, peace pill, lovely, and green) is an illicit drug manufactured as a tablet, capsule, liquid, flake, spray, or crystal-like white powder that can be swallowed, smoked, sniffed, or injected. Sometimes it is sprinkled on crack, marijuana, tobacco, or parsley, and smoked. A fine-powdered form of PCP can be snorted or injected. Once PCP was thought to have medicinal value as an anesthetic, but its side effects, including delirium and hallucinations, now make it unacceptable for medical use.

PCP use peaked in the 1970s, but it remains a popular drug of abuse in both inner-city ghettos and suburban high schools. Users often think that the PCP they take together with another illegal psychoactive substance, such as amphetamines, coke, or hallucinogens, is responsible for the highs they feel, so they seek it out specifically.

How Users Feel. The effects of PCP are utterly unpredictable. It may trigger violent behavior or irreversible psychosis the first time it is used, or the twentieth time, or never. In low doses, PCP produces changes—from hallucinations or euphoria to feelings of emptiness or numbness—similar to those produced by other psychoactive drugs. Higher doses may produce a stupor that lasts several days, increased heart rate and blood pressure, flushing, sweating, dizziness, and numbness.

Risks. The behavioral changes associated with PCP intoxication, which can develop within minutes, include belligerence, aggressiveness, impulsiveness, unpredictability, agitation, poor judgment, and impaired functioning at work or in social situations. The physical symptoms of PCP intoxication include involuntary eye movements, increased blood pressure or heart rate, numbness or diminished responsiveness to pain, impaired coordination and speech, muscle rigidity, seizures, and a painful sensitivity to sound. Some people experience repetitive motor movements (such as facial grimacing), hallucinations, and paranoia. Suicide is a definite risk. Intoxication typically lasts four to six hours, but some effects can linger for several days. Delirium may occur within 24 hours of taking PCP or after recovery from an overdose and can last as much as a week.

Inhalants

Inhalants or **deleriants** are chemicals that produce vapors with psychoactive effects. The most commonly abused inhalants are solvents, aerosols, model-airplane glue, cleaning fluids, and petroleum products like kerosene and butane. Some anesthetics and nitrous oxide (laughing gas) are also abused. Almost 21 percent of eighth graders surveyed have used household products, such as glue, solvents, and aerosols, to get high.[51]

How Users Feel. Inhalants very rapidly reach the lungs, bloodstream, and other parts of the body. At low doses, users may feel slightly stimulated; at higher doses, they may feel less inhibited. Intoxication often occurs within five minutes and can last more than an hour. Inhalant users do not report the intense rush associated with other drugs, nor do they experience the perceptual changes associated with LSD. However, inhalants interfere with thinking and impulse control, so users may act in dangerous or destructive ways.

Often there are visible external signs of use: a rash around the nose and mouth; breath odors; residue on face, hands, and clothing; redness, swelling, and tearing of the eyes; and irritation of throat, lungs, and nose that leads to coughing and gagging. Nausea and headache also may occur.

Risks. Regular use of inhalants leads to tolerance, so the sniffer needs more and more to attain the desired effects. Younger children who use inhalants several times a week may develop dependence. Older users who become dependent may use the drugs many times a day. They are likely to have used many different substances as adolescents, and to have gradually turned to inhalants as their preferred substance.

Although some young people believe inhalants are safe, this is far from true. Inhalation of butane from cigarette lighters displaces oxygen in the lungs, causing suffocation. Users also can suffocate while covering their heads with a plastic bag to inhale the substance, or from inhaling vomit into their lungs while high. According to the International Institute on Inhalant Abuse, the effects of inhalants are unpredictable, and even a single episode can trigger asphyxiation or cardiac arrhythmia, leading to disability or death. Abusers also can develop difficulties with memory and abstract reasoning, problems with coordination, and uncontrollable movements of the extremities.

◾ Treating Drug Dependence and Abuse

An estimated 6.1 million Americans are in need of drug treatment, but the vast majority—some 5 million—never get treatment.[52] The most difficult step for a drug user is to admit that he or she *is* in fact an addict. If drug abusers are not forced to deal with their problem through some unexpected trauma, such as being fired or going bankrupt, those who care—family, friends, coworkers, doctors—may have to confront them and insist that they do something about their addiction. Often this *intervention* can be the turning point for addicts and their families. Treatment has proven equally successful for young people and for older adults.[53]

Treatment may take place in an outpatient setting, a residential facility, or a hospital. Increasingly, treatment thereafter is tailored to address coexisting or dual diagnoses. A personal treatment plan may consist of individual psychotherapy, marital and family therapy, medication, and behavior therapy. Once an individual has made the decision to seek help for substance abuse, the first step usually is detoxification, which involves clearing the drug from the body. An exception is methadone maintenance, discussed earlier in this chapter, which does not rely on complete detoxification.

Controlled and supervised withdrawal within a medical or psychiatric hospital may be recommended if an individual has not been able to stop using drugs as an outpatient or in a residential treatment program. Detoxification is most likely to be complicated in a polysubstance abuser, who may require close monitoring and treatment of potentially fatal withdrawal symptoms. Other reasons for inpatient treatment include lack of psychosocial support for maintaining abstinence and the absence of a drug-free living environment. Restrictions on insurance coverage may limit the number of days of inpatient care. Increasingly, once individuals complete detoxification, they continue treatment in residential programs or as outpatients.

Medications are used in detoxification to alleviate withdrawal symptoms and prevent medical and psychiatric complications. Once withdrawal is complete, these medications are discontinued, so the individual is in a drug-free state. However, individuals with mental disorders may require appropriate psychiatric medication to manage their symptoms and reduce the risk of relapse. For example, a person suffering from major depression or panic disorder may require ongoing treatment with antidepressant medication.

The aim of chemical dependence treatment is to help individuals establish and maintain their recovery from alcohol and drugs of abuse. Recovery is a dynamic process of personal growth and healing in which the drug user makes the transition from a lifestyle of active substance use to a drug-free lifestyle.

Whatever their setting, chemical dependence treatment programs initially involve some period of intensive treatment followed by one or two years of continuing aftercare. Most freestanding programs (those not affiliated with a hospital) follow what is known as the *Minnesota model,* a treatment approach developed at Hazelden Recovery Center in Center City, Minnesota, more than 30 years ago. Its key principles include a focus on drug use as the primary problem, not as a symptom of underlying emotional problems; a multidisciplinary approach that addresses the physical, emotional, spiritual, family, and social aspects of the individual; a supportive community; and a goal of abstinence and health.

Outpatient programs for substance abuse, offered by freestanding centers, hospitals, and community mental health centers, often run four or five nights a week for four to eight weeks, or in daily eight-hour sessions for seven to eight days, followed by weekly group therapy. These outpatient programs allow recovering drug users to go on with their daily lives and learn to deal with day-to-day work and family stresses. Mental health professionals in private practice also offer individually structured outpatient treatment.

Therapy groups provide an opportunity for individuals who have often been isolated by their drug use to participate in normal social settings. Small groups with other former drug users can be especially valuable because they all share the experience of drug use. Group members can confront one another with frankness and cut through lies and rationalizations. A professional therapist keeps members of the group from ganging up on one person. After their discharge from inpatient treatment, individuals who became involved in self-help groups are less likely to use drugs, cope better with stress, and develop richer friendship networks.

12-Step Programs

Since its founding in 1935, Alcoholics Anonymous (AA)—the oldest, largest, and most successful self-help program in the world—has spawned a worldwide movement. As many as 200 different recovery programs are based on the spiritual **12-step program** of AA. Participation in 12-step programs for drug abusers, such as Substance Anonymous, Narcotics Anonymous, and Cocaine Anonymous, is of fun-

Based on the Alcoholics Anonymous model, 12-step programs have helped many people overcome addictions. The one requirement for membership is a desire to stop following a pattern of addictive behavior.

damental importance in promoting and maintaining long-term abstinence.

The basic precept of 12-step programs is that members have been powerless when it comes to controlling their addictive behavior on their own. These programs don't recruit members. The desire to stop must come from the individual, who can call the number of a 12-step program, listed in the telephone book, and find out when and where the next nearby meeting will be held. A representative may offer to send someone to the caller's house to talk about the problem and to escort him or her to the next meeting.

Meetings of various 12-step programs are held daily in almost every city in the country. (Some chapters, whose members often include the disabled or those in remote areas, meet via Internet chat rooms or electronic bulletin boards.) There are no dues or fees for membership. Many individuals belong to several programs because they have several problems, such as alcoholism, substance abuse, and pathological gambling. All have only one requirement for membership: a desire to stop an addictive behavior.

To get the most out of a 12-step program:

:: Try out different groups until you find one you like and in which you feel comfortable.

:: Once you find a group in which you feel comfortable, go back several times (some recommend a minimum of six meetings) before making a final decision on whether to continue.

:: Keep an open mind. Listen to other people's stories and ask yourself if you've had similar feelings or experiences.

:: Accept whatever feels right to you and ignore the rest. One common saying in 12-step programs is "Take what you like and leave the rest."

Relapse Prevention

The most common clinical course for substance abuse disorders involves a pattern of multiple relapses over the course of a lifespan. It is important for individuals with these problems and their families to recognize this fact. When relapses do occur, they should be viewed as neither a mark of defeat nor evidence of moral weakness. While painful, they do not erase the progress that has been achieved and ultimately may strengthen self-understanding. They can serve as reminders of potential pitfalls to avoid in the future.

One key to preventing relapse is learning to avoid obvious cues and associations that can set off intense cravings. This means staying away from the people and places linked with past drug use. Some therapists use conditioning techniques to give former users some sense of control over their urge to use the drug. The theory behind this approach, which is called *extinction* of conditioned behavior, is that with repeated exposure—for example, to videotapes of dealers selling crack cocaine—the arousal and craving will diminish. While this technique by itself cannot ward off relapses, it does seem to enhance the overall effectiveness of other therapies.

Another important lesson that therapists emphasize is that every lapse does not have to lead to a full-blown relapse. Users can turn to the skills acquired in treatment—calling people for support or going to meetings—to avoid

STRATEGIES FOR PREVENTION

Relapse-Prevention Planning

The following steps, from Terence Gorski and Merlene Miller's *Staying Sober: A Guide for Relapse Prevention*, can lower the likelihood of relapses:

1. *Stabilization and self-assessment.* Get control of yourself. Find out what's going on in your head, heart, and life.

2. *Education.* Learn about relapse and what to do to prevent it.

3. *Warning-sign identification and management.* Make a list of your personal relapse warning signs. Learn how to interrupt them before you lose control.

4. *Inventory training.* Learn how to become consciously aware of warning signs as they develop.

5. *Review of the recovery program.* Make sure your recovery program is able to help you manage your warning signs of relapse.

6. *Involvement of significant others.* Teach them how to help you avoid relapses.

a major relapse. Ultimately, users must learn much more than how to avoid temptation; they must examine their entire view of the world and learn new ways to live in it without turning to drugs. This is the underlying goal of the recovery process.

Outlook

Whatever the drug, recovery from dependence and abuse is a process of immense inner change that involves every aspect of a person's life. It does not follow a straight, even course, but moves back and forth between denial—of dependence, of loss of control, or of the severity of the problem—and awareness, ignorance and knowledge, craving and commitment. It often starts with a feeling of great relief, followed by a deep sense of emptiness. Individuals who have abused or become dependent on drugs must form a new identity, stop living in the past or future, give up their search for a quick fix, change the way they relate to family and old friends, find new things to do with the time they previously spent on their drug habit, learn new behaviors, and adopt new attitudes. Through treatment, education, and a reevaluation of what is meaningful in life, drug users can find a better way of living.

Codependence

Codependence refers to the tendency of the spouses, partners, parents, and friends of individuals who use drugs or alcohol to allow, or *enable,* their loved ones to continue their drug use and self-destructive behavior. (Codependence is also discussed in Chapter 11.)

Codependents Anonymous, founded in 1986 for "men and women whose common problem is an inability to maintain functional relationships," sponsors support programs throughout the country. Nar-Anon provides groups for people affected by drug abuse. Local chapters are in the white pages of the telephone directory.

If someone you love has a drug problem, get as much information as you can so that you understand what you—and your loved one—are up against. Also get some intervention training. Specially trained counselors work at most chemical-dependency units; some offer advice by phone. Here are some specific recommendations:

:: Confront the user. Along with other loved ones and, if possible, a professional counselor, detail incident after incident in which the drug abuse affected or hurt you, other members of your family, or the user.

:: Don't expect a drug abuser to quit without help. Chemical dependence is a medical and psychological disorder that requires professional treatment. Offer your support, but make it clear that you expect your loved one to undergo therapy.

:: If your loved one agrees to treatment, make sure that the program is based on a complete evaluation, checking for medical and emotional problems, as well as chemical dependency.

:: Don't believe abusers who say they've learned to control their drug use. Abstinence is a cornerstone of any good rehabilitation program.

:: Encourage a user to attend support groups, such as Cocaine Anonymous or Narcotics Anonymous, for at least one year after rehabilitation. Get help for yourself. Most hospitals and chemical-dependency programs offer educational programs for codependents.

The Bottom Line ▼
Living Drug-Free

When you're anxious, bored, restless, or confused, when drugs seem all too appealing as a "quick fix," there are real solutions, "positive addictions" that can help you solve your problems without creating new and bigger ones. A positive addiction—whether it is exercising, mountain-climbing, or listening to music—can produce very real "highs." But there's a crucial difference between this sort of stimulation and drug dependency: one is real, the other is chemical. With one, you're in control; with the other, drugs are.

Here are some examples:

:: If you feel a need for physical relaxation, if you want more energy or distraction from physical discomforts, you can turn to athletics, exercise (including walking and hiking), dance, or outdoor hobbies.

:: If you want to stimulate your senses, enhance sexual stimulation, or magnify the sensations of sight, sound, and touch, train yourself to be more sensitive to nature and beauty. Take time to appreciate the sensations you experience when you're walking in the woods or embracing a person you love. Through activities like sailing or sky-diving you can literally fill up your senses without relying on chemicals.

:: If you have psychological troubles, if you're anxious or depressed, if you feel inhibited or uptight, if you don't know how to solve complex personal problems and want relief from emotional pain, turn to people who can offer lasting help: in some cases, friends; in others, professional counselors or support groups.

:: If you want peer acceptance, if you'd like to overcome your shyness, if you want to communicate and relate more effectively, you can join expertly managed sensitivity or encounter groups, enroll in confidence-building seminars, seek counseling, or volunteer in programs in which you can assist others and not focus only on your self-consciousness.

:: If you want to escape mental boredom, gain new understanding of the world around you, study better, experiment with your levels of awareness, or indulge your intellectual curiosity, challenge your mind through reading, classes, creative games, discussion groups, memory training, or travel.

:: If you want to enhance your creativity or your appreciation of the arts, pursue training in music, art, singing, gardening, or writing. Sign up for a nongraded course in art history or music appreciation. Attend more concerts, ballets, museum shows.

:: If you want to promote political or social change, defy the establishment, change drug legislation, or gain power, you can volunteer in political campaigns, work on nonpartisan projects, or join lobbying and political action groups.

:: If you want to find meaning in life, to understand the nature of the universe, or expand your personal awareness, explore various philosophical theories through classes, seminars, and discussion groups. Study different religious orientations, including mysticism, or try yoga and meditation.

:: If you're looking for kicks, adventure, danger, and excitement, sign up for an "Outward Bound" wilderness survival course. Take up an adventurous sport, like hang-gliding or parachuting. Set a challenging professional or personal goal and direct your energies to meeting it.

CNN After watching the CNN video segment, discuss the following question. Why is there a growing trend in ritalin abuse among college students?

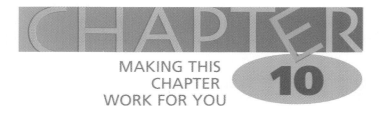

MAKING THIS CHAPTER WORK FOR YOU **10**

1. Which of the following statements about drugs is *false?*
   a. A potentiating drug interaction is one in which one drug neutralizes or blocks the effects of another drug.
   b. Drugs can be injected into the body intravenously, intramuscularly, or subcutaneously.

c. Drug misuse is the taking of a drug for a purpose other than that for which it was medically intended.
   d. An individual's response to a drug can be affected by the setting in which the drug is used.

2. To help ensure that an over-the-counter or prescription drug is safe and effective,
   a. take smaller dosages than indicated in the instructions.
   b. test your response to the drug by borrowing a similar medication from a friend.
   c. ask your doctor or pharmacist about possible interactions with other medications.
   d. buy all of your medications online.

3. Which of the following drugs does not cause withdrawal symptoms?
   a. caffeine
   b. marijuana
   c. heroin
   d. aspirin

4. Individuals with substance use disorders
   a. are usually not physically dependent on their drug of choice.
   b. have a compulsion to use one or more addictive substances.
   c. require less and less of the preferred drug to achieve the desired effect.
   d. suffer withdrawal symptoms when they use the drug regularly.

5. Amphetamine is very similar to which of the following in its effects on the central nervous system?
   a. marijuana
   b. heroin
   c. cocaine
   d. alcohol

6. Which of the following statements about marijuana is *false?*
   a. People who have used marijuana may experience psychoactive effects for several days after use.
   b. Marijuana has shown some effectiveness in treating chemotherapy-related nausea.
   c. Unlike long-term use of alcohol, regular use of marijuana does not have any long-lasting health consequences.
   d. Depending on the amount of marijuana used, its effects can range from a mild sense of euphoria to extreme panic.

7. Cocaine dependence can result in all of the following *except*
   a. stroke.
   b. paranoia and violent behavior.

c. heart failure.

d. enhanced sexual performance.

8. Which of the following statements about club drugs is true?
   a. The main ingredient of GHB is an industrial solvent used to strip floors.
   b. Most club drugs do not pose the same health dangers as "hard" drugs such as heroin.
   c. MDMA is the street name for ecstasy.
   d. When combined with extended physical exertion, club drugs can lead to hypothermia (lowered body temperature).

9. The opioids
   a. are not addictive if used in a prescription form such as codeine or Demerol.
   b. produce an immediate but short-lasting high and feeling of euphoria.
   c. include morphine, which is typically used for cough suppression.

d. are illegal in the United States, although they are allowed in other countries to help control severe pain.

10. Which of the following statements about drug dependence treatment is *false?*
    a. Chemical dependence treatment programs usually involve medications to alleviate withdrawal symptoms.
    b. Detoxification is usually the first step in a drug treatment program.
    c. Relapses are not uncommon for a person who has undergone drug treatment.
    d. The 12-step recovery program associated with Alcoholics Anonymous has been shown to be ineffective with individuals with drug dependence disorders.

Answers to these questions can be found on p. 652.

Critical Thinking

1. Some argue that marijuana should be a legal drug like alcohol and tobacco. What is your opinion on this issue? Defend your position.

Critical Thinking

2. Some Web enthusiasts oppose any kind of government regulations on the Internet. Do you agree or disagree? How would you address the problems associated with distributing drugs online?

Critical Thinking

3. Suppose that a close friend is using amphetamines to keep her energy levels high so that she can continue to attend school full-time and hold down a job to pay her school expenses. You fear that she is developing a substance abuse disorder. What can you do to help her realize the dangers of her behavior? What resources are available at your school or in your community to help her deal with both her drug problem and her financial needs?

Profile Plus

Drug dependency robs you of enjoying a full, happy life. Are you concerned about your drug use? Begin the process of change with this activity on your Profile Plus CD-ROM:

Profile Plus

• Is it a substance abuse problem?

Profile Plus

Sites and Bytes

National Institute on Drug Abuse
www.nida.nih.gov

This government site—a virtual clearinghouse of information for students, parents, teachers, researchers, and health professionals—features current treatment and research, as well as a comprehensive database on common drugs of abuse.

Sites and Bytes

Addiction Alternatives
www.addictionalternatives.com

This site features information on a variety of addictions, including alcohol, drugs, food, gambling, and personal interactive quizzes on alcohol, drugs, sex, sleep, attention/concentration, personality, and emotional quotient. Tools to change behavior as well as consultations and information on self-help and professional therapy are available.

Sites and Bytes

Partnership for a Drug-Free America
www.drugfreeamerica.org

This site features current resources and photographs on a variety of drugs, including a special section on ecstasy and club drugs. It also includes resources, several video clips, and true-life stories revealing the consequences of drug use.

InfoTrac College Edition

Activity

Sigel, Eric. "Club Drugs: Nothing to Rave About." *Contemporary Pediatrics,* Vol. 19, No. 10, October 2002, p. 47(12).

1. What are the psychological and physiological effects of ecstasy?
2. What are the neurological effects of GHB and how does this con-

InfoTrac College Edition

tribute to its use as the "date rape" drug of choice?
3. What are the short-term health effects of using methamphetamine?

You can find additional readings related to drug abuse with InfoTrac College Edition, an online library of more than 900 journals and publications. Follow the instructions that

InfoTrac College Edition

were packaged with your textbook; then search for articles using a key word search.

For additional links, resources, and suggested readings on InfoTrac College Edition, visit our Health & Wellness Resource Center at **http://health.wadsworth.com**.

Key Terms

The terms listed are used on the page indicated. Definitions of the terms are in the Glossary at the end of this book.

Key Terms

addiction 330
additive 325
amphetamines 344
antagonistic 325
barbiturates 348
benzodiazepines 347
club drugs 342
cocaine 345
codependence 354
deleriants 351
drug 324
drug abuse 324
drug misuse 324
ecstasy (MDMA) 342
generic 328

Key Terms

GBL(gamma butyrolactone) 343
GHB (gamma hydroxybutyrate) 343
hallucinogens 350
hashish 337
inhalants 351
intoxication 333
intramuscular 324
intravenous 324
marijuana 337
nonopioids 348
opioids 348
over-the-counter (OTC) drugs 325

Key Terms

PCP(phencyclidine) 351
physical dependence 331
polyabuse 333
potentiating 325
psychoactive 330
psychological dependence 331
psychotropic 329
stimulant 329
subcutaneous 324
synergistic 325
toxicity 324
12-step program 352
withdrawal 333

References

1. "U.N. Report: Synthetic Drugs Could Become Severe Problem." *Alcoholism & Drug Abuse Weekly,* Vol. 15, No. 16, April 21, 2003, p. 7.
2. Eisenberg, M., and H. Wechsler. "Substance Use Behaviors Among College Students with Same-Sex and Opposite-Sex Experience: Results from a National Study." *Addictive Behaviors,* Vol. 28, No. 6, 2003, p. 899.
3. Lewis, Carol. "The Impact of Direct-to-Consumer Advertising." FDA Consumer, Vol. 37, No. 2, March–April 2003. www.fda.gov.
4. Meadows, Michelle. "Prescription Drug Abuse: FDA and SAMHSA Join Forces." *FDA Consumer,* Vol. 37, No. 2, March–April 2003. www.fda.gov.
5. DEA Congressional Testimony by John B. Brown, III, Acting Administrator, March 20, 2003.
6. Paluska, S. A. "Caffeine and Exercise." *Current Sports Medical Report,* Vol. 2, No. 4, 2003, p. 213.
7. Scott, William H., Jr., et al. "Effects of Caffeine on Performance of Low Intensity Tasks." *Perceptual and Motor Skills,* Vol. 94, No. 2, April 2002, p. 521.
8. Cerrato, Paul. "Caffeine May Protect Women from Parkinson's." *Contemporary OB/GYN,* Vol. 47, No. 5, May 2002, p. 168.
9. "U.N. Report: Synthetic Drugs Could Become Severe Problem." *Alcoholism and Drug Abuse Weekly,* Vol. 15, No. 16, April 21, 2003, p. 7.
10. Frances, Richard. Personal interview.
11. Wilens, T. E., et al. "Does Stimulant Therapy of Attention-Deficit/Hyperactivity Disorder Beget Later Substance Abuse? A Meta-Analytic Review of the Literature." *Pediatrics,* Vol. 111, No. 1, 2003, p. 179.
12. "Parental Attitudes, History Affect Children's Drug Use." *Alcoholism & Drug Abuse Weekly,* Vol. 13, No. 32, August 20, 2001, p. 7.
13. Martin, Kimberly. "Youths' Opportunities To Experiment Influence Later Use of Illegal Drugs." *Research News,* Vol. 17, No. 5, January 2003.
14. "Heroin, Cocaine, Alcohol Most Cited in Drug Deaths." *Alcoholism and Drug Abuse Weekly,* Vol. 15, No. 10, March 10, 2003, p. 3.
15. Zickler, Patrick. "Teen Drug Use Declined in 2002, Report Shows." *Research News,* Vol. 17, No. 5, January 2003.
16. Johnston, L. D., et al. *Monitoring the Future National Results on Adolescent Drug Use.* Bethesda, MD: National Institute on Drug Abuse, 2003. http://monitoringthefuture.org.
17. Strote, J., et al. "Increasing MDMA Use Among College Students: Results of a National Survey." *Journal of Adolescent Health,* Vol. 30, January 2002, p. 64.
18. Yacoubian, George, et al. "Correlates of Ecstasy Use Among Students Surveyed Through the 1997 College Alcohol Study." *Journal of Drug Education,* Vol. 33, No. 1, January 2003, p. 61.
19. Bon, Rebecca, et al. "Normative Perceptions in Relation to Substance Use and HIV-Risky Sexual Behaviors of College Students." *Journal of Psychology,* Vol. 135, No. 2, March 2001, p. 165.
20. Jones, Sherry, et al. "Binge Drinking Among Undergraduate College Students in the United States: Implications for Other Substance Use." *Journal of American College Health,* Vol. 50, No. 1, July 2001, p. 33.
21. Boyd, C. J., et al. "Ecstasy Use Among College Undergraduates: Gender, Race, and Sexual Identity." *Substance Abuse Treatment,* Vol. 24, No. 3, April 2003, p. 209.
22. McCabe, S. E., et al. "Sexual Identity and Substance Use Among Undergraduate Students." *Substance Abuse,* Vol. 24, No. 2, June 2003, p. 77.
23. Eisenberg and Wechsler, "Substance Use Behaviors."
24. Hanson, Glen. NIDA Research Report Series: Marijuana Abuse. www.nida.nih.gov/Research Reports/Marijuana/
25. Ibid.
26. "Government of Canada Adopts Interim Policy on the Provision of Marihuana for Medical Purposes." News Release, Health Canada, July 9, 2003.
27. National Institute on Drug Abuse, www.nida.nih.gov.
28. Henry, John, et al. "Comparing Cannabis with Tobacco: Smoking Cannabis, Like Smoking Tobacco, Can be a Major Public Health Hazard." *British Medical Journal,* Vol. 326, No. 7396, May 3, 2003, p. 942.
29. "Marijuana," www.drugfreeamerica.org.
30. Mittleman, Murray. "Triggering Myocardial Infarction by Marijuana." *Journal of the American Medical Association,* Vol. 286, No. 6, August 8, 2001, p. 655.
31. "Marijuana May Boost Heart Attack Risk." *Alcoholism & Drug Abuse Weekly,* Vol. 13, No. 37, October 1, 2001, p. 7.
32. Walling, Anne. "Marijuana Use During Pregnancy." *American Family Physician,* Vol. 63, No. 12, June 15, 2001, p. 2463.
33. Hanson, Glen. "Testimony Before the Subcommittee on Criminal Justice, Drug Policy, and Human Resources Committee on Government Reform, United States House of Representatives—Research on MDMA," September 19, 2002.
34. Yacoubian et al., "Correlates of Ecstasy Use."
35. Walters, Scott, et al. "The Agony of Ecstasy: Responding to Growing MDMA Use Among College Students." *Journal of American College Health,* Vol. 51, No. 3, November 2002, p. 139.
36. National Institute on Drug Abuse, www.nida.nih.gov.
37. "Ecstasy." *Psychiatric Services,* Vol. 53, No. 6, June 2002, p. 667.
38. "Long-Term Ecstasy Use Impairs Memory." *Science News,* Vol. 159, No. 18, May 5, 2001, p. 280.
39. "Can Ecstasy's Effects Be Passed on to Offspring?" *Brown University Child and Adolescent Behavior Letter,* Vol. 17, No. 8, August 2001, p. 1.
40. *Drugs of Abuse.* Washington, DC: U.S. Department of Justice, Drug Enforcement Administration, February 2003.
41. "New Form of Methamphetamine Seen in California Dance Clubs." *Alcoholism and Drug Abuse Weekly,* Vol. 14, No. 37, September 30, 2002, p. 8.
42. *Drugs of Abuse.*
43. Ibid.
44. Volkow, Nora, et al. "Higher Cortical and Lower Subcortical Metabolism in Detoxified Methamphetamine Abusers." *American Journal of Psychiatry,* Vol. 158, March 2001, p. 383.
45. Boschert, Sherry. "Chest Pain in Young May Mean Cocaine Use." *Family Practice,* Vol. 33, No. 6, March 15, 2003, p. 16.
46. Little, Karley, et al. "Loss of Striatal Vesicular Monoamine Transporter Protein in Human Cocaine Users." *American Journal of Psychiatry,* Vol. 160, No. 1, January 2003, p. 47.

References

47. "Cocaine May Reduce Immune System Response." *Alcoholism and Drug Abuse Weekly,* Vol. 15, No. 10, March 10, 2003, p. 7.
48. "Stimulants May Have Long Lasting Effects." *Alcoholism and Drug Abuse Weekly,* Vol. 15, No. 10, March 24, 2003, p. 3.

References

49. DEA Congressional Testimony by John B. Brown.
50. "Heroin." National Institute on Drug Abuse, www.nida.nih.gov.
51. National Institute on Drug Abuse, www.nida.nih.gov/Research Reports/Inhalants/Inhalants.html.
52. National Institute on Drug Abuse, www.nida.nih.gov.

References

53. "Youth Treatment Study Shows Good Results, Parallels Findings for Adult Outcomes." *Alcoholism & Drug Abuse Weekly,* Vol. 13, No. 27, July 16, 2001, p. 1.

Alcohol Use, Misuse, and Abuse

It was just another Friday night at the frat house. The drinking started early and usually didn't stop until dawn. One of the brothers, a popular easy-going guy named Ryan—not usually much of a drinker—was celebrating a big birthday: his twenty-first. Egged on by the hooting crowd, Ryan bolted down one drink after another, after another, after another.

By the time Ryan reached twelve, he was slurring his words. As he kept chugging drinks, his face looked flushed; he started sweating heavily. When Ryan lurched to his feet, he swayed unsteadily for a few moments and then collapsed. At first everyone laughed. Then two of his buddies tried to revive him. They couldn't.

"He's not breathing!" one of them shouted. Someone called 911, and paramedics rushed Ryan to the nearest hospital. His blood alcohol concentration was several times above the legal limit. Despite intensive efforts by the medical team, nothing helped. Ryan's twenty-first birthday was his last.

As Ryan's tragic death shows, alcohol, when not used responsibly, can take an enormous toll. No medical conditions, other than heart disease, cause more disability and premature death than alcohol-related problems. No mental or medical disorders touch the lives of more families. No other form of disability costs individuals, employers, and the government more for treatment, injuries, reduced worker productivity, and property damage. The costs in emotional pain and in lost and shattered lives because of irresponsible drinking are beyond measure.

This chapter provides information about alcohol, its impact on the body, brain, behavior, and society, patterns of drinking, drinking on campus, binge drinking, and the recognition, understanding, and treatment of drinking problems and of alcoholism.

© DTF Productions/The Image Bank/Getty Images

After studying the material in this chapter, you should be able to:

- **Describe** the factors affecting a drinker's response to alcohol consumption.
- **List** the effects of alcohol on the body systems.

- **Describe** the impact of alcohol misuse among college students, and **define** binge drinking.
- **Define** alcohol abuse, dependence, and alcoholism, and **list** their symptoms.
- **List** the negative consequences to individuals, and to our society, from alcohol abuse.
- **Explain** the common treatment methods for alcoholism.

361

Alcohol and Its Effects

Pure alcohol is a colorless liquid obtained through the fermentation of a liquid containing sugar. **Ethyl alcohol,** or *ethanol,* is the type of alcohol in alcoholic beverages. Another type—methyl, or wood, alcohol—is a poison that should never be drunk. Any liquid containing 0.5 to 80 percent ethyl alcohol by volume is an alcoholic beverage. However, different drinks contain different amounts of alcohol. (See Figure 11-1.)

One drink can be any of the following:

:: One bottle or can (12 ounces) of beer, which is 5 percent alcohol.

:: One glass (4 ounces) of table wine, such as burgundy, which is 12 percent alcohol.

:: One small glass (2½ ounces) of fortified wine, which is 20 percent alcohol.

:: One shot (1 ounce) of distilled spirits (such as whiskey, vodka, or rum), which is 50 percent alcohol.

All of these drinks contain close to the same amount of alcohol—that is, if the number of ounces in each drink is multiplied by the percentage of alcohol, each drink contains the equivalent of approximately ½ ounce of 100 percent ethyl alcohol. With distilled spirits (such as bourbon, scotch, vodka, gin, and rum), alcohol content is expressed in terms of **proof,** a number that is twice the percentage of alcohol: 100-proof bourbon is 50 percent alcohol; 80-proof gin is 40 percent alcohol.

But the words *bottle* and *glass* can be deceiving in this context. Drinking a 16-ounce bottle of malt liquor, which is 6.4 percent alcohol, is not the same as drinking a 12-ounce glass of 3.2 percent beer. Two bottles of high-alcohol wines (such as Cisco), packaged to resemble much less powerful wine coolers, can lead to alcohol poisoning, especially in those who weigh less than 150 pounds. This is one reason alcoholic drinks are a serious danger for young people.

How Much Alcohol Can I Drink?

The best way to figure how much you can drink safely is to determine the amount of alcohol in your blood at any given time, or your **blood-alcohol concentration (BAC).** BAC is expressed in terms of the percentage of alcohol in the blood and is often measured from breath or urine samples.

Law enforcement officers use BAC to determine whether a driver is legally drunk. The federal Department of Transportation has called on states to set 0.08 percent—the BAC that a 150-pound man would have after consuming about three mixed drinks within an hour—as the threshold at which a person can be cited for drunk driving. (See Figure 11-2.) In the past, 0.1 percent was often the legal limit. According to the National Institute on Alcohol Abuse and Alcoholism, lowering the BAC can lead to a significant drop in fatal car crashes related to alcohol.[1]

A BAC of 0.05 percent indicates approximately 5 parts alcohol to 10,000 parts other blood components. Most people reach this level after consuming one or two drinks and experience all the positive sensations of drinking—relaxation, euphoria, and well-being—without feeling intoxicated. If they continue to drink past the 0.05 percent BAC level, they start feeling worse rather than better, gradually losing control of speech, balance, and emotions. At a BAC of 0.2 percent, they may pass out. At a BAC of 0.3 percent, they could lapse into a coma; at 0.4 percent, they could die.

For some people, even very low blood alcohol concentrations can cause a headache, upset stomach, or dizziness. These reactions often are inborn. People who have suffered brain damage, often as a result of head trauma or encephalitis, may lose all tolerance for alcohol, either temporarily or permanently, and behave abnormally after drinking small amounts. The elderly, as well as those who are unusually fatigued or have a debilitating physical illness, may also have a low tolerance for alcohol and respond inappropriately to a small amount.

Your Body's Response to Alcohol

Many factors affect an individual's BAC and response to alcohol, including the following:

:: **How much and how quickly you drink.** The more alcohol you put into your body, the higher your BAC. If you chug drink after drink, your liver, which

Figure 11-1 THE ALCOHOL CONTENT OF DIFFERENT DRINKS

	Light beer (12-oz can)	Regular beer (12-oz bottle)	Wine (4-oz glass)	Most cocktails (mixed drinks)
Percentage of alcohol by volume	2.4%–4.8%	3.2%–5.0%	12%	40%–50%
Amount of alcohol per serving	0.29–0.58 oz	0.38–0.60 oz	0.48 oz	1 oz

Men	Approximate blood alcohol percentage										
	Body weight in pounds										
Drinks	100	120	140	160	180	200	220	240			
0	.00	.00	.00	.00	.00	.00	.00	.00	Only safe driving limit		
1	.04	.03	.03	.02	.02	.02	.02	.02	Impairment begins		
2	.08	.06	.05	.05	.04	.04	.03	.03	Driving skills significantly affected		
3	.11	.09	.08	.07	.06	.06	.05	.05			
4	.15	.12	.11	.09	.08	.08	.07	.06	Possible criminal penalties		
5	.19	.16	.13	.12	.11	.09	.09	.08			
6	.23	.19	.16	.14	.13	.11	.10	.09			
7	.26	.22	.19	.16	.15	.13	.12	.11			
8	.30	.25	.21	.19	.17	.15	.14	.13	Legally intoxicated		
9	.34	.28	.24	.21	.19	.17	.15	.14	Criminal penalties		
10	.38	.31	.27	.23	.21	.19	.17	.16			

Subtract .01% for each 40 minutes of drinking
One drink is 1.25 oz. of 80 proof liquor, 12 oz. of beer, or 5 oz. of table wine.

Women	Approximate blood alcohol percentage										
	Body weight in pounds										
Drinks	90	100	120	140	160	180	200	220	240		
0	.00	.00	.00	.00	.00	.00	.00	.00	.00	Only safe driving limit	
1	.05	.05	.04	.03	.03	.03	.02	.02	.02	Impairment begins	
2	.10	.09	.08	.07	.06	.05	.05	.04	.04	Driving skills significantly affected	
3	.15	.14	.11	.10	.09	.08	.07	.06	.06		
4	.20	.18	.15	.13	.11	.10	.09	.08	.08	Possible criminal penalties	
5	.25	.23	.19	.16	.14	.13	.11	.10	.09		
6	.30	.27	.23	.19	.17	.15	.14	.12	.11		
7	.35	.32	.27	.23	.20	.18	.16	.14	.13		
8	.40	.36	.30	.26	.23	.20	.18	.17	.15	Legally intoxicated	
9	.45	.41	.34	.29	.26	.23	.20	.19	.17	Criminal penalties	
10	.51	.45	.38	.32	.28	.25	.23	.21	.19		

Subtract .01% for each 40 minutes of drinking
One drink is 1.25 oz. of 80 proof liquor, 12 oz. of beer, or 5 oz. of table wine.

Figure 11-2 ALCOHOL IMPAIRMENT CHART

Source: Adopted from data supplied by the Pennsylvania Liquor Control Board.

tains water, juice, or milk, the rate of absorption will be slowed. However, carbon dioxide—whether in champagne, ginger ale, or a cola—whisks alcohol into your bloodstream. Also, the alcohol in warm drinks—such as a hot rum toddy or warmed sake—moves into your bloodstream more quickly than the alcohol in chilled wine or scotch on the rocks.

:: **Your size.** If you're a large person (whether due to fat or to muscle), you'll get drunk more slowly than someone smaller who's drinking the same amount of alcohol at the same rate. Heavier individuals have a larger water volume, which dilutes the alcohol they drink.

:: **Your gender.** Women have lower quantities of a stomach enzyme that neutralizes alcohol, so one drink for a woman has the impact that two drinks have for a man. Hormone levels also affect the impact of alcohol. Women are more sensitive to alcohol just before menstruation, and birth control pills and other forms of estrogen can intensify alcohol's impact. (See the section "Alcohol and Gender" later in this chapter.)

:: **Your age.** The same amount of alcohol produces higher BACs in older drinkers, who have lower volumes of body water to dilute the alcohol than younger drinkers do.

:: **Your race.** Many members of certain ethnic groups, including Asians and Native Americans, are unable to break down alcohol as quickly as Caucasians. This can result in higher BACs, as well as uncomfortable reactions, such as flushing and nausea, when they drink.

:: **Other drugs.** Some common medications—including aspirin, acetaminophen (Tylenol), and ulcer

metabolizes about ½ ounce of alcohol an hour, won't be able to keep up—and your BAC will soar.

:: **What you're drinking.** The stronger the drink, the faster and harder the alcohol hits. Straight shots of liquor and cocktails such as martinis will get alcohol into your bloodstream faster than beer or table wine. Beer and wine not only contain lower concentrations of alcohol, but they also contain nonalcoholic substances that slow the rate of **absorption** (passage of the alcohol into your body tissues). If the drink conmedications—can cause blood-alcohol levels to increase more rapidly. Individuals taking these drugs can be over the legal limit for blood-alcohol concentration after as little as a single drink.

:: **Family history of alcoholism.** Some children of alcoholics don't develop any of the usual behavioral symptoms that indicate someone is drinking too much. It's not known whether this behavior is genetically caused or is a result of growing up with an alcoholic.

:: **Eating.** Food slows the absorption of alcohol by diluting it, by covering some of the membranes through which alcohol would be absorbed, and by prolonging the time the stomach takes to empty.

:: **Expectations.** In various experiments, volunteers who believed they were given alcoholic beverages but were actually given nonalcoholic drinks acted as if they were guzzling the real thing and became more talkative, relaxed, and sexually stimulated.

:: **Physical tolerance.** If you drink regularly, your brain becomes accustomed to a certain level of alcohol. You may be able to look and behave in a seemingly normal fashion, even though you drink as much as would normally intoxicate someone your size. However, your driving ability and judgment will still be impaired.

Once you develop tolerance, you may drink more to get the desired effects from alcohol. In some people, this can lead to abuse and alcoholism. On the other hand, after years of drinking, some people become exquisitely sensitive to alcohol. Such reverse tolerance means that they can become intoxicated after drinking only a small amount of alcohol.

How Much Alcohol Is Too Much?

Federal health authorities at the National Institute of Alcohol Abuse and Alcoholism (NIAAA) recommend that men have no more than two drinks a day and women, no more than one. The American Heart Association (AHA) advises that alcohol account for no more than 15 percent of the total calories consumed by an individual every day, up to an absolute maximum of 1.75 ounces of alcohol a day—the equivalent of three beers, two mixed drinks, or three and a half glasses of wine.

Your own limit may well be less, depending on your gender, size, and weight. Some people—such as women who are pregnant or trying to conceive; individuals with problems, such as ulcers, that might be aggravated by alcohol; those taking medications such as sleeping pills or antidepressants; and those driving or operating any motorized equipment—shouldn't drink at all.

The dangers of alcohol increase along with the amount you drink. Heavy drinking destroys the liver, weakens the heart, elevates blood pressure, damages the

brain, and increases the risk of cancer. Individuals who drink heavily have a higher mortality rate than those who have two or fewer drinks a day. However, the boundary between safe and dangerous drinking isn't the same for everyone. For some people, the upper limit of safety is zero: Once they start, they can't stop.

Intoxication

If you drink too much, the immediate consequence is that you get drunk—or, more precisely, intoxicated. According to the American Psychiatric Association's definition, **intoxication** consists of "clinically significant maladaptive behavioral or psychological changes," such as inappropriate sexual or aggressive behavior, mood changes, and impaired judgment and social and occupational functioning. Alcohol intoxication, which can range from mild inebriation to loss of consciousness, is characterized by at least one of the following signs: slurred speech, poor coordination, unsteady gait, abnormal eye movements, impaired attention or memory, stupor, or coma. Medical risks of intoxication include falls, hypothermia in cold climates, and increased risk of infections because of suppressed immune function.

Time and a protective environment are the recommended treatments for alcohol intoxication. Anyone who passes out after drinking heavily should be monitored regularly to ensure that vomiting (the result of excess alcohol irritating the stomach) doesn't block the breathing airway. Always make sure that an unconscious drinker is lying on his or her side, with the head lower than the body. Intoxicated drinkers can slip into shock, a potentially life-threatening condition characterized by a weak pulse, irregular breathing, and skin-color changes. This is an emergency, and professional medical care should be sought immediately.

The Impact of Alcohol

Unlike drugs in tablet form or food, alcohol is directly and quickly absorbed into the bloodstream through the stomach walls and upper intestine. The alcohol in a typical drink reaches the bloodstream in 15 minutes and rises to its peak concentration in about an hour. The bloodstream carries the alcohol to the liver, heart, and brain. (See Figure 11-3.)

Most of the alcohol you drink can leave your body only after metabolism by the liver, which converts about 95 percent of the alcohol to carbon dioxide and water. The other 5 percent is excreted unchanged, mainly through urination, respiration, and perspiration.

Alcohol affects the major organ systems of the body, and its effects are cumulative. Light alcohol intake (no more than one drink a day for women and two for men) is associated with lower mortality than abstinence, but mortality rates increase with the amount of alcohol consumed. The mortality rate for alcoholics is two and a half times higher than for nonalcoholics of the same age.

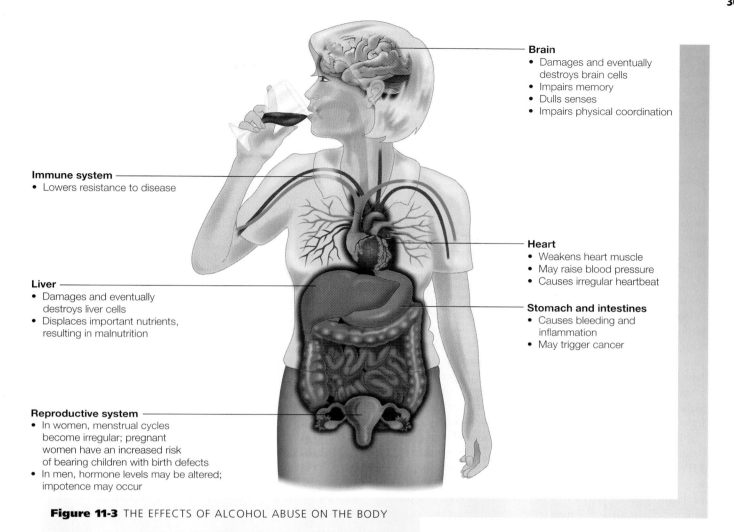

Brain
- Damages and eventually destroys brain cells
- Impairs memory
- Dulls senses
- Impairs physical coordination

Immune system
- Lowers resistance to disease

Heart
- Weakens heart muscle
- May raise blood pressure
- Causes irregular heartbeat

Liver
- Damages and eventually destroys liver cells
- Displaces important nutrients, resulting in malnutrition

Stomach and intestines
- Causes bleeding and inflammation
- May trigger cancer

Reproductive system
- In women, menstrual cycles become irregular; pregnant women have an increased risk of bearing children with birth defects
- In men, hormone levels may be altered; impotence may occur

Figure 11-3 THE EFFECTS OF ALCOHOL ABUSE ON THE BODY

Alcohol is a diuretic, a drug that speeds up the elimination of fluid from the body, so drink water when you drink alcohol to maintain your fluid balance. And alcohol lowers body temperature, so you should never drink to get or stay warm.

Digestive System

Alcohol reaches the stomach first, where it is partially broken down. The remaining alcohol is absorbed easily through the stomach tissue into the bloodstream. In the stomach, alcohol triggers the secretion of acids, which irritate the stomach lining. Excessive drinking at one sitting may result in nausea; chronic drinking may result in peptic ulcers (breaks in the stomach lining) and bleeding from the stomach lining.

The alcohol in the bloodstream eventually reaches the liver. The liver, which bears the major responsibility of fat metabolism in the body, converts this excess alcohol to fat. After a few weeks of four or five drinks a day, liver cells start to accumulate fat. Alcohol also stimulates liver cells to attract white blood cells, which normally travel throughout the bloodstream engulfing harmful substances and wastes. If white blood cells begin to invade body tissue, such as the liver, they can cause irreversible damage.

Weight and Waists

At 7 calories per gram, alcohol has nearly as many calories as fat (9 calories per gram) and significantly more than carbohydrates or protein (which have 4 calories per gram). Since a standard drink contains 12–15 grams of alcohol, the alcohol in a single drink adds about 100 calories to your daily intake. A glass of wine contains as many calories as some candy bars; you would have to walk a mile to burn them off. In addition to being a calorie-dense food, alcohol stimulates the appetite so you're likely to eat more.[2]

"Beer bellies" earn their name. In a study of men and women over age 20 in Copenhagen, those who drank the most beer or spirits had wider waists on a ten-year followup. Wine did not have a similar impact. In another study of the waist-hip ratio and body mass index of French adults who consumed varying amounts of alcohol, drinking was linked to an increase in both waist circumference and waist-to-hip ratio in both men and women.[3]

Cardiovascular System

Alcohol gets mixed reviews regarding its effects on the cardiovascular system. As several studies have shown, people who drink moderate amounts of alcohol have lower mortality rates after a heart attack, as well as a lower risk of heart attack compared to abstainers and heavy drinkers.

In one of the most recent studies of alcohol and cardiovascular health, men in Harvard's long-term Health Professionals Follow-Up Study who consumed moderate amounts of alcohol (less than two 12-ounce bottles of beer, three 4-ounce glasses of wine, or two shots of liquor) three or more days a week were about a third less likely to have heart attacks over a 12-year period than men who never drank. Unlike in earlier French studies, heart attack protection was most strongly associated with beer and liquor consumption and most weakly linked to red wine.[4]

How does alcohol enhance heart health? Researchers believe that it boosts beneficial high-density lipoproteins (HDL), lowers the risk of blood clots, and also may have an anti-inflammatory effect. According to recent studies, alcohol may lower two blood components, C-reactive protein and fibrinogen, that indicate increased heart disease risk (discussed in Chapter 14).[5]

Some cardiologists contend that the benefits of moderate drinking may be overstated, especially because of alcohol's contribution to the epidemic of obesity around the world.[6] Heavy or abusive drinking accounts for more than 100,000 deaths in the United States each year.[7] Heavier drinking triggers the release of harmful oxygen molecules called free radicals, which can increase the risk of heart disease, stroke, and cirrhosis of the liver. Alcohol use can weaken the heart muscle directly, causing a disorder called cardiomyopathy. The combined use of alcohol and other drugs, including tobacco and cocaine, greatly increases the likelihood of damage to the heart.

Breast Cancer

According to analysis of data from many large studies, women who take two or more drinks per day are 40 percent more likely to develop breast cancer than women who don't drink at all. The risk occurs with all forms of alcohol—beer, wine, and spirits—and increases the more women drink.

In the Nurses' Health Study, breast cancer rates rose slightly even in women who took as little as half a drink per day. A single daily drink of 1 ounce of spirits, such as whiskey, gin, or vodka, or 3 ounces of wine increases a woman's breast cancer risk slightly—perhaps 3 or 4 percent. Every additional daily drink increases the risk by 7 percent. By four drinks a day, a woman's risk increases 30 percent.[8]

A non-drinking woman's lifetime risk of breast cancer by age 80 is 1 in 11. A heavy drinker has about a 1 in 7 chance of developing breast cancer by age 80, regardless of her race, education, family history, use of hormone replacement therapy, or other risk factors.[9] In another study of postmenopausal women on estrogen or combination hormone therapy, an average intake of less than one drink a day did not increase the risk of breast cancer. However, there was an elevated risk with 1.5 to 2 drinks a day.

Scientists don't know how alcohol increases breast cancer risk. In some studies, alcohol raised levels of estrogen, perhaps by decreasing the body's ability to metabolize the hormone or by promoting its release into the bloodstream. But other studies have not shown increased estrogen levels in women who drink. Alcohol may also interact with carcinogens (cancer-causing agents), perhaps inhibiting the body's capacity to detoxify carcinogens or activating carcinogens directly.[10]

Immune System

Chronic alcohol use can inhibit the production of both white blood cells, which fight off infections, and red blood cells, which carry oxygen to all the organs and tissues of the body. Alcohol may increase the risk of infection with human immunodeficiency virus (HIV), by altering the judgment of users so that they more readily engage in activities, such as unsafe sexual practices, that put them in danger. If you drink when you have a cold or the flu, alcohol interferes with the body's ability to recover. It also increases the chance of bacterial pneumonia in flu sufferers.

Brain and Behavior

At first, when you drink, you feel up. In low dosages, alcohol affects the regions of the brain that inhibit or control behavior, so you feel looser and act in ways you might not otherwise. However, you also experience losses of concentration, memory, judgment, and fine motor control; and you have mood swings and emotional outbursts. Moderate and heavy drinkers show signs of impaired intelligence, slowed-down reflexes, and difficulty remembering. As recent research has shown, heavy drinking also depletes the brain's supplies of crucial chemicals, including dopamine, gamma aminobutyric acid, opioid peptides, and serotonin, that are responsible for our feelings of pleasure and well-being. At the same time, it promotes the release of stress chemicals, such as corticotropin releasing factor (CRF), that create tension and depression.

Heavy alcohol use may pose special dangers to the brains of drinkers at both ends of the age spectrum.

Adolescents who drink regularly show impairments in their neurological and cognitive functioning. Elderly people who drink heavily appear to have more brain shrinkage, or atrophy, than those who drink lightly or not at all. In general, moderate drinkers have healthier brains and a lower risk of dementia than those who don't drink and those who drink to excess.[11]

Because alcohol is a central nervous system depressant, it slows down the activity of the neurons in the brain, gradually dulling the responses of the brain and nervous system. One or two drinks act as a tranquilizer or relaxant. Additional drinks result in a progressive reduction in central nervous system activity, leading to sleep, general anesthesia, coma, and even death. Moderate amounts of alcohol can have disturbing effects on perception and judgment, including the following:

:: **Impaired perceptions.** You're less able to adjust your eyes to bright lights because glare bothers you more. Although you can still hear sounds, you can't distinguish between them or judge their direction well.

:: **Dulled smell and taste.** Alcohol itself may cause some vitamin deficiencies, and the poor eating habits of heavy drinkers result in further nutrition problems.

:: **Diminished sensation.** On a freezing winter night, you may walk outside without a coat and not feel the cold.

:: **Altered sense of space.** You may not realize, for instance, that you have been in one place for several hours.

:: **Impaired motor skills.** Writing, typing, driving, and other abilities involving your muscles are impaired. This is why law enforcement officers sometimes ask suspected drunk drivers to touch their nose with a finger or to walk a straight line. Drinking large amounts of alcohol impairs reaction time, speed, accuracy, and consistency, as well as judgment.

:: **Impaired sexual performance.** While drinking may increase your interest in sex, it may also impair sexual response, especially a man's ability to achieve or maintain an erection. As Shakespeare wrote, "It provokes the desire, but it takes away the performance."

Increased Risk of Dying

Alcohol kills. Alcohol is responsible for 100,000 deaths each year and is the third leading cause of death after tobacco and improper diet and lack of exercise. The leading alcohol-related cause of death is injury. Alcohol plays a role in at least half of all traffic fatalities, half of all homicides, and a quarter of all suicides. The second leading cause of alcohol-related deaths is cirrhosis of the liver, a chronic disease that causes extensive scarring and irreversible damage. In addition, as many as half of patients admitted to hospitals and 15 percent of those making office visits seek or need medical care because of the direct or indirect effects of alcohol.

Young drinkers—teens and those in their early twenties—are at highest risk of dying from injuries, mostly car accidents. Older drinkers over age 50 face the greatest danger of premature death from cirrhosis of the liver, hepatitis, and other alcohol-linked illnesses.

Most studies of the relationship between alcohol consumption and death from all causes show that moderate drinkers—those who consume approximately seven drinks per week—have a lower risk of death than abstainers, while heavy drinkers have a higher risk than either group. (See Table 11-1.) In one ten-year study, never-drinkers showed no elevated risk of dying, while consistent heavier drinkers were at higher risk of dying of any cause than other men. New drinkers who had previously abstained did not improve their chances for longevity by starting to drink. However, heavier drinking men who cut down on alcohol consumption did increase their longevity.[12]

Interaction with Other Drugs

Alcohol can interact with other drugs—prescription and nonprescription, legal and illegal. Of the 100 most frequently prescribed drugs, more than half contain at least one ingredient that interacts adversely with alcohol. Because alcohol and other psychoactive drugs may work on the same areas of the brain, their combination can produce an effect much greater than that expected of either drug by itself. The consequences of this synergistic interaction can be fatal. (See Savvy Consumer: "Alcohol and Drug Interactions.") Alcohol is particularly dangerous

TABLE 11-1	**Weighing the Effects of Light to Moderate Drinking**
Positive effects of light to moderate drinking—no more than 1 drink per day for women or 2 drinks/day for men	**Negative effects of light to moderate drinking**
Lower risk of heart attack than abstinence	Higher risk of breast cancer in women
Lower mortality than abstinence	Possible interaction with prescription and nonprescription drugs
Lower risk of dementia	Impaired perceptions
	Diminished smell, taste, and sensation
	Impaired motor skills
	Impaired sexual performance
	Possible weight gain

Savvy Consumer

ALCOHOL AND DRUG INTERACTIONS

Drug	Possible Effects of Interaction
Analgesics (painkillers)	
Narcotic (Codeine, Demerol, Percodan)	Increase in central nervous system depression, possibly leading to respiratory failure and death.
Nonnarcotic (aspirin, acetaminophen)	Irritation of stomach resulting in bleeding and increased susceptibility to liver damage.
Antabuse	Nausea, vomiting, headache, high blood pressure, and erratic heartbeat.
Antianxiety drugs (Valium, Librium)	Increase in central nervous system depression; decreased alertness and impaired judgment.
Antidepressants	Increase in central nervous system depression; certain antidepressants in combination with red wine could cause a sudden increase in blood pressure.
Antihistamines (Actifed, Dimetap, and other cold medications)	Increase in drowsiness; driving more dangerous.
Antibiotics	Nausea, vomiting, headache; some medications rendered less effective.
Central nervous system stimulants (caffeine, Dexedrine, Ritalin)	Stimulant effects of these drugs may reverse depressant effect of alcohol but do not decrease its intoxicating effects.
Diuretics (Diuril, Lasix)	Reduction in blood pressure resulting in dizziness upon rising.
Sedatives (Dalmane, Nembutal, Quaalude)	Increase in central nervous system depression, possibly leading to coma, respiratory failure, and death.

when combined with depressants and antianxiety medications.

Aspirin, long used to prevent or counter alcohol's effects, may actually enhance its impact by significantly lowering the body's ability to break down alcohol in the stomach. In a study of healthy men between the ages of 30 and 45, volunteers who took two extra-strength aspirin tablets an hour before drinking a glass and a half of wine had a 30 percent higher BAC than when they drank alcohol alone. This increase could make a difference in impairment for individuals driving cars or operating machinery.

If you want to drink while taking medication, be sure you read the warnings on nonprescription-drug labels or prescription-drug containers; ask your doctor about possible alcohol–drug interactions; and check with your pharmacist if you have any questions about your medications, especially over-the-counter (OTC) products.

✸ Drinking in America

According to the most recent statistics available from the National Institute on Alcohol Abuse and Alcoholism, about 60 percent of American adults use alcohol, although they vary in how much and how often they drink. Whites are more likely to be daily or near-daily drinkers than non-whites. Men tend to drink more and more often than women. Young people between the ages of 21 and 34 are most likely to drink, and alcohol use typically declines with age.

Why People Drink

The most common reason people drink alcohol is to relax. Because it depresses the central nervous system, alcohol can make people feel less tense. Other motivations for drinking include the following:

:: **Celebration.** Unless alcohol use violates family, ethnic, or religious values, people raise their glasses together on life's important occasions—births, graduations, weddings, promotions.

:: **Friendship.** When friends visit, they may have a drink, or they may meet somewhere "for a drink." Young people are much more likely to experiment with alcohol if their friends drink.

:: **Social ease.** When people use alcohol, they may seem bolder, wittier, sexier. At the same time, they become more relaxed and seem to enjoy each other's

Alcohol can be part of many enjoyable social situations, as long as individuals know when to say "no more." Many people are increasingly substituting non-alcoholic drinks.

company more. Because alcohol lowers inhibitions, some people see it as a prelude to seduction.

:: **Self-medication.** Like other drugs, alcohol may be the means some people use to treat—or escape from—painful feelings or bad moods.

:: **Role models.** Athletes, some of the most admired celebrities in our country, have a long history of appearing in commercials for alcohol. Many advertisements feature glamorous women holding or sipping alcoholic beverages.

:: **Advertising.** Brewers and beer distributors spend $15 to $20 million a year promoting the message: If you want to have fun, have a drink. Adolescents may be especially responsive to such sales pitches. Nearly two dozen national groups, including the American Medical Association, have petitioned the Federal Trade Commission to ban alcohol advertisements that link drinking to risky activities (such as driving, water skiing, and skydiving) and that target youth.

Patterns of Alcohol Use

Patterns of alcohol consumption tend to change over time, especially among younger people. In one 15-year study, most increases in consumption took place among moderate drinkers and most decreases took place among heavy drinkers. Overall, abstainers and moderate drinkers showed greater stability than did heavy drinkers.[13]

Drinking patterns vary with the seasons. Researchers have documented a phenomenon called "the January effect." Regardless of gender or race, people are more likely to report recent heavy drinking in the first month of the year than any other time. In general, drinking also rises

in the summer and slumps in spring and fall.[14] There are racial variations on this seasonal pattern. Drinking peaks in January for black and white men and women and Hispanic women, but in June for Hispanic men. Asians, who typically drink less than other minorities, reveal no significant monthly variations.

Although there are no standard definitions for drinking patterns, the following are generally recognized as most common:

:: **Abstinence.** Because of concern about alcohol's health effects, increasing numbers of Americans are choosing not to drink. With alcohol consumption in the United States at its lowest level in 30 years, nonalcoholic beverages have grown in popularity. They appeal to drivers, boaters, pregnant women, individuals with health problems that could worsen with alcohol, those who are older and can't tolerate alcohol, anyone taking medicines that interact with alcohol (including antibiotics, antidepressants, and muscle relaxers), and everyone interested in limiting alcohol intake. Under federal law, these drinks can contain some alcohol, but a much smaller amount than regular beer or wine. Nonalcoholic beers and wines on the market also are lower in calories than alcoholic varieties.

:: **Light drinking.** This is defined as having fewer than three alcoholic drinks a week. (A drink equals 1 ounce of spirits, a 4-ounce glass of table wine, or a 12-ounce can of beer, each of which contains approximately 12 grams of absolute alcohol.)

:: **Infrequent drinking.** This term refers to frequency, not quantity. Infrequent drinkers have less than one drink a month but drink at least once a year. Some "low maximum" infrequent drinkers drink one to three times a month but never have five or more drinks at a sitting. "High maximum" infrequent drinkers do not drink more often, but they occasionally have five or more drinks at a sitting.

:: **Moderate drinking.** Moderate drinking generally is defined as having an upper limit of four standard drinks on any day, on no more than three days a week. For women, the upper limit is three drinks a day, on no more than three days a week.

:: **Social drinking.** This term—used by laypeople rather than health-care professionals or researchers—refers to drinking patterns that are accepted by friends and peers. If your friends drink only on special occasions, you may think that having one glass of wine at a party is social drinking. On the other hand, if the people you socialize with drink regularly and heavily, you may mistakenly think that having a six-pack of beer every night is social drinking.

:: **Problem drinking.** Any kind of drinking that interferes with a major aspect of life, such as sleep, energy, family relationships, health, or safety, qualifies as problem drinking. Some of the problems associated with drinking—getting into fights, unwanted sexual activity, car accidents—are obvious. Others, such as alcohol-related damage to the digestive system, heart, liver or brain, may remain invisible for years.

:: **Binge drinking.** When applied to alcohol, a binge consists of having five or more drinks at a single sitting for a man or four drinks at a single sitting for a woman.

Binge drinking is on the rise, with 1.5 billion episodes occurring every year. Binge drinkers are 14 times more likely to drive drunk than non-binge-drinkers. They also are at risk for a long list of adverse health outcomes, including injuries from falls, drowning, hypothermia, and burns; heart attacks; suicide; violence to others; and unplanned pregnancy and sexually transmitted infection.[15] As discussed later in this chapter, binge drinking is common in college.

Drinking is often part of the college social and athletic scene—friends have a strong influence on their peers.

© Uwe Krejci/Taxi/Getty Images

Teen Drinking

Alcohol is the leading drug of abuse among teenagers: 78 percent of high school students say they have tried alcohol, 30 percent—some 5 million—admit to binge drinking at least once a month. Individuals who begin drinking before age 15 are four times more likely to become alcohol dependent than those who do not drink before age 21.[16] Those who start drinking younger than 19 also are more likely to become alcohol-dependent or frequent heavy drinkers.[17]

Underage drinkers consume about 20 percent of the 4.21 billion alcohol drinks consumed every month in the United States. Based on these estimates, underage drinkers spend $22.5 billion a year on alcohol. Together underage drinkers and adult excessive drinkers (those consuming more than two drinks a day) are responsible for about half of the alcohol consumed and the money spent on alcohol in this country.[18]

 Drinking in College

Drinking has long been part of the college experience. For the majority of students, alcohol usually does not interfere with their school and work responsibilities.[19] However, alcohol use can—and too often does—become problematic and even tragic. A single episode, combined with poor judgment or bad luck, can lead to life-altering and sometimes life-threatening consequences.

Every year students spend $5.5 billion on alcohol, mostly beer—more than they spend on books, soda pop, coffee, juice, and milk combined. The total amount of alcohol consumed by college students each year is 430 million gallons, enough for every college and university in the United States to fill an Olympic-size swimming pool.

 How Common Is Drinking on College Campuses?

In the last decade, patterns in college drinking have changed in some ways, but not in others. More students abstain—19.3 percent, up from 16.4 percent in 1993.[20] However, more students now say that they drink primarily for the purpose of getting drunk. While fewer students attend or drink heavily at fraternity and sorority parties than a decade ago, more are drinking heavily at off-campus parties. College women are as likely to drink, but men drink more heavily. About half of college men and a third of college women report drinking to excess.[21] (See Fact or Fiction? "More Canadian . . .")

Students drink more at certain colleges, such as those located along the Mexican border,[22] and in certain locations, such as off-campus parties and bars and fraternity and sorority parties.[23] Heavy drinking is most likely to occur at events where many people become intoxicated, illicit drugs are available, and drinking games are played. More college sports fans drink alcohol, engage in binge drinking, have a heavy drinking style, and report alcohol-related problems compared with non-fans.[24]

Two in five students, 44 percent, report at least occasional binge drinking. Schools with large fraternity systems and rural colleges typically report more heavy drinking, while Christian and women's colleges have less drinking. However, heavy drinking has become more prevalent on most campuses. An estimated 10 percent of college students drink more than 15 alcoholic beverages per week.[25]

From 50 to 62 percent of undergraduates report playing drinking games in the preceding month. More than 500 different drinking games—such as tongue twisters or drinking whenever a certain phrase is mentioned in a song or on a TV program—are popular on college campuses. They are dangerous because they can result in high levels of intoxication in a short period of time.[26]

Why College Students Drink

Students' motives for drinking—whether to feel more at ease socially, to cope with stress, or to enhance well-being—as well as their friend's drinking motives affect how much and how often they drink.[27] Most college students drink for the same reasons undergraduates have always turned to alcohol: Away from home, often for the first time, many are excited by and apprehensive about their newfound independence. When new pressures seem overwhelming, when they feel awkward or insecure, when they just want to let loose and have a good time, they reach for a drink.

Freshmen may be especially vulnerable to dangerous drinking as they struggle to adapt to an often bewildering new world. Many who were nondrinkers as high school seniors start to drink in college. They are less likely to do so if friends discourage them from drinking.

Studies have also linked alcohol consumption with where students live on campus and what they perceive as the norm for acceptable drinking.[28] Stress-related drinking is common. Students in competitive academic environments may turn to alcohol to reduce their anxiety and the pressure to perform. Athletes have higher drinking rates than nonathletes.[29] Members of sororities and fraternities rated all drinking norms as more extreme and perceived fraternity drinking as particularly heavy. Fraternity leaders are among the heaviest drinkers and the most out-of-control partygoers, with the highest incidence of heavy drinking and bingeing.

The most dramatic increases in college drinking have been among women: Eight in ten female undergraduates say they drink; one in four get drunk three or more times in a month. (See The X & Y File: "Why Men and Women Drink.")

Binge Drinking on Campus

Binge drinking—defined as the consumption of five or more alcoholic drinks in a row by men and four or more by women—is the leading cause of preventable death among undergraduates and the most serious threat to their intellectual, physical, and psychological development.

In spite of great efforts across U.S. college campuses to decrease binge drinking, the national average—two out of five students report bingeing—has remained steady for the last 15 to 20 years.[30] According to the Harvard School of Public Health's College Alcohol Study, which has conducted four national surveys of students at 119 colleges, 40 to 45 percent of college students report binge drinking. This percentage has remained stable in the last decade—despite greater awareness, more efforts at prevention, and demands for greater accountability.[31]

The number of frequent binge drinkers has increased somewhat in the last decade, even though fewer undergraduates say they were binge drinkers in high school.[32] Frequent binge drinkers account for almost 70 percent of all alcohol consumed by college students.[33] Students in four-year colleges are more likely to binge than those in two-year colleges. Many more of those living in fraternity or sorority houses (65.9 percent) report bingeing than students living elsewhere (38.1 percent).[34] The students least likely to binge drink were African American or Asian, aged 24 years or older, married, and had not been binge drinkers in high school.[35]

More women now binge. At coed schools, 41.2 percent report at least one binge within the previous two weeks; 17.4 percent are frequent bingers. At all-female colleges, binge drinking has jumped 25 percent, from 24.5 percent in 1993 to 32.1 percent in 2001.[36] Unplanned sexual activities, date rape, and sexual assault are 150 percent more likely among women who drink than among

the XY & file   *Why Men and Women Drink*

In recent years, researchers have been comparing and contrasting the reasons why men and women drink. Undergraduate women and men are equally likely to drink for stress-related reasons; both perceive alcohol as a means of tension relaxation. Some psychologists theorize that men engage in *confirmatory drinking,* that is, they drink to reinforce the image of masculinity associated with alcohol consumption. Both genders may engage in *compensatory drinking,* consuming alcohol to heighten their sense of masculinity or femininity.

Here are some other reasons why men, women, or both drink:

:: **Inherited susceptibility.** In both women and men, genetics accounts for 50 to 60 percent of a person's vulnerability to a serious drinking problem. Female alcoholics are more likely than males to have a parent who abused drugs or alcohol, who had psychiatric problems, or who attempted suicide.

:: **Childhood traumas.** Female alcoholics often report that they were physically or sexually abused as children or suffered great distress because of poverty or a parent's death.

:: **Depression.** Women are more likely than men to be depressed prior to drinking and to suffer from both depression and a drinking problem at the same time. Young men who do not drink, as well as those who drink heavily, have high levels of depression and distress.

:: **Relationship issues.** Single, separated, or divorced men and women drink more and more often than married ones.

:: **Psychological factors.** Both men and women may drink to compensate for feelings of inadequacy. Women who tend to ruminate or mull over bad feelings may find that alcohol increases this tendency and makes them feel more distressed.

:: **Employment.** Women who work outside the home are less likely to become problem drinkers or alcoholics than those without paying jobs. The one exception: women in occupations still dominated by men, such as engineering, science, law enforcement, and top corporate management.

:: **Self-medication.** More so than men, some women feel it's permissible to use alcohol as if it were a medicine. As long as they're taking it for a reason, it seems acceptable to them, even if they're drifting into a drinking problem.

those who do not. Sophomore, junior, and senior women are much less likely to engage in heavy episodic drinking than freshman women.[37] (See Fact or Fiction? "College students account . . .")

Why do Students Binge?

Young people who came from, socializes within, or were exposed to "wet" environments—setting in which alcohol is cheap and accessible and drinking is prevalent—are more likely to engage in binge drinking. Students who reported drinking at least once a month during their final year of high school were over three times more likely to binge drink in college than those who drank less frequently in high school.[38]

The factors that most influence students to binge drink are:

:: **Low price** for alcohol.

:: **Easy access to alcohol.** In one study, the density of alcohol outlets (such as bars) near campus affected the drinking of students.[39]

:: **Attending a school** or living in a residence with many binge drinkers.

:: **Belief** that close friends were likely to binge.

FACT OR FICTION? ?????????????????

College students account for most binge-drinking.

Fiction: According to an analysis of lifestyle habits of adults over age 20 by the Centers for Disease Control and Prevention, neither college students nor alcoholics account for the bulk of binge drinking. Most binge drinking is done by moderate drinkers (men who usually average two or less drinks a day and women who average one). They do not binge as often as heavier drinkers, but because there are far more of them than college students or alcoholics, the numbers add up. The consequences of binge drinking are similar for all: injuries from car accidents, drowning, burns, and hypothermia, heart attacks, suicide, violence to others, sexually transmitted infections, and unwanted pregnancy.

Source: "Binge Drinking: Not Just About Teenagers." *Tufts University Health & Nutrition Letter,* Vol. 20, No. 12, February 2003, p. 2.

Binge drinkers can get into—and cause—trouble. Dangerously large amounts of alcohol can cause death, and heavy party drinking often results in violence.

:: **Parents who drank** or did not disapprove of their children drinking.

:: **Recreational drinking** before age 16.

Some educators view bingeing as a product of the college environment. More students binge drink at the beginning of the school year and then cut back as the semester progresses and academic demands increase. Binge drinking also peaks following exam times, during home football weekends, and during spring break. Many new students engage in binge drinking for the first time very soon after they arrive on campus. Binges become less common in their subsequent years at school and almost always end with education. Real life, one educator notes, is "a strong disincentive" to this type of drinking.[40]

Underage Drinking on Campus

Students under age 21 drink less often than older students, but tend to drink more heavily and to experience more negative alcohol-related consequences. While fewer underage students report drinking on 10 or more occasions in the past 30 days, more report being drunk on three or more occasions in the past 30 days. More underage students also report drinking "to get drunk" and drinking at binge levels when they consumed alcohol. Among the younger men, 57.8 percent reported that they usually had five or more drinks per drinking occasion, compared with 41.9 percent of older students. Similar rates were found among female students, with 32.4 of underage women versus 20.5 percent of those over 21 reporting binge drinking.

Underage students are more likely than students of legal age to experience a host of negative drinking-related consequences, including doing something they regretted; forgetting where they were or what they did; causing property damage; getting into trouble with police; and being hurt or injured. However, underage students are less likely than older students to drink and drive, miss a class, or engage in unprotected sex because of their alcohol use.

The drinking behavior of underage students also depends on their living arrangements. Those in controlled settings, such as their parents' home or a substance-free dorm, are less likely to binge drink. Students living in fraternities or sororities were most likely to binge drink, regardless of age.[41]

Students under age 21 in states with tough laws against underage drinking are less likely to drink than those in states with fewer restrictions. When they drink, underage students are more likely to drink to excess than older ones—possibly because they feel greater pressure to drink quickly before some authority cuts off their alcohol supply or they get caught.[42]

The Toll of College Drinking

Each year more than 2 million college students aged 18–24 drive after drinking; more than 3 million ride in motor vehicles with drinking drivers; over one half million are injured because of drinking; and 1,400 die from alcohol-related unintentional injuries, most sustained in alcohol-related traffic crashes.[43] (See Student Snapshot: "The Consequences of College Drinking.")

According to the Commission on Substance Abuse at Colleges and Universities, alcohol is involved in two-thirds of college student suicides, nine of ten rapes, and 95 percent of violent crimes on campus.[44] According to a national survey released by the Higher Education Center for Alcohol and Other Drug Prevention, 75 to 90 percent of all violence on college campuses is alcohol-related. About 300,000 of today's college students will eventually die from alcohol-related causes, including drunk-driving accidents, cirrhosis of the liver, various cancers, and heart disease, estimates the Core Institute, an organization that studies college drinking.

Drinking also increases sexual risks for college students. (See Figure 11-4.) Heavy drinking has been correlated with increased casual sex without condoms, an increased number of sex partners, and sexual attacks on women. According to a 2002 survey, half of 15- to 24-year-olds mix alcohol, drugs, and sex "a lot." Alcohol and drug use can lead to earlier sexual initiation, unprotected sexual intercourse, multiple sex partners, and increased risk of sexually transmitted infections.[45]

Four in ten college students have experienced alcohol-related blackouts that led to risky behaviors in the past year, according to a survey at Duke University. During

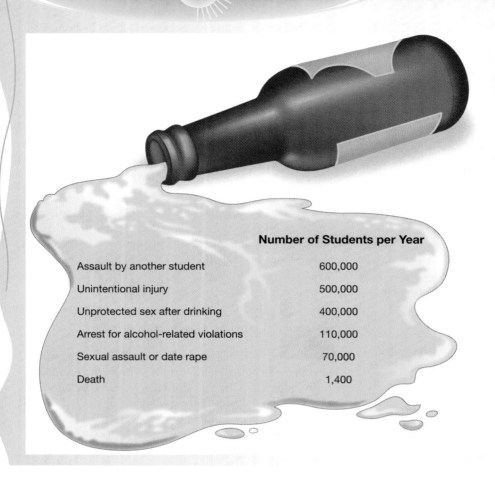

Student Snapshot — **The Consequences of College Drinking**

	Number of Students per Year
Assault by another student	600,000
Unintentional injury	500,000
Unprotected sex after drinking	400,000
Arrest for alcohol-related violations	110,000
Sexual assault or date rape	70,000
Death	1,400

Source: www.collegedrinkingprevention.gov.

these blackouts, students often participated in behaviors such as unprotected sexual intercourse, vandalizing property or driving. Female students were at greater risk of engaging in risky behavior during blackouts than male students.[46]

Surveys consistently show that students who engage in binge drinking, particularly those who do so more than once a week, experience a far higher rate of problems than other students. Frequent binge drinkers are likely to miss classes, vandalize property, and drive after drinking. (See Table 11-2.) Frequent binge drinkers are also more likely to experience five or more different alcohol-related problems and to use other substances, including nicotine, marijuana, cocaine, and LSD.[47]

Students on campuses with many binge drinkers report higher rates of secondhand problems caused by others' alcohol use, compared with students on campuses with lower rates of binge drinking. These problems include loss of sleep, interruption of studies, assaults, vandalism, and unwanted sexual advances. Students living on campuses with high rates of binge drinking are two or more times as likely to experience these secondhand effects as those living on campuses with low rates.[48]

The impact of student drinking spills beyond campus borders. Neighbors living within a mile of a college are much more likely to experience disturbances such as vandalism, assault, noise, litter, and drunkenness than those living farther away.[49] Support for tougher restrictions on alcohol has grown on some campuses. Laws restricting underage drinking or governing the volume of sales and consumption of alcohol are associated with less drinking among underage students.[50]

Alcohol Problems on Campus

According to researchers from Harvard Medical School, students generally fall into four categories based on their patterns of drinking behavior:

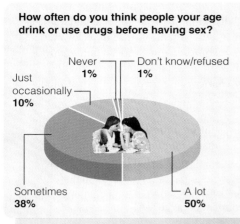

How often do you think people your age drink or use drugs before having sex?

Never 1%
Don't know/refused 1%
Just occasionally 10%
Sometimes 38%
A lot 50%

How concerned are you personally that you might do more sexually than you had planned because you are drinking or using drugs?

Don't know/refused 1%
Very concerned 21%
Not at all concerned 37%
Not too concerned 19%
Somewhat concerned 22%

Figure 11-4 SUBSTANCE ABUSE AND RISKY SEXUAL BEHAVIOR

Source: Henry J. Kaiser Family Foundation.

:: **"Abstainers"** report consuming no alcohol during the prior year.

:: **"Nonheavy episodic drinkers"** report drinking in the past year, but no heavy drinking episodes in the past 2 weeks.

TABLE 11-2	Alcohol-Related Problems Among Students Who Drink Alcohol
Alcohol-Related Problem	**Percentage of Students Reporting the Problem**
Miss a class	29.5
Get behind in school work	21.6
Do something you regret	35.0
Forget where you were or what you did	26.8
Argue with friends	22.9
Engage in unplanned sexual activities	21.3
Not use protection when you had sex	10.4
Damage property	10.7
Get into trouble with the campus or local police	6.5
Get hurt or injured	12.8
Require medical treatment for an overdose	0.8
Drive after drinking	29.0

Source: Henry Wechsler et al. "Trends in College Binge Drinking During a Period of Increased Prevention Efforts." *Journal of American College Health*, Vol. 50, No. 5, March 2002, p. 203.

:: **"Occasional heavy episodic drinkers"** report heavy episodic or binge drinking (5 drinks/occasion for males, 4 drinks/occasion for females) on one or two occasions during the past 2 weeks.

:: **"Heavy episodic drinkers"** report heavy episodic drinking on three or more occasions in the past two weeks.

According to the researchers, 31.6 percent of the students meet the diagnostic standards for alcohol abuse, 6.3 percent, for alcohol dependence. More than half (53.7 percent) of male students under 24 years of age reported at least one symptom.

Other risky behaviors associated with an alcohol-use diagnosis were using marijuana in the past 30 days, smoking cigarettes, and having multiple sexual partners. Students who drank heavily in high school or reported getting drunk before age 16 were more likely to be diagnosed, as were students whose parents drank or whose parents were problem drinkers. Students who said parties were important to them, who belonged to a fraternity or sorority, lived with a roommate, had five or more friends, socialized four or more hours per day, watched television three or more hours per day, studied fewer than five hours per day, or played intercollegiate sports more than one hour per day were more likely to be diagnosed with alcohol abuse or dependence. Living in an alcohol-free dorm slightly reduced the risk of having abuse but not dependence; living on an alcohol-free campus had no significant effect on either diagnosis.[51]

Changing Drinking Patterns on Campus

At many schools, a growing number of students almost never engage in heavy drinking. Even those who drank heavily as freshmen often curtail their alcohol use either before or after graduation. This is the result both of personal changes in behavior and in college policies.

Stages of Personal Change

In a study at Ohio State University, researchers classified student heavy drinkers according to the stages of change:[52]

:: **Pre-Contemplation.** Nearly two-thirds of the students continued to drink heavily and had no intention of changing their behavior. These students drank an average of 12.5 alcoholic beverages a week.

:: **Contemplation:** 12 percent of the students were still drinking heavily but considering changing their drinking behavior.

:: **Action:** 14 percent of the students had stopped their pattern of heavy drinking.

:: **Maintenance:** 9 percent of the students had avoided heavy alcohol use for at least six months. They drank an average of one alcoholic drink a month. These students no longer drank heavily, even though they felt that such drinking was the norm on their campus. However, they saw more risks and fewer benefits associated with alcohol use.

Such change is not unusual, even among students who continued heavy drinking throughout their college years. Despite their heavy drinking as undergraduates, within three years of graduation, students who had been members of fraternities and sororities drink no more than students who did not join Greek houses. Heavy drinking may be the result of students' perceptions that excessive alcohol use is normal in Greek houses, along with the encouragement of peers.[53]

College Alcohol Policies

Colleges and universities, which have been held legally liable for the deaths of students from alcohol poisoning, are establishing tough new policies to crack down on underage and heavy drinking and change the "drinking culture" on campus. Some have banned alcohol from events in freshman dorms or prohibited delivery of beer kegs to dorms, fraternities, and sororities. Others have rearranged academic schedules to require more Friday classes or have established a policy of notifying parents if students break drinking rules.[54] Colleges and universities are required to provide a copy of their alcohol policies to students. Some schools post their policies online, but in many cases they are difficult to find among all of the other information on a school's web site.[55] Can you find the policy for your school?

A number of colleges are trying a social-norms approach, spreading the message to students that their peers drink less than they think, in an attempt to make heavy drinking less socially acceptable.[56]

Fewer than 10 percent of frequent binge drinkers experience any disciplinary action as a result of their drinking.[57] Support for tougher campus restrictions has grown among students, particularly those who do not

binge drink and who have experienced the negative consequences of others' drinking, such as violence and vandalism.[58] According to studies of schools that have lowered binge drinking rates, a combination of social and environmental approaches has the greatest impact on reducing binge drinking. Key elements are involvement of students and development of alternatives, such as alcohol-free parties and events.[59]

The U.S. Department of Education has begun highlighting innovative antidrinking practices on campus; Mothers Against Drunk Driving (MADD) is planning to rank colleges based on how well they curb student drinking. There has been an increase in on-campus chapters of national support groups such as AA, Al-Anon, Adult Children of Alcoholics, and a peer-education program called BACCHUS: Boost Alcohol Consciousness Concerning the Health of University Students.

⚫ Drinking and Driving

Alcohol impairs driving-related skills regardless of the age of the driver or the time of day it is consumed.[60] However, younger drinkers and drivers are at greatest risk. Underage drinkers are more likely to drive after drinking, to ride with intoxicated drivers, and to be injured after drinking—at least in part because they believe that people can drive safely and legally after drinking.[61]

Drunk driving is the most frequently committed crime in the United States. In the last two decades, families of the victims of drunk drivers have organized to change the way the nation treats its drunk drivers. Because of the efforts of MADD (Mothers Against Drunk Driving), SADD (Students Against Destructive Decisions), and other lobbying groups, cities, counties, and states are cracking down on drivers who drink. Since courts have held establishments that serve alcohol liable for the consequences of allowing drunk customers to drive, many bars and restaurants have joined the campaign against drunk driving. Many communities also provide free rides home on holidays and weekends for people who've had too much to

 drink. Designated drivers can help save lives—if they refrain from drinking. In one study of college students, female designated drivers had lower Blood Alcohol Concentrations than males.[62]

To keep drunk drivers off the road, many cities have set up checkpoints to stop automobiles and inspect drivers for intoxication. The U.S. Supreme Court has ruled that a driver's refusal to submit to a blood-alcohol concentration test at checkpoints or at any other time can be used as evidence to prosecute him or her for drunk driving. An increasing number of states have toughened their enforcement of drunk-driving penalties. Some suspend a driver's license for several months for a first offense; repeat offenders can lose their license for a year or more.

STRATEGIES FOR PREVENTION

How to Prevent Drunk Driving

- When going out in a group, always designate one person who won't drink at all to serve as the driver.

- Never get behind the wheel if you've had more than two drinks within two hours, especially if you haven't eaten.

- Never let intoxicated friends drive home. Call a taxi, drive them yourself, or arrange for them to spend the night in a safe place.

The National Highway Traffic Safety Administration estimates that setting the legal age limit for drinking at 21 has saved 16,500 lives in traffic crashes alone since 1975. The majority of states have made it illegal for people younger than 21 to drive with a measurable amount of alcohol in their blood. Research comparing states that adopted such zero tolerance laws to those that did not have such laws found that zero tolerance states experienced 20 percent declines in the proportions of fatal single-vehicle, night crashes (the type most often alcohol-related) involving young drivers. Nationwide, alcohol-related traffic deaths among 15- to 20-year-olds have declined.

:: Alcohol and Race

Experts in alcohol treatment are increasingly recognizing racial and ethnic differences in risk factors for drinking problems, patterns of drinking,

Public awareness campaigns like this one for designated drivers can help prevent the high incidence of fatalities caused by drunk drivers.

and most effective types of treatment. Increases in drinking have been traced to stresses related to immigration, acculturation, poverty, racial discrimination, and powerlessness. Environmental factors, such as aggressive marketing and advertising of alcoholic beverages in minority neighborhoods, also play a role. On campus white students report the highest rates of heavy drinking; black students, the lowest. Hispanic students are intermediate.

African-American Community

Overall, African Americans consume less alcohol per person than whites, yet twice as many blacks die of cirrhosis of the liver each year. In some cities, the rate of cirrhosis is ten times higher among African-American than white men. Alcohol also contributes to high rates of hypertension, esophageal cancer, and homicide among African-American men.

Drinking patterns among African Americans are more extreme than those of white drinkers, with more abstinence, but also more occasions of heavy drinking. While the average weekly consumption of alcohol is similar in African Americans and whites, the average amount consumed over a 24-hour period is significantly different. Both African American men and women drink more during a single occasion compared to their white counterparts.[63]

The makers of alcoholic beverages aggressively market their products to African Americans, and there are many more liquor stores (per capita) in many African-American neighborhoods than in white communities. Peer pressure to drink, the easy accessibility of alcohol, and socioeconomic frustrations increase the likelihood of alcohol problems among African Americans. Moreover, recovery can be especially difficult because of the lack of treatment programs and role models in the African-American community and ongoing pressures to resume drinking.

Hispanic Community

The various Hispanic cultures tend to discourage any drinking by women but encourage heavy drinking by men as part of machismo, or feelings of manhood. According to the Department of Health and Human Services, Hispanic men have higher rates of alcohol use and abuse than the general population and suffer a high rate of cirrhosis. Moreover, American-born Hispanic men drink more than those born in other countries.

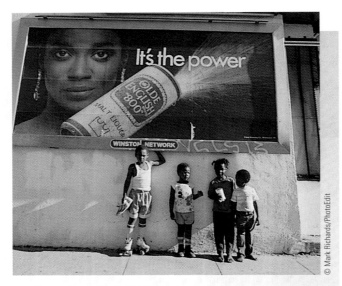

The makers of alcoholic beverages aggressively market their products in poor urban neighborhoods, where liquor stores and bars are common.

Few Hispanics enter treatment, partly because of a lack of information, language barriers, and poor community-based services. Hispanic families generally try to resolve problems themselves, and their cultural values discourage the sharing of intimate personal stories, which characterizes Alcoholics Anonymous and other support groups. Churches often provide the most effective forms of help.

Native American Community

European settlers introduced alcohol to Native Americans. Because of the societal and physical problems resulting from excessive drinking, at the request of tribal leaders, the U.S. Congress in 1832 prohibited the use of alcohol by Native Americans. Many reservations still ban alcohol use, so Native Americans who want to drink may have to travel long distances to obtain alcohol, which may contribute to the high death rate from hypothermia and pedestrian and motor-vehicle accidents among Native Americans. (Injuries are the leading cause of death among this group.)

Certainly, not all Native Americans drink, and not all who drink do so to excess. However, they have three times the general population's rate of alcohol-related injury and illness. Cirrhosis of the liver is the fourth-leading cause of death among this cultural group. While many Native American women don't drink, those who do have high rates of alcohol-related problems, which affect both them and their children. Their rate of cirrhosis of the liver is 36 times that of white women. In some tribes, 10.5 out of every 1,000 newborns have fetal alcohol syndrome, compared with 1 to 3 out of 1,000 in the general population.

(See the discussion on fetal alcohol syndrome in the next section.)

Both a biological predisposition and socioeconomic conditions may contribute to alcohol abuse by Native Americans. In addition, alcoholism is not a physical disease according to their cultural beliefs, but a spiritual disorder, making it less likely that they'll seek appropriate treatment.

Asian-American Community

Asian Americans tend to drink very little or not at all, in part because of an inborn physiological reaction to alcohol that causes facial flushing, rapid heart rate, lowered blood pressure, nausea, vomiting, and other symptoms. A very high percentage of women of all Asian-American nationalities abstain completely. Some sociologists have expressed concern, however, that as Asian Americans become more assimilated into American culture, they'll drink more—and possibly suffer very adverse effects from alcohol.

▶ Alcohol and Gender

According to conventional gender stereotypes, drinking is a symbol of manliness. In the past, far more men than women drank. In the United States today, both genders are likely to consume alcohol. However, there are well-documented differences in how often and how much men and women drink. In general, men drink more frequently, consume a larger quantity of alcohol per drinking occasion, and report more problems related to drinking. More than half of women drink: Of these, 45 percent are light drinkers; 3 percent, moderate drinkers; 2 percent, heavy drinkers; and 21 percent, binge drinkers.

 College women are as likely to drink as men and, increasingly to drink in the same dangerous ways. According to the College Alcohol Study findings, approximately two in five undergraduates—female as well as male—report binge drinking.[64] At women's colleges fewer women students (about one in three) binge, but this represents a major increase from a decade ago.

Women and men vary in the reasons why and the ways in which they drink. (See "The X&Y File: "Why Men and Women Drink" on page 372.) Depression affects drinking in both sexes. Major depressive episodes increased the risk of harmful drinking among women.[65] Both not drinking and driving heavily are characteristic of young men with high levels of depression and emotional distress.[66]

Their bodies also respond to alcohol in different ways. Because they have a far smaller quantity of a protective enzyme in the stomach to break down alcohol before it's absorbed into the bloodstream, women absorb about 30 percent more alcohol into their bloodstream than men. The alcohol travels through the blood to the brain, so women become intoxicated much more quickly. And because there's more alcohol in the bloodstream to break down, the liver may also be adversely affected. In alcoholic women, the stomach seems to completely stop digesting alcohol, which may explain why women alcoholics are more likely to suffer liver damage than men.

Both men and women experience blackouts after heavy drinking, but women black out after consuming half as much alcohol as men. Women also may be more susceptible to alcohol-induced memory problems when given comparable amounts of alcohol.[67] In addition, they are at greater risk of engaging in risky behavior, including unprotected sex, than men. Drinking games increase the risks for women, particularly of sexual assault, rape, and attempted rape.[68]

Recent research, discussed earlier in this chapter, has revealed a connection between women's alcohol consumption and their risk of breast cancer. Other gender-specific health problems caused by alcohol include:

:: **Reproductive and sexual dysfunction.** Alcohol interferes with male sexual function and fertility through direct effects on testosterone and the testicles. In half of alcoholic men, increased levels of female hormones lead to breast enlargement and a feminine pubic hair pattern. Damage to the nerves in the penis by heavy drinking can lead to impotence. In women who drink heavily, a drop in female hormone production may cause menstrual irregularity and infertility. Women who binge, particularly white women, are at greater risk of unintended pregnancies.[69]

:: **Fetal Alcohol Effects and Fetal Alcohol Syndrome.** Binge drinking during pregnancy also increases the risk of Sudden Infant Death Syndrome.[70] In a recent study, 15 percent of women drank alcohol while pregnant; most reported having one drink or less per day. Even light consumption of alcohol can lead to **Fetal Alcohol Effects (FAE):** low birth-weight, irritability as newborns, and permanent mental impairment.

The babies of women who consume three or more ounces of alcohol (the equivalent of six or seven cocktails) are at risk of more severe problems. One of every 750 newborns has a cluster of physical and mental defects called **Fetal Alcohol Syndrome (FAS):** small head, abnormal facial features, jitters, poor muscle tone, sleep disorders, sluggish motor development, failure to thrive, short stature, delayed speech, mental retardation, and hyperactivity.

:: **Osteoporosis.** As women age, their risk of osteoporosis, a condition characterized by calcium loss and bone thinning, increases. Alcohol can block the absorption of many nutrients, including calcium, and heavy drinking may worsen the deterioration of bone tissue.

:: **Heart disease.** Women who are very heavy drinkers are more at risk of developing irreversible heart disease than men who drink even more.

A child with fetal alcohol syndrome (FAS) has distinctive facial characteristics that vary with the severity of the disease, including droopy eyelids, a thin upper lip, and a wide space between the nose and upper lip.

© K. L. Jones/LLR Research

Alcohol Problems

About 20 percent of Americans are at-risk drinkers whose alcohol consumption exceeds the limits recommended by government studies (two drinks a day for men, one for women). These individuals are at increased risk of high blood pressure, stroke, violence, motor vehicle accidents, injury, and certain types of cancer.

By the simplest definition, problem drinking is the use of alcohol in any way that creates difficulties, potential difficulties, or health risks for an individual. Like alcoholics, problem drinkers are individuals whose lives are in some way impaired by their drinking. The only difference is one of degree. Alcohol becomes a problem, and a person becomes an alcoholic, when the drinker can't "take it or leave it." He or she spends more and more time anticipating the next drink, planning when and where to get it, buying and hiding alcohol, and covering up secret drinking. (See Table 11-3.)

Alcohol abuse involves continued use of alcohol despite awareness of social, occupational, psychological, or physical problems related to drinking, or drinking in dangerous ways or situations (before driving, for instance). A diagnosis of alcohol abuse is based on one or more of the following occurring at any time during a 12-month period:

:: A failure to fulfill major role obligations at work, school, or home (such as missing work or school).

TABLE 11-3	Recognizing the Warning Signs of Alcoholism		
• Experiencing the following symptoms after drinking: frequent headaches, nausea, stomach pain, heartburn, gas, fatigue, weakness, muscle cramps, irregular or rapid heartbeats. • Needing a drink in the morning to start the day.	• Denying any problem with alcohol. • Doing things while drinking that are regretted afterward. • Dramatic mood swings, from anger to laughter to anxiety. • Sleep problems.	• Depression and paranoia. • Forgetting what happened during a drinking episode. • Changing brands or going on the wagon to control drinking. • Having five or more drinks a day.

:: The use of alcohol in situations in which it is physically hazardous (such as before driving).

:: Alcohol-related legal problems (such as drunk-driving arrests).

:: Continued alcohol use despite persistent or recurring social or interpersonal problems caused or exacerbated by alcohol (such as fighting while drunk).

Alcohol dependence is a separate disorder in which individuals develop a strong craving for alcohol because it produces pleasurable feelings or relieves stress or anxiety. Over time they experience physiological changes that lead to *tolerance* of its effects; this means that they must consume larger and larger amounts to achieve intoxication. If they abruptly stop drinking, they suffer *withdrawal,* a state of acute physical and psychological discomfort. A diagnosis of alcohol dependence is based on three or more of the following symptoms occurring during any 12-month period:

:: Tolerance, as defined by either a need for markedly increased amounts of alcohol to achieve intoxication or desired effect, or a markedly diminished effect with continued drinking of the same amount of alcohol as in the past.

:: Withdrawal, including at least two of the following symptoms: sweating, rapid pulse, or other signs of autonomic hyperactivity; increased hand tremor; insomnia; nausea or vomiting; temporary hallucinations or illusions; physical agitation or restlessness; anxiety; or grand mal seizures.

:: Drinking to avoid or relieve the symptoms of withdrawal.

:: Consuming larger amounts of alcohol, or drinking over a longer period than was intended.

:: Persistent desire or unsuccessful efforts to cut down or control drinking.

:: A great deal of time spent in activities necessary to obtain alcohol, drink it, or recover from its effects.

:: Important social, occupational, or recreational activities given up or reduced because of alcohol use.

:: Continued alcohol use despite knowledge that alcohol is likely to cause or exacerbate a persistent or recurring physical or psychological problem.

More than 8 million Americans are alcohol-dependent; an additional 5.6 million abuse alcohol.[71] According to a survey of more than 14,000 undergraduates at four-year colleges, 6 percent of college students met criteria for a diagnosis of alcohol dependence or alcoholism, 31 percent for alcohol abuse. More than two of every five students reported at least one symptom of these conditions and were at increased risk of developing a true alcohol disorder. Few reported seeking treatment since coming to college.

Alcoholism, as defined by the National Council on Alcoholism and Drug Dependence and the American

Alcohol dependence may spring from the perception that alcohol relieves stress or creates a pleasant feeling. Daytime drinking and drinking alone can be a sign of a serious problem, even though the drinker may otherwise appear to be in control.

Society of Addiction, is a primary, chronic disease in which genetic, psychosocial, and environmental factors influence its development and manifestations. The disease is often progressive and fatal. Its characteristics include an inability to control drinking, a preoccupation with alcohol, continued use of alcohol despite adverse consequences, and distorted thinking, most notably denial. Like other diseases, alcoholism is not simply a matter of insufficient willpower, but a complex problem that causes many symptoms, can have serious consequences, yet can improve with treatment.

A lack of obvious signs of alcoholism can be deceiving. A person who doesn't drink in the morning but feels that he or she must always have a drink at a certain time of the day may have lost control over his or her drinking. A person who never drinks alone but always drinks socially with others may be camouflaging loss of control. A person who is holding a job or taking care of the family may still spend every waking hour thinking about that first drink at the end of the day (preoccupation).

Probably fewer than 5 percent of alcoholics and problem drinkers are "skid-row drunks." The other 95 percent are all around us, every day. (See Self-Survey: "Do You Have a Drinking Problem?") Alcoholism generally first appears between the ages of 20 and 40, although even children and young teenagers can become alcoholics. It takes 5 to 15 years of heavy drinking for an adult to become alcoholic, but just 6 to 18 months for an adolescent to develop the disease.

Types of Alcoholism

Mental health professionals have developed different theoretical models to explain alcoholism. Although these models are used mainly by researchers and clinicians, they offer individuals with drinking problems and those close to them some insight into various personality and drinking patterns.

According to one long-established model, there are two primary types of alcoholics. *Type I*, or milieu-limited, alcoholics generally start heavy drinking, often in response to setbacks, losses, or other external circumstances, after age 25. They can abstain for long periods of time and frequently feel loss of control, guilt, and fear about their alcoholism. They also have characteristic personality traits: they tend to be anxious, shy, pessimistic, sentimental, emotionally dependent, rigid, reflective, and slow to anger. Because alcohol reduces their anxiety level, it serves as a positive reinforcer for continued use and contributes to the development of alcohol dependence.

Type II alcoholics are close relatives of an alcoholic male and become heavy drinkers before age 25. They drink regardless of what is going on in their lives; have frequent fights and arrests; and do not usually experience guilt, fear, or loss of control over their drinking. Unlike Type I alcoholics, they are impulsive and aggressive risk-

takers, curious, excitable, quick-tempered, optimistic, and independent. Alcohol reinforces their feelings of euphoria and pleasant excitement. Often they abuse drugs as well as alcohol.

Newer research on male and female alcoholics classifies alcoholics as *Type A* or *Type B*. Type A alcoholism is a milder form, characterized by onset later in life, fewer childhood risk factors, less severe dependence, fewer alcohol-related physical and social consequences, fewer symptoms of other mental disorders, and less interference with work and family. Type B alcoholism is linked with childhood and familial risk factors, begins at an earlier age, involves more severe dependence and abuse of other substances, leads to more serious consequences, and often occurs along with other mental disorders. Type B alcoholics are younger, more inclined to experiment with other drugs and are more anxious, and of lower occupational status than Type A alcoholics.

What Causes Alcohol Dependence and Abuse?

Although the exact cause of alcohol dependence and abuse is not known, certain factors—including biochemical imbalances in the brain, heredity, cultural acceptability, and stress—all seem to play a role. They include the following:

:: **Genetics.** Scientists who are working toward mapping the genes responsible for addictive disorders have not yet been able to identify conclusively a specific gene that puts people at risk for alcoholism. However, epidemiological studies have shown evidence of heredity's role. Studies of twins—identical, who share the same genes, and fraternal, who like other siblings share about half their genes—suggest that heredity accounts for two-thirds of the risk of becoming alcoholic in both men and women. An identical twin of an alcoholic is twice as likely as a fraternal twin to have an alcohol-related disorder. The incidence of alcoholism is four times higher among the sons of Caucasian alcoholic fathers, regardless of whether they grow up with their biological or adoptive parents. The sons of alcoholic fathers have characteristic changes in brain wave activity.

:: **Stress and traumatic experiences.** Many people start drinking heavily as a way of coping with psychological problems. About half of all individuals who abuse or are dependent on alcohol also have another mental disorder. Alcohol often is linked with depressive and anxiety disorders. Men and women with these problems may start drinking in an attempt to alleviate their anxiety or depression.

:: **Parental alcoholism.** According to researchers, alcoholism is four to five times more common among the

Self Survey   **Do You Have a Drinking Problem?**

This self-assessment, the Michigan Alcoholism Screening Test (MAST), is widely used to identify potential problems. This test screens for the major psychological, sociological, and physiological consequences of alcoholism.

To complete it, simply answer Yes or No to the following questions, and add up the points shown in the right column for your answers.

	Yes	No	Points
1. Do you enjoy a drink now and then?			(0 for either)
2. Do you think that you're a normal drinker? (By normal, we mean that you drink less than or as much as most other people.)			(2 for no)
3. Have you ever awakened the morning after some drinking the night before and found that you couldn't remember part of the evening?			(2 for yes)
4. Does your wife, husband, a parent, or other near relative ever worry or complain about your drinking?			(1 for yes)
5. Can you stop drinking without a struggle after one or two drinks?			(2 for no)
6. Do you ever feel guilty about your drinking?			(1 for yes)
7. Do friends or relatives think that you're a normal drinker?			(2 for no)
8. Do you ever try to limit your drinking to certain times of the day or to certain places?			(0 for either)
9. Have you ever attended a meeting of Alcoholics Anonymous?			(2 for yes)
10. Have you ever gotten into physical fights when drinking?			(1 for yes)
11. Has your drinking ever created problems for you and your wife, husband, a parent, or other relative?			(2 for yes)

	Yes	No	Points
12. Has your wife, husband, or other family members ever gone to anyone for help about your drinking?			(2 for yes)
13. Have you ever lost friends because of your drinking?			(2 for yes)
14. Have you ever gotten into trouble at work or school because of your drinking?			(2 for yes)
15. Have you ever lost a job because of your drinking?			(2 for yes)
16. Have you ever neglected your obligations, your family, or your work for two or more days in a row because of drinking?			(2 for yes)
17. Do you drink before noon fairly often?			(1 for yes)
18. Have you ever been told you have liver trouble? cirrhosis?			(2 for yes)
19. After heavy drinking, have you ever had delirium tremens (DTs) or severe shaking, or heard voices or seen things that weren't actually there?			(2 for yes*)
20. Have you ever gone to anyone for help about your drinking?			(5 for yes)
21. Have you ever been in a hospital because of your drinking?			(5 for yes)
22. Have you ever been a patient in a psychiatric hospital or on a psychiatric ward of a general hospital where drinking was part of the problem that resulted in hospitalization?			(2 for yes)

children of alcoholics, who may be influenced by the behavior they see in their parents. The sons and daughters of alcoholics share certain characteristics, including early onset of problem drinking with severe social consequences, an unstable family, poor academic and social performance in school, and antisocial behavior. By some estimates, one of five college students comes from an alcoholic home and may be at increased risk of developing a drinking problem. More than two of every five students report at least one symptom of alcohol abuse or dependence and are at increased risk of developing a true alcohol disorder.[72]

:: **Drug abuse.** Alcoholism is also associated with the abuse of other psychoactive drugs, including mari-

juana, cocaine, heroin, amphetamines, and various antianxiety medications. Adults under age 30 and adolescents are most likely to use alcohol plus several drugs of abuse, such as marijuana and cocaine. Middle-aged men and women are more likely to combine alcohol with benzodiazepines, such as antianxiety medications or sleeping pills, which may be prescribed for them by a physician. Whatever the reason they start, some people keep drinking out of habit. Once they develop physical tolerance and dependence—the two hallmarks of addiction—they may not be able to stop drinking on their own.

Self Survey | **Do You Have a Drinking Problem?**

Yes   No   Points

23. Have you ever been seen at a psychiatric or mental health clinic or gone to any doctor, social worker, or clergyman for help with any emotional problem where drinking was part of the problem? _____ _____ (2 for yes)

24. Have you ever been arrested for drunk driving, driving while intoxicated, or driving under the influence of alcoholic beverages? _____ _____ (2 for yes)

25. Have you ever been arrested, or taken into custody, even for a few hours, because of drunken behavior? _____ _____ (2 for yes)
(If Yes, How many times? _____ **)

*Five points for delirium tremens

**Two points for each arrest

Scoring:
In general, five or more points places you in an alcoholic category; four points suggests alcoholism; while three or fewer points indicates that you're *not* alcoholic.

Your Health Change Plan
for Responsible Drinking

:: **Don't drink alone.** Cultivate friendships with non-drinkers and responsible moderate drinkers.

:: **Don't use alcohol as a medicine.** Rather than reaching for a drink to put you to sleep, help you relax, or relieve tension, develop alternative means of unwinding, such as exercise, meditation, or listening to music.

:: **Develop a party plan.** Set a limit on how many drinks you'll have before you go out—and stick to it.

:: **Alternate alcoholic and nonalcoholic drinks.** At a social occasion, have a nonalcoholic beverage to quench your thirst.

:: **Drink slowly.** Never have more than one drink an hour.

:: **Eat before and while drinking.** Choose foods high in protein (cheese, meat, eggs, or milk) rather than salty foods, like peanuts or chips, that increase thirst.

:: **Be wary of mixed drinks.** Fizzy mixers, like club soda and ginger ale, speed alcohol to the blood and brain.

:: **Don't make drinking the primary focus of any get-together.** Cultivate other interests and activities that you can enjoy on your own or with friends.

:: **Learn to say no.** A simple "Thank you, but I've had enough" will do.

:: **Stay safe.** During or after drinking, avoid any tasks, including driving, that could be affected by alcohol.

Medical Complications of Alcohol Abuse and Dependence

Excessive alcohol use adversely affects virtually every organ system in the body, including the brain, the digestive tract, the heart, muscles, blood, and hormones (look back at Figure 11-3). In addition, because alcohol interacts with many drugs, it can increase the risk of potentially lethal overdoses and harmful interactions. Among the major risks and complications are:

:: **Liver disease.** Because the liver is the organ that breaks down and metabolizes alcohol, it is especially vulnerable to its effects. Chronic heavy drinking can lead to alcoholic hepatitis (inflammation and destruction of liver cells) and, in the 15 percent of people who continue drinking beyond this stage, cirrhosis (irreversible scarring and destruction of liver cells). The liver eventually may fail completely, resulting in coma and death.

:: **Cardiovascular disease.** Heavy drinking can weaken the heart muscle (causing cardiac myopathy), elevate blood pressure, and increase the risk of stroke. The combined use of alcohol and tobacco greatly increases the likelihood of damage to the heart.

:: **Cancer.** Heavy alcohol use may contribute to cancer of the liver, stomach, and colon, as well as malignant melanoma, a deadly form of skin cancer. Alcohol, in combination with tobacco use, also increases the risk of cancer of the mouth, tongue, larynx, and

Mark Nielsen (both)

A normal liver (top) compared to one with cirrhosis.

esophagus. Regular drinkers significantly increase their risk of rectal cancer, but that risk is reduced if wine makes up a third or more of weekly consumption.[73]

:: **Brain damage.** Chronic brain damage resulting from alcohol consumption is second only to Alzheimer's disease as a cause of cognitive deterioration in adults. Long-term heavy drinkers may suffer memory loss, and be unable to think abstractly, recall names of common objects, and follow simple instructions.

:: **Vitamin deficiencies.** Alcoholics often tend to have very poor nutrition. Alcoholism is associated with vitamin deficiencies, especially of thiamin (B_1), which may be responsible for certain diseases of the neurological, digestive, muscular, and cardiovascular systems. Lack of thiamin may result in Wernicke-Korsakoff syndrome, which is characterized by disorientation, memory failure, hallucinations, and jerky eye movements, and can be disabling enough to require lifelong custodial care.

:: **Digestive problems.** Alcohol triggers the secretion of acids in the stomach that irritate the mucous lining and cause gastritis. Chronic drinking may result in peptic ulcers (breaks in the stomach lining) and bleeding from the stomach lining.

:: **Accidents and injuries.** Alcohol may contribute to almost half of the deaths caused by car accidents, burns, falls, and choking. Nearly half of those convicted and jailed for criminal acts committed these crimes while under the influence of alcohol.

:: **Higher mortality.** As discussed earlier, the mortality rate for alcoholics is two to three times higher than that for nonalcoholics of the same age. Injury is the leading alcohol-related cause of death, chiefly in auto accidents involving a drunk driver. Digestive disease, most notably cirrhosis of the liver, is second. Alcohol is a factor in about 30 percent of all suicides. Alcoholics who attempt suicide may have other risk factors, including major depression, poor social support, serious medical illness, and unemployment.

◼ Alcoholism Treatments

Almost 600,000 Americans undergo treatment for alcohol-related problems every year. Until recent years, the only options for professional alcohol treatment were, as one expert puts it, "intensive, extensive, and expensive," such as residential programs at hospitals or specialized treatment centers. Today individuals whose drinking could be hazardous to their health may choose from a variety of approaches. Treatment that works well for one person may not work for another. As research into the outcomes of alcohol treatments has grown, more attempts have been made to match individuals to approaches tailored to their needs and more likely to help them overcome their alcohol problems.

Men and women who have seriously remained sober for more than a decade credit a variety of approaches, including Alcoholics Anonymous (AA), individual psychotherapy, and other groups, such as Women for Sobriety. There is no one sure path to sobriety,—a wide variety of treatments may offer help and hope to those with alcohol-related problems. In one of the few studies to follow adolescents for four years after alcohol treatment, about half either completely stopped drug and alcohol involvement or substantially reduced their use. Very few abstained entirely from any substances; over a third of youth treated showed fluctuations in their usage patterns over four years.[74]

Detoxification

The first phase of treatment for alcohol dependence focuses on **detoxification,** the gradual withdrawal of alcohol from the body. For 90 to 95 percent of alcoholics, withdrawal symptoms are mild to moderate. They include sweating; rapid pulse; elevated blood pressure; hand tremor; insomnia; nausea or vomiting; malaise or weakness; anxiety; depressed mood or irritability; headache; and temporary hallucinations or illusions. Withdrawal can be life-threatening when accompanied by medical problems, such as grand mal seizures, pneumonia, liver failure, or gastrointestinal bleeding.

Alcohol withdrawal delirium, commonly known as **delirium tremens,** or **DTs,** is most common in chronic heavy drinkers who also suffer from a physical illness, fatigue, depression, or malnutrition. Delirium tremens are characterized by agitated behavior, delusions, rapid heart rate, sweating, vivid hallucinations, trembling hands, and fever. The symptoms usually appear over several days after heavy drinking stops. Individuals frequently report terrifying visual hallucinations, such as seeing insects all over their bodies. With treatment, most cases subside after several days, although delirium tremens has been known to last as long as four or five weeks. In some cases, complications such as infections or heart arrhythmias prove fatal.

Are There Medications That Treat Alcoholism?

Antianxiety and antidepressive drugs are sometimes used in early treatment for alcoholism, especially for those with underlying mental disorders. Several medications, including certain antidepressant drugs that increase the neurotransmitter serotonin, are being studied as medical interventions to reduce cravings or prevent relapses. Two new medications, naltrexone and acamprosate, also have shown promise. Vitamin supplements, especially thiamin and folic acid, can help overcome some of the nutritional deficiencies linked with alcoholism.

The drug disulfiram (Antabuse), given to deter drinking, causes individuals to become nauseated and acutely ill when they consume alcohol. Antabuse interrupts the removal of acetaldehye by the liver, so this toxic substance accumulates and causes nausea or vomiting. If individuals taking Antabuse drink at all or consume foods with alcoholic content, they become extremely ill. They must avoid foods cooked or marinated in wine and cough syrup preparations containing alcohol. Some individuals have reactions to the alcohol in after-shave lotion. A large amount of alcohol can make them dangerously ill; fatalities have occurred. Side effects are usually mild and include drowsiness, bad breath, skin rash, and temporary impotence. Because Antabuse does not reduce cravings for alcohol, psychotherapy and support groups remain a necessary part of treatment.

Inpatient or Residential Treatment

In the past, 28-day treatment programs in a medical or psychiatric hospital or a residential facility were the cornerstone of early recovery treatment. According to outcome studies, inpatient treatment was effective, with as many as 70 percent of "graduates" remaining abstinent or stable, nonproblem drinkers for five years after. However, because of cost pressures from the insurance industry, the length of stay has been reduced, and there's been increasing emphasis on outpatient care.

Outpatient Treatment

Outpatient treatment may involve group therapy, individual supportive therapy, marital or family therapy, regular attendance at Alcoholics Anonymous (AA) or another support group, brief interventions, and relapse prevention. According to outcome studies, intensive outpatient treatment at a day hospital (with individuals returning home every evening) are as effective as inpatient care. Outpatient therapy continues for at least a year, but many individuals continue to participate in outpatient programs for the rest of their lives.

Brief Interventions

These methods include individual counseling, group therapy, and training in specific skills—such as assertiveness—all packed into a six- to eight-week period. Offered at a growing number of centers, brief interventions may be most helpful for problem drinkers who are not physically dependent on alcohol. They have proven effective in reducing alcohol consumption up to one year compared with no intervention or standard care. However, at ten years, there is no difference in alcohol consumption among those who had a brief intervention and those who did not. This indicates the need for follow-up advice and counseling.[75]

Moderation Training

Highly controversial, this approach uses cognitive-behavioral techniques, such as keeping a diary to chart drinking patterns and learning "consumption management" techniques, such as never having more than one drink an hour.

Treatment programs in other countries, such as Great Britain and Canada, have long offered moderation training for problem drinkers who consume too much alcohol. However, most experts agree that the best—and perhaps only—hope for recovery for chronic alcoholics who are physically dependent on alcohol is complete abstinence.

Self-Help Programs

The best-known and most commonly used self-help program for alcohol problems is Alcoholics Anonymous (AA), which was founded more than 60 years ago and which has grown into an international organization that includes 2 million members and 185,000 groups worldwide. Acknowledging the power of alcohol, AA offers support from others struggling with the same illness, from a sponsor available at any time of the day or night, and from fellowship meetings that are held every day of the year. Because anonymity is a key part of AA, it has been difficult for researchers to study its success, but it is generally believed to be a highly effective means of overcoming alcoholism and maintaining abstinence. Its 12 steps, which emphasize honesty, sobriety, and acknowledgment of a "higher power," have become the model for self-help groups for other addictive behaviors, including drug abuse (discussed in Chapter 10) and compulsive eating.

The average age of entry into AA is 30; about 60 percent of the members are men. Members encompass a wide range of ages, occupations, nationalities, and socioeconomic classes. People generally attend 12-step meetings every day when they first begin recovery; most programs recommend 90 meetings in 90 days. Many people taper off to one or two meetings a week as their recovery progresses. No one knows exactly how 12-step programs help people break out of addictions. Some individuals stop their drinking, or other destructive behavior, simply on the basis of the information they get at meetings. Others bond to the group and use it as a social support and refuge while they explore and release their inner feelings—a process similar to what happens in psychotherapy.

Alternatives to AA

Secular Organizations for Sobriety (SOS) was founded in 1986 as an alternative for people who couldn't accept the spirituality of AA. Like AA, SOS holds confidential meetings, celebrates sobriety anniversaries, and views recovery as a one-day-at-a-time process.

Rational Recovery, which also emphasizes anonymity and total abstinence, focuses on the self rather than spirituality. Members use reason instead of prayer and learn to control the impulse to drink by learning how to control the emotions that lead them to drink.

One of the most effective programs for women is Women for Sobriety, founded in 1975 by sociologist Jean Kirkpatrick, Ph.D. Its meetings focus on building self-esteem, self-confidence, and responsibility. "AA was started by men, and its message is very disempowering for women," said Kirkpatrick. "We view members as competent women who are struggling with issues that all women must face. Women don't need to recall the painful process of becoming alcoholics. They need to put the past behind them and move on, upward and onward."[76]

Recovery

Recovery from alcoholism is a lifelong process of personal growth and healing. The first two years are the most difficult, and relapses are extremely common. By some estimates, more than 90 percent of those recovering from substance use will use alcohol or drugs in any one 12-month period after treatment. However, approximately 70 percent of those who get formal treatment stop drinking for prolonged periods. Even without treatment, 30 percent of alcoholics are able to stop drinking for long periods. Those most likely to remain sober after treatment have the most to lose by continuing to drink: they tend to be employed, married, and upper-middle class.

Most recovering alcoholics experience urges to drink, especially during early recovery when they are likely to feel considerable stress. These urges are a natural consequence of years of drinking and diminish with time. Mood swings are common during recovery, and individuals typically describe themselves as alternately feeling relieved or elated and then discouraged or tearful. Such disconcerting ups and downs also decrease over time. Patience—learning to take "one day at a time"—is crucial.

Increasingly, treatment programs focus on **relapse prevention,** which includes the development of coping strategies and learning techniques that make it easier to live with alcohol cravings and rehearsal of various ways of saying "no" to offers of a drink. According to outcomes research, social skills training—a combination of stress management therapy, assertiveness and communication skills training, behavioral self-control training, and behavioral marital therapy—has proven effective in decreasing the duration and severity of relapses after one year in a group of alcoholics.

◼ Alcoholism's Impact on Relationships

Alcoholism shatters families and creates unhealthy patterns of communicating and relating. Separation and divorce rates are high among alcoholics. Another common occurrence is **codependence,** a term used to describe the behavior of close family members or friends who act in ways that enable their spouses, parents, or friends to continue their self-destructive behavior.

Codependence and Enabling

Codependent spouses of alcoholics follow a predictable pattern of behavior: While trying to control the drinkers, they act in ways that enable the drinkers to keep drinking. If an alcoholic finds it hard to get up in the morning, his wife wakes him up, pulls him out of bed and into the shower, and drops him off at work. If he is late, she makes excuses to his boss. By helping him evade his responsibilities, his wife is helping him continue drinking. Indeed, he might not be able to keep up his habit without her cooperation.

Such behavior is harmful for individuals who are dependent on alcohol because it reinforces their denial. They do not feel out of control or powerless over alcohol because the person or persons closest to them are constantly protecting them from the consequences of their actions. Every crisis—a missed deadline, a forgotten appointment, a child's disappointment when a parent doesn't come to an important event—should be seen as a chance for the individual to recognize what alcohol is doing to the lives of all those close to him or her. If family members let their loved one experience the consequences of drinking, the person may be able to come to the moment of truth concerning alcohol.

Codependents often need help in acknowledging their own feelings and needs. National self-help organizations, such as Al-Anon, help adult family members recognize dysfunctional behaviors in their relationships and start looking at their own problems. Similar self-help groups, such as Alateen, provide support for the teenaged children of alcoholics. These organizations also help family members cope with their loved one's alcoholism—whether or not codependence is a problem.

Growing Up with an Alcoholic Parent

An estimated 28 million children in the United States (or one of every four) are living in a household with an alcoholic adult.[77] Parental alcoholism increases the likelihood of childhood ADHD, conduct disorder, and anxiety disorders. The experience often leads youngsters to play certain roles: The adjuster or "lost child" does whatever the parent says. The responsible child, or "family hero," typically takes over many household tasks and responsibilities. The acting-out child, or "scapegoat," shows his or her anger early in life by causing problems at home or in school and taking on the role of troublemaker. The "mascot" disrupts tense situations by focusing attention on himself or herself, often by clowning. Regardless of which roles they assume, the children of alcoholics are prone to learning disabilities, eating disorders, and addictive behavior.

Numerous studies have linked child abuse and neglect to parental drinking. Children of women who are problem drinkers have twice the risk of serious injury as children of mothers who don't drink. Children with two parents who are problem drinkers are at even higher risk. As teenagers, children of alcoholics are more likely to report early sexual intercourse and face a greater risk of adolescent pregnancy.

Adult Children of Alcoholics

Growing up with an alcoholic parent can have a long-lasting effect. Adult children of alcoholics are at risk for many problems. Some try to fill the emptiness inside with alcohol, drugs, or addictive habits. Others find themselves caught up in destructive relationships that repeat the patterns of their childhood. They are likely to have difficulty solving problems, identifying and expressing their feelings, trusting others, and being intimate. In addition to their own increased risk of addictive behavior, they are likely to marry individuals with some form of addiction and keep on playing out the roles of their childhood. They may feel inadequate, not know how to set limits or recognize normal behavior, be perfectionistic, and want to control all aspects of their lives. However, not all adult children are alike or necessarily suffer from psychological problems or face an increased risk of substance abuse themselves.

Because the impact of alcoholism can be so enduring, support groups—such as Adult Children of Alcoholics, Children of Alcoholics, and Adult Children of Dysfunctional Families—have spread throughout the country in the last decade. These organizations provide adult children of alcoholics a mutually supportive group setting to discuss their childhood experiences with alcoholic parents and the emotional consequences they carry into adult life. Through such groups or other forms of therapy, individuals may learn to move beyond anger and blame, see the part they themselves play in their current state of unhappiness, and create a future that is healthier and happier than their past.

STRATEGIES FOR CHANGE

If Someone Close to You Drinks Too Much

- Try to remain calm, unemotional, and factually honest in speaking about the drinker's behavior. Include the drinker in family life.

- Discuss the situation with someone you trust: a member of the clergy, social worker, friend, or someone who has experienced alcoholism directly.

- Never cover up or make excuses for the drinker, or shield him or her from the consequences of drinking. Assuming the drinker's responsibilities undermines his or her dignity and sense of importance.

- Refuse to ride with the drinker if he or she is driving while intoxicated.

- Encourage new interests and participate in leisure-time activities that the drinker enjoys.

- Try to accept setbacks and relapses calmly.

The Bottom Line ▼
Taking Charge of Your Alcohol Use

Problems with drinking aren't just the serious ones such as drunk driving and alcoholism. They can start with minor problems, such as missing classes and term paper deadlines. Or they can start with the belief that a party is no fun unless there is a bottle or a six-pack.

As you decide about the role alcohol should play in your life, you might want to follow these guidelines, proposed by BACCHUS, a volunteer college student organization that promotes responsible alcohol-related behavior:

:: Set a limit on how many drinks you're going to have ahead of time—and stick to it.

:: When you're mixing a drink, measure the alcohol.

:: Alternate non-alcoholic and alcoholic drinks.

:: Drink slowly; don't guzzle.

:: Eat before and while drinking.

:: Develop alternatives to drinking so you don't turn to alcohol whenever you're depressed or upset. Exercise is a wonderful release for tension; meditation or relaxation techniques can also help you cope.

:: Avoid performing tasks that require skilled reactions during or after drinking.

:: Don't encourage or reinforce others' irresponsible behavior.

Above all, keep in mind that drinking should not be the primary focus of any activity. Responsible drinking is a matter of you controlling your drinking rather than the drinking controlling you.

CNN. After watching the CNN video segment, discuss the following questions. Based on the information you have read in the chapter, is Odansetron a viable candidate for long-term treatment? What other therapeutic methods could produce successful treatment?

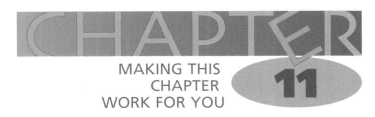

MAKING THIS
CHAPTER
WORK FOR YOU   **11**

1. An individual's response to alcohol depends on all of the following *except*

  a. the rate at which the drink is absorbed into the body's tissues.
  b. the blood alcohol concentration.
  c. socioeconomic status.
  d. gender and race.

2. Which of the following statements about the effects of alcohol on the body systems is true?
  a. In most individuals, alcohol sharpens the responses of the brain and nervous system, enhancing sensation and perception.
  b. Moderate drinking may have a positive effect on the cardiovascular system.
  c. French researchers have found that drinking red wine with meals may have a positive effect on the digestive system.
  d. The leading alcohol-related cause of death is liver damage.

3. Responsible drinking includes which of the following behaviors?
  a. avoiding eating while drinking because eating speeds up absorption of alcohol
  b. limiting alcohol intake to no more than four drinks in an hour
  c. taking aspirin while drinking to lower your risk of a heart attack
  d. socializing with individuals who limit their alcohol intake

4. Which of the following statements about drinking on college campuses is true?
  a. The percentage of students who abstain from alcohol has increased.
  b. The number of women who binge drink has decreased.
  c. Because of peer pressure, students in fraternities and sororities tend to drink less than students in dormitories.
  d. Students who live in substance-free dormitories tend to binge drink when alcohol is available.

5. Racial and ethnic patterns related to alcohol use include which of the following?
  a. Asian-American women tend to have higher rates of alcoholism than Asian-American men.
  b. Socioeconomic conditions increase the likelihood of alcohol problems in African Americans and Native Americans.
  c. White Americans tend to have higher rates of cirrhosis of the liver than African Americans or Native Americans.
  d. The Latino culture discourages men from drinking because heavy drinking indicates a lack of machismo.

6. Women who have drinking problems
  a. often have suffered from fetal alcohol syndrome as a result of their mothers' alcohol consumption.

b. are less likely to have an alcoholic parent than men with drinking problems.

c. are at higher risk for osteoporosis than women who are not heavy drinkers.

d. are less likely to suffer liver damage than men.

7. Alcoholism

a. is considered a chronic disease with genetic, psychosocial, and environment components.

b. is characterized by a persistent lack of willpower.

c. may be classified as either Type A, which affects people who are high-strung, or Type B, which affects people who are more mild mannered.

d. is easily controlled by avoiding exposure to social situations where drinking is common.

8. Which of the following statements about alcohol abuse and dependence is *false?*

a. Alcohol dependence involves a persistent craving for and an increased tolerance to alcohol.

b. An individual may have a genetic predisposition for developing alcoholism.

c. Alcoholics often abuse other psychoactive drugs.

d. Alcohol abuse and alcohol dependence are different names for the same problem.

9. Health risks of alcoholism include all of the following *except*

a. hypertension.

b. lung cancer

c. peptic ulcers.

d. hepatitis.

10. Which of the following statements about alcoholism treatment is true?

a. Inpatient treatment has been shown to be more effective than outpatient treatment.

b. Alcoholism can be cured by detoxifying or ridding the body of all traces of alcohol.

c. Antabuse is a medication given to alcoholics with underlying mental disorders.

d. A combination of medical, behavioral, and self-help approaches may be necessary to treat alcohol abuse and dependence.

Answers to these questions can be found on page 652.

Critical Thinking

1. Driving home from his high school graduation party, 18-year-old Rick has had too much to drink. As he crosses the dividing line on the two-lane road, the driver of an oncoming car—a young mother with two young children in the backseat—swerves to avoid an accident. She hits a concrete wall and dies instantly, but her children survive. Rick has no record of drunk driving. Should he go to prison? Is he guilty of manslaughter? How would you feel if you were the victim's husband? If you were Rick's friend?

2. Some groups concerned about alcohol abuse advocate greater restrictions on availability, such as prohibiting the sale of alcoholic beverages in supermarkets, convenience stores, and gas stations. They would like to see a ban on advertisements, especially those aimed at young people. Opponents argue that laws have never been effective in controlling alcohol abuse. Do you think our society is too permissive in the way we allow alcohol to be promoted or sold? Would you support anti-alcohol laws? Why or why not?

3. Have you ever been around people who have been intoxicated when you have been sober? What did you think of their behavior? Were they fun to be around? Was the experience not particularly enjoyable, boring, or difficult in some way? Have you ever been intoxicated? How do you behave when you are drunk? Do you find the experience enjoyable? What do the people around you think of your actions when you are drunk?

4. What effects has alcohol use had in your life? Try making a list of the positive and negative effects your own alcohol use has had. Be specific. If you continue to drink at your current rate, what positive and negative effects do you think it will have on your future? What effects has other people's drinking had on your life? List family members and friends who drink regularly, and how their drinking has affected you.

Profile Plus

Excessive drinking can cause long-term health problems. How is alcohol affecting you? Find out with these activities on your Profile Plus CD-ROM:

Profile Plus

• Do You Have a Drinking Problem?

Profile Plus

• Addictive Behavior Questionnaires

Sites and Bytes

Facts On Tap: Alcohol and Your College Experience
www.factsontap.org

The Children of Alcoholics Foundation and the American Council for Drug Education, two of the nation's leaders in substance abuse prevention education, sponsor this excellent website written specifically for college students. The interactive site features activities and straightforward information, including alcohol and the college experience, the effects of alcohol on the nondrinker, alcohol and the family, and a true/false quiz to test your knowledge about alcohol and its effects.

Sites and Bytes

Students Against Destructive Decisions (SADD)
www.saddonline.com

This site features resources and relevant information to empower students to help their peers understand the consequences of destructive decisions related to alcohol use and abuse, and to live safe and happy lives.

Sites and Bytes

BACCHUS & GAMMA Peer Education Network for Colleges
www.bacchusgamma.org

This site designed for college students and health services professionals features information on college and university peer health education programs focusing on alcohol abuse prevention and other student health and safety issues.

InfoTrac College Edition

Activity

Hingson, Ralph, et al. "Early Age of First Drunkenness as a Factor in College Students' Unplanned and Unprotected Sex Attributable to Drinking." *Pediatrics,* Vol. 111, No. 1, January 2003, p. 34(8).

1. What is the relationship between age of first alcohol use and 1) the rate of alcohol dependency later in life and 2) the rate of unplanned sexual activity?

InfoTrac College Edition

2. What variables that are significantly related to age of first intoxication were measured by this study and what was the correlation?

3. According to the researchers, what factors should be considered when interpreting the results of this study?

InfoTrac College Edition

You can find additional readings related to alcohol use with InfoTrac College Edition, an online library of more than 900 journals and publications. Follow the instructions for access that were packaged with your textbook; then search for articles using a key word search.

For additional links, resources, and suggested readings on InfoTrac College Edition, visit our Health & Wellness Resource Center at **http://health.wadsworth.com**.

Key Terms

The terms listed are used on the page indicated. Definitions of the terms are in the Glossary at the end of this book.

absorption 363
alcohol abuse 379
alcohol dependence 380
alcoholism 380
binge drinking 371
blood-alcohol
    concentration
    (BAC) 362

codependence 386
delirium tremens
    (DTs) 384
detoxification 384
ethyl alcohol 362
fetal alcohol effects
    (FAE) 379

fetal alcohol syndrome
    (FAS) 379
intoxication 364
proof 362
relapse prevention 386

References

1. National Institute on Alcohol Abuse and Alcoholism, www.niaaa.nih.gov.
2. "Alcohol and Your Waistline." *Harvard Men's Health Watch,* July 2003, p. 1.
3. "Alcohol Consumption and Waist Circumference." *Nutrition Research Newsletter,* Vol. 22, No. 5, May 2003, p. 5.
4. "Regular Alcohol Consumption is Good for the Heart." *Harvard Health Letter,* Vol. 28, No. 6, April 2003, p. 1.
5. Kuritzky, Louis. "Relation Between Alcohol Consumption and C-Reactive Protein Levels in the Adult United States Population." *Clinical Oncology Alert,* Vol. 18, No. 3, March 2003, p. 5.
6. "To Drink or Not to Drink?" *Internal Medicine Alert,* Vol. 25, No. 6, March 29, 2003, p. 44.
7. Jancin, Bruce. "Cardiovascular Benefits of Alcohol Challenged." *Family Practice News,* Vol. 33, No. 6, March 15, 2003, p. 12.
8. "Alcohol and Hormone Therapy Increase the Risk of Breast Cancer." *OB/GYN Clinical Alert,* January 2003, p. 68.
9. "Drinking Increases Risk." *Women's Health Weekly,* February 6, 2003, p. 2.
10. Robb-Nicholson, Celeste. "Alcohol and Breast Cancer." *Harvard Women's Health Watch,* Vol. 10, No. 9, May 2003, p. 1.
11. Mukamai, Kenneth, et al. "Prospective Study of Alcohol Consumption and Risk of Dementia in Older Adults." *Journal of the American Medical Association,* Vol. 289, No. 11, March 19, 2003, p. 1405.
12. Fillmore, Kaye, et al. "Changes in Drinking Status, Serious Illness and Mortality." *Journal of Studies on Alcohol,* Vol. 64, No. 2, March 2003, p. 278.
13. "Drinking Pattern, Alcohol Severity Studied." *The Brown University Digest of Addiction Theory and Application,* Vol. 22, No. 4, April 2003, p. S1.

14. Carpenter, Christopher. "Seasonal Variation in Self-Reports of Recent Alcohol Consumption: Racial and Ethnic Differences." *Journal of Studies on Alcohol,* Vol. 64, No. 3, May 2003, p. 415.
15. "Binge Drinking: Not Just About Teenagers." *Tufts University Health & Nutrition Letter,* Vol. 20, No. 12, February 2003, p. 2.
16. "Underage Drinkers and Adult Excessive Drinkers Account for Half of Consumption in U.S." *Medical Letter on the CDC & FDA,* March 23, 2003, p. 4.
17. Hingston, Ralph, et al. "Age of First Intoxication, Heavy Drinking, Driving and Drinking and Risk of Unintentional Injury Among U.S. College Students." *Journal of Studies on Alcohol,* Vol. 64, No. 1, January 2003, p. 23.
18. "Alcohol Consumption and Waist Circumference."
19. Schulenberg, John, and Jennifer Maggs. "A Developmental Perspective on Alcohol Use and Heavy Drinking During Adolescence and the Transition to Young Adulthood." *Journal of Studies on Alcohol,* Vol. 63, No. 2, March 2002, p. 54.
20. Wechsler, Henry, et al. "Trend in College Binge Drinking During a Period of Increased Prevention Efforts." *Journal of American College Health,* Vol. 50, No. 5, March 2002, p. 203.
21. www.hsph.harvard.edu/cas.
22. McKinnon, Sarab, et al. "Increased Risk of Alcohol Abuse Among College Students Living on the U.S.-Mexico Border: Implications for Prevention." *Journal of American College Health,* Vol. 51, No. 4, January 2003, p. 149.
23. Harford, T. C., et al. "Attendance and Alcohol Use at Parties and Bars in College: A National Survey of Current

Drinkers." *Journal of Studies on Alcohol,* Vol. 63, No. 6, November 2002, pp. 726–733.
24. Nelson, T. F., and H. Wechsler. "School Spirits: Alcohol and Collegiate Sports Fans." *Addictive Behaviors,* Vol. 28, No. 1, 2003, p. 1.
25. Anding, Jenna, et al. "Dietary Intake, Body Mass Index, Exercise, and Alcohol." *Journal of American College Health,* Vol. 49, January 2001, p. 167.
26. Borsari, Brian, et al. "Self-Reported Drinking Game Participation of Incoming College Students." *Journal of American College Health,* Vol. 51, No. 4, January 2003, p. 149.
27. Hussong, A. M. "Social Influences in Motivated Drinking Among College Students," *Psychology of Addictive Behaviors,* Vol. 17, No. 2, June 2003, p. 142.
28. Wood, Mark, et al. "Social Influence Processes and College Student Drinking: The Mediational Role of Alcohol Outcome Expectancies." *Journal of Studies on Alcohol,* Vol. 62, No. 1, January 2001, p. 32.
29. Hildebran, Kathryn, and Dewaynef Johnson. "Comparison of Patterns of Alcohol Use Between High School and College Athletes and Nonathletes." *Research Quarterly for Exercise and Sport,* Vol. 72, No. 1, March 2001, p. A-30.
30. Glassman, Tavis. "The Failure of Higher Education to Reduce the Binge Drinking Rate." *Journal of American College Health,* Vol. 51, No. 3, November 2002, p. 143.
31. Wechsler et al. "Trend in College Binge Drinking During a Period of Increased Prevention Efforts."

References

32. Harford, T. C., et al. "The Impact of Current Residence and High School Drinking on Alcohol Problems Among College Students." *Journal of Studies on Alcohol*, Vol. 63, No. 3, May 2002, p. 271.

33. "NIAAA Study Finds Extensive Damage from College Drinking." *Alcoholism & Drug Abuse Weekly*, Vol. 14, No. 15, April 15, 2002, p. 6.

34. "Binge Drinkers More Likely to Abuse Additional Substances." *Brown University Digest of Addiction Theory and Application*, Vol. 21, No. 3, March 2002, p. 2.

35. Wechsler, Henry, et al. "Binge Drinking on America's College Campuses." Harvard School of Public Health, 2001. Available at www.hsph.harvard.edu/cas.

36. Wechsler et al. "Trend in College Binge Drinking During a Period of Increased Prevention Efforts."

37. Cariati, Sophia. "More Young Women Drinking, Suffering Disproportionate Consequences." News Release, Society for Women's Health Research, April 12, 2002.

38. Weitzman, Elissa, et al. "Taking Up Binge Drinking in College: The Influences of Person, Social Group, and Environment." *Journal of Adolescent Health*, Vol. 32, No. 1, January 2003, p. 26.

39. Weitzman, Elissa, et al. "The Relationship of Alcohol Outlet Density to Heavy and Frequent Drinking and Drinking-Related Problems Among College Students at Eight Universities." *Health and Place*, Vol. 9, 2003, p. 1.

40. Brower, Aaron. "Are College Students Alcoholics?" *Journal of American College Health*, Vol. 50, No. 5, March 2002, p. 253.

41. Wechsler, H., et al. "Underage College Students' Drinking Behavior, Access to Alcohol, and the Influence of Deterrence Policies: Findings from the Harvard School of Public Health College Alcohol Study." *Journal of American College Health*, Vol. 50, 2002, pp. 223–236.

42. Ibid.

43. Hingston et al., "Age of First Intoxication, Heavy Drinking, Driving after Drinking, and Risk of Unintentional Injury."

44. Jones, Sherry, et al. "Binge Drinking Among Undergraduate College Students in the United States: Implications for Other Substance Use." *Journal of American College Health*, Vol. 50, No. 1, July 2001, p. 33.

45. *Substance Use and Risky Sexual Behavior*. Menlo Park, CA: Henry J. Kaiser Family Foundation, 2002.

46. Steinman, Kenneth. "College Students' Early Cessation from Episodic Heavy Drinking: Prevalence and Correlates." *Journal of American College Health*, Vol. 51, No. 5, March 2003, p. 197.

47. Jones et al., "Binge Drinking Among Undergraduate College Students in the United States."

48. Wechsler, Henry, et al. "Drinking Levels, Alcohol Problems, and Secondhand Effects in Substance-Free College Residences: Results of a National Study." *Journal of Studies on Alcohol*, Vol. 62, No. 1, January 2001, p. 23.

49. Wechsler, Henry, et al. "Secondhand Effects of Student Alcohol Use Reported by Neighbors of Colleges." *Social Science & Medicine*, Vol. 55, No. 3, July 2002, p. 425.

50. Ziemelis, Andris, et al. "Prevention Efforts Underlying Decreases in Binge Drinking at Institutions of Higher Education." *Journal of American College Health*, Vol. 50, No. 5, March 2002, p. 238.

51. "Survey Reveals High Prevalence of AIDs among students," *The Brown University Digest of Addiction Theory and Application*, Vol. 22, No. 3, March 2003, p. 4.

52. Steinman, "College Students' Early Cessation."

53. Wilenz, Pam. "Greek Membership Does Not Predict Post-College Drinking Levels." *American Psychological Association*, March 1, 2001.

54. "Colleges Work to Reduce Heavy Drinking Among Students." *Alcoholism and Drug Abuse Weekly*, Vol. 15, No. 15, April 14, 2003, p. 8.

55. Faden, Vivian, and Marcy Baskin. "An Evaluation of College Online Alcohol-Policy Information." *Journal of American College Health*, Vol. 51, No. 3, November 2002, p. 101.

56. Minto, Scott, et al. "A New Approach to Student Alcohol Abuse at Georgetown University." *Journal of American College Health*, Vol. 51, No. 2, September 2002, p. 81.

57. "Report Gives Colleges Failing Grades for Reducing College Binge Drinking." *Alcoholism & Drug Abuse Weekly*, Vol. 14, No. 13, April 1, 2002, p. 1.

58. "Colleges Report More Alcohol, Drug Violations." *Alcoholism & Drug Abuse Weekly*, Vol. 14, No. 14, April 8, 2002, p. 7.

59. Harris, Rebecca. "Party Patrol: Squad Fights for Alcohol-Free Fun." *Careers & Colleges*, Vol. 22, No. 4, March 2002, p. 5.

60. Dalrymple, John, et al. "The Effects of Alcohol on Driving-Related Sensorimotor Performance Across Four Times of Day." *Journal of Studies on Alcohol*, Vol. 64, No. 1, January 2003, p. 93.

61. Hingston et al., "Age of First Intoxication, Heavy Drinking, Driving after Drinking, and Risk of Unintentional Injury."

62. Timmerman, M. A., et al. "Do the Designated Drivers of College Students Stay Sober?" *Journal of Safety Research*, Vol. 34, No. 2, 2003, p. 127.

63. Sempos, C. T., et al. "Average Volume of Alcohol Consumption and All-Cause Mortality in African Americans: The NHEFS Cohort." *Alcoholism, Clinical and Experimental Research*, Vol. 27, No. 1, 2003, p. 88.

64. www.hsph.harvard.edu/cas.

65. "Female Drinkers and Drug Users Tend to Have More Depressive Disorders." *Women's Health Weekly*, March 20, 2003, p. 4.

66. Caldwell, T. M., et al. "Young Men Who Do Not Drink, as Well as Those Who Drink Heavily, Have High Levels of Depression and Distress." *Evidence-Based Mental Health*, Vol. 6, No. 1, 2003, p. 13.

67. White, Aaron, et al. "Prevalence and Correlates of Alcohol-Induced Blackouts among College Students: Results of an E-Mail Survey." *Journal of American College Health*, Vol. 51, No. 3, November 2002, p. 117.

68. Borsari et al., "Self-Reported Drinking Game Participation."

69. "Binge Drinking Linked to Unintended Pregnancies." *The Brown University Digest of Addiction Theory and Application*, Vol. 22, No. 6, June 2003, p. 51.

70. "Binge Drinking and SIDS." *Family Practice News*, Vol. 33, No. 6, March 15, 2003, p. 40.

71. Foster, Susan, et al. "Alcohol Consumption and Expenditures for Underage Drinking and Adult Excessive Drinking." *Journal of the American Medical Association*, Vol. 289, No. 6, February 26, 2003, p. 989.

References

72. O'Malley, Patrick, et al. "Epidemiology of Alcohol and Other Drug Use Among American College Students." *Journal of Studies on Alcohol,* Vol. 63, No. 2, March 2002, p. 23.
73. "Alcohol and Rectal Cancer Risk." *The Lancet,* Vol. 361, No. 9370, May 17, 2003, p. 1713.

References

74. Brown, Sandra, et al. "Four-Year Outcomes from Adolescent Alcohol and Drug Treatment." *Journal of Studies on Alcohol,* Vol. 62, No. 3, May 2001, p. 381.
75. Wutzke, S. "At 10 Year Follow Up, Brief Interventions Had No Effect on Harmful Alcohol Consumption." *Evidence-Based*

References

Mental Health, Vol. 6, No. 1, February 2003, p. 31.
76. Kirkpatrick, Jean. Personal interview.
77. "When Parents Have a Drinking Problem." *Contemporary Pediatrics,* Vol. 18, No. 1, January 2001, p. 67.

Tobacco Use, Misuse, and Abuse

Andrea didn't really want her first cigarette. Her tent mate at camp had snatched one from a counselor's pack, and the two of them had climbed to a remote rock to share it. Andrea hated everything about her first drag: the taste, the smell, the horrible burning in her throat and lungs. But she loved feeling more grown-up and sophisticated than other seventh graders. By the time she reached high school, Andrea would sneak off to smoke with friends at least once a week. By graduation, she was smoking daily.

As a college freshmen, Andrea discovered that she was part of an unpopular minority. Even though her dorm didn't ban smoking, her roommate declared their room a smoke-free zone. Her college didn't allow smoking in any classrooms or public areas. And many of her new friends reacted as if smoking was a sign of impaired intelligence. Andrea has decided to quit, but she's discovered that nicotine dependence is very difficult to overcome. "I just wish I'd never started smoking in the first place," she says.

According to the National Household Survey on Drug Abuse, 25 percent of Americans age 12 and older—some 56 million persons—smoked part or all of a cigarette during the past month. College-age young adults have the highest percentage of smokers.[1] The more and the longer they smoke, the greater their risks of heart disease, respiratory problems, several types of cancer, and a shortened lifespan.[2]

Despite widespread awareness of the dangers of tobacco, smoking continues to kill more people than AIDS, alcohol, drug abuse, car crashes, murders, suicides, and fires combined. Nationally, smoking results in more than 5 million years of potential life lost each year.

This chapter discusses the effects of tobacco on the body, smoking patterns, tobacco dependence, quitting smoking, smokeless tobacco, and environmental tobacco smoke. The information it provides may help you to breathe easier today—and may help ensure cleaner air for others to breathe tomorrow.

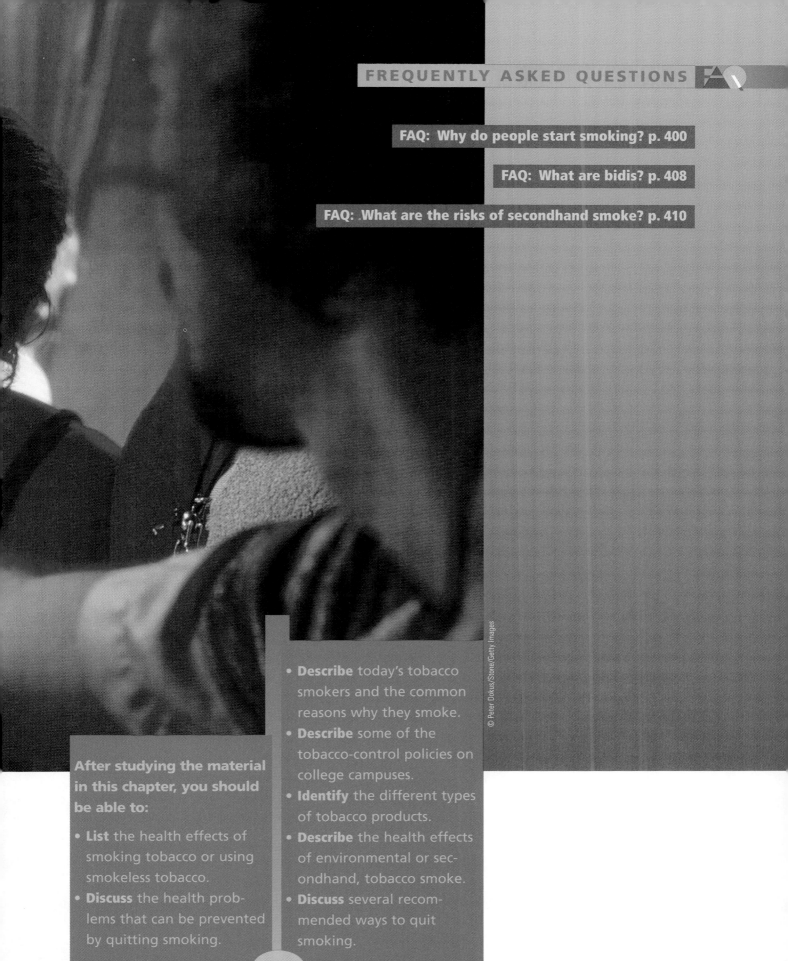

© Peter Dakus/Stone/Getty Images

- **Describe** today's tobacco smokers and the common reasons why they smoke.
- **Describe** some of the tobacco-control policies on college campuses.
- **Identify** the different types of tobacco products.
- **Describe** the health effects of environmental or secondhand, tobacco smoke.
- **Discuss** several recommended ways to quit smoking.

After studying the material in this chapter, you should be able to:

- **List** the health effects of smoking tobacco or using smokeless tobacco.
- **Discuss** the health problems that can be prevented by quitting smoking.

Tobacco's Immediate Effects

Tobacco, an herb that can be smoked or chewed, directly affects the brain. While its primary active ingredient is nicotine, tobacco smoke contains almost 400 other compounds and chemicals, including gases, liquids, particles, tar, carbon monoxide, cadmium, pyridine, nitrogen dioxide, ammonia, benzene, phenol, acrolein, hydrogen cyanide, formaldehyde, and hydrogen sulfide.

How Nicotine Works

A colorless, oily compound, **nicotine** is poisonous in concentrated amounts. If you inhale while smoking, 90 percent of the nicotine in the smoke is absorbed into your body. Even if you draw smoke only into your mouth and not into your lungs, you still absorb 25 to 30 percent of the nicotine. The FDA has concluded that nicotine is a dangerous, addictive drug that should be regulated.

Faster than an injection, smoking speeds nicotine to the brain in seconds. (See Figure 12-1.) Nicotine affects the brain in much the same way as cocaine, opiates, and amphetamines, triggering the release of dopamine, a neurotransmitter associated with pleasure and addiction, as well as other messenger chemicals. Because nicotine acts on some of the same brain regions stimulated by interactions with loved ones, smokers come to regard cigarettes as friends that they turn to when they're stressed, sad, or mad.[3]

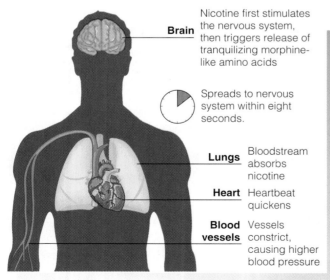

Figure 12-1 THE IMMEDIATE EFFECTS OF NICOTINE ON THE BODY

The primary active ingredient in tobacco is nicotine, a fast-acting and potent drug.

Sources: American Cancer Society, National Cancer Institute.

Nicotine may enhance smokers' performance on some tasks but leaves other mental skills unchanged. Nicotine also acts as a sedative. How often you smoke and how you smoke determine nicotine's effect on you. If you're a regular smoker, nicotine will generally stimulate you at first, then tranquilize you. Shallow puffs tend to increase alertness because low doses of nicotine facilitate the release of the neurotransmitter *acetylcholine,* which makes the smoker feel alert. Deep drags, on the other hand, relax the smoker because high doses of nicotine block the flow of acetylcholine.

Nicotine stimulates the adrenal glands to produce adrenaline, a hormone that increases blood pressure, speeds up the heart rate by 15 to 20 beats a minute, and constricts blood vessels (especially in the skin). Nicotine also inhibits the formation of urine, dampens hunger, irritates the membranes in the mouth and throat, and dulls the taste buds so foods don't taste as good as they would otherwise. Nicotine is a major contributor to heart and respiratory diseases.

Tar and Carbon Monoxide

As it burns, tobacco produces **tar,** a thick, sticky dark fluid made up of several hundred different chemicals—many of them poisonous, some of them *carcinogenic* (enhancing the growth of cancerous cells). As you inhale tobacco smoke, tar and other particles settle in the forks of the branchlike bronchial tubes in your lungs, where precancerous changes are apt to occur. In addition, tar and smoke damage the mucus and the cilia in the bronchial tubes, which normally remove irritating foreign materials from your lungs.

Smoke from cigarettes, cigars, and pipes also contains **carbon monoxide,** the deadly gas that comes out of the exhaust pipes of cars, in levels 400 times those considered safe in industry. Carbon monoxide interferes with the ability of the hemoglobin in the blood to carry oxygen, impairs normal functioning of the nervous system, and is at least partly responsible for the increased risk of heart attacks and strokes in smokers.

Health Effects of Cigarette Smoking

Figure 12-2 shows a summary of the physiological effects of tobacco and the other chemicals in tobacco smoke. If you're a smoker who inhales deeply and started smoking before the age of 15, you're trading a minute of future life for every minute you now spend smoking. On average smokers die nearly seven years earlier than nonsmokers.[4] Smoking not only eventually kills, it also ages you: Smokers get more wrinkles than nonsmokers.

Brain
- Alters mood-regulating chemicals
- Stimulates cravings for more nicotine

Mouth and throat
- Dulls taste buds
- Irritates the membranes

Lungs
- Damages the air sacs, which affects the lungs' ability to bring in oxygen and remove carbon dioxide
- Increases mucus secretion in the bronchial tubes, which narrows air passages

Heart
- Increases heart rate Increases blood pressure by constricting blood vessels
- Affects the oxygen-carrying ability of hemoglobin so less oxygen reaches the heart

Adrenal glands
- Stimulates adrenaline production

Kidneys
- Inhibits formation of urine

Figure 12-2 SOME EFFECTS OF SMOKING ON THE BODY

But the effects of smoking are far more than skin-deep. A cigarette smoker is 10 times more likely to develop lung cancer than a nonsmoker, and 20 times more likely to have a heart attack. Moreover, the danger of lung cancer skyrockets when smokers are also exposed to other carcinogens, such as asbestos. This double threat increases the risk of lung cancer to as much as 92 times that for non-smokers not exposed to asbestos.

Heart Disease and Stroke

The toxic chemicals in tobacco signal the heart to beat faster and harder. Blood vessels constrict, forcing blood to travel through a narrower space. Blood pressure increases—temporarily at first. Over time smokers develop chronic high blood pressure. Smoking also increases harmful cholesterol (LDL) and lowers beneficial cholesterol (HDL), the buildup of plaques, or fatty deposits within the arteries, the hardening of the arteries, and the risk of blood clots.[5]

Although a great deal of publicity has been given to the link between cigarettes and lung cancer, heart attack is actually the leading cause of deaths for smokers. Smoking doubles the risk of heart disease and increases the risk of sudden death two to four times. The effect of smoking on risk of heart attack is greater in younger smokers.[6]

Smokers who suffer heart attacks have only a 50 percent chance of recovering. Smokers have a 70 percent higher death rate from heart disease than nonsmokers, and those who smoke heavily have a 200 percent higher death rate.

The federal Office of the Surgeon General blames cigarettes for one of every ten deaths attributable to heart disease. Smoking is more dangerous than the two most notorious risk factors for heart disease: high blood pressure and high cholesterol. If smoking is combined with one of these, the chances of heart attack are four times greater. Women who smoke and use oral contraceptives have a ten times higher risk of suffering heart attacks than women who do neither.

Smoking also causes a condition called *cardiomyopathy*, which weakens the heart's ability to pump blood and results in the death of about 10,000 people a year.

Smoking doubles your risk of heart disease and stroke.

Although researchers don't know precisely how smoking poisons the heart muscle, they speculate that either nicotine or carbon monoxide has a direct toxic effect.

Other coronary diseases may be associated with smoking. *Aortic aneurysm* is a bulge in the aorta (the large artery attached to the heart) caused by a weakening of its walls. *Pulmonary heart disease* is a heart disorder caused by changes in blood vessels in the lungs.

Even people who have smoked for decades can reduce their risk of heart attack if they quit smoking. However, studies indicate some irreversible damage to blood vessels. Progression of atherosclerosis (hardening of the arteries) among former smokers continues at a faster pace than among those who never smoked.

In addition to contributing to heart attacks, cigarette smoking increases the risk of stroke two to three times in men and women, even after other risk factors are taken into account.

The risk of heart disease drops about 50 percent after one year's abstinence and continues to decline gradually. After 5 to 10 years, an ex-smoker's risk of heart disease or stroke is similar to that of a person who has never smoked.[7]

Cancer

The American Cancer Society estimates that tobacco smoking is the cause of 28 percent of all deaths from cancer and the cause of more than 85 to 90 percent of all cases of lung cancer. The more people smoke, the longer they smoke, and the earlier they start smoking, the more likely they are to develop lung cancer.

Smoking causes 130,000 lung cancer deaths each year.[8] Smokers of two or more packs a day have lung cancer mortality rates 15 to 25 times greater than nonsmok-

ers. If smokers stop smoking before cancer has started, their lung tissue tends to repair itself, even if there were already precancerous changes. Former smokers who haven't smoked for 15 or more years have lung cancer mortality rates only somewhat above those for nonsmokers.

Chemicals in cigarette smoke and other environmental pollutants switch on a particular gene in the lung cells of some individuals. This gene produces an enzyme that helps manufacture powerful carcinogens, which set the stage for cancer. The gene seems more likely to be activated in some people than others, and people with this gene are at much higher risk of developing lung cancer. However, smokers without the gene still remain at risk, because other chemicals and genes also may be involved in the development of lung cancer.

Smokers who are depressed are more likely to get cancer than nondepressed smokers. Although researchers don't know exactly how smoking and depression may work together to increase the risk of cancer, one possibility is that stress and depression cause biological changes that lower immunity, such as a decline in natural killer cells that fight off tumors.

Using a new online interactive prediction tool, physicians can assess a longtime smoker's risk based on a person's age, sex, and smoking history. Screening with low-dose computed tomography (CT) scans can help diagnose the disease earlier than in the past.[9] Yet despite some advances in treating lung cancer, the prognosis for sufferers is not good. Even with vigorous therapy, fewer than 10 percent survive for five years after diagnosis. This is one of the lowest survival rates of any type of cancer. And if the cancer has spread from the lungs to other parts of the body, only 1 percent survive for five years after diagnosis.

Respiratory Diseases

Smoking quickly impairs the respiratory system, including the cough reflex, a vital protective response.[10] Even some teenage smokers show signs of respiratory difficulty— breathlessness, chronic cough, excess phlegm production— when compared with nonsmokers of the same age. Cigarette smokers are up to 18 times more likely than nonsmokers to die of noncancerous diseases of the lungs.

Cigarette smoking is the major cause of chronic obstructive lung disease (COLD), which includes emphysema and chronic bronchitis. COLD is characterized by progressive limitation of the flow of air into and out of the lungs. In emphysema, the limitation of air flow is the result of disease changes in the lung tissue, affecting the bronchioles (the smallest air passages) and the walls of the alveoli (the tiny air sacs of the lung). Eventually, many of the air sacs are destroyed, and the lungs become much less able to bring in oxygen and remove carbon dioxide. As a result, the heart has to work harder to deliver oxygen to all organs of the body.

Healthy nonsmoker's lung (left) and smoker's lung (right). Healthy lungs are pink, with a smooth but porous texture. Smokers' lungs show obvious signs of impairment—bronchial tubes are inflamed, air passages are constricted, and tar coats the bronchial tubes.

In chronic bronchitis, the bronchial tubes in the lungs become inflamed, thickening the walls of the bronchi, and the production of mucus increases. The result is a narrowing of the air passages. Smoking is more dangerous than any form of air pollution, at least for most Americans, but exposure to both air pollution and cigarettes is particularly harmful. Although each may cause bronchitis, together they have a synergistic effect—that is, their combined impact exceeds the sum of their separate effects.

Other Smoking-Related Problems

Smokers are more likely than nonsmokers to develop gum disease, and they lose significantly more teeth. Even those who quit have worse gum problems than people who never smoked at all. Smoking may also contribute to the loss of teeth and teeth supporting bone, even in individuals with good oral hygiene.

Cigarette smoking is associated with stomach and duodenal ulcers; mouth, throat, and other types of cancer; and cirrhosis of the liver. Smoking may worsen the symptoms or complications of allergies, diabetes, hypertension, peptic ulcers, and disorders of the lungs or blood vessels. Some men who smoke ten cigarettes or more a day may experience erectile dysfunction.[11] Cigarette smokers also tend to miss work one-third more often than nonsmokers, primarily because of respiratory illnesses. In addition, each year cigarette-ignited fires claim thousands of lives.

Smoking is an independent risk factor for high-frequency hearing loss and also adds to the danger of hearing loss for those exposed to noise.[12] (See Chapter 19.) Cigarette smoking also may increase the likelihood of anxiety, panic attacks, and social phobias.

Smoking and Medication

Smokers use more medications—aspirin, painkillers, sleeping pills, tranquilizers, antihistamines, cough medicines, stomach medicines, laxatives, diuretics, and antibiotics—than nonsmokers do. According to the American Pharmaceutical Association, nicotine and other tobacco ingredients speed up the process by which the body uses and eliminates drugs, so they may not be able to do what they're intended to do. As a result, smokers may have to take a medication more frequently than do nonsmokers. If you smoke, let your physician know so that he or she can adjust any prescriptions, if necessary.

◗ The Impact of Tobacco

Tobacco use, particularly cigarette smoking, is the leading preventable cause of death in the United States, claiming approximately 440,000 lives each year.[13] It accounts for about one in every five deaths in the United States and between $50 billion and $73 billion in medical expenses. Globally some 1.2 billion people smoke, three-quarters in developing countries. Tobacco consumption claims 4.9 million lives a year, a toll that is expected to double by 2020.

In rich countries, after years of advertising restrictions and campaigns warning of the health risks of smoking, consumers are starting to kick the habit. But consumption is still growing strongly in poorer countries. According to WHO (World Health Organization), 50,000 Asian

STRATEGIES FOR PREVENTION

Why Not to Light Up

Before you start smoking—before you ever face the challenge of quitting—think of what you have to gain by *not* smoking:

- A significantly reduced risk of cancer of the lungs, larynx, mouth, esophagus, pancreas, and bladder.

- Half the risk of heart disease that smokers face.

- A lower risk of stroke, chronic obstructive lung disease (COLD), influenza, ulcers, and pneumonia.

- A lower risk of having a low-birthweight baby.

- A longer lifespan.

- Potential savings of tens of thousands of dollars that you would otherwise spend on tobacco products and medical care.

teenagers start smoking each day. In the Philippines, more than half of children aged seven to 17 smoke.[14]

Financial Cost of Smoking

Tobacco costs society almost three times as much as any other category of drug.[15] (See Fact or Fiction? "American taxpayers pay . . .") The total cost of cigarette smoking to American society includes greater work absenteeism, higher insurance premiums, increased disability payments, and the training costs to replace employees who die prematurely from smoking. In the course of a lifetime, the average smoker can expect to spend tens of thousands of dollars on cigarettes—but that's only the beginning. The potential costs for medical services for a man between the ages of 35 and 39 who smokes heavily may run $60,000 or higher. But the greatest toll—the pain and suffering of cancer victims and their loved ones—obviously cannot be measured in dollars and cents.

Why Do People Start Smoking?

Most people are aware that an enormous health risk is associated with smoking, but many don't know exactly what that risk is or how it might affect them.

The two main factors linked with the onset of a smoking habit are age and education. The vast majority of white men with less than a high school education are current or former daily cigarette smokers. White women with a similar educational background are also very likely to smoke or to have smoked every day. Hispanic men and women without a high school education are less likely to be or become daily smokers. Other factors associated with

the reasons for smoking are discussed in the following sections.

Genetics

Researchers speculate that genes may account for about 50 percent of smoking behavior, with environment playing an equally important role.[16] Studies have shown that identical twins, who have the same genes, are more likely to have matching smoking profiles than fraternal twins. If one identical twin is a heavy smoker, the other is also likely to be; if one smokes only occasionally, so does the other.

According to Swedish research that has followed 25,000 pairs of same-sex twins since 1886, smoking patterns in men suggested both genetic and environmental influences. The smoking patterns in female twins, however, were quite different. Among those born before 1925, when smoking was socially unacceptable for women, the overall rate of smoking was low and the genetic influence was absent. However, among those born after 1940, when smoking had become much more acceptable for women, rates of tobacco use increased and the role of genetic influences rose as well—essentially to the same level as that among men. This suggests that some individuals do have a strong genetic predisposition toward tobacco use. However, when smoking is strongly discouraged, they do not express that genetic tendency. On the other hand, if smoking is socially acceptable, the genetic tendency to smoke emerges.

Parental Role Models

Children who start smoking are 50 percent more likely than youngsters who don't smoke to have at least one smoker in their family. A mother who smokes seems a

FACT OR FICTION? ??????????????

American taxpayers pay a higher price for every pack of cigarettes sold in the United States than the smoker who buys it.

Fact: Every purchase of a pack of cigarettes adds $7.18 to the nation's tax bill to cover medical costs and lost productivity due to smoking. This works out to $3,391 per smoker per year. Since about 22 billion packs of cigarettes are sold in the United States each year, the health-related economic costs come to an estimated $157 million a year.

Source: "What Others' Smoking Costs You." *Vibrant Living,* Vol. 19, No. 1, January–February 2003, p. 7.

A parent's smoking habit influences the way a child thinks about smoking.

© Peter Poulides/Stone/Getty Images

particularly strong influence on making smoking seem acceptable. The majority of youngsters who smoke say that their parents also smoke and are aware of their own tobacco use.

Adolescent Experimentation and Rebellion

For teenagers, smoking may be a coping mechanism for dealing with boredom and frustration; a marker of the transition into high school or college; a bid for adult status; a way of gaining admission to a peer group; or a way to have fun, reduce stress, or boost energy. The teenagers most likely to begin smoking are those least likely to seek help when their emotional needs are not met. They might smoke as a means of gaining social acceptance or to self-medicate when they feel helpless, lonely, or depressed. Adolescents are more likely to smoke, express an intention to smoke, or smoke longer if their parents smoked. Depressed teens are more susceptible to cigarette ads than their counterparts. For example, one recent study showed that depressed teens are more likely to have a favorite cigarette ad or own clothing with cigarette logos.[17]

Teens often misjudge the addictive power of cigarettes. Many, sure that they'll be able to quit any time they want, figure that smoking for a year or two won't hurt them. But when they try to quit, they can't. Like older smokers, most young people who smoke have tried to quit at least once.

Depression and Smoking

The relationship between depression and smoking is complex. Smokers are more likely to be depressed, while adults who are depressed are 40 to 50 percent more likely to smoke than adults who are not depressed. Recent research has identified biological connections between smoking and depression, suggesting a biological similarity between substance use and depressive disorders.[18]

Limited Education

People who have graduated from college are much less likely to smoke than high school graduates; those with fewer than 12 years of education are more likely to smoke. An individual with 8 years or less of education is 11 times more likely to smoke than someone with postgraduate training.

Weight Control

Concern about weight is a significant risk factor for smoking among young women.[19] Daily smokers are two to four times more likely to fast, use diet pills, and purge to control their weight than nonsmokers. Although black girls smoke at substantially lower rates than white girls, the common factor in predicting daily smoking among all girls, regardless of race, is concern with weight.[20]

Aggressive Marketing

Cigarette companies spend billions of dollars each year on advertisements and promotional campaigns, with manufacturers targeting ads especially at women, teens, minorities, and the poor. Most controversial are cigarette advertisements in magazines and media aimed at teenagers and even younger children.

Stress

In studies that have analyzed the impact of life stressors, depression, emotional support, marital status, and income, researchers have concluded that an individual with a high stress level is approximately 15 times more likely to be a smoker than a person with low stress. About half of smokers identify workplace stress as a key factor in their smoking behavior.

Addiction

Nicotine addiction is as strong, or stronger than, addiction to drugs such as cocaine and heroin.[21] According to recent research, the first symptoms of nicotine addiction can begin within a few days of starting to smoke and after just a few cigarettes, particularly in teenagers.[22] The findings, based on a study of almost 700 adolescents, challenges the conventional belief that nicotine dependence is a gradual process that takes hold after prolonged daily smoking.

Why People Keep Smoking

Whatever the reasons for lighting up that first cigarette, very different factors keep cigarettes burning pack after pack, year after year. In national polls, seven in ten smokers say that they want to quit but can't. The reason isn't a lack of willpower. Medical scientists have recognized tobacco dependence as an addictive disorder that may be more powerful than heroin dependence and that may affect more than 90 percent of all smokers.

Pleasure

According to the American Cancer Society, nine in ten regular smokers find smoking pleasurable. Nicotine—the addictive ingredient in tobacco—is the reason. Researchers have shown that nicotine reinforces and strengthens the desire to smoke by acting on brain chemicals that influence feelings of well-being. This drug also can improve memory, help in performing certain tasks, reduce anxiety, dampen hunger, and increase pain tolerance.

Mental Disorders

Individuals with mental disorders are twice as likely to smoke as others, and people with mental illness may account for nearly one-half of the tobacco market in the United States. Heavy smoking also is linked with an almost elevenfold risk of anxiety disorders in early adulthood.

Smokers with a history of depression are about half as likely to quit as others. Even after a recovery from major depression, smokers often continue to report some symptoms of depression. Smokers who are depressed tend to smoke more cigarettes than other smokers, are less successful in their efforts to stop smoking, and are more prone to depression after quitting. The longer people smoke, the more likely they are to develop symptoms of depression and anxiety.[23]

Fear of Weight Gain

Smokers burn up an extra 100 calories a day—the equivalent of walking a mile—probably because nicotine increases metabolic rate. Once they start smoking, many individuals say they cannot quit because they fear they'll gain weight. The CDC estimates that women who stop smoking gain an average of 8 pounds, while men put on an average of 6 pounds. One in eight women and one in ten men who stop smoking put on 29 pounds or more. The reasons for this weight gain include nicotine's effects on metabolism as well as emotional and behavioral factors, such as the habit of frequently putting something into one's mouth. Yet as a health risk, smoking a pack and a half to two packs a day is a greater danger than carrying 60 pounds of extra weight.

Weight gain for smokers who quit is not inevitable. Aerobic exercise helps increase metabolic rate, and limiting alcohol and foods high in sugar and fat can help smokers control their weight as they give up cigarettes.

Dependence

Nicotine has a much more powerful hold on smokers than alcohol does on drinkers. Whereas about 10 percent of alcohol users lose control of their intake of alcohol and become alcoholics, as many as 80 percent of all heavy smokers have tried to cut down on or quit smoking but cannot overcome their dependence.

Nicotine causes dependence by at least three means:

:: It provides a strong sensation of pleasure.

:: It leads to fairly severe discomfort during withdrawal.

:: It stimulates cravings long after obvious withdrawal symptoms have passed.

Few drugs act as quickly on the brain as nicotine does. It travels through the bloodstream to the brain in seven seconds—half the time it takes for heroin injected into a blood vessel to reach the brain. And a pack-a-day smoker gets 200 hits of nicotine a day—73,000 a year.

After a few years of smoking, the most powerful incentive for continuing to smoke is to avoid the discomfort of withdrawal. Generally, ten cigarettes a day will prevent withdrawal effects. For many who smoke heavily, signs of withdrawal, including changes in mood and performance, occur within two hours after smoking their last cigarette. Smokeless tobacco users also get constant doses of nicotine. However, absorption of nicotine by the lungs is more likely to lead to dependence than absorption through the linings of the nose and mouth. As with other drugs of abuse, continued nicotine intake results in tolerance (the need for more of a drug to maintain the same effect), which is why only 2 percent of all smokers smoke just a few cigarettes a day, or smoke only occasionally. (See Self-Survey: "Are You Addicted to Nicotine?")

Use of Other Substances

Many smokers also drink or use drugs. According to the Addiction Research Foundation in Canada, tobacco smokers say cigarettes are harder to abandon than other drugs, even when they find them less pleasurable than their preferred drug of abuse. Individuals who drink excessively also find their cigarette habit a hard one to break.

Smoking in America

Tobacco use remains the most serious and widespread addictive behavior in the world and the major cause of preventable deaths in our society. One of the national health objectives for 2010 is to reduce the prevalence of cigarette smoking among adults to 12 percent. We have a way to go. Almost twice as many adults—23.4 percent—smoke.[24] (See Figure 12-3 on page 404.)

 "Current smokers" report having smoked at least 100 cigarettes during their lifetime and smoke every day or some days. "Some day" smokers do not smoke every day. In the last five years "some-day" smoking has increased significantly among those with some college education or a college degree. The proportion of "light smokers," who smoke less than 15 cigarettes per day, also has increased, particularly among adolescents, college students, pregnant women, and some minorities.[25]

According to the "Monitoring the Future" survey, teen smoking has declined sharply. Following increases in

Self Survey   **Are You Addicted to Nicotine?**

Answer the following questions as honestly as you can by placing a check mark in the appropriate column:

	Yes	No
1. Do you smoke every day?	___	___
2. Do you smoke because of shyness and to build up self-confidence?	___	___
3. Do you smoke to escape from boredom and worries or while under pressure?	___	___
4. Have you ever burned a hole in your clothes, carpet, furniture, or car with a cigarette?	___	___
5. Have you ever had to go to the store late at night or at another inconvenient time because you were out of cigarettes?	___	___
6. Do you feel defensive or angry when people tell you that your smoke is bothering them?	___	___
7. Has a doctor or dentist ever suggested that you stop smoking?	___	___
8. Have you ever promised someone that you would stop smoking, then broken your promise?	___	___
9. Have you ever felt physical or emotional discomfort when trying to quit?	___	___
10. Have you ever successfully stopped smoking for a period of time, only to start again?	___	___
11. Do you buy extra supplies of tobacco to make sure you won't run out?	___	___
12. Do you find it difficult to imagine life without smoking?	___	___

	Yes	No
13. Do you choose only those activities and entertainments during which you can smoke?	___	___
14. Do you prefer, seek out, or feel more comfortable in the company of smokers?	___	___
15. Do you inwardly despise or feel ashamed of yourself because of your smoking?	___	___
16. Do you ever find yourself lighting up without having consciously decided to?	___	___
17. Has your smoking ever caused trouble at home or in a relationship?	___	___
18. Do you ever tell yourself that you can stop smoking whenever you want to?	___	___
19. Have you ever felt that your life would be better if you didn't smoke?	___	___
20. Do you continue to smoke even though you are aware of the health hazards posed by smoking?	___	___

If you answered Yes to one or two of these questions, there's a chance that you are addicted or are becoming addicted to nicotine. If you answered Yes to three or more of these questions, you are probably already addicted to nicotine.

Source: Nicotine Anonymous World Services, San Francisco.

Your Health Change Plan

for Kicking the Habit

Here's a six-point program to help you or someone you love quit smoking. (*Caution:* Don't undertake the quit-smoking program until you have a two- to four-week period of relatively unstressful work and study schedules or social commitments.)

1. *Identify your smoking habits.* Keep a daily diary (a piece of paper wrapped around your cigarette pack with a rubber band will do) and record the time you smoke, the activity associated with smoking (after breakfast, in the car), and your urge for a cigarette (desperate, pleasant, or automatic). For the first week or two, don't bother trying to cut down; just use the diary to learn the conditions under which you smoke.

2. *Get support.* It can be tough to go it alone. Phone your local chapter of the American Cancer Society, or otherwise get the names of some ex-smokers who can give you support.

3. *Begin by tapering off.* For a period of one to four weeks, aim at cutting down to, say, 12 or 15 cigarettes a day; or change to a lower-nicotine brand, and concentrate on not increasing the number of cigarettes you smoke. As indicated by your diary, begin by cutting out those cigarettes you smoke automatically. In addition, restrict the times you allow yourself to smoke. Throughout this period, stay in touch, once a day or every few days, with your ex-smoker friend(s) to discuss your problems.

4. *Set a quit date.* At some point during the tapering-off period, announce to everyone—friends, family, and ex-smokers—when you're going to quit. Do it with flair. Announce it to coincide with a significant date, such as your birthday or anniversary.

5. *Stop.* A week before Q-day, smoke only five cigarettes a day. Begin late in the day, say after 4:00 P.M. Smoke the first two cigarettes in close succession. Then, in the evening, smoke the last three, also in close succession,

(Continued)

Self Survey | **Are You Addicted to Nicotine?—continued**

about 15 minutes apart. Focus on the negative aspects of cigarettes, such as the rawness in your throat and lungs. After seven days, quit and give yourself a big reward on that day, such as a movie or a fantastic meal or new clothes.

6. *Follow up.* Stay in touch with your ex-smoker friend(s) during the following two weeks, particularly if anything stressful or tense occurs that might trigger a

return to smoking. Think of the person you're becoming—the very person cigarette ads would have you believe smoking makes you. Now that you're quitting smoking, you're becoming healthier, sexier, more sophisticated, more mature, and better looking—and you've earned it!

Sources: American Cancer Society; National Cancer Institute.

the early 1990s, the rates of current and daily smoking among middle and high school students have fallen but remain higher than in adults: 27.7 percent of female high school students and 29.2 percent of male high school students smoke. The reasons for the decline include higher prices, less tobacco advertising pitched to young people, more antismoking ads, and much more negative publicity about the tobacco industry. More teenagers now see smoking as dangerous and have become less accepting of smoking and being around smokers. More than seven in ten teens, girls and boys, say they would prefer to date nonsmokers.[26]

Tobacco Use on Campus

Tobacco use has fallen off slightly among college students after increasing steadily during the 1990s. About 25 percent of undergraduates smoke.

Some began smoking in high school. However, more than half of student smokers begin or increase the amount they smoke after entering college.

One reason may be that young adults between ages 18 and 24 are the youngest legal targets of tobacco marketing. Increasingly, tobacco makers have focused on attracting new smokers, not only by direct advertising, but by sponsoring social events where free cigarettes are distributed.[27] Some young men start to smoke as a coping mechanism during the stressful transition from high school to college. The immediate danger for students who start smoking, even light smoking, in college is nicotine dependence.[28]

In an online survey of 224 college students, researchers concluded that four elements contribute to undergraduate smoking: a tendency toward risk-taking, depression, social norms that tolerate or encourage smoking, and a lack of self-efficacy in resisting pressure to smoke.[29]

Today's students also use a broader range of tobacco products: cigarettes, cigars, pipes, and smokeless tobacco. In a recent survey of students at four-year colleges and universities in Massachusetts, one-third had used a tobacco product, mostly cigarettes, in the past month; 46.4 percent had used tobacco in the past year.[30]

Among African-American students, almost half have tried smoking (that is, smoked at least one cigarette but less than 100 during their lifetime); about one in ten were "lifetime smokers" (smoked more than 100 cigarettes during their lifetime). More black women than men have tried smoking.[31]

College men and women have nearly identical rates for cigarette smoking, but more men used cigars and smokeless tobacco. White students use more cigarettes and smokeless tobacco than Hispanics, African Americans, or Asians.

Students who use tobacco are more likely to smoke marijuana, binge drink, have more sexual

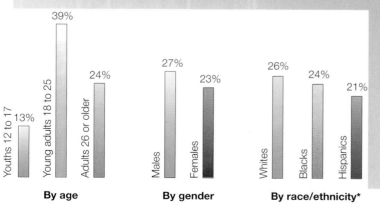

Figure 12-3 WHO SMOKES IN AMERICA?

Source: National Household Survey on Drug Abuse. *The NHSDA Report: Cigarette Brand Preferences,* U.S. Department of Health and Human Services, July 11, 2003.

By age: Youths 12 to 17 — 13%; Young adults 18 to 25 — 39%; Adults 26 or older — 24%

By gender: Males — 27%; Females — 23%

By race/ethnicity*: Whites — 26%; Blacks — 24%; Hispanics — 21%

partners, have lower grades, rate parties as important, and spend more time socializing with friends. They are less likely than nonusers to rate athletics or religion as important. Tobacco use is lower in western colleges. Unlike cigarette smokers, cigar users rate fraternities, sororities, and sporting events as important. College students who use smokeless tobacco tend to be white men attending schools in rural areas.

College Tobacco-Control Policies

Other than religious institutions, colleges and universities have traditionally had few smoking restrictions. This has changed. Several national health organizations, including the American College Health Association and National Center on Addiction and Substance Abuse, have recommended that colleges ban smoking in and around all campus buildings, including student housing, and prohibit the sale, advertisement, and promotion of tobacco products on campus. Although some schools, particularly large public universities, have made progress in adopting such policies, most still fall short of the national recommendations.[32]

A growing number of public and private schools provide completely smoke-free student housing, a dramatic increase from a decade ago. (See Student Snapshot: "Smoke-Free Housing.") Two-thirds did not allow tobacco sales on campus; a third of student newspapers did not allow tobacco advertising. None specifically banned tobacco industry sponsorships and promotions on college property. Less than a fifth of colleges' student health plans covered visits and medications for tobacco cessation. In general, schools in the West have done the most to implement tobacco policies. Those in the South, particularly in the major tobacco-growing states, have done the least.[33]

In a survey of 393 colleges and universities, 85 percent of student health center directors considered student smoking a problem or a major problem. Those at public institutions were more likely to perceive smoking as a major problem, while those at religiously affiliated schools were less likely to do so. Most schools—97 percent—restricted smoking in some way, usually in public areas but not in offices or student residences.

An estimated 44 percent of students live in smoke-free dorms, while another 29 percent who don't would like to move into one. Freshmen who did not smoke regularly in high school and who live in smoke-free dorms are 40 percent less likely to take up smoking than those in unrestricted housing, according to a study of the smoking behavior of 4,495 students at 101 schools.[34]

Despite concern about student smoking, more than 40 percent of schools do not offer smoking cessation programs to students who want to quit. Those that do primarily refer students to campus support groups or community-based programs like Nicotine Anonymous; they report little student demand for these options. Colleges are much less likely to offer individualized support, medical screening and assistance, or FDA-approved cessation products. Few provide smoking awareness programs, peer education, or quitting incentive programs.[35]

Smoking and Race

Cigarette smoking is a major cause of disease and death in all population groups. However, tobacco use varies within and among racial and ethnic minority groups. Among adults, Native Americans and Alaska Natives have the highest rates of tobacco use—37.9 percent of the men smoke cigarettes, compared with about 25 percent of adults in the overall U.S. population. African-American men (32.1 percent) and Southeast Asian men also have a high smoking rate. Asian-American and Hispanic women have the lowest rates of smoking. Tobacco use is significantly higher among white college students than among Hispanic, African-American, and Asian students.[36]

Tobacco has taken the greatest toll on the health of African Americans. Middle-aged and older African Americans are far more likely than their counterparts in other major racial and ethnic minority groups to die from coronary heart disease, stroke, or lung cancer. In the 1970s and 1980s, death rates from respiratory cancers (mainly lung cancer) increased among both African-American men and women. In the last decade, these rates declined substantially among African-American men and leveled off in African-American women.

As several studies have shown, many African-American adolescents experiment with smoking but then stop. Among black college students, the risk factors for smoking include friends who smoke, parents who smoked, and a view of religion as unimportant. For lifetime smoking, being single, having had no or few childhood friends who smoked, and having no current friends who smoke decrease the likelihood that an African American would continue to smoke.[37]

African-American teens who smoke are at greater risk of developing long-term consequences than other youths, even when they smoke less. The reason for their increased susceptibility to asthma, allergies, and depression may be potential differences in the way ethnic groups metabolize nicotine.[38]

Tobacco is the substance most abused by Hispanic youth, whose smoking rates have soared in the last ten years.[39] In general, smoking rates among Hispanic adults increase as they adopt the values, beliefs, and norms of American culture. Recent declines in the prevalence of smoking have been greater among Hispanic men with at

Student Snapshot **Smoke-Free Housing**

Increase in smoke-free housing at 50 U.S. public universities

30%
2002-03

13%
1999-2000

2%
1994-95

Student Housing

Source: Abigail Halperin and Nancy Rigotti. "US Public Universities' Compliance with Recommended Tobacco-Control Policies." *Journal of American College Health,* Vol. 51, No. 5, March 2003, p. 181.

least a high school education than among those with less education.

According to the U.S. Surgeon General, "adverse infant health outcomes," such as low-birthweight babies, sudden infant death syndrome (SIDS), and infant mortality, are especially high for African Americans, Native Americans, and Alaska Natives who smoke. Cigarette smoking also increases these risks, especially for SIDS, among Asian Americans, Pacific Islanders, and Hispanics.

❒ Smoking and Gender

In the past, men were far more likely than women to smoke—and to suffer the health consequences. More women today, particularly young women, smoke. According to the Centers for Disease Control and Prevention, 28 percent of men and 22 percent of women are smokers. Among teens, more girls than boys smoke.

Male and female smokers share certain characteristics: Most start smoking as teenagers; the lower their educational level, the more likely they are to smoke. But there are gender differences in tobacco use. In the last decade, smoking rates among adult women stopped their previous

decline and have risen sharply among teenage girls. Men of all ages are more likely than women to use other forms of tobacco, such as cigars and chewing tobacco.

Women with less than a high school education are three times more likely to smoke than those with a college degree.[40] Girls making the transition from high school to college show the largest increase in smoking, drinking, and marijuana use. Those who drink coffee are significantly likelier than girls and women who do not to become smokers.[41]

The genders smoke for different reasons. Men smoke to decrease boredom and fatigue and to increase arousal and concentration. Women smoke to control their weight and to decrease stress, anger, and other negative feelings.

Men respond more intensely to the pleasurable and painkilling effects of nicotine on brain chemistry. While nicotine affects appetite and weight in both genders, its effects are more pronounced in women. Yet accumulating evidence shows that, for women, nicotine intake may be less important in smoking behavior than it is for men. Women take fewer and shorter puffs from cigarettes and are less sensitive to some of nicotine's effects, but they may be more sensitive to external stimuli, such as the presence of a lit cigarette or the smell of smoke. (See the X&Y File: "Which Gender Finds It Harder to Quit?")

According to the U.S. Surgeon General, women account for 39 percent of smoking-related deaths each

the X & Y file   *Which Gender Finds It Harder to Quit?*

Breaking the cigarette habit is tough. Nicotine addiction may be as difficult to overcome as dependence on any other drug. Some contend it's even harder—especially for women.

Like other smokers, women want to quit. Most try, and try, and try again. Many men do the same, but the odds of a man's successful quitting remain higher. Why? The reasons may have to do both with nicotine and with the behaviors associated with smoking.

Nicotine replacement therapy, which supplies ex-smokers with lower levels of nicotine in the form of a gum or patch, has proven more beneficial for men than women—particularly with higher doses of nicotine. Men who receive more nicotine achieve a higher quit rate than men getting lower doses. For women, the nicotine "dose" does not have an impact on successful quitting. They are no more likely to stop smoking with high doses than with lower ones, indicating that they may be less dependent on nicotine than men.

Compared with men, women seem to have a higher behavioral dependence on cigarettes. For them, wearing a nicotine patch or chewing nicotine gum does not substitute for the "hand-to-mouth" behaviors associated with smoking, such as lighting a cigarette, inhaling, and handling the cigarette. Some investigators have found that women are more likely to quit successfully when they receive a combination of nicotine replacement and the use of a device like a nicotine inhaler to substitute for smoking behaviors.

Women may face other barriers to quitting. Because of fear of weight gain, they may relapse if they put on even a pound or two. Withdrawal symptoms may be more intense at certain times of the menstrual cycle. And women may not be able to use nicotine replacement products or medications such as Zyban because they are pregnant or trying to conceive.

But there is good news for women who do manage to quit: According to the federal Lung Health Study, women's lung function improves significantly more than men's after five cigarette-free years—although both sexes show clear improvement.

---

year, a proportion that has doubled since 1965. Each year, American women lose an estimated 2.1 million years of life due to premature deaths attributable to smoking. If she smokes, a woman's annual risk of dying more than doubles after age 45 compared with a woman who has never smoked.

Lung cancer now claims more women's lives than breast cancer.[42] In men, cigarette smoking increases the risk of aggressive prostate cancer.[43]

Smoking is a risk factor for developing rheumatoid arthritis for men, but not for women.[44] Women who smoke are more likely to develop osteoporosis, a bone-weakening disease. They tend to be thin, which is a risk factor for osteoporosis, and they enter menopause earlier, thus extending the period of jeopardy from estrogen loss.

High nicotine intake may affect male hormones, including testosterone. Smoking also can reduce blood flow to the penis, impairing a man's sexual performance and increasing the likelihood of erectile dysfunction.[45] Smoking directly affects women's reproductive organs and processes. Women who smoke are less fertile and experience menopause one or two years earlier than women who don't smoke. Smoking also greatly increases the possible risks associated with taking oral contraceptives. Older women who smoke are weaker, have poorer balance, and are at greater risk of physical disability than nonsmokers.

Women who smoke during pregnancy increase their risk of miscarriage and pregnancy complications, including

bleeding, premature delivery, and birth defects such as cleft lip or palate. Women who smoke are twice as likely to have an ectopic pregnancy (in which a fertilized egg develops in the fallopian tube rather than in the uterus) and to have babies of low birthweight as those who have never smoked. However, women who stop smoking before pregnancy reduce their risk of having a low-birthweight baby to that of women who don't smoke. Even those who quit three or four months into the pregnancy have babies with higher birthweights than those who continue smoking throughout pregnancy. Almost 60 percent of the women who had quit smoking during pregnancy resumed the habit within 6 months after delivery.[46]

:¦ Other Forms of Tobacco

Some 10.7 million Americans smoke cigars; 7.6 million use smokeless tobacco, and 2.1 million smoke pipes.[47] Ingesting tobacco may be less deadly than smoking cigarettes, but it is dangerous. Smoking cigars, clove cigarettes, and pipes, and chewing or sucking on smokeless tobacco all put the user at risk of cancer of the lip, tongue, mouth, and throat, as well as other diseases and ailments.

Cigars

Cigar use has declined in the last few years. However, after cigarettes, cigars are the tobacco product most widely used by college students. According to the first national survey to report on undergraduate cigar use, more than a third reported ever smoking a cigar (more than half of men and a quarter of women); 23 percent had smoked a cigar within the past year and 8.5 percent had smoked one within the previous 30 days. About one in five students smoked both cigars and cigarettes. Most cigar use was occasional; fewer than 1 percent of current cigar users on campus smoked daily. Cigar use was similar in white and black students but lower in Hispanics and Asians. In contrast to the ratio for men, more African-American than white women reported smoking cigars (6.8 versus 4 percent).[48]

Cigar smoking is as dangerous even though smokers do not inhale. Cigars are known to cause cancer of the lung and the digestive tract. The risk of death related to cigars approaches that of cigarettes, as the number of cigars smoked and the amount of cigar smoke inhaled increases. (See Figure 12-4.) Cigar smoking can lead to nicotine addiction, even if the smoke is not inhaled. The nicotine in the smoke from a single cigar can vary from an amount roughly equivalent to that in a single cigarette to that in a pack or more of cigarettes.

Clove Cigarettes

Sweeteners have long been mixed with tobacco, and clove, a spice, is the latest ingredient to be added to the recipe for cigarettes. Clove cigarettes typically contain two-thirds tobacco and one-third clove. Consumers of these cigarettes are primarily teenagers and young adults.

Many users believe that clove cigarettes are safer because they contain less tobacco, but this isn't necessarily the case. The CDC reports that people who smoke clove cigarettes may be at risk of serious lung injury. Smoking clove cigarettes during a mild upper respiratory tract illness can lead to severe breathing difficulty. And clove cigarette smokers, like other cigarette smokers, can become addicted to the tobacco.

Clove cigarettes may be more harmful than conventional cigarettes. They deliver twice as much nicotine, tar, and carbon monoxide as moderate-tar American brands. Eugenol, the active ingredient in cloves (which dentists have used as an anesthetic for years), deadens sensation in the throat, allowing smokers to inhale more deeply and hold smoke in their lungs for a longer time. Chemical relatives of eugenol can produce the kind of damage to cells that may lead to cancer.

What Are Bidis?

Skinny, sweet-flavored cigarettes called **bidis** (pronounced "beedees") have become a smoking fad among teens and young adults. For centuries, bidis were popular in India, where they are known as the poor man's cigarette and sell for less than five cents a pack. They look strikingly like clove cigarettes or marijuana joints, and are available in flavors like grape, strawberry, and mandarin orange. Bidis are legal for adults and even minors in some states, and are sold on the Internet as well as in stores.

Although bidis contain less tobacco than regular cigarettes, their unprocessed tobacco is more potent. Smoke from bidis has about three times as much nicotine and

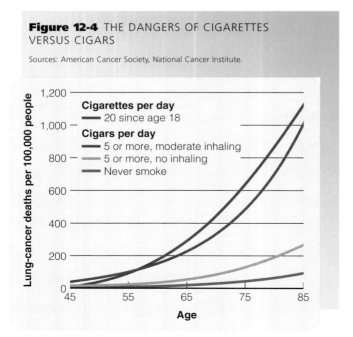

Figure 12-4 THE DANGERS OF CIGARETTES VERSUS CIGARS

Sources: American Cancer Society, National Cancer Institute.

Lung-cancer deaths per 100,000 people

Cigarettes per day
— 20 since age 18

Cigars per day
— 5 or more, moderate inhaling
— 5 or more, no inhaling
— Never smoke

Age

AP/Wide World Photos

The smoke produced by bidis—skinny, flavored cigarettes—can contain higher concentrations of toxic chemicals than the smoke from regular cigarettes.

carbon monoxide and five times as much tar as smoke from regular filtered cigarettes.[49] Because bidis are wrapped in nonporous brownish leaves, they don't burn as easily as cigarettes, and smokers have to inhale harder and more often to keep them lit. In one study, smoking a single bidi required 28 puffs, compared to 9 puffs for cigarettes. (See Fact or Fiction? "Additive-free cigarettes . . .")

Health authorities view bidis as "cigarettes with training wheels," products that can lead to a lifetime of nicotine addiction because they are easy to buy and lack the health-warning labels required of cigarettes. Unlike regular cigarettes, which are smoked mostly by white youths, bidis also are popular among young Hispanics and blacks.

Pipes

Many cigarette smokers switch to pipes to reduce their risk of health problems. But former cigarette smokers may continue to inhale, even though pipe smoke is more irritating to the respiratory system than cigarette smoke. People who have smoked only pipes and who do not inhale are much less likely to develop lung and heart disease than cigarette smokers. However, they are as likely as cigarette smokers to develop—and die of—cancer of the mouth, larynx, throat, and esophagus.

Smokeless Tobacco

The consumption of smokeless tobacco products is rising, particularly among young males. These substances include snuff, finely ground tobacco that can be sniffed or placed inside the cheek and sucked, and chewing tobacco,

Chewing smokeless tobacco can damage the tissues of the mouth and lead to cancer of the larynx, esophagus, kidney, pancreas, and bladder.

Leonard Morse/Medical Images

tobacco leaves mixed with flavoring agents such as molasses. With both, nicotine is absorbed through the mucous membranes of the nose or mouth.

Every day approximately 2,200 U.S. youths, ages 11 to 19, try smokeless tobacco for the first time. About 830 become regular users. Many are emulating professional baseball players who keep wads of tobacco jammed in their cheeks. These young users often lack awareness of its dangers. Smokeless tobacco can cause cancer and noncancerous oral conditions and lead to nicotine addiction and dependence. Smokeless tobacco users are more likely than nonusers to become cigarette smokers. Powerful carcinogens in smokeless tobacco include nitrosamines, polycyclic aromatic hydrocarbons, and radiation-emitting polonium. Its use can lead to the development of white patches on the mucous membranes of the mouth, particularly on the site where the tobacco is placed. Most lesions of the mouth lining that result from the use of smokeless tobacco dissipate six weeks after the use of the tobacco products is stopped, according to a U.S. Air Force study. However, when first found, about 5 percent of these lesions are cancerous or exhibit changes that progress to cancer within ten years if not properly treated. Cancers of the lip, pharynx, larynx, and esophagus have all been linked to smokeless tobacco.

More than 7 million people, many of them young, use snuff and chewing tobacco. In a national survey of 5,894 men and women from 72 colleges and universities, 22 percent of college men and 2 percent of college women used smokeless tobacco. The lowest percentage was in the northeast, the highest in the south-central region. In different regions, 8 to 36 percent of male high school students were regular users. Even when they spot lesions in their mouths, most do not seek medical help but continue to use smokeless tobacco.

In recent years, there has been a decline in chewing tobacco, but an increase in the use of moist snuff, a product that is higher in nicotine and potential cancer-causing chemicals. The use of snuff increases the likelihood of oral cancer by more than four times. Other effects include bad breath, discolored or missing teeth, cavities, gum disease, and nicotine addiction. In a study by the Oregon Research Institute, dental patients were three times more likely to quit snuff and chewing tobacco after hygienists taught them that smokeless tobacco was responsible for their mouth sores, bleeding gums, and receding gums.

"Safer" Cigarettes

Tobacco companies are producing "lower-risk" cigarettes that they claim reduce secondhand smoke and have fewer carcinogens and less nicotine. For example, "Eclipse" cigarettes heat rather than burn tobacco inside a cigarette-like tube to reduce the release of carbon monoxide, a big contributor to heart disease. Users of another product, "Accord," insert special cigarettes into a small electronic device about the size of a pager that ignites the cigarette when the smoker puffs and sucks up secondhand smoke. Other brands claim to use genetic engineering or a chemical process to remove major carcinogens. Currently under development are very low-nicotine cigarettes that may help smokers wean themselves from their habit.[50]

Are these products truly safer? Public health officials are skeptical. The only proven way to avoid smoking-related risks of disease and death is to stop smoking.

Environmental Tobacco Smoke

Maybe you don't smoke—never have, never will. That doesn't mean you don't have to worry about the dangers of smoking, especially if you live or work with people who smoke. **Environmental tobacco smoke,** or secondhand cigarette smoke, the most hazardous form of indoor air pollution, ranks behind cigarette smoking and alcohol as the third-leading preventable cause of death.

On average, a smoker inhales what is known as **mainstream smoke** eight or nine times with each cigarette, for a total of about 24 seconds. However, the cigarette burns for about 12 minutes, and everyone in the room (including the smoker) breathes in what is known as **sidestream smoke.**

According to the American Lung Association, incomplete combustion from the lower temperatures of a smoldering cigarette makes sidestream smoke dirtier and chemically different from mainstream smoke. It has twice as much tar and nicotine, five times as much carbon monoxide, and 50 times as much ammonia. And because the particles in sidestream smoke are small, this mixture of

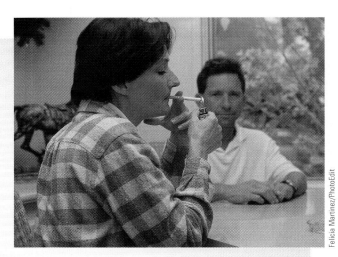

Secondhand smoke is the most hazardous form of indoor air pollution.

irritating gases and carcinogenic tar reaches deeper into the lungs. If you're a nonsmoker sitting next to someone smoking seven cigarettes an hour, even in a ventilated room, you'll take in almost twice the maximum amount of carbon monoxide set for air pollution in industry—and it will take hours for the carbon monoxide to leave your body.

What Are the Risks of Secondhand Smoke?

Even a little secondhand smoke is dangerous. According to the Centers for Disease Control and Prevention, every year environmental tobacco smoke causes 3,000 deaths from lung cancer. In a ten-year Harvard University study that tracked 10,000 healthy women who never smoked, regular exposure to other people's smoke at home or work almost doubled the risk of heart disease. On the basis of their findings, the researchers estimated that up to 50,000 Americans may die every year of heart attacks from environmental tobacco smoke, and another 3,000 to 4,000 die of other forms of heart disease caused by secondhand smoke.[51] As a cancer-causing agent, secondhand smoke may be twice as dangerous as radon gas and more than a hundred times more hazardous than outdoor pollutants regulated by federal law. Secondhand smoke also increases the sick leave rates among employees.[52]

Families of Smokers: Living Dangerously

Just thirty minutes of exposure to secondhand smoke at home may have a substantial impact on health. The most vulnerable nonsmokers are the spouses and children of smokers. Numerous epidemiological and autopsy studies have linked environmental tobacco smoke with lung cancer and other disorders. The nonsmoking spouses of smokers, for instance, are 30 percent more likely to die of heart disease than other nonsmokers.

Prenatal exposure to tobacco can have significant effects that may extend from infancy into adulthood. Smoking during pregnancy affects a child's growth, cognitive development, and behavior both before and after birth. Birthweight decreases in direct proportion to the number of cigarettes smoked. The babies of teenage mothers who smoke have lower birthweight, length, head circumference, and chest circumference.[53] As they grow, children of smokers tend to be shorter and weigh less than children of nonsmokers.[54]

A mother's smoking during pregnancy may have cognitive and behavioral effects as well. These include abnormal neurological responses, such as more tremors and startles. Among older children, researchers have found deficits in language and reading abilities and poorer visual perception. Youngsters whose mothers smoked during pregnancy also tend to have problems with hyperactivity, inattention, and impulsivity. Some of these behavior problems persist through the teenage years and even into adulthood. At ages 16 to 18, children exposed to prenatal smoking have higher rates of conduct disorder, substance use, and depression than others.

Even if their mothers don't smoke, children exposed to secondhand smoke before birth also are likely to weigh less and to perform more poorly on tests of speech, language skills, intelligence, and visual-spatial abilities and to develop behavior problems. These youngsters perform at a level between that of children of active smokers and children of nonsmokers.

Exposure to smoke after birth increases the risk of sudden infant death syndrome (SIDS) and is associated with lower IQ scores and deficits in cognitive development.

Children who breathe environmental tobacco smoke suffer from more asthma, wheezing, and bronchitis than children in smoke-free homes. They also face increased risk of lung cancer, heart disease, and stroke.

 The negative effects of childhood exposure to environmental tobacco smoke persist even after youngsters leave home. In recent research at Ohio State University, college students who grew up in a smoking household had higher blood pressure and resting heart rates at rest and during psychological stress than those who grew up in smoke-free homes.

✖ The Politics of Tobacco

The World Health Organization's Framework Convention on Tobacco Control, signed by 171 countries in 2003, supports restrictions on tobacco advertising, increasing taxes, government financing of tobacco control programs, and holding tobacco companies liable for costs related to tobacco use. It also encourages countries to set taxes at a level that will discourage smoking, and to pass laws holding the tobacco industry to account for medical and other costs.[55]

More than three decades after U.S. government health authorities began to warn of the dangers of cigarette smoking, tobacco remains a politically hot topic. A survey of U.S. adults shows that a majority of people support tobacco control strategies, including creation of smoke-free environments, an increase in cigarette excise taxes, more funds to prevent people from smoking and to help smokers quit, and restriction of youth access to tobacco.[56]

"Big Tobacco"

After many years of difficult negotiations, the tobacco industry and attorneys general from nearly 40 states reached a historic settlement. Major tobacco companies have agreed to pay more than $200 billion to settle smoking-related lawsuits filed by 46 states, to finance antismoking campaigns, to restrict marketing, to permit federal regulation of tobacco, and to pay fines if tobacco use by minors does not decline.

The funds from the U.S. state tobacco settlement, won in 1998, were supposed to support antismoking programs, but the majority of that funding is not being spent on anything related to smoking. Those few states, such as Massachusetts, that are spending the funds on cessation programs report some success in reducing cigarette consumption.[57]

Increasing the price of cigarettes by 10 percent reduces the number of smokers by about 2 percent. Many states have raised taxes on cigarettes; some now charge more than a dollar a pack.[58] Although personal health warnings are not particularly effective, new in-your-face warning labels are grabbing smokers' attention; for example, extra-large Canadian cigarette labels show rotting lungs and decaying teeth. According to a Canadian Cancer Society study, 44 percent of smokers said the gory warning increased their motivation to quit.

The Fight for Clean Air

Nonsmokers, realizing that their health is being jeopardized by environmental tobacco smoke, have increasingly turned to legislative and administrative measures to clear the air and protect their rights. (See Figure 12-5.) Thousands of cities, towns, and counties now restrict smoking in public places and/or regulate the sale of tobacco to minors. Nationally, the airlines have banned smoking on domestic flights. Many institutions, including medical centers and some universities, no longer allow

Nonsmoker's Bill of Rights

Nonsmokers Help Protect the Health, Comfort, and Safety
of Everyone by Insisting on the Following Rights:

The Right to Breathe Clean Air

*Nonsmokers have the right to breathe clean air, free from harmful and irritating
tobacco smoke. This right supersedes the right to smoke when the two conflict.*

The Right to Speak Out

*Nonsmokers have the right to express — firmly but politely — their discomfort
and adverse reactions to tobacco smoke. They have the right to voice their objections
when smokers light up without asking permission.*

The Right to Act

*Nonsmokers have the right to take action through legislative means — as
individuals or in groups — to prevent or discourage smokers from polluting the
atmosphere and to seek the restriction of smoking in public places.*

Figure 12-5 NONSMOKER'S BILL OF RIGHTS

smoking on their premises. Some cities restrict smoking in bars, restaurants, and other public places.[59]

Supporters of smoking restrictions argue that no one should be subjected involuntarily to the dangers of environmental tobacco smoke. (See Savvy Consumer: "How Nonsmokers Can Clear the Air.") Besides the health hazards, smokers jeopardize nonsmokers by increasing the danger of fire.

Opponents of smoking restrictions contend that banning smoking on the job might impair rather than

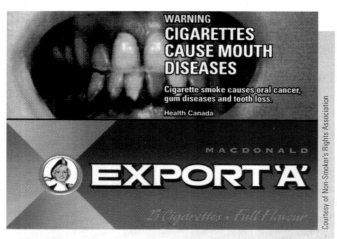

Graphic warning labels on cigarette packages in Canada have discouraged smoking.

enhance productivity, because employees would take more frequent breaks to go to lounges where smoking is permitted—or else would suffer the negative effects of nicotine withdrawal. When workplaces become smoke-free, workers almost immediately smoke 29 percent fewer cigarettes per day.[60]

Quitting

Smoking is a remarkably difficult habit to kick. About 70 percent of smokers want to quit, but only about 5 percent succeed, according to the American Lung Association.

About half of whites who have smoked were able to kick the habit, compared with 45 percent of Asian Americans, 43 percent of Hispanics, and 37 percent of African Americans. Men and women with college and graduate degrees were much more likely to quit successfully than high-school dropouts.[61]

Most people who eventually quit on their own have already tried other methods. Nicotine withdrawal symptoms can behave like characters in a bad horror flick: Just when you think you've killed them, they're back with a vengeance. In recent studies, some people who tried to quit smoking reported a small improvement in withdrawal symptoms over two weeks, but then their symptoms leveled off and persisted. Others found that their symptoms intensified rather than lessened over time. For reasons scientists cannot yet explain, former smokers who start smoking again put their lungs at even greater jeopardy than smokers who never quit.[62]

Once a former smoker takes a single puff, the odds of a relapse are 80 to 85 percent. Smokers are most likely to quit in the third, fourth or fifth attempt.[63] The good news is that half of all living Americans who ever smoked have managed to quit. And thanks to new products and programs, it may be easier now than ever before to become an ex-smoker.

Quitting on Your Own

More than 90 percent of former smokers quit on their own—by throwing away all their cigarettes, by gradually cutting down, or by first switching to a less potent brand. One characteristic of successful quitters is that they see themselves as active participants in health maintenance and take personal responsibility for their own health. Often they experiment with a variety of strategies, such as learning relaxation techniques. In women, exercise has proven especially effective for quitting and avoiding weight gain. Making a home a smoke-free zone also increases a smoker's likelihood of successfully quitting.

Stop-Smoking Groups

Joining a support group doubles your chances of quitting for good. The American Cancer Society's FreshStart program runs about 1,500 stop-smoking clinics, each with about 8 to 18 members meeting for eight two-hour sessions over four weeks. Instructors explain the risks of smoking, encourage individuals to think about why they smoke, and suggest ways of unlearning their smoking habit. A quitting day is set for the third or fourth session.

The American Lung Association's Freedom from Smoking program consists of eight one- to two-hour sessions over seven weeks. The approach is similar to the American Cancer Society's, but smokers keep diaries and team up with buddies. Ex-smokers serve as advisers on quitting day. Both groups estimate that 27 or 28 percent of their participants successfully stop smoking.

Stop-smoking classes are also available through health-science departments and student-health services on many college campuses, as well as through community public health departments. The Seventh-Day Adventists sponsor a four-week Breathe Free Plan, in which smokers commit themselves to clean living (no smoking, alcohol, tea, or coffee, along with a balanced diet and regular exercise).

Many businesses sponsor smoking-cessation programs for employees, which generally follow the approaches of professional groups. Motivation may be even higher in these programs than in programs outside the workplace because some companies offer attractive incentives to participants, such as lower rates on their health insurance.

Some smoking-cessation programs rely primarily on **aversion therapy,** which provides a negative experience every time a smoker has a cigarette. This may involve taking drugs that make tobacco smoke taste unpleasant, undergoing electric shocks, having smoke blown at you, or rapid smoking (the inhaling of smoke every six seconds until you're dizzy or nauseated).

Telephone-counseling "quit lines," which advise smokers on how to restructure their lives and deal with urges, are also helpful because people can get counseling without leaving their homes.[64]

Nicotine Replacement Therapy

This approach uses a variety of products that supply low doses of nicotine in a way that allows smokers to taper off gradually over a period of months. Nicotine replacement therapies include nonprescription products (nicotine gum and nicotine patches) and prescription products (nicotine nasal spray and nicotine inhaler). The nasal spray, dispensed from a pump bottle, delivers nicotine to the nasal membranes and reaches the bloodstream faster than any other nicotine replacement therapy product. The inhaler delivers nicotine into the mouth and enters the bloodstream much more slowly than the nicotine in cigarettes.

Antismoking drugs can help smokers quit, but they are not a runaway success. The steady, continuous dose of nicotine from patches and gums does not compare to the nearly instantaneous impact of inhaled nicotine, so smokers may return to cigarettes. Because nicotine is a powerful, addictive substance, using nicotine replacements for a prolonged period is not advised. Pregnant women and individuals with heart disease shouldn't use them.

The most effective approaches combine medication—nicotine patches or Zyban, for instance—with psychological intervention. Each doubles a person's chance of quitting successfully.

Nicorette gum, when chewed, gradually releases a nicotine resin and helps some smokers break their habit. Nicorette is available without a prescription.

Nicotine Gum

Nicotine gum, sold as Nicorette, contains a nicotine resin that's gradually released as the gum is chewed. Absorbed through the mucous membrane of the mouth, the nicotine doesn't produce the same rush as a deeply inhaled drag on a cigarette. However, the gum maintains enough nicotine in the blood to diminish withdrawal symptoms. A month's supply of Nicorette costs roughly $45.

Although this gum is lightly spiced to mask nicotine's bitterness, many users say that it takes several days to become accustomed to its unusual taste. Its side effects include mild indigestion, sore jaws, nausea, heartburn, and stomachache. Also, because Nicorette is heavier than regular chewing gum, it may loosen fillings or cause problems with dentures. Drinking coffee or other beverages may block absorption of the nicotine in the gum; individuals trying to quit smoking shouldn't ingest any substance immediately before or while chewing nicotine gum. You have to chew nicotine gum until you get a tingling sensation, and then place it between the cheek and gum.[65]

Most people use nicotine gum as a temporary crutch and gradually taper off until they can stop chewing it relatively painlessly. However, 5 to 10 percent of users transfer their dependence from cigarettes to the gum. When they stop using Nicorette, they experience withdrawal symptoms, although the symptoms tend to be milder than those prompted by quitting cigarettes. Intensive counseling to teach smokers coping methods can greatly increase the success rates.

Nicotine skin patch

Nicotine inhaler

Counseling

Nicotine nasal spray

Nicotine gum

Bupropion sustained release

Figure 12-6 HOW TO QUIT
Combining one of the four nicotine replacement therapies (or bupropion/Zyban) with counseling is the most effective strategy to quit smoking.

Source: Department of Medicine, Center for Tobacco Research and Intervention, University of Wisconsin Medical School, Madison. Correspondence to Douglas E. Jorenby, PhD, University of Wisconsin Medical School, 1930 Monroe St, Suite 200, Madison WI 53711. (*Circulation*. 2001; 104:e51–e52.) © 2001 American Heart Association, Inc.

Nicotine Patches

Nicotine transdermal delivery system products, or patches, provide nicotine, their only active ingredient, via a patch attached to the skin by an adhesive. Like nicotine gum, the nicotine patch minimizes withdrawal symptoms, such as intense craving for cigarettes. Nicotine patches

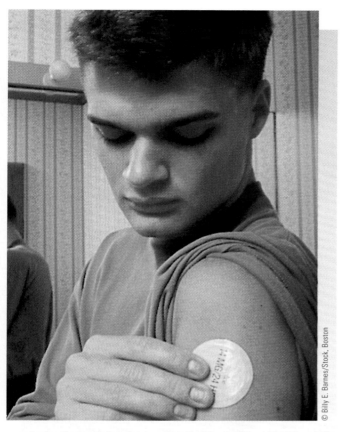

A nicotine patch releases nicotine transdermally (through the skin) in measured amounts, which are gradually decreased over time.

Nicotrol Inhaler

Available only by prescription, the Nicotrol Inhaler consists of a mouthpiece and a cartridge containing a nicotine-impregnated plug. The smoker inhales through the mouthpiece, using either shallow or deep puffs. The inhaled air becomes saturated with nicotine, which is absorbed mainly through the tissues of the mouth. The Inhaler releases less nicotine per puff than a cigarette and does not contain a cigarette's harmful tars, carbon monoxide, and smoke. Treatment is recommended for three months with a gradual reduction over the next six to twelve weeks. Total treatment should not exceed six months.[66]

Bupropion (Zyban)

An alternative to the patch is **bupropion,** a drug initially developed to treat depression, that is marketed in a slow-release form for nicotine addiction as Zyban. In studies that have combined Zyban with nicotine replacement and counseling, 40 to 60 percent of those treated have remained smoke-free for at least a year after completing the program. This success rate is much higher than the 10 to 26 percent reported among smokers who try to quit

help nearly 20 percent of smokers quit entirely after six weeks, compared with 7 percent on a placebo patch. Some insurance programs pay for patch therapy. Nicotine patches, which cost between $3.25 and $4 each, are replaced daily during therapy programs that run between 6 and 16 weeks. There is no evidence that continuing their use for more than 8 weeks provides added benefit.

Some patches deliver nicotine around the clock and others for just 16 hours (during waking hours). Those most likely to benefit from nicotine patch therapy are people who smoke more than a pack a day, are highly motivated to quit, and participate in counseling programs. While using the patch, 37 to 77 percent of people are able to abstain from smoking. When combined with counseling, the patch can be about twice as effective as a placebo, enabling 26 percent of smokers to abstain for six months.

Patch wearers who smoke or use more than one patch at a time can experience a nicotine overdose; some users have even suffered heart attacks. Occasional side effects include redness, itching, or swelling at the site of the patch application; insomnia; dry mouth; and nervousness.

THE CUTTING EDGE

An Anti-Nicotine Vaccine

Scientists are testing a vaccine that would block nicotine's action on the brain. Rather than generating an immune response that clears away nicotine, the anti-nicotine vaccine would create antibodies that bind nicotine in the blood and prevent it from crossing the blood-brain barrier. The result: Nicotine would not be able to stimulate the brain's reward centers. In other words, smokers would not feel a "buzz," which would leave little, if any, reason to smoke.

In laboratory studies, animals given the vaccine were interested less in self-administering intravenous nicotine. However, it is not clear if the vaccines will work against the faster and stronger effect of nicotine delivered by smoking. So far, human trials have measured only safety, yet investigators are hopeful that the vaccines could be especially helpful in blocking relapses. With a vaccine, even if an ex-smoker lights up, nicotine won't reach the brain, and cravings may not be activated. As one investigator put it, the ex-smoker "might as well be smoking lettuce."

Source: Mignon Fogarty. "Depending on Cigarettes, Counting on Science: Understanding How Specific Genes Work Could Keep Smokers from Coveting That Next Hit or Lighting Up in the First Place." *The Scientist,* Vol. 17, No. 6, March 24, 2003, p. 21.

using nicotine replacement alone. The combination of Zyban and nicotine replacement also prevented the initial weight gain that often accompanies quitting.[67] Other medications used to treat nicotine addiction are clonidine, mecamylamine, and buspirone.

Other Ways to Quit

Hypnosis may help some people quit smoking. Hypnotherapists use their techniques to create an atmosphere of strict attention and give smokers in a mild trance positive suggestions for breaking their cigarette habit.

Acupuncture, in which a circular needle or staple is inserted in the flap in front of the opening to the ear, has also had some success. When smokers feel withdrawal symptoms, they gently move the needle or staple, which may increase the production of calming chemicals in the brain.

Since 1976, a November day has been set aside in the United States for the annual Great American Smoke-Out, an idea promoted by the American Cancer Society to encourage smokers to give up cigarettes for 24 hours. As many as 36 percent of American smokers have given up cigarettes on Smoke-Out Day; about 5 to 6 percent have quit permanently; 15 percent reduced smoking for extended periods. In addition, the World Health Organization has established World No-Tobacco Days in May to call on nations to urge tobacco users to abstain for at least one day and perhaps quit for good.

The Bottom Line ▼
Living Smoke-Free

If you smoke—even just a few cigarettes a few times a week—you are at risk of nicotine addiction. Here is how to get back into control:

:: *Use delaying tactics.* Have your first cigarette of the day 15 minutes later than usual, then 15 minutes later than that the next day, and so on.

:: *Distract yourself.* When you feel a craving for a cigarette, talk to someone, drink a glass of water, or get up and move around.

:: *Establish nonsmoking hours.* Instead of lighting up at the end of a meal, for instance, get up immediately, brush your teeth, wash your hands, or take a walk.

:: *Never smoke two packs of the same brand in a row.* Buy cigarettes only by the pack, not by the carton.

:: *Make it harder to get to your cigarettes.* Lock them in a drawer, wrap them in paper, or leave them in your coat or car.

:: *Change the way you smoke.* Smoke with the hand you don't usually use. Smoke only half of each cigarette.

:: *Keep daily records.* Chart your daily cigarette tally to see what progress you're making.

:: *Stop completely for just one day at a time.* Promise yourself 24 hours of freedom from cigarettes; when the day's over, make the same commitment for one more day. At the end of any 24-hour period, you can go back to smoking and not feel guilty.

:: *Spend more time in places where you can't smoke.* Take up bike-riding or swimming. Shower often. Go to movies or other places where smoking isn't allowed.

:: *Go cold turkey.* If you're a heavily addicted smoker, try a decisive and complete break. Smokers who quit completely are less likely to light up again than those who gradually decrease their daily cigarette consumption, switch to low-tar and low-nicotine brands, or use special filters and holders.

 Kids and Tobacco Addictions. After watching the CNN video segment, discuss the following question. Why are teen smokers at a greater risk for cancer and other diseases?

MAKING THIS
CHAPTER
WORK FOR YOU

12

1. Which of the following statements about tobacco and its components is *true*?
    a. Nicotine affects the central nervous system in 8 seconds.
    b. Tobacco stimulates the kidneys to form urine.
    c. Carbon monoxide contained in tobacco smoke is an addictive substance.
    d. The tar in burning tobacco impairs oxygen transport in the body.

2. Cigarette smokers
    a. are more likely to die of lung cancer than heart disease.
    b. usually develop lung problems after years of tobacco use.
    c. have two to three times the risk of suffering a stroke than nonsmokers.

d. may completely reverse the damage to their blood vessels if they quit smoking.

3. Which of the following statements about smoking is *false?*
   a. Smoking behavior may have a genetic component.
   b. People who graduate college are less likely to smoke than those who complete only high school.
   c. Most regular smokers enjoy smoking.
   d. Smoking two packs of cigarettes daily is as dangerous as carrying 40 pounds of extra weight.

4. Tobacco use on college campuses
   a. is most often in the form of smokeless tobacco products used by students to avoid detection.
   b. is more prevalent among those students who also use marijuana, binge drink, and spend more time socializing with friends.
   c. has decreased in the past 10 years because almost all schools have adopted a no-smoking policy on their premises.
   d. is considered a minor problem by most student health center directors, since less than a third of students smoke.

5. Which of the following statements about smoking and minorities is true?
   a. Hispanic men are less likely to smoke than Hispanic women.
   b. Native American women who smoke are at low risk of having babies with health problems.
   c. African Americans are at greater risk for dying from heart disease, lung cancer, and stroke than those of other population groups.
   d. Smoking is culturally unacceptable among Southeast Asian men.

6. Women smokers
   a. tend to be less successful than men in quitting smoking.
   b. are more likely to die from breast cancer than lung cancer.

c. experience menstruation earlier than women who don't smoke.
   d. who smoke low-nicotine cigarettes lower their risk of having a heart attack to the same level as women who don't smoke.

7. Which of the following statements is *false?*
   a. Using chewing tobacco can lead to lesions on the mucous membranes of the mouth.
   b. Bidis come in several flavors.
   c. The active ingredient in cloves lowers sensation in the throat, so clove-cigarette smokers inhale more deeply.
   d. Smoking cigars is safe if you don't inhale.

8. Secondhand tobacco smoke is
   a. the smoke inhaled by a smoker.
   b. more hazardous than outdoor pollution as a cancer-causing agent.
   c. less hazardous than mainstream smoke.
   d. less likely to cause serious health problems in children than in adults.

9. Quitting smoking
   a. usually results in minor withdrawal symptoms.
   b. will do little to reverse the damage to the lungs and other parts of the body.
   c. can be aided by using nicotine replacement products.
   d. is best done by cutting down on the number of cigarettes you smoke over a period of months.

10. Ways to help yourself quit include all of the following except
    a. join a support group.
    b. make your home a smoke-free zone.
    c. try acupuncture.
    d. switch to bidis.

Answers to these questions can be found on page 652.

Critical Thinking

1. Has smoking become unpopular among your friends or family? What social activities continue to be associated with smoking? Can you think of any situation in which smoking might be frowned upon?

Critical Thinking

2. How would you motivate someone you care about to stop smoking? What reasons would you give for them to stop? Describe your strategy.

Critical Thinking

3. According to the chapter, environmental tobacco smoke is even more dangerous than mainstream smoke. If you're a nonsmoker, how would you react to someone who's smoking in the same room as you? Define the rights of smokers and nonsmokers.

Profile Plus

Tobacco use is the leading cause of preventable death in the United States. Learn how you might "breathe easier" with these activities on your Profile Plus CD-ROM.

Profile Plus

• Are You Addicted to Nicotine?

Profile Plus

• Smoking Cessation Questionnaire

Sites and Bytes

Centers for Disease Control: Tobacco Information & Prevention Source (TIPS)

www.cdc.gov/tobacco

This site features comprehensive educational materials on smoking, quitting tips, surgeon general reports, research data on tobacco use among specific populations and minority groups, and helpful information for educators and youth.

Sites and Bytes

Joe Chemo Antismoking Site
www.joechemo.org

Based on the character Joe Chemo, an antismoking parody of Joe Camel, this site is highly interactive and allows visitors to test their "Tobacco IQ," get a personalized "Smoke-o-Scope," and send free Joe Chemo E-Cards. There is also extensive information for teachers, antismoking activists, health-care providers, journalists, and smokers who wish to quit.

Sites and Bytes

American Lung Association Tobacco Control
www.lungusa.org/tobacco/index.html

This site features information on smoking cessation, including seven steps to a smoke-free life, as well as information on tobacco control, smoking and special populations, and several fact sheets on secondhand smoke, data and statistics, and current news events.

InfoTrac College Edition

Activity

Biasco, Frank, and James P. Hartnett. *College Student Journal,* Vol. 36, No. 3, September 2002, p. 442(6).

1. According to the various studies cited in this article, what characteristics of college students were associated with higher rates of smoking?

InfoTrac College Edition

2. What factors contribute to college students' attitudes toward smoking and how do these attitudes translate into smoking behaviors?

3. Based on the study, what are college students' attitudes regarding the social, health, interpersonal, legal, and modeling aspects about smoking?

You can find additional readings relating to tobacco use with InfoTrac

InfoTrac College Edition

College Edition, an online library of more than 900 journals and publications. Follow the instructions for accessing InfoTrac that were packaged with your textbook; then search for articles using a keyword search.

For additional links, resources, and suggested readings on InfoTrac College Edition, visit our Health & Wellness Resource Center at **http://health.wadsworth.com**.

Key Terms

The terms listed are used on the page indicated. Definitions of the terms are in the Glossary at the end of this book.

Key Terms

aversion therapy 413
bidis 408
bupropion 415
carbon monoxide 396

Key Terms

environmental tobacco smoke 410
mainstream smoke 410
nicotine 396

Key Terms

sidestream smoke 410
tar 396

References

1. National Household Survey on Drug Abuse. *The NHSDA Report: Cigarette Brand Preferences,* U.S. Department of Health and Human Services, July 11, 2003.
2. Parmet, Sharon. "Smoking and the Heart." *Journal of the American Medical Association,* Vol. 290, No. 1, July 2, 2003, p. 146.
3. Fogarty, Mignon. "Depending on Cigarettes, Counting on Science: Understanding How Specific Genes Work Could Keep Smokers From Coveting That Next Hit or Lighting Up in the First Place." *The Scientist,* Vol. 17, No. 6, March 24, 2003, p. 21.
4. "Reducing Tobacco Use: The Quest to Quit." *Facts of Life: Issue Briefing for Health Reporters,* Vol. 6, No. 3, March–April 2001.
5. Parmet, "Smoking and the Heart."
6. Sutherland, G. "Smoking: Can We Really Make a Difference?" *Heart,* Vol. 89, No. 5, May 2003, p. ii25.
7. Critchley, Julia, and Simon Capewell. "Mortality Risk Reduction Associated with Smoking Cessation in Patients with Coronary Heart Disease." *Journal of the American Medical Association,* Vol. 290, No. 1, July 2, 2003, p. 86.
8. "Study Finds Risk for Lung Cancer Varies Among Smokers." *Cancer Weekly,* April 8, 2003, p. 95.
9. Ibid.
10. Laloo, Umesh. "The Cough Reflex and the 'Healthy Smoker.'" *Chest,* Vol. 123, No. 3, March 2003, p. 660.
11. Yap, Ronald, and Kevin McVary. "Smoking and Erectile Dysfunction: How Strong a Link?" *Contemporary Urology,* Vol. 15, No. 3, March 2003, p. 34.
12. Mizoue, T., et al. "Combined Effect of Smoking and Occupational Exposure to Noise on Hearing Loss in Steel Factory Workers." *Occupational and Environmental Medicine,* Vol. 60, No. 1, January 2003, p. 56.
13. "Prevalence of Current Cigarette Smoking Among Adults and Changes in Prevalence of Current and Some Day Smoking—United States, 1996–2001." *Morbidity and Mortality Weekly Report,* Vol. 52, No. 14, April 11, 2003, p. 303.
14. "Killjoy Woz Here; The World Health Organisation." *The Economist (US),* Vol. 366, No. 8314, March 8, 2003.
15. "Social Costs of Smoking Are Triple Those of Illicit Drugs." *British Medical Journal,* Vol. 326, No. 7383, February 1, 2003, p. 242.
16. Fogarty, "Depending on Cigarettes, Counting on Science."

17. Johnston, Lloyd, et al. *Monitoring the Future: National Results on Adolescent Drug Use.* Bethesda, MD: National Institute on Drug Abuse, 2003.
18. Vogel, Julie, et al. "The Relationship Between Depression and Smoking in Adolescents." *Adolescence,* Vol. 38, No. 149, Spring 2003, p. 57.
19. Fogarty, "Depending on Cigarettes, Counting on Science."
20. Delnevo, Christine, et al. "Relationships Between Cigarette Smoking and Weight Control in Young Women." *Family and Community Health,* Vol. 26, No. 2, April–June 2003, p. 140.
21. Sutherland, "Smoking."
22. DiFranza, Joseph. "Initial Symptoms of Nicotine Dependence in Adolescents." *Tobacco Control,* Vol. 9, 2000.
23. Fiske, Susan. "Butt Out?" *Psychology Today,* March/April 2003, p. 41.
24. "Prevalence of Current Cigarette Smoking Among Adults."
25. Okuyemi, K. S., et al. "Light Smokers: Issues and Recommendations." *Nicotine and Tobacco Research,* Vol. 4, No. 2, 2002, p. 103.
26. Johnston et al., *Monitoring the Future.*
27. Halperin, Abigail, and Nancy Rigotti. "US Public Universities' Compliance with Recommended Tobacco-Control Policies." *Journal of American College Health,* Vol. 51, No. 5, p. 181.
28. Gaffney, K. F., et al. "Smoking Among Female College Students: A Time for Change." *Journal of Obstetrics, Gynecology, and Neonatal Nursing,* Vol. 31, No. 5, September–October 2002, p. 502.
29. Kear, M. E. "Psychosocial Determinants of Cigarette Smoking Among College Students." *Journal of Community Health Nursing,* Vol. 19, No. 4, Winter 2002, p. 245.
30. Rigotti, N. A., et al. "Tobacco Use by Massachusetts Public College Students: Long Term Effect of the Massachusetts Tobacco Control Program." *Tobacco Control,* Vol. 11, No. 2, June 2002, p. ii20.
31. Hestick, Henrietta, et al. "Trial and Lifetime Smoking Risks Among African-American College Students." *Journal of American College Health,* Vol. 49, No. 5, March 2001, p. 205.
32. Halperin and Rigotti, "US Public Universities' Compliance with Recommended Tobacco-Control Policies."
33. Ibid.
34. Wechsler, Henry, et al., "College Smoking Policies and Smoking Cessation

Programs: Results of a Survey of College Health Center Directors." *Journal of American College Health,* Vol. 49, No. 5, March 2001, p. 205.
35. Mooney, Debra. "Facilitating Student Use of Campus Smoking Cessation Services." *Journal of American College Health,* Vol. 50, No. 3, November 2001, p. 137.
36. Rigotti, Nancy, et al. "US College Students' Use of Tobacco Products: Results of a National Survey." *Journal of the American Medical Association,* Vol. 284, No. 6, August 9, 2000.
37. Hestick et al., "Trial and Lifetime Smoking Risks Among African-American College Students."
38. "African-American Teens at High Risk from Smoking." *Alcoholism & Drug Abuse Weekly,* Vol. 13, No. 10, March 5, 2001, p. 8.
39. Guinn, Bobby, et al. "Association of Tobacco Use with Acculturative Status, Knowledge, and Attitudes Among Early Adolescent Mexican Americans." *Research Quarterly for Exercise and Sport,* Vol. 72, No. 1, March 2001, p. A-29.
40. *Women and Smoking: A Report of the Surgeon General—2001.* Washington, DC: U.S. Department of Health and Human Services, 2001.
41. *The Formative Years: Pathways to Substance Abuse Among Girls and Young Women Ages 8 to 22.* Available at www.casacolumbia.org.
42. "New Evidence Links Smoking and Lung Cancer in Women." *Women's Health Weekly,* January 9, 2003, p. 18.
43. Sullivan, Michelle. "Smoking Can Lead to More Serious Prostate Cancer." *Family Practice News,* Vol. 33, No. 2, January 15, 2003, p. 25.
44. Krishnan, E., et al. "Smoking-Gender Interaction and Risk for Rheumatoid Arthritis." *Arthritis Research Therapy,* Vol. 5, No. 3, 2003, p. R158.
45. Bacon, C. G., et al. "Sexual Function in Men Older than 50 years of Age: Results from the Health Professionals Follow-up Study." *Annals of Internal Medicine,* Vol. 139, No. 3, August 5, 2003, p. I22.
46. "More Women Quit Smoking During Pregnancy but not Before and After." *Medical Letter on the CDC & FDA,* February 9, 2003, p. 33.
47. "HHS Report Shows Drug Use Rates Stable, Youth Tobacco Use Declines." *Medical Letter on the CDC & FDA,* October 21, 2001, p. 2.
48. Rigotti et al., "U.S. College Students' Use of Tobacco Products."

References

49. Malson, Jennifer, et al. "Comparison of the Nicotine Content of Tobacco Used in Bidis and Conventional Cigarettes." *Tobacco Control,* Vol. 10, No. 2, June 2001, p. 181.
50. "Can Science Make Cigarettes Safer?" *The Scientist,* Vol. 17, No. 6, March 24, 2003, p. 24.
51. Glantz, Stanton, and William Parmley. "Even a Little Secondhand Smoke Is Dangerous." *Journal of the American Medical Association,* Vol. 286, No. 4, July 25, 2001, p. 436.
52. Heloma, Antero, et al. "The Short-Term Impact of National Smoke-Free Workplace Legislation on Passive Smoking and Tobacco Use." *American Journal of Public Health,* Vol. 91, No. 9, September 2001, p. 1416.
53. England, Lucinda, et al. "Effects of Smoking Reduction During Pregnancy on the Birth Weight of Term Infants." *American Journal of Epidemiology,* Vol. 154, No. 8, October 15, 2001, p. 694.

References

54. "Tobacco Exposure Linked with Long-term Adverse Effects." *Brown University Digest of Addiction Theory and Application,* Vol. 20, No. 10, October 2001, p. 3.
55. "Killjoy Woz Here; The World Health Organisation."
56. "Public Supports Tobacco Control Strategies Outlined by American Lung Association." *Medical Letter on the CDC & FDA,* February 2, 2003, p. 28.
57. Robbins, Leslie. "Balancing Smokers, Nonsmokers and Health Concerns: Delaware and California Have Banned All Public Smoking." *State Legislatures,* Vol. 29, No. 1, January 2003, p. 27.
58. Fogarty, Mignon. "Public Health and Smoking Cessation: What Helps, What Doesn't." *The Scientist,* Vol. 17, No. 6, March 24, 2003, p. 21.
59. Robbins, "Balancing Smokers, Nonsmokers, and Health Concerns."

References

60. Glantz and Parmley. "Even a Little Secondhand Smoke Is Dangerous."
61. Centers for Disease Control and Prevention, www.cdc.gov.
62. "Study Shows Dangers of Resuming Smoking." *Alcoholism & Drug Abuse Weekly,* Vol. 13, No. 40, October 22, 2001, p. 8.
63. Fiske, Susan. "Sad Facts." *Psychology Today,* March/April 2003, p. 41.
64. James-Enger, Kelly. "Giving Up Smoking for Good: Use These Strategies to Help You Stop Smoking." *Diabetes Forecast,* Vol. 56, No. 2, February 2003, p. 84.
65. Ibid.
66. www.nicotrol.com.
67. Hales, Robert, and Dianne Hales. *The Mind-Mood Pill Book.* New York: Bantam Books, 2001.

SECTION V

PROTECTING YOUR HEALTH

EVERY day you make choices that affect both the quantity and the quality of your life. The right choices aren't always easy to make or to sustain. The chapters in this section can help by providing information you can use in making and implementing healthful decisions. By understanding the risks to your health, you can prepare to overcome them—and not simply live life, but celebrate it every day.

© Lori Adamski Peek/Stone/Getty Images

421

Preventing Infectious Diseases

There's something I have to tell you." Anise knew, just by the sound of her boyfriend's voice, that the "something" wasn't good news.

"My herpes is back."

Stunned, Anise tried to absorb all the information packed into this short sentence: She'd had no idea that the man she'd been sleeping with for several months had a sexually transmitted infection (STI). How did he get it? What else hadn't he told her about his past? What did he mean that it was "back"? Could she have caught it? And, finally, she asked the all-too-human question: How could this have happened to me?

By their very nature, infectious diseases take people by surprise. Throughout history, they have claimed more lives than any military conflict or natural disaster. Although modern medicine has won many victories against the agents of infection, we remain vulnerable to a host of infectious illnesses. Drug-resistant strains of tuberculosis and *Staphylococcus* bacteria challenge current therapies. New infectious diseases, such as SARS, are emerging and traveling around the world. Agents of infection also can be used as weapons of bioterrorism.[1]

Some of today's most common and dangerous infectious illnesses spread primarily through sexual contact, and their incidence has skyrocketed. The federal government estimates that 65 million Americans have a sexually transmitted infection.[2] These diseases cannot be prevented in the laboratory. Only you, by your behavior, can prevent and control them.

This chapter is a lesson in self-defense against all forms of infection. The information it provides can help you boost your defenses, recognize and avoid enemies, protect yourself from sexually transmitted infections, and realize when to seek help.

Steve Allen/Brand X Pictures/Getty Images

After studying the material in this chapter, you should be able to:

- **Explain** how the different agents of infection spread disease.
- **Describe** how your body protects itself from infectious disease.
- **List** and **describe** some common infectious diseases.

- **Identify** the sexually transmitted infections and the symptoms and treatment for each.
- **List** the methods of STI transmission.
- **Define** HIV infection and **describe** its symptoms.
- **Explain** some practical methods for preventing HIV infection and other sexually transmitted infections.

Understanding Infection

We live in a sea of microbes. Most of them don't threaten our health or survival; some, such as the bacteria that inhabit our intestines, are actually beneficial. Yet in the course of history, disease-causing microorganisms have claimed millions of lives. The twentieth century brought the conquest of infectious killers such as cholera and scarlet fever. Although modern science has won many victories against the agents of infection, infectious illnesses remain a serious health threat.

Infection is a complex process, triggered by various **pathogens** (disease-causing organisms) and countered by the body's own defenders. Physicians explain infection in terms of a **host** (either a person or a population) that contacts one or more agents in an environment. A **vector**—a biological or physical vehicle that carries the agent to the host—provides the means of transmission.

Agents of Infection

The types of microbes that can cause infection are viruses, bacteria, fungi, protozoa, and helminths (parasitic worms).

Viruses

The tiniest pathogens—**viruses**—are also the toughest; they consist of a bit of nucleic acid (DNA or RNA, but never both) within a protein coat. Unable to reproduce on its own, a virus takes over a body cell's reproductive machinery and instructs it to produce new viral particles, which are then released to enter other cells.

The most common viruses are these types:

:: Rhinoviruses and adenoviruses, which get into the mucous membranes and cause upper-respiratory tract infections and colds.

:: Coronaviruses, named for their corona or halo-like appearance, are second only to rhinoviruses in causing the common cold, and other respiratory infections. A coronavirus is the prime suspect in severe acute respiratory syndrome (SARS).

:: Influenza viruses, which can change their outer protein coats so dramatically that individuals resistant to one strain cannot fight off a new one.

:: Herpes viruses, which take up permanent residence in the cells and periodically flare up.

:: Papilloma viruses, which cause few symptoms in women and almost none in men, but may be responsible, at least in part, for a rise in the incidence of cervical cancer among younger women.

:: Hepatitis viruses, which cause several forms of liver infection, ranging from mild to life threatening.

:: Slow viruses, which give no early indication of their presence but can produce fatal illnesses within a few years.

:: Retroviruses, which are named for their backward (*retro*) sequence of genetic replication compared to other viruses. One retrovirus, human immunodeficiency virus (HIV), causes acquired immune deficiency syndrome (AIDS).

:: Filoviruses, which resemble threads and are extremely lethal.

The problem in fighting viruses is that it's difficult to find drugs that harm the virus and not the cell it has commandeered. **Antibiotics** (drugs that inhibit or kill bacteria) have no effect on viruses. **Antiviral drugs** don't completely eradicate a viral infection, although they can decrease its severity and duration. Because viruses multiply very quickly, antiviral drugs are most effective when taken before an infection develops or in its early stages.

Bacteria

Simple one-celled organisms, **bacteria** are the most plentiful microorganisms as well as the most pathogenic. Most kinds of bacteria don't cause disease; some, like certain strains of *Escherichia coli* that aid in digestion, play important roles within our bodies. Even friendly bacteria, however, can get out of hand and cause acne, urinary tract infections, vaginal infections, and other problems.

Bacteria harm the body by releasing either enzymes that digest body cells or toxins that produce the specific effects of such diseases as diphtheria or toxic shock syndrome. In self-defense the body produces specific proteins (called *antibodies*) that attack and inactivate the invaders. Tuberculosis, tetanus, gonorrhea, scarlet fever, and diphtheria are examples of bacterial diseases.

Because bacteria are sufficiently different from the cells that make up our bodies, antibiotics can kill them without harming our cells. Antibiotics work only against specific types of bacteria. If your doctor thinks you have a bacterial infection, tests of your blood, pus, sputum, urine, or stool can identify the particular bacterial strain.

Fungi

Single-celled or multicelled organisms, **fungi** consist of threadlike fibers and reproductive spores. Fungi lack chlorophyll and must obtain their food from organic material, which may include human tissue. Fungi release enzymes that digest cells and are most likely to attack hair-covered areas of the body, including the scalp, beard, groin, and external ear canals. They also cause athlete's foot. Treatment consists of antifungal drugs.

Protozoa

These single-celled, microscopic animals release enzymes and toxins that destroy cells or interfere with their function. Diseases caused by **protozoa** are not a major health problem in this country, primarily because of public health measures. Around the world, however, some 2.24 billion people (more than 40 percent of the world's population) are at risk for acquiring malaria—a protozoan-caused disease. Up to 3 million die from this disease annually. Many more come down with amoebic dysentery. Treatment for protozoa-caused diseases consists of general medical care to relieve the symptoms, replacement of lost blood or fluids, and drugs that kill the specific protozoan.

The most common disease caused by protozoa in the United States is *giardiasis,* an intestinal infection caused by microorganisms in human and animal feces. It has become a threat at day-care centers, as well as among campers and hikers who drink contaminated water. Symptoms include nausea, lack of appetite, gas, diarrhea, fatigue, abdominal cramps, and bloating. Many people recover in a month or two without treatment. However, in some cases the microbe causes recurring attacks over many years. Giardiasis can be life-threatening in small children and the elderly, who are especially prone to severe dehydration from diarrhea. Treatment usually consists of antibiotics.

Helminths (Parasitic Worms)

Small parasitic worms that attack specific tissues or organs and compete with the host for nutrients are called **helminths.** One major worldwide health problem is *schistosomiasis,* a disease caused by a parasitic worm, the fluke, that burrows through the skin and enters the circulatory system. Infection with another helminth, the tapeworm, may be contracted from eating undercooked beef, pork, or fish containing larval forms of the tapeworm. Helminthic diseases are treated with appropriate medications.

How Do You Catch an Infection?

The major vectors, or means of transmission, for infectious disease are animals and insects, people, food, and water.

Animals and Insects

Disease can be transmitted by house pets, livestock, and wild animals. Insects also spread a variety of diseases. The housefly may spread dysentery, diarrhea, typhoid fever, or trachoma (an eye disease rare in the United States but

(a)
© Omikron/Photo Researchers, Inc.

(b)
© John Durham/SPL/Photo Researchers, Inc.

(c)
© David Philips/Visuals Unlimited

(d)
Howard Sochurek/Medichrome

(e)
© Biophoto Associates/Photo Researchers, Inc.

Examples of the major categories of organisms that cause disease in humans. Except for the helminths (parasitic worms), pathogens are microorganisms that can be seen only with the aid of a microscope. (a) Viruses: common cold, (b) Fungi: yeast, (c) Protozoa: trichomonas, (d) Bacteria: syphilis, (e) Helminths: tapeworm.

common in other parts of the world). Other insects, including mosquitoes, ticks, mites, fleas, and lice, can transmit such diseases as malaria, yellow fever, encephalitis, dengue fever (a growing threat in Mexico), and Lyme disease.

New threats in the United States include West Nile virus (WNV), which can be spread to humans by mosquitoes that bite infected birds, and monkeypox virus, carried by various animals, including prairie dogs.[3] (Both of these illnesses are discussed later in this chapter.)

People

The people you're closest to can transmit pathogens through the air, through touch, or through sexual contact. To avoid infection, stay out of range of anyone who's coughing, sniffling, or sneezing, and don't share food or dishes. Carefully wash your dishes, utensils, and hands, and abstain from sex or make self-protective decisions about sexual partners. (See "Sexually Transmitted Infections" later in this chapter.)

Food

Every year foodborne illnesses strike millions of Americans, sometimes with fatal consequences. Bacteria account for two-thirds of foodborne infections, and thousands of suspected cases of infection with *Escherichia coli* bacteria in undercooked or inadequately washed food have been reported.

Every year as many as 4 million Americans have a bout with *Salmonella* bacteria, which have been found in about a third of all poultry sold in the United States. These infections can be serious enough to require hospitalization and can lead to arthritis, neurological problems, and even death. Consumers can greatly reduce the number of salmonella infections by proper handling, cooking, and refrigeration of poultry.

A deadly food disease, *botulism,* is caused by certain bacteria that grow in improperly canned foods. Although its occurrence is rare in commercial products, botulism is a danger in home canning. Another uncommon threat is *trichinosis,* caused by the larvae of a parasitic roundworm in uncooked meat. This infection, which causes nausea, vomiting, diarrhea, fever, thirst, profuse sweating, weakness, and pain, can be avoided by thoroughly cooking meat.

Water

Waterborne diseases, such as typhoid fever and cholera, are still widespread in less developed areas of the world. They have been rare in the United States, although outbreaks caused by inadequate water purification have occurred.

The Process of Infection

If someone infected with the flu sits next to you on a bus and coughs or sneezes, tiny viral particles may travel into your nose and mouth. Immediately the virus finds or creates an opening in the wall of a cell, and the process of infection begins. During the **incubation period,** the time between invasion and the first symptom, you're unaware of the pathogen multiplying inside you. In some diseases, incubation may go on for months, even years; for most, it lasts several days or weeks.

The early stage of the battle between your body and the invaders is called the *prodromal period.* As infected cells die, they release chemicals that help block the invasion. Other chemicals, such as *histamines,* cause blood vessels to dilate, thus allowing more blood to reach the battleground. During all of this, you feel mild, generalized symptoms, such as headache, irritability, and discomfort. You're also highly contagious. At the height of the battle—the typical illness period—you cough, sneeze, sniffle, ache, feel feverish, and lose your appetite.

Recovery begins when the body's forces gain the advantage. With time, the body destroys the last of the invaders and heals itself. However, the body is not able to develop long-lasting immunity to certain viruses, such as colds, flu, or HIV.

How Your Body Protects Itself

Various parts of your body safeguard you against infectious diseases by providing **immunity,** or protection, from these health threats. Your skin, when unbroken, keeps out most potential invaders. Your tears, sweat, skin oils, saliva, and mucus contain chemicals that can kill bacteria. Cilia, the tiny hairs lining your respiratory passages, move mucus, which traps inhaled bacteria, viruses, dust, and foreign matter, to the back of the throat, where it is swallowed; the digestive system then destroys the invaders.

When these protective mechanisms can't keep you infection-free, your body's immune system, which is on constant alert for foreign substances that might threaten the body, swings into action. The immune system includes structures of the lymphatic system—the spleen, thymus gland, lymph nodes, and lymph vessels—that help filter impurities from the body. (See Figure 13-1.) More than a dozen different types of white blood cells (lymphocytes) are concentrated in the organs of the lymphatic system or patrol the entire body by way of the blood and lymph vessels.

Some of these white blood cells are generalists and some are specialists. The generalists include *macrophages,* which are large scavenger cells with insatiable appetites for foreign cells, diseased and run-down red blood cells, and other biological debris (see photo on p. 428). The specialists are the *B cells* and *T cells,* which respond to specific invaders.

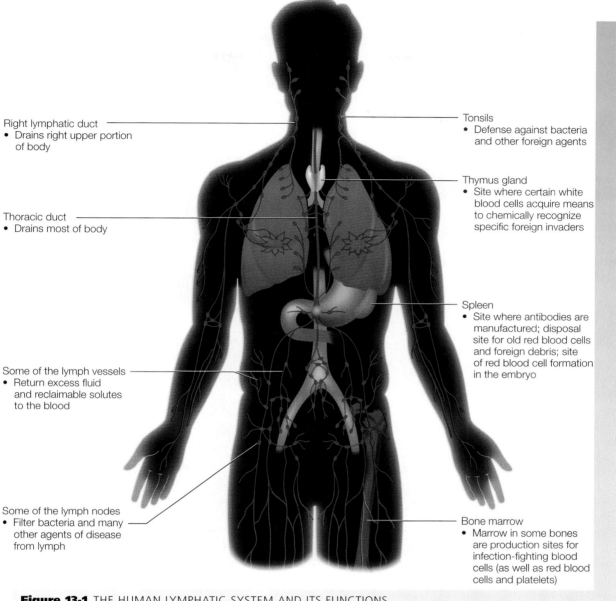

Right lymphatic duct
• Drains right upper portion of body

Thoracic duct
• Drains most of body

Some of the lymph vessels
• Return excess fluid and reclaimable solutes to the blood

Some of the lymph nodes
• Filter bacteria and many other agents of disease from lymph

Tonsils
• Defense against bacteria and other foreign agents

Thymus gland
• Site where certain white blood cells acquire means to chemically recognize specific foreign invaders

Spleen
• Site where antibodies are manufactured; disposal site for old red blood cells and foreign debris; site of red blood cell formation in the embryo

Bone marrow
• Marrow in some bones are production sites for infection-fighting blood cells (as well as red blood cells and platelets)

Figure 13-1 THE HUMAN LYMPHATIC SYSTEM AND ITS FUNCTIONS
The lymphatic system helps filter impurities from the body.

An *antigen* is any substance the white blood cells recognize as foreign. B cells create antibodies, which are proteins that bind to antigens and mark them for destruction by other white blood cells. Antigens are specific to the pathogen, and the antibody to a particular antigen binds only to that antigen (see Figure 13-2). Once the human body produces antibodies against a specific antigen—the mumps virus, for instance—you're protected against that antigen for life. If you're again exposed to mumps, the antibodies previously produced prevent another episode of the disease. This protection is called **antibody–mediated immunity** (or humoral immunity). Antibody-mediated immunity is generally effective against bacterial or viral infections.

But you don't have to suffer through an illness to acquire immunity. Inoculation with a vaccine containing synthetic or weakened antigens can give you the same protection. The type of long-lasting immunity in which the body makes its own antibodies to a pathogen is called *active immunity.* Immunity produced by the injection of **gamma globulin,** the antibody-containing part of the blood from another person or animal that has developed antibodies to a disease, is called *passive immunity.*

The various types of T cells are responsible for **cell-mediated immunity.** T cells are lymphocytes manufactured in the bone marrow and carried to the thymus for maturation. Cell-mediated immunity mainly protects against parasites, fungi, cancer cells, and foreign tissue. Thousands of different T cells work together to ward off

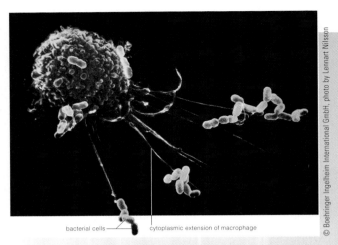

bacterial cells —   cytoplasmic extension of macrophage

Electron micrograph of macrophage (red), with extensions that are making contact with bacterial cells (green). Bacteria are engulfed by this type of white blood cell.

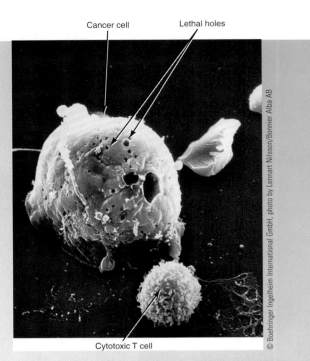

Cancer cell   Lethal holes

Cytotoxic T cell

Electron micrograph of a T cell touch-killing a cancer cell. The T cell releases toxic substances that puncture the cancer cell's membrane, move into the cell, and kill it.

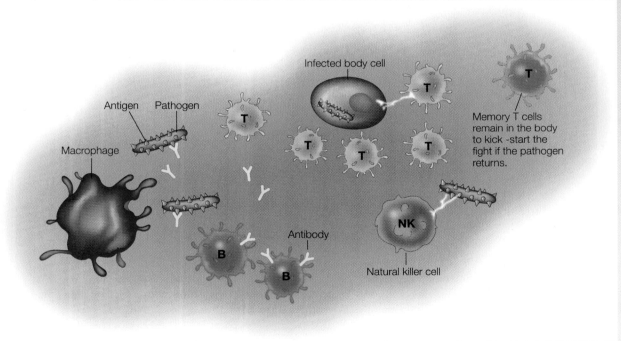

Antigen   Pathogen

Macrophage

Infected body cell

Memory T cells remain in the body to kick -start the fight if the pathogen returns.

Antibody

NK

Natural killer cell

Figure 13-2 THE IMMUNE RESPONSE

Some T cells can touch-kill infected body cells, and B cells churn out antibodies to tag the pathogen for destruction by macrophages and other white blood cells.

disease. Different T cells have differing functions, including the activation of other immune cells, help in antibody-mediated responses, and the suppression of lymphocyte activity.

Immune Response

Attacked by pathogens, the body musters its forces and fights. Sometimes the invasion is handled like a minor border skirmish; other times a full-scale battle is waged throughout the body. Together, the immune cells work like an internal police force. When an antigen enters the body, the T cells aided by macrophages engage in combat with the invader. Certain T cells (cytotoxic T cells) can destroy infected body cells or tumor cells by "touch-killing." Meanwhile, the B cells churn out antibodies, which rush to the scene and join in the fray. Also busy at surveillance are natural killer cells that, like the elite forces of a SWAT team, seek out and destroy viruses and cancer cells. (See Figure 13-2.)

The **lymph nodes,** or glands, are small tissue masses in which some protective cells are stored. If pathogens invade your body, many of them are carried to the lymph nodes to be destroyed. This is why your lymph nodes often feel swollen when you have a cold or the flu.

If the microbes establish a foothold, the blood supply to the area increases, bringing oxygen and nutrients to the fighting cells. Tissue fluids, as well as antibacterial and antitoxic proteins, accumulate. You may develop redness, swelling, local warmth, and pain—the signs of **inflammation.** As more tissue is destroyed, a cavity, or **abscess,** forms, and fills with fluid, battling cells, and dead white blood cells (pus). If the invaders aren't killed or inactivated, the pathogens are able to spread into the bloodstream and cause what is known as **systemic disease.**

Some people have an **immune deficiency**—either inborn or acquired. A very few children are born without an effective immune system; their lives can be endangered by any infection. Although still experimental, therapy to implant a missing or healthy gene may offer new hope for a normal life.

Immunity and Stress

Whenever we confront a crisis, large or small, our bodies produce powerful hormones that provide extra energy. However, this stress response dampens immunity, reducing the number of some key immune cells and the responsiveness of others.

Stress affects the body's immune system in different ways, depending on two factors: the controllability or uncontrollability of the stressor and the mental effort required to cope with the stress. An uncontrollable stressor that lasts longer than 15 minutes may interfere with cytokine interleukin-6, which plays an essential role in

activating the immune defenses. Uncontrollable stressors also produce high levels of the hormone cortisol, which suppress immune system functioning. The mental efforts required to cope with high-level stressors produce only brief immune changes that appear to have little consequence for health. However, stress has been shown to slow pro-inflammatory cytokine production, which is essential for wound healing.

Immune Disorders

Sometimes our immune system overreacts to certain substances, mistakes the body's own tissues for enemies, or doesn't react adequately. The result is an immune disorder such as allergies and autoimmune disorders.

Allergies

An **allergy** represents a hypersensitivity to a substance in our environment or diet. According to the American College of Allergy, Asthma, and Immunology, allergies affect about 38 percent of all Americans—almost twice as many as allergy experts once believed—and millions of them suffer unnecessarily because they don't know about effective treatment options, such as allergy shots (immunotherapy).

Allergy sufferers run annual tabs of up to $2 billion in doctor visits, diagnostic tests, prescriptions, and decreased productivity. Every year they account for more than 10 million workdays missed; every day they keep 10,000 children out of school.

Allergies are common on campus. In one study of 251 college seniors, more than half (58 percent) reported some allergy symptoms during the previous year. More than nine in ten took medications for relief—prescription drugs, over-the-counter agents, or a combination of both. Even though more than half of allergy sufferers described the effects of medications as comparable to three or four drinks of alcohol, about a third reported taking over-the-counter antihistamines, with or without prescription drugs prior to a test.[4]

Allergy symptoms are many and miserable: itching, nasal congestion, eye irritation, coughing, wheezing, hives, vomiting, and diarrhea (from food allergies), even sudden, life-threatening collapse (from anaphylaxis, the most extreme allergic reaction). While victims seldom die of allergies, they just as rarely recover. And when individuals try to outrun allergies by moving away from one region's irritants, they often end up acquiring new sensitivities on their new home ground.

A list of allergic triggers, or allergens, reads like an inventory of creation, including life's pleasures (such as foods and flowers), perils (insect stings and poison ivy), and

STRATEGIES FOR PREVENTION

Fighting Hidden Allergens

- *Switch to feather pillows.* Researchers in the United Kingdom found significantly higher levels of house dust mite allergens in synthetic pillows.

- *Use bleach rather than detergent.* Very low concentrations of bleach are more effective in removing allergens from various surfaces around the house than other common cleaners.

- *Cover mattresses and pillows with tightly woven fabrics.* These materials, compared with non-woven or semipermeable synthetic fabrics, effectively block cat and dust allergens even after repeated washings.

- *Store clothing in sealed containers with moth-killing products.* Products such as moth balls or crystals and lavandin oil packets also kill house dust mites and their eggs.

- *Put comforters in the clothes dryer.* An hour of dry heat in a home dryer dramatically reduces the number of house dust mites in comforters and duvets filled with synthetic materials.

inescapable realities (like mold and dust). The very air we breathe can be a danger. The symptoms of allergy and of its more sinister sister-disease, asthma, increase along with pollutants, such as diesel fumes, and the number of small particles in the environment.

Thanks to breakthroughs in treatments allergy sufferers no longer have to choose between feeling better or feeling alert. Treatment options include non-sedating oral medications, nasal sprays, and **immunotherapy,** which consists of a series of injections of small but increasing doses of an allergen.

Immunotherapy has proven to have long-term, perhaps permanent, benefits. In one study, traditional allergen immunotherapy with a grass-pollen extract, administered for three to four years, induced a clinical remission that persisted for at least three years after treatment. Immunotherapy in patients allergic to insect stings also induces long-lasting immunologic changes and reduces their risk of potentially fatal reactions. Immunotherapy has the greatest benefit, relative to the investment of time and cost, for allergies that persist for more than one season or throughout the year.

Autoimmune Disorders

For unknown reasons, the immune system sometimes declares war on the cells, tissues, or organs it normally protects. This misfiring can cause more than 80 **autoimmune disorders,** including rheumatoid arthritis, myasthenia gravis, and systemic lupus erythematosus. Striking women three times as often as men, these illnesses afflict some 14 to 22 million Americans and rank among the top ten killers and top four disablers of women under age 65.[5] See The X&Y File: "Diseases That Discriminate."

Genetics accounts for about half of vulnerability to autoimmune disorders, which tend to cluster in families. Environmental factors—drugs, chemicals, bacteria and viruses—also may play a role. Recent research has led to new understanding of why the body sometimes turns on itself as well as breakthroughs in diagnosis and treatment.

"A new era is beginning," says rheumatologist Jill Buyon, M.D., of New York University, coauthor of *The Autoimmune Connection.* "Better tests may allow us to diagnose autoimmune disorders before they damage organs, and new treatments may make these diseases easier to manage and maybe even stop them in their tracks."[6] New biological agents target specific proteins involved in inflammation. Stem cell transplants destroy a patient's immune system, usually with high-dose chemotherapy, and then reinfuse stem cells, either removed previously from the patient or from another person. Because of potentially fatal risks, stem cells usually are transplanted only in life-or-death cases when other therapies fail.

✖ Immunization: The Key to Prevention

One of the great success stories of modern medicine has been the development of vaccines that provide protection against many infectious diseases. Immunization has reduced cases of measles, mumps, tetanus, whooping cough, and other life-threatening illnesses by more than 95 percent.

Immunizations for Children

The number of vaccines recommended for children has grown from four—diphtheria, tetanus, pertussis (whooping cough), and smallpox—in the 1950s to more than twenty today, with more on the horizon. Federal health officials and medical organizations currently recommend immunization against diphtheria, tetanus, pertussis, measles, mumps, rubella, polio, *Haemophilus influenzae* type b (Hib), hepatitis B (Hep B), varicella (chickenpox), and *S. pneumoniae.* Most are given in combined vaccines.[7]

In the past, these diseases infected hundreds of thousands of children and claimed many lives every year. Public health officials estimate that every dollar spent on childhood immunizations saves $10 to $14 in preventing future diseases. Yet only about three-quarters of young children are fully immunized. The American College of Preventive *the X & Y file* *Diseases That Discriminate*

Autoimmune Diseases	Characteristics	Prevalence in Women vs. Men	Common Symptoms
Graves' disease	A thyroid condition characterized by an overactive thyroid gland, which produces too much thyroid hormone.	7:1	Nervousness and irritability; weight loss; fast/irregular heart rate; heat intolerance/increased perspiration; increased appetite; sleep disturbances (such as insomnia); muscle weakness; trembling hands; irregular menstrual periods; exophthalmos (bulging eyes); appearance of a goiter (a swelling in the neck caused by enlargement of the thyroid gland).
Systematic lupus erythematosus (lupus)	A chronic autoimmune disorder that can affect any tissue or organ system including the joints, kidneys, heart, lungs, brain, blood or skin.	6:1	Achy joints. frequent fever of 100 degrees F or higher; anemia; fatigue; arthritis; skin rash; butterfly-shaped rash across cheek and nose; hair loss.
Scleroderma	Proliferation of immune cells that produce scar tissue in the skin, some internal organs and small blood vessels.	3:1	Reynaud's phenomenon, a condition characterized by decreased blood flow, usually to the fingers, and often brought on by cold temperatures; swelling and puffiness of the fingers or hands, followed by skin thickening a few months later; skin ulcers on the fingers; joint stiffness in the hands; sore throat; diarrhea.
Rheumatoid arthritis	Develops when the immune system attacks the synovium (the membranes that surround joints) causing inflammation, which gradually destroys cartilage, making movement of the joints painful and difficult. May also affect muscles, lungs and liver.	2.5:1	Inflamed, swollen and tender joints that may eventually become deformed; weakness or loss of function of joints; morning stiffness, fatigue or general sense of malaise. Often affects joints in a symmetrical pattern: if one knee or hand is affected, the other one usually also is impaired.
Multiple sclerosis	Occurs when immune system attacks the myelin sheath—the fatty insulation surrounding nerve cells in the brain and spinal cord. The myelin sheath enables high speed transmission of messages between these centers and the rest of the body; gradually as scar tissue develops in different areas of myelin, nerve messages are disrupted, affecting the body in a variety of ways.	2:1	Fatigue; short-term memory problems; temporary weakness, tingling or paralysis in one or more limbs; loss of coordination or unsteady gait; balance problems; blurred vision; difficulty swallowing; any or all symptoms may appear and then subside, then appear again, weeks, months or years later.

Sources: American Autoimmune Related Diseases Association, Inc.; American Diabetes Association; American Thyroid Association; Lupus Foundation of America; National Graves' Disease Foundation; National Institute of Diabetes and Digestive and Kidney Diseases; National Institute of Arthritis and Musculoskeletal and Skin Diseases; National Multiple Sclerosis Society.

Medicine has called for expansion of immunization to all children.[8]

Large numbers of children in urban centers and a disproportionately high number of African-American youngsters, haven't been properly immunized. While there has been progress in protecting most American children against infectious diseases, many children are going without the booster shots necessary for complete immunization.[9]

:: ***Hepatitis B (HepB).*** The U.S. Public Health Service recommends immunization against hepatitis B for infants as a way of preventing a disease (discussed later in this chapter) that infects an estimated 200,000 people in the United States and kills 4,000 to 5,000 Americans each year. However, some object to hepatitis B vaccinations for children, because the potential risks associated with the vaccine are greater than the odds of a child contracting what is primarily an adult disease. Public health professionals counter by saying that children under age 5, although they constitute a

Immunizations are an important protection against childhood diseases. Neighborhood clinics in urban centers offer immunizations to those children at particular risk.

small minority of those with hepatitis B, face the highest risk of death from cirrhosis and liver cancer.

A problem with delaying immunization until the teen years is a lower compliance rate among some groups of adolescents. A new vaccine against both hepatitis A and hepatitis B has proven to be effective over long periods (at least five years) in both children and adults.

:: *Diphtheria, tetanus, and acellular pertussis (DTaP).* Diphtheria, a dangerous disease, is rare because of immunization. An average of fewer than three cases per year have been reported in the last decade. Adults as well as children should get booster shots every 10 years.

Tetanus is an uncommon disease transmitted via a variety of injuries. Since the tetanus germ cannot grow in the presence of air, puncture wounds, such as those caused by stepping on a nail or gardening rake, pose the greatest danger. Tetanus is often called lockjaw, because the characteristic symptom is a stiffening of the jaws so severe that the patient is unable to open his or her mouth. Everyone should get booster inoculations for tetanus at least once every 10 years.

Pertussis (whooping cough), a bacterial infection that can develop into pneumonia, is potentially fatal. *Acellular* pertussis vaccines, made of only a few parts of the pertussis cell, have proven effective against pertussis and produce fewer side effects than earlier vaccines.

:: **Haemophilus influenzae *type B (Hib).*** In the United States, Hib was once a cause of bacterial *meningitis,* a life-threatening infection of the lining of the brain and spinal cord. A vaccine that protects children has nearly eliminated this potentially deadly disease.

:: *Inactivated Polio.* Polio, spread from person to person by the oral-fecal route, can lead to paralysis and even death. Immunization has greatly reduced its incidence.

:: *Measles, mumps, and rubella (MMR).* The number of cases of measles has fallen to an all-time low. However, the Centers for Disease Control (CDC) recommends continued vigilance and immunizations.

Symptoms of measles include a rash on the face and body, runny nose, high fever, cough, eye inflammation, and fatigue. Ten to 15 percent of measles patients develop serious complications, such as ear infections, diarrhea, or pneumonia. One out of every 1,000 develops encephalomyelitis, an inflammation of the brain that can be fatal or lead to mental retardation, or to movement, behavioral, or neurological disorders.

Mumps, caused by a virus, can lead to deafness, meningitis, and painful swelling of the ovaries and testicles.

Rubella (German measles) is another serious threat. Recent outbreaks among newborns have been blamed on the lack of routine rubella screening and follow-up vaccination of susceptible women of childbearing age.

About 85 percent of adults are immune to rubella, even if they have no history of the disease. The most serious consequence of this mild disease is the destructive effect it has on an unborn baby—including blindness—if the mother is infected in early pregnancy.

:: *Varicella (Chickenpox).* A vaccine against chickenpox, a common childhood disease that causes itchy red pustules, seems more effective when given alone rather than in combination with MMR vaccine.

:: **S. pneumoniae.** This vaccine protects children from the leading cause of bacterial meningitis, a potentially fatal illness.

:: *Hepatitis A.* This vaccine is recommended for children and adolescents in selected states and regions where they may be at higher risk because of contaminated water or the high number of local cases.

:: *Influenza.* This annual vaccine is recommended for children with certain illnesses, including asthma, diabetes, heart disease, sickle cell disease, and HIV, or who are living with household members at high risk. It is also recommended for healthy children between the ages of 6 and 23 months, a peak time for influenza-related hospitalizations.

A new nasal vaccine, FluMist, delivers protection via a squirt up the nose instead of a shot in the arm. The FDA has approved its use for healthy people age 5 to 49, but not for toddlers, the elderly, and people with asthma or some other chronic diseases.

Immunizations for Adolescents and Young Adults

Although many people think that vaccines are only for children, they remain an important part of protection throughout life. All adolescents and young adults should have the following vaccinations:

:: *Varicella* (chickenpox), for those who have not had chickenpox or been vaccinated against it. Adults are 10 times more likely than children to be hospitalized with the severe consequences of chickenpox, including pneumonia and encephalitis (inflammation of the brain). The American Academy of Pediatrics recommends that 13- to 18-year-olds receive two doses, the second one given four to eight weeks after the first.

:: *Hepatitis B,* for those who did not receive the vaccine as infants. Hepatitis B virus, which is easily transmitted by simple contact with a toothbrush or hand towel, primarily infects teenagers and young adults. The vaccine is given in a series of three shots.

:: *Measles, mumps, and rubella,* for those who did not receive two doses of the vaccine. A second dose has been required since 1989, after several serious measles outbreaks. About 95 percent of people develop immunity after one dose of the vaccine; about 99 percent after two doses of the vaccine.

CDC officials estimate that 5 to 15 percent of college students are susceptible to measles because they were vaccinated at 12 months of age rather than the currently recommended 15 months, or did not receive a second dose of the vaccine between ages 4 and 12. Others were given immune globulin, which was intended to lower the risk of reaction but which also reduced the vaccine's effectiveness. Many colleges are requiring students to submit proof of measles immunization before allowing them to enroll. In all, some 3 million Americans, aged 20 to 37, are at risk.

:: *Tetanus and diphtheria.* Since most children complete their initial series of diphtheria and tetanus vaccinations (given as part of the combination vaccine called DTaP) at four to six years of age, they should get their next booster dose during adolescence. The American Academy of Pediatrics recommends that teenagers receive a special preparation of the tetanus and diphtheria vaccines (known as Td).

College students living in dormitories are at increased risk of infection with the meningococcus bacterium, which causes meningitis, an inflammation of the lining of the brain. The pros and cons of vaccination are discussed on page 437.

Immunizations for Adults

Table 13-1 shows the recommended immunizations for adults. If you're uncertain about your past immunizations, check with family members or your doctor. If you can't find answers, a blood test can show whether you carry antibodies to specific illnesses.

If you're pregnant or planning to get pregnant within the next three months, do not get a measles, mumps, rubella, or polio vaccination. If you're allergic to neomycin, consult your doctor before getting a measles, mumps, rubella, or intramuscular polio vaccination. Those with egg allergies should also check with a doctor before getting a measles, mumps, or flu vaccination. Also, never get a vaccination when you have a high fever.

■ Infectious Diseases

An estimated 500 microorganisms cause disease; no effective treatment exists for about 200 of these illnesses. Although infections can be unavoidable at times, the more you know about their causes, the more you can do to protect yourself.

■ Who Is at Highest Risk of Infectious Diseases?

Like human bullies, the viruses responsible for the most common infectious illnesses tend to pick on those least capable of fighting back. Among the most vulnerable are the following groups:

:: *Children and their families.* Youngsters get up to a dozen colds annually; adults average two a year. When a flu epidemic hits a community, about 40 percent of school-age boys and girls get sick, compared with only 5 to 10 percent of adults. But parents get up to six times as many colds as other adults.

:: *The elderly.* Statistically, fewer older men and women are likely to catch a cold or flu, yet when they do, they face greater danger than the rest of the population. People over 65 who get the flu have a one in ten chance of being hospitalized for pneumonia or other respiratory problems, and a one in fifty chance of dying from the disease.

:: *The chronically ill.* Lifelong diseases, such as diabetes, kidney disease, or sickle-cell anemia, decrease an individual's ability to fend off infections. Individuals taking medications that suppress the immune system, such as steroids, are more vulnerable to infections, as are those with medical conditions that impair immunity, such as infection with HIV.

:: *Smokers and those with respiratory problems.* Smokers are a high-risk group for respiratory infections and serious complications, such as pneumonia. Chronic breathing disorders, such as asthma and emphysema, also greatly increase the risk of respiratory infections.

:: *Those who live or work in close contact with someone sick.* Health-care workers who treat high-risk patients, nursing home residents, and others living in close quarters—such as students in dormitories—face greater odds of catching others' colds and flus.

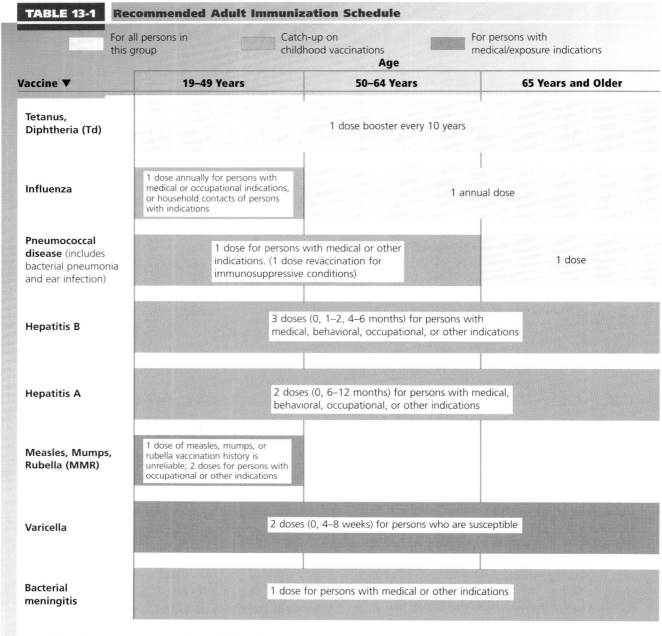

TABLE 13-1 **Recommended Adult Immunization Schedule**

	For all persons in this group	Catch-up on childhood vaccinations	For persons with medical/exposure indications

	Age		
Vaccine ▼	**19–49 Years**	**50–64 Years**	**65 Years and Older**
Tetanus, Diphtheria (Td)	1 dose booster every 10 years		
Influenza	1 dose annually for persons with medical or occupational indications, or household contacts of persons with indications	1 annual dose	
Pneumococcal disease (includes bacterial pneumonia and ear infection)	1 dose for persons with medical or other indications. (1 dose revaccination for immunosuppressive conditions)		1 dose
Hepatitis B	3 doses (0, 1–2, 4–6 months) for persons with medical, behavioral, occupational, or other indications		
Hepatitis A	2 doses (0, 6–12 months) for persons with medical, behavioral, occupational, or other indications		
Measles, Mumps, Rubella (MMR)	1 dose of measles, mumps, or rubella vaccination history is unreliable; 2 doses for persons with occupational or other indications		
Varicella	2 doses (0, 4–8 weeks) for persons who are susceptible		
Bacterial meningitis	1 dose for persons with medical or other indications		

Sources: Advisory Committee on Immunization Practices (ACIP), American College of Obstetricians and Gynecologists (ACOG), and the American Academy of Family Physicians (AAFP as found at www.cdc.gov/mmwr/preview/mmwrhtml.mm5140a5.htm).

:: ***Residents or workers in poorly ventilated buildings.***
Building technology has helped spread certain air-borne illnesses, such as tuberculosis, via recirculated air. Indoor air quality can be closely linked with disease transmission in winter, when people spend a great deal of time in tightly sealed rooms.

Common Cold

There are more than 200 distinct cold viruses, including a recently discovered metapneumovirus.[10] Although in a single season you may develop a temporary immunity to one

or two, you may then be hit by a third. Americans come down with 1 billion colds annually.

Every year, about 25 million cold-sufferers in the United States visit their family doctors with uncomplicated upper respiratory infections. The common cold results in about 20 million days of absence from work and 22 million days of absence from school.[11]

Colds can strike in any season, but different cold viruses are more common at different times of years. Rhinoviruses cause most spring, summer, and early fall colds, and tend to cause more symptoms above the neck (stuffy nose, headache, runny eyes). Adenoviruses, parain-

One of the telltale symptoms of a cold is sneezing.

fluenza viruses, coronaviruses, influenza viruses, and others that strike in the winter are more likely to get into the bronchi and trachea (the breathing passages) and cause more fever and bronchitis.

Cold viruses spread by coughs, sneezes, and touch. Cold-sufferers who sneeze and then touch a doorknob or countertop leave a trail of highly contagious viruses behind them. The best preventive tactics are frequent hand-washing, replacing toothbrushes regularly, exercising regularly, and avoiding stress overload. High levels of stress increase the risk of becoming infected by respiratory viruses and developing cold symptoms. People who feel unable to deal with everyday stresses have an exaggerated immune reaction that may intensify cold or flu symptoms once they've contracted a virus. Those with a positive emotional outlook are less vulnerable.[12]

Until scientists develop truly effective treatments, experts advise against taking aspirin and acetaminophen (Tylenol), which may suppress the antibodies the body produces to fight cold viruses and increase symptoms such as nasal stuffiness. A better alternative for achiness is ibuprofen (brand names include Motrin, Advil, and Nuprin), which doesn't seem to affect immune response. Children, teenagers, and young adults should never take aspirin for a cold or flu because of the danger of Reye's syndrome, a potentially deadly disorder that can cause convulsions, coma, swelling of the brain, and kidney damage.

The main drawback of antihistamines, the most widely used cold remedy, is drowsiness, which can impair a person's ability to safely drive or operate machinery. Another common ingredient, pseudoephedrine, opens and drains sinus passages without drowsiness but can speed up heart rate and cause complications for individuals with high blood pressure, diabetes, heart disease, or thyroid disorders. Nasal sprays clear a stuffy nose, but they invariably cause a rebound effect.

In general, doctors recommend treating specific symptoms—headache, cough, chest congestion, sore throat—

rather than taking a multisymptom medication. For a cough, the ingredient to look for in any suppressant is dextromethrophan, which turns down the brain's cough reflex. In expectorants, the only medicine the FDA has deemed effective is guaifenesin, which helps liquefy secretions so you can bring up mucus from the chest. Unless you're coughing up green or foul yellow mucus (signs of a secondary bacterial infection), antibiotics won't help. They have no effect against viruses and may make your body more resistant to such medications when you develop a bacterial infection in the future.[13]

Many Americans try alternative remedies for colds. Vitamin C and extracts of the plant *echinacea* are widely used to prevent the common cold, but there is no conclusive evidence that they help.[14] In a recent carefully controlled study of college students, echinacea tablets proved no more effective than placebos in reducing the duration or severity of a cold. (See Fact or Fiction? "Echinacea can help . . .")[15]

Zinc lozenges, another popular alternative treatment in recent years, have not proven to be clearly beneficial. In at least ten studies that have evaluated the benefits of zinc, some have found no benefit, whereas others have found significant reductions in the severity or duration of cold symptoms. Almost all have been criticized for various reasons, such as the size of the sample or the formulation of zinc used.

Although colds and sore throats—a frequent cold symptom—are caused by viruses, many people seek treatment with antibiotics, which are effective only against bacteria. An estimated 5 to 17 percent of sore throats in adults

---

FACT OR FICTION? ???????????

Echinacea can help fight the common cold.

Fiction: In a recent study, 148 college students at the University of Wisconsin, Madison, took echinacea or placebos when they came down with colds. Every day the students completed a detailed questionnaire about the presence and severity of symptoms such as dry cough, sore throat, and runny nose. The echinacea capsules had no effect on either the duration or severity of cold symptoms. Students in both groups continued to sniffle and suffer for about six days. This randomized, double-blind, placebo-controlled trial was more scientifically rigorous than previous studies, which had yielded contradictory findings.

Source: Richard Sadovsky. "Unrefined Echinacea Does Not Ease Common Cold Symptoms." *American Family Physician*, Vol. 67, No. 7, April 1, 2003, p. 1589.

are caused by bacteria *(Group A streptococci)*. The inappropriate use of antibiotics contributes to the growing problem of bacteria becoming resistant to the antibiotics that previously were able to kill them.[16]

 Colds are common among college students, many of whom do not recognize their signs or respond effectively to their symptoms. In a survey of 425 students at three college campuses in Louisiana and Indiana, 10 percent said they would see a physician for a cold; 41 percent believed that antibiotics were an effective treatment. More students said they would use antibiotics if their symptoms included a fever or discolored nasal discharge.[17]

Your own immune system can do something modern science cannot: cure a cold. All it needs is time, rest, and plenty of fluids. Usually cold symptoms last for one to two weeks, although chest colds (bronchitis) may last two or three weeks.[18] Warmth is important because the aptly named "cold" viruses replicate at lower temperatures. Hot soups and drinks (particularly those with a touch of something pungent, like lemon or ginger) raise body temperature and help clear the nose.[19] Tea may enhance the immune system.[20] Even more important is getting off your feet. Taking it easy reduces demands on the body, which helps speed recovery.

FACT OR FICTION? ??????????????

Tea may help keep infections at bay.

Fact: In a small controlled study, researchers at Harvard's Brigham and Women's Hospital have shown that ordinary tea may enhance the immune system by increasing the body's output of an infection fighter called interferon gamma. Coffee does not have the same effect. Doctors still do not know whether a particular type of tea—black, green, or oolong—may be more effective in fending off bacteria and other pathogens. The volunteers in the study drank 20 ounces of black tea for two weeks and doubled or tripled their interferon gamma levels. Other studies have suggested additional possible benefits for tea-lovers, including protection from various forms of cancer, cardiovascular disease, Alzheimer's, Parkinson's, and rheumatoid arthritis.

Source: Arati Kamath, et al. "Antigens in Tea-Beverage Prime Human V2V2 T Cells *In Vitro* and *In Vivo* for Memory and Nonmemory Antibacterial Cytokine Responses." *Proceedings of the National Academy of the Sciences*, Vol. 100, No. 10, May 13, 2003, p. 6009.

Influenza

Although similar to a cold, **influenza**—or the flu—causes more severe symptoms that last longer. Every year 10 to 20 percent of Americans develop influenza, 114,000 are hospitalized, and 36,000 die. (www.cdc.gov.)

Flu viruses, transmitted by coughs, sneezes, laughs, and even normal conversation, are extraordinarily contagious, particularly in the first three days of the disease. The usual incubation period is two days, but symptoms can hit hard and fast. Two varieties of viruses—influenza A and influenza B—cause most flus. In recent years, the deadliest flu epidemics have been caused by various forms of influenza A viruses.

A vaccine against the flu is available, but it is not foolproof. "Because the flu virus is constantly changing, you need a new shot every year," explains Edwin Kilbourne, M.D., of New York Medical College, who decides the components of each year's flu vaccine. "And because it takes the body time to manufacture antibodies to the new viruses, you should get a vaccination at least 10 to 14 days before an outbreak hits your area."[21]

Flu shots now are advised for almost everyone. The Center for Infectious Diseases of the CDC recommends a yearly flu shot for people older than age 50, residents of nursing homes and other long-term care facilities, adults and children with chronic illnesses or weakened immune systems, women who will be more than three months pregnant during the flu season, and, when feasible, young, otherwise healthy children between the ages of 6 and 23 months.[22] In older individuals, flu shots may offer significant protection against strokes and heart disease.[23] The only individuals who should steer clear are those allergic to eggs, since the inactivated flu viruses are grown in chick embryos.

A new alternative to flu shots is FluMist, an intranasal spray containing a live, attenuated influenza virus vaccine. The aerosol vaccine significantly reduces flu severity, days lost from work, health-care visits, and the use of over-the-counter medication. The spray represents a particular advantage for children since more than 30 percent of youngsters get the flu, but most don't receive a flu shot.

For those who don't get vaccinated this year, anti-viral drugs, such as Relenza (zanamivir) and Tamiflu (oseltamivir), are the next best line of defense. These *neuraminidase inhibitors* are designed to block a protein (neuraminidase) that allows the flu virus to escape from one cell and infect others. A small handheld oral inhaler, used twice a day for five days, delivers Relenza to the surface of the lungs, the primary site of flu infection. Tamiflu, taken twice a day for five days, comes in pill form. These agents act against both influenza A and influenza B viruses and cause few side effects. In research trials, they shortened the duration of flu by up to two days and decreased the likelihood of complications such as bronchitis, sinusitis, and ear infections. However, to be effective, treatment with either medication must begin within 36 to 48 hours of the first flu symptom. Although approved only for use as a treatment, antiviral drugs also can prevent flu from spreading through a family, workplace, or school.[24]

Meningitis

Meningitis, or invasive meningococcal disease, attacks the membranes around the brain and spinal cord and can result in hearing loss, kidney failure, and permanent brain damage. An estimated 2,400 to 3,000 cases occur every year; approximately 10 percent are fatal. One of the most common types is caused by the bacterium *Neisseria meningitidis,* which is spread through coughing; kissing; sharing drinks, eating utensils, or cigarettes; or prolonged exposure to infected individuals. Viral meningitis is typically less severe.

 Most common in the first year of life, the incidence of bacterial meningitis rises in young people between ages 15 and 24. College students are generally not at greater risk, except freshmen living in dormitories (see Table 13-2).[25] In an analysis of data from 50 state health departments and 231 college health centers, CDC researchers found that the risk of meningitis is three times greater for freshmen in dorms than for other college students.[26]

Early symptoms of meningitis include rash, fever, severe headache, nausea, vomiting, and lethargy. A telltale symptom in many, but not all, cases is stiffness of the neck when bending forward. Meningitis progresses rapidly, often in as little time as 12 hours. If untreated, it can lead to permanent hearing loss, brain damage, seizures, or death. If it is caught early and treated with antibiotics, however, it is usually curable.

Should I get vaccinated for meningitis?

 The Advisory Committee on Immunization Practices of the CDC and the American Academy of Pediatrics have recommended that all college freshmen be informed that

TABLE 13-2	Incidence of Meningitis in College Students
Population Studied	**Rate of Meningitis**
Students between ages 18 and 23	0.7 per 100,000
Nonstudents between ages 18 and 23	1.4 per 100,000
Freshmen living in dormitories	5.1 per 100,000

Source: Michael Bruce, et al. "Risk Factors for Meningococcal Disease in College Students." *Journal of the American Medical Association,* Vol. 286, No. 6, August 8, 2001, p. 286.

vaccination is effective against 70 percent of the bacterial meningitis strains found on campuses and could prevent 80 percent or more of cases among undergraduates.[27] Immunization is recommended primarily for freshmen living in dormitories, who make up 4 percent of the total college population but 31 percent of those diagnosed with meningitis. Other factors increasing meningitis risk are smoking and alcohol consumption, especially binge drinking. Smokers, who cough more, and drinkers, who often share glasses, are at higher risk of transmitting and contracting meningitis. Peak incidence for bacterial meningitis is November to March.

Some experts disagree on whether colleges should recommend or require vaccination.[28] According to CDC statistics, only about five deaths as a result of meningitis would be expected annually among the 520,000 freshmen who live in dormitories. By comparison, binge drinking, car accidents, and suicide claim many more lives. Some contend that colleges should devote their limited resources to fighting these threats.[29] Others argue that students should do everything possible to avoid any potential threat to their health.[30]

 At most schools, the cost of vaccination ranges from $50 to $75. Research into the success of meningococcal vaccination programs on college campuses has shown that women are more likely than men to be vaccinated and that vaccination rates for all nonwhite ethnic groups are somewhat lower than rates for whites. Students majoring in science-oriented fields have higher vaccination rates than those majoring in the humanities. More younger students living on campus than older ones get vaccinations, possibly because of greater parental influence or because they see themselves as being at higher risk.[31]

The current vaccine protects against the most common strains for the *N. meningitidis* bacterium but does not provide complete protection and remains effective for only about three years.[32] More effective vaccines that confer long-lasting immunity and could be administered with other routine infant immunizations have been developed. Some have been introduced in the United Kingdom and other European countries.

Hepatitis

An estimated 500,000 Americans contract hepatitis each year. At least five different viruses, referred to as **hepatitis A, B, C, Delta, and E,** can cause this inflammation of the liver. Newly identified viruses also may be responsible for some cases of what is called "non-A, non-B" hepatitis.

All forms of hepatitis target the liver, the body's largest internal organ. Symptoms include headaches, fever, fatigue, stiff or aching joints, nausea, vomiting, and diarrhea. The liver becomes enlarged and tender to the touch; sometimes the yellowish tinge of jaundice develops. Treatment consists of rest, a high-protein diet, and the avoidance of alcohol and drugs that may stress the liver. Alpha interferon, a protein that boosts immunity and prevents viruses from replicating, may be used for some forms.

Most people begin to feel better after two or three weeks of rest, although fatigue and other symptoms can linger. As many as 10 percent of those infected with hepatitis B and up to two-thirds of those with hepatitis C become carriers of the virus for several years or even life. Some have persistent inflammation of the liver, which may cause mild or severe symptoms and increase the risk of liver cancer.

Hepatitis A

Hepatitis A, a less serious form, is generally transmitted by poor sanitation, primarily fecal contamination of food or water, and is less common in industrialized nations than in developing countries. Among those at highest risk in the United States are children and staff at day-care centers, residents of institutions for the mentally handicapped, sanitation workers, and workers who handle primates such as monkeys. Gamma globulin can provide short-term immunity; vaccines against hepatitis A have been approved by the FDA. The CDC has recommended routine immunization against hepatitis A in 11 Western states with high rates.

Hepatitis B

Hepatitis B, a potentially fatal disease transmitted through the blood and other bodily fluids, infects an estimated 350,000 people around the world each year. Once spread mainly by contaminated tattoo needles, needles shared by drug users, or transfusions of contaminated blood, hepatitis B is now transmitted mostly through sexual contact. It can cause chronic liver infection, cirrhosis, and liver cancer.

Hepatitis B is a particular threat to young people; 75 percent of new cases are diagnosed in those between ages 15 to 39. They usually contract hepatitis B through high-risk behaviors such as multiple sex partners and use of injected drugs. Individuals who have tattoos or body piercing may also be at risk if procedures are not done under regulated conditions. At highest risk are male homosexuals, heterosexuals with multiple sex partners, health-care workers with frequent contact with blood, injection drug users, and infants born to infected mothers. Vaccination can prevent hepatitis B and is recommended for all children and teens, and adults at high risk.

Hepatitis C

Hepatitis C virus (HCV) is four times as widespread as HIV, infecting about 2 percent of Americans.[33] A simple blood test can show if you are infected with HCV. However, few of the estimated 3 to 4 million carriers in the U.S. realize they are infected. 80 percent of those infected with HCV have no symptoms.[34]

The risk factors for HCV infection are blood transfusion or organ transplant before 1992, exposure to infected blood, illegal drug use, tattoos, or body piercing.[35] (See Savvy Consumer: "Before You Get a Tattoo or Piercing.") Hepatitis C virus is not spread by casual contact, such as hugging, kissing, or sharing food utensils. There is controversy over whether HCV also can be transmitted sexually.[36]

About three-quarters of those infected with HCV develop chronic or long-term hepatitis. About one-quarter develop progressive, irreversible liver damage, with scar tissue (cirrhosis) gradually replacing healthy liver tissue.

The most common treatment for Hepatitis C is a combination of interferon, which stops the virus from making copies of itself; and ribavirin, an antiviral medication. If the liver no longer functions adequately, a patient may require liver transplantation.[37]

Mononucleosis

You can get **mononucleosis** through kissing—or any other form of close contact. "Mono" is a viral disease that targets people 15 to 24 years old. Its symptoms include a sore throat, headache, fever, nausea, and prolonged weakness. The spleen is swollen and the lymph nodes are enlarged. You may also develop jaundice or a skin rash similar to German measles.

The major symptoms usually disappear within two to three weeks, but weakness, fatigue, and often depression may linger for at least two more weeks. The greatest danger is from physical activity that might rupture the spleen, resulting in internal bleeding. The liver may also become inflamed. A blood test can determine whether you have mono. However, there's no specific treatment other than rest.

Chronic Fatigue Syndrome (CFS)

An estimated 200,000 to 500,000 Americans have the array of symptoms known as **chronic fatigue syndrome (CFS)** which was discussed in Chapter 2. Diagnosis of CFS remains difficult, although numerous studies have found significant immune abnormalities, such as high levels of certain immune cells (B lymphocytes and cytokines) that act as if they were constantly battling a viral infection. Researchers are working to develop a blood test that will definitively diagnose CFS.

Pneumonia

An inflammation of the lungs, **pneumonia** fills the fine, spongy networks of the lungs' tiny air chambers with fluid. It can be caused by bacteria, viruses (including flu), or for-

Savvy Consumer

BEFORE YOU GET A TATTOO OR PIERCING

"Body art"—tattoos and piercings—may seem harmless, but health officials warn of hidden risks, including Hepatitis B and C infection and transmission of HIV. In a survey of undergraduates at a university in New York, 51 percent reported body piercings, and 23 percent had gotten tattoos. Almost one in five of those with piercings reported medical complications. Bacterial infection was the most common, followed by bleeding and injury or tearing at the site.

With no state or federal regulations of "body artists," unsafe tattooing and piercing practices can put consumers in danger. In one survey of "skin-penetration operators," only half said that they followed governmental guidelines for infection control. Many were not knowledgeable about standard infection-control principles and practices.

Epidemiologists have identified tattooing as a strong, independent risk factor for testing positive for hepatitis C virus (HCV), but not with development of acute hepatitis. In other words, individuals with tattoos may acquire HCV but may not develop symptoms themselves. This does not mean that they will never become symptomatic or that they cannot transmit HCV to others.

Even so-called "temporary tattooing" with henna is not without risk. Dermatologists have reported an increasing number of skin reactions. The culprit is an ingredient in many henna preparations called paraphenyllenediamine (PPD). Allergic reactions to henna itself can occur, but are much rarer. Piercings of the tongue, lips, or cheeks present different dangers, including recessed gums; loose, chipped, or fractured teeth; pain; infection; inflammation; nerve damage; and tooth loss.

You may think you're safe if you go to a licensed tattoo or piercing salon. However, there are no formal schools, no certification requirements, and no diplomas for these practitioners. In many states it is possible to get a license without the benefit of any kind of training. Your best assurance of quality is making sure that basic safety principles are followed:

- *Ask to see certification that the autoclave, a high-temperature pressure cooker used for medical instruments, has been sterilized.* Ask to see the autoclave itself. Is it clean? More importantly, are the shop personnel happy to show it to you, or do they seem to have something to hide? Autoclaves need to be regularly tested to ensure that they are working property. Ask to see the results of their latest spore test. Check the date. The results should be no more than two months old.

- *Make sure the artist is wearing standard medical latex gloves.* Check the fit. If the gloves are too big or too small, the artists runs the risk of either poking a hole in the gloves or tearing them. All it takes is a pinhole to run the risk of cross-contamination.

- *Find out if the artist is vaccinated for Hepatitis B.* As this infection has spread, vaccination has become essential for a tattoo artist's own safety as well as that of clients. If artists claim to be vaccinated, never just take their word for it. Can they show you proof, such as a doctor's record, that they were vaccinated? If they tell you they don't remember if they've been vaccinated, they're probably lying. Most people vividly remember the vaccinations.

- *Make sure the artist uses only new sterile needles.* The needles should not be removed from the autoclave bag, the sort of pouch you see in dentists' offices, until you are ready for your tattoo. Ask to see the sterile confirmation logo on the bag itself. Usually the name of the company that made the bag will be visible on the front of the bag only when the equipment has been properly autoclaved. To determine if the needles are new and not just sterilized after previous use, check the color. They should be bright silver, not stained with ink or brownish looking.

- *Ask how the artist disposes of used needles.* They should be placed in a sharps container, a plastic container, usually red, with a biohazard symbol on the outside, and removed in a timely manner.

- *Always ask to see photos of the artist's finished work.* Examine the designs up close to check precision and skill. If you have the time, watch the artist work on another client before you go ahead with your tattoo.

- *If you require prophylactic antibiotics for dental cleanings or other procedures, do not get a tattoo.* Consumers with rheumatic heart disease and other conditions that increase their risk have died as a result of bacterial infection contracted from a tattoo.

eign material in the lungs (such as smoke). The symptoms of classic bacterial pneumonia are fever, shortness of breath, and general weakness. Along with influenza, pneumonia is the fifth-leading killer of Americans and the most common infectious cause of death.

The typical signs of pneumonia include cough, a fever of more than 101°F, difficulty breathing, chills, and excessive yellow-green phlegm. Symptoms of pneumonia can develop either gradually or else so quickly that a person's life is in danger within hours. Antibiotics can control bacterial pneumonia, but they must be given before microbes erode local tissues and spread through the blood elsewhere in the body, causing a condition known as septicemia, or blood poisoning. Because of the dangers of pneumonia, you should see a doctor if there's any chance you have it. Severe cases may require hospitalization and high doses of antibiotics.

Vaccination against pneumonia is recommended for those who've had pneumonia in the past, those with impaired immune function, and those over age 65. The pneumonia vaccine greatly reduces the risk of this disease, especially for women and those with impaired immunity.

Tuberculosis

A bacterial infection of the lungs that was once the nation's leading killer, **tuberculosis (TB)** claims the lives of more people than any acute infectious disease other than pneumonia (Figure 13-3). One-third of the world's population is infected with the TB organism, although not all develop active disease. Each year the infection spreads to another 8 million people. In the United States, TB cases, after declining for decades, increased from the mid-1980s to the early 1990s. The reasons include immigration from countries where TB is common, poverty, homelessness, alcoholism and drug abuse, the HIV/AIDS epidemic, and the emergence of resistant strains of TB. Some cities have reported a decline in TB, thanks to better infection control and greater monitoring to ensure completion of treatment.

Although TB is most prevalent among high-risk groups, the overall danger increases as more people develop active disease because TB is highly contagious. TB outbreaks have occurred throughout the country in hospitals, nursing homes, prisons, and office buildings, where inadequate ventilation increases the risk of infection.

Most TB patients recover completely after six months of taking a combination of three different medicines. Drug-resistant forms of the tuberculosis microorganism strike mostly patients who start drug treatment but don't follow through with it. Because they don't take enough of the medication to kill all the TB bacteria in their system, those that survive become resistant. Even with full treatment, the risk of dying from drug-resistant tuberculosis is 50 percent. HIV infection greatly increases susceptibility to infection with TB and the risk of dying if infected with treatment-resistant forms.[38]

If you think you may have been exposed to TB or if you develop suspicious symptoms (loss of appetite and weight, low-grade fever, fatigue, chills, night sweats, coughing), see your doctor for a TB test. This consists of an injection just under the skin. The area of the arm where the test was administered should be checked by a health-care professional to determine the presence of the TB bacteria; further tests confirm the diagnosis. If the skin test is positive, indicating that TB is present, you'll be monitored with yearly chest X rays. You may also require treatment with a drug such as rifampin or isoniazid (also called INH).

Group A and Group B Strep Infection

Sore throats are common winter complaints, but those caused by group A streptococcus bacteria—"strep throats"—are more than a trivial threat. If not treated promptly with antibiotics, strep bacteria can travel to the kidneys, the liver, or the heart, where they can cause rheumatic fever—an inflammation of the heart that can cause weakness, shortness of breath, joint pain, and an abnormal heartbeat. In recent years clusters of rheumatic fever have sprung up in several major cities. Pediatricians are urging parents to consult their doctors if a youngster complains of a sore throat or if strep is widespread in the community. Rapid new diagnostic tests can identify strep within minutes. If the test is positive, treatment with penicillin or a similar antibiotic is indicated. Brief treatment (five days) with Omnicef, a new antibiotic, has proven as effective as ten days of oral penicillin.

Toxic streptococcal shock syndrome, or toxic strep, is an invasive form of the disease in which strep gains access to the blood and causes a drop in blood pressure, a very high fever, and the production of exotoxins (substances that can attack various organs, such as the kidneys, heart or, in rare cases, flesh). Toxic strep is rather rare and usually doesn't occur with strep throats. Prompt treatment is critical.

When someone with active tuberculosis exhales, coughs, or sneezes, tuberculosis is expelled in tiny airborne droplets that others may inhale.

The TB bacteria lodge mainly in the lungs, where they slowly multiply, creating patches, then cavities, in the lungs.

Other parts of the lung are affected, including bronchi and the lining of the lung.

Figure 13-3 HOW TUBERCULOSIS SPREADS
If untreated, TB can eventually spread to and damage the brain, bone, eyes, liver and kidneys, spine, and skin.

Group B streptococcus (GBS), the leading cause of life-threatening perinatal infections in the United States, is primarily a threat to newborns. Because some 15 to 40 percent of pregnant women carry GBS but have no symptoms, the American Academy of Pediatrics has called for universal screening of expectant mothers. Each year 12,000 newborns are infected, most of them during childbirth; more than 1,600 die, and another 1,600 suffer permanent brain damage from meningitis. Women at high risk of infecting their newborns with GBS are those who have premature labor, early rupture of their amniotic membranes, fever, and a high group B strep count before or during pregnancy, or who have previously borne an infant infected with GBS. Also at risk are diabetics, poor women, and those under age 20.

Toxic Shock Syndrome

As discussed in Chapter 8, **toxic shock syndrome (TSS)** is a potentially deadly disease associated with the use of tampons, particularly high-absorbency types. It is caused by *Staphylococcus aureus* and group A *Streptococcus pyogenes* bacteria that release toxins (poisonous waste products) into the bloodstream. Symptoms include a high fever; a rash that leads to peeling of the skin on the fingers, toes, palms, and soles; dizziness; dangerously low blood pressure; and abnormalities in several organ systems (the digestive tract and the kidneys) and in the muscles and blood.

In addition to women who use high-absorbency tampons, or leave their tampons in too long, those who have given birth within the preceding six to eight weeks are at greater risk. Children (including newborns), men, and postmenopausal women also have developed TSS, which usually has been traced to bacteria in skin abscesses, boils, cuts, or postsurgical wounds.

Without prompt treatment, TSS can cause severe and permanent damage, including muscle weakness, partial paralysis, amnesia, disorientation, an inability to concentrate, and impaired lung and kidney function. Sometimes toxic shock weakens the blood vessels, increasing the risk of heart problems. Victims can enter the life-threatening crisis called shock, in which blood flow throughout the body is inadequate to sustain life. Treatment usually consists of immediate hospitalization, intravenous administration of fluids, medications to raise blood pressure, and powerful antibiotics; intravenous administration of immunoglobins that attack the toxins produced by these bacteria may also be beneficial.

Insect and Animal Borne Infections

Common insects and animals, including ticks and mosquitoes, can transmit dangerous infections. Lyme disease is the most widespread in the United States, while West Nile

Virus continues to spread. The first outbreak of animal-borne monkeypox virus occurred in 2003.

Lyme Disease

Lyme disease, a bacterial infection, is spread by ticks carrying a particular bacterium—the spirochete *Borrelia burgdorferi*. An infected person may have various symptoms, including joint inflammation, heart arrhythmias, blinding headaches, and memory lapses. The disease can also cause miscarriages and birth defects. Lyme disease is by far the most commonly reported vector-borne infectious disease in the United States. The vast majority of all reported cases have occurred in just ten states; those leading the list are New York, New Jersey, Connecticut, Pennsylvania, and Wisconsin.

The FDA has licensed a vaccine to prevent Lyme disease in individuals 15 to 70 years old. LYMErix, like most vaccines, stimulates the immune system to produce antibodies, in this case against the bacteria that cause Lyme disease. But the vaccine, administered in three doses over a one-year period, is not 100 percent effective and should not be considered a substitute for protective clothing and tick repellent. Administration must be timed so the second and third doses are given at the beginning of the tick transmission season, usually April in the Northeastern United States. It is not known how long protection against Lyme disease lasts after vaccination. Vaccination is recommended for individuals at very high risk of Lyme disease, such as park rangers, others who spend much time in wooded areas, and people who live where Lyme disease is exceptionally prevalent.

The primary culprit in most cases of Lyme disease is the deer tick, although other ticks, including the Western black-legged tick, the dog tick, and the Lone Star tick, also may transmit the bacterium that causes Lyme disease as well as organisms that transmit other diseases, such as Rocky Mountain spotted fever and babesiosis.

Hunters and campers are more likely to test positive for Lyme disease. Pet owners are not at additional risk. The most important preventive step is to check yourself for

© Scott Camazine/Photo Researchers, Inc.

Ticks are responsible for the spread of Lyme disease. If you spot a tick, remove it as soon as possible with tweezers or small forceps. Put it in a plastic bag or sealed bottle and save it. If you develop a rash or other symptoms, take it with you to the doctor.

ticks whenever you come in from the outdoors. However, detecting some types of ticks can be difficult. In their nymphal stage, when they're most likely to bite, ticks are about the size of a poppyseed. Even as adults, some ticks are no bigger than a sesame seed.

Regardless of whether or not they've spotted a tick, residents of infested areas should check regularly for signs of a bite. About two-thirds of those bitten develop some skin changes from two days to four weeks afterward. The classic skin lesion is a small, clear-centered red doughnut that expands, but most people simply have a red blotch or two blotches. However, the rash always expands, usually to about 2 inches in diameter. In some cases, it may cover a person's entire chest or thigh; others develop rashes far from the bite, caused by spirochetes that travel through the bloodstream. More sensitive diagnostic tests allow detection of extremely low numbers of spirochetes and make earlier diagnosis possible.

Guidelines issued by the Infectious Diseases Society of America do not recommend routine use of blood testing or antibiotics after a tick bite. However, experts do recommend antibiotic treatment if a tick may have been attached for more than 48 hours (which can be determined by the engorgement of the tick with blood) and monitoring of individuals who have removed ticks. However, prolonged antibiotic treatment does not appear to help patients with Lyme disease who do not respond to the initial antibiotic treatment.

A rash similar to that of Lyme disease has been reported in southeastern and south-central states and traced to the bite of the lone star tick. Treatment for Southern tick-associated rash illness (STARI) consists of antibiotics.[39]

West Nile Virus

West Nile Virus (WNV) is transmitted by a mosquito that feeds on an infected bird and then bites a human. The first cases in the United States occurred in 1999. Experts now see WNV as a seasonal epidemic that flares up in the summer and continues into the fall.[40] WNV also can be spread through blood transfusions, organ transplants, breastfeeding, and from mother to fetus during pregnancy.[41]

WNV interferes with normal central nervous system functioning and causes inflammation of brain tissue. The risk of catching WNV is low. Relatively few mosquitoes carry WNV, and less than 1 percent of people who are bitten by mosquitoes experience any symptoms.[42] Approximately 80 percent of individuals infected with WNV develop no symptoms at all. Most others display mild symptoms, such as fever, headache and body aches, nausea, vomiting, swollen glands or a skin rash on the chest, stomach, and back. They usually disappear in a few days.[43]

About one in 150 infected people develop severe symptoms, including high fever, headache, neck stiffness, stupor, disorientation, coma, tremors, convulsions, muscle

STRATEGIES FOR PREVENTION

Protecting Yourself from Insect-Borne Diseases

- Apply insect repellent containing DEET (N,N-diethyl-meta-toluamide), which provides the longest-lasting protection against bites, when you're outdoors.

- When possible, wear long-sleeved clothes and long pants treated with repellents containing permethrin or DEET since insects may bite through thin clothing. Do not apply repellents containing permethrin directly to exposed skin. If you spray your clothing, there is no need to spray repellent containing DEET on the skin under your clothing.

- Consider staying indoors at dawn, dusk, and in the early evening, which are peak mosquito-biting times.

- After spending time outdoors, examine yourself for ticks or bites every day. Check less obvious places, such as the scalp and behind the ears.

- If you do spot a tick, remove it right away. Using tweezers or forceps, grasp the tick firmly as close to its head and as near to your skin as possible. Gently pull backward, without squeezing the tick's body, until its hold is released. Wash your hands thoroughly. Treat the wound with rubbing alcohol.

weakness, vision loss, numbness, and paralysis. People over 50 are more likely to develop serious symptoms and to die if they do get sick. Symptoms may last several weeks and cause permanent neurological damage.[44]

The FDA has approved a test for WNV.[45] There is no specific treatment for WNV infection. People with more severe cases usually require hospitalization and supportive treatment, including intravenous fluids and help with breathing. An antiviral drug, interferon, which might lessen the symptoms and duration of the illness in infected patients, is undergoing testing.

Monkeypox Virus

This rare viral disease occurs mainly in Africa, where it was first identified in monkeys. Researchers have since recovered monkeypox from other animals, including rats, mice, and rabbits, as well as humans. In 2003 several dozen people in Wisconsin, Indiana, Illinois, Missouri, Kansas, and Ohio got sick after contact with pet prairie dogs infected with monkeypox. This was the first outbreak of monkeypox in the United States.[46]

The signs and symptoms of monkeypox are similar to those of smallpox, but milder. People can catch monkeypox from an infected animal's bite, blood, or body fluids. It can spread from person to person during long periods of face-to-face contact or by touching the body fluids of a sick person or bedding or clothing contaminated with the virus. There is no specific treatment.[47]

New Infectious Threats

The 21st century has ushered in new agents of infection and new apprehension about the potential use of infectious diseases as instruments of terror and mass destruction. When it emerged in 2003, the virus that causes Severe Acute Respiratory Syndrome (SARS), traveled rapidly around the globe, virtually shutting down certain regions. Other infectious agents could become global threats if used as weapons of biological terrorism.

What Is SARS?

Severe Acute Respiratory Syndrome (SARS) became a new global health threat in 2003, with major outbreaks in several Asian countries, including China and Hong Kong and in Toronto. In its first six months, SARS infected more than 8,400 people and killed at least 513, according to WHO estimates.[48]

Researchers suspect that a newly recognized coronavirus causes SARS.[49] It spreads by close face-to-face contact, most often by droplets expelled into the air when an infected person coughs or sneezes. The virus is believed capable of living outside the body for at least 24 hours. A few persons may be especially infectious and are more

Surgical masks do not offer complete protection against the SARS virus.

likely to spread the SARS virus to others in the same airplane, household, school, workplace, or hospital.[50] Doctors do not know how long a person remains contagious.

The average incubation period for SARS is six to ten days. Symptoms include fever, coughing, headache, chills, muscle aches, and shortness of breath.[51] There are no specific treatments for SARS. Patients receive supportive care, such as fluids to prevent dehydration and ventilators to aid breathing. Scientists are developing possible vaccines and antiviral agents.

The best defenses against SARS are avoiding travel to regions with high numbers of cases and frequent, thorough handwashing with soap and water. Although many people in areas of SARS outbreaks wore surgical masks as protection during the 2003 outbreaks, the CDC does not recommend their routine use because they are not 100 percent effective in blocking the SARS virus.

WHO officials pronounced the global SARS outbreak "contained" by the summer of 2003 but caution— based on what experts know about other members of the coronavirus family—that SARS could be a seasonal disease and return in the winter months.

Bioterror Infections

Americans have learned firsthand that certain infectious agents can be used as weapons of terrorism and war.[52] Bioterror agents, such as anthrax and, potentially, smallpox or botulism, have been added to the ranks of emerging infectious diseases. (See Table 13-3.) Federal and state governments have launched new bioterrorism preparedness programs.[53]

Anthrax

Anthrax, which is found naturally in wild and farm animals, can also be produced in a laboratory. The disease is spread through exposure to anthrax spores, not through exposure to an infected person. Anthrax in the mail threatened thousands of postal workers and others in 2001 and killed five people.

Smallpox

Smallpox is a serious, contagious, and sometimes fatal infectious disease. Smallpox was eradicated decades ago after a successful worldwide vaccination program. The last case of smallpox in the United States was in 1949. The last naturally occurring case in the world was in Somalia in 1977. There is no treatment, and up to 30 percent of those infected with smallpox die.[54]

Because of fear that terrorists might use smallpox as a biological weapon, the U.S. government has stockpiled enough vaccine to inoculate everyone in the event of an emergency. Most individuals vaccinated before 1972, when

TABLE 13-3	Biological Threats			
Disease	**Germ**	**Symptoms**	**Mortality**	**Treatment**
Smallpox	Variola virus	Fever, aches, pustules on face and torso	30%	Vaccination within three days after exposure; no treatment later
Inhalation anthrax	*Bacillus anthracis*	Fever, chest pain, difficulty breathing	90%	Cipro floxacin and other antibodies
Pneumonic plague	*Yersinia pestis*	Fever after 2–4 days, then pneumonialike symptoms	50–90%	Antibiotics such as streptomycin, tetracycline, and doxycycline
Botulism	*Clostridium botulinum*	Progressive paralysis, respiratory failure	5%	Botulism antitoxins
Tularemia	*Francisella tularensis*	Fever, sore throat, weakness, weight loss	30–60%	Antibiotics such as streptomycin and gentamicin
Viral Hemorrhagic fevers	Several viruses	Vary, but include bleeding, shock, coma	Varies	Some, such as Ebola, have no cure; the antiviral ribavirin helps others

Source: Information from "Recognition and Management of Bioterrorism Infections." from the February 15, 1999 issue of *American Family Physician.*

mandated smallpox immunization ended in the United States, retain some immunity for many years, some for up to 75 years.[55] However, half of all Americans have never received the smallpox vaccine, and many scientists believe protection wanes over time for those who did. Those vaccinated in the past can safely be revaccinated for optimum protection.[56]

In 2003 military forces and health workers began receiving vaccinations against smallpox.[57] The risks associated with these inoculations have ranged from mild rashes to potentially fatal cardiac infections and a rare fatal brain inflammation (encephalitis).[58] An Institute of Medicine committee has recommended against vaccinating the entire population at this time.[59]

◼ Reproductive and Urinary Tract Infections

Reproductive and urinary tract infections are very common. Many are not spread exclusively by sexual contact, so they are not classified as sexually transmitted diseases.

Vaginal Infections

The most common vaginal infections are trichomoniasis, candidiasis, and bacterial vaginosis.

Protozoa *(Trichomonas vaginalis)* that live in the vagina can multiply rapidly, causing itching, burning, and discharge—all symptoms of **trichomoniasis.** Male carriers usually have no symptoms, although some may develop urethritis or an inflammation of the prostate and seminal vesicles. Anyone with this infection should be screened for syphilis, gonorrhea, chlamydia, and HIV. Sexual partners must be treated with oral medication (metronidazole, trade name Flagyl), even if they have no symptoms, to prevent reinfection.

Populations of a yeast called *Candida albicans*—normal inhabitants of the mouth, digestive tract, and vagina—are usually held in check. Under certain conditions, however (such as poor nutrition, stress, or antibiotic use), the microbes multiply, causing burning, itching, and a whitish discharge, and producing what is commonly known as a yeast infection. Common sites for **candidiasis,** which is also called *moniliasis,* are the vagina, vulva, penis, and mouth. The women most likely to test positive for candidiasis have never been pregnant, use condoms for birth control, have sexual intercourse more than four times a month, and have taken antibiotics in the previous 15 to 30 days. Vaginal medications, such as GyneLotrimin and Monistat, are nonprescription drugs that provide effective treatment. Male sexual partners may be advised to wear condoms during outbreaks of candidiasis. Women should keep the genital area dry and wear cotton underwear.

Bacterial vaginosis is characterized by alterations in the microorganisms that live in the vagina, including depletion of certain bacteria and overgrowth of others. It typically causes a white or gray vaginal discharge with a distinctive fishy odor similar to that of trichomoniasis. Its underlying cause is unknown, although it occurs most frequently in women with multiple sex partners. Long-term dangers include pelvic inflammatory disease (PID, discussed later in this chapter) and pregnancy complications. Metronidazole, either in the form of a pill or a vaginal gel, is the primary treatment. According to CDC guidelines, treatment for male sex partners appears to be of little benefit, but some health practitioners recommend treatment for both partners in cases of recurrent infections.

Urinary Tract Infections

A urinary tract infection (UTI) can be present in any of the three parts of the urinary tract: the urethra, the bladder, or the kidneys. An infection involving the urethra is known as **urethritis.** If the bladder is also infected, it's called **cystitis.** If it reaches the kidneys, it's called **pyelonephritis.**

An estimated 40 percent of women report having had a UTI at some point in their lives. Three times as many women as men develop UTIs, probably for anatomical reasons. A woman's urethra is only 1.5 inches long; a man's is 6 inches. Therefore, bacteria, the major cause of UTIs, have a shorter distance to travel to infect a woman's bladder and kidneys. About one-fourth to one-third of all women between ages 20 and 40 develop UTIs, and 80 percent of those who experience one infection develop recurrences.

Conditions that can set the stage for UTIs include irritation and swelling of the urethra or bladder as a result of pregnancy, bike riding, irritants (such as bubble bath, douches, or a diaphragm), urinary stones, enlargement in men of the prostate gland, vaginitis, and stress. Early diagnosis is critical because infection can spread to the kidneys and, if unchecked, result in kidney failure. Symptoms include frequent burning, painful urination, chills, fever, fatigue, and blood in the urine.

Recurrent UTIs, a frequent problem among young women, have been linked with a genetic predisposition, sexual intercourse, and the use of diaphragms. Post-intercourse treatment with antibiotics can lower the risk. Frequent recurrence of symptoms may not be caused by infection but by interstitial cystitis, a little-understood bladder inflammation that afflicts an estimated 450,000 Americans, almost all of them women.

◼ Sexually Transmitted Infections

Venereal diseases (from the Latin *venus,* meaning *love* or *lust*) are called **sexually transmitted infections (STIs)** or sexually transmitted diseases (STDs). Around the world, some 50 million cases of curable STIs occur each year (not

including HIV and herpes).[60] Almost 700,000 people are infected every day with one of the over 20 STIs tracked by world health officials. The highest rates of sexually transmitted infections occur among 16- to 24-year-olds, particularly older teenagers.[61] STIs are much more widespread in developing nations because of lack of adequate health standards, prevention practices, and access to treatment.[62]

More Americans are infected with STIs now than at any other time in history. According to the Institute of Medicine, the odds of acquiring an STI during a lifetime are one in four. STIs are among the top ten most frequently reported diseases in the United States, and their annual economic cost is $17 billion. The major cause of preventable sterility in America, STIs have tripled the rate of ectopic (tubal) pregnancies, which can be fatal if not detected early. STI complications, including miscarriage, premature delivery, and uterine infections after delivery, annually affect more than 100,000 women. Moreover, infection with an STI greatly increases the risk of HIV transmission (discussed later in this chapter). The incidence of STIs is highest in young adults and homosexual men. Others affected by STIs include unborn and newborn children who can "catch" potentially life-threatening infections in the womb or during birth.

Although each STI is a distinct disease, all STI pathogens like dark, warm, moist body surfaces, particularly the mucous membranes that line the reproductive organs; they hate light, cold, and dryness. (See Figure 13-4.) It is possible to catch or have more than one STI at a time. Curing one doesn't necessarily cure another, and treatments don't prevent another bout with the same STI. (See Table 13-4 on page 448.)

Many STIs, including early HIV infection and gonorrhea in women, may not cause any symptoms. As a result, infected individuals may continue their usual sexual activity without realizing that they're jeopardizing others' well-being.

In a national survey of physicians, fewer than one-third routinely screened men or women for STIs. When they did diagnose an STI, many failed to report to public health officials, as required by law. Screening and reporting were lowest for chlamydia, the most common of all bacterial STIs.[63]

STIs in Adolescents and Young Adults

Nearly two-thirds of the people who acquire STIs in the United States are under age 25. The most common bacterial STI is chlamydia, with two of the highest rates of chlamydia occurring among adolescents in general and among young adult women. Cases of genital herpes among white adolescents have increased five times, and cases among white people in their twenties have doubled over the past few years.

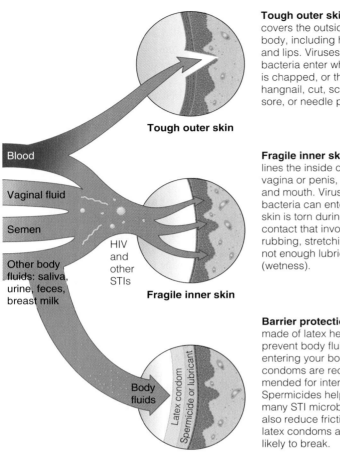

Tough outer skin
covers the outside of your body, including hands and lips. Viruses and bacteria enter when skin is chapped, or through a hangnail, cut, scrape, sore, or needle puncture.

Tough outer skin

Fragile inner skin
lines the inside of your vagina or penis, anus, and mouth. Viruses and bacteria can enter when skin is torn during sexual contact that involves rubbing, stretching, or not enough lubrication (wetness).

Blood

Vaginal fluid

Semen

Other body fluids: saliva, urine, feces, breast milk

HIV and other STIs

Fragile inner skin

Barrier protection
made of latex helps prevent body fluids from entering your body. Latex condoms are recommended for intercourse. Spermicides help kill many STI microbes. They also reduce friction so latex condoms are less likely to break.

Body fluids

Latex condom

Spermicide or lubricant

Figure 13-4 HOW HIV INFECTION AND OTHER STIS ARE SPREAD
Most STIs are spread by viruses or bacteria carried in certain body fluids.

The college years are a prime time for contracting STIs. According to the American College Health Association, chlamydia and HPV have reached epidemic levels at many schools—although many of those infected aren't even aware of it.

In one study of college-age women, cases of human papilloma virus (HPV) infections increased from 26 percent to 43 percent over a three-year period. Contracting STIs may increase the risk of being infected with HIV, and half of new HIV infections occur in people under age 25. Because college students have more opportunities to have different sexual partners and may use drugs and alcohol more often before sex, they are at greater risk. Many college students misjudge the number of people with HIV who live in Africa and who live in the United States.[64] More than half of 13- to 24-year-old women with HIV are infected heterosexually.[65]

Even when high school and college students have generally accurate knowledge about STIs, they don't necessarily practice safe sex. According to research, those students with

the greatest number of sexual partners are least likely to use condoms. Other studies have shown that proximity to a high-density AIDS epicenter (such as San Francisco) has no impact on HIV/AIDS knowledge and attitudes, and that religious affiliation does not decrease risky sexual behavior, at least among religious students who are sexually active. College students admit to engaging in behaviors that put them at risk of HIV and other STIs but believe that they are not at risk (See Student Snapshot: "Unsafe Sex on Campus.")

According to a survey of 410 students at a public university in the Southeast, students engaged in more unprotected intercourse and oral sex when they were not under the influence of drugs or alcohol—but were more likely to engage in sexual activity with someone they'd just met when drunk or high. However, the undergraduates perceived that the "average" student engaged in risky behaviors more frequently under any circumstance.[66]

Various factors put young people at risk of STIs, including:

:: *Feelings of invulnerability,* which lead to risk-taking behavior. Even when they are well informed of the risks, adolescents may remain unconvinced that anything bad can or will happen to them.

:: *Multiple partners.* In surveys of students, a significant minority report having had four or more sexual partners during their lifetime.

:: *Failure to use condoms.* Among those who reported having had sexual intercourse in the previous three months, fewer than half reported condom use.[67] Students who'd had four or more sexual partners were significantly less likely to use condoms than those who'd had fewer partners.

:: *Substance abuse.* Teenagers who drink or use drugs are more likely to engage in sexually risky behaviors, including sex with partners whose health status and history they do not know, and unprotected intercourse.

Although young adulthood is the age of greatest risk for acquiring STIs, the likelihood that men and women will receive information about prevention declines after they graduate from high school. The media, particularly television, is by far the most common source of health information for young men. In a recent survey, about one-third of young adult men said they received no information about AIDS or STIs from any other source.[68]

Race and ethnicity also affect risk in the young. Young African-American men, who are more likely to be sexually active and to have more partners than young white men, also have higher STI infection rates. While

Student Snapshot **Unsafe Sex on Campus**

Based on an online survey of 516 college students in the United States by the Society for Adolescent Medicine

Source:www. adolescenthealth.org

College

68% of students who have had unprotected sex don't believe they are at risk of STIs

73% of sexually active students report having unprotected sex

56% of college students not living at home are sexually active

the chlamydia rate for Hispanics is almost three times that of whites, the rate for blacks is ten times that of whites. The gonorrhea rate for African-American males aged 20 to 24 is 40 times that of whites. Although HIV infection rates have declined for all men, they are falling at a slower rate for African-American men.

Early communication about AIDS and STIs also affects risk later in life. Several studies have shown that discussing sexual risks with parents or counseling by physicians can promote changes in condom use and sexual behavior.[69] Although parents believe that talking to children about sex is important, adolescents say that their parents do not talk to them early enough about sexual issues.

Prevention and Protection

Abstinence is the best way of preventing young people being "engulfed" by sexually transmitted infections. This is the conclusion of researchers who surveyed abstinence education projects in several countries, including the United States and Uganda. In Africa ABC programs (Abstain, Be faithful, or wear a Condom) have helped lower rates of sexual activity—and of STIs.[70] By choosing not to be sexually active with a partner, individuals can safeguard their physical health, their fertility, and their future.

For men and women who are sexually active, a mutually faithful sexual relationship with just one healthy partner is the safest option. For those not in such relationships, safer-sex practices are essential for reducing risks. However, no "protection" is 100 percent "safe." For instance, nonoxynol-9, the most widely used spermicide in the world, does not protect women from gonorrhea or chlamydia.[71]

© LWA/CORBIS

Talking openly about STIs and being tested with your partner will protect your health and foster a sense of trust and commitment.

TABLE 13-4	**Common Sexually Transmitted Infections (STIs): Mode of Transmission, Symptoms, and Treatment**		
STI	**Transmission**	**Symptoms**	**Treatment**
Chlamydia	The *Chlamydia trachomatis* bacterium is transmitted primarily through sexual contact. It can also be spread by fingers from one body site to another.	In women, PID (pelvic inflammatory disease) caused by chlamydia may include disrupted menstrual periods, pelvic pain, elevated temperature, nausea, vomiting, headache, infertility, and ectopic pregnancy. In men, chlamydial infection of the urethra may cause a discharge and burning during urination. Chlamydia-caused epididymitis may produce a sense of heaviness in the affected testicle(s), inflammation of the scrotal skin, and painful swelling at the bottom of the testicle.	Doxycycline, azithromycin, ofloxacin, levofloxacin
Gonorrhea ("clap")	The *Neisseria gonorrhoeae* bacterium ("gonococcus") is spread through genital, oral-genital, or genital-anal contact.	The most common symptoms in men are a cloudy discharge from the penis and burning sensations during urination. If disease is untreated, complications may include inflammation of scrotal skin and swelling at base of the testicle. In women, some green or yellowish discharge is produced but commonly remains undetected. Later, PID may develop.	Dual therapy of a single dose of ceftriaxone, cefixime, ciprofloxacin, ofloxacin, or levofloxacin for seven days or a single dose of azithromycin
Non-gonococcal urethritis (NGU)	Primary causes are believed to be the bacteria *Chlamydia trachomatis* and *Ureaplasma urealyticum,* most commonly transmitted through coitus. Some NGU may result from allergic reactions or from *Trichomonas* infection.	Inflammation of the urethral tube. A man has a discharge from the penis and irritation during urination. A woman may have a mild discharge of pus from the vagina but often shows no symptoms.	A single dose of azithromycin or doxycycline for seven days
Syphilis	The *Treponema pallidum* bacterium ("spirochete") is transmitted from open lesions during genital, oral-genital, or genital-anal contact.	*Primary stage:* A painless chancre appears at the site where the spirochetes entered the body. *Secondary stage:* The chancre disappears and a generalized skin rash develops. *Latent stage:* There may be no visible symptoms. *Tertiary stage:* Heart failure, blindness, mental disturbance, and many other symptoms occur. Death may result.	Benzathine penicillin G, doxycycline, erythromycin, or ceftriaxone
Herpes simplex	The genital herpes virus (HSV-2) seems to be transmitted primarily by vaginal, anal, or oral-genital intercourse. The oral herpes virus (HSV-1) is transmitted primarily by kissing.	Small, painful red bumps (papules) appear in the genital region (genital herpes) or mouth (oral herpes). The papules become painful blisters that eventually rupture to form wet, open sores.	No known cure. A variety of treatments may reduce symptoms; acyclovir, famciclovir or valacyclovir promote healing and suppress recurrent outbreaks.
Chancroid	The *Haemophilus ducrevi* bacterium is usually transmitted by sexual interaction.	Small bumps (papules) in genital regions eventually rupture and form painful, soft, crater-like ulcers that emit a foul-smelling discharge.	Single doses of either ceftriaxone or azithromycin, or seven days of erythromycin
Human papilloma virus (HPV) (genital warts)	The virus is spread primarily through vaginal, anal, or oral-genital sexual interaction.	Hard and yellow-gray on dry skin areas; soft, pinkish-red, and cauliflowerlike on moist areas.	Freezing; application of topical agents like trichloroacetic acid or podofilox; cauterization, surgical removal, or vaporization by carbon dioxide laser

Many factors affect women's decisions about safer sex practices, including race and ethnicity. African–American women are more likely to make contraceptive decisions without the influence of partners and to focus on pregnancy rather than STI prevention. European–American and Hispanic women are more likely to be influenced by their partners in making decisions about safer sex and STI protection. Women who had an STI are much more vigilant about

TABLE 13-4	Common Sexually Transmitted Infections (STIs): Mode of Transmission, Symptoms, and Treatment (continued)		
STI	**Transmission**	**Symptoms**	**Treatment**
Pubic lice ("crabs")	*Phthirus pubis,* the pubic louse, is spread easily through body contact or through shared clothing or bedding.	Persistent itching. Lice are visible and may often be located in pubic hair or other body hair.	1% permethrin cream for body areas; 1% Lindane shampoo for hair
Scabies	*Sarcoptes scabiei* is highly contagious and may be transmitted by close physical contact, sexual and nonsexual.	Small bumps and a red rash that itch intensely, especially at night.	5% permethrin lotion or cream
Acquired immune-deficiency syndrome (AIDS)	Blood and semen are the major vehicles for transmitting HIV, which attacks the immune system. It appears to be passed primarily through sexual contact, or needle sharing among injection drug users.	Vary with the type of cancer or opportunistic infections that afflict an infected person. Common symptoms include fevers, night sweats, weight loss, chronic fatigue, swollen lymph nodes, diarrhea and/or bloody stools, atypical bruising or bleeding, skin rashes, headache, chronic cough, and a whitish coating on the tongue or throat.	Commence treatment early after a positive HIV test with a combination of three or more antiretroviral drugs (HAART) plus other specific treatment(s), if necessary, of opportunistic infections and tumors.
Viral hepatitis	Hepatitis A seems to be primarily spread via the fecal-oral route, but oral-anal sexual contact is a common mode for sexual transmission. The hepatitis B virus can be transmitted by blood, semen, vaginal secretions, and saliva. Manual, oral, or penile stimulation of the anus are strongly associated with the spread of this virus.	Vary from nonexistent to mild, flulike symptoms to an incapacitating illness characterized by high fever, vomiting, and severe abdominal pain.	No specific therapy for A and B types; treatment generally consists of bed rest and adequate fluid intake. Combination therapy with interferon and ribavarin may be effective for hepatitis C infections.
Bacterial vaginosis	The most common causative agent, the *Gardnerella vaginalis* bacterium, is sometimes transmitted through coitus.	In women, a fishy- or musty-smelling, thin discharge, like flour paste in consistency and usually gray. Most men are asymptomatic.	Metronidazole (Flagyl) by mouth or intravaginal applications of topical metronidazole gel or clindamycin cream
Candidiasis (yeast infection)	The *Candida albicans* fungus may accelerate growth when the chemical balance of the vagina is disturbed; it may also be transmitted through sexual interaction.	White, "cheesy" discharge; irritation of vaginal and vulval tissues.	Vaginal suppositories or topical cream, such as clotrimazole and miconazole, or oral fluconazole
Trichomoniasis	The protozoan parasite *Trichomonas vaginalis* is usually passed through genital sexual contact.	White or yellow vaginal discharge with an unpleasant odor; vulva is sore and irritated.	Metronidazole (Flagyl) for both women and men

Sources: Robert L. Crooks, and Karla Baur. *Our Sexuality,* 8th ed. Pacific Grove, CA: Wadsworth, 2002; Karl Miller, et al. "Update on Prevention and Treatment of Sexually Transmitted Diseases." *American Family Physician,* Vol. 67, No. 9, May 1, 2003, p. 1915.

using methods to prevent disease and pregnancy.[72] In a survey of 123 sexually experienced African–American undergraduate women, 38 percent reported at least one previous diagnosis of an STI, yet only 24 percent said that they always used condoms. Early age at first intercourse and a greater number of sexual partners increased a woman's likelihood of having an STI.[73]

Self Survey   **How Much Do You Know About STIs?**

1. Which of the following STIs can be transmitted EVEN when you use a condom?
   a. chlamydia
   b. HIV
   c. gonorrhea
   d. genital warts

2. True or False: Cold sores and genital herpes are not the same thing, so oral sex is safe when my partner has a cold sore.
   True
   False

3. Hepatitis B is ___ times more infectious than HIV.
   a. 20
   b. 100
   c. 50
   d. 10

4. The STI below is known as the "silent" epidemic.
   a. HIV
   b. genital herpes
   c. chlamydia
   d. public lice ("crabs")

5. True or False: It's estimated that at least half of all new HIV infections in the United States are among people under 25.
   True
   False

6. What do Pope Alexander VI, Ivan the Terrible, Henry VIII, and Al Capone have in common?
   a. They all lost their virginity after the age of 30.
   b. They all had taken a vow of celibacy.
   c. They all died virgins.
   d. They all died of syphillis.

7. By age 24, at least one in ___ sexually active people will have contracted an STI.
   a. 10
   b. 20
   c. 3
   d. 5

8. True or False: "My girlfriend has a Pap smear every year, so I know I'm clean."
   True
   False

9. It takes up to ___ months for people infected with HIV to develop enough antibodies for their HIV status to be accurately detected by testing.
   a. 6
   b. 12
   c. 3
   d. 9

10. True or False: You are doomed, you may as well walk around in a latex bodysuit and never touch another person again!
    True
    False

Scoring:

Question 1: d. genital warts
Unlike the other three infections, genital warts, caused by certain strains of the human papilloma virus, are transmitted by direct skin-to-skin contact. If your partner has a genital wart on an exposed area and your skin comes in contact with it, transmission is likely. Even scarier, HPV is one of the most common STIs among young, sexually active people, with an estimated 5.5 million people becoming infected with HPV each year. Using condoms is still a good idea though, because condom use may reduce exposure to HPV. Like all STIs, the best way to prevent infection is to limit your number of sex partners, practice sexual abstinence, and avoid sexual contact if you think your partner is infected.

Question 2: False
Absolutely not! The herpes simplex virus (HSV) 1 and 2 look similar and either one can infect the mouth or genitals. Usually, HSV-1 occurs above the waist and HSV-2 occurs below the waist, but it is possible that HSV-1 can cause genital herpes. Herpes is a lifelong disease once infected, so it's not worth the risk! Because the virus can linger in body fluids long after a sore is gone, if you or your partner have either type of herpes the absolute best protection is to use dental dams or condoms every time you have sex or oral sex.

Question 3: b. 100
Yep, Hepatitis B is 100 times more infectious than HIV. Hepatitis B is a viral disease that attacks the liver and can cause extreme illness, even death. But the good news is that this is a 100-percent preventable disease! There is a safe and effective vaccine against hepatitis B, which is usually available at your student health center. This is the only STI vaccine that you can protect yourself with, so what are you waiting for?

Question 4: c. chlamydia
Crabs may be silent, but chlamydia is considered to be the "silent" epidemic because three-quarters of women and half of men with the disease have no symptoms. Possible symptoms include discharge from the penis or vagina and a burning sensation when urinating. This "silent" epidemic can lead to devastating results if untreated. Genital chlamydia can cause preventable infertility and ectopic pregnancy.

Question 5: True
This means that every hour, two Americans between the ages of 13 and 24 contract HIV. In 2002, the Centers for Disease Control report that there have been 27,880 cases of AIDS reported for people in the U.S. aged 20–24. This includes college students. It's important to realize that AIDS is an epidemic that affects everyone, not just IV-drug users and promiscuous homosexuals. The only way to protect yourself is to use a condom EVERY time. It's just that simple.

Question 6: They all died of syphilis.
These guys don't just have fame in common—they also all died from syphilis. HIV and Hepatitis B aren't the only deadly STIs. Syphilis progresses in stages, and during the first stage, a single sore may appear on the genitals or mouth, but often there are no symptoms. If untreated, the symptoms may disappear, but the infection stays in the body and progresses into the third stage, causing damage to the brain, heart, and nervous system, and even death.

Question 7: c. 3
There are approximately 10 million new cases of STIs each year among people aged 15–24 in the United States; that means that one in three sexually active people will have contracted an STI by age 24. So you can't go by looks, clothes, or how much money somebody has to determine if they have an STI. Remember, you're not just having sex with that person, but with everyone they've slept with, and everyone they've slept with . . . .

Question 8: False
Many people assume STI screening is a standard part of a routine Pap smear, but it isn't. Men and women should have yearly physical exams, and at that time should ask their doctor to screen them for STIs. This may seem like common sense, but getting screened through your partner does not mean you're safe. Not everyone develops an STI when exposed, so it's important you get tested.

Question 9: a. 6
A negative HIV result means that no HIV antibodies were found at the time that the blood was drawn. In most instances that means a person does not have HIV; however, it might mean you were tested too soon after infection. Your best bet is to get tested every six months, just to make sure. It's better to know now and get treated, than not know and infect people you love.

Question 10: False
Yes, sex can be scary these days, but it doesn't mean you can't enjoy yourself. If you are responsible about using a condom EVERY time you have intercourse, the chances of ending up with something nasty are slim. Free love comes with a price, one that you won't have to pay if you act responsibly. If you make STI screening a routine part of your physical, know your partner's status, and use a condom and dental dam every time you have sex, you are doing "it" right!

Your Health Change Plan

for Coping with STIs

More than 25 infections are spread by sexual activity. Here are some practical steps that reduce—but do not eliminate—the risks as well as recommendations for what to do if you contract a sexually transmitted infection and for informing a potential partner:

What You Can Do to Lower the Risk

:: Use a new condom each and every time you engage in any form of intercourse. Men should try different brands to find the ones they like best.

:: When putting on a condom, men should pinch its tip as they unroll it (all the way down!) to prevent an air bubble from forming in the reservoir tip. They must hold onto the base of their condom as they withdraw so it doesn't slip off.

:: Do not use spermicide containing nonoxynol-9. Contrary to past advice, experts now advise against choosing safer sex products with nonoxynol-9. According to recent research, nonoxynol-9 without condoms is ineffective against HIV transmission. Even with condoms, it does not protect women from the bacteria that cause gonorrhea and chlamydia.

:: If a condom fails during vaginal or anal intercourse, remove it.

:: After potential exposure to an STI, men may give themselves a little extra protection by urinating and washing their genitals with an antibacterial soap.

:: Oral sex can transmit various STIs, including herpes, gonorrhea, syphilis, and HIV. Safer-sex barriers, including latex condoms (without nonoxynol-9) for fellatio and either saran wrap or **dental dams** for cunnilingus, can lower the risk.

:: Because bacteria can be transmitted by hand, wash your hands with hot water and antibacterial soap after sex.

What to Do If You Have an STI

:: If you suspect that you have an STI, don't feel too embarrassed to get help through a physician's office or a clinic. Treatment relieves discomfort, prevents complications, and halts the spread of the disease.

:: Following diagnosis, take oral medication (which may be given instead of or in addition to shots) exactly as prescribed.

:: Try to figure out from whom you got the STI. Be sure to inform that person, who may not be aware of the problem.

:: If you have an STI, never deceive a prospective partner about it. Tell the truth—simply and clearly. Be sure your partner understands exactly what you have and what the risks are.

(Continued)

Self Survey **How Much Do You Know About STIs? (continued)**

Telling a Partner You Have an STI

Even though the conversation can be awkward and embarrassing, you need to talk honestly about any STI that you may have been exposed to or contracted. What you don't say can be hazardous to your partner's health. Here are some guidelines:

:: **Talk before you become intimate.** A good way to start is simply by saying, *"There is something we need to talk over first."*

:: **Be honest.** Don't downplay any potential risks.

:: **Don't blame.** Even if you suspect that your partner was the source of your infection, focus on the need for medical attention.

:: **Be sensitive to your partner's feelings.** Anger and resentment are common reactions when someone feels at risk. Try to listen without becoming defensive.

:: **Seek medical attention.** Do not engage in sexual intimacies until you obtain a doctor's assurance that you are no longer contagious.

Source: From www.smartersex.org, the Bacchus and Gamma Peer Education Network

---

How can you tell if someone you're dating or hope to date has been exposed to an STI? The bad news is you can't. But the good news is it doesn't matter—as long as you avoid sexual activity that could put you at risk of infection. Ideally, before engaging in any such behavior, both of you should talk about your prior sexual history (including number of partners and sexually transmitted infections) and other high-risk behavior, such as the use of injection drugs. If you know someone well enough to consider having sex with that person, you should be able to talk about STIs. If the person is unwilling to talk, you shouldn't have sex.

Chlamydia

The most widespread sexually transmitted bacterium in the United States is *Chlamydia trachomatis,* which causes an estimated 3 million cases of **chlamydia** each year.[74] Chlamydial infections are more common in younger than in older women, in African-American than in white women, and in unmarried than in married pregnant women. They also occur more often in both men and women with gonorrhea.

Those at greatest risk of chlamydial infection are individuals 25 years old or younger who engage in sex with more than one new partner within a two-month period and women who use birth control pills or other nonbarrier contraceptive methods. The U.S. Preventive Services Task Forces recommend regular screening for chlamydia for all sexually active women under age 25 and for older women with multiple sexual partners, a history of STIs, or inconsistent use of condoms.[75]

As many as 75 percent of women and 50 percent of men with chlamydia have no symptoms or symptoms so mild that they don't seek medical attention. Without treatment, up to 40 percent of cases of chlamydia can lead to pelvic inflammatory disease, a serious infection of the woman's fallopian tubes that can also damage the ovaries and uterus. Also, women infected with chlamydia may have

three to five times the risk of getting infected with HIV if exposed. Babies exposed to chlamydia in the birth canal during delivery can be born with pneumonia or with an eye infection called conjunctivitis, both of which can be dangerous unless treated early with antibiotics. Symptomless women who are screened and treated for chlamydial infection are almost 60 percent less likely than unscreened women to develop pelvic inflammatory disease.

Traditional methods of screening require a health professional to collect a swab sample of genital secretions. In the past, the sample had to be cultured in a laboratory to look for *C. trachomatis,* and results could take three days or more. Today, a number of tests are available to supplement or sometimes replace the relatively expensive and slow traditional culture. The three major types of nonculture tests are:

:: Direct fluorescent antibody test (DFA), which uses a scientific method called staining to make chlamydia easier to spot under a microscope. DFA can give quicker results than a culture and can be performed on specimens taken from the eye, cervix, or penis.

:: Enzyme immunoassays, available in some forms that don't require special lab equipment. Results are more rapid than with culture, and costs can be lower.

:: Tests to detect the genes of *C. trachomatis* in urine and in genital samples, which can accurately identify even very small numbers of genes in a specimen. While expensive, they are easy to perform and have a high level of accuracy.

According to CDC guidelines, the treatment of choice for uncomplicated chlamydia infections is a seven-day regimen of two daily doses of doxycycline or a single, 1-gram dose of azithromycin (Zithromax). Because chlamydia often occurs along with gonorrhea, some health practitioners prescribe seven days of ofloxacin, a drug effective against both chlamydial and gonorrheal infections. The use of condoms with spermicide can reduce, but not eliminate, the risk of chlamydial infection.[76] Sexual partners should be examined and treated if necessary. The

CDC, in its most recent guidelines, recommends that all women with chlamydia be rescreened three to four months after treatment is completed. The reason is that re-infection, which often happens because a patient's sex partners were not treated, increases the risk of pelvic inflammatory disease and other complications.[77]

Pelvic Inflammatory Disease

Infection of a woman's fallopian tubes or uterus, called **pelvic inflammatory disease (PID),** is not actually an STI, but rather a complication of STIs. About one in every seven women of reproductive age has PID; half of all adult women may have had it. Each year, about 1 million new cases are reported.

Ten to 20 percent of initial episodes of PID lead to scarring and obstruction of the fallopian tubes severe enough to cause infertility. Other long-term complications are ectopic pregnancy and chronic pelvic pain. The risk of these complications rises with subsequent PID episodes, bacterial vaginosis (discussed earlier in this chapter), and use of an IUD. Smoking also may increase the likelihood of PID. Two bacteria—gonococcus (the culprit in gonorrhea) and chlamydia—are responsible for one-half to one-third of all cases of PID. Other organisms are responsible for the remaining cases.

Most cases of PID occur among women under age 25 who are sexually active. Gonococcus-caused cases tend to affect poor women; those caused by chlamydia range across all income levels. One-half to one-third of all cases are transmitted sexually, and others have been traced to some IUDs that are no longer on the market. Several studies have shown that women with PID are more likely to have used douches than those without the disease. Consistent condom use may decrease PID risk.[78]

PID is a silent disease that, in half of all cases, often produces no noticeable symptoms as it progresses and causes scarring of the fallopian tubes. Experts are encouraging women with mild symptoms, such as abdominal pain or tenderness, to seek medical evaluation, and also encouraging physicians to test these patients for infections. Urine testing is a cost-effective method of detecting gonorrhea and chlamydia in young women and can prevent development of PID. For women with symptoms, magnetic resonance imaging (MRI) is highly accurate in establishing a diagnosis of PID and detecting other diseases that may be responsible for the symptoms.

Women may learn that they have PID only after discovering that they cannot conceive or after they develop an ectopic pregnancy (see Chapter 9). PID causes an estimated 15 to 30 percent of all cases of infertility every year, and about half of all cases of ectopic pregnancy. Most women do not experience any symptoms, but some may develop abdominal pain, tenderness in certain sites during pelvic exams, or vaginal discharge. Treatment may require hospitalization and intensive antibiotics therapy.

Gonorrhea

Gonorrhea (sometimes called "the clap" in street language) is one of the most common STIs in the United States and is increasing in occurrence, reversing a downward trend in the previous two decades. By some estimates, there may be approximately 1 million new cases every year. The incidence is highest among teenagers and young adults. Sexual contact, including oral-genital sex, is the primary means of transmission.

Most men who have gonorrhea know it. Thick, yellow-white pus oozes from the penis and urination causes a burning sensation. These symptoms usually develop two to nine days after the sexual contact that infected them. Men have a good reason to seek help: It hurts too much not to. Women also may experience discharge and burning on urination. However, as many as eight out of ten infected women have no symptoms.

Gonococcus, the bacterium that causes gonorrhea, can live in the vagina, cervix, and fallopian tubes for months, even years, and continue to infect the woman's sexual partners. Approximately 5 percent of sexually active American women have positive gonorrhea cultures but are unaware that they are silent carriers.

If left untreated in men or women, gonorrhea spreads through the urinary-genital tract. In women, the inflammation travels from the vagina and cervix, through the uterus, to the fallopian tubes and ovaries. The pain and fever are similar to those caused by stomach upset, so a woman may dismiss the symptoms. Eventually these symptoms diminish, even though the disease spreads to the entire pelvis. Pus may ooze from the fallopian tubes or ovaries into the peritoneum (the lining of the abdominal cavity), sometimes causing serious inflammation. However, this, too, can subside in a few weeks. Gonorrhea, the leading cause of sterility in women, can cause PID. In pregnant women, gonorrhea becomes a threat to the newborn. It can infect the infant's external genitals and cause a serious form of conjunctivitis, an inflammation of the eye that

A cloudy discharge is symptomatic of gonorrhea.

© Science VU/Visuals Unlimited

may lead to blindness. As a preventive step, newborns may have penicillin dropped into their eyes at birth.

In men, untreated gonorrhea can spread to the prostate gland, testicles, bladder, and kidneys. Among the serious complications are urinary obstruction and sterility caused by blockage of the vas deferens (the excretory duct of the testis). In both sexes, gonorrhea can develop into a serious, even fatal, bloodborne infection that can cause arthritis in the joints, attack the heart muscle and lining, cause meningitis, and attack the skin and other organs.

Although a blood test has been developed for detecting gonorrhea, the tried-and-true method of diagnosis is still a microscopic analysis of cultures from the male's urethra, the female's cervix, and the throat and anus of both sexes.

Because gonorrhea often occurs along with chlamydia, practitioners often prescribe an agent effective against both, such as ofloxacin. In some parts of the United States, gonorrhea has become so resistant to certain antibiotics that they are no longer advised for use in its treatment. Antibiotics taken for other reasons may not affect or cure the gonorrhea because of their dosage or type. And you can't develop immunity to gonorrhea; within days of recovering from one case, you can catch another.

Nongonococcal Urethritis

The term **nongonococcal urethritis (NGU)** refers to any inflammation of the urethra that is not caused by gonorrhea. NGU is the most common STI in men, accounting for 4 million to 6 million visits to a physician every year. Three microorganisms—*Chlamydia trachomatis, Ureaplasma urealyticum,* and *Mycoplasma genitalium*—are the primary causes; the usual means of transmission is sexual intercourse. Other infectious agents, such as fungi or bacteria, allergic reactions to vaginal secretions, or irritation by soaps or contraceptive foams or gels may also lead to NGU.

In the United States, NGU is more common in men than gonoccocal urethritis. The symptoms in men are similar to those of gonorrhea, including discharge from the penis (usually less than with gonorrhea) and mild burning during urination. Women frequently develop no symptoms or very mild itching, burning during urination, or discharge. Symptoms usually disappear after two or three weeks, but the infection may persist and cause cervicitis or PID in women and, in men, may spread to the prostate, epididymis, or both. Treatment usually consists of doxycycline or azithromycin and should be given to both sexual partners after testing.

Syphilis

A corkscrew-shaped, spiral bacterium called *Treponema pallidum* causes **syphilis.** This frail microbe dies in seconds if dried or chilled but grows quickly in the warm, moist tissues of the body, particularly in the mucous membranes of the genital tract. Entering the body through any tiny break in the skin, the germ burrows its way into the bloodstream. Sexual contact, including oral sex or intercourse, is a primary means of transmission. Genital ulcers caused by syphilis may increase the risk of HIV infection, while individuals with HIV may be more likely to develop syphilis.

Public education programs, expanded screening and surveillance, increased tracing of contacts, and condom promotion have helped control the spread of syphilis in some areas. Syphilis rates have fallen to the lowest ever reported in the United States. The decline has been particularly significant in African Americans.

Syphilis has clearly identifiable stages:

::   *Primary syphilis.* The first sign of syphilis is a lesion, or *chancre* (pronounced "shanker"), an open lump or crater the size of a dime or smaller, teeming with bacteria. The incubation period before its appearance ranges from 10 to 90 days; three to four weeks is average. The chancre appears exactly where the bacteria entered the body: in the mouth, throat, vagina, rectum, or penis. Any contact with the chancre is likely to result in infection.

::   *Secondary syphilis.* Anywhere from one to twelve months after the chancre's appearance, secondary-stage symptoms may appear. Some people have no symptoms. Others develop a skin rash or a small, flat rash in moist regions on the skin; whitish patches on the mucous membranes of the mouth or throat; temporary baldness; low-grade fever; headache; swollen glands; or large, moist sores around the mouth and genitals. These are loaded with bacteria; contact with them, through kissing or intercourse, may transmit the infection. Symptoms may last for several days or several months. Even without treatment, they eventually disappear as the syphilis microbes go into hiding.

::   *Latent syphilis.* Although there are no signs or symptoms, no sores or rashes at this stage, the bacteria are invading various organs inside the body, including the heart and brain. For two to four years, there may be recurring infectious and highly contagious lesions of the skin or mucous membranes. However, syphilis loses its infectiousness as it progresses: After the first two years, a person rarely transmits syphilis through intercourse.

After four years, even congenital syphilis is rarely transmitted. Until this stage of the disease, however, a pregnant woman can pass syphilis to her unborn child. If the fetus is infected in its fourth month or earlier, it may be disfigured or even die. If infected late in pregnancy, the child may show no signs of infection for months or years after birth, but may then become disabled with the symptoms of tertiary syphilis.

::   *Tertiary syphilis.* Ten to twenty years after the beginning of the latent stage, the most serious symptoms of syphilis emerge, generally in the organs in which the bacteria settled during latency. Syphilis that has progressed to this stage has become increasingly rare. Victims of tertiary syphilis may die of a ruptured aorta or of other heart damage, or may have progressive brain or spinal cord damage, eventually leading to blindness, insanity, or paralysis. About a third of those who are not treated during the first three stages of syphilis enter the tertiary stage later in life.

Health experts are urging screening for syphilis for everyone who seeks treatment for an STI, especially adolescents; for everyone using illegal drugs; and for the partners of these two groups. They also recommend that anyone diagnosed with syphilis be screened for other STIs and be counseled about voluntary testing for HIV.

Early diagnosis of syphilis can lead to a complete cure. The most widely used diagnostic techniques are the Venereal Disease Research Laboratory (VDRL) test or the rapid-plasma-reagin (RPR) test. However, these may be positive only during the secondary stage of the disease, when the bacteria have reached the bloodstream. A positive finding always requires additional information, including a physical exam and other laboratory tests, to confirm the diagnosis and plan treatment.

Penicillin is the drug of choice for treating primary, secondary, and latent syphilis. The earlier treatment begins, the more effective it is. Those allergic to penicillin may be treated with doxycycline, ceftriaxone, or erythromycin. An added danger of not getting treatment for syphilis is an increased risk of HIV transmission.

Herpes

Herpes (from the Greek word that means *to creep*) collectively describes some of the most common viral infections in humans. Characteristically, **herpes simplex** causes blisters on the skin or mucous membranes. Herpes simplex exists in several varieties. *Herpes simplex virus 1 (HSV-1)* generally causes cold sores and fever blisters around the mouth. *Herpes simplex virus 2 (HSV-2)* may cause blisters on the penis, inside the vagina, on the cervix, in the pubic area, on the buttocks, or on the thighs. With the increase of oral-genital sex, some doctors report finding type 2 herpes lesions in the mouth and throat.

About 1.6 million new herpes simplex virus cases are acquired every year.[79] An estimated 135 million Americans age 12 or over carry HSV-1, the most common herpes virus. The prevalence of HSV-2 has increased 30 percent since the late 1970s. According to the CDC, one in five American adolescents and adults is now infected, but 80 to 90 percent of these individuals do not realize they carry the virus because they never develop genital lesions, or they experience only very subtle symptoms. Men and women ages 20 to 29 have higher rates of infection than other age groups.[80]

Research has shown that individuals without any obvious symptoms shed the virus subclinically, whether or not they have lesions. Most people with herpes contract it from partners who were not aware of any symptoms or of their own contagiousness. Standard methods of diagnosing genital herpes in women, which rely primarily on physical examination and viral cultures, may miss as many as two-thirds of all cases. Newly developed blood tests are more effective in detecting unrecognized and subclinical infections with HSV-2.

In the past, patients and most doctors thought people with herpes could safely have unprotected sex when they had no symptoms. The herpes virus is present in genital secretions even when patients do not notice any signs of the disease, and people infected with genital herpes can spread it even between flare-ups when they have no symptoms. There is growing evidence that genital herpes promotes the spread of HIV.

HSV transmission occurs through close contact with mucous membranes or abraded skin. Condoms help prevent infection but aren't foolproof. When herpes sores are present, the infected person is highly contagious and should avoid bringing the lesions into contact with someone else's body through touching, sexual interaction, or kissing.

A newborn can be infected with genital herpes while passing through the birth canal, and the frequency of mother-to-infant transmission seems to be increasing. Most infected infants develop typical skin sores, which should be cultured to confirm a herpes diagnosis. Some physicians recommend treatment with acyclovir. Because of the risk of severe damage and possible death, caesarean delivery may be advised for a woman with active herpes lesions.

The virus that causes herpes never entirely goes away; it retreats to nerves near the lower spinal cord, where it remains for the life of the host. Herpes sores can return without warning weeks, months, or even years after their

(a) **(b)**

(a) Herpes simplex virus (HSV-1) as a mouth sore (b) Herpes simplex virus (HSV-2) as a genital sore.

first occurrence, often during menstruation or times of stress, or with sudden changes in body temperature. Of those who experience HSV recurrence, 10 to 35 percent do so frequently—that is, about six or more times a year. In most people, attacks diminish in frequency and severity over time. Herpes, like other STIs, can trigger feelings of shame, guilt, and depression.

Antiviral drugs, such as acyclovir (Zovirax), have proven effective in treating and controlling herpes. Available as an ointment, in capsules, and in injection form, acyclovir relieves the symptoms but doesn't kill the virus. Whereas the ointment works only for the initial bout with herpes, acyclovir in injectable and pill form dramatically reduces the length and severity of herpes outbreaks. Continuing daily oral acyclovir can reduce recurrences by about 80 percent. However, its safety in pregnant women has not been established. Infection with herpes viruses resistant to acyclovir is a growing problem, especially in individuals with immune-suppressing disorders.

Various treatments—compresses made with cold water, skim milk, or warm salt water; ice packs; or a mild anesthetic cream—can relieve discomfort. Herpes sufferers should avoid heat, hot baths, or nylon underwear. In recent years physicians have tried a host of therapies, including topical ointments, various vaccines, exposure to light, and ultrasonic waves—all with little success. Some physicians have used laser therapy to vaporize the lesions. Clinical trials of an experimental vaccine to protect people from herpes infections are underway.

Can stress trigger a flare-up of genital herpes? To test this common assumption, for six months researchers followed 58 women, aged 20 to 44, with a history of herpes; they assessed stress, mood, life changes, and diary reports of herpes recurrences. The researchers found that single stressful events and temporary bad moods were not related to recurrence of the disease, but long-term stresses (lasting more than seven days) were. The more intense the long-term stress, the greater the likelihood of a herpes flare-up.[81]

College-age women are among those at greatest risk of acquiring HPV infection. In various studies conducted in college health centers, 10 to 46 percent of female students (mean age 20 to 22) had a cervical HPV infection—and increased risk of precancerous cell changes. Risk factors include smoking, use of oral contraceptives, multiple sex partners, anal as well as vaginal intercourse, alcohol consumption at the time of engaging in vaginal intercourse, and sex partners with a history of HPV.

In a survey of 1,000 women, fewer than half knew that HPV is the main cause of cervical cancer and only a third knew that genital warts, also caused by types of HPV, do not themselves cause the disease. Most believed that condoms protect against infection with the virus, although the evidence for this is not clear. Only half knew that the contraceptive pill does not protect against infection.[83]

HPV infections in young women tend to be of short duration. In a three-year study, 60 percent of 608 college women became infected with the virus; the average duration of infection was eight months. According to the researchers, many young women who get HPV may not require treatment because the condition often regresses on its own.

HPV is transmitted primarily through vaginal, anal, and oral-genital sex. More than half of HPV-infected individuals do not develop any symptoms. After contact with an infected individual, genital warts may appear from three weeks to eighteen months, with an average period of about three months. The warts are treated by freezing, cauterization, chemicals, or surgical removal. Recurrences are common because the virus remains in the body.

HPV infection may invade the urethra and cause urinary obstruction and bleeding. It greatly increases a woman's risk of developing a precancerous condition called *cervical intraepithelial neoplasia,* which can lead to cervical cancer. There also is a strong association between HPV infections and cancer of the vagina, vulva, urethra, penis, and anus.

What Is Human Papilloma Virus?

Infection with **human papilloma virus (HPV),** a pathogen that can cause *genital warts,* is the most common viral STI. By some estimates, 20 million or more women in the United States are infected with HPV, as are three out of four of their male sexual partners. Young women who engage in sexual intercourse at an early age are more likely than those with later sexual debuts to become infected with HPV. Their risk also increases if they have multiple sexual partners or a history of a sexually transmitted disease, use drugs, or have partners with multiple sexual partners.[82]

© Marazzi/Photo Researchers, Inc.

Human papilloma virus, which causes genital warts, is the most common viral STI.

HPV may be the single most important risk factor in 95 percent of all cases of cervical cancer. Adolescent girls infected with HPV appear to be particularly vulnerable to developing cervical cancer. It is not known if HPV itself causes cancer or acts in conjunction with cofactors (such as other infections, smoking, or suppressed immunity). HPV transmission may be the reason women are five to eleven times as likely to get cervical cancer if their steady sexual partner has had 20 or more previous partners.

Women who have had an HPV infection should examine their genitals regularly and get an annual Pap smear. However, this standard diagnostic test for cervical cancer doesn't identify HPV infection. A new laboratory test can detect the presence of HPV, including the high-risk types associated with the development of cervical cancer. The HPV DNA test does not test for cancer, but for the HPV viruses that can cause cell changes in the cervix. If left untreated, these changes can eventually lead to cancer in some women. Surgery or laser therapy can prevent further damage.

HPV may also cause genital warts in men and increase the risk of cancer of the penis. HPV-infected men, who may not develop any symptoms, can spread the infection to their partners. People with visible genital warts also may have asymptomatic or subclinical HPV infections that are extremely difficult to treat.

No form of therapy has been shown to completely eradicate HPV, nor has any single treatment been uniformly effective in removing warts or preventing their recurrence. CDC guidelines suggest treatments that focus on the removal of visible warts—cryotherapy (freezing) and topical applications of podofilox, podophyllin, or trichloroacetic acid—and then eradication of the virus. At least 20 to 30 percent of treated individuals experience recurrence. In experimental studies, interferon, a biologic substance produced by virus-infected cells that inhibits viral replication, has proven helpful.

Chancroid

A **chancroid** is a soft, painful sore or localized infection caused by the bacterium *Haemophilus ducrevi* and usually acquired through sexual contact. Half of the cases heal by themselves. In other cases, the infection may spread to the lymph glands near the chancroid, where large amounts of pus can accumulate and destroy much of the local tissue. The incidence of this STI, widely prevalent in Africa and tropical and semitropical regions, is rapidly increasing in the United States, with outbreaks in several states, including Louisiana, Texas, and New York. Chancroids, which may increase susceptibility to HIV infection, are believed to be a major factor in the heterosexual spread of HIV. This infection is treated with antibiotics (ceftriaxone, azithromycin, or erythromycin) and can be prevented by keeping the genitals clean and washing them with soap and water in case of possible exposure.

Actual size

A pubic louse, or "crab."

Pubic Lice and Scabies

These infections are sometimes, but not always, transmitted sexually. *Pubic lice* (or "crabs") are usually found in the pubic hair, although they can migrate to any hairy areas of the body. Lice lay eggs called nits that attach to the base of the hair shaft. Irritation from the lice may produce intense itching. Scratching to relieve the itching can produce sores. *Scabies* is caused by a mite that burrows under the skin, where they lay eggs that hatch and undergo many changes in the course of their life cycle, producing great discomfort, including intense itching.

Lice and scabies are treated with applications of permethrin cream and Lindane shampoo to all the areas of the body where there are concentrations of body hair (genitals, armpits, scalp). You must repeat treatment in seven days to kill any newly developed adults. Wash or dry-clean clothing and bedding.

:•: HIV and AIDS

Thirty years ago, no one knew about **human immunodeficiency virus (HIV).** No one had ever heard of **acquired immune deficiency syndrome (AIDS).** Once seen as an epidemic affecting primarily gay men and injection drug users, AIDS has taken on a very different form. Today, heterosexuals in developing countries have the highest rates of infection and mortality. And HIV infection continues to spread, doubling at an estimated rate of every ten years. About 40 million people worldwide are infected with HIV; 15,000 more individuals are infected every day.

AIDS has surpassed tuberculosis and malaria as the leading infectious cause of death and has become the fourth-largest killer worldwide. The cumulative death toll for AIDS exceeds 22 million. The region that has been hardest hit is sub-Saharan Africa, the site of seven of every ten of the world's cases of HIV infection and nine of every ten deaths due to AIDS. In the two hardest-hit countries, Zimbabwe and Botswana, one of every four adults is infected, and AIDS has cut the average life expectancy by nearly 20 years. In Asia, the total number of people infected is expanding rapidly, even though the rate of new infection remains relatively low. Russia, China, and India are experiencing dramatic increases in AIDS cases.[84]

According to CDC estimates, between 850,000 and 950,000 people are living with HIV in the United States; nearly 385,000 of these men and women have full-blown AIDS. The annual number of new HIV infections, which had held steady at about 40,000 for a decade, has been rising, particularly among gay and bisexual men.[85]

At least half of new HIV infections occur in people under age 25, mainly by sexual contact. HIV is the fifth leading cause of death for Americans between the ages of 25 and 44. Among African-American women in this age group, HIV infection is the third leading cause of death, and among African-American men, it's the leading cause of death.[86]

Federal health officials fear that a new generation may not be using adequate safer sex precautions because they have grown complacent about the dangers of HIV/AIDS.[87] Efforts to prevent sexual transmission of HIV have taken a new focus: counseling those who already have HIV in an attempt to get them to stop spreading it.

Revolutionary new drugs are indeed allowing HIV-infected people to live longer. However, new dangers have emerged. Up to 15 percent of new HIV cases in the country may stem from drug-resistant strains of the virus. "Superinfection" with more than one strain of HIV seems more common than previously thought. As a result, HIV-infected people who initially were doing well without drugs may become ill after contracting a second strain of the AIDS virus.

Efforts to prevent nonsexual forms of HIV transmission have been very effective. Screening the blood supply has reduced the rate of transfusion-associated HIV transmission by 99.9 percent. Treatment with antiretroviral drugs during pregnancy and birth has reduced transmission by about 90 percent in optimal conditions. Among drug users in some settings, programs that combine addiction treatment and needle exchange reduced the incidence of HIV infection by 30 percent.

The Spread of HIV

HIV came to the United States in the late 1970s. Several factors—including frequent sexual activity with multiple, anonymous partners and high-risk sexual practices, such as anal intercourse—may have caused its quick spread through gay communities in the 1980s. As more became known about HIV transmission, many homosexual men adopted safer ways of sexual expression, reduced the number of sexual partners, or entered into monogamous relationships. As a result, the spread of HIV among gay men, especially older men in metropolitan areas, slowed.

In the 1980s, HIV also spread among injection drug users who, by sharing contaminated needles, injected the virus directly into their bloodstream. Injection drug use has been the number-one source of HIV infection in heterosexual men and women in this country. Sex with an infected injection drug user is also a major cause of HIV infection.

The percentage of individuals who acquired HIV through heterosexual contact has increased from about 2 percent in 1985 to about 15 percent. However, many heterosexual adults are not aware of their partners' HIV status and may not see themselves as at risk of HIV infection. According to the CDC, about a third of the HIV-infected individuals in the United States have not been diagnosed.[88]

Although HIV/AIDS is often seen as a threat to men, 30 percent of new HIV infections in the United States occur among women. About a quarter of Americans living with HIV/AIDS are women. Women of color, particularly African Americans, have been hardest hit. While African-American women make up just 13 percent of the female population of the United States, they account for 63 percent of newly diagnosed cases. HIV/AIDS is most prevalent among women in their childbearing years.[89]

Half of the world's 39 million adults with HIV/AIDS are women, according to a report of the latest data on the epidemic. Women also made up half of the 2.5 million adults who died of AIDS in 2002 and half of the 4.2 million adults who were newly infected during that year. In Sub-Saharan Africa, where HIV spreads mainly through heterosexual activity, 58 percent of HIV-positive adults are women.[90]

Reducing the Risk of HIV Transmission

HIV/AIDS can be so frightening that some people have exaggerated its dangers, whereas others understate them. The fact is that although no one is immune to HIV, you can reduce the risk if you abstain from sexual activity, remain in a monogamous relationship with an uninfected partner, and do not inject drugs. If you're not in a long-term monogamous relationship with a partner you're sure is safe, and you're not willing to abstain from sex, there are things you can do to lower your risk of HIV infection. Remember that the risk of HIV transmission depends on sexual behavior, not sexual orientation. Among young men, the prevalence and frequency of sexual risk behaviors are similar regardless of sexual orientation, ethnicity, or age. Homosexual, heterosexual, and bisexual individuals all need to know about the kinds of sexual activity that increase their risk.

Here's what you should know about HIV transmission:

:: Casual contact does *not* spread HIV infection. You cannot get HIV infection from drinking from a water fountain, contact with a toilet seat, or touching an infected person.

:: Compared to other viruses, HIV is extremely difficult to get.

:: HIV can live in blood, semen, vaginal fluids, and breast milk.

:: Many chemicals, including household bleach, alcohol, and hydrogen peroxide, can inactivate HIV.

:: In studies of family members sharing dishes, food, clothing, and frequent hugs with people with HIV infection or AIDS, those who have contracted the virus have shared razor blades, toothbrushes, or had other means of blood contact.

:: You cannot tell visually whether a potential sexual partner has HIV. A blood test is needed to detect the antibodies that the body produces to fight HIV, thus indicating infection.

:: HIV can be spread in semen and vaginal fluids during a single instance of anal, vaginal, or oral sexual contact between heterosexuals, bisexuals, or homosexuals. The risk increases with the number of sexual encounters with an infected partner.

:: Teenage girls may be particularly vulnerable to HIV infection because the immature cervix is easily infected.

:: Anal intercourse is an extremely high-risk behavior because HIV can enter the bloodstream through tiny breaks in the lining of the rectum. HIV transmission is much more likely to occur during unprotected anal intercourse than vaginal intercourse.

:: Other behaviors that increase the risk of HIV infection include having multiple sexual partners, engaging in sex without condoms or virus-killing spermicides, sexual contact with persons known to be at high risk (for example, prostitutes or injection drug users), and sharing injection equipment for drugs.

:: Individuals are at greater risk if they have an active sexual infection. Sexually transmitted infections, such as herpes, gonorrhea, and syphilis, facilitate transmission of HIV during vaginal or rectal intercourse.

:: No cases of HIV transmission by deep kissing have been reported, but it could happen. Studies have found blood in the saliva of healthy people after kissing; other lab studies have found HIV in saliva. Social (dry) kissing is safe.

:: Oral sex can lead to HIV transmission. The virus in any semen that enters the mouth could make its way into the bloodstream through tiny nicks or sores in the mouth. A man's risk in performing oral sex on a woman is smaller because an infected woman's genital fluids have much lower concentrations of HIV than does semen.

:: HIV infection is not widespread among lesbians, although there have been documented cases of possible female-to-female HIV transmission. In each instance, one partner had had sex with a bisexual man or male injection drug user, or had injected drugs herself.

HIV Infection

HIV infection refers to a spectrum of health problems that results from immunologic abnormalities caused by the virus when it enters the bloodstream. In theory, the body may be able to resist infection by HIV. In reality, in almost all cases, HIV destroys the cell-mediated immune system, particularly the CD4+ T-lymphocytes (also called *T4 helper cells*). The result is greatly increased susceptibility to various cancers and opportunistic infections (infections that take hold because of the reduced effectiveness of the immune system).

Researchers now know that HIV triggers a state of all-out war within the immune system. Almost immediately following infection with HIV, the immune system responds aggressively by manufacturing enormous numbers of CD4+ cells. It eventually is overwhelmed, however, as the viral particles continue to replicate, or multiply. The intense war between HIV and the immune system indicates that the virus itself, not a breakdown in the immune system, is responsible for disease progression.

Shortly after becoming infected with HIV, individuals may experience a few days of flulike symptoms, which most ignore or attribute to other viruses. Some people

Electron micrograph of a white blood cell being attacked by HIV (*blue light particles*), the virus that causes AIDS.

develop a more severe mononucleosis-type syndrome. After this stage, individuals may not develop any signs or symptoms of disease for a period ranging from weeks to more than 12 years.

HIV symptoms, which tend to increase in severity and number the longer the virus is in the body, may include any of the following:

:: Swollen lymph nodes.

:: Fever, chills, and night sweats.

:: Diarrhea.

:: Weight loss.

:: Coughing and shortness of breath.

:: Persistent tiredness.

:: Skin sores.

:: Blurred vision and headaches.

:: Development of other infections, such as certain kinds of pneumonia.

HIV infection is associated with a variety of HIV-related diseases, including different cancers and dangerous infections, including tuberculosis. HIV-infected individuals may develop persistent generalized lymphadenopathy, enlargement of the lymph nodes at two or more different sites in the body. This condition typically persists for more than three months without any other illness to explain its occurrence. Diminished mental function may appear before other symptoms. Tests conducted on infected but apparently healthy men have revealed impaired coordination, problems in thinking, or abnormal brain scans.

HIV Testing

Nearly 50 percent of American adults younger than 65 have been tested for HIV. In general, women are more likely to have sought testing than men.[91] About 10,000 facilities provide publicly funded HIV testing and counseling in the United States; approximately 2.6 million tests are performed annually at these sites. The CDC now recommends that all sexually active gay and bisexual men be tested at least once a year for HIV, as well as for chlamydia, syphilis, and gonorrhea. The rates of bacterial STIs in HIV-positive gay and bisexual men are increasing.[92]

All HIV tests measure antibodies, cells produced by the body to fight HIV infection. A negative test indicates no exposure to HIV. It can take three to six months for the body to produce the telltale antibodies, however, so a negative result may not be accurate, depending on the timing of the test.

HIV testing can be either confidential or anonymous. In confidential testing, a person's name is recorded along with the test results, which are made available to medical personnel and, in 32 states, the state health department. In anonymous testing, no name is associated with the test results. Anonymous testing is available in 39 states.

Different groups of individuals at risk prefer different tests. Asian–Pacific Islander and white men who have sex with men are most likely to choose anonymous testing; African-American men who have sex with men are much more likely to choose confidential testing. Consumers must be wary of bogus HIV tests offered via the Internet.

The following HIV tests are currently available in the United States:

:: **EIA** (Enzyme Immune Assay) or **ELISA** (Enzyme-Linked ImmunoSorbent Assay). These standard blood tests are the most commonly used HIV screens. A health-care provider draws a blood sample, which is analyzed for antibodies produced to fight against HIV particles. Results are available within a few days to two weeks.

:: **Oral HIV tests.** These tests have become available in some doctors' offices and health clinics. A health-care worker swabs a tissue sample from the inside of the mouth. The only oral test approved by the Food and Drug Administration (FDA) is the OraSure.

:: **Rapid Tests.** Different types, such as the OraQuick Rapid HIV-1 Antibody Test, can detect HIV antibodies in blood. The advantage is fast results—usually in 20 or 30 minutes.

:: **Western blot.** This more accurate and expensive test is used to confirm the results of a positive HIV test.

:: **HomeAccess.** This test—the only home HIV test approved by the FDA—is available in drug stores for $40 to $50. An individual draws a blood sample by pricking a finger and sends it to a laboratory along with a personal identification number. Results are given over the phone by a trained counselor, usually within several days.

:: **Urine Test.** This alternative to a blood test must be ordered by a physician. A urine sample is screened by a laboratory. Results are generally available in a few days to two weeks.[93]

Newly developed blood tests can determine how recently a person was infected with HIV and distinguish between long-standing infections and those contracted within the previous four to six months. Health officials recommend HIV testing for the following individuals:

:: Men who have had sex with other men, regardless of whether they consider themselves homosexual.

:: Anyone who uses injection drugs or has shared needles.

:: Anyone who has had sex with someone who uses injection drugs or has shared needles.

:: Women who have had sex with bisexual men.

:: Anyone who has had sex with someone from an area with a high incidence of HIV infection.

:: Individuals who have had sex with people they do not know well.

:: Anyone who received blood transfusions or blood products between 1978 and 1985, their sexual partners, and, if they are new mothers, their infants.

Diagnosing AIDS

A diagnosis of AIDS applies to anyone with HIV whose immune system is severely impaired, as indicated by a CD41 count of less than 200 cells per cubic millimeter of blood, compared to normal CD41 cell counts in healthy people not infected with HIV of 800 to 1,200 per cubic millimeter of blood. In addition, AIDS is diagnosed in persons with HIV infection who experience recurrent pneumonia, invasive cervical cancer, or pulmonary tuberculosis.

People with AIDS also may experience persistent fever, diarrhea that persists for more than one month, or involuntary weight loss of more than 10 percent of normal body weight. Generalized lymphadenopathy may persist. Neurological disease—including dementia (confusion and impaired thinking) and other problems with thinking, speaking, movement, or sensation—may occur. Secondary infectious diseases that may develop in people with AIDS include *Pneumocystis carinii* pneumonia, tuberculosis, or oral candidiasis (thrush). Secondary cancers associated with HIV infection include Kaposi's sarcoma and cancer of the cervix.

Treating HIV/AIDS

New forms of therapy have been remarkably effective in boosting levels of protective T cells and reducing *viral load*—the amount of HIV in the bloodstream. People with high viral loads are more likely to progress rapidly to AIDS than people with low levels of the virus.

The current "gold-standard" approach to combating HIV is known as HAART (Highly Active AntiRetroviral Therapies), which dramatically reduces viral load even though it does not eradicate the virus. This complex regimen uses one of 250 different combinations of three or more antiretroviral drugs. Since the development of HAART, the number of deaths among persons with AIDS in the United States has declined substantially, and the number of those living with AIDS has risen. After recent declines, the number of U.S. AIDS cases has remained stable at approximately 10,000 per quarter.[94] An increasing proportion of people living with AIDS in the United States are heterosexual, black or Hispanic, female, and residents of the South.

A year of HAART treatment costs more than $10,000, which is not always covered by health insurance and which has restricted the use of HAART in poor nations. Its success depends on consistent adherence to the drug regimen over a prolonged period of time. However, as many as 30 to 70 percent of patients do not strictly adhere to their schedules. Another drawback is serious side effects, including anemia, mouth ulcers, diarrhea, respiratory difficulties, digestive problems, liver damage, and skin rashes. There also is concern about emerging resistance to some antiretroviral medications. Researchers are continuing to work toward development of more effective and less toxic treatments as well as a vaccine against HIV. However, the first AIDS vaccine to undergo clinical trials of its efficacy failed to provide protection against the virus in the general population.[95]

The Bottom Line ▼
The Best Defense

Some day medical science may develop vaccines or other means of providing total protection against infectious diseases. Until then your best defense is to take commonsense steps to promote well-being and reduce the risks of infection. Here are some basic principles of self-defense:

:: *Eat a balanced diet* to be sure you get essential vitamins and minerals. Severe deficiencies in vitamins B_6, B_{12}, and folic acid impair immunity. Keep up your iron and zinc intake. Iron influences the number and vigor of certain immune cells, whereas zinc is crucial for cell repair. Too little vitamin C may also increase susceptibility to infectious diseases.

:: *Avoid fatty foods.* A low-fat diet can increase the activity of immune cells that hunt down and knock out cells infected with viruses.

:: *Get enough sleep.* Without adequate rest, your immune system cannot maintain and renew itself.

:: *Exercise regularly.* Aerobic exercise stimulates the production of an immune-system booster called interleukin-2.

:: *Don't smoke.* Smoking decreases the levels of some immune cells and increases susceptibility to respiratory infections.

:: *Control your alcohol intake.* Heavy drinking interferes with normal immune responses and lowers the number of defender cells.

:: Wash your hands frequently with hot water and soap. In a public restroom, use a paper towel to turn off the faucet after you wash your hands, and avoid touching the doorknob. Wash objects used by someone with a cold.

:: Don't share food, drinks, silverware, glasses, and other objects that may carry infectious microbes.

:: During cold and flu season, spend as little time as possible in crowds, especially closed places, such as elevators and airplanes. When out, keep your distance from sneezers and coughers.

:: Don't touch your eyes, mouth, and nose after being with someone who has cold symptoms.

:: Use tissues rather than cloth handkerchiefs, which may harbor viruses for hours or days.

:: Try to avoid irritating air pollutants.

:: Always use safer sex practices.

:: If you have any reason to suspect that you may have been exposed to an STI, get tested immediately.

 After watching the CNN video segment, discuss the following question. How large is the threat of emerging or re-emerging infectious diseases?

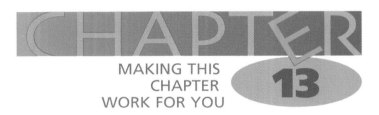

MAKING THIS
CHAPTER
WORK FOR YOU

13

1. Which of the following statements about disease-causing microbes is *false?*
   a. Helminths cause malaria, one of the major worldwide diseases.
   b. AIDS is caused by a retrovirus.
   c. In the United States, the most common protozoan disease is giardiasis.
   d. Salmonella and botulism are foodborne illnesses caused by bacteria.

2. Which of the following statements about the immune system is *false?*
   a. The immune system has two types of white blood cells: B cells, which produce antibodies that fight bacteria and viruses, and T-cells, which protect against parasites, fungi, and cancer cells.
   b. Immune system structures include the spleen, tonsils, thymus gland, and lymph nodes located throughout the body.
   c. Inoculation with a vaccine confers active immunity.
   d. The effect of stress on the human immune system depends on whether you can control the stressor and on the mental effort required to cope.

3. Booster immunizations are recommended for all of the following diseases *except*
   a. diphtheria
   b. tetanus

   c. measles
   d. pertussis

4. Which of the following statements about the common cold and influenza is true?
   a. Influenza is just a more severe form of the common cold.
   b. Aspirin should be avoided by children and young adults who have a cold or influenza.
   c. The flu vaccine is also effective against most of the viruses that cause the common cold.
   d. Antibiotics are appropriate treatments for colds but not for influenza.

5. Which of the following statements about specific infectious diseases is *false?*
   a. Yeast infections can be treated with nonprescription drugs.
   b. Symptoms of UTIs include burning urination, chills, fever, and blood in the urine.
   c. Hepatitis A is usually transmitted through contaminated needles, transfusions, and sexual contact.
   d. College freshmen are at higher risk for contracting meningitis than the general population of young people between the ages of 18 and 23.

6. Sexually transmitted infections
   a. are the major cause of preventable sterility in the United States.
   b. can result in a severe kidney disease called pylonephritis.
   c. have declined in incidence in developing nations due to improving health standards.
   d. do not increase the risk of being infected with HIV.

7. Bacterial agents cause all of the following STIs except for
   a. genital warts
   b. syphilis
   c. chlamydia
   d. gonorrhea

8. Viral agents cause all of the following STIs except for
   a. herpes
   b. genital warts
   c. hepatitis B
   d. candidiasis

9. Which of the following statements about HIV transmission is true?
   a. Individuals are not at risk for HIV if they are being treated for chlamydia or gonorrhea.
   b. HIV can be transmitted between lesbians.
   c. Heterosexual men who do not practice safe sex are at less risk for contracting HIV than homosexual men who do practice safe sex.
   d. HIV cannot be spread in a single instance of sexual intercourse.

10. A person with AIDS
    a. has a low viral load and a high number of T4 helper cells.
    b. can no longer pass HIV to a sexual partner.
    c. may suffer from secondary infectious diseases and cancers.
    d. will not respond to treatment.

Answers to these questions can be found on page 652.

Critical Thinking

1. Before you read this chapter, describe what you did to avoid contracting infectious disease. Now that you have read the chapter, will you be making any changes in your practices? Briefly explain the convenience, advantages, and disadvantages of each practice that you have and/or will be using to prevent infection.

Critical Thinking

2. The U.S. military and some employers routinely screen personnel for HIV. Some hospitals test patients and note their HIV status on their charts. Some insurance companies test for HIV before selling a policy. Do you believe that an individual has the right to refuse to be tested for HIV? Should a physician be able to order an HIV test without a patient's consent? Can a surgeon refuse to operate on an HIV-infected patient or one who refuses HIV testing? Do patients have the right to know if their doctors, dentists, or nurses are HIV-positive?

Critical Thinking

3. A man who developed herpes sued his former girlfriend. A woman who became sterile as a result of pelvic inflammatory disease (PID) took her ex-husband to court. A woman who contracted HIV infection from her dentist, who had died of AIDS, filed suit against his estate. Do you think that anyone who knowingly transmits a sexually transmitted disease should be held legally responsible? Do you think such an act should be a criminal offense?

Profile Plus

Practice self-defense against all forms of infection. Use the following activities from your Profile Plus CD-ROM to assess your risks.

Profile Plus

• STD Attitude Scale

Profile Plus

• Self-Quiz on HIV and AIDS

Sites and Bytes

Centers for Disease Control and Prevention
www.cdc.gov

This comprehensive governmental site sponsored by the U.S. Department of Health and Human Services features information on bioterrorism, travel medicine, infectious diseases, immunization, statistics, and a comprehensive list of health topics.

Sites and Bytes

National Institute of Allergy and Infectious Diseases
www.niaid.nih.gov

The Microbiology and Infectious Diseases section of this site features a variety of infectious diseases, including emerging infectious diseases, influenza, sexually transmitted infections, and tuberculosis, as well as information on vaccines and the U.S. Biodefense Program.

Sites and Bytes

Immunization Action Coalition
www.immunize.org

This site features comprehensive vaccination information for children, adolescents, and adults. Vaccine information sheets in English and Spanish are available for measles, rubella, tetanus, hepatitis A & B, influenza, chickenpox, polio, diphtheria, and more.

InfoTrac College Edition

Activity

Holtgrave, D. R., and R. A. Crosby. "Social Capital, Poverty, and Income Inequality as Predictors of Gonorrhea, Syphilis, Chlamydia and AIDS Case Rates in the United States." *Sexually Transmitted Infections,* Vol. 79, No. 1, February 2003, p. 62(3).

InfoTrac College Edition

1. What are four important public health variables that are correlated with social capital?

2. Explain the causal mechanisms that have been postulated for the linkages between social capital and health.

3. Describe the correlation of social capital, poverty, and income inequality to the prevalence of gonorrhea, syphilis, chlamydia, and AIDS.

InfoTrac College Edition

You can find additional readings related to infectious diseases with InfoTrac College Edition, an online library of more than 900 journals and publications. Follow the instructions that were packaged with your textbook; then search for articles using a key word search.

For additional links, resources, and suggested readings on InfoTrac College Edition, visit our Health & Wellness Resource Center at **http://health.wadsworth.com**.

Key Terms

The terms listed are used on the page indicated. Definitions of the terms are in the Glossary at the end of this book.

Key Terms

abscess 429
acquired immune deficiency syndrome (AIDS) 457
allergy 429
antibiotics 424
antibody-mediated immunity 427
antiviral drug 424
autoimmune disorder 430
bacteria 424
bacterial vaginosis 444
candidiasis 444
cell-mediated immunity 427
chanchroid 457
chlamydia 452
chronic fatigue syndrome (CFS) 438
cystitis 445

Key Terms

dental dam 451
fungi 424
gamma globulin 427
gonorrhea 453
helminth 425
hepatitis 437
herpes simplex 455
host 424
human immunodeficiency virus (HIV) 457
human papilloma virus (HPV) 456
immune deficiency 429
immunity 426
immunotherapy 430
incubation period 426
inflammation 429
influenza 436
Lyme disease 441
lymph nodes 429
meningitis 437

Key Terms

mononucleosis 438
nongonococcal urethritis (NGU) 454
pathogen 424
pelvic inflammatory disease (PID) 453
pneumonia 438
protozoa 425
pyelonephritis 445
sexually transmitted infections (STIs) 445
syphilis 454
systemic disease 429
toxic shock syndrome (TSS) 441
trichomoniasis 444
tuberculosis (TB) 440
urethritis 445
vector 424
virus 424

References

1. Elliott, Victoria. "Infectious Disease Outbreaks Signal Need to Think Globally." amednews.com, April 7, 2003. www.ama-assn.org/amnews.

2. Centers for Disease Control and Prevention, www.cdc.gov.

3. Ibid.
4. Howland, Jonathan, et al. "Prevalence of Allergy Symptoms and Associated

References

Medication Use in a Sample of College Seniors." *Journal of American College Health,* Vol. 51, No. 2, September 2002, p. 67.

5. Autoimmune Diseases Coordinating Committee. *Autoimmune Diseases Research Plan.* Washington, DC: Department of Health and Human Services, 2003.

6. Baron-Faust, Rita, and Jill P. Buyon. *The Autoimmune Connection.* New York: McGraw-Hill, 2003.

7. Adetunji, Yemisi, et al. "American College of Preventive Medicine Practice Policy Statement." *American Journal of Preventive Medicine,* Vol. 25, No. 2, August 2003, p. 69.

8. Ibid.

9. "One More Visit Could Close Demographic Gaps in Infant Immunization Efforts." Media Release, National Center for HIV, STD, and TB Prevention, Office of Communication, April 20, 2001.

10. Heikkinen, Terho, and Asko Jarvin. "The Common Cold." *Lancet,* Vol. 361, No. 9351, January 4, 2003, p. 51.

11. "Information From Your Family Doctor. Flu and Colds." *American Family Physician,* Vol. 67, No. 4, February 15, 2003, p. 793.

12. Cohen, S., et al. "Emotional Style and Susceptibility to the Common Cold." *Psychosomatic Medicine,* Vol. 65, No. 4, July–August, 2003, p. 652.

13. Wooten, James. "Teach Patients to Read Their Cold Remedy Labels." *RN,* Vol. 66, No. 1, January 2003, p. 94.

14. Sadovsky, Richard. "Unrefined Echinacea Does Not Ease Common Cold Symptoms." *American Family Physician,* Vol. 67, No. 7, April 1, 2003, p. 1589.

15. Barrett, B. P., et al. "Treatment of the Common Cold with Unrefined Echinacea. A Randomized, Double-Blind, Placebo-Controlled Trial." *American Family Physician,* Vol. 67, No. 7, April 1, 2003, p. 1589.

16. "Misconceptions About Cause of Colds and Health Service Use." *American Family Physician,* Vol. 67, No. 11, June 1, 2003, p. 2384.

17. Zoorob, Roger, et al. "Use and Perceptions of Antibiotics for Upper Respiratory Infections Among College Students." *Journal of Family Practice,* Vol. 50, No. 1, January 2001, p. 32.

18. Torpy, Janet. "Coughs, Colds, and Antibiotics." *Journal of the American Medical Association,* Vol. 289, No. 20, May 28, 2003, p. 2750.

19. Hopkins, A. B. "Chicken Soup Cure May Not Be a Myth." *Nurse Practitioner,* Vol. 28, No. 6, June 2003, p. 16.

20. Kamath, Arati, et al. "Antigens in Tea-Beverage Prime Human V2V2 T Cells *In Vitro* and *In Vivo* for Memory and Nonmemory Antibacterial Cytokine Responses." *Proceedings of the National Academy of the Sciences,* Vol. 100, No. 10, May 13, 2003, p. 6009.

21. Kilbourne, Edwin. Personal Interview.

22. "Prevention and Control of Influenza, Recommendations of the Advisory Committee on Immunization Practices (ACIP)." *Morbidity and Mortality Weekly Report,* Vol. 51, No. RR-3, April 12, 2002, p. 1.

23. Nichol, Kristin, et al. "Influenza Vaccination and Reduction in Hospitalizations for Cardiac Disease and Stroke among the Elderly." *New England Journal of Medicine,* Vol. 348, No. 14, April 3, 2003, p. 1322.

24. Montalto, Norman. "An Office-Based Approach to Influenza: Clinical Diagnosis and Laboratory Testing." *American Family Physician,* Vol. 67, No. 1, January 1, 2003, p. 111.

25. "Meningitis on Campus." National Meningitis Association. www.nmaus.org.

26. Bruce, Michael, et al. "Risk Factors for Meningococcal Disease in College Students." *Journal of the American Medical Association,* Vol. 286, No. 6, August 8, 2001, p. 286.

27. "Parents Urged to Learn About Campus Meningitis Risk." *TB & Outbreaks Week,* September 17, 2002, p. 15.

28. Manchester, Ralph. "Reaction to the September Viewpoint on Meningococcal Vaccine." *Journal of American College Health,* Vol. 51, No. 4, January 2003, p. 171.

29. Grace, Ted. "Response to the Critique of the September Meningococcal Vaccine Viewpoint." *Journal of American College Health,* Vol. 51, No. 4, January, 2003, p. 171.

30. Nice, Ruth. "Meningitis, Life and Death, and Why We Do What We Do." *Journal of American College Health,* Vol. 50, No. 6, May 2002, p. 313.

31. Paneth, Nigel, et al. "Predictors of Vaccination Rates During a Mass Meningococcal Vaccination Program on a College Campus." *Journal of American College Health,* Vol. 49, No. 1, July 2000.

32. Kelleher, J. A., and M. A. Raebel. "Meningococcal Vaccine Use in College Students." *Annals of Pharmacotherapy,* Vol. 36, No. 11, November 2002, p. 1776.

33. Flamm, Steven. "Chronic Hepatitis C Virus Infection." *Journal of the American Medical Association,* Vol. 289, No. 18, May 14, 2003, p. 2413.

34. "Hepatitis C Fact Sheet." CDC, www.cdc.gov/hepatitis.

35. Haley, Robert, and Paul Fischer. "Are Studies of Acute Hepatitis Adequate to Identify Routes of Transmission of Subclinical Hepatitis C Infection?" *Archives of Internal Medicine,* Vol. 163, 2003, p. 1095.

36. Flamm, "Chronic Hepatitis C Virus Infection."

37. Torpy, Janet, et al. "Hepatitis C." *Journal of the American Medical Association,* Vol. 289, No. 18, May 14, 2003, p. 2450.

38. Corbett, Elisabeth, et al. "The Growing Burden of Tuberculosis: Global Trends and Interactions With the HIV Epidemic." *Archives of Internal Medicine,* Vol. 163, 2003, pp. 1009–1021.

39. Centers for Disease Control and Prevention, www.cdc.gov.

40. Torpy, Janet, et al. "West Nile Virus." *Journal of the American Medical Association,* Vol. 290, 2003, p. 558.

41. Mitka, Mike. "As West Nile Virus Season Heats Up, Blood Safety Testing Lags Behind." *Journal of the American Medical Association,* Vol. 289, No., 18, May 14, 2003, p. 2341.

42. Bren, Linda. "West Nile Virus: Reducing the Risk." *WORLD,* March 2003, p. 6(2).

43. Petersen, Lyle, et al. "West Nile Virus." *Journal of the American Medical Association,* Vol. 290, 2003, p. 524.

44. Sejvar, James, et al. "Neurologic Manifestations and Outcome of West Nile Virus Infection." *Journal of the American Medical Association,* Vol. 290, No. 4, July 23, 2003, pp. 511–515.

45. "FDA Clears First Test for West Nile Virus." *American Family Physician,* Vol. 67, No. 4, February 15, 2003.

References

46. Centers for Disease Control and Prevention. "Update: Multistate Outbreak of Monkeypox—Illinois, Indiana, Kansas, Missouri, Ohio, and Wisconsin, 2003." *Journal of the American Medical Association,* Vol. 290, No. 1, July 2, 2003, p. 30.

47. "What You Should Know about Monkeypox." *CDC Fact Sheet,* Centers for Disease Control and Prevention, June 12, 2003.

48. Stephenson, Joan. "Sayonara to SARS—for Now." *Journal of the American Medical Association,* Vol. 290, No. 6, August 13, 2003, p. 740.

49. Rados, Carol. "SARS: Protecting against a Deadly Disease." *FDA Consumer,* July–August 2003, www.fda.gov/fdac/features.

50. Gerberding, Julie. "Faster . . . but Fast Enough? Responding to the Epidemic of Severe Acute Respiratory Syndrome." *New England Journal of Medicine,* Vol. 348, No. 20, May 15, 2003, p. 2030.

51. Centers for Disease Control and Prevention SARS Investigative Team. "Outbreak of Severe Acute Respiratory Syndrome—Worldwide, 2003." *Journal of the American Medical Association,* Vol. 289, No. 14, April 9, 2003, p. 1775.

52. O'Brien, Karl, et al. "Recognition and Management of Bioterrorism Infections." *American Family Physician,* Vol. 67, No. 9, May 1, 2003, p. 1927.

53. Henderson, Donald, et al. *Bioterrorism: Guidelines for Medical and Public Health Management.* Chicago: AMA Press, 2003.

54. Meadows, Michelle. "An Update on Smallpox." *FDA Consumer Magazine,* March–April 2003, www.fda.gov/fdac/features.

55. Hammarlund, E., et al. "Duration of Antiviral Immunity after Smallpox Vaccination." *Nature Medicine,* published online: August 17, 2003, doi:10.1038/nm917.

56. Frey, Sharon, et al. "Response to Smallpox Vaccine in Persons Immunized in the Distant Past." *Journal of the American Medical Association,* Vol. 289, No. 24, June 25, 2003, p. 327.

57. Grabenstein, John, and William Winkenwerder. "US Military Smallpox Vaccination Program Experience." *Journal of the American Medical Association,* Vol. 289, No. 24, June 25, 2003, p. 3278.

58. "Update: Cardiac-Related Events during the Smallpox Vaccination Program—United States, 2003." *Journal of the American Medical Association,* Vol. 290, No. 1, July 2, 2003, p. 31.

59. Committee on Smallpox Vaccination Program Implementation. *Review of the Centers for Disease Control and Prevention's Smallpox Vaccination Program Implementation, Letter Report #4.* Washington, DC: Institute of Medicine, August 12, 2003.

60. Panchaud, Christine, et al. "Sexually Transmitted Diseases Among Adolescents in Developed Countries." *Family Planning Perspectives,* Vol. 32, No. 1, January 2000.

61. "The Truth About STDs." *SIECUS Fact Sheet,* March 2003.

62. Beyer, Chris. "Hidden Epidemic of Sexually Transmitted Diseases in China." *Journal of the American Medical Association,* Vol. 289, No. 11, March 12, 2003, p. 1303.

63. "Check STD Screening: Room for Improvement?" *Contraceptive Technology Update,* January 2003, p. 5.

64. Dowd, Timothy. "College Students Perceptions of the HIV Epidemic." Presentation, American Psychological Society, New Orleans, July 2002.

65. Bon, Rebecca, et al. "Normative Perceptions in Relation to Substance Use and HIV-Risky Sexual Behaviors of College Students." *Journal of Psychology,* Vol. 135, No. 2, March 2001, p. 165.

66. Ibid.

67. Buunk, Bram, et al. "The Double-Edge Sword of Providing Information About Safer Sex." *Journal of Applied Social Psychology,* Vol. 32, No. 4, April 2002, p. 684.

68. Bradner, Carolyn, et al. "Older, But Not Wiser: How Men Get Information about AIDS and Sexually Transmitted Diseases After High School." *Family Planning Perspectives,* Vol. 32, No. 1, January 2000.

69. "Counseling Can Help Correct Misconceptions About Sexually Transmitted Diseases." *Medical Letter on the CDC & FDA,* October 8, 2000.

70. Stammers, Trevor. "Abstinence Under Fire." *Postgraduate Medical Journal,* Vol. 79, August 2003, p. 365.

71. "Nonoxynol-9 Found Ineffective Against STDs." *Contemporary OB/GYN,* Vol. 47, No. 7, July, 2002, p. 33.

72. Wyatt, Gail. "Factors Affecting HIV Contraceptive Decision-Making Among Women." *Sex Roles: A Journal of Research,* April 2000.

73. Lewis, Lisa, et al. "Factors Influencing Condom Use and STD Acquisition Among African-American College Women." *Journal of American College Health,* Vol. 49, No. 1, July 2000.

74. "Check STD Screening."

75. "Chlamydia Screening for Young Women." *American Journal of Preventive Medicine,* Vol. 20, April 2001, p. 90.

76. Roddy, Ronald, et al. "Effect of Nonoxynol-9 Gel on Urogenital Gonorrhea and Chlamydial Infection." *Journal of the American Medical Association,* Vol. 287, No. 9, March 6, 2002, p. 1117.

77. Centers for Disease Control and Prevention. "New CDC Treatment Guidelines Critical to Preventing Health Consequences of Sexually Transmitted Diseases." May 9, 2002.

78. Ross, Jonathan. "Pelvic Inflammatory Disease." *British Medical Journal,* Vol. 322, No. 7287, March 17, 2001, p. 658.

79. Brown, Zane, et al. "Effect of Serologic Status and Cesarean Delivery on Transmission Rates of Herpes Simplex Virus from Mother to Infant." *Journal of the American Medical Association,* Vol. 289, No. 2, January 8, 2003, p. 203.

80. Armstrong, Gregory, et al. "Herpes." *American Journal of Epidemiology,* Vol. 153, May 2001, p. 912.

81. Cohen, Frances. "Persistent Stress As a Predictor of Genital Herpes Recurrence." *Archives of Internal Medicine,* Vol. 282, No. 11, March 15, 2000.

82. Rosenberg, J. "Age at First Sex and Human Papillomavirus Infection Linked Through Behavioral Factors and Partner's Traits." *Perspectives on Sexual and Reproductive Health,* Vol. 34, No. 3, May–June 2002, p. 171.

83. Waller, J., et al. "Awareness of Human Papillomavirus among Women Attending a Well Woman Clinic." *Sexually Transmitted Infections,* Vol. 79, 2003, p. 320.

References

84. Stephenson, Joan. "At International HIV/AIDS Conference, Daunting Challenges Mixed with Hope." *Journal of the American Medical Association,* Vol. 288, No. 6, August 14, 2002.

85. Northridge, Mary. "HIV Returns." *American Journal of Public Health,* Vol. 93, 2003, p. 860.

86. Gross, Michael. "When Plagues Don't End." *American Journal of Public Health,* Vol. 93, No. 6, June 1, 2003, p. 861.

87. Beck, A., et al. "Psychosocial Predictors of HIV/STI Risk Behaviours in a Sample of Homosexual Men." *Sexually Transmitted Infections,* Vol. 79, No. 2, April 2003, p. 142(5). www.cdc.gov.

88. Klevens, R. Monina, et al. "Many Heterosexuals Unaware of their HIV Risk." *American Journal of Preventive Medicine,* April 2001.

References

89. "Women and HIV/AIDS Fact Sheet." Menlo Park, CA: Henry J. Kaiser Family Foundation, May 2001.

90. *Joint United Nations Programme on HIV/AIDS (UNAIDS) and World Health Organization (WHO), AIDS Epidemic Update:* Geneva: UNAIDS and WHO, 2002.

91. *Morbidity and Mortality Weekly Report,* Vol. 52, 2003, pp. 540–544.

92. Malebranche, David. "Black Men Who Have Sex with Men and the HIV Epidemic: Next Steps for Public Health." *American Journal of Public Health,* Vol. 93, 2003, pp. 862–865.

References

93. "HIV Testing in the United States." *HIV/AIDS Policy Fact Sheet,* Kaiser Family Foundation, June 2003.

94. "Number of U.S. AIDS Cases Remains Stable After Recent Declines." Office of Communications, National Center for HIV, STD, and TB Prevention, Centers for Disease Control and Prevention, July 7, 2002.

95. Elliott, Victoria. "AIDS Vaccine Trial Called Disappointing, But Not Futile." amednews.com, March 17, 2003. www.ama-assn.org/amnews.

Keeping Your Heart Healthy

Jamal never forgot the terror he felt when his Dad had his first heart attack. Only ten, he couldn't understand why this towering giant of a man had fallen to the ground, his face twisted in pain, his fist pressed against his chest. His father seemed different when he came home from the hospital, as if something had gone out of him. But his face would still light up with an impish grin, especially when he'd sneak a cigarette and wink at Jamal so he wouldn't tell his mother. The second heart attack came four years later. This time Jamal's Dad didn't come home.

Jamal promised his mother that he'd take better care of his heart. He wouldn't smoke; he'd watch his blood pressure and weight; he'd keep tabs on his diet; he'd exercise regularly. Jamal didn't forget these promises as time passed. But like many college students, he felt invincible. He was shocked when a sports physical revealed that his blood pressure was high and his levels of the most dangerous type of cholesterol were elevated. But he

also felt lucky: "I got my wake-up call," he explains. "And I'm not going to ignore it."

As Jamal realizes, it's never too soon, or too late, to start being heart smart. Cardiovascular disease remains the nation's top killer, but death rates have dropped by 60 percent since 1950, one of the major U.S. health achievements of the twentieth century. The medical advances described in this chapter have contributed to this decline, but much of the credit goes to lifestyle changes, such as quitting smoking and making dietary changes that lower blood pressure and cholesterol levels.

Yet we still have a long way to go to keep the hearts of all Americans healthy. One of every two men and one of every three women in the United States will develop some form of cardiovascular illness. Each year an estimated one million Americans suffer a heart attack; nearly half of them die.

Heart-related disorders account for almost as many deaths as the *combined* total for cancer, accidents, influenza, pneumonia, AIDS, and all other causes. Cardiovascular disease is increasing rapidly around the globe. By 2020 disorders of the heart and blood vessels will overtake infectious illnesses as the world's leading cause of death and disability.[1]

This chapter provides the information you need about risk factors, silent dangers such as high blood pressure and cholesterol, and medical advances that can improve your chances to have a healthier heart and a longer life.

© Peter Beavis/Taxi/Getty Images

After studying the material in this chapter, you should be able to:

- **Explain** how the heart functions.
- **Identify** the risk factors for cardiovascular disease that you can control and those that you cannot control.
- **Define** hypertension, and **discuss** why it is dangerous and ways to prevent it.

- **Describe** the types of cholesterol that compose your lipoprotein profile and the effects of each on heart health.
- **Explain** how coronary artery disease occurs, and **list** effective treatments for it.
- **Explain** what happens during a myocardial infarction (MI) (heart attack) and what can be done to prevent and treat such attacks.
- **Define** stroke and transient ischemic attacks (TIAs), and **explain** their cause, prevention, and treatment.

How the Heart Works

The heart is a hollow, muscular organ with four chambers that serve as two pumps (see Figure 14-1). It is about the size of a clenched fist. Each pump consists of a pair of chambers formed of muscles. The upper two—each called an **atrium**—receive blood, which then flows through valves into the lower two chambers, the **ventricles,** which contract to pump blood out into the arteries through a second set of valves. A thick wall divides the right side of the heart from the left side; even though the two sides are separated, they contract at almost the same time. Contraction of the ventricles is called **systole;** the period of relaxation between contractions is called **diastole.** The heart valves, located at the entrance and exit of the ventricular chambers, have flaps that open and close to allow blood to flow through the chambers of the heart.

The *myocardium* (heart muscle) consists of branching fibers that enable the heart to contract or beat between 60 and 80 times per minute, or about 100,000 times a day. With each beat, the heart pumps about 2 ounces of blood. This may not sound like much, but it adds up to nearly 5 quarts of blood pumped by the heart in one minute, or about 75 gallons per hour.

The heart is surrounded by the *pericardium,* which consists of two layers of a tough membrane. The space between the two contains a lubricating fluid that allows the heart muscle to move freely. The *endocardium* is a smooth membrane lining the inside of the heart and its valves.

Blood circulates through the body by means of the pumping action of the heart, as shown in Figure 14-2. The right ventricle (on your own right side) pumps blood, via the *pulmonary arteries,* to the lungs, where it picks up oxygen (a gas essential to the body's cells) and gives off carbon dioxide (a waste product of metabolism). The blood returns from the lungs via the *pulmonary veins* to the left side of the heart, which pumps it, via the **aorta,** to the arteries in the rest of the body.

The arteries divide into smaller and smaller branches, and finally into **capillaries,** the smallest blood vessels of all (only slightly larger in diameter than a single red blood cell). The blood within the capillaries supplies oxygen and nutrients to the cells of the tissues, and takes up various waste products. Blood returns to the heart via the veins: The blood from the upper body (except the lungs) drains into the heart through the *superior vena cava,* while blood from the lower body returns via the *inferior vena cava.*

The workings of this remarkable pump affect your entire body. If the flow of blood to or through the heart or to the rest of the body is reduced, or if a disturbance occurs in

Superior vena cava

Right pulmonary artery

Right pulmonary veins

Right atrium

Right coronary artery

Right ventricle

Inferior vena cava

Aorta

Left pulmonary artery

Left pulmonary veins

Left atrium

Left coronary artery

Left ventricle

Pericardium

(a)

Right atrium

Right ventricle

Left atrium

Left ventricle

Myocardium

Pericardium

(b)

Figure 14-1 THE HEALTHY HEART

(a) The heart muscle is nourished by blood from the coronary arteries, which arise from the aorta. (b) The cross section shows the four chambers and the myocardium, the muscle that does the heart's work. The pericardium is the outer covering of the heart.

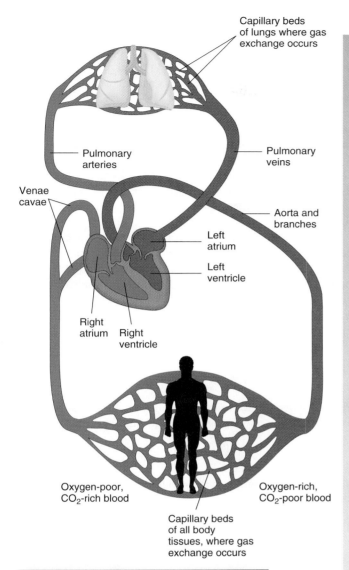

Capillary beds of lungs where gas exchange occurs

Pulmonary arteries

Pulmonary veins

Venae cavae

Aorta and branches

Left atrium

Left ventricle

Right atrium   Right ventricle

Oxygen-poor, CO₂-rich blood

Oxygen-rich, CO₂-poor blood

Capillary beds of all body tissues, where gas exchange occurs

© Charles Gupton/Stock, Boston

Figure 14-2 THE PATH OF BLOOD FLOW

Blood is pumped from the right ventricle into the pulmonary arteries, which lead to the lungs, where gas exchange (oxygen for carbon dioxide) occurs. Oxygenated blood returning from the lungs drains into the left atrium and is then pumped into the left ventricle, which sends the blood into the aorta and its branches. The oxygenated blood flows through the arteries, which extend to all parts of the body. Again, gas exchange occurs in the body tissues; this time oxygen is "dropped off" and carbon dioxide "picked up." The photo depicts a computer-enhanced image of a healthy heart.

the small bundle of highly specialized cells in the heart that generate electrical impulses to control heartbeats, the result may at first be too subtle to notice. However, without diagnosis and treatment, these changes could develop into a life-threatening problem.

Perhaps the biggest breakthrough in the field of cardiology has been not a test or a treatment, but a realization: Heart disease is not inevitable. We can keep our hearts healthy for as long as we live, but the process of doing so must start early and continue throughout life.

Preventing Heart Problems

Heart disease, contrary to a common misperception (See Fact or Fiction? "Heart attacks often strike . . ."), generally does not occur without warning. According to recent research, 80 to 90 percent of those who develop heart disease and 95 percent of those who suffer a fatal heart attack have at least one major risk factor.[2] Recognition of the risk factors for heart disease (discussed in this chapter) has helped prevent many heart-related problems and saved countless lives.[3] Yet many people, including college students and other young adults, are unaware of habits and conditions that put their hearts at risk.[4]

FACT OR FICTION? ???????????????

Heart attacks often strike out of the blue.

Fiction: For years conventional wisdom held that half of heart attack victims had no previous symptoms of heart disease and never saw trouble coming. But new research suggests that most heart attack patients have at least one major risk factor such as high cholesterol, smoking, or hypertension. In a study of individuals between ages 40 and 50 who suffered nonfatal heart attacks, 92 percent of men and 87 percent of women had at least one risk factor. An analysis of 14 earlier studies involving 122,458 adults found that 84.6 percent of women and 80.6 percent of men with heart disease also had one or more unrecognized risk factors.

Sources: John Canto and Ami Iskandrian. "Major Risk Factors for Cardiovascular Disease: Debunking the 'Only 50%' Myth." *Journal of the American Medical Association*, Vol. 290, No. 7, August 20, 2003, p. 947. Philip Greenland et al. "Major Risk Factors as Antecedents of Fatal and Nonfatal Coronary Heart Disease Events." *Journal of the American Medical Association*, Vol. 290, No. 7, August 20, 2003, p. 891.

📢 Why Should I Worry About Heart Disease?

Young people, even those who smoke, are overweight, or have diabetes, often assume heart attacks and stroke happen only to folks who are much older.[5] But heart disease is the third leading cause of death among adults aged 25 to 44. Many behaviors that endanger a heart's health begin in adolescence and early adulthood, including tobacco use, high-fat diets, sedentary lifestyles, and high stress.

Even college students who indicate that they're aware of cardiovascular risks often behave in ways that do not reflect their knowledge. In one study of 226 students at a New Jersey college, half or more ate a high-fat diet or reported moderate to severe stress. (See Table 14-1.) Many did not exercise frequently; some already had high cholesterol or high blood pressure.[6]

College students also underestimate their risk of heart problems. In a study of 341 undergraduates enrolled in physical activity classes at a large university, 68 percent rated their risk of heart disease as lower or much lower than that of their peers, reflecting what researchers called "a clear optimistic bias." (See Student Snapshot: "How Students Rate Their Heart Disease Risk.") The undergraduates who exercised regularly rated their risk as lower than those who did not. Women perceived several risk factors, such as high-fat foods and smoking, to be more potent than men did, but students of both genders did not realize that diabetes, family history, and other risk, factors increase their likelihood of heart disease.[7]

When researchers have studied the hearts of young people—age 15 to 34—who died as a result of accidents, murder, or suicide, those with cardiovascular risk factors were significantly more likely to show signs of atherosclerosis, such as fatty streaks.[8] According to another report, the teenagers with the highest blood pressure and weights had thicker arteries at age 30 and a greater risk of heart disease.[9]

People under 40 who are diagnosed with coronary artery disease have a dramatically increased risk of death.[10] In a study of 843 young adult heart patients (with an average age of 35 for women and 36 for men) who were diagnosed with one or more coronary artery blockages, a third died by age 50. For those with diabetes, the death rate was almost two out of three. Smoking also greatly increased the risk of death.[11]

Young athletes face special risks. Each year seemingly healthy youngsters die suddenly on playing fields and courts. The culprit in one of every three cases of sudden cardiac death in young athletes is a silent condition called hypertrophic cardiomyopathy (HCM), an excessive thickness of the heart muscle. Because of HCM, the heart is more prone to dangerous heart irregularities.

Physical Activity

Physical activity prevents or reduces many of the risk factors for heart disease discussed later in this chapter by:

:: reducing body weight

:: reducing blood pressure

:: reducing harmful low-density-lipoprotein (LDL) and total cholesterol

:: increasing beneficial high-density lipoprotein (HDL) cholesterol

:: increasing insulin sensitivity (and lowering the risk of diabetes).[12]

Sometimes exercise alone can lower an individual's risk of heart problems; in other cases exercise enhances the benefits of other treatments, such as cholesterol-lowering medications.[13]

To maintain cardiovascular fitness, many medical groups, including the American Heart Association, American College of Sports Medicine, and the CDC, recommend 30 minutes or more of moderate-intensity physical activity such as brisk walking on most, if not all, days of the week. Simply meeting this recommendation for activity would reduce heart disease by 30 to 40 percent.[14] As noted in Chapters 4 and 6, the Institute of Medicine has called for 60 minutes of daily physical activity to counter the epidemic of obesity in the United States.

While these recommendations may seem contradictory, experts agree that some exercise is better than none in lowering heart disease risks. The greatest cardiovascular gains occur in people who go from being sedentary to engaging in low-intensity to moderate activities, such as gardening, walking, and housecleaning. Their blood pressure falls; they lose weight; their hearts function more effi-

TABLE 14-1	Heart Disease Risk Factors on Campus

In a study of 226 college students, ages 18 to 26, these were the top five risk factors reported by the students.

Risk Factor	Percentage of Students
Moderate to extreme stress	54
Diet high in saturated fat	52
Diet with high cholesterol or high blood pressure	50
Exercise fewer than two times a week	36
Undesirable total cholesterol levels	29

Source: Leslie Spencer. "Results of a Heart Disease Risk-Factor Screening Among Traditional College Students." *Journal of American College Health,* Vol. 50, No. 6, May 2002, p. 291.

Student Snapshot — How Students Rate Their Heart Disease Risk

These answers, which researchers describe as overly optimistic, were given by 341 undergraduates enrolled in physical activity classes at a large state university.

Source: John Green et al. "Heart Disease Risk Perception in College Men and Women." *Journal of American College Health,* Vol. 51, No. 5, March 2003, p. 207.

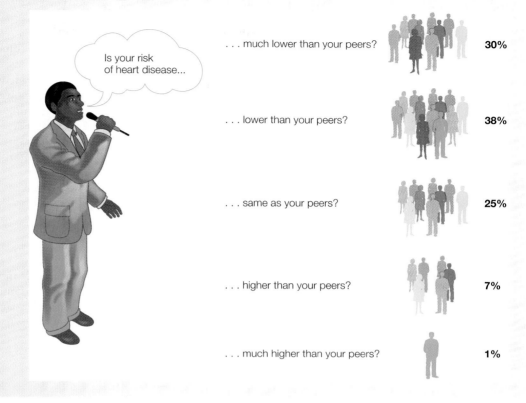

Is your risk of heart disease...

. . . much lower than your peers? **30%**

. . . lower than your peers? **38%**

. . . same as your peers? **25%**

. . . higher than your peers? **7%**

. . . much higher than your peers? **1%**

ciently. According to Japan's National Institute on Health and Nutrition, just 60 to 90 minutes of aerobic exercise a week reduces high blood pressure—an average of 12 mm Hg systolic and 8 mm Hg diastolic (blood pressure readings are explained on page 475).[15]

The greater the exercise "dose," the more benefits it yields. In studies that compared individuals of different fitness levels, the least fit were at much greater risk of dying. (See Fact or Fiction? "Exercise can do . . .") In men, more rigorous exercise, such as jogging, produces greater protection against heart disease and boosts longevity.[16] (See Chapter 4 on exercise.)

Heart-Healthy Nutrition

A balanced, low-fat diet is the best recipe for a healthy heart. Fruits and vegetables, in particular, are associated with a reduced risk of cardiovascular disease, including lower blood pressure.

The American Heart Association also recommends including cholesterol-lowering foods, such as oats, barley, soy protein, and nuts, in your daily diet. Debate continues over the role of other foods, alcohol, and dietary supplements in threatening or protecting our hearts.

FACT OR FICTION? ????????????????

Exercise can do more harm than good.

Fiction: During exercise, there is a small, temporary increase in the odds of a heart-related problem, such as a rhythm disorder (arrhythmia) or heart attack. However, the risk is small: one in 400,000 to 800,000 hours of exercise for people without heart disease and one in 62,000 hours for those with heart disease. Sedentary individuals are at fifty times greater risk of such problems than those who work out five times a week. Contrary to a common misbelief, nine in ten heart attacks occur while people are at rest, not during physical exercise.

Source: Jonathan Myers. "Exercise and Cardiovascular Health." *Circulation,* Vol. 107, January 2003.

One definite dietary heart-helper is fish. Eating fish two times a week, as the AHA recommends, can reduce blood pressure, decrease levels of the blood fats known as triglycerides, and increase HDL ("good") cholesterol levels. The more fish you eat, the slower your heart beats. This may protect against the fast irregular heart beats that can lead to sudden death.[17] People who regularly eat fish may also tend to do other healthy things, such as exercise, not smoke, or eat more fruits and vegetables.

Federal researchers have concluded that the evidence is insufficient to recommend for or against the use of supplements of vitamins A, C, or E; multivitamins with folic acid; or antioxidant combinations for the prevention of cardiovascular disease. They also advise against the use of beta-carotene supplements.[18]

Risk Factors for Cardiovascular Disease

The best way of identifying individuals in potential danger of heart disease is by looking for risk factors.[19] About 35 percent of adults over age 25 have no elevated risk factors and can be categorized as low risk. Roughly 40 percent with one or more elevated risk factors are at intermediate risk. They should undergo regular testing by a physician. Approximately 25 percent of adults have multiple risk factors, some form of heart disease, or type 2 diabetes. They are considered at high risk and should work with their physicians on specific strategies to protect their hearts.

Risk Factors You Can Control

The choices you make and the habits you follow can have a significant impact on whether or not your heart remains healthy. You can choose to avoid the following potential risks for the sake of your heart's health.

An increasing danger to hearts and health is "the lifestyle syndrome," a term medical experts have coined for a cluster of conditions and diseases that result from consuming too many calories; ingesting too much saturated fat, sodium, and alcohol; not burning up enough calories; and smoking or being exposed to tobacco smoke. The consequences of these behaviors include hypertension, metabolic syndrome, obesity, high cholesterol, cardiovascular disease, cancer, osteoarthritis, depression, sexual dysfunction, and diabetes mellitus.[20]

Physical Inactivity

Most Americans get too little physical activity. About one-quarter of U.S. adults are sedentary and another third are not active enough to reach a healthy level of fitness.

Physical inactivity is more common among women than men, among blacks and Hispanics than whites, among older than younger adults, and among the less affluent than the more affluent. The risk for heart disease is 1.5 to 2.4 times higher for people who are inactive compared with those who engage in regular physical activity.[21]

As noted earlier, even some activity is better than none. According to one study, even walking for a minimum of half an hour a day reduces a women's risk of coronary heart disease.[22] However, in men, more rigorous exercise produced greater protection against heart disease.[23] Those who ran for an hour or more per week reduced their risk of heart disease by 42 percent, compared with an 18 percent reduction for those who walked briskly for a half-hour per day or more. With walking, pace, not duration, was linked with lower danger of heart disease.[24]

Tobacco

Smoking may be the single most significant risk factor for cardiovascular disease—and quitting may do more to reduce the risk of mortality among heart disease patients who smoke than any other intervention or treatment.[25] Each year smoking causes more than 250,000 deaths from cardiovascular disease—far more than it causes from cancer and lung disease. Smokers who have heart attacks are more likely to die from them than are nonsmokers. Smoking is the major risk factor for *peripheral vascular disease,* in which the vessels that carry blood to the leg and arm muscles become hardened and clogged.

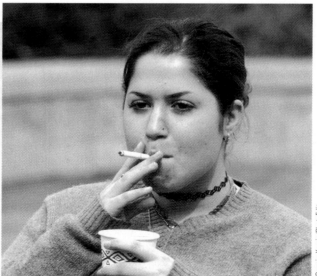

© Bonnie Kamin/PhotoEdit

You can lower your risk of heart disease by not smoking, maintaining a healthy weight, and exercising.

Cigar smoking causes a moderate, but significant increase in an individual's risk for coronary artery disease, as well as for cancers of the upper digestive tract and chronic obstructive pulmonary disease.

Both active and passive smoking accelerate the process by which arteries become clogged and increase the risk of heart attacks and strokes. The American Heart Association estimates that 37,000 to 40,000 nonsmokers die each year from cardiovascular diseases as a result of exposure to environmental tobacco smoke. Overall, nonsmokers exposed to environmental tobacco smoke are at a 25 percent higher relative risk of developing coronary heart disease than nonsmokers not exposed to environmental tobacco smoke.

Cigarette smoking and secondhand smoke can damage the heart in several ways:

:: The nicotine may repeatedly overstimulate the heart.

:: Carbon monoxide may take the place of some of the oxygen in the blood, which reduces the oxygen supply to the heart muscle.

:: Tars and other smoke residues may damage the lining of the coronary arteries, making it easier for cholesterol to build up and narrow the passageways.

:: Smoking increases blood clotting, leading to a higher incidence of clotting in the coronary arteries and subsequent heart attack. Clotting in the peripheral arteries is also increased, which can cause leg pain with walking and, ultimately, stroke.

:: Even ex-smokers may have irreversible damage to their arteries.

In various studies, quitting has reduced the risk of heart disease and subsequent death among patients with heart disease by as much as 50 percent. After 18 years without cigarettes, the risk of dying among ex-smokers is no greater than that of never-smokers.[26]

Obesity

Obesity has emerged as an increasingly common and dangerous risk factor for cardiovascular disease, increasing the risk for hypertension, diabetes, coronary artery disease, and congestive heart failure in both men and women. Body mass index (BMI) and measurement of waist circumference, both discussed in Chapter 4, are good indicators of increased risk.

According to the National Heart, Lung, and Blood Institute (NHLBI), losing weight at any age can help reduce the risk of heart problems. For women, obesity is as great a cause of death and disability from heart disease as smoking and heavy drinking. Even mild to moderately obese women are more likely to suffer chest pain or a heart attack than thinner women. Weight loss significantly reduces high blood pressure, another risk factor for heart disease. (See Chapter 6 for a discussion of weight control.)

High Blood Pressure (Hypertension)

Blood pressure is a result of the contractions of the heart muscle, which pumps blood through your body, and the resistance of the walls of the vessels through which the blood flows. Each time your heart beats, your blood pressure goes up and down within a certain range. It's highest when the heart contracts; this is called *systolic blood pressure.* It's lowest between contractions; this is called *diastolic blood pressure.* A blood pressure reading consists of the systolic measurement "over" the diastolic measurement, recorded in millimeters of mercury (mm Hg) by a sphygmomanometer (see Figure 14–3).

High blood pressure, or **hypertension,** occurs when the artery walls become constricted so that the force exerted as the blood flows through them is greater than it should be. Physicians see blood pressure as a continuum: The higher the reading, the greater the risk of stroke and heart disease. New guidelines have lowered the levels considered dangerous and identified *prehypertension* as a potential threat to the heart's health.[27] (See the discussion of high blood pressure later in this chapter.)

As a result of the increased work in pumping blood, the heart muscle of a person with hypertension can become stronger and also stiffer. This stiffness increases resistance to filling up with blood between beats, which can cause shortness of breath with exertion. Hypertension can also act on the kidney arteries, which can lead to kidney failure in some cases. In addition, hypertension accelerates the development of plaque buildup within the arteries. Especially when combined with obesity, smoking, high cholesterol levels, or diabetes, hypertension increases the risks of cardiovascular problems several times. However, you can control high blood pressure through diet, exercise, and medication (if necessary).

Blood Fats

Cholesterol is a fatty substance found in certain foods and also manufactured by the body. The measurement of cholesterol in the blood is one of the most reliable indicators of the formation of plaque, the sludgelike substance that builds up on the inner walls of arteries. You can lower blood cholesterol levels by cutting back on high-fat foods and exercising more, thereby reducing the risk of a heart attack. According to the NHLBI, for every 1 percent drop in blood cholesterol, studies show a 2 percent decrease in the likelihood of a heart attack.[28]

Lipoproteins are compounds in the blood that are made up of proteins and fat. The different types are classified by their size or density. The heaviest are *high-density lipoproteins,* or HDLs, which have the highest portion of protein. These "good guys," as some cardiologists refer to them, pick up excess cholesterol in the blood and carry it back to the liver for removal from the body. An HDL level of 40 mg/dL or lower substantially increases the risk of

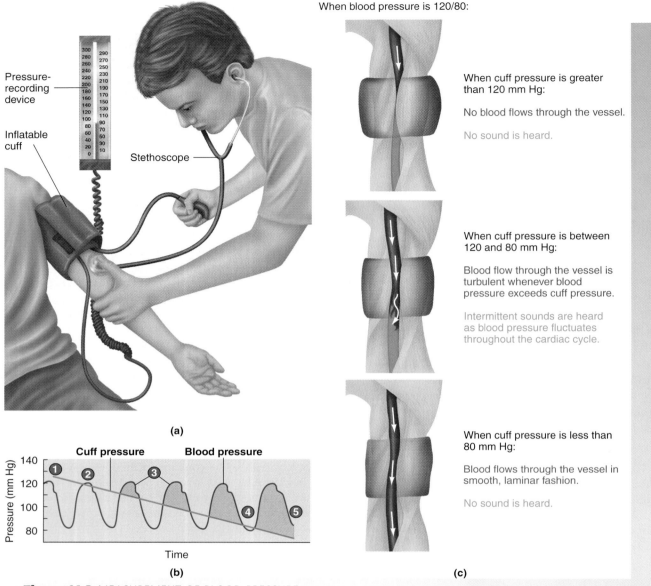

When blood pressure is 120/80:

When cuff pressure is greater than 120 mm Hg:

No blood flows through the vessel.

No sound is heard.

When cuff pressure is between 120 and 80 mm Hg:

Blood flow through the vessel is turbulent whenever blood pressure exceeds cuff pressure.

Intermittent sounds are heard as blood pressure fluctuates throughout the cardiac cycle.

When cuff pressure is less than 80 mm Hg:

Blood flows through the vessel in smooth, laminar fashion.

No sound is heard.

(a)

(b)

(c)

Figure 14-3 MEASUREMENT OF BLOOD PRESSURE
The three steps in measuring blood pressure.

heart disease. (Cholesterol levels are measured in milligrams of cholesterol per deciliter of blood—mg/dL.) The average HDL for men is about 45 mg/dL; for women, it is about 55 mg/dL. *Low-density lipoproteins,* or LDLs, and very low-density lipoproteins (VLDLs) carry more cholesterol than HDLs and deposit it on the walls of arteries—they're the "bad guys." The higher your LDL cholesterol, the greater your risk for heart disease. If you are at high risk of heart disease, any level of LDL higher than 100 mg/dL may increase your danger. (See "Your Lipoprotein Profile" later in this chapter.)

Triglycerides are fats that flow through the blood after meals and have been linked to increased risk of coronary artery disease, especially in women. Triglyceride levels

tend to be highest in those whose diets are high in calories, sugar, alcohol, and refined starches. High levels of these fats may increase the risk of obesity, and cutting back on these foods can reduce high triglyceride levels.

Metabolic Syndrome

Metabolic syndrome, also known as Syndrome X or insulin-resistant syndrome, is a cluster of medical abnormalities that increases the risk of heart disease and diabetes. Genetics, lack of exercise, and overeating are its probable causes. According to the National Institutes of Health, three or more of the following symptoms indicate metabolic syndrome:

:: Waist measurement of 40 inches or more in men and 35 inches or more in women. (In one recent study, waist circumference proved the best indicator of increased heart risk.)[29]

:: Levels of triglycerides of 150 mg/dL or more.

:: Levels of high-density lipoprotein—"good" cholesterol—of less than 40 mg/dL in men or 50 mg/dL in women.

:: Blood pressure of 130 mm Hg systole over 85 mm Hg diastole (130/85), or higher.

:: Fasting blood sugar of 110 mg/dL or higher.[30]

Diabetes Mellitus

Diabetes mellitus, a disorder of the endocrine system, increases the likelihood of hypertension and atherosclerosis, thereby increasing the risk of heart attack and stroke. A physician can detect diabetes and prescribe a diet, exercise program, and, if necessary, medication to keep it in check. Even before developing diabetes, individuals at high risk for this disease—those who are overweight, have a family history of the disease, have mildly elevated blood pressure and blood sugar levels, and above-ideal levels of harmful blood fats—may already be at increased risk of heart disease. Up to one-half of diabetics also have hypertension, another risk factor.

Individuals with diabetes who have never had a heart attack are as likely to experience what physicians call a "cardiac event" as nondiabetics who have had heart attacks.[31] Diabetics who develop heart disease are more likely to die if they suffer a heart attack or develop heart failure. Two-thirds of people with diabetes die from cardiovascular disease.

 Type 2 diabetes, a strong risk factor for coronary heart disease in all women, is especially common in black women. If combined with other risk factors, it puts them at very high risk of cardiovascular disease.[32] Researchers report that a combination of lifestyle changes, including a Mediterranean diet (discussed in Chapter 5), stress-management training, exercise, group support, and smoking cessation, can reduce their risks and improve their quality of life.[33]

Other Risk Factors

Psychosocial Factors. How we respond to everyday sources of stress can affect our hearts as well as our overall health. While we may not be able to control the sources of stress, we can change how we habitually respond to it.

Researchers classify psychological risk factors for heart disease into three categories: chronic, episodic, and acute. Chronic factors, such as Type A behavior, play an important role in the build-up of artery-clogging plaque.

Episodic factors, such as depression, can last from several weeks to two years and may lead to the creation of "unstable" plaque (discussed later in this chapter), which is more likely to break off and block a blood vessel within the heart. Short-term or acute psychological risk factors, such as an angry outburst, can directly trigger a heart attack in people with underlying heart disease.[34]

These factors may act alone or combine and exert different effects at different ages and stages of life. They may influence behaviors such as smoking, diet, alcohol consumption, and physical activity, as well as directly cause changes in physiology.

Although Type A behavior—especially anger—has long been linked with heart disease, a recent review of all prospective studies of its effects found no increased risk for Type A patients with coronary heart disease. However, women who bottle up their anger may be more likely to have a heart attack by age 60 than other women. According to a ten-year study of 200 women, those who conceal their anger or are concerned about their public appearance may have rising heart rates, elevated stress hormones, and high blood pressure—all associated with thickening of the carotid arteries.

Depression and heart disease often occur together. While about one in twenty Americans experiences depression in any given year, the number goes up to one in five of those who experience heart attacks.[35] Patients who suffer heart attacks and develop clinical depression have higher rates of complications and an increased risk of dying.[36]

Job stress also can be hard on the heart, particularly for employees who have little control over their work. A lack of social supports also seems to increase risk, possibly because intimate, caring relationships may buffer the effect of other stressors in life.

Illegal Drug Use. Illegal drugs, which were discussed in depth in Chapter 10, pose many dangers. One of the most serious is their potentially deadly impact on the cardiovascular system. An estimated one in four heart attacks in individuals between the ages of 18 and 45 can be linked to cocaine use.[37]

Cocaine, ecstasy, and amphetamines have similar harmful effects on the heart. They can cause a sudden rise in blood pressure, heart rate, and contractions of the left ventricle (the pumping chamber) of the heart, which can increase the risk of a heart attack. These drugs also tightly squeeze, or constrict, the coronary arteries that feed blood to the heart. If the artery constricts, blood flow to the heart and brain can be obstructed, causing a heart attack or stroke.

The hallucinogens lysergic acid diethylamide (LSD) and psilocybin (psychoactive mushrooms) also have the potential for triggering irregular heartbeats and heart attacks, although less serious cardiac complications, such as a temporary rise in blood pressure, are more common. Morphine and heroin, which account for almost half of drug-related deaths, can lower blood pressure and affect the heart rate. Inhalants can produce fatal heartbeat irregularities.[38] Marijuana, the most widely used illegal drug among young adults, can affect blood pressure and heart rate, but it is not known whether it can trigger a heart attack.[39]

Risk Factors You Can't Control

Heredity

Anyone whose parents, siblings, or other close relatives suffered heart attacks before age 50 is at increased risk of developing heart disease. Certain risk factors, such as abnormally high blood levels of lipids, can be passed down from generation to generation. Although you can't rewrite your family history, individuals with an inherited vulnerability to cardiovascular disease can lower the danger by changing the risk factors within their control. Your heart's health depends to a great extent on your behavior, including the decisions you make about the foods you eat or the decision not to smoke. As an added preventive step, cardiologists may prescribe a small daily dose of aspirin to individuals with a history of coronary artery disease who are at risk of forming clots that could block blood supplies to the heart, brain, and other organs. (Note: Daily aspirin is not advised for individuals who are not at risk because of their age or health history.)

Race and Ethnicity

African Americans are twice as likely to develop high blood pressure as whites. African Americans also suffer strokes at an earlier age and of greater severity. Poverty may be an unrecognized risk factor for members of this minority group, who are less likely to receive medical treatments or undergo corrective surgery. Family history, lifestyle, diet, and stress may also play a role, starting early in life. However, researchers have found no single explanation for why African-American youngsters, like their parents, tend to have higher blood pressure than white children.

Black women are twice as likely as white women to suffer heart attacks and to die from heart disease, according to a four-year study of 2,700 women nationwide.[40] Common risk factors—high blood pressure, diabetes, and high cholesterol—account for this increased jeopardy. In addition, black women are less likely to receive common medications, such as aspirin and cholesterol-lowering drugs to lower their risk.[41]

Age

Almost four out of five people who die of a heart attack are over age 65. Heart disease accounts for more than 40 percent of deaths among people between 65 and 74, and

almost 60 percent at age 85 and above. However, the risk factors that are likely to cause heart disease later in life, including high blood pressure and high levels of "bad" cholesterol, may begin to develop in childhood. Nevertheless, although cardiovascular function declines with age, heart disease is not an inevitable consequence of aging. Many 80- and 90-year-olds have strong, healthy hearts.

Gender

Men have a higher incidence of cardiovascular problems than women before age 45. The onset of heart disease in women lags behind that in men by 10 to 15 years. However, for the U.S. population as a whole, as many women as men eventually die of heart disease. (See The X&Y File: "His Heart, Her Heart.") Although the same risk factors jeopardize the hearts of men and women, each gender also faces some unique heart-related issues, including male pattern baldness and menopause.

Male pattern baldness (the loss of hair at the vertex, or top, of the head) is associated with increased risk of heart attack in men under age 55. A study of 1,437 men showed a "modest" increased risk for those men who'd lost hair at the top of their heads but not for those with receding hairlines. The speed at which men lose their hair also may be an indicator of risk. Scientists speculate that men with male pattern baldness who lose their hair quickly may metabolize male sex hormones differently than others, thereby increasing the likelihood of heart disease.[42] Although it's premature to say that baldness is definitely bad news for the heart, health experts advise bald men to follow basic guidelines, such as not smoking and controlling their cholesterol levels, to lower any possible risk.

Heart disease is the fourth leading cause of death among women aged 30 to 34, third among women aged 35 to 39, second among women aged 40 to 64, and first among women over age 65. A woman's risk increases sharply after menopause (discussed in Chapter 17).

Researchers long believed that postmenopausal hormone replacement therapy (HRT) protected women from heart disease. However, recent studies have shown this not to be true.[43] A major long-term study, the Women's Health Initiative, has shown that women on HRT actually have an increased risk of heart attack and stroke.[44] In the Women's Angiographic Vitamin and Estrogen (WAVE) trial, the women taking HRT and vitamin supplements were most likely to have heart attacks, including fatal ones.[45] As in previous studies, HRT showed no cardiovascular benefits and appears more harmful than helpful, at least in the short term.[46]

the X&Y file   *His Heart, Her Heart*

Many people still think of heart disease as a "guy problem." However, in every year since 1984, heart disease has claimed the lives of more females than males. Cardiovascular diseases are the number-one killer of women as well as men. Yet most women are far more afraid of breast cancer (the cause of 1 in 27 female deaths) than heart disease (which is responsible for almost 1 in 2 female deaths).

The same risk factors—high cholesterol, high blood pressure, and obesity—endanger both sexes, but they play out differently in women than in men. Women with an HDL under 45 mg/dL are at greater risk, while men don't seem to be at risk unless their HDL dips below 40. Chest pain, or angina, is much more likely to predict coronary artery disease in men than women. About 50 to 60 percent of women with chest pain go on to develop heart disease, compared to 80 to 99 percent of men.

High blood pressure is more common in older women, but treating it may not be as beneficial for women as it is for men. In men, reducing blood pressure by any means reduces the mortality risk by 15 percent. The use of blood pressure medications to lower mild to moderate hypertension actually increases women's overall risk of dying.

For women, extra pounds spell extra danger. Even those who are moderately overweight (10 to 20 percent above their ideal weight) may have twice the risk of leaner women—particularly if they put on weight after age eighteen. In both men and women, the risk of heart disease increases if their extra pounds lodge around the waist rather than in the hips and thighs. Mid-torso fat seems more likely to move to the bloodstream, where it can build up and clog arteries.

Standard diagnostic tests are less precise in detecting heart disease in women. The traditional treadmill or exercise stress test, the gold standard for evaluating men, produces a high rate of false positive results in women. A thallium stress test also is less accurate than in men.

If tests indicate a problem, the next step is an "invasive" diagnostic procedure called angiography or cardiac catheterization. Women are much less likely to undergo angiography—a critical prerequisite for angioplasty (balloon surgery to unclog arteries) or coronary bypass surgery.

Women who have heart attacks are less likely than men to survive over both the short and the long term. A woman's risk of dying within a month of a heart attack is up to 75 percent higher than a man's, in part because women typically take an hour longer to get to the hospital than men. Women also have more complications than men during hospitalization and a higher death rate. Men are more likely to receive therapy with aspirin, beta-blockers, or angiotensin-converting enzyme inhibitors and to undergo angioplasty or bypass surgery.

Both men and women benefit from cardiac rehabilitation—an option that cardiologists often didn't even suggest for women in the past. Given the same opportunity to strengthen their hearts, women continue to show improvements for three years after they start an exercise program; men reach a certain performance plateau within months.

Bacterial Infection

Unlike the illnesses discussed in Chapter 13, heart disease was never viewed as an illness caused by an infectious agent. However, recent investigations suggest that certain bacteria may indeed put the heart at risk. *Streptococcus sanguis,* the bacterium found in dental plaque, has been implicated in the buildup of atherosclerotic plaque.[47] Individuals with periodontal disease are at increased risk of heart disease and stroke. Regular brushing, flossing, and dental visits can reduce this danger.

The link between gum disease and heart disease has been disputed by researchers who found that toothless individuals do not have a lower risk of heart disease. The American Heart Association advises, "It is not reasonable at this time to look at people's mouth and aggressively treat their periodontal disease—which usually involves antibiotics and surgery and other risks—for the sole purpose of reducing coronary disease risk. . . . You should treat your teeth for your teeth, not for your heart."[48]

Another common bacterium, *Chlamydia pneumoniae,* long linked to respiratory infections, also may threaten the heart. Individuals with high levels of antibodies to this bacteria are more likely to suffer a heart-related problem. Researchers have reported that antibiotics, taken to treat common infections, may protect against first-time heart attacks. A national clinical trial to determine whether antibiotics can reduce the risk of heart attack and stroke is underway.

◼ High Blood Pressure (Hypertension)

Blood pressure refers to the force of blood against the walls of arteries. When blood pressure remains elevated over time—a condition called hypertension—it forces the heart to pump harder than is healthy. Because the heart must force blood into arteries that are offering increased resistance to blood flow, the left side of the heart becomes enlarged. If untreated, high blood pressure can cause a variety of cardiovascular complications, including heart attack and stroke—two of the three leading causes of death among U.S. adults—as well as kidney failure and blindness. (See Figure 14-4.)

The World Health Organization estimates that hypertension causes one in every eight deaths globally, making it the third leading killer in the world.[49] In the United States, high blood pressure is responsible for 35 percent of cardiovascular problems like heart attack or stroke, 19 percent of all episodes of heart failure, and 24 percent of all premature deaths.[50] Rates of hypertension are 60 percent higher in Europe, regardless of gender and age, than in the United States and Canada.[51]

More than 50 million adults in the United States—about one in every four—have hypertension; an estimated 31 percent are not aware of this problem.[52] Blood pressure often increases with age. Even people who have normal blood pressure at age 55 have a 90 percent chance of developing hypertension as they get older unless they actively take steps to prevent it.

However, the ideal time to start caring about blood pressure is in your teens, twenties, and thirties. In a young person even mild hypertension can cause organs such as the heart, brain, and kidneys to start to deteriorate. By age 50 or 60, the damage may be irreversible.

 Different races suffer different consequences of high blood pressure. An African American with the same elevated blood pressure reading as a Caucasian faces a greater risk of stroke, heart disease, and kidney problems.

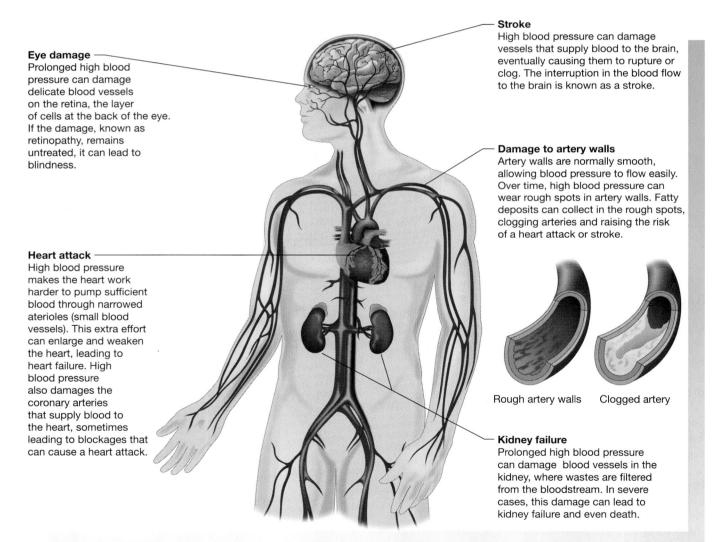

Stroke
High blood pressure can damage vessels that supply blood to the brain, eventually causing them to rupture or clog. The interruption in the blood flow to the brain is known as a stroke.

Eye damage
Prolonged high blood pressure can damage delicate blood vessels on the retina, the layer of cells at the back of the eye. If the damage, known as retinopathy, remains untreated, it can lead to blindness.

Damage to artery walls
Artery walls are normally smooth, allowing blood pressure to flow easily. Over time, high blood pressure can wear rough spots in artery walls. Fatty deposits can collect in the rough spots, clogging arteries and raising the risk of a heart attack or stroke.

Heart attack
High blood pressure makes the heart work harder to pump sufficient blood through narrowed aterioles (small blood vessels). This extra effort can enlarge and weaken the heart, leading to heart failure. High blood pressure also damages the coronary arteries that supply blood to the heart, sometimes leading to blockages that can cause a heart attack.

Rough artery walls   Clogged artery

Kidney failure
Prolonged high blood pressure can damage blood vessels in the kidney, where wastes are filtered from the bloodstream. In severe cases, this damage can lead to kidney failure and even death.

Figure 14-4 CONSEQUENCES OF HIGH BLOOD PRESSURE
If left untreated, elevated blood pressure can damage blood vessels in several areas of the body and lead to serious health problems.

No one knows shy African Americans are more vulnerable, although some speculate that overweight or dietary factors may contribute.

 Family history also plays a role. "If you study healthy college students with normal blood pressures, those who have one parent with hypertension will have blood pressure that's a little higher than average," notes Rose Marie Robertson, M.D., of the American Heart Association. "If two parents have high blood pressure, their levels will be a little higher, and they're destined to go higher still. If your parents have high blood pressure, have yours checked regularly.[53]

Men and women are equally likely to develop hypertension, but in women, blood pressure tends to rise around the time of menopause. Half of all women over age 45 have hypertension. For individuals who smoke, are overweight, don't exercise, or have high cholesterol levels, hypertension multiplies the risk of heart disease and stroke. At ultrahigh risk are people with diabetes or kidney disease.

Preventing Hypertension

Prevention pays off when it comes to high blood pressure. The most effective preventive measures involve lifestyle changes. Losing weight is the best approach for individuals with high normal values. Exercise may be effective in lowering mildly elevated blood pressure. As noted earlier, just 60 to 90 minutes of aerobic activity a week can reduce both systolic and diastolic blood pressure.[54] Among the approaches that have not proven effective are dietary supplements, such as calcium, magnesium, potassium, and fish oil.

The National Heart, Lung, and Blood Institute has developed what is known as the DASH diet. Following DASH, which stands for Dietary Approaches to Stop Hypertension, has proven as effective as drug therapy in lowering blood pressure. An additional benefit: The DASH diet also lowers harmful blood fats, including cholesterol and low-density lipoprotein, and the amino acid homocysteine (one of the new suspects in heart disease risk).[55]

Restriction of sodium intake also helps. Most Americans consume more salt than they need. The current federal recommendation is to limit sodium to less than 2.4 grams (2,400 milligrams) a day. That equals 6 grams (about a teaspoon) of salt a day, including salt used in cooking and at the table. Doctors may advise those with high blood pressure to eat less salt. According to recent research, diets of less than 1,500 milligrams of sodium produce even greater benefits and help blood pressure medicines work better.

The lower the amount of sodium in the diet, the lower the blood pressure for both those with and those without hypertension, and for both genders and all racial and ethnic groups. However, reducing dietary sodium has

STRATEGIES FOR PREVENTION
Reducing Sodium in Your Diet

- Buy fresh, plain frozen, or canned "with no salt added" vegetables.
- Use fresh poultry, fish, and lean meat, rather than canned or processed types.
- Use herbs, spices, and salt-free seasoning blends in cooking.
- Check labels and choose "convenience" foods that are lower in sodium.
- Avoid frozen dinners, pizza, packaged mixes, canned soups or broths, and salad dressings, which often have large amounts of sodium.

an even greater effect on blood pressure in blacks than whites, in women than men, and in individuals with hypertension.[56]

What Is a Healthy Blood Pressure?

The answer to this question has changed. The past standard for normal—120/80 millimeters of mercury (mm Hg)—is no longer considered low enough to prevent serious health consequences. New guidelines, released in 2003 (see Table 14-2), categorize a reading of 120/80 as **prehypertension,** a condition that is likely to worsen in time. A healthy reading is 115/75 mm Hg. Once blood pressure rises about this threshold, the risk of cardiovascular disease may increase.[57]

In healthy adults, blood pressure screening should begin at age 21, with repeat evaluations at least every two years, or more often depending on your current health, medical history and risk factors for cardiovascular disease.

To get an accurate blood pressure reading, you should visit the doctor's office at least twice and have your blood pressure taken two or more times while you're seated. The average of those measurements determines how your blood pressure is classified.

Prehypertension

Prehypertension is a systolic pressure (top number) ranging from 120 to 139 or a diastolic pressure (bottom number) ranging from 80 to 90. An individual can have prehypertension even if just one of the two numbers is elevated, for

TABLE 14-2		What Your Blood Pressure Means		
Top Number (systolic)		**Bottom Number (diastolic)**	**Your Group**	**What To Do**
Below 120	and	Below 80	Normal blood pressure	Maintain a healthy lifestyle
120–139	or	80–89	Prehypertension	Adopt a healthy lifestyle
140–159	or	90–99	Stage 1 hypertension	Adopt a healthy lifestyle; take medication
160 or more	or	100 or more	Stage 2 hypertension	Adopt a healthy lifestyle; take more than one medication

Source: Seventh Report of the Joint National Committee on Prevention, Detection, Evaluation and Treatment of High Blood Pressure, 2003. Numbers are expressed in millimeters of mercury (mm Hg).

instance, a systolic pressure of 115 but a diastolic pressure of 85. If you have prehypertension but are otherwise healthy, lifestyle modifications, such as cutting back on sodium in your diet and exercising more, may be enough to reduce your blood pressure to less than 120/80 mm Hg.

The Stages of Hypertension

The new guidelines classify hypertension into two categories:

:: **Stage 1.** This consists of a systolic pressure ranging from 140 to 159 or a diastolic pressure ranging from 90 to 99.

:: **Stage 2.** The most severe form of hypertension occurs with a systolic pressure of 160 or higher or a diastolic reading of 100 or higher.

Only one of the numbers—the top or bottom—needs to be high to meet these criteria. In people over age 50, systolic pressure is more important than diastolic. If it rises to 140 mm Hg or higher, doctors advise treatment regardless of the diastolic pressure.

Lifestyle changes are a first-line weapon in the fight against high blood pressure. Rather than making a single change, a combination of behavioral changes, including losing weight, eating heart-healthy foods, reducing sodium, and exercising more, yields the best results.

Making healthy lifestyle modifications can help reduce Stage 1 hypertension, but most people also require a medication. Those with Stage 2 hypertension typically need at least two types of high blood pressure medications (antihypertensives) to reduce blood pressure to a safer level. The goal for most people with hypertension is to reduce blood pressure to below 140/90 mm Hg.

Controlling High Blood Pressure

Only about one-third of people with hypertension have it effectively controlled—below 140/90 mm Hg. Yet the higher your blood pressure, the higher your risk of heart attack, heart failure, stroke, and kidney disease. For those between 40 and 70 years old, each increase of 20 mm Hg in systolic pressure and 10 mm Hg in diastolic pressure doubles the risk of cardiovascular complications, starting at 115/75 mm Hg. This means that a blood pressure of 135/85—technically considered only prehypertension—doubles the risk of a heart attack or stroke compared with a blood pressure of 115/75. Certain high-risk medical conditions, such as diabetes, require more aggressive treatment to help prevent these conditions from worsening or to avoid developing other cardiovascular diseases.

Reducing systolic blood pressure 12 mm Hg for 10 years can prevent one death in every 11 people treated for hypertension. In those with existing cardiovascular disease or organ damage, such as kidney disease, that reduction has an even bigger benefit, preventing one death in every nine people treated. Although a wide range of anti-hypertensive medications is available, thiazide diuretics, the least expensive, are among the most effective.[58] Lifestyle changes also are effective in treating and preventing hypertension.[59] These include increasing physical activity, losing weight if overweight, quitting smoking, limiting alcohol consumption, and following a heart-healthy eating plan, such as the DASH diet.

Your Lipoprotein Profile

Medical science has changed the way it views and targets the blood fats that endanger the healthy heart. In the past, the focus was primarily on total cholesterol in the blood. The higher this number was, the greater the risk of heart disease. In 2001, the NHLBI's National Cholesterol Education Program revised federal guidelines and recommended more comprehensive testing, called a *lipoprotein profile,* for all individuals age 20 or older.[60] (See Savvy Consumer: "What You Need to Know About Testing Lipoproteins.")

Savvy Consumer

WHAT YOU NEED TO KNOW ABOUT TESTING LIPOPROTEINS

- Go to your primary health-care provider to get a lipoprotein profile. Although cholesterol tests at shopping malls or health fairs can help identify people at risk, the analyzers are often not certified technicians, and the readings may be inaccurate. In addition, without a health expert to counsel them, some people may be unnecessarily frightened by a high reading—or falsely reassured by a low one.

- Ask about accuracy. Even at first-rate laboratories, cholesterol readings are often inaccurate. Find out if the lab is using the National Institutes of Health standards, and ask about the lab's margin for error (which should be less than 5 percent).

- Fast beforehand. Lipoprotein tests are most accurate after a 9- to 14-hour fast. Schedule the test before breakfast if you can. Women may not want to get tested at the end of their menstrual cycles, when minor elevations in cholesterol levels occur because of lower estrogen levels. Cholesterol levels can also rise 5 to 10 percent during periods of stress. Reschedule the test if you come down with an intestinal flu because the viral infection could interfere with the absorption of food and thus with cholesterol levels. Let your doctor know if you're taking any drugs. Common medications, including birth control pills and hypertension drugs, can affect cholesterol levels.

- Sit down before allowing blood to be drawn or your finger to be pricked; fluids pool differently in the body when you're standing than when you're sitting. Don't let a technician squeeze blood from your finger, which forces fluid from cells, diluting the blood sample and possibly leading to a falsely low reading.

- Get real numbers. Don't settle for "normal" or "high" because laboratories can inaccurately label results. Find out exactly what your reading is. Find out your HDL/LDL ratio, and HDL and LDL levels.

- Get two tests in the same month and average the result. A person's cholesterol levels vary so much from day to day that a single measurement may not be significant.

This blood test, which should be performed after a 9- to 12-hour fast and repeated at least once every five years, provides readings of:

:: Total cholesterol.

:: LDL (bad) cholesterol, the main culprit in the buildup of plaque within the arteries.

:: HDL (good or Healthy) cholesterol, which helps prevent cholesterol buildup.

:: Triglycerides, which are blood fats released into the bloodstream after a meal.

What Is a Healthy Cholesterol Reading?

The answer to this question has become more complex. In general, a total cholesterol reading of less than 200 mg/dL is considered healthy. However, one single cholesterol count no longer applies to everyone. (See Table 14–3.)

The greatest threat to your heart's health is LDL cholesterol. The degree of danger of a higher reading depends, not just on the number itself, but on whether or not you have other risk factors for heart disease. These include age (over 45 in men, over 55 in women), smoking, high blood pressure, high blood sugar, diabetes, abdominal obesity ("belly" fat), and a family history of heart disease. Depending on your individual risk, your doctor may recommend lifestyle changes or medications that lower cholesterol.

An optimal LDL reading of less than 100 mg/dL should be the goal of those at highest risk of heart disease. Those at moderate risk should keep their LDL level under 130 mg/dL; those at low risk should keep their LDL level at or below 160 mg/dL.

HDL, good cholesterol, also is important, particularly in women. Federal guidelines define an HDL reading of less than 40 mg/dL as a major risk factor for developing heart disease. HDL levels of 60 mg/dL or more are protective and lower the risk of heart disease.

© Will & Deni McIntyre/Photo Researchers, Inc.

Getting a cholesterol test is a quick, simple, and relatively painless procedure.

TABLE 14-3	What Do Your Cholesterol Numbers Mean?*
Total Cholesterol Level	**Category**
Less than 200 mg/dL	Desirable
200–238 mg/dL	Borderline high
240 mg/dL and above	High
LDL ("Bad") Cholesterol	**Category**
Less than 100 mg/dL	Optimal
100–129 mg/dL	Near optimal/above optimal
130–159 mg/dL	Borderline high
160–189 mg/dL	High
190 mg/dL and above	Very high

HDL ("Good") Cholesterol

For HDL, higher numbers are better. A level less than 40 mg/dL is considered a major risk factor because it increases your risk for developing heart disease. An HDL level of 60 mg/dL or more helps lower your risk for heart disease.

Triglycerides

Triglycerides can also raise heart disease risk. Levels that are borderline high (150–199 mg/dL) or high (200 mg/dL or more) may need treatment in some people.

*Cholesterol levels are measured in milligrams (mg) of cholesterol per deciliter (dL) of blood.
Source: "High Blood Cholesterol: What You Need to Know." National Cholesterol Education Program, 2001.

A lipoprotein profile also measures triglycerides, the free-floating molecules that transport fats in the bloodstream. Ideally this should be below 150 mg/dL. Individuals with readings of 150 to 199 mg/dL, considered borderline, as well as those with higher readings, may benefit from weight control, physical activity, and, if necessary, medication.

Lowering Cholesterol

According to federal guidelines, about one in five Americans may require treatment to lower their cholesterol level and the risk of dying from heart disease. The National Cholesterol Education Program (NCEP) estimates that some 36 million Americans should be watching their diet and exercising more. Another 65 million should be taking cholesterol-lowering drugs. Depending on your lipoprotein profile and an assessment of other risk factors, your physician may recommend that you take steps to lower your LDL cholesterol. For some people, therapeutic life changes can make a difference. Simply eating more often may have an effect on cholesterol. According to several small studies, "grazers" who eat small meals six or more times a day tend to have lower cholesterol levels than "gorgers" who eat three times a day.

Therapeutic Life Changes (TLC)

Some individuals with elevated cholesterol can improve their lipoprotein profile with lifestyle changes:

:: ***Dietary changes.*** In the past, dietary changes reduced cholesterol by only 4 to 13 percent, relatively modest improvements compared to the effects of medications, which can cut cholesterol by as much as 35 percent. However, a diet consisting of cholesterol-lowering foods, including nuts, soy, oats, and plant sterols (in margarine and green leafy vegetables), reduced LDL cholesterol by about 30 percent. An added benefit: a reduction in C-reactive protein, discussed on page 485.[61] Researchers are recommending this diet as an effective first treatment for individuals with high cholesterol levels, particularly when coupled with exercise and weight loss.[62]

:: ***Weight management.*** For individuals who are overweight, losing weight can help lower LDL. This is especially true for those with high triglyceride levels and/or low HDL levels and those who have a large waist measurement (more than 40 inches for a man and more than 35 inches for a woman).

:: ***Physical activity.*** The recommended amount is 30 minutes on most, if not, all days. Regular activity can help lower LDL, lower blood pressure, reduce triglycerides, and, particularly importantly, raise HDL. Again, these benefits are especially important for those with high triglyceride levels or large waist measurements.

Medications

The last decade has seen a revolution in treatment for high cholesterol, thanks to a new class of drugs called statins—better known by brand names such as Lipitor, Mevacor, Pravachol, and Zocor. These medications, which block cholesterol production in the liver, can cut the risk of dying of a heart attack by as much as 40 percent. Initially tested in men, statins have proven equally beneficial for women, including those whose cholesterol levels rise after menopause. Depending on your lipoprotein profile and other risk factors, your doctor may suggest one of the following or a combination of medications:

:: ***Statins.*** These medications, among the most widely prescribed drugs in the United States, inhibit an enzyme called HMB-CoA reductase, which controls the rate of cholesterol production in the body. They thereby slow down cholesterol production and increase the liver's ability to remove the LDL cholesterol already in the blood. In several large studies, statins produced large reductions in total and LDL cholesterol—and in heart attacks and heart disease deaths. In some patients, statins can reduce LDL cholesterol by 20 to 60 percent. They also reduce elevated triglyceride levels and produce a modest increase in

HDL cholesterol. In individuals with normal cholesterol levels but high levels of C-reactive protein, an indicator of inflammation, statins also have proven effective in lowering the risk of "coronary events," such as heart attacks. Serious side effects, such as liver abnormalities and muscle problems, are rare. More common complaints include stomach upset, gas, constipation, and abdominal pain or cramps.

:: **Bile acid sequestrants.** These drugs bind with bile acids that contain cholesterol and remove them in a person's stool. They generally lower LDL cholesterol by 10 to 20 percent. Often these agents are combined with statins to produce a greater reduction in LDL cholesterol. Side effects include constipation, bloating, nausea, and gas.

:: **Nicotinic acid (niacin).** This B vitamin, taken in high doses and in various release forms, can lower LDL cholesterol, total cholesterol, and triglyceride levels. The niacin preparations used to lower cholesterol should be taken only under a doctor's supervision because of the danger of serious side effects. These include flushing, hot flashes, nausea, indigestion, gas, vomiting, diarrhea, peptic ulcers, gout, liver problems, and high blood pressure.

:: **Fibrates.** These agents—Gemfibrozil is the most widely used—are most effective in lowering triglycerides and, to a lesser extent, increasing HDL cholesterol. Digestive complaints are the most common side effect. Fibrates also may increase the likelihood of gallstones and may increase the effects of blood-thinning medications.

Novel Risk Factors

To identify more individuals in danger, researchers have been investigating other potential cardiovascular villains. Most cardiologists do not test these "novel" risk factors routinely, but for some patients, they can provide an additional warning of potential risk.

C-Reactive Protein (CRP)

C-reactive protein is a marker of inflammation in the blood vessels, which may make atherosclerotic plaque more likely to rupture. A simple and inexpensive blood test called hs-CRP (for high-sensitivity CRP) that measures very low levels of CRP can detect inflammation within blood vessels and indicate increased danger of heart disease.

The CDC and American Heart Association have not endorsed CRP testing as a standard screening tool for the general public but recommend it for those at intermediate risk of developing coronary heart disease in the next 10 years. The test can help a cardiologist decide on further evaluations and the need for more aggressive therapy to prevent cardiovascular disease. The test may be especially useful in evaluating heart disease risk in women.

Testing for CRP usually requires two blood tests two weeks apart. C-reactive protein is measured in milligrams per liter (mg/L) of blood, and the results indicate:

:: **Low risk:** Less than 1 mg/L
:: **Average risk:** 1 to 3 mg/L
:: **High risk:** Over 3 mg/L

To lower CRP and potential heart risks, physicians recommend a low-fat diet, exercise, losing weight, and stopping smoking, sometimes along with aspirin and cholesterol-lowering statins. There is no evidence that lowering CRP itself reduces heart attack risk. However, statin therapy does seem to lower the danger of dying as a result of heart disease.

Lipoprotein (a)

About 10 percent of the population have elevated levels of the fat-carrying particle called lipoprotein (a) [Lp(a)]. They are at two to three times greater risk of heart attack, coronary heart disease and stroke. Unlike cholesterol, lipoprotein (a) levels, primarily genetically determined, are not easily lowered with diet or lifestyle changes. There is no specific therapy for a high Lp (a), but lowering LDL levels is crucial because high LDL multiplies the danger. Niacin also can help bring down Lp (a) levels.

Lipoprotein Particle Size and Density

For some individuals, the size and density of their lipoprotein particles may be as important as their number. About 30 percent of Americans tend to have higher-than-normal concentrations of small LDL particles, which may multiple the risk of heart attack in some people. A tendency to small particle size is inherited, but diet and weight loss can make a difference. Niacin, or nicotinic acid, also can help increase particle size. However, there is no evidence that doing so lowers the risk of heart disease.

Homocysteine

Elevated levels of the amino acid **homocysteine** have been associated with greater risk of heart disease, including congestive heart failure and stroke.[63] A diet rich in fruits, vegetables, whole grains, poultry, fish, and low-fat dairy products can significantly reduce homocysteine. A folate supplement also helps lower homocysteine, but it does not reduce the rate of heart attacks or strokes. Currently physicians do not recommend its use.

Fibrinogen

This protein, which circulates in the blood, plays a role in blood clotting. Fibrinogen levels tend to be higher in smokers and in people with diabetes, hypertension, obesity, and sedentary lifestyles.[64]

:◼: Crises of the Heart

Coronary Artery Disease

The general term for any impairment of blood flow through the blood vessels, often referred to as "hardening of the arteries," is **arteriosclerosis.** The most common form is **atherosclerosis,** a disease of the lining of the arteries in which **plaque**—deposits of fat, fibrin (a clotting material), cholesterol, other cell parts, and calcium—narrows the artery channels. (See Figure 14-5.)

Atherosclerosis

Atherosclerosis, or atherosclerotic vascular disease (ASVD), is the most common form of cardiovascular disease. While it may begin in childhood, atherosclerosis worsens with the continued buildup of plaque on the arterial lining. The arteries lose their ability to expand and contract. Blood moves with increasing difficulty through the narrowed channels, making it easier for a clot (thrombus) to form, perhaps blocking the channel and depriving vital organs of blood. When such a blockage is in a coronary artery, the result is coronary thrombosis, one form of heart attack. When the clot occurs in the brain, the result is cerebral thrombosis, one form of stroke (discussed later in this chapter).

Unstable Plaque

Extra cholesterol deposited on an artery wall creates a "bump" covered by a hard scar. This plaque narrows the space in the arteries, and the heart may not receive an adequate supply of oxygen-carrying blood, which may lead to chest pain (angina) or a heart attack.

Cardiologists long believed that the most dangerous plaques were the largest ones, which were most likely to cause total blockage of the coronary arteries. However, small plaques are now thought to be very unstable and more likely to burst or rupture, spewing cholesterol into the bloodstream. This triggers blood clotting, which blocks the artery, stops blood flow, and leads to a heart attack.

Lowering cholesterol can make plaque more stable and less prone to rupture. A possible early warning of unstable plaque is an elevated level of C-reactive protein (see page 485).

Unclogging the Arteries

For years, heart specialists said that, once clogged, arteries couldn't be unclogged. However, research has now shown that it is possible to reverse the buildup of plaque inside the arteries by means of cholesterol-lowering drugs and a low-fat diet. A strict program of dietary and lifestyle change without any medication, developed by Dean Ornish, M.D., of the University of California, San Francisco, also has proven effective in reversing coronary artery disease. The following are the key elements of this approach:

:: A very low-fat, vegetarian diet, including nonfat dairy products and egg whites, keeping fat intake to below 8 percent of total calories consumed. Ornish's recommended diet allows no meat, poultry, fish, butter, cheese, ice cream, or any form of oil.

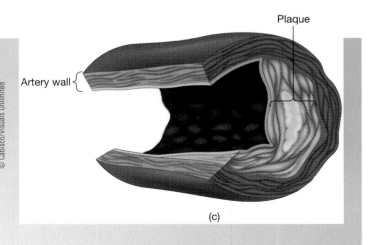

Figure 14-5 PLAQUE IN THE ARTERIES
(a) A healthy coronary artery. (b) An artery partially blocked by the buildup of atherosclerotic plaque. (c) Cross-section of plaque and artery.

:: Moderate exercise, consisting of an hour of aerobic activity three times a week. Walking is recommended because more rigorous exercise might be dangerous for heart patients, who may develop increased risk of blood clots, irregular heartbeats, or coronary artery spasms during exertion.

:: Stress counseling. Ornish's patients learn how the body's stress response can cause a rapid heartbeat and narrowing of the arteries, and how stress reduction can reduce cholesterol levels.

:: An hour a day of yoga, meditation, breathing, and progressive relaxation. Some patients use visualization, for instance, imagining their arteries being cleared by a tunneling machine.

Angina Pectoris

A temporary drop in the supply of oxygen to the heart tissue causes feelings of pain or discomfort in the chest known as **angina pectoris.** Some people suffer angina only when the demands on their hearts increase, such as during exercise or when under stress. Many people have angina for years and yet never suffer a heart attack; in some, the angina even disappears. However, angina should be considered a warning of danger if it becomes more severe or more frequent, occurs with less activity or exertion, begins to waken a person from a sound sleep at night, persists for more than ten to fifteen minutes, or causes unusual perspiration.

Angina is most commonly treated with beta-blockers, calcium channel blockers, or nitrates. The American College of Cardiology, the American Heart Association, and the American College of Physicians have issued guidelines that call for daily aspirin, sublingual (under the tongue) nitroglycerine, and appropriate medications for lowering of cholesterol and control of diabetes.

Coronary Artery Spasms

Sometimes the arteries tighten suddenly or go into a spasm, cutting off or reducing blood flow. Spasms can produce heart attacks, as well as angina, and can be fatal. Several factors may trigger spasms in the heart, including the following:

:: ***Clumping of platelets.*** When *platelets* (a type of blood cell) clump together, they produce a substance called thromboxane A-2, which causes the narrowing of a blood vessel.

:: ***Smoking.*** When some angina victims stop smoking, their chest pain declines or disappears.

:: ***Stress.*** No one knows exactly how stress may lead to spasms, but many heart specialists believe that it's a culprit.

:: ***Increased calcium flow.*** Calcium regularly flows into smooth muscle cells; too much calcium, however, may lead to a spasm. (This calcium flow is not regulated by the amount of calcium in your diet.)

Heart Attack (Myocardial Infarction)

Each year, about 1.1 million Americans suffer a heart attack. About 460,000 are fatal. Half of the deaths occur within an hour of the start of symptoms and before the person reaches the hospital.[65] The medical name for a heart attack, or coronary, is **myocardial infarction (MI).** The *myocardium* is the cardiac muscle layer of the wall of the heart. It receives its blood supply, and thus its oxygen and other nutrients, from the coronary arteries. If an artery is blocked by a clot or plaque, or by a spasm, the myocardial cells do not get sufficient oxygen, and the portion of the myocardium deprived of its blood supply begins to die. (See Figure 14-6.) Although such an attack may seem sudden, usually it has been building up for years, particularly if the person has ignored risk factors and early warning signs.

How Do I Know It's a Heart Attack?

Individuals should seek immediate medical care if they experience the following symptoms:

:: A tight ache, heavy, squeezing pain, or discomfort in the center of the chest, which may last for 30 minutes or more and is not relieved by rest.

:: Chest pain that radiates to the shoulder, arm, neck, back, or jaw.

:: Anxiety.

:: Sweating or cold, clammy skin.

:: Nausea and vomiting.

:: Shortness of breath.

:: Dizziness, fainting, or loss of consciousness.

If you're with someone who's exhibiting the classic signs of heart attack, and if they last for two minutes or more, act at once. Expect the person to deny the possibility of anything as serious as a heart attack, but insist on taking prompt action.

Time is of the essence when a heart attack occurs. If you develop symptoms or if you're with someone who does, call the emergency system (911 in most places) immediately. The sooner emergency personnel get to a heart attack and administer cardiac life support, the greater the odds of survival. Yet according to the American Heart Association, most patients wait three hours after the initial symptoms begin before seeking help. By that time, half of the affected heart muscle may already be lost.

Figure 14-6 HEART ATTACK

If blood flow within a coronary artery is blocked, the lack of blood supply causes cells in that area of the heart to die. This blockage is most often caused by plaque breaking loose, and a blood clot forms and blocks the artery. A coronary artery spasm can also stop the flow of blood.

Individuals trained in **cardiopulmonary resuscitation (CPR),** a combination of mouth-to-mouth breathing and chest compression, should use this technique only after calling or having someone else call for help. Survival rates increase by 3 to 4 to 6 to 10 percent per minute, depending on when paramedics arrive. CPR offers no advantage when ambulances respond within five minutes but does provide benefits when more than five minutes pass before the paramedics arrive.[66]

Treatments That Save Hearts

State-of-the-art treatments for heart attacks include clot-dissolving drugs, early administration of medications to thin the blood, intravenous nitroglycerin, and, in some cases, a beta-blocker (which blocks many of the effects of adrenaline in the body, particularly its stimulating impact on the heart).

Clot-dissolving drugs called thrombolytic agents are the treatment of choice for acute myocardial infarction in most clinical settings. Administered through a *catheter* (flexible tube) threaded through the arteries to the site of the blockage (the more effective method of delivery) or injected intravenously (the faster, cheaper method of delivery), these agents can save lives and dissolve clots, but don't remove the underlying atherosclerotic plaque.

Two clot-thinning drugs may be better than one for treating heart attacks. One drug, called a thrombolytic, dissolves blood clots. The second drug, a platelet receptor blocker, keeps platelets from clumping and forming the blood clots that can obstruct blood flow and thereby trigger a heart attack or stroke. The platelet blockers, sometimes called "super aspirin," are more potent than aspirin. They are also administered through an intravenous drip or infusion. Patients receiving such therapy may require further procedures, such as bypass surgery or angioplasty, which can reduce their risk of another heart attack or death. In a coronary bypass, an artery from the patient's leg or chest wall is grafted onto a coronary artery to detour blood around the blocked area.

Emergency balloon **angioplasty** has shown greater effectiveness than clot-dissolving medication in restoring blood flow in arteries immediately after an attack.[67] With this approach, arteries are less likely to close down again and patients have shorter hospital stays and fewer hospital readmissions. Angioplasty patients also are less likely to die of the heart attack or to experience repeat attacks. However, most American hospitals do not perform angioplasty, and not all can do it on an emergency basis.

Self Survey

Check Your Cholesterol and Heart Disease IQ

Instructions

Test your knowledge about high blood cholesterol. Mark each statement true or false.

1. High blood cholesterol is one of the risk factors for heart disease that you can do something about. _____
2. To lower your blood cholesterol level, you must stop eating meat altogether. _____
3. Any blood cholesterol level below 240 mg/dL is desirable for adults. _____
4. Fish oil supplements are recommended to lower blood cholesterol. _____
5. To lower your blood cholesterol level, you should eat less saturated fat, total fat, and cholesterol, and lose weight if you are overweight. _____
6. Saturated fats raise your blood cholesterol levels more than anything else in your diet. _____
7. All vegetable oils help lower blood cholesterol levels.
8. Lowering blood cholesterol levels can help people who have already had a heart attack. _____
9. All children need to have their blood cholesterol levels checked. _____
10. Women don't need to worry about high blood cholesterol and heart disease. _____
11. Reading food labels can help you eat the heart healthy way. _____

Answers

1. **True.** High blood cholesterol is one of the risk factors for heart disease that a person can do something about. High blood pressure, cigarette smoking, diabetes, being overweight, and physical inactivity are the others.
2. **False.** Although some red meat is high in saturated fat and cholesterol, which can raise your blood cholesterol, you do not need to stop eating it or any other single food. Red meat is an important source of protein, iron, and other vitamins and minerals. You should, however, cut back on the amount of saturated fat and cholesterol that you eat. One way to do this is by choosing lean cuts of meat with the fat trimmed. Another way is to watch your portion sizes and eat no more than 6 ounces of meat a day. Six ounces is about the size of two decks of playing cards.
3. **False.** A total blood cholesterol level under 200 mg/dL is desirable and usually puts you at a lower risk for heart disease. A blood cholesterol level of 240 mg/dL is high and increases your risk of heart disease. If your cholesterol level is high, your doctor will want to check your level of LDL-cholesterol ("bad" cholesterol). A *high* level of LDL-cholesterol increases your

risk of heart disease, as does a *low* level of HDL-cholesterol ("good" cholesterol). An HDL-cholesterol level below 35 mg/dL is considered a risk factor for heart disease. A total cholesterol level of 200–239 mg/dL is considered borderline-high and usually increases your risk for heart disease. All adults 20 years of age or older should have their blood cholesterol level checked at least once every five years.

4. **False.** Fish oils are a source of omega-3 fatty acids, which are a type of polyunsaturated fat. Fish oil supplements generally do not reduce blood cholesterol levels. Also, the effect of the long-term use of fish oil supplements is not known. However, fish is a good food choice because it is low in saturated fat.
5. **True.** Eating less fat, especially saturated fat, and cholesterol can lower your blood cholesterol level. Generally your blood cholesterol level should begin to drop a few weeks after you start on a cholesterol-lowering diet. How much your level drops depends on the amounts of saturated fat and cholesterol you used to eat, how high your blood cholesterol is, how much weight you lose if you are overweight, and how your body responds to the changes you make. Over time, you may reduce your blood cholesterol level by 10–50 mg/dL or even more.
6. **True.** Saturated fats raise your blood cholesterol level more than anything else. So, the best way to reduce your cholesterol level is to cut back on the amount of saturated fats that you eat. These fats are found in largest amounts in animal products such as butter, cheese, whole milk, ice cream, cream, and fatty meats. They are also found in some vegetable oils—coconut, palm, and palm kernel oils.
7. **False.** Most vegetable oils—canola, corn, olive, safflower, soybean, and sunflower oils—contain mostly monounsaturated and polyunsaturated fats, which help lower blood cholesterol when used in place of saturated fats. However a few vegetable oils—coconut, palm, and palm kernel oils—contain more saturated fat than unsaturated fat. Limit the total amount of any fats or oils, since even those that are unsaturated are rich sources of calories.
8. **True.** People who have had one heart attack are at much higher risk for a second attack. Reducing blood cholesterol levels can greatly slow down (and, in some people, even reverse) the buildup of cholesterol and fat in the wall of the coronary arteries and significantly reduce the chances of a second heart attack. If you have had a heart attack or have coronary heart disease, your LDL level should be around 100 mg/dL which is even lower than the recommended level of less than 130 mg/dL for the general population.

(continued)

9. False. Children from high-risk families, in which a parent has high blood cholesterol (240 mg/dL or above) or in which a parent or grandparent has had heart disease at an early age (at 55 years or younger), should have their cholesterol levels tested. If a child from such a family has a cholesterol level that is high, it should be lowered under medical supervision, primarily with diet, to reduce the risk of developing heart disease as an adult. For most children, who are not from high-risk families, the best way to reduce the risk of adult heart disease is to follow a low saturated fat, low cholesterol eating pattern.

10. False. Blood cholesterol levels in both men and women begin to go up around age 20. Women before menopause have levels that are lower than men of the same age. After menopause, a woman's LDL-

cholesterol level goes up—and so her risk for heart disease increases. For both men and women, heart disease is the number one cause of death.

11. True. Food labels have been changed. Look on the nutrition label for the amount of saturated fat, total fat, cholesterol, and total calories in a serving of the product. Use this information to compare similar products. Also, look for the list of ingredients. Here, the ingredient in the greatest amount is first and the ingredient in the least amount is last. So to choose food low in saturated fat or total fat, go easy on products that list fats or oil first, or that list many fat and oil ingredients.

Source: National Institutes of Health. www.nhlbi.nih.gov/health/public/heart or the online personal heart risk calculator at http://hin.nhlbi.nih.gov/atpiii/calculator.asp?usertype=pub.

Your Health Change Plan

for Lowering Heart Disease Risk

1. **Maintain a healthy weight**
   - Check with your health care provider to see if you need to lose weight.
   - If you do, lose weight slowly using a healthy eating plan and engaging in physical activity.

2. **Be physically active**
   - Engage in physical activity for a minimum of 30 minutes on most days of the week.
   - Combine everyday chores with moderate-level sporting activities, such as walking, to achieve your physical activity goals.

3. **Follow a healthy eating plan**
   - Set up a healthy eating plan with foods low in saturated fat, total fat, and cholesterol, and high in fruits, vegetables, and low fat dairy foods.
   - Write down everything that you eat and drink in a food diary. Note areas that are successful or need improvement.

   - If you are trying to lose weight, choose an eating plan that is lower in calories.

4. **Reduce sodium in your diet**
   - Choose foods that are low in salt and other forms of sodium.
   - Use spices, garlic, and onions to add flavor to your meals without adding more sodium.

5. **Drink alcohol only in moderation**
   - In addition to raising blood pressure, too much alcohol can add unneeded calories to your diet.
   - If you drink alcoholic beverages, have only a moderate amount—one drink a day for women, two drinks a day for men.

6. **Take prescribed drugs as directed**
   - If you need drugs to help lower your blood pressure or cholesterol, you still must follow the lifestyle changes mentioned above.
   - Use notes and other reminders to help you remember to take your drugs.

Source: NHLBI

Arrhythmias (Heart Rate Abnormalities)

The heart has its own electrical system, which produces an evenly timed, regular beat. When relaxed, most adults have a heart rate of between 60 and 80 beats per minute—slower if they're in good physical condition. During strenuous activity or stress, the heart beats faster. Sometimes the heart seems to skip a beat or experience premature (or early) heartbeats. In many cases, these irregularities or **arrhythmias,** are no cause for alarm; but they can be dan-

gerous in an MI victim. Caffeine, long suspected of triggering irregular heartbeats, doesn't seem to be a culprit.

A very fast heart rate (over 100 beats per minute) is known as **tachycardia;** a very slow one (under 60 beats per minute) is **bradycardia.** Resting heart rates of under 60 beats per minute aren't necessarily signs of illness, even though they meet the definition of bradycardia; in fact, they may reflect excellent physical condition. Portable monitors that patients wear around the clock are most likely to catch the heart in an irregular pattern. One, the Holter monitor, provides a continuous 24-hour record of the heart rate. Another is a "loop" recorder or event monitor that "lies in ambush" for an attack.[68]

The pacemaker can be surgically implanted in the chest to deliver electrical impulses that normalize a weak or irregular heartbeat.

Treatment options include medications, an artificial pacemaker about the size of a small beeper (to ensure that the heart keeps beating regularly), and radio frequency ablation, a nonsurgical procedure that has revolutionized arrhythmia therapy. In this treatment, cardiologists thread a catheter with an electrode at its tip into the blood vessels of the heart. Using drugs to trigger an irregular heartbeat, they pinpoint its source and administer pulses of radio frequency energy (similar to microwave heat) that destroy the cells sending errant signals. The risks are low, and more than 90 percent of patients report a complete cure.

As both sexes age, other arrhythmias, often linked with coronary artery disease, increase—and become increasingly perilous. Half of all deaths associated with coronary artery disease are due to arrhythmias.

More than 680 Americans each day die because their hearts suddenly stop beating. Cardiac arrest, which results from the extremely rapid, chaotic quivering of the heart's lower chambers (a condition called ventricular fibrillation), often is reversible—if treated within a few minutes with an electric shock to the heart from a defibrillator, a device that can allow a normal rhythm to resume.

More doctors' offices, airlines, and public meeting places, such as casinos, are purchasing heart defibrillators. This life-saving equipment may seem expensive, at an estimated $3,500, but the cost of defibrillators and training teams of nurses in their use comes to only about a nickel per paying patient.

Mitral-Valve Prolapse

Mitral-valve prolapse (MVP) is a condition in which a valve in the heart is abnormally long and floppy. Normally, after blood rushes from the left atrium to the left ventricle, the valve between the two chambers slaps shut. But in some people, the closed valve bulges or prolapses back into the atrium. This often occurs because the valve doesn't close completely and blood leaks back into the atrium. This leakage, also called regurgitation, is what doctors may hear as a murmur when listening to your heart.

In the past doctors calculated that up to 30 percent of otherwise healthy young people had MVP. However, this problem is substantially less common and less serious than

THE CUTTING EDGE

The Big Chill

When the heart stops beating, the flow of blood to other vital organs, including the brain, stops. Even if revived from cardiac arrest, survivors often suffer permanent brain damage because of the lack of oxygen. However, cooling the body temperature—therapeutic hypothermia—may protect the brain by decreasing demand for oxygen, reducing the release of nerve-killing chemicals, suppressing inflammation, and stabilizing cell membranes.

According to two major studies, cooling the body temperature by a few degrees may protect the heart itself from further damage as well as the brain and other organs. Doctors have known for some time that reducing a person's body temperature *before* the heart stops—such as when open-heart surgery is performed—can help prevent brain damage. The new research shows cooling *after* oxygen has been cut off also is beneficial.

Researchers in Europe used ice bags and a special mattress with a cover that blew air over the body to cool cardiac arrest victims for 24 hours. In an Australian study, paramedics applied ice packs to patients' heads and torsos, with ice applications continuing in the hospital for 12 more hours. With both methods, cooling slowed the chemical reactions that cause inflammation and possible neurological damage. Cooling therapy carries a slightly increased risk of bleeding, infection, and abnormal heart rhythms. However, the American Heart Association and an international research council have endorsed research and application of hypothermia to save brains, hearts, and lives.

Source: J. P. Nolan, et al. "Therapeutic Hypothermia After Cardiac Arrest: An Advisory Statement by the Advanced Life Support Task Force of the International Liaison Committee on Resuscitation." *Circulation: Journal of the American Heart Association*, Vol. 108, No. 1, July 8, 2003, p. 118.

previously believed. According to recent estimates, MVP affects about 2 percent of the population rather than the 5 to 35 percent of the population previously believed. MVP, once thought to be more common in women, affects men and women equally.

In addition to being thought to have a high prevalence rate, MVP was seen as a disease with frequent and serious complications, including stroke and heart failure. New data show that these complications do not occur at higher rates among patients with mitral-valve prolapse compared to those patients without prolapse.

Congestive Heart Failure

When the heart's pumping power is well below normal capacity, fluid begins to collect in the lungs, hands, and feet. The heart is then said to be in failure. As blood fluids accumulate in the lungs, pulmonary congestion occurs, causing shortness of breath. In other parts of the body, fluid seeps through the thin capillary walls and causes swelling (edema), especially in the ankles and legs. **Congestive heart failure** usually results from myocardial infarction but can also be the result of rheumatic fever, birth defects, hypertension, or atherosclerosis. As many as 4.7 million Americans develop congestive heart failure, which causes 250,000 deaths a year. It is treated by reducing the workload on the heart, modifying salt intake, administering drugs that rid the body of excess fluid, and using medications (such as digitalis) to improve the heart's pumping efficiency. Adding the medication spironolactone, a standard diuretic, can reduce heart failure deaths by 30 percent.

Rheumatic Fever

Rheumatic fever, which strikes most often between the ages of 5 and 15, is a disease that causes painful, swollen joints; skin rashes; and heart damage in half its victims. It is always preceded by a streptococcal infection (see Chapter 13 on infectious diseases). A new strain of streptococcal bacteria has caused a resurfacing of rheumatic fever, which had been considered a disease of the past. The first step to prevention is early identification of the streptococcal infection; the second is treatment with antibiotics to avoid permanent scarring of the heart valves.

Congenital Defects

Approximately 8 out of every 1,000 children born in the United States have congenital heart disease. The most common defects are holes in the ventricular septum, the wall dividing the lower chambers of the heart. Holes may also occur in the atrial septum, the wall between the upper chambers. Sometimes the arteries delivering blood to the body and lungs are transposed and thus attached to the wrong ventricles. Such babies have a bluish color because their blood isn't carrying sufficient oxygen.

✖ Heart Savers

A generation ago physicians had no way of detecting problems before the symptoms of heart disease began and could offer little more than bed rest as a therapy after they struck. Tremendous progress has been made in the diagnosis and treatment of heart problems. Today men and women with heart problems can learn of possible dangers much earlier than in the past and undergo treatments that may add years to their lives.

Diagnostic Tests

The **electrocardiogram (ECG, EKG),** a recording of the electrical activity of the heart, is the traditional method of evaluating the heart's health. (See Figure 14-7.) An exercise ECG—or *stress test*—is one method of finding out whether an area of the heart begins to run out of blood during the stress of an athletic workout. The subject walks or jogs on a treadmill while the ECG monitors the heart's

Figure 14-7 ECG READINGS
(a) A recording of normal electrical activity in the heart. (b) Grossly irregular activity seen in an acute heart attack.

response. This test is less accurate in women because of a high rate of false positives.

Thallium scintigraphy uses radioactive isotopes that are injected into the bloodstream. A special imaging device called a *scintillation,* or gamma camera, picks up the rays emitted by the isotopes; a computer translates these signals into images of the heart as it pumps. The test can be performed while the patient is either resting or exercising on a treadmill or bicycle. Adding a thallium scan to an exercise ECG increases the probability of detecting existing heart disease by 70 to 90 percent. A stress echocardiogram uses ultrasound to study the heart.[69]

In **coronary angiography,** the most complete and accurate diagnostic test for heart problems, a thin tube is threaded through the blood vessels of the heart, a radiopaque dye is injected, and X rays are taken to detect any blockage of the arteries. Angiography is extremely precise, but it's also costly and risky: About one of every 1,500 patients dies as a result of the test.

New methods of diagnosing the heart include ultrafast scans that can capture the heart as it beats: electron beam computed tomography (EBCT) and multidetector computed tomography (MDCT). The 10-minute scans are simple and convenient, requiring no special preparations. Patients lie still, holding their breath for 10 to 30 seconds. However, it is not yet clear how beneficial heart scans are for healthy individuals. A "positive" test indicates calcifications in the walls of the coronary arteries, a condition called subclinical coronary artery disease. However, there is controversy about whether such calcification indicates increased risk of angina, myocardial infarction, or sudden cardiac death. A negative test indicates very low risk of a coronary event over the next two to five years.[70]

Treatments

Most people with heart disease can be treated successfully with medications. Other alternatives are bypass surgery, balloon angioplasty, heart transplants, and external and implanted mechanical devices. Patients who respond positively, remain optimistic, and are conscientious in taking prescribed medications significantly reduce their risk of death, a subsequent heart attack, or another coronary event.

Aspirin Therapy

Daily aspirin is recommended as a preventive step for people at high risk of cardiovascular disease because it reduces the stickiness of platelets (cells that cause blood clotting). This lowers the risk of blood clots, which can block a blood vessel and trigger a heart attack or stroke. Several research studies, such as the Hypertension Optimal Treatment study, have demonstrated an association between aspirin use and reductions in heart attacks and strokes. Aspirin lowers the risk of death from any cause, not just

heart disease. Its protective effects are strongest in the elderly and those with heart disease.[71] People who regularly take other painkillers, such as ibuprofen, may not benefit from aspirin.[72]

Only 26 percent of patients who could have benefited from aspirin therapy have ever used it. Aspirin can produce side effects, including gastrointestinal bleeding, allergic reactions, and peptic ulcers. However, the very low doses recommended for heart disease prevention generally do not cause serious problems. They are not advised for people taking anticlotting medication, who have stomach ulcers, or who have kidney or liver disease.

Medications

The main types of drugs used to treat high blood pressure and heart disease include diuretics; beta-blockers; calcium channel blockers; and angiotensin-converting enzyme (ACE) inhibitors, which block the hormone angiotensin that strongly influences blood pressure. Side effects range from lethargy and fatigue to an increased risk of chest pain and heart attack if certain drugs are discontinued abruptly. Calcium channel blockers and ACE inhibitors have become more popular, even though they have not proved more effective than older medications such as diuretics and beta-blockers. Unlike the older drugs, the new ones are less likely to cause side effects such as impotence, insomnia, lethargy, and depression. The newer drugs can be taken in lower doses with negligible side effects.

However, reports have found dangers associated with several widely used heart medications, including a modestly increased risk of heart attack in patients taking some calcium channel blockers, which are used to lower blood pressure, raise cardiac output in heart failure, relieve various forms of angina, and control arrhythmias. They work by countering the flow of calcium ions into the heart muscle cells; calcium is believed to stimulate and contract heart muscle, occasionally causing a sudden spasm that can completely close an artery.

Beta-blockers lower the heart's demand for blood by producing changes in the autonomic (involuntary) nervous system. A variety of beta-blockers are widely used for medical problems, including migraine headaches and glaucoma (a serious eye disease), as well as heart disease. Other cardiac medications include thrombolytic drugs and antiarrythmics. These drugs are not risk-free, and there have been recent reports that some may actually increase the likelihood of a heart attack.

Surgical Procedures and Mechanical Aids

A **coronary bypass** is a procedure in which an artery from the patient's leg or chest wall is grafted onto a coronary artery to detour blood around the blocked area. Each

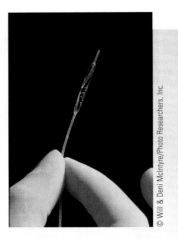

A catheter with a tiny balloon is used in balloon angioplasty to widen a clogged artery.

year hundreds of thousands of coronary bypasses are performed in the United States; about 1 to 5 percent of these patients die as a result of surgical complications. Surgery or angioplasty to improve blood flow in patients with moderate to severe levels of blood flow restriction to the heart reduces the risk of cardiac death more than drugs alone. However, patients with little or no blood flow restriction fared better on medical treatment than on surgery.[73]

For many patients, the results of bypass surgery are positive. But about one out of five patients suffers subtle, long-lasting impairment of mental performance, including problems concentrating and learning, remembering new information, and performing mental tasks as quickly as before the surgery. About 20 percent remain depressed a year after their operations; their mood changes may stem from damage sustained in the surgery.

Coronary bypasses do not extend life for individuals with mild to moderate angina unless the left main coronary artery was the one that was blocked. If drugs fail to control angina, a coronary bypass can eliminate pain. But surgery is not a cure for the atherosclerotic process that caused the blockage; indeed, in as many as 80 percent of bypass patients, the grafts themselves develop blockages within ten years.

Percutaneous transluminal coronary angioplasty (PTCA), also called balloon angioplasty, is the most often performed heart operation. Less costly and less risky than bypass surgery, PTCA opens blood vessels in the heart that are narrowed but not completely blocked. PTCA involves a precise, time-consuming technique called *cardiac catheterization*—the threading of a narrow tube or catheter through an artery to the heart. An X ray taken with a special dye injected into the arteries reveals the location and extent of a blockage. By inflating a tiny balloon at the tip of the catheter, physicians can break up the clog and widen the narrowed artery. When they deflate the balloon, circulation is restored. Balloon angioplasties are not without risks, however; and balloon-opened arteries can clog up again.

For a variety of heart disorders in which the heart muscle has become so damaged that it can no longer effectively pump blood throughout the body, the only hope is a heart transplant. In recent years the survival rates for transplant recipients have improved dramatically. *Left-ventricular-assist devices (LVADs)* enhance the pumping action of the heart. Used as external, temporary measures

until a donor heart becomes available, fully implantable models may someday serve as permanent blood-pumping devices.

✴ Stroke

When the blood supply to a portion of the brain is blocked, a cerebrovascular accident, or **stroke,** occurs. Someone in the United States suffers a stroke every 53 seconds; more than a quarter are under age 65. An estimated 20 percent of stroke victims die within three months; 50 to 60 percent are disabled. About half of those who have a stroke are partially paralyzed on one side of their body; between a quarter and a half are partially or completely dependent on others for daily living; a third become depressed; a fifth cannot walk.

Strokes rank third, after heart disease and cancer, as a cause of death in this country. Worldwide, stroke is second only to heart disease as a cause of death.[74] After decades of steady decline, the number of strokes per year has begun to rise. The main reasons seem to be that more people in the United States are living longer, advanced medical care is allowing more people to survive heart disease, and doctors are better able to diagnose and detect strokes. Yet 80 percent of strokes are preventable, and key risk factors can be modified through either lifestyle changes or drugs. The most important steps are treating hypertension, not smoking, managing diabetes, lowering cholesterol, and taking aspirin.

Strokes continue to occur 40 percent more often in the Southeast (the so-called Stroke Belt) than in other regions of the United States. However, stroke rates have fallen in Mississippi and Alabama while they've increased in Oregon, Washington, and Arkansas. The decline in deaths among stroke victims has been greatest in white men and smallest among black men.[75]

▣ What Causes a Stroke?

There are two types of stroke: *ischemic stroke,* which is the result of a blockage that disrupts blood flow to the brain, and *hemorrhagic stroke,* which occurs when blood vessels rupture. One of the most common causes of ischemic stroke is the blockage of a brain artery by a thrombus, or blood clot—a *cerebral thrombosis.* Clots generally form around deposits sticking out from the arterial wall. Sometimes a wandering blood clot (embolus), carried in the bloodstream, becomes wedged in one of the cerebral arteries. This is called a *cerebral embolism,* and it can completely plug up a cerebral artery.

In hemorrhagic stroke, a diseased artery in the brain floods the surrounding tissue with blood. The cells nourished by the artery are deprived of blood and can't function, and the blood from the artery forms a clot that may interfere with brain function. This is most likely to occur if the patient suffers from a combination of hypertension and atherosclerosis. Hemorrhage (bleeding) may also be caused by a head injury or by the bursting of an aneurysm, a blood-filled pouch that balloons out from a weak spot in the wall of an artery.

Brain tissue, like heart muscle, begins to die if deprived of oxygen, which may then cause difficulty speaking and walking, and loss of memory. These effects may be slight or severe, temporary or permanent, depending on how widespread the damage and whether other areas of the brain can take over the function of the damaged area. About 30 percent of stroke survivors develop dementia, a disorder that robs a person of memory and other intellectual abilities.

The following symptoms should alert you to the possibility that you or someone with you has suffered a stroke:

:: Sudden weakness or loss of strength.

:: Numbness of face, arm, or leg.

:: Loss of speech, or difficulty speaking or understanding speech.

:: Dimness or loss of vision, particularly double vision in one eye.

:: Unexplained dizziness.

:: Change in personality.

:: Change in pattern of headaches.

Transient Ischemic Attacks (TIAs)

Sometimes a person will suffer **transient ischemic attacks (TIAs),** "little strokes" that cause minimal damage but serve as warning signs of a potentially more severe stroke. One of three people who suffer TIAs will have a stroke during the following five years if they don't get treatment. The two major types of TIAs are:

:: *Transient monocular blindness.* Blurring, a blackout or whiteout of vision, a sense of a shade coming down, or another visual disturbance in one eye.

:: *Transient hemispheral attack.* Diminished blood flow to one side of the brain, causing numbness or weakness of one arm, leg, or side of the face, or problems speaking or thinking.

Many TIAs are caused by a narrowing of blood vessels in the neck (carotid arteries) because of a buildup of plaque. Specialists can diagnose this problem by feeling and listening to the arteries, by ultrasound, by measuring the pressure or circulation rate from the carotid arteries to the eyes, or by arterial angiography (injection of a dye into the arteries as X rays are taken), a procedure that can be dangerous, even deadly, or lifesaving.

Surgery to widen the carotid arteries may be recommended for individuals under age 60 with significant narrowing (50 to 80 percent or more). For other patients, aspirin and other drugs that make platelets less sticky and interfere with clotting may be effective.

Risk Factors for Strokes

People who've experienced transient ischemic attacks (TIAs) are at the highest risk for stroke. Other risk factors, like those for heart disease, include some that can't be changed (such as gender and race) and some that can be controlled:

:: *Gender.* Men have a greater risk of stroke than women. However, women are at increased risk at times of marked hormonal changes, particularly pregnancy and childbirth. Past studies have shown an association between oral contraceptive use and stroke, particularly in women over age 35 who smoke. The newer low-dose oral contraceptives have not shown an increased stroke risk among women ages 18 to 44. A woman's stroke risk may increase markedly at menopause.

:: *Race.* The incidence of strokes is two to three times greater in blacks than whites in the same communities.[76] Hispanics also are more likely to develop hemorrhagic strokes than whites.

:: *Age.* A person's risk of stroke more than doubles every decade after age 55.

:: *Hypertension.* Detection and treatment of high blood pressure are the best means of stroke prevention.

:: *High red blood cell count.* A moderate to marked increase in the number of a person's red blood cells increases the risk of stroke.

:: *Heart disease.* Heart problems can interfere with the flow of blood to the brain; clots that form in the heart can travel to the brain, where they may clog an artery.

:: *Blood fats.* Although the standard advice from cardiologists is to lower harmful LDL levels, what may be more important for stroke risk is a drop in the levels of protective HDL.

:: *Diabetes mellitus.* Diabetics have a higher incidence of stroke than nondiabetics.

Treatments for Strokes

A small ("baby") aspirin a day cuts in half the risk of strokes caused by abnormal heartbeats, which strike 75,000 Americans each year. Extremely rapid beating of the heart's upper chambers causes blood clots to form; they may enter the bloodstream and travel to the brain, where they can get stuck and choke off the blood supply. In the past, the only way to prevent such strokes was regular use of a medication called warfarin, which inhibits blood clotting and therefore increases the risk of severe bleeding. However, aspirin proved as effective as warfarin—without that dangerous side effect.[77]

Increasingly, surgeons are operating on carotid arteries that may have been narrowed by a buildup of atherosclerotic plaque—a condition that contributes to 20 to 30 percent of strokes, some in individuals with no symptoms—by cleaning them out in a procedure called *carotid endartectomy*. This procedure has been shown to be effective in preventing stroke in patients with and without early symptoms of stroke. An alternative is brain angioplasty, in which surgeons thread a catheter tipped with a tiny inflatable balloon into an artery and gently inflate it to restore blood flow.

It now seems possible to save brain cells for a brief time after a thrombotic stroke occurs. Thrombolytic drugs such as tissue-type plasminogen activator (tPa), can restore brain blood flow after a thrombotic stroke; other medications called heparinoids can reduce the blood's tendency to clot. For thrombolytic drugs to be effective, they must be administered within three hours after the stroke; heparinoids must be given within 24 hours. However, the average person does not seek help for 22 hours or longer. As a result, only 3.4 percent of stroke patients may receive tPa.[78]

In addition, drugs such as nimodipine and other agents undergoing clinical testing at major medical centers, are being used to protect brain cells from damage. Clinicians also are experimenting with ways to tie off tiny, bleeding, cranial arteries with tiny clothespins or to suction off blood that is exerting pressure on the brain. Using stereotactic radio imagery, which relies on a three-dimensional imaging system, surgeons can focus an X-ray beam on a clot or hemorrhage and destroy it.

The Bottom Line ▼
Heart-Smart Strategies for Life

:: **Don't smoke.** There's no bigger favor you can do your heart—and lungs!

:: **Watch your weight.** Even relatively modest gains can have a big effect on your risk of heart disease.

:: **Cut down on saturated fats and cholesterol.** This can help prevent high blood cholesterol levels, obesity, and heart disease.

:: **Get moving.** Engage in regular physical activity. A little is better than none; more is even better.

:: **Lower your stress levels.** If too much stress is a problem in your life, try the relaxation techniques described in Chapter 3.

:: **Know your family history.** Inheriting a predisposition to high blood pressure or heart disease means that your heart needs extra preventive care.

:: **Get your blood pressure checked regularly.** Knowing your numbers can alert you to a potential problem long before you develop any symptoms.

:: **Tame your temper.** Hostility can be hazardous to the heart. Look for other ways of releasing anger and frustration.

:: **Get a lipoprotein profile.** You can't know if your heart is in danger unless you know your cholesterol and lipoprotein levels. Get a blood test at your next physical, and discuss the results with your physician.

:: **Take appropriate medications.** Those with high cholesterol or high blood pressure should seek their physicians' advice.

 After watching the CNN video segment, discuss the following question. What are the greatest risk factors for heart disease?

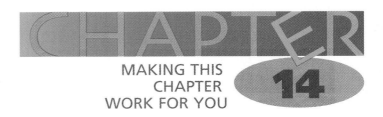

MAKING THIS CHAPTER WORK FOR YOU

14

1. The heart
   a. has four chambers, which are responsible for pumping blood into the veins for circulation through the body.
   b. pumps blood first to the lungs where it picks up oxygen and discards carbon dioxide.
   c. beats about 10,000 times and pumps about 75 gallons of blood per day.
   d. has specialized cells that generate electrical signals to control the amount of blood that circulates through the body.

2. You can help maintain a healthy heart by doing all the following *except*
   a. getting regular moderate levels of exercise every day.
   b. stopping smoking and avoiding regular exposure to secondhand smoke.
   c. eating a diet high in levels of free radicals.
   d. controlling your blood pressure.

3. Which of the following statements about blood pressure is true?
   a. blood pressure increases when the heart relaxes.
   b. systolic blood pressure is the pressure of the blood entering the atrium of the heart.
   c. high blood pressure is usually the cause of sudden cardiac death in young athletes.
   d. blood pressure decreases during diastole.

4. Risk factors for heart disease that cannot be controlled include
   a. male pattern baldness
   b. diabetes mellitus
   c. sedentary lifestyle
   d. blood fat cells

5. Your lipoprotein profile
   a. provides a breakdown of the different types and levels of blood fats circulating in your body.
   b. is best obtained at a health fair where the results are uniformly accurate.
   c. will give a total cholesterol level, which is the amount of triglycerides and LDL cholesterol levels added together.
   d. should be evaluated after eating a full meal.

6. Hypertension
   a. is diagnosed when blood pressure is consistently less than 130/85 mm Hg.
   b. may be treated with dietary changes, which include eating low-fat foods and avoiding sodium.
   c. can cause fatty deposits to collect on the artery walls.
   d. usually does not respond to medication, especially in severe cases.

7. Which of the following statements about coronary artery disease is *false*?
   a. In atherosclerosis, arteries are narrowed by deposits of plaques on the arterial walls.
   b. One successful approach to treatment combines a very low-fat diet, moderate exercise, and stress reduction.
   c. Once plaque appears in the arteries, it is impossible to reverse the effects of coronary artery disease.

   d. A coronary thrombosis may occur if a coronary artery is blocked by a blood clot.

8. A heart attack
   a. occurs when the myocardium receives an excessive amount of blood from the coronary arteries.
   b. is typically suffered by individuals who have irregular episodes of atherosclerosis.
   c. can be treated successfully up to four hours after the event.
   d. occurs when the myocardial cells are deprived of oxygen-carrying blood, causing them to die.

9. Treatments for heart disease include all the following *except*
   a. daily aspirin to reduce the risk of blood clots.
   b. coronary bypass surgery to detour blood around a blocked artery.
   c. electrocardiogram to normalize the electrical activity of the heart.
   d. balloon angioplasty to open narrowed blood vessels.

10. Which of the following statements about stroke is true?
    a. A stroke occurs when the blood supply to the aorta is blocked.
    b. Ischemic stroke is usually caused by a blood clot in the brain.
    c. Little strokes, also called transient ischemic attacks, can cause permanent blindness and paralysis of one side of the body.
    d. Risk factors for stroke include gender and occupation.

Answers to these questions can be found on page 652.

Critical Thinking

1. Have you had your blood pressure checked lately? If your reading was high, what steps are you now taking to help reduce your blood pressure?

2. Have you had a lipoprotein profile lately? Do you think it's necessary for you to obtain one? If your reading was/is borderline or high, what lifestyle changes can you make to help control your cholesterol level?

Critical Thinking

3. The costs for a heart transplant are over $100,000. The annual price tag for a year's worth of cyclosporine, the drug that prevents rejection and must be taken for the rest of a transplant recipient's life, is about $5,000. The total medical bill can come to hundreds of thousands of dollars—enough to fund programs to

Critical Thinking

improve the nutrition of poor pregnant women, to treat alcoholism, or to provide regular preventive care. Does treatment of any single individual justify such huge costs? Should our society try to balance the costs versus the benefits of such heroic measures as heart transplants? How would you go about making such decisions?

Profile Plus

Assess your risks for cardiovascular disease with the activity on your Profile Plus CD-ROM:

Profile Plus

• Cardiovascular Risk

Profile Plus

Sites & Bytes

American Heart Association
www.americanheart.org

This comprehensive site features a searchable database of all major cardiovascular diseases, plus information on healthy lifestyles, current research, CPR, cardiac warning signs, risk awareness, low-cholesterol diets, and family health. The interactive Heart Profiler provides personalized information about treatment options for common cardiovascular conditions such as hypertension, heart failure, and cholesterol.

Sites and Bytes

National Heart, Lung, and Blood Institute—National Cholesterol Education Program
www.nhlbi.nih.gov/chd/

This interactive site describes the new 2001 cholesterol guidelines and has sites that allow you to create a heart healthy diet or take a heart disease quiz, print tipsheets, or find other heart resources.

Sites and Bytes

HeartSite.com
www.heartsite.com

This site, developed by two prominent cardiologists at the Medical College of Georgia, features many color diagrams to illustrate cardiac disease, including diagnostic tests, procedures, and treatment. The site also features a multimedia lecture on heart disease and heart failure with slides and accompanying audio lecture.

InfoTrac College Edition

Activity

"The Latest News on Preventing Heart Disease: Inflammation May Be Worse For Your Heart Than High Cholesterol, According To Recent Reports. Here's What To Do." *Natural Health,* Vol. 33, No. 2, March 2003, p. 19(1).

1. Describe how the blood test C-Reactive Protein potentially can predict heart disease risk.

InfoTrac College Edition

2. How can inflammation cause a heart attack? Name three cardiac risk factors that promote inflammation.

3. According to the authors, name three dietary modifications that are likely to reduce inflammation.

You can find additional readings related to heart disease with InfoTrac College Edition, an online library of

InfoTrac College Edition

more than 900 journals and publications. Follow the instructions that were packaged with your textbook; then search for articles using a key word search.

For additional links, resources, and suggested readings on InfoTrac College Edition, visit our Health & Wellness Resource Center at **http://health.wadsworth.com**.

Key Terms

The terms listed are used on the page indicated. Definitions of the terms are in the Glossary at the end of this book.

Key Terms

angina pectoris 487
angioplasty 488
aorta 470
arrhythmia 490
arteriosclerosis 486
atherosclerosis 486
atrium 470
bradycardia 490
capillary 470
cardiopulmonary
   resuscitation
   (CPR) 488
cholesterol 475
congestive heart
   failure 492

Key Terms

coronary
   angiography 493
coronary bypass 493
diabetes mellitus 477
diastole 470
electrocardiogram
   (ECG, EKG) 492
homocysteine 485
hypertension 475
lipoprotein 475
male pattern
   baldness 478
metabolic syndrome 476
mitral valve prolapse 491
myocardial infarction
   (MI) 487

Key Terms

percutaneous
   transluminal coronary
   angioplasty
   (PTCA) 494
plaque 486
prehypertension 481
stroke 494
systole 470
tachycardia 490
thallium scintigraphy 493
transient ischemic attack
   (TIA) 495
triglyceride 476
ventricle 470

References

1. Hackam, Daniel, and Sonia S. Anand. "Emerging Risk Factors for Atherosclerotic Vascular Disease: A Critical Review of the Evidence." *Journal of the American Medical Association,* Vol. 290, No. 7, August 20, 2003, p. 932.
2. Khot, Umesh, et al. "Prevalence of Conventional Risk Factors in Patients With Coronary Heart Disease." *Journal of the American Medical Association,* Vol. 290, No. 7, August 20, 2003, p. 898.
3. Torpy, Janet, et al. "Risk Factors for Heart Disease." *Journal of the American Medical Association,* Vol. 290, No. 7, August 20, 2003, p. 980.
4. Greenland, Philip. "Improving Risk of Coronary Heart Disease." *Journal of the American Medical Association,* Vol. 289, No. 17, May 7, 2003, p. 2270.
5. "Young People Put Themselves at Risk of Heart Disease with Lack of Fitness." *Heart Disease Weekly,* March 23, 2003, p. 6.
6. Spencer, Leslie. "Results of a Heart Disease Risk-Factor Screening Among Traditional College Students." *Journal of American College Health,* Vol. 50, No. 6, May 2002, p. 291.
7. Green, John, et al. "Heart Disease Risk Perception in College Men and Women." *Journal of American College Health,* Vol. 51, No. 5, March 2003, p. 207.
8. McCarthy, Michael. "Heart Disease Prevention Should Start with the Young, Studies Suggest." *Lancet,* Vol. 357, No. 9260, March 24, 2001, p. 939.

9. Vos, Lydia, et al. "Adolescent Blood Pressure and Blood Pressure Tracking into Young Adulthood Are Related to Subclinical Atherosclerosis: The Atherosclerosis Risk in Young Adults (ARYA) Study." *American Journal of Hypertension,* Vol. 16, No. 7, July 2003, p. 549.
10. "Young Adults with Heart Disease Have Dramatically Increased Risk of Death." *Heart Disease Weekly,* February 2, 2003, p. 11.
11. Cole, J. H., et al. "Long-Term Follow-Up of Coronary Artery Disease Presenting in Young Adults." *Journal of the American College of Cardiology,* Vol. 41, No. 4, February 2003, p. 521.
12. Myers, Jonathan. "Exercise and Cardiovascular Health." *Circulation,* Vol. 107, January 7/14, 2003, p. 2.
13. Thompson, Paul, et al. "Exercise and Physical Activity in the Prevention and Treatment of Atherosclerotic Cardiovascular Disease." *Circulation,* May 2003, Vol. 107, p. 3109.
14. Myers, "Exercise and Cardiovascular Health."
15. Ishikawa-Takata, Kazuko, et al. "How Much Exercise is Required to Reduce Blood Pressure in Essential Hypertension: A Dose-Response Study." *American Journal of Hypertension,* Vol. 23, August 2003, p. 629.

16. Marcovitch, Harvey. "Light Exercise Doesn't Protect Against Heart Disease." *British Medical Journal,* Vol. 327, No. 7407, July 19, 2003, p. 125.
17. Dallongeville, Jean, et al. "Fish Consumption Is Associated With Lower Heart Rates." *Circulation,* Vol. 108, 2003, pp. 820–825.
18. U.S. Preventive Services Task Force. *Routine Vitamin Supplementation to Prevent Cancer and Cardiovascular Disease.* Rockville, MD; Agency for Healthcare Research and Quality, 2003.
19. Greenland, Philip. "Major Risk Factors as Antecedents of Fatal and Nonfatal Coronary Heart Disease Events." *Journal of the American Medical Association,* Vol. 290, No. 7, August 20, 2003, p. 891.
20. Kottke, Thomas, et al. "JNC 7—It's More Than High Blood Pressure." *Journal of the American Medical Association,* Vol. 289, No. 19, May 21, 2003, p. 2573.
21. "Heart Disease and Stroke Statistics—2003." American Heart Association, 2003.
22. Weemering, Mary Lynne. "Physical Activity and Coronary Heart Disease in Women: Is "No Pain, No Gain" Passé?" *The Association of Perioperative Registered Nurses Journal,* Vol. 76, No. 2, August, 2002, p. 331.

References

23. Bauer, Jeff. "Intensity of Exercise Is What Counts When It Comes to Reducing Heart Disease Risk." *RN,* Vol. 66, No. 1, January 2003, p. 97.

24. Tanasescu, Mihaela, et al. "Exercise Type and Intensity in Relation to Coronary Heart Disease in Men." *Journal of the American Medical Association,* Vol. 288, No. 16, October 23, 2002, p. 1994.

25. Canto, John, and Ami Iskandrian. "Major Risk Factors for Cardiovascular Disease: Debunking the 'Only 50%' Myth." *Journal of the American Medical Association,* Vol. 290, No. 7, August 20, 2003, p. 947.

26. Critchley, Julia, and Simon Capewell. "Mortality Risk Reduction Associated with Smoking Cessation in Patients with Coronary Artery Disease." *Journal of the American Medical Association,* Vol. 290, No. 1, July 2, 2003, p. 86.

27. Chobanian, Aram, et al. "The Seventh Report of the Joint National Committee on Prevention, Detection, Evaluation, and Treatment of High Blood Pressure, the JNC 7 Report." *Journal of the American Medical Association,* Vol. 289, No. 19, May 21, 2003, p. 2560.

28. National Cholesterol Education Program Expert Panel on Detection, Evaluation, and Treatment of High Blood Cholesterol in Adults. "Prevalence of Metabolic Syndrome Based on Results of NHANES III." *Nutrition Research Newsletter,* Vol. 21, No. 2, February 2002, p. 7.

29. Siani, Alfonso, et al. "The Relationship of Waist Circumference to Blood Pressure: The Olivetti Heart Study." *American Journal of Hypertension,* Vol. 15, No. 9, September 2002, p. 780.

30. National Cholesterol Education Program Expert Panel on Detection, Evaluation, and Treatment of High Blood Cholesterol in Adults. "Prevalence of Metabolic Syndrome Based on Results of NHANES III."

31. Canto and Iskandrian, "Major Risk Factors for Cardiovascular Disease."

32. Amend, Allison, et al. "Diabetes Control and Cardiac Risk Factors among Urban Black American Women." *Diabetes,* Vol. 52, No. 6, June 2003, p. A490(1).

33. Toobert, Deborah, et al. "Results of a Lifestyle Change Program to Prevent CHD among Women with Diabetes." *Diabetes,* Vol. 52, No. 6, June 2003, p. A420.

34. Kop, Willem. "The Integration of Cardiovascular Behavioral Medicine and Psychoneuroimmunology: New Developments Based on Converging Research Fields." *Brain, Behavior, and Immunity,* Vol. 17, No. 4, August 2003, p. 233.

35. Parmet, Sharon. "Depression and Heart Disease." *Journal of the American Medical Association,* Vol. 288, No. 6, August 14, 2002, p. 792.

36. Watkins, L. L., et al. "Cognitive and Somatic Symptoms of Depression Are Associated with Medical Comorbidity in Patients After Acute Myocardial Infarction." *American Heart Journal,* Vol. 146, July 2003, p. 48.

37. Lange, Richard, and David Hillis. "Cardiovascular Complications of Cocaine Use." *New England Journal of Medicine,* Vol. 345, No. 5, August 2, 2001, p. 351.

38. Ghuran, A., et al. "Cardiovascular Complications of Recreational Drugs." *British Medical Journal,* Vol. 323, No. 7311, September 1, 2001, p. 844.

39. Mittleman, Murray. "Triggering Myocardial Infarction by Marijuana." *Journal of the American Medical Association,* Vol. 286, No. 6, August 8, 2001, p. 655.

40. Jha, Ashish, et al. "Differences in Medical Care and Disease Outcomes Among Black and White Women with Heart Disease." *Circulation,* Vol. 108, No. 9, September 2003, p. 1089.

41. Ibid.

42. Lotufo, Paolo, et al. "Male Pattern Baldness and Coronary Heart Disease." *Journal of the American Medical Association,* Vol. 160, No. 2, January 24, 2000.

43. Bailar, John. "Hormone-Replacement Therapy and Cardiovascular Diseases." *New England Journal of Medicine,* Vol. 349, No. 6, August 7, 2003, p. 521.

44. Herrington, David, and Timothy Howard. "From Presumed Benefit to Potential Harm—Hormone Therapy and Heart Disease." *New England Journal of Medicine,* Vol. 349, No. 6, August 7, 2003, p. 519.

45. Manson, Joanne. "Estrogen Plus Progestin and the Risk of Coronary Heart Disease." *New England Journal of Medicine,* Vol. 349, No. 6, August 7, 2003, p. 523.

46. Hodis, Howard. "Hormone Therapy and the Progression of Coronary-Artery Atherosclerosis in Postmenopausal Women." *New England Journal of Medicine,* Vol. 349, No. 6, August 7, 2003, p. 535.

47. Fahdi, Ibrahim, et al. "Inflammation, Infection, and Atherosclerosis." *Brain, Behavior, and Immunity,* Vol. 17, No. 4, August 2003, p. 238.

48. Larkin, Marilynn. "Link Between Gum Disease and Heart Disease." *Lancet,* Vol. 358, No. 9278, July 28, 2001, p. 303.

49. Kottke et al., "JNC7—It's More Than High Blood Pressure."

50. "High Blood Pressure Is on the Rise in U.S." *Diabetes,* Vol. 52, No. 6, June 2003, p. 490.

51. Wolf-Maier, Katharina, et al. "Hypertension Prevalence and Blood Pressure Levels in 6 European Countries, Canada, and the United States." *Journal of the American Medical Association,* Vol. 289, No. 18, May 14, 2003, p. 2363.

52. "High Blood Pressure Is on the Rise in U.S."

53. Robertson, Rose Marie. Personal interview.

54. Ishikawa-Takata et al., "How Much Exercise Is Required to Reduce Blood Pressure in Essential Hypertension."

55. "DASH Hypertension Diet Also Lowers Cholesterol." NIH News Release, June 21, 2001.

56. Greenland, Philip. "Beating High Blood Pressure with Low-Sodium DASH." *New England Journal of Medicine,* Vol. 344, No. 1, January 4, 2001.

57. Chobanian et al., "The Seventh Report of the Joint National Committee on Prevention, Detection, Evaluation, and Treatment of High Blood Pressure."

58. Psaty, Bruce, et al. "Health Outcomes Associated with Various Antihypertensive Therapies Used as First Line Agents." *Journal of the American Medical Association,* Vol. 289, No. 19, May 21, 2003, p. 2534.

59. Kottke, et al., "JNC7—It's More Than High Blood Pressure."

60. Expert Panel on Detection, Evaluation, and Treatment of High Blood Cholesterol in Adults. "Executive Summary of the Third Report of the National Cholesterol Education Program (NCEP) Expert Panel on Detection, Evaluation, and Treatment of High Blood Cholesterol in Adults." *Journal of the American Medical Association,* Vol. 285, No. 19, May 16, 2001, p. 2486.

References

61. Jenkins, David, et al. "Effects of a Dietary Portfolio of Cholesterol-Lowering Foods vs. Lovastatin on Serum Lipis and C-Reactive Protein." *Journal of the American Medical Association,* Vol. 290, No. 4, July 23/30, 2003, p. 502.

62. Anderson, James. "Diet First, Then Medication for Hypercholesteremia." *Journal of the American Medical Association,* Vol. 290, No. 4, July 23/30, 2003, p. 531.

63. Vasan, Ramachandran, et al. "Plasma Homocysteine and Risk for Congestive Heart Failure in Adults without Prior Myocardial Infarction." *Journal of the American Medical Association,* Vol. 289, No. 10, March 12, 2003, p. 1251.

64. Hackam, Daniel, and Sonia S. Anand. "Emerging Risk Factors for Atherosclerotic Vascular Disease: A Critical Review of the Evidence." *Journal of the American Medical Association,* Vol. 290, No. 7, August 20, 2003, p. 932.

65. www.nhlbi.nih.gov/actintime/aha/aha.htm

66. Wik, Lars, et al. "Delaying Defibrillation to Give Basic Cardiopulmonary Resuscitation to Patients with Out-of-Hospital Ventricular Fibrillation." *Journal of the American Medical Association,* Vol. 289, No. 11, March 19, 2003, p. 1389.

References

67. Anderson, Henning, et al. "A Comparison of Coronary Angioplasty with Fibrinolytic Therapy in Acute Myocardial Infarction." *New England Journal of Medicine,* Vol. 349, No. 8, August 21, 2003, p. 733.

68. Huikun, Heikki, et al. "Prediction of Sudden Cardiac Death: Appraisal of the Studies and Methods Assessing the Risk of Sudden Arrhythmic Death." *Circulation,* Vol. 108, July 8, 2003, pp. 110–115.

69. DiCarli, Marcelo, and Sharmila Dorbala. "Exercise Testing and Nuclear Scanning," *Circulation,* Vol. 107, No. 16, April 29, 2003, p. e100.

70. Hoffmann, Udo, et al. "Use of New Imaging Techniques to Screen for Coronary Artery Disease." *Circulation,* Vol. 108, August 26, 2003, p. 50.

71. Gum, Patricia, et al. "Aspirin Use and All-Cause Mortality Among Patients Being Evaluated for Known or Suspected Coronary Artery Disease: A Propensity Analysis." *Journal of the American Medical Association,* Vol. 286, No. 10, September 10, 2001, p. 1187.

72. Cross, P. L. "Effect of Ibuprofen on Cardioprotective Effect of Aspirin." *Lancet,* Vol. 361, No. 9368, May 3, 2003, p. 1560.

References

73. "Surgery Better Than Drugs?" *Lancet,* Vol. 361, No. 9372, May 31, 2003, p. 1877.

74. Staessen, Jan, et al. "Hypertension, Prevalence, and Stroke Mortality across Populations." *Journal of the American Medical Association,* Vol. 289, No, 18, May 14, 2003, p. 2420.

75. Sacco, Ralph. "Preventing Stroke among Blacks." *Journal of the American Medical Association,* Vol. 289, No. 22, June 11, 2003, p. 3005.

76. Ibid.

77. Gorelick, Philip, et al. "Aspirin and Ticlopidine for Prevention of Recurrent Stroke in Black Patients." *Journal of the American Medical Association,* Vol. 289, No. 22, June 11, 2003, p. 2947.

78. Mitka, Mike. "Tensions Remains over tPa for Stroke." *Journal of the American Medical Association,* Vol. 289, No. 11, March 19, 2003, p. 1363.

Lowering Your Risk of Cancer and Other Major Diseases

Celine knows that she inherited her mother's brown eyes and buoyant sense of humor. She wonders whether she's also inherited "the bad gene"—the cancer-causing one that killed her grandmother and great-grandmother. Celine's mother was 42 years old when she learned that she, too, had cancer. She died two years later, leaving behind eight sisters. Within the next decade, six had developed breast or ovarian cancer.

Unlike most college students, Celine never thinks of cancer as something that affects only people much older than she. Three of her five sisters have tested positive for what is called "the breast cancer gene." Celine is struggling to decide whether she too will undergo testing.

An estimated 10 percent of cancers are hereditary, but no one is immune from the threat of cancer or other serious diseases. Yet you do have some control over your risk of disease. About one-third of annual cancer deaths are related to lifestyle choices and could be prevented.[1]

Prevention and health promotion hold great promise for cancer and for the other noninfectious illnesses discussed in this chapter: diabetes mellitus; epilepsy; respiratory diseases; anemias; liver disorders; kidney problems; digestive diseases; disorders of the muscles, joints, and bones; and skin disorders. This chapter also explains the causes, risk factors, development, diagnosis, and treatment of these disorders and discusses special needs related to differences in physical and mental abilities.

© Steve Smith/Taxi/Getty Images

After studying the material in this chapter, you should be able to:

- **Explain** how cancer develops and how cancers are classified.
- **List** the risk factors for cancer, and **describe** ways you can reduce your risk of cancer.

- **Discuss** the most common types of cancer, and **describe** the treatments for each.
- **Explain** the disease process of diabetes mellitus, and **describe** the early symptoms and treatment for this disease.
- **Describe** common major respiratory, liver, kidney, digestive, skeletal-muscular, and skin diseases.

503

☒ Understanding Cancer

The uncontrolled growth and spread of abnormal cells causes cancer. Normal cells follow the code of instructions embedded in DNA (the body's genetic material); cancer cells do not. Think of the DNA within the nucleus of a cell as a computer program that controls the cell's functioning, including its ability to grow and reproduce itself. If this program or its operation is altered, the cell goes out of control. The nucleus no longer regulates growth. The abnormal cell divides to create other abnormal cells, which again divide, eventually forming **neoplasms** (new formations), or tumors.

How Cancer Begins

For decades researchers have tried to figure out exactly how a normal cell turns into a cancer cell. They've made dramatic progress in unraveling this mystery by studying **oncogenes,** normal genes that control growth but have gone awry. For reasons that scientists don't yet understand, the DNA in these genes changes and cells proliferate at a very rapid rate. In addition, other genes, called **tumor suppressor genes,** which normally control cell growth, fail to stop cells from dividing before they become cancerous. More than half of all known types of cancer, including those of the colon, brain, lung, breast, bone, and blood, have been linked to defects in one particular tumor suppressor gene: *p53*. Mismatch/repair genes correct mistakes in a cell's DNA when it is copied. If they do not function properly, mutations can occur in other genes, including oncogenes and tumor suppressor genes.

How Cancer Spreads

Tumors can be either *benign* (slightly abnormal, not considered life-threatening) or *malignant* (cancerous). The only way to determine whether a tumor is benign is by microscopic examination of its cells. Cancer cells have larger nuclei than the cells in benign tumors, they vary more in shape and size, and they divide more often.

At one time cancer was thought to be a single disease that attacked different parts of the body. Now scientists believe that cancer comes in countless forms, each with a genetically determined

molecular "fingerprint" that indicates how deadly it is. With this understanding, doctors can identify how aggressively a tumor should be treated.

Without treatment, cancer cells continue to grow, crowding out and replacing healthy cells. This process is called **infiltration,** or invasion. Cancer cells may also **metastasize,** or spread to other parts of the body via the bloodstream or lymphatic system. (See Figure 15-1.) For many cancers, as many as 60 percent of patients may have metastases (which may be too small to be felt or seen without a microscope) at the time of diagnosis.

Cancer Staging

Once they diagnose a cancer, oncologists (specialists in cancer care) calculate the extent of the disease or the spread of cancer from the site of origin. This process, called staging, is essential in determining therapy and assessing prognosis. A cancer's stage is based on the primary tumor's size and location and whether it has spread to other areas of the body. According to one staging system, if cancer cells have not spread to other parts of the affected organ or elsewhere in the body, the stage is "in situ." If cancer cells have spread beyond the original layer of tissue, then the cancer is considered invasive. If it has traveled to distant parts of the body, it has metastasized.

☒ ☒ Who Is at Risk for Developing Cancer?

Everyone and anyone can develop cancer. However, since the occurrence of cancer increases over time, most cases affect adults who are middle-aged or older. (See Table 15-1.) In the United States, men have a one in two life-

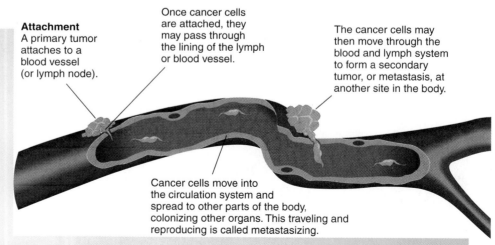

Attachment
A primary tumor attaches to a blood vessel (or lymph node).

Once cancer cells are attached, they may pass through the lining of the lymph or blood vessel.

The cancer cells may then move through the blood and lymph system to form a secondary tumor, or metastasis, at another site in the body.

Cancer cells move into the circulation system and spread to other parts of the body, colonizing other organs. This traveling and reproducing is called metastasizing.

Figure 15-1 METASTASIS, OR SPREAD OF CANCER
Cancer cells can travel through the blood vessels to spread to other organs, or through the lymphatic system to form secondary tumors.

the X & Y file *Sex Differences in Cancer**

Estimated New Cases*		Estimated Deaths	
Male	Female	Male	Female
Prostate 220,900 (33%)	Breast 211,300 (32%)	Lung and bronchus 88,400 (31%)	Lung and bronchus 68,800 (25%)
Lung and bronchus 91,800 (14%)	Lung and bronchus 80,100 (12%)	Prostate 28,900 (10%)	Breast 39,800 (15%)
Colon and rectum 72,800 (11%)	Colon and rectum 74,700 (11%)	Colon and rectum 28,300 (10%)	Colon and rectum 28,800 (11%)
Urinary bladder 42,200 (6%)	Uterine Corpus 40,100 (6%)	Pancreas 14,700 (5%)	Pancreas 15,300 (6%)
Melanoma of the skin 29,900 (4%)	Ovary 25,400 (4%)	Non-Hodgkin's lymphoma 12,200 (4%)	Ovary 14,300 (5%)
Non-Hodgkin's lymphoma 28,300 (4%)	Non-Hodgkin's lymphoma 25,100 (4%)	Leukemia 12,100 (4%)	Non-Hodgkin's lymphoma 11,200 (4%)
Kidney 19,500 (3%)	Melanoma of the skin 24,300 (3%)	Esophagus 9,900 (4%)	Leukemia 9,800 (4%)
Oral cavity 18,200 (3%)	Thyroid 16,300 (3%)	Liver 9,200 (3%)	Uterine Corpus 6,800 (3%)
Leukemia 17,900 (3%)	Pancreas 15,800 (2%)	Urinary bladder 8,600 (3%)	Brain 5,800 (2%)
Pancreas 14,900 (2%)	Urinary bladder 15,200 (2%)	Kidney 7,400 (3%)	Multiple myeloma 5,500 (2%)
All sites 675,300 (100%)	All sites 658,800 (100%)	All sites 285,900 (100%)	All sites 270,600 (100%)

Half of all men—compared to a third of women—develop cancer. Smoking, which for many years was much more prevalent among men, accounts for some of this difference. As more women became smokers in the last thirty years, lung cancer rates in women have doubled.

*Excludes basal and squamous cell skin cancers and in situ carcinoma except urinary bladder. Percentages may not total 100% due to rounding.

Source: ©2003, Data from American Cancer Society, Inc., 2003, Surveillance Research.

time risk of developing cancer; for women, the risk is one in three.[2] (See The X & Y File: "Sex Differences in Cancer.")

The term **relative risk** compares the risk of developing cancer in people with a certain exposure or trait to the risk in those who do not have this exposure or trait. Smokers, for instance, have a ten-times-greater relative risk of developing lung cancer than nonsmokers. Most relative risks are smaller. For example, women who have a first-degree (mother, sister, or daughter) family history of breast cancer have about a twofold increased risk of developing breast cancer compared with women who do not have a family history of the disease. This means that they are about twice as likely to develop breast cancer.

TABLE 15-1	Age and the Risk of Cancer (All Sites)	
	Men	**Women**
Birth to age 39	1 in 64	1 in 51
Ages 40 to 59	1 in 12	1 in 11
Ages 60 to 79	1 in 3	1 in 4
Birth to death	1 in 2	1 in 3

Source: *Cancer Facts & Figures 2003*. Atlanta, GA: American Cancer Society, 2003.

Heredity

An estimated 13 to 14 million Americans may be at risk of a hereditary cancer. In hereditary cancers, such as retinoblastoma (an eye cancer that strikes young children) or certain colon cancers, a specific cancer-causing gene is passed down from generation to generation. The odds of any child with one affected parent inheriting this gene and developing the cancer are fifty-fifty.

Other people are born with genes that make them susceptible to having certain cells grow and divide uncontrollably, which may contribute to cancer development. The most well-known are mutations of the BRCA gene, linked with increased risk of breast, colon, and ovarian cancer. Researchers recently recognized an even more common inherited cancer susceptibility gene, known as TGFRB1*6A, carried by nearly one in eight people, that increases cancer risk by 26 percent.[3]

Genetic tests can identify some individuals who are born with an increased susceptibility to cancer. By spotting a mutated gene in an individual, doctors can sometimes detect cancer years earlier through increased cancer screening. The most likely sites for inherited cancers to develop are the breast, brain, blood, muscles, bones, and adrenal glands. The telltale signs of inherited cancers include:

:: **Early development.** Genetic forms of certain diseases strike earlier than noninherited cancers. For example, the average age of women diagnosed with breast cancer is 62. But if breast cancer is inherited, the average age at diagnosis is 44, an 18-year difference.

:: **Family history.** Anyone with a close relative (mother, father, sibling, child) with cancer has about three times the usual chance of getting the same type of cancer.

:: **Multiple targets.** The same type of hereditary cancer often strikes more than once—in both breasts or both kidneys, for instance, or in two separate parts of the same organ.

:: **Unusual gender pattern.** Genes may be responsible for cancers that generally don't strike a certain gender—for example, breast cancer in a man.

:: **Cancer family syndrome.** Some families, with unusually large numbers of relatives affected by cancer, seem clearly cancer-prone. For instance, in Lynch syndrome (a form of colon cancer), more than 20 percent of the family members in at least two generations develop cancer of both the colon and the endometrium.

Racial and Ethnic Groups

The American Cancer Society estimates that about 1.3 million cases of cancer are diagnosed each year, with more cases in black Americans than in any other racial or ethnic group.[4] Blacks are 30 percent more likely to die of cancer than whites. African-American women have the highest incidence of colorectal and lung cancers of any ethnic group, while black men have the highest rates of prostate, colorectal, and lung cancer. African Americans also have higher rates of incidence and deaths from other cancers, including those of the mouth, throat, esophagus, stomach, pancreas, and larynx.

Cancer rates also vary in other racial and ethnic groups. Hispanics have six times lower risk of developing melanoma than Caucasians, yet tend to have a worse prognosis than Caucasians when they do develop this skin cancer.[5] The incidence of female breast cancer is highest among white women and lowest among Native American women.[6]

Obesity

Long recognized as threats to cardiovascular health, overweight and obesity may play a role in an estimated 90,000 cancer deaths each year. According to American Cancer Society researchers who examined the relationship between body mass index (BMI) and risk of dying from cancer, 14 percent of cancer deaths in men and 20 percent of cancer deaths in women may stem from excess weight.

The higher an individual's BMI, the greater the likelihood of dying of cancer. A woman with a BMI of 25 to 30 faces a 30 percent higher risk of breast cancer, while the risk is 63 percent higher for women with BMIs in the 30 to 35 range and 70 percent higher for those with a BMI between 35 and 40. The heaviest men had a 52 percent higher death rate from all cancers, while the heaviest women had a 62 percent higher death rate.[7]

© Michael Doolittle/The Image Works

By age 39, 1 in 64 men and 1 in 51 women will have cancer. Look at your risk factors and lifestyle—what do you think are your odds?

Eating at least five servings of fruits and vegetables a day can help reduce your cancer risk.

An unhealthy body weight increases the risk of many types of cancer, including breast (in postmenopausal women), colon and rectum, kidney, cervix, ovary, uterus, esophagus, gallbladder, stomach (in men), liver, pancreas, prostate, non-Hodgkin lymphoma, and multiple myeloma. Yet in an ACS survey, only 1 percent of Americans identified maintaining a healthy weight as a way to reduce their cancer risk.

The degree to which extra pounds affect cancer risk varies by site. Obesity elevates the risk of esophageal cancer fivefold; increases the risk of breast or uterine cancer by two to four times, and boosts the risk for colon cancer by 35 percent to twofold.[8]

Infectious Agents

Several cancers have been linked with infectious agents, including human papilloma virus (HPV) with cervical cancer and *Helicobacter pylori* with stomach cancer. Viruses have been implicated in certain leukemias (cancers of the blood system) and lymphomas (cancers of the lymphatic system), cancers of the nose and pharynx, liver cancer, and cervical cancer. Human immune deficiency virus (HIV) can lead to certain lymphomas and leukemias and to a type of cancer called Kaposi's sarcoma.

Generally the presence of a bacterium or a virus, per se, is not enough to cause cancer. A predisposing environment and other cofactors—most still unknown, are needed for cancer development and growth.[9]

▰▰ ⬚ How Can I Reduce My Cancer Risk?

Environmental factors may cause between 80 and 90 percent of cancers. At least in theory, these cancers can be prevented by avoiding cancer-causing substances (such as

tobacco and sunlight) or using substances that protect against cancer-causing factors (such as antioxidants and vitamin D). How do you start protecting yourself? Simple changes in lifestyle—smart eating, losing excess weight, not smoking, protecting yourself from the sun, exercising regularly—are essential.

Physical activity reduces the risk of breast cancer by 10 to 25 percent and colon cancer by 25 to 50 percent.[10]

Cancer-Smart Nutrition

Diets high in antioxidant-rich fruits and vegetables have long been linked with lower rates of esophageal, lung, colon, and stomach cancer. At least in theory, antioxidants—substances that prevent the damaging effects of oxidation in cells—can block genetic damage induced by free radicals that could lead to some cancers. However, scientific studies have not proven conclusively that any specific antioxidant, particularly in supplement form, can prevent cancer. The U.S. Preventive Services Task Force advises against the use of beta-carotene supplements because of a risk of increased mortality from lung cancer.[11]

Eating as many different types of fruits and vegetables as possible—for a total of five to nine servings a day—remains a standard recommendation. However, a low-fat diet rich in fruit, vegetables, and fiber does not influence the risk of recurrence of colorectal polyps. Some studies have found a correlation between very high consumption of fruits and vegetables and lower risk of breast cancer, but the overall findings have been inconclusive.

Another way to lower your cancer risk is to reduce the fat in your diet. There is solid evidence that cutting back on fat can lower the risks of colon, ovarian, and pancreatic cancer.

It's also important to pay attention to food processing and preparation. Whenever possible, select foods close to their natural state, grown locally and without pesticides. Avoid cured, pickled, or smoked meats. When cooking, try not to fry or barbecue often; these cooking methods can produce mutagens that induce cancer in animals. The process of smoking or charcoal-grilling releases carcinogenic tar that may increase the risk of cancer of the stomach and esophagus.

Tobacco Smoke

Cigarette smoking is the single most devastating and preventable cause of cancer deaths in the United States. People who smoke two or more packs of cigarettes a day are 15 to 25 times more likely to die of cancer than nonsmokers. Cigarettes cause most cases of lung cancer and increase the risk of cancer of the mouth, pharynx, larynx, esophagus, pancreas, and bladder. Pipes, cigars, and smokeless tobacco also increase the danger of cancers of the mouth and throat.

Environmental tobacco smoke can increase the risk of cancer even among those who've never smoked. For example, exposure to others' tobacco smoke for as little as three hours a day can increase the risk of developing cancer. (See the discussion of environmental tobacco smoke in Chapter 12.)

Environmental Risks

Although it may not be possible to avoid all possible **carcinogens** (cancer-causing chemicals), you can take steps to minimize your danger. Many chemicals used in industry, including nickel, chromate, asbestos, and vinyl chloride, are carcinogens; employees as well as people living near a factory that creates smoke, dust, or gases are at risk. If your job involves their use, follow safety precautions at work. If you are concerned about possible hazards in your community, check with local environmental protection officials.

Women and men who frequently dye their hair, particularly with very dark shades of permanent coloring, may be at increased risk for leukemia (cancer of blood-forming cells), non-Hodgkin's lymphoma (cancer of the lymph system), multiple myeloma (cancer of the bone marrow), and, in women, ovarian cancer. Lighter shades and less permanent tints do not seem to be a danger. (Chapter 19 discusses pesticides, toxic wastes, and other environmental threats.)

Early Detection

Proven methods of cancer prevention and early detection could save more than 60,000 lives a year.[12] Screening examinations, conducted regularly by a health-care professional, can lead to early diagnosis of cancers of the breast, colon, rectum, cervix, prostate, testicles, and oral cavity, and can improve the odds of successful treatment. (See Your Health Change Plan for Early Detection of Cancer on page 510.) Self-examinations for cancers of the breast, testicles, and skin may also result in detection of tumors at earlier stages. The five-year relative survival rate for all these cancers is about 81 percent. If all Americans participated in regular cancer screenings, this rate could increase to more than 95 percent.[13]

Chemoprevention

Chemoprevention uses natural or laboratory-made substances to reduce the risk of cancer by halting or reversing the process by which a cell becomes cancerous.

The first medication that proved effective in preventing a major cancer is **tamoxifen,** a modified or "designer" estrogen that belongs to a group of medications called selective estrogen receptor modulators (SERMs), which have different effects in various parts of the body. In the breast, they block estrogen's harmful effects and lower cancer risk; in the skeleton, they mimic estrogen's beneficial impact and maintain bone density. Tamoxifen's primary disadvantage is an increased risk of three rare but potentially life-threatening problems: endometrial cancer, deep vein thrombosis (a blood clot in a large vein), and pulmonary embolism (a clot in the lung) in women over age 50.

A second SERM—raloxifene (Evista), FDA-approved to prevent osteoporosis—also may lower breast cancer risk without such serious side effects. NCI's ongoing STAR (Study of Tamoxifen and Raloxifene) trial aims to find the answer. However, there is considerable debate over giving any drug that can cause significant side effects to healthy women.

NCI also is investigating the possible chemopreventive benefits of finasteride (Proscar), a drug used to treat benign swelling of the prostate, a common problem in older men. Unlike tamoxifen, it does not increase the risk of other cancers, but it does have side effects, including sexual dysfunction.

◖ Common Types of Cancer

Cancer refers to a group of more than a hundred diseases characterized by abnormal cell growth. Although all cancers have similar characteristics, each is distinct. Some cancers are relatively simple to cure, whereas others are more threatening and mysterious. The earlier any cancer is found, the easier it is to treat and the better the patient's chances of survival.

Cancers are classified according to the type of cell and the organ in which they originate, such as the following:

:: **Carcinoma,** the most common kind, which starts in the epithelium, the layers of cells that cover the body's surface or line internal organs and glands.

:: **Sarcoma,** which forms in the supporting, or connective, tissues of the body: bones, muscles, blood vessels.

:: **Leukemia,** which begins in the blood-forming tissues (bone marrow, lymph nodes, and the spleen).

:: **Lymphoma,** which arises in the cells of the lymph system, the network that filters out impurities.

Skin Cancer

Sunlight is the primary culprit in the 1 million new cases of skin cancer that develop every year. Once scientists thought exposure to the B range of ultraviolet light (UVB), the wavelength of light responsible for sunburn, posed the greatest danger. However, longer-wavelength UVA, which penetrates deeper into the skin, also plays a major role in skin cancers. An estimated 80 percent of total

lifetime sun exposure occurs during childhood, so sun protection is especially important in youngsters. Tanning salons
and sunlamps also increase the risk of skin cancer because
they produce ultraviolet radiation. A half-hour dose of
radiation from a sunlamp can be equivalent to the amount
you'd get from an entire day in the sun.

The most common skin cancers are *basal-cell* (involving the base of the epidermis, the top level of the skin) and
squamous-cell (involving cells in the epidermis). (See Figure
15-2.) Every year more than 5 million Americans develop
skin lesions known as actinic keratoses (AKs), rough red or
brown scaly patches that develop in the upper layer of the
skin, usually on the face, lower lip, bald scalp, neck, and
back of the hands and forearms. Forty percent of squamous cell carcinomas, the second leading cause of skin
cancer deaths, begin as AKs. Treatments include surgical
removal, cryosurgery (freezing the skin), electrodesiccation
(heat generated by an electric current), topical chemotherapy, and removal with lasers, chemical peels, or
dermabrasion.

Smoking and exposure to certain hydrocarbons in
asphalt, coal tar, and pitch may increase the risk of squamous-cell skin cancer. Other risk factors include occupational exposure to carcinogens and inherited skin
disorders, such as xeroderma pigmentosum and familial
atypical multiple-mole melanoma.

**The "healthy" glow of tanned skin may be the precursor
to a severe, even fatal, case of skin cancer.**

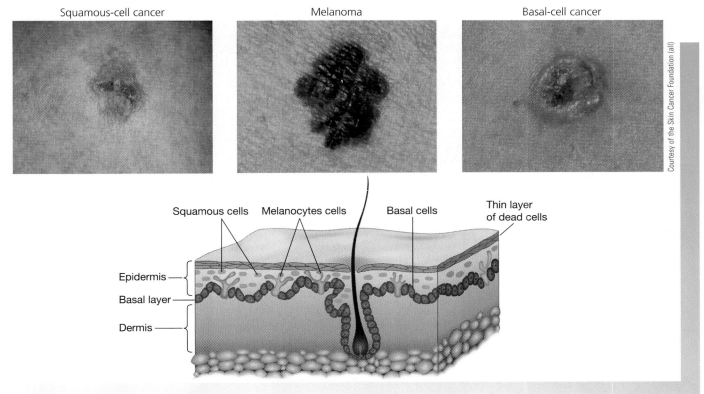

Squamous-cell cancer   Melanoma   Basal-cell cancer

Squamous cells   Melanocytes cells   Basal cells   Thin layer of dead cells

Epidermis

Basal layer

Dermis

Figure 15-2 THREE TYPES OF SKIN CANCER
Squamous-cell cancer arises from the squamous cells in the epidermis. Malignant
melanoma, the deadliest form of skin cancer, arises from malanocyte cells. Basal-
cell cancer arises from the basal cells.

Self Survey   **Are You at Risk of Cancer?**

Answer the following questions:

1. Do you protect your skin from overexposure to the sun? _____
2. Do you abstain from smoking or using tobacco in any form? _____
3. If you're over 40 or if family members have had colon cancer, do you get routine digital rectal exams? _____
4. Do you eat a balanced diet that includes the recommended Daily Value for vitamins A, B, and C? _____
5. If you're a woman, do you have regular Pap tests and pelvic exams? _____
6. If you're a man over 40, do you get regular prostate exams? _____
7. If you have burn scars or a history of chronic skin infections, do you get regular checkups? _____
8. Do you avoid smoked, salted, pickled, and high-nitrite foods? _____
9. If your job exposes you to asbestos, radiation, cadmium, or other environmental hazards, do you get regular checkups? _____

10. Do you limit your consumption of alcohol? _____
11. Do you avoid using tanning salons or home sunlamps? _____
12. If you're a woman, do you examine your breasts every month for lumps? _____
13. Do you eat plenty of vegetables and other sources of fiber? _____
14. If you're a man, do you perform regular testicular self-exams? _____
15. Do you wear protective sunglasses in sunlight? _____
16. Do you follow a low-fat diet? _____
17. Do you know the cancer warning signs? _____

Scoring:

If you answered no to any of the questions, your risk for developing various kinds of cancer may be increased.

Your Health Change Plan

for Early Detection of Cancer

Site	Recommendation
Breast	Women 40 and older should have an annual mammogram, an annual clinical breast examination (CBE) by a health-care professional, and should perform monthly breast self-examinations (BSE). Ideally the CBE should occur before the scheduled mammogram. Women ages 20–39 should have a CBE by a health-care professional every 3 years and should perform BSE monthly.

© Bill Crump/Brand X Pictures/PictureQuest

STRATEGIES FOR PREVENTION

Seven Warning Signs of Cancer

If you note any of the following seven warning signs, immediately schedule an appointment with your doctor:

- Change in bowel or bladder habits.
- A sore that doesn't heal.
- Unusual bleeding or discharge.
- Thickening or lump in the breast, testis, or elsewhere.
- Indigestion or difficulty swallowing.
- Obvious change in a wart or mole.
- Nagging cough or hoarseness.

Malignant *melanoma,* the deadliest type of skin cancer, causes 1 to 2 percent of all cancer deaths. During the 1930s, the lifetime risk of melanoma was about 1 in 1,500. Today it is 1 in 75. This increase in risk is due mostly to overexposure to UV radiation. The use of a tanning bed ten times or more a year doubles the risk for individuals over age 30. For those younger than 30, this type of exposure increases the risk by a factor of 7.7.[14]

Both the amount and the intensity of lifetime sun exposure play key roles in determining risk for melanoma. People living in areas where the sun's ultraviolet rays reach the earth with extra intensity, such as tropical or high-altitude regions, are at increased risk.[15] Although melanoma occurs more often among people over 40, it is increasing in younger people, particularly those who had severe sunburns in childhood. The rate of increase in melanoma also has risen more in men (4.6 percent a year)

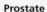

Self Survey   **Are You at Risk of Cancer? (Continued)**

Site	Recommendation
Colon and Rectum	Beginning at age 50 men and women should follow one of the examination schedules below: • A fecal occult blood test (FOBT) every year • A flexible sigmoidoscopy (FSIG) every 5 years • Annual fecal occult blood test and flexible sigmoidoscopy every five years* • A double-contrast barium enema every 5 years • A colonoscopy every 10 years* *Combined testing is preferred over either annual FOBT, or FSIG every 5 years, alone. People who are at moderate or high risk for colorectal cancer should talk with a doctor about a different testing schedule.*
Prostate	The PSA test and the digital rectal examination should be offered annually, beginning at age 50, to men who have a life expectancy of at least 10 years. Men at high risk (African American men and men with a strong family history of one or more first-degree relatives diagnosed with prostate cancer at an early age) should begin testing at age 45. For both men at average risk and high risk, information should be provided about what is known and what is uncertain about the benefits and limitations of early detection and treatment of prostate cancer so that they can make an informed decision about testing.
Uterus	**Cervix:** Screening should begin approximately three years after a woman begins having vaginal intercourse, but no later than 21 years of age. Screening should be done every year with regular Pap tests or every two years using liquid-based tests. At or after age 30, women who have had three normal test results in a row may get screened every 2–3 years. However, doctors may suggest a woman get screened more often if she has certain risk factors, such as HIV infection or a weak immune system. Women 70 years and older who have had three or more consecutive normal Pap tests in the last 10 years may choose to stop cervical cancer screening. Screening after total hysterectomy (with removal of the cervix) is not necessary unless the surgery was done as a treatment for cervical cancer. **Endometrium:** The American Cancer Society recommends that all women should be informed about the risks and symptoms of endometrial cancer, and strongly encouraged to report any unexpected bleeding or spotting to their physicians. Annual screening for endometrial cancer with endometrial biopsy beginning at age 35 should be offered to women with or at risk for hereditary nonpolyposis colon cancer (HNPCC).
Cancer-related checkup	For individuals undergoing periodic health examinations, a cancer-related checkup should include health counseling, and depending on a person's age, might include examinations for cancers of the thyroid, oral cavity, skin, lymph nodes, testes, and ovaries, as well as for some nonmalignant diseases.

than for women (3.2 percent). Men are more likely than women to be diagnosed with melanoma after age 40.[16]

Individuals with any of the following characteristics are at increased risk:

:: *Fair skin,* light eyes, or fair hair.

:: *A tendency to develop freckles* and to burn instead of tan.

:: *A history of childhood sunburn* or intermittent, intense sun exposure.

:: *A personal or family history* of melanoma.

:: *A large number of* **nevi,** or moles (200 or more, or 50 or more if under age 20), or dysplastic (atypical) moles.

Detection

The most common predictor for melanoma is a change in an existing mole or development of a new and changing pigmented mole. The most important early indicators are change in color, an increase in diameter, and changes in the borders of a mole. (See Figure 15-3.) An increase in height signals a corresponding growth in depth under the skin. Itching in a new or long-standing mole also should not be ignored.[17]

Treatment

If caught early, melanoma is highly curable, usually with surgery alone. Once it has spread, chemotherapy with a single drug or a combination can temporarily shrink tumors in some people. However, the five-year survival rate for metastatic melanoma is 14 percent.

Asymmetry: One half doesn't match the other half

Border irregularity: The edges are ragged, notched, or blurred

Color: Rather than uniform pigmentation, there are shades of tan, brown, and black, with possible dashes of red, white, and blue.

Diameter: The mole is larger than 6 mm (about the size of a pencil eraser). (The melanoma shown here is magnified about 20 times its actual size.)

Figure 15-3 ABCD: THE WARNING SIGNS OF MELANOMA

An estimated 95 percent of cases of melanoma arise from an existing mole. A normal mole is usually round or oval, less than 6 millimeters (about 1/4 inch) in diameter, and evenly colored (black, brown, or tan). Seek prompt evaluation of any moles that change in ways shown in the photo.

Breast Cancer

Every 3 minutes a woman in the United States learns that she has breast cancer. Every 12 minutes a woman dies of breast cancer. Many women misjudge their own likelihood of developing breast cancer, either overestimating or underestimating their susceptibility. In a national poll, one in every ten surveyed considered herself at no risk at all. This is never the case. "Every woman is at risk for breast cancer simply because she's female," says Leslie Ford, M.D., associate director for early detection at the National Cancer Institute (NCI).[18]

However, not all women's risks are equal. NCI has developed a computerized Breast Cancer Risk Assessment Tool, based on data from more than 280,000 women, that allows a woman to sit down with her doctor and discuss her own odds of developing breast cancer within the next five years and over her entire lifetime. A report on risk factors in Marin County, California, which has the highest breast cancer rate in the country, found that women with breast cancer differ from cancer-free women in various ways: They were thinner, never used birth control pills, averaged two or more drinks per day, and were more likely to be smokers.[19]

The most common risk factors include the following:

:: **Age.** As shown in Figure 15-4, at 25, a woman's chance of developing breast cancer is 1 in 19,608; at

STRATEGIES FOR PREVENTION

Scanning Your Skin

Here's how to screen yourself for possible changes that may indicate skin cancer:

■ Once a month, stand in front of a full-length mirror to examine your front and back, and your left and right sides with your arms raised. Check the backs of your legs, the tops and soles of your feet, and the surfaces between your toes. Use a hand mirror to check the back of your neck, behind your ears, and your scalp.

■ Watch for changes in the size, color, number, and thickness of moles. Suspicious moles are likely to be asymmetrical (one half doesn't match the other), with ragged, notched, or blurred edges. Also look for any signs of darkly pigmented growth, oozing, scaliness, bleeding, or a change in sensation, itchiness, tenderness, or pain.

■ Don't put too much faith in sunscreens. Wearing sunscreen (with a Sun Protection Factor, or SPF, of at least 15) is good, but protective clothing is better—and staying in the shade is best. Check your shadow. One simple guideline for reducing the risk of skin cancer is avoiding the sun anytime your shadow is shorter than you are. According to NCI, this shadow method—based on the principle that the closer the sun comes to being directly overhead, the stronger its ultraviolet rays—works for any location and at any time of year.

■ Check for photosensitivity. If you are taking any drugs, ask your doctor or pharmacist to see if the medication could make you more sensitive to sun damage. Be especially cautious about sun exposure if you have been using a synthetic preparation derived from vitamin A (Retin A) as an acne or anti-wrinkle treatment; it can increase your susceptibility.

45, 1 in 93; at 65, 1 in 17; at 85, 1 in 9. By age 90 to 95, 1 in 8 women will have developed breast cancer. The mean age at which women are diagnosed is 63.

:: **Family history.** The overwhelming majority of breast cancers—90 to 95 percent—are not due to strong genetic factors. However, having a first-degree relative—mother, sister or daughter—with breast cancer does increase risk, and if the relative developed breast cancer before menopause, the cancer is more likely to be hereditary. Genetic testing, controversial but sometimes recommended for women in cancer-prone families, can identify these defects. However, it's not yet clear how many women with a defective gene actually will develop breast cancer; estimates range from 50 to

By age 25	1 in 19,608	By age 60	1 in 24
By age 30	1 in 2,525	By age 65	1 in 17
By age 35	1 in 622	By age 70	1 in 14
By age 40	1 in 217	By age 75	1 in 11
By age 45	1 in 93	By age 80	1 in 10
By age 50	1 in 50	By age 85	1 in 9
By age 55	1 in 33	Ever	1 in 8

Figure 15-4 A WOMAN'S RISK OF DEVELOPING BREAST CANCER

Source: Surveillance Program, National Cancer Institute.

80 percent, or higher in families with many affected members.

:: **Age at menarche.** Women who had their first period before age 12 are at greater risk than women who began menstruating later. The reason is that the more menstrual cycles a woman has, the longer her exposure to estrogen, a hormone known to increase breast cancer danger. For similar reasons, childless women, who menstruate continuously for several decades, are also at greater risk.

:: **Age at birth of first child.** An early pregnancy—in a woman's teens or twenties—changes the actual maturation of breast cells and decreases risk. But if a woman has her first child in her forties, precancerous cells may actually flourish with the high hormone levels of the pregnancy.

:: **Breast biopsies.** Even if laboratory analysis finds no precancerous abnormalities, women who require such tests are more likely to develop breast cancer. Fibrocystic breast disease, a term often used for "lumpy" breasts, is not a risk factor.

:: **Race.** Breast cancer rates are lower in Hispanic and Asian populations than in whites, but higher in African-American women up to age 50. In postmenopausal African-American women, rates are lower. Nonetheless, African-American women are still more likely to die of breast cancer than whites. Scientists don't know if that's because they don't have equal access to care, if they don't get optimal care, or if the disease itself is more aggressive in black women.

:: **Occupation.** Based on two decades of following more than a million women, Swedish researchers have developed a list of jobs linked with a high risk of breast cancer. These include pharmacists, certain types of teachers, schoolmasters, systems analysts and programmers, telephone operators, telegraph and radio operators, metal platers and coaters, and beauticians.

:: **Alcohol.** As discussed in Chapter 11, women's risk of breast cancer increases with the amount of alcohol they drink. Those who take two or more drinks per day are 40 percent more likely to develop breast cancer than women who don't drink at all. For a nondrinking woman, the lifetime risk of breast cancer by age 80 is 1 in 11. For heavy drinkers it's about 1 in 7, regardless of race, education, family history, use of hormone replacement therapy, or other risk factors.[20] Scientists don't know how alcohol increases breast cancer risk. In some studies, alcohol raised levels of estrogen, either by decreasing the body's ability to metabolize the hormone or by promoting its release into the bloodstream. But other studies have not shown increased estrogen levels in women who drink. Alcohol may also interact with carcinogens (cancer-causing agents), either inhibiting the body's capacity to detoxify carcinogens or even activating carcinogens directly.[21]

Hormone Replacement Therapy

After years of debate over postmenopausal hormone replacement therapy (HRT), several studies confirmed an increased risk with a combination of estrogen and progestin, particularly in women who use combination HRT for five years or longer.[22] Women taking combination HRT are more likely to have abnormal mammograms requiring further testing and to be diagnosed at a more advanced stage of breast cancer. Researchers theorize that estrogen and progestin may stimulate breast cancer growth and hinder cancer diagnosis by increasing breast density.[23] Women using only estrogen did not have an elevated rate of breast cancer, even after 25 years of use.[24] (See Chapter 17 for a more extensive discussion of menopause and hormone replacement.)

Detection

Doctors long advised women to perform monthly breast self-exams after their periods (Figure 15-5). According to a recent study, breast self-examination (BSE) does *not* appear to decrease the number of deaths from breast cancer. Highly motivated women practicing BSE, the researchers found, are more likely to find benign tumors and undergo expensive and unnecessary testing.[25] Based on the new findings, rather than spending time teaching BSE, physicians have been urged to educate women about breast cancer symptoms and spend a little longer on the clinical breast exam.[26]

In its newest guidelines, the American Cancer Society describes BSE as "an option" for women starting in their twenties and urges all women to report any breast changes promptly.[27] It recommends a breast exam by a trained practitioner every three years for women in their 20s and 30s and every year for women 40 and over and a yearly mammogram for all women, starting at age 40.[28]

Looking

Stand in front of a mirror with your upper body unclothed. Look for changes in the shape and size of the breast, and for dimpling of the skin or "pulling in" of the nipples. Any changes in the breast may be made more noticeable by a change in position of the body or arms. Look for any of the above signs or for changes in shape from one breast to the other.

1. Stand with your arms down.

2. Raise your arms overhead.

3. Place your hands on your hips and tighten your chest and arm muscles by pressing firmly.

Feeling

1. Lie flat on your back. Place a pillow or towel under one shoulder, and raise that arm over your head. With the opposite hand, you'll feel with the pads, not the fingertips, of the three middle fingers, for lumps or any change in the texture of the breast or skin.

2. The area you'll examine is from your collarbone to your bra line and from your breastbone to the center of your armpit. Imagine the area divided into vertical strips. Using small circular motions (the size of a dime), move your fingers up and down the strips. Apply light, medium, and deep pressure to examine each spot. Repeat this same process for your other breast.

3. Gently squeeze the nipple of each breast between your thumb and index finger. Any discharge, clear or bloody, should be reported to your doctor immediately.

Figure 15-5 BREAST SELF-EXAM
The best time to examine your breasts is after your menstrual period every month.

The best tool for early detection is the diagnostic X-ray exam called **mammography.** Overall, screening mammograms could reduce breast cancer deaths by 25 percent. Mammograms can detect a tumor two to three years before it can be detected by manual exam. According to a recent report, annual mammography for women in their forties is more cost-effective than Pap smear tests for cervical cancer and installation of airbags and seat belts in vehicles.

Recent reviews of mammography's impact on breast cancer mortality have triggered disagreements about the benefits of routine mammograms.[29] Some experts have concluded there isn't enough evidence to support the claim that routine mammography lessens deaths from breast cancer.[30] Others, including the American Cancer Society, continue to recommend regular screening for women age 40 and older, not just women 50 and older.

Mammography is more likely to detect early-stage disease in white than black and Hispanic women, possibly because of lack of insurance coverage for the screening tests.[31]

Hispanic women undergo these potentially live-saving tests less often than white and African-American women and appear less likely than other women to seek follow-up mammograms in the recommended time frame.

Treatment

Breast cancer can be treated with surgery, radiation, and drugs (chemotherapy and hormonal therapy). Doctors may use one of these options or a combination, depending on the type and location of the cancer and whether the disease has spread.

Most women undergo some type of surgery. **Lumpectomy** or breast-conserving surgery removes only the cancerous tissue and a surrounding margin of normal tissue. A modified radical **mastectomy** includes the entire breast and some of the underarm lymph nodes. Radical mastectomy, in which the breast, lymph nodes, and chest wall muscles under the breast are removed, is rarely performed today because modified radical mastectomy has proven just as effective. Removing underarm lymph nodes is important to determine if the cancer has spread, but a technique called sentinel node biopsy allows physicians to pinpoint the first lymph node into which a tumor drains (the sentinel node) and remove only the nodes most likely to contain cancer cells.

Radiation therapy is treatment with high-energy rays or particles to destroy cancer. In almost all cases, lumpectomy is followed by six to seven weeks of radiation. Chemotherapy is used to reach cancer cells that may have spread beyond the breast—in many cases even if no cancer is detected in the lymph nodes after surgery.

The use of the drugs paclitaxe (Taxol) or docetaxel (Taxotere), which inhibit cell division, in addition to standard chemotherapy, can significantly lower the risk of recurrence. A new biological therapy—a monoclonal antibody that zeros in on cancer cells like a miniature guided missile—also has shown promise against some aggressive breast tumors. The drug Herceptin targets a defective growth-promoting gene (HER-2/neu) found in about 30 percent of women with breast cancer. The combination of Herceptin and standard chemotherapy has significantly improved survival rates in women with this gene.

Cervical Cancer

An estimated 12,200 cases of invasive cervical cancer are diagnosed in the United States every year, with about 4,100 annual deaths from this disease. The highest incidence rate occurs among Vietnamese women; Alaskan Native, Korean, and Hispanic women also have higher rates than the national average. The mortality rate for African-American women is more than twice that of whites, largely because of a high number of deaths among older black women.

The primary risk factor for cervical cancer is infection with certain types of the human papilloma virus (HPV), discussed in Chapter 13. HPV occurs in more than 99.7 percent of cervical cancer cases. However, not every HPV infection becomes cervical cancer, and while HPV infection is very common, cervical cancer is not. Other risk factors for cervical cancer include early age of first intercourse, multiple sex partners, genital herpes, and smoking or significant exposure to passive smoking.

The standard screening test for cervical cancer is the Pap smear. New, more precise forms of Pap testing and new screening tests for HPV may help detect cases of cervical cancer at earlier stages. A vaccine against HPV, currently in development, might prevent 450,000 new cases of cervical cancer a year.[32]

Warning signs for cervical cancer include irregular bleeding or unusual vaginal discharge. In precancerous stages, cervical cells can be destroyed by laser surgery or freezing in a doctor's office.

The National Cancer Institute recommends a combination of chemotherapy and radiation rather than the standard use of radiation alone for invasive tumors. For women whose cervical cancer is detected early, cryotherapy (use of extreme cold), electrocoagulation (intense heat), or surgery are standard treatments.

Ovarian Cancer

Ovarian cancer is the leading cause of death from gynecological cancers, with 23,400 new cases diagnosed and 13,900 deaths each year. Risk factors include a family history of ovarian cancer; personal history of breast cancer; obesity; infertility (because the abnormality that interferes with conception may also play a role in cancer development); and low levels of transferase, an enzyme involved in the metabolism of dairy foods. Often women develop no obvious symptoms until the advanced stages, although they may experience painless swelling of the abdomen, irregular bleeding, lower abdominal pain, digestive and urinary abnormalities, fatigue, backache, bloating, and weight gain.

The lifetime risk of ovarian cancer in a woman with no affected relatives is 1 in 70. The risk for a woman with one first-degree relative with ovarian cancer is 1 in 20, and the risk increases with additional affected relatives. For women who may have a hereditary ovarian cancer syndrome and have mutations in genes BRCA-1 or BRCA-2, the lifetime risk may be as high as 1 in 2. Routine screening is not recommended for women who are not at known risk. For those at increased risk, an NIH consensus panel has recommended annual pelvic and rectal exams, and ultrasound imaging of the pelvic region and a blood test for a substance called CA125 every six months. In cases of very high risk, some oncologists (cancer specialists) recommend prophylactic removal of the ovaries when childbearing is completed or by no later than age 35. Treatment involves surgery, radiation therapy, and chemotherapy. The five-year survival rate is 53 percent.

Colon and Rectal Cancer

Colon and rectal, or colorectal, cancer is the third most common cancer and accounts for 10 percent of cancer deaths. Most cases occur after age 50. Both age and gender influence the risk of colon cancer. Older individuals and men are more likely to develop *polyps* (nonmalignant growths that may turn cancerous at some point) and tumors in the colon than young people and women.

Risk factors include age (over 50), personal or family history of colon and rectal cancer, polyps in the colon or rectum, ulcerative colitis, smoking, alcohol consumption, high-fat or low-fiber diet, and inadequate intake of fruits and vegetables. Nonsteroidal anti-inflammatory drugs, such as aspirin and ibuprofen, and regular exercise may reduce the risk.

New guidelines recommend screening for colon cancer beginning at age 50, earlier for those at higher risk based on personal, family, or medical history.[33] The initial screening is crucial because it detects the largest, most dangerous polyps, which can then be removed.[34] Debate over the relative merits and limitations of sigmoidoscopy and colonoscopy continues.[35] Medical organizations have not found one screening strategy superior to others but instead emphasize the importance of screening itself.[36]

The simplest test for colon cancer, the fecal occult blood test, detects blood in a person's stool. It involves placing a small sample of feces on a card and then adding a chemical solution. If the result indicates blood, further testing is needed to detect its source. While simple and easy, it does not detect all colon cancers.[37]

Flexible sigmoidoscopy places a lighted tube into the lowest part of the colon after enemas to cleanse the lower part of the bowel. Even a single sigmoidoscopy reduces mortality from cancers in the areas examined by two-thirds. Its primary limitation is inability to screen about half of the bowel, so half of potentially cancerous polyps might not be detected. An estimated 1 to 3 percent of adults have cancerous growths that would not be detected

by sigmoidoscopy alone.[38] Current recommendations call for repeat sigmoidoscopies every five years, but some researchers recommend a shorter time interval of every three years.[39]

In a colonoscopy, a physician inserts a lighted tube with a camera at its end through the rectum after laxative solutions have cleared feces from the bowel. The colonoscope can be used to sample suspicious areas in the colon and to remove polyps (small growth) that may be precancerous. Colonoscopy is more sensitive and specific than sigmoidoscopy or fecal blood testing, but it also is more expensive and entails greater risks. This screening test should be repeated every ten years. (See Figure 15-6.)

Other forms of screening for colorectal cancer include a specific type of X ray called a double-contrast barium enema and "virtual colonoscopy," a still-experimental technique that uses data from CT or MRI scans to generate 2- or 3-dimensional images of the colon.[40]

Early signs of colorectal cancer are bleeding from the rectum, blood in the stool, or a change in bowel habits. Treatment may involve surgery, radiation therapy, and/or chemotherapy.

Prostate Cancer

After skin cancer, prostate cancer is the most common form of cancer in American men. The risk of prostate cancer is 1 in 6; the risk of death due to metastatic prostate cancer is 1 in 30.[41] More than a quarter of men diagnosed with cancer have prostate cancer. The disease strikes African-American men more often than white; Asian and American Indian men are affected less often.[42]

The risk of prostate cancer increases with age, family history, exposure to the heavy metal cadmium, high number of sexual partners, and history of frequent sexually transmitted diseases. An inherited predisposition may account for 5 to 10 percent of cases. A purported link between vasectomy and prostate cancer has been disproven.[43]

The development of a simple annual screening test that measures levels of a protein called prostate-specific antigen (PSA) in the blood has revolutionized the diagnosis of prostate cancer. PSA testing is recommended for men at high risk (African Americans and men with close relatives with prostate cancer) starting at age 45 and for all men at age 50. It remains controversial, however. Some

Transverse colon

Ascending colon

Appendix

☐ Sigmoidoscopy
■ Colonoscopy

Sigmoid colon

Rectum

Figure 15-6 SCREENING FOR COLON CANCER
Flexible sigmoidoscopy examines about half of the colon—the sigmoid colon and rectum. In a colonoscopy the physician examines the entire colon.

claim that PSA testing saves lives; others, that it leads to unnecessary and potentially harmful treatments.[44]

Treatment may include hormones, chemotherapy, and radiation. The five-year survival rate is 97 percent.

Testicular Cancer

In the last 20 years the incidence of testicular cancer has risen 51 percent in the United States—from 3.61 to 5.44 per 100,000. It is not clear why testicular cancer is on the rise, although researchers speculate that changing environmental or socioeconomic risk factors could have a role. Testicular cancer occurs mostly among young men between the ages of 18 and 35, who are not normally at risk of cancer. At highest risk are men with an undescended testicle (a condition that is almost always corrected in childhood to prevent this danger). To detect possibly cancerous growths, men should perform monthly testicular self-exams, as shown in Figure 15-7.

 Although college-age men are among those at highest risk of testicular cancer, three in four do not know how to perform a testicular self-examination. Only 8 to 14 percent examine their testicles regularly.[45]

Often the first sign of this cancer is a slight enlargement of one testicle. There also may be a change in the way it feels when touched. Sometimes men with testicular cancer report a dull ache in the lower abdomen or groin, along with a sense of heaviness or sluggishness. Lumps on the testicles also may indicate cancer.

A man who notices any abnormality should consult a physician. If a lump is indeed present, a surgical biopsy is necessary to find out if it is cancerous. If the biopsy is positive, a series of tests generally is needed to determine whether the disease has spread.

Treatment for testicular cancer generally involves surgical removal of the diseased testis, sometimes along with radiation therapy, chemotherapy, and the removal of nearby lymph nodes. The remaining testicle is capable of maintaining a man's sexual potency and fertility. Only in rare cases is removal of both testicles necessary. Testosterone injections following such surgery can maintain potency. The chance for a cure is very high if testicular cancer is spotted early.

Leukemia

Risk factors for this cancer of the blood include Down syndrome and other inherited abnormalities and excessive exposure to radiation or certain chemicals, such as benzene. Leukemia can be difficult to detect early because its symptoms are often similar to those of less serious conditions, such as influenza. Diagnosis is based on blood tests and a bone-marrow biopsy. Treatment may involve chemotherapy, drugs, blood transfusions, and bone-marrow transplants.

Lung Cancer

Cigarettes cause most cases of lung cancer, which is the leading cause of cancer deaths in women and in men. Risk factors include cigarette smoking; exposure to certain industrial substances, particularly asbestos; radiation or

Figure 15-7 TESTICULAR SELF-EXAM
The best time to examine your testicles is after a hot bath or shower, when the scrotum is most relaxed. Place your index and middle fingers under each testicle and the thumb on top, and roll the testicle between the thumb and fingers. If you feel a small, hard, usually painless lump or swelling, or anything unusual, consult a urologist.

© Lawrence Migdale

Two-pack-a-day smokers are 15 to 25 times more likely to die of cancer than nonsmokers.

radon exposure; and environmental tobacco smoke. A smoker's risk of developing lung cancer drops almost to that of a nonsmoker within ten years after his or her last cigarette, although the lungs may still be damaged.

Warning signs include a persistent cough, sputum streaked with blood, chest pain, recurring bronchitis, or pneumonia. Diagnosis is based on a chest X ray, sputum cytology (cell) testing, and fiber-optic bronchoscopy (direct examination of the lungs by means of a specially lighted tube). The use of CT scans, which can detect tiny tumors, and molecular markers in sputum can lead to earlier diagnosis and might improve survival rates. Treatment generally involves surgery, chemotherapy, and/or radiation. The five-year survival rate for all stages combined is just 15 percent.

Oral Cancer

Heavy smoking of cigarettes, cigars, or pipes; excessive drinking; and the use of chewing tobacco increase the risk of oral cancer. Those who drink as well as smoke are particularly vulnerable. More young Americans are being diagnosed with oral and tongue cancer.

Early signs include a mouth sore that bleeds easily and doesn't heal; a lump or thickening; a reddish or whitish patch; and difficulty chewing, swallowing, or moving the tongue or jaws. Regular exams by your dentist or primary care physician can detect oral cancers. Surgery and radiation are the standard treatments.

New Hope Against Cancer

A variety of treatments have had a dramatic effect on improving the prognosis and decreasing mortality rates for most major cancers. Conventional cancer therapies include:

:: *Surgery* to remove a tumor and surrounding cells. The oldest and most widely used approach, surgery is most effective for small, localized cancers.

:: *Radiation therapy,* which exposes the involved area of the body to powerful radiation, which destroys cancer cells. Radiation therapy is sometimes used as an adjuvant, or supplementary, treatment along with surgery or chemotherapy.

:: *Chemotherapy,* which uses powerful drugs or hormones, taken orally or through injection, to interfere with the reproduction of fast-multiplying cancer cells.

:: *Biological Therapies.* New drugs that target specific molecular abnormalities in cancer cells hold promise as extremely potent weapons against various cancers. Some researchers have described these medications as having the potential to change the way doctors treat cancer in much the same way the discovery of antibiotics changed the way doctors treated infections.[46]

Some of these agents block signals that instruct a cancer cell to grow out of control. Others drive cancer cells to self-destruct or keep tumors from building new blood vessels to supply themselves with food and oxygen.

However, cancer therapy remains a challenging experience for patients and their families, and many turn to unproven alternative therapies. (See Savvy Consumer: "Alternative Cancer Treatments.")

The FDA accelerates approval of new treatments that give people suffering from serious or life-threatening diseases earlier access to promising new drugs. These include the first in a new class of anticancer agents known as proteasome inhibitors for multiple myeloma, a cancer of the bone marrow, and a single agent treatment for people with the most common form of lung cancer in the United States.

Bone-marrow transplantation involves extremely high doses of radiation or, increasingly, chemotherapy to kill cancer cells; however, the marrow in the patient's body is also destroyed. The patient then receives healthy bone-marrow cells, either his or her own (which may have undergone treatment in a laboratory) or a carefully matched donor's. *Autologous* transplants (those using the person's own blood) have produced long-term survival rates of more than 50 percent for certain leukemias and lymphomas (cancer of the immune system). Most patients with leukemia and other life-threatening cancers who survive the initial recovery period following bone marrow transplants have survival rates that approach that of the general population.

Cancer treatments affect normal, healthy cells as well as cancerous ones. Most vulnerable to radiation and chemotherapy are the fastest-growing body cells: hair cells, cells of the gastrointestinal tract, cells in the reproductive organs, and cells of the blood-producing tissue, the bone marrow.

Promising advances in cancer treatment that may save lives in the future include **gene therapy,** the insertion of genes into a patient, as a possible cancer treatment, and the development of cancer vaccines. Immunotherapy uses substances such as interferons (proteins produced by cells to resist viruses) and interleukins (proteins released by certain white blood cells to support the growth of others) to attack cancer cells.

Using the Mind to Help the Body

The powers of the mind also can be a powerful resource for cancer patients. In fact, knowledge itself can be powerful. Cancer patients who participate in educational programs that explain their disease and treatment have significantly higher survival rates. Support groups also affect both the quality and quantity of life. Patients with melanoma who attended support groups did much better

Savvy Consumer

ALTERNATIVE CANCER TREATMENTS

About one-third of cancer patients use alternative medicine, such as meditation, reflexology, herbal medicine, food supplements, or homeopathy. None of these can cure cancer, but some may help ease patient suffering when used to complement mainstream treatments. Nonetheless, alternative therapies that are overused or used in lieu of mainstream treatments can be dangerous to a patient's health. Keep these points in mind when evaluating unconventional treatments for cancer:

- Special diets, especially those rich in high-antioxidant foods, may help prevent cancer. No diet can cure cancer.

- Vitamins, even in very high doses, cannot cure cancer. Excessive amounts of vitamins and minerals can be harmful and may even speed tumor growth.

- Over-the-counter herbal remedies for cancer can be contaminated or diluted with useless leaves.

- Detoxification regimens, such as high colonic irrigation to remove toxins thought to cause cancer, can be dangerous and have resulted in infection and death.

- Among the alternative therapies that can decrease pain and improve the quality of a cancer patient's life are relaxation techniques, massage, and aromatherapy.

- Patients should never put their trust in an alternative practitioner who encourages them to avoid or stop conventional cancer therapy.

- Many websites offering cancer information, particularly about unproven or alternative therapies, are unreliable. Always check that the website creators are clearly identified, that their credentials are reputable, and that the posting date is recent.

both on psychological tests and on measures of tumor-fighting immune cells. Melanoma patients with strong religious and spiritual beliefs also were able to cope with their illness better and to view it in a positive, meaningful way.

Cancer Survivorship

The estimated 8.9 million cancer survivors make up one of the fastest growing groups in the American population.[47] Many have had no evidence of cancer for years; others are in remission, a state in which the spread of cancerous cells is presumed to be temporarily stopped. (See Fact or Fiction? "A cancer diagnosis . . . .")

But for millions of men, women, and children who "win" their battle against cancer, survival, even when they live past the milestone five-year mark, does not mark the end of their cancer experience. Many cancer survivors encounter difficulties that persist for years after initial diagnosis and treatment. These include physical problems, such as pain and fatigue, that can stem from the cancer itself or from cancer treatments. Sexual problems are a common consequence, affecting as many as 50 percent of women surviving breast and gynecologic cancers and as many as 70 percent of men surviving prostate cancer. Coping with cancer also causes psychological and emotional difficulties that can lead to depression, posttraumatic stress disorder, and profound fear of recurrence. Another source of anxiety is the cost of medical treatments, which, along with the loss of wages or a job, can be financially devastating.

Cancer survivors also are at risk of another bout with cancer. Of the 1.3 million new cancer cases diagnosed each year, almost 100,000 are second cancers. Patients surviving one cancer have almost twice the risk of developing a second cancer as the general population has of developing an initial cancer. Children under age 15 who have survived cancer have eight times the risk. Young women

FACT OR FICTION? ???????????????

A cancer diagnosis usually is a death sentence.

Fiction: The majority of people diagnosed with all types of cancer—62 percent—survive for at least five years. For many cancers, particularly those detected early, survival rates are much higher. Among women with local breast cancer that has not spread to the lymph nodes, 97 percent live for five years. For men diagnosed in the earliest stages of prostate cancer, the survival rate is 100 percent. Even the most lethal form of skin cancer, melanoma, has a 96 percent survival rate when caught early. The cancers with the lowest survival rates affect the pancreas, liver, and lungs.

Source: *Cancer Facts and Figures—2003.* Atlanta: American Cancer Society, 2003.

treated with radiation for Hodgkin disease remain at exceptionally high risk of breast cancer for 25 or more years and require lifetime surveillance.[48]

✖ Diabetes Mellitus

About 100 million people around the world, including nearly 16 million people in the United States, have **diabetes mellitus,** a disease in which the body doesn't produce or respond properly to insulin, a hormone essential for daily life. In those who have diabetes, the pancreas, which produces insulin (the hormone that regulates carbohydrate and fat metabolism) doesn't function as it should. When the pancreas either stops producing insulin or doesn't produce sufficient insulin to meet the body's needs, almost every body system can be damaged.

Understanding Diabetes

Glucose is the primary form of sugar that the body cells use for energy. When a healthy person eats a meal, the level of glucose in the blood rises, triggering the production and release of insulin by special cell clusters in the pancreas called the islets of Langerhans. Insulin enhances the movement of glucose into various body cells, bringing down the level of glucose in the blood. In those who have diabetes, however, insulin secretion is either nonexistent (referred to as type 1 or *insulin-dependent diabetes*) or deficient (referred to as type 2 or *non–insulin-dependent diabetes*). Without sufficient insulin, the glucose in the blood is unable to enter most body cells, so the cells' energy needs aren't met. The levels of glucose in the blood rise higher and higher after each meal. This unused glucose eventually passes through the kidneys, which are unable to process the excessive glucose, and out of the body in urine.

Deprived of the fuel it needs, the body begins to break down stored fat as a source of energy. This process produces weak acids, called ketones. A buildup of ketones leads to ketoacidosis, an upheaval in the body's chemical balance that brings on nausea, vomiting, abdominal pain, lethargy, and drowsiness. Severe ketoacidosis can lead to coma and eventual death.

✍ Who Is at Risk for Developing Diabetes?

One in three Americans with diabetes is not aware of having an illness that increases the risk of blindness, kidney failure, cardiovascular disease, and premature death. The incidence of this potential killer, which jumped about a third in the last decade, is growing so fast that Dr. Allen Spiegel, director of the National Institute of Diabetes and Digestive and Kidney Diseases (NIDDK), describes it as "a

definite epidemic."[49] There has been a particularly dramatic rise in type 2 diabetes in children and adolescents, especially among minority populations. "The fact that kids just past puberty are getting type 2 diabetes blows us out of the water compared to what we were taught in medical school, which was that type 2 diabetes was a disease of aging," says Dr. Spiegel.

Uncontrolled glucose levels slowly damage blood vessels throughout the body, thus individuals who become diabetic early in life may face devastating complications even before they reach middle age. "Diabetes is already the number one cause of blindness, nontraumatic amputations, and kidney failure, and diabetes increases by two or three times the risk of heart attack or stroke," says Dr. Robert Sherwin of Yale University, president of the American Diabetes Association, who estimates that the disease may affect 22 million Americans within the next two decades.[50]

Lifestyle factors, especially a lack of physical activity, greatly increase the risk for type 2 diabetes.[51] Television watching, more than other sedentary activities such as sewing, reading, writing, and driving, is strongly associated with weight and obesity, a risk factor for diabetes in both children and adults. In a ten-year study of 1,058 individuals with type 2 diabetes, watching television for 2 to 10 hours a week increased the risk of diabetes 66 percent; 21 to 40 hours per week more than doubled the risk; more than 40 hours a week nearly tripled the risk.[52]

To identify individuals with this disease as early as possible, the American Diabetes Association now recommends screening every three years for all men and women beginning at age 45. Those at highest risk include relatives of diabetics (whose risk is two and a half times that of others), obese persons (85 percent of diabetics are or were obese), older persons (four out of five diabetics are over

STRATEGIES FOR PREVENTION

Lowering the Risk of Diabetes

- Eat a diet rich in complex carbohydrates (bread and other starches) and high-fiber foods, and low in sodium and fat.

- Eat fruits and vegetables that are rich in antioxidants, substances that prevent oxygen damage to cells.

- Keep your weight down. Weight loss for those who are overweight can sometimes decrease or eliminate the need for insulin or oral drugs. For individuals at high risk of developing type 2 diabetes, losing just half the pounds needed to reach their ideal weight can prevent the onset of the disease.

- Exercise regularly. Regular, vigorous aerobic activity reduces the risk of type 2 diabetes in men and women.

Individuals with type 1 or insulin-dependent diabetes control their disease by injecting insulin.

age 45), and mothers of large babies (an indication of maternal prediabetes). A child of two parents with type 2 diabetes faces an 80 percent likelihood of also becoming diabetic.

The early signs of diabetes are frequent urination, excessive thirst, a craving for sweets and starches, and weakness. Diagnosis is based on tests of the sugar level in the blood. Researchers are working to develop a test that would help identify telltale antibodies in the blood; this could indicate that pancreas cells are being destroyed years before the first signs of diabetes.

Dangers of Diabetes

Before the development of insulin injections, diabetes was a fatal illness. Today diabetics can have normal life spans. However, both types of diabetes can lead to devastating complications, including increased risk of heart attack or stroke, blindness, and loss of circulation to the extremities. Diabetes is the most common cause of kidney failure.[53]

Diabetic women who become pregnant face higher risks of miscarriage and babies with serious birth defects; however, precise control of blood sugar levels before conception and in early pregnancy can lower the likelihood of these problems. The development of diabetes during pregnancy, called *gestational diabetes,* may pose potentially serious health threats to mother and child years later. Women who develop gestational diabetes are more than three times as likely to develop type 2 diabetes if they have a second pregnancy; their infants may be at increased risk of cardiovascular disease later in life.

Diabetes and Ethnic Minorities

Several minority groups, especially African Americans, Native Americans, and Hispanics, are at high risk of developing diabetes. One in every ten African Americans and Hispanics has this disease. The members of some Native American tribes are 300 percent more likely to develop diabetes than the general population. For many, obesity and unhealthy food choices increase the risk. Researchers now believe that the interaction of environmental factors and genes varies among different racial and ethnic groups.

Treatment

The goal for diabetics is to keep blood sugar levels as stable as possible to prevent complications, such as kidney damage. Home glucose monitoring allows diabetics to check their blood sugar levels as many times a day as necessary and to adjust their diet or insulin doses as appropriate.

An estimated 6 to 7 million Americans use insulin or insulin analogues.[54] Newer insulin therapies help patients with diabetes maintain better control of blood sugar levels around the clock.[55] Types of insulin differ in how long it takes to start working after injection (onset), when it works hardest (peak), and how long it lasts in the body (duration). Individuals with diabetes may use different types in various combinations, depending on time of day and timing of meals.[56]

Those with type 1 diabetes require daily doses of insulin via injections, an insulin infusion pump, or oral medication. Those with type 2 diabetes can control their disease through a well-balanced diet, exercise, and weight management. However, insulin therapy may be needed to keep blood glucose levels near normal or normal, thereby reducing the risk of damage to the eyes, nerves, and kidneys.

Medical advances hold out bright hopes for diabetics. Laser surgery, for instance, is saving eyesight. Bypass operations are helping restore blood flow to the heart and feet. Dialysis machines and kidney and pancreas transplants save many lives. Researchers are exploring various approaches to prevention, including early low-dose insulin therapy, oral insulin to correct immune intolerance, and immunosuppressive drugs. A true cure may come through transplanting insulin-producing cells from healthy pancreases. In preliminary trials, this procedure has helped patients become insulin-independent.

⬛ Other Major Illnesses

Other noninfectious diseases besides cancer and diabetes have a debilitating effect on many people. But most of the diseases discussed in this section can be controlled, if not cured.

Epilepsy and Seizure Disorders

About 10 percent of all Americans will have at least one seizure at some time. Between 0.5 and 1 percent of all Americans have recurrent seizures. Derived from the Greek word for seizure, **epilepsy** is the term used to refer to a variety of neurological disorders characterized by sudden attacks (seizures) of violent muscle contractions and unconsciousness. Epilepsy is rarely fatal; the primary danger to life is to suffer an attack while driving or swimming.

Seizures can be major, referred to as *grand mal;* minor, referred to as *petit mal;* or psychomotor. In a grand-mal seizure, the person loses consciousness, falls to the ground, and experiences convulsive body movements. Petit-mal seizures are brief, characterized by a loss of consciousness for 10 to 30 seconds, by eye or muscle flutterings, and occasionally by a loss of muscle tone. About 90 percent of all epileptics have grand-mal seizures; 40 percent suffer both petit-mal and grand-mal seizures. The frequency of attacks defines the severity of the epilepsy. Diagnosis is based on a history of recurring attacks and a study of the brain's electrical activity, called an electroencephalogram (EEG).

About half of all cases of epilepsy have no known cause and are therefore classified as *idiopathic.* All others stem from conditions that affect the brain, such as trauma, tumors, congenital malformations, or inflammation of the membranes covering the brain. Idiopathic epilepsy usually begins between the ages of 2 and 14. Seizures before age 2 are usually related to developmental defects, birth injuries, or a metabolic disease affecting the brain. (Fever-induced convulsions are not related to epilepsy.) Seizures after age 14 are generally symptoms of brain disease or injury.

Seizure disorders don't reflect or affect intellectual or psychological soundness; people who suffer from them have normal intelligence. Therapy with anticonvulsant drugs can control seizures in most people, and once seizures are under control, epileptics can live full, normal lives by continuing to take their medications. However, about 10 to 20 percent of the 120,000 people who develop epilepsy every year continue to have seizures despite medical therapy. Early treatment of seizures by paramedics with benzodiazepines can prevent serious neurologic damage.

Technological advances have allowed doctors to identify more accurately where seizures originate in the brain; and surgery, though risky and expensive, is offering new hope to many epileptics.

If you're with a person who suffers a grand-mal seizure, make sure he or she isn't injured during the attack. Don't try to restrain the person or interfere with his or her movements, and don't try to force anything into the person's mouth.

Respiratory Diseases

See Chapter 13 for the major infectious respiratory diseases and Chapter 12 for smoking-induced problems. In addition to the diseases treated below, chronic bronchitis and emphysema can also be causes of disability and death.

⬛ What Is Asthma?

Asthma is a disease characterized by constriction of the breathing passages. As with allergy, asthma rates have skyrocketed in the last two decades. Asthma-related problems account for more than half a million hospital stays each year and 14 deaths each day in the United States, according to the Asthma and Allergy Foundation of America.

 The Centers for Disease Control and Prevention (CDC) estimates that approximately 17 million people in the United States, or 6.4 percent of the population, say they have asthma. Asthma is more common among blacks and other inner-city residents. The disease disproportionately affects African Americans. A black man in New York City is 11 times more likely to die from asthma than other men in the city.[57]

While asthma is not always linked to allergy, the two are related. Among people with asthma, 90 percent of the children, 70 percent of young adults, and 50 percent of older adults also have allergies. According to epidemiologic research, 23 percent of youngsters diagnosed with allergies by age 1 develop asthma by age 6. Of those diagnosed after age 1, 13 percent eventually become asthmatic. Symptoms include wheezing, coughing, shortness of breath, and chest tightness. If the symptoms are untreated or undertreated, they can worsen and damage the lungs.

The number of people with asthma continues to increase into adulthood. However, as shown by a study that followed college students for 23 years, most report that their symptoms improve or disappear.[58] (See Student Snapshot: "Asthma in College—and Beyond.")

The two main approaches to asthma treatment are control of the underlying inflammation by means of anti-inflammatory drugs, such as corticosteroids, cromolyn sodium, and nedocromil, and short-term relief of symptoms with bronchodilators, such as albuterol, which expand the breathing passages. In its most recent official guidelines, the National Heart, Lung, and Blood Institute encouraged more frequent use of inhaled steroids and less reliance on bronchodilators, which have little effect on the underlying inflammation.

Student Snapshot — Asthma in College—and Beyond

In their initial study, researchers evaluated 1,837 freshman at Brown University for medical conditions, including asthma and allergy. Some 23 years later, 1,601 alumni completed a detailed question-naire about asthma and allergies. The prevalence of asthma continues to increase until age 40 or 42. However, of the alumni with active asthma at follow-up, asthma symptoms had either improved or disappeared in three-fourths. Of the remaining fourth, most said their symptoms were unchanged; only a small number reported worsening of their symptoms.

Source: Helen Skolnick and Robert Wood. "Natural History of Asthma: A 23-Year Follow-Up of College Students. *Pediatrics,* Vol. 198, No. 2, August 2001, p. 547.

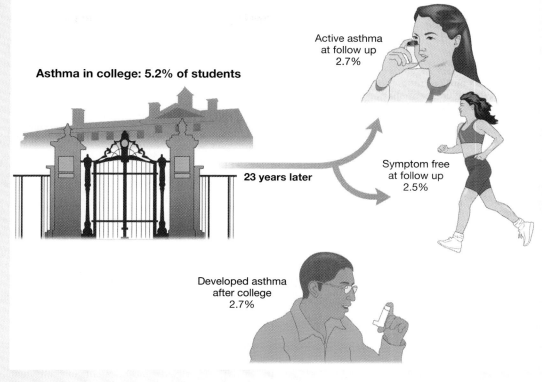

Asthma in college: 5.2% of students

23 years later

Active asthma at follow up 2.7%

Symptom free at follow up 2.5%

Developed asthma after college 2.7%

Although medications can help relieve asthma symptoms in the short term, prolonged use of the most popular drugs, the short-acting beta-agonists, actually can produce the opposite effect by closing air passages. Many people with severe asthma use more medication as their symptoms worsen—but the drugs actually exacerbate their condition. The reason, researchers theorize, may be that continuous use of asthma medications changes how the airway contracts in ways that intensify the constriction and make breathing more difficult.[59]

Chronic Obstructive Lung Disease (COLD)

Chronic obstructive lung disease (COLD), also called chronic obstructive pulmonary disease (COPD), is characterized by progressively more limited flow of air into, and out of, the lungs. COLD consists of two separate but closely related conditions: chronic bronchitis and emphysema. Most COLD patients develop both forms. The major cause is cigarette smoking, although air pollution may also play a role.

In chronic bronchitis, the bronchial passageways are constantly inflamed, and individuals develop a persistent, sputum-producing cough; shortness of breath; and wheezing. They must stop smoking, lose excess weight, exercise, and avoid or reduce contact with air pollutants.

Chronic bronchitis can lead to emphysema, a deterioration of the lungs that may begin in adolescence. Eventually, the alveoli, tiny air sacs in the lungs, tear, reducing the lungs' ability to exhale. This condition can lead to heart failure.

Anemias

The **anemias** are diseases affecting the oxygen-carrying capacity of the blood. Usually there's a reduced number of red blood cells or a reduced amount of hemoglobin, the oxygen-carrying component of red blood cells. Anemia

Biological Photo Service (both)

(a)   (b)

Sickle-cell anemia. (a) Normal mature red blood cells are disk-shaped and concave. (b)In sickle-cell anemia, the red blood cells are crescent-shaped and jagged, causing them to pile up and obstruct small blood vessels. Areas of the body are thus deprived of oxygen and nutrients.

can be caused by nutritional inadequacies; loss of blood, including heavy menstrual bleeding; deficiencies in red-cell production; or genetic disorders. Iron-deficiency anemia is a form of anemia caused by a lack of dietary iron, an essential component of the hemoglobin molecule that carries oxygen. It's the most common form of anemia and often goes undiagnosed in women.

:: *Sickle-cell anemia* is a genetic blood disorder that occurs when the hemoglobin contained in the red blood cells is abnormal. The red blood cells become crescent or sickle-shaped and unable to supply oxygen to body tissues (see photos above). This disease causes crippling, severe pain, and premature death. About 8 to 10 percent of African Americans carry the gene for sickle-cell anemia.

:: *Pernicious anemia* results from a lack of vitamin B_{12} (cobalamine), which causes a deficiency in the formation of red blood cells. Although B_{12} is usually present in the diet, some people lack a substance needed to absorb it into their blood. Injections of B_{12} can control this condition.

:: *Aplastic anemia,* most common in young adults and adolescents, interferes with the bone marrow's ability to form blood. Usually it results from ingesting a toxic agent, often a medication; symptoms include multiple internal hemorrhages. Whole-blood transfusions are the primary therapy, but the condition is usually fatal.

Liver Disorders

Cirrhosis is characterized by significant loss of liver cells and the formation of scar tissue that can interfere with circulation in the liver. The major cause of one of the most common forms of cirrhosis, Laennec's cirrhosis, is chronic alcoholism. Each year, about 30,000 Americans die of alcohol-related liver disorders. (See also Chapter 11.)

Early signs of liver damage include an enlarged liver (which your doctor can feel during a physical exam) and tiny, spiderlike blood vessels on the surface of the skin.

Blood tests may show abnormal levels of certain enzymes or enlarged red blood cells. Even people with advanced liver disease feel better and live longer once they've stopped drinking alcohol. Cirrhosis symptoms, which occur only in the advanced stages of the disease, include yellow discoloration of the skin and eyes (jaundice), accumulation of fluid in the abdomen, and mental confusion.

Liver transplants are the only hope for those with advanced liver disease. With improvements in surgical techniques and the use of antirejection drugs (including cyclosporin, a combination of cyclosporin and an antifungal medication, and a drug called FK-506), 70 percent or more of liver-transplant recipients—including some in their sixties and seventies—now live for at least a year. Some liver transplant recipients have lived longer than 20 years.

Kidney Diseases

A wide range of diseases can affect the kidneys and their ability to process fluids and waste. Some are acute, temporary problems; others are chronic, progressive illnesses that permanently impair kidney function.

Nephrosis refers to a cluster of symptoms indicating chronic damage to the kidneys, including chronic proteinuria (the loss of more than 1 gram of protein a day in the urine), hypercholesteremia (high levels of fats in the blood), and edema (fluid retention). The kidney damage can be the result of diabetes, heavy metal poisoning, allergic reactions to insect stings, or other disorders.

Kidney stones can form either from calcium salts or from minerals (the causes are unknown). Most stones eventually pass out of the body in urine, which can be extremely painful. They don't usually obstruct the flow of urine or interfere with kidney function. However, infection can develop behind a stone. Larger stones can be surgically removed or painlessly shattered into harmless fragments by high-frequency sound waves.

The various chronic and inflammatory diseases of the kidney can all lead to kidney failure. A mechanical process of clearing waste fluids from the body, called *dialysis,* can do the kidneys' job temporarily. Another alternative is a kidney transplant, either from a living, related donor or from a cadaver whose kidney has been carefully tissue-matched to the recipient to minimize the risk of rejection. On average, a transplanted kidney continues to function for only nine years. Kidneys that came from cadaver donors are especially likely to deteriorate slowly but steadily. The antirejection drugs that transplant recipients must take may themselves cause side effects and impair the functioning of the new kidney over time. High blood pressure and high glucose and cholesterol levels also can be harmful. A lack of organ donors remains a critical obstacle to performing more of these lifesaving operations.

Digestive Diseases

Most disorders of the digestive tract affect only one section: either the esophagus, the stomach and duodenum, the small intestine, the large intestine, the liver, the pancreas, the gallbladder, or the rectum. The most dangerous are Crohn's disease and ulcerative colitis. According to the National Digestive Diseases Advisory Board, almost half of the U.S. population will suffer a digestive problem at some time in their lives.

Ulcers

Open sores, often more than an inch wide, that develop in the lining of the stomach or the duodenum (the first part of the small intestine) are called **ulcers.** They are caused by excessive acidic digestive juices. The major symptom is a burning pain felt throughout the upper abdomen. The pain may come and go, lasting up to three hours. It may begin either right after eating or several hours later.

One in five men and one in ten women get ulcers of the stomach or duodenum, but the number of ulcers is declining. Risk factors include heavy use of cigarettes, alcohol, or caffeine; the ingestion of large amounts of painkillers that contain aspirin or ibuprofen; and advanced age. Bleeding is not common but may be dangerous, even life-threatening. An untreated stomach ulcer can lead to serious weight loss and anemia.

Researchers have identified a bacterium, *Helicobacter pylori* that may infect the digestive system and set the stage for ulcers. According to various studies, most ulcer patients carry this organism. One theory is that infection leads to an inflammation of the stomach lining called gastritis, which increases vulnerability to other stressors, such as smoking, alcohol, or anxiety.

H. pylori can be detected in several ways. A blood test can reveal the presence of infection by detecting antibodies against *H. pylori.* However, a blood test can be positive

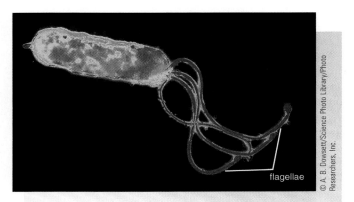

The bacterium *Helicobacter pylori* has flagellae that enable it to tunnel beneath the protective layer coating the stomach lining.

flagellae

© A. B. Dowsett/Science Photo Library/Photo Researchers, Inc.

even if someone has long been free of the bacteria. The most definitive test requires endoscopy, a procedure in which a physician examines the lining of the stomach or duodenum by passing a thin flexible tube (an endoscope) down the patient's throat and snips a small bit of tissue for laboratory analysis to detect bacteria. Researchers are experimenting with a simpler diagnostic breath test in which patients drink a special liquid that triggers a response by *H. pylori* bacteria in the stomach. Treatment with antibiotics leads to improvement in most patients.

Conventional therapy for ulcers includes self-help measures, such as avoiding aspirin; eating small, frequent meals; taking antacids; and not smoking or drinking alcohol or caffeine. Drugs such as cimetidine, ranitidine, and sucralfate can reduce the amount of acid produced by the stomach and relieve ulcer symptoms. If a stomach ulcer doesn't heal after six to eight weeks of drug treatment, physicians may recommend surgery to remove the ulcer.

Inflammatory Bowel Disease (IBD)

As many as 2 million Americans—many in the prime of life—suffer from one of the two forms of **inflammatory bowel disease (IBD):** *Crohn's disease,* which causes inflammation anywhere in the digestive tract, and *ulcerative colitis,* which creates severe ulcers in the inner lining of the colon and rectum. Both illnesses can trigger frequent and intense diarrhea, abdominal pain, gas, fever, and rectal bleeding.

The specific causes of IBD remain unknown, but scientists speculate that some irritating substance—perhaps a bacterium, virus, or chemical or environmental agent—somehow leaks through the intestine's thin lining into the bowel's deep inner wall. Inflammation develops, setting into motion a chain of harmful reactions by the body's protective immune system and causing swelling, pain, and damage to the intestinal wall. Ulcers (small perforations or holes) may form, exposing cells and tissues to destructive intestinal bacteria and enzymes. Blood and fluid from body tissues may leak into the intestines, showing up as diarrhea or blood in the stool. Twenty percent of cases involve a genetic or familial predisposition.

Treatment for IBD consists primarily of drugs, including powerful steroids, antibiotics, and medications that fight inflammation. Dietary changes can also help. Crohn's patients who don't improve on medication or who develop life-threatening complications, such as a severe intestinal blockage, may undergo surgery to remove or bypass the diseased part of the intestine and reconnect two healthy segments. However, the disease very often recurs in another part of the intestinal tract. For those with ulcerative colitis, removal of the entire colon brings an end to troubling symptoms—and to the increased risk of colon cancer that these individuals face. Most gastroenterologists advise patients with ulcerative colitis to undergo annual colonoscopies to detect precancerous changes in cells.

Irritable Bowel Syndrome

Irritable bowel syndrome (also called irritable colon or spastic colon) is a common problem caused by intestinal spasms. The muscular contractions that move waste material through the intestines become irregular and uncoordinated, causing frequent feelings of a need to defecate, nausea, cramping, pain, gas, and a sensation that the rectum is never emptied.

Diagnostic tests, including X rays, stool samples, and sigmoidoscopy, can rule out colon cancer and other problems. Travel, stress, changes in diet, and smoking often worsen these symptoms. Many people respond well to a high-fiber diet; others prefer a bland diet. There's no standard medical treatment for irritable bowel syndrome; some physicians prescribe stool softeners, laxatives, or drugs to reduce intestinal spasms.

Gallstones

An estimated 25 million Americans—about 10 percent of the population—have **gallstones:** clumps of solid material, usually cholesterol, that form in bile stored in the gallbladder. One-third to one-half of all gallstones produce no symptoms. However, some gallstones, carried out of the liver with bile, get stuck in the bile duct and cause intense pain that lasts for several hours. Ultrasound and special X rays called cholecystograms can detect gallstones.

During an attack of gallstone pain, a physician may recommend a painkiller. Some gallstones can be dissolved by long-term drug treatment. Another alternative to traditional gallbladder surgery is laparoscopic surgery, in which gallstones are removed without having to cut through the major abdominal muscles.

Disorders of the Muscles, Joints, and Bones

Because they're constantly being used, muscles, joints, and bones are more susceptible to damage from injury than are most other parts of the body.

Arthritis

More than 22 million people suffer from some form of **arthritis,** an inflammatory disease of the joints that takes over a hundred forms. Rheumatoid arthritis is an autoimmune disease in which the body attacks its own connective tissue; it's fairly common among younger people. Degenerative arthritis, or osteoarthritis, characterized by changes in bone tissue and cartilage, primarily at the joints, seems to be the result of normal wear and tear.

Women are generally affected by arthritis three times more often than are men, until the seventh or eighth

Those who suffer arthritis pain may tend to minimize movement in their joints, but moderate activity can help functioning in muscles that stabilize the joints.

David Young-Wolff/PhotoEdit

decade of life. Race and occupation don't seem to be factors; climate affects symptoms but not causes.

Aggressive treatment of arthritis pays off, but to be successful, early diagnosis before cartilage destruction occurs is critical. The most effective therapies include anti-inflammatory agents, which prevent or delay joint destruction and new drugs called COX-2 inhibitors. An educational arthritis self-help course can reduce physician visits by 40 percent and pain perception by about 20 percent. Relaxation training and cognitive-behavioral techniques also have proven highly effective in controlling arthritis pain.

The goal of all treatments for arthritis is to maintain the patient's ability to function. Drugs can relieve pain and reduce inflammation; surgical treatments, including total joint replacement, and physical therapy are also used to maintain motion and strength, and to correct deformities.

Hernias

A **hernia** is a bulge of soft tissue that forces its way through or between strained or weakened muscles. Hernias can occur in many parts of the body, but they're most common in the abdominal wall. A surgeon can push the protruding tissue back into place and tighten or sew together the loose muscles.

Backaches

Back woes, which rank second only to headaches among modern miseries, eventually afflict seven of every ten adults. Anyone from a college athlete to a retired grandparent can suffer a back injury, but the risks increase with time as the deeper muscles and tendons surrounding the

FACT OR FICTION????????????????

College athletes are at greater risk for lower back pain later in life.

Fiction: About one in three intercollegiate rowers develop back pain during their college career, and they often worry that they will continue to have back problems throughout life. This is not the case. In a study of 1561 former competitive rowers who had graduated a mean of 13 years previously, rowers—even those who develop back pain during college—are no more likely than the general population to have episodic back pain or to miss work because of back pain. Rowers who do not develop back pain in college have significantly lower rates of back pain as they age than the general population.

Source: Carol Teitiz, et al. "Back Pain in Former Intercollegiate Rowers: A Long-Term Follow-Up Study." *American Journal of Sports Medicine,* Vol. 31, No. 4, July–August 2003, p. 590.

spine become less resilient. Yet age itself is rarely the only factor in a disabling back attack; almost always tense, injured, or weak muscles are to blame. Other risk factors include extra pounds, particularly if stuffed into a pot belly; lack of exercise; poor posture; and bending from the waist to hoist a heavy load. (See Fact or Fiction? "College athletes are at greater risk . . . .")

Strain from use or abuse accounts for 80 percent of back ailments. Most vulnerable is the lower, or lumbar, part of the spine, which bears the greatest pressure when bending and lifting. Five to 10 percent of back problems involve the discs between the vertebrae. Most common is the protrusion (or herniation) of the soft center of a disc through the casing so that it presses on spinal nerves. Another 10 percent of back problems involve structural defects, which may be the result of injuries, tumors, arthritis, congenital malformations, osteoporosis (the weakening of the bones), or scoliosis (side-to-side curving of the spine). Sometimes a sore back is a symptom of diseases of other organs, such as the kidneys, gallbladder, or stomach. A physical exam and various tests, including electrodiagnostic studies, X rays, CT scans, and MRIs (magnetic resonance imaging), may be necessary to pinpoint the problem.

Bed rest, supplemented by moist heat or other muscle relaxants and anti-inflammatory drugs, eases most backaches. However, the days when doctors advised two weeks of bed rest for a bad back are gone. After two or three days, most back patients are urged to get up, start walking, and resume light activity.

STRATEGIES FOR PREVENTION

Preventing Back Problems

- When standing, shift your weight from one foot to the other. If possible, place one foot on a stool, step, or railing 4 to 6 inches off the ground. Hold in your stomach, tilt your pelvis toward your back, and tuck in your buttocks to provide crucial support for the lower back.

- Because sitting places more stress on the lower back than standing, try to get up from your seat at least once an hour to stretch or walk around. Whenever possible, sit in a straight chair with a firm back. Avoid slouching in overstuffed chairs or dangling your legs in midair. When driving, keep the seat forward so that your knees are raised to hip level; your right leg should not be fully extended. A small pillow or towel can help support your lower back.

- Sleep on a flat, firm mattress. The best sleep position is on your side, with one or both knees bent at right angles to your torso. The pillow should keep your head in line with your body so that your neck isn't bent forward or to the side.

- When lifting, bend at the knees, not from the waist. Get close to the load. Tighten your stomach muscles, but don't hold your breath. Let your leg muscles do the work.

- Don't smoke. Smoking may interfere with circulation to the lower back; and a chronic smoker's cough can be so irritating that it provokes a back spasm.

Back specialists tailor treatment programs to an individual's needs. Different forms of physical therapy—including specific exercises, massage, heat, ultrasound, and electrical stimulation—often relieve pain and speed recovery. COX-2 inhibitors, which include drugs like Vioxx, could benefit migraine and back pain sufferers as well as those with arthritis.[60]

Back pain may account for 40 percent of visits to chiropractors, 20 percent of visits to massage therapists, and 14 percent of visits to acupuncturists. Do these alternative treatments work? According to recent analysis, spinal manipulation is not found any more effective than traditional back pain management.[61] The effectiveness of acupuncture for back pain remains unclear, but massage has proven effective in relieving persistent back pain."[62] (See Chapter 16 for a comprehensive discussion of complementary and alternative medicine.)

Skin Disorders

Your skin is the largest organ of your body. Because of its visibility, none of its problems may seem trivial. Two serious skin diseases are discussed below.

Eczema and Dermatitis

Dermatitis is any inflammation of the skin. *Eczema,* a specific type of dermatitis usually caused by allergies, is a skin inflammation that results from internal processes. Symptoms of eczema include redness, flaking, blistering, and thickening of the skin. Self-help treatments include avoiding irritants, such as dishwater, and using steroid creams containing 0.5 percent hydrocortisone.

Psoriasis

In **psoriasis,** the rate of skin cell production is speeded up. As skin cells pile up faster than they can be shed, they produce scaly, deep pink, raised patches on the skin. Triggers of psoriasis are stress, skin damage, and illness. Self-help measures include sunbathing or using ultraviolet light to clear up the psoriasis. Physicians usually prescribe ointments, creams, or pastes, including some steroid preparations, or ultraviolet treatment.

Special Needs for Different Abilities

About 49 million Americans have physical or mental impairments, including blindness, deafness, disorders of the muscles or nerves, paralysis, loss of limbs, or mental retardation, that substantially limit one or more major life activities. Most are the result of illnesses, such as strokes, arthritis, or heart disease, and affect the ability to walk, speak, or live independently. Some congenital disorders, such as cerebral palsy, cause speech problems, muscular weakness, and mental retardation. Accidents are responsible for other disabilities, including paralysis.

Individuals with special needs and abilities can live full, happy, and productive lives. Famous people who've made major contributions to the world despite disabilities include the composer Ludwig van Beethoven, who wrote some of his most famous music after becoming deaf; the inventor Thomas A. Edison, who was deaf throughout much of his life; and President Franklin D. Roosevelt, who became paralyzed in both legs at the age of 39.

Few such problems can be cured, but a great deal can be done to overcome them. **Rehabilitation medicine,** the specialty dedicated to improving the condition of the disabled, can provide treatments such as surgery for certain types of blindness or deafness, medications to ease the crip-

pling pain of arthritis, and physical therapy, including special exercises to build up endurance and muscle strength. Mechanical devices, such as electric wheelchairs, artificial limbs, and hearing aids, can open up wider worlds to people with disabilities. Occupational therapy teaches skills to help them gain confidence, and vocational training prepares them to find employment.

Individuals with special needs face special challenges in their daily lives. Some are primarily physical, such as difficulty bathing, lifting groceries, opening cans and bottles, or going someplace. They also face many social and economic challenges. Because some people feel uncomfortable about disabilities, they may not treat individuals with special needs with the same acceptance and respect that they show to others. This can lead to discrimination from employers.

The Americans with Disabilities Act protects people with disabilities from discrimination by private employers, requires wheelchair access to public buildings and mass transportation, and orders telephone companies to provide telephone relay services that allow people with impaired speech or hearing to make and receive calls. Many states require insurers to provide coverage for high-risk individuals such as cancer survivors. The names of many of the organizations that help the disabled, such as the National Coalition for Cancer Survivorship and the National Library Service for the Blind and Physically Handicapped, are in "Your Health Almanac" at the back of the book.

The Bottom Line ▼
Protecting Yourself from Cancer and Major Illnesses

You may not be able to control every risk factor in your life or environment, but you can protect yourself from the obvious ones.

:: *Avoid excessive exposure to ultraviolet light.* If you spend a lot of time outside, you can protect your skin by using sunscreen and wearing long-sleeve shirts and a hat. Also, wear sunglasses to protect your eyes. Don't purposely put yourself at risk by binge-sunbathing or by using sunlamps.

:: *Avoid obvious cancer risks.* Besides ultraviolet light, other environmental factors that have been linked with cancer include tobacco, asbestos, and radiation.

:: *Eat a variety of healthful foods, with an emphasis on whole foods and plant sources.* Populations that eat diets high in vegetables and fruit and low in animal fat, meat, and/or calories have reduced risk of some of the most common cancers.

:: *Keep moving.* Physical activity may reduce the risk of certain cancers as well as provide other important health benefits.

:: ***Watch your weight.*** Overweight and obesity are associated with increased risk for cancers at several sites: breast (among post-menopausal women), colon, endometrium, adenocarcinoma of the esophagus, and kidney.

:: ***If you drink alcoholic beverages, limit consumption.*** The risk of cancers of the mouth, pharynx, larynx, esophagus, liver, and breast increases substantially with intake of more than 2 drinks per day for men or one drink for women.

:: ***Be alert to changes in your body.*** You know your body's rhythms and appearance better than anyone else, and only you will know if certain things aren't right. Changes in bowel habits, skin changes, unusual lumps or discharges—anything out of the ordinary—may be clues that require further medical investigation.

CNN After watching the CNN video segment, discuss the following question. Can phytochemicals found in fruit, vegetables and whole grain stop the growth of cancer cells?

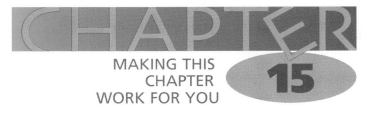

MAKING THIS
CHAPTER
WORK FOR YOU **15**

1. Which of the following statements about cancer is true?
   a. When cancer cells spread to another part of the body, the process is called infiltration.
   b. Cancer occurs when abnormal cells grow and spread uncontrollably until they form an ectoplasm.
   c. Those cancers that have been shown to be triggered by viruses are contagious.
   d. In some sense, all cancers are caused by genetic abnormalities.

2. Signs that a cancer might be inherited include all of the following *except*
   a. family history
   b. late development of the disease
   c. a diagnosis of retinoblastoma
   d. unusual gender pattern in the incidence of the disease

3. You can protect yourself from certain types of cancer by
   a. eating a diet rich in antioxidants.
   b. avoiding people who have had cancer.
   c. wearing sunscreen with an SPF of less than 15.
   d. using condoms during sexual intercourse.

4. Which of the following statements about skin cancer is true?
   a. Individuals with a large number of moles are at decreased risk for melanoma.
   b. The most serious type of skin cancer is squamous-cell carcinoma.
   c. The safest way to get a tan and avoid skin cancer is to use tanning salons and sunlamps instead of sunbathing in direct sunlight.
   d. Individuals with a history of childhood sunburn are at increased risk for melanoma.

5. A woman's risk of developing breast cancer increases if
   a. she is African American under the age of 50.
   b. she had her first child when in her teens or twenties.
   c. her husband's mother had breast cancer.
   d. she began menstruating when she was 15 or 16.

6. Prostate cancer
   a. occurs mostly among men between the ages of 18 and 35.
   b. is usually more aggressive in white men.
   c. has a low survival rate.
   d. can be detected through a screening test that measures the levels of prostate-specific antigen in the blood.

7. Which of the following statements about diabetes mellitus is *false?*
   a. The two types of diabetes are insulin-dependent and non–insulin-dependent.
   b. The incidence of diabetes has decreased in the last decade, especially among African Americans, Native Americans, and Latinos.
   c. Individuals with diabetes must measure the levels of glucose in their blood to ensure that it does not rise to unsafe levels.
   d. Untreated or uncontrolled diabetes can lead to coma and eventual death.

8. With asthma,
   a. the most common symptom is a persistent, sputum-producing cough.
   b. the recommended treatments include antibiotics to eliminate the underlying infection and bronchodilators to expand the breathing passages.
   c. an individual experiences wheezing and shortness of breath because of constricted breathing passages.
   d. if the disease is untreated, it may lead to emphysema.

9. Major disorders of the digestive system include all of the following *except*
   a. irritable bowel disease
   b. Crohn's disease
   c. gallstones
   d. abdominal hernia

10. Which of the following statements is *false?*
   a. Psoriasis is the most severe form of dermatitis.
   b. In rheumatoid arthritis, the body attacks its own connective tissue.

c. Sickle-cell anemia is a fatal genetic blood disorder of African Americans.
d. Cirrhosis of the liver is commonly caused by chronic alcoholism.

Answers to these questions can be found on page 652.

Critical Thinking

1. Do you have family members who have had cancer? Were these individuals at risk for cancer because of specific environmental factors, such as long-term exposure to tobacco smoke? If no particular cause was identified, what other factors could have triggered their diseases? Are you concerned that you might have inherited a genetic predisposition to any particular type of cancer because of your family history?

2. A friend of yours, Karen, discovered a small lump in her breast during a routine self-examination. When she mentions it, you ask if

Critical Thinking

she has seen a doctor. She tells you that she hasn't had time to schedule an appointment; besides, she says she's not sure it's really the kind of lump one has to worry about. It's clear to you that Karen is in denial and procrastinating about seeing a doctor. What advice would you give her?

3. Because of advances in antirejection treatment, organ transplants have proven highly successful in helping many people who otherwise might have died. Even elderly patients have clearly benefited from donated kidneys and livers.

Critical Thinking

However, because the demand for organs to transplant greatly exceeds the supply, health experts have debated setting priorities. Should a 30-year-old be placed higher on the waiting list for a particular organ than a 70-year-old? Should a nurse who needs a liver because she contracted hepatitis on the job get priority over an alcoholic whose liver has been destroyed by cirrhosis? Who, if anyone, should make such decisions? Would a lottery be a fair way to determine who receives an available organ?

Profile Plus

The vast majority of cancers are caused by lifestyle and environmental factors. Determine your risks with this activity on your Profile Plus CD-ROM.

Profile Plus

• Cancer Risk

Profile Plus

Sites & Bytes

American Cancer Society
www.cancer.org

The site features comprehensive information about different kinds of cancer: statistics, early detection, prevention, treatment options, alternative treatments, and coping strategies for families. In addition, you can type in your zip code and find local resources or order books from the online bookstore.

Sites and Bytes

The Susan G. Komen Breast Cancer Foundation
www.komen.org

This site features an excellent personal breast cancer risk analysis and a multimedia library, including a self-exam video and a mammogram video.

Sites and Bytes

American Diabetes Association
www.diabetes.org

Here you will find the latest information on both type 1 and type 2 diabetes mellitus, including suggestions regarding diet and exercise. The online bookstore features meal planning guides, cookbooks, and self-care guides. Type in your zip code to find community resources.

InfoTrac College Edition

Activity

Drab, Scott. "Diabetes: Past, Present, and Future." *Diabetes Forecast,* Vol. 55, No. 11, November 2002, p. 11(1).

1. What led to the discovery of the cause of diabetes?

2. Describe three mechanisms of action of the current medications used to treat diabetes.

InfoTrac College Edition

3. What current research will hopefully result in a cure of diabetes?

You can find additional readings related to cancer with InfoTrac College Edition, an online library of more than 900 journals and publications. Follow the instructions that were packaged

InfoTrac College Edition

with your textbook; then search for articles using a key word search.

For additional links, resources, and suggested readings on InfoTrac College Edition, visit our Health & Wellness Resource Center at **http://health.wadsworth.com**.

Key Terms

The terms listed are used on the page indicated. Definitions of the terms are in the Glossary at the end of this book.

Key Terms

anemia 523
arthritis 526
asthma 522
bone-marrow
     transplantation 518
carcinogen 508
chemoprevention 508
chronic obstructive lung
     disease (COLD) 523
cirrhosis 524
dermatitis 528
diabetes mellitus 520
epilepsy 522

Key Terms

gallstones 526
gene therapy 518
hernia 526
infiltration 504
inflammatory bowel
     disease (IBD) 525
irritable bowel
     syndrome 526
kidney stones 524
lumpectomy 515
mammography 514
mastectomy 514
metastasize 504

Key Terms

neoplasm 504
nephrosis 524
oncogene 504
psoriasis 528
rehabilitation
     medicine 528
relative risk 505
tamoxifen 508
tumor suppressor
     gene 504
ulcer 525

References

1. *Cancer Facts & Figures—2003.* Atlanta: American Cancer Society, 2003.
2. Wizeman, Theresa, and Mary-Lou Pardue. *Exploring the Biological Contributions to Human Health: Does Sex Matter?* Washington, DC: National Academy Press, 2001.
3. Kaklamani, Virginia. "TGFBR1*6A and Cancer Risk," *Journal of Clinical Oncology,* Vol. 21, No. 17, September 1, 2003, p. 3236.
4. *Cancer Facts & Figures for African Americans—2003–2004.* Atlanta: American Cancer Society, 2003.
5. *Cancer Facts & Figures for Hispanics/Latinos—2003.* Atlanta: American Cancer Society, 2003.
6. *Cancer Facts & Figures—2003.*
7. Calle, Eugenia, et al. "Overweight, Obesity, and Mortality from Cancer in a Prospectively Studied Cohort of U.S. Adults." *New England Journal of Medicine,* Vol. 348, No. 17, April 24, 2003, p. 1625.
8. *Fulfilling the Potential of Cancer Prevention and Early Detection.* Washington, DC: National Academy of Sciences, 2003.
9. Mariani, Sara. "Highlights From the 2003 Annual Meeting of the American Association for Cancer Research." Washington, DC, July, 2003. www.medscape.com/viewarticle/458995
10. *Fulfilling the Potential of Cancer Prevention and Early Detection.*
11. U.S. Preventive Services Task Force. *Routine Vitamin Supplementation to Prevent Cancer and Cardiovascular Disease.* Rockville, MD: Agency for Healthcare Research and Quality, 2003.
12. *Fulfilling the Potential of Cancer Prevention and Early Detection.*
13. *Cancer Facts & Figures—2003.*
14. Goldstein, Beth, and Adam Goldstein. "Diagnosis and Management of Malignant Melanoma." *American Family Physician,* Vol. 63, No. 7, April 1, 2001, p. 1101.
15. Gorgos, Diana. "Intensity of Lifetime Sun Exposure Tied to Melanoma Risk." *Dermatology Nursing,* Vol. 15, No. 3, June 2003, p. 288.
16. Beddingfield, Frederick. "Melanoma Strikes Men and Women Differently." Presentation, Society for Investigative Dermatory, Annual Meeting, Washington, DC, May 12, 2001.
17. Goldstein and Goldstein, "Diagnosis and Management of Malignant Melanoma."
18. Ford, Leslie. Personal interview.

19. Wrensch, Margaret, et al. "Risk Factors for Breast Cancer in a Population With High Incidence Rates." *Breast Cancer Research,* Vol. 5, No. 4, July 2003, p. 88.
20. "Drinking Increases Risk." *Women's Health Weekly,* February 6, 2003, p. 2.
21. Robb-Nicholson, Celeste. "Alcohol and Breast Cancer." *Harvard Women's Health Watch,* Vol. 10, No. 9, May 2003, p. 1.
22. Li, Christopher, et al. "Relationship Between Long Durations and Different Regimens of Hormone Therapy and Risk of Breast Cancer." *Journal of the American Medical Association,* Vol. 289, No. 24, June 25, 2003, p. 3254.
23. Gann, Peter, and Monica Morrow. "A Single-Edged Sword." *Journal of the American Medical Association,* Vol. 289, No. 24, June 25, 2003, p. 3304.
24. Chlebowski, Rowan, et al. "Influence of Estrogen Plus Progestin on Breast Cancer and Mammography in Healthy Postmenopausal Women." *Journal of the American Medical Association,* Vol. 289, No. 24, June 25, 2003, p. 3243.
25. Thomas, David B., et al. "Randomized Trial of Breast Self-Examination in Shanghai: Final Results." *Journal of National Cancer Institute,* Vol. 94, No. 19, October 2, 2002, p. 1445.
26. Harris, Russell, and Linda Kinsinger. "Routinely Teaching Breast Self-Examination Is Dead. What Does This Mean?" *Journal of National Cancer Institute,* Vol. 94, No. 19, October 2, 2002, p. 1420.
27. Smith, R. A. "Screening Mammography." *Ca—A Cancer Journal for Clinicians,* Vol. 53, No. 3, 2003, p. 141.
28. "American Cancer Society Issues Updated Breast Cancer Screening Guidelines," News Release, May 15, 2003.
29. Christensen, Damaris. "A Decades-Old Debate: Do Mammograms Save Lives?" *Consumers Research Magazine,* Vol. 85, No. 7, July, 2002, p. 26.
30. Duffy, Stephen, et al. "The Impact of Organized Mammography Service Screening on Breast Carcinoma Mortality in Seven Swedish Counties." *Cancer,* Vol. 95, No. 3, August 1, 2002, p. 458.
31. Jacobellis, Jillian, and Gary Cutter. "Mammography Screening and Differences in Stage of Disease by Race/Ethnicity." *American Journal of Public Health,* Vol. 92, No. 7, July 2002, p. 1144.
32. Mariani, "Highlights from the 2003 Annual Meeting of the American Association for Cancer Research."

33. U.S. Multisociety Task Force on Colorectal Cancer. "Screening Guidelines for Colorectal Cancer." *Gastroenterology,* Vol. 124, February 2003, p. 544.
34. Mitka, Mike. "Colon Cancer Screening Guidelines Stress Initial Test's Importance." *Journal of the American Medical Association,* Vol. 289, No. 10, March 12, 2003, p. 1334.
35. Walsh, Judith, and Jonathan Terdiman. "Colorectal Cancer Screening: Scientific Review." *Journal of the American Medical Association,* Vol. 289, No. 10, March 12, 2003, p. 1288.
36. Walsh, Judith, and Jonathan Terdiman. "Colorectal Cancer Screening: Clinical Applications." *Journal of the American Medical Association,* Vol. 289, No. 10, March 12, 2003, p. 1414.
37. Torpy, Janet. "Colon Cancer Screening." *Journal of the American Medical Association,* Vol. 289, No. 10, March 12, 2003, p. 1089.
38. Fletcher, Robert. "Screening Sigmoidoscopy—How Often and How Good?" *Journal of the American Medical Association,* Vol. 290, No. 1, July 2, 2003, p. 106.
39. Schoen, Robert, et al. "Results of Repeat Sigmoidoscopy 3 Years after a Negative Examination." *Journal of the American Medical Association,* Vol. 290, No. 1, July 2, 2003, p. 41.
40. Walsh and Terdiman, "Colorectal Cancer Screening: Scientific Review."
41. Nelson, William. "Prostate Cancer." *New England Journal of Medicine,* Vol. 349, No. 4, July 24, 2003, p. 366.
42. "Prostate Cancer: New Test Identifies Aggressive and Less Aggressive Forms." *Cancer Weekly,* July 9, 2002, p. 25.
43. Strayer, Scott. "Vasectomy Not a Risk Factor for Prostate Cancer." *Journal of Family Practice,* Vol. 51, No. 9, September 2002, p. 791.
44. Sirovich, Brenda, et al. "Screening Men for Prostate and Colorectal Cancer in the United States." *Journal of the American Medical Association,* Vol. 289, No. 10, March 12, 2003, p. 1334.
45. Courtenay, Will. "Behavioral Factors Associated with Disease, Injury, and Death Among Men: Evidence and Implications for Prevention." *Journal of Men's Studies,* Vol. 9, No. 1, Fall 2000, p. 81.
46. McCarthy, Michael. "Targeted Drugs Take Center Stage at US Cancer Meeting." *Lancet,* Vol. 357, No. 9268, May 19, 2001, p. 1593.

References

47. *Cancer Facts & Figures—2003.*

48. Travis, Lois, et al. "Breast Cancer Following Radiotherapy and Chemotherapy Among Young Women With Hodgkin Disease." *Journal of the American Medical Association,* Vol. 290, No. 4, July 23, 2003, p. 529.

49. Spiegel, Allen. Personal interview.

50. Sherwin, Robert. Personal interview.

51. Hu, Frank, et al. "Diet, Lifestyle, and the Risk of Type 2 Diabetes Mellitus in Women." *New England Journal of Medicine,* Vol. 345, No. 11, September 13, 2001, p. 790.

52. Ibid.

53. Parmer, Sharon. "Diabetes and the Kidney." *Journal of the American Medical Association,* Vol. 289, No. 24, June 25, 2003, p. 3372.

54. DeWitt, Dawn, and Irl Hirsch. "Outpatient Insulin Therapy in Type 1 and Type 2 Diabetes Mellitus." *Journal of the American Medical Association,* Vol. 289, No. 17, May 7, 2003, p. 2254.

References

55. DeWitt, Dawn, and David Dugdale. "Using New Insulin Strategies in the Outpatient Treatment of Diabetes." *Journal of the American Medical Association,* Vol. 289, No. 17, May 7, 2003, p. 2265.

56. Parmer, Sharon. "Insulin." *Journal of the American Medical Association,* Vol. 289, No. 17, May 7, 2003, p. 2254.

57. Hopkins, Janice. "Asthma 'Crisis' for Black Americans." *British Medical Journal,* Vol. 323, No. 7308, August 11, 2001, p. 302.

58. Skolnick, Helen, and Robert Wood. "Natural History of Asthma: A 23-Year Follow-up of College Students." *Pediatrics,* Vol. 108, No. 2, August 2001, p. 547.

59. Shore, Stephanie, and Jeffrey Drazen. "β-Agonists and Asthma: Too Much of a Good Thing?" *Journal of Clinical Investigation,* Vol. 112, August 2003, p. 495.

References

60. "COX-2 Inhibitors Aid Back Pain Sufferers." *Clinician Reviews,* Vol. 13, No. 7, July 2003, p. 34(2).

61. Assendelft, W. J., et al. "Spinal Manipulative Therapy for Low Back Pain: A Meta-Analysis of Effectiveness Relative to Other Therapies." *Annals of Internal Medicine,* Vol. 138, June 3, 2003, p. 871.

62. Cherkin, D. C., et al. "A Review of the Evidence for the Effectiveness, Safety, and Cost of Acupuncture, Massage Therapy, and Spinal Manipulation for Back Pain." *Annals of Internal Medicine,* Vol. 138, June 3, 2003, p. 898.

16 Health-Care Consumerism and Complementary/ Alternative Medicine

Long after she immigrated to the United States from India, Tapu's grandmother refused to go to Western doctors. She preferred practitioners who used the herbs and techniques she had relied on in her homeland. Tapu's father, an American-trained physician, would argue with his mother-in-law about what he considered her old-fashioned views. As a doctor's son, Tapu grew up believing in the superiority of Western medicine.

In his sophomore year at college, Tapu found out that he needed oral surgery. To his surprise, the oral surgeon suggested an alternative method of controlling post-operative pain: acupuncture. "My

dad's never going to approve," he said. "And he's the one who's still paying my medical bills." The doctor referred Tapu—and his father—to recent studies conducted by National Institute of Health researchers on acupuncture's efficacy in relieving postsurgical pain. After doing more research online, Tapu agreed to try acupuncture following his operation.

Like Tapu, millions of Americans are turning to complementary and alternative medicine (CAM), a term that includes a broad range of healing philosophies, approaches, and therapies not traditionally taught in

medical schools or provided in hospitals. But consumers are learning that they have to be just as savvy—and skeptical—about these therapies and practitioners as they are with any other form of health care.

Because there are so many health-care choices, you face a greater responsibility for your personal well-being. Whether you are monitoring your blood pressure, considering elective surgery, or deciding whether to try an alternative therapy, you need to gather information, ask questions, weigh advantages and disadvantages, and take charge of your health. The reason: No one cares more about your health than you do, and no one will do more to promote your well-being than you.

© Lightscapes Photography, Inc./CORBIS

After studying the material in this chapter, you should be able to:

- **List** ways of becoming an informed health-care consumer.
- **Discuss** strategies for self-care, as well as how to get the best possible health care.
- **Describe** common medical exam procedures and medical tests.

- **Identify** strategies for maintaining good oral health.
- **List** your rights as a medical consumer.
- **Describe** the different types of complementary and alternative therapies and **explain** what research has shown about their effectiveness.
- **Compare** and **contrast** the different types of health-care practitioners and health-care facilities.
- **Explain** what managed care is.

✖ Becoming a Savvy Health-Care Consumer

Americans are the world's foremost health-care consumers. We see more health practitioners, undergo more surgery, take more prescription drugs, and spend more time in hospitals than the citizens of any other nation. Not surprisingly, we also spend more money on health care.

Yet not every American receives good, or even adequate, medical care. Consumers have long complained about insensitive treatment, lack of comprehensive care, and far too little emphasis on the prevention of disease. Because of recent efforts to curb spending, health-care providers may seem to pay greater attention to cost than caring. And because of a lack of insurance, millions of people have limited access, or no access at all, to needed health services.

It's up to you. Knowing how to spot health problems, how to evaluate health news, what to expect from health-care professionals, and where to turn for appropriate treatment can help you keep your own costs down while ensuring the best possible care.

Health Care and the College Student

All of the more than 14 million men and women enrolled in institutions of higher learning need some health-care services, regardless of their age or general health. The Preventive Services Task Force of the U.S. Public Health Service recommends that all adolescents and young adults have periodic screenings for high blood pressure, obesity, and problem alcohol consumption and that they receive regular counseling concerning the use of drugs, tobacco, and alcohol; sexually transmitted infections; effective contraception; a healthy diet; exercise; oral health; and prevention of motor vehicle injuries and other accidents.[1]

In addition to the medical services available at student health centers, colleges provide health information. According to a CDC survey of approximately 4,600 undergraduates at 136 colleges and universities, about three-quarters of undergraduates have received some form of health information.[2] About half of all students surveyed had been given some information on prevention of alcohol and drug use and HIV infection and AIDS.

Black students were more likely than white students to say they'd been taught about AIDS and HIV in college classes. African-American, Hispanic, or students of other racial and ethnic groups also were more likely than whites to report receiving information on any health topic. More traditional full-time students between ages 18 and 24 who have never been married and were not working full-time had received health information, compared to part-time, older, nontraditional students.

Because undergraduates are remarkably diverse, they also vary in their health beliefs and practices, particularly when born outside the United States in countries with different medical traditions. A recent study that compared the health beliefs of undergraduates born in the United States, China, and India found unexpected similarities and differences. Regardless of their origins, students identified the same four factors as very important for keeping healthy: enough rest and sleep, physical exercise, proper weight, and eating proper foods. The students also agreed on the need for rest and sleep in recovering from an illness. Only 20 percent of American-born students—compared with 40 percent of those born in China and 48 percent of those born in India—said seeing a nurse or doctor promptly was very important for recovering from illness. More of the India-born students placed great importance on eating proper foods, taking vitamins, and religious faith for recovery. The largest proportion of each group placed their greatest faith in doctors and in their families to help them when sick.[3] [See Student Snapshot: "Health Beliefs of Students," p. 537.]

Informing Yourself

Knowledge is power. In the case of health care, knowledge gives you the power to make the best possible decisions about your well-being.

☞ How Can I Evaluate Online Health Advice?

The Internet has become a major source of health information—and misinformation—with more than 10,000 health-related sites. According to a national survey, approximately 40 percent of Americans with Internet access occasionally use it to obtain health information or advice. About two-thirds of respondents with no chronic health problems reported that the Internet had improved their understanding of symptoms, treatments, or conditions. However, the Internet had little impact on patients' calls or visits to doctors.[4] (See Fact or Fiction? "The Internet and e-mail. . . ." on page 537)

The Internet permits ease of access to cutting-edge medical knowledge and bridges the communication gap created by high-tech medicine. However, it also has serious drawbacks. Simple queries for terms such as obesity or depression often lead to irrelevant sites, relevant sites with incomplete information, or sites that are difficult for most consumers to understand.[5] Many sites are used to promote products or people. Some chat rooms can lead to encoun-

Student Snapshot — Health Beliefs of Students Born in the U.S., China and India

Factors Students See as Very Important in Recovering from Sickness

Source: Data from William Rothstein and Sushama Rajapaksa. "Health Beliefs of College Students Born in the United States, China, and India," *Journal of American College Heath,* Vol. 51, No. 5, March 2003, p. 189.

Factors Students See as Very Important In Recovering from Sickness

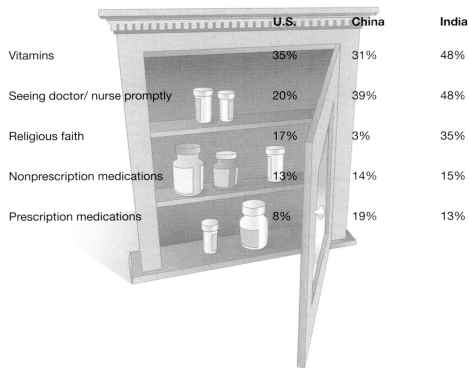

	Birthplace		
	U.S.	China	India
Vitamins	35%	31%	48%
Seeing doctor/ nurse promptly	20%	39%	48%
Religious faith	17%	3%	35%
Nonprescription medications	13%	14%	15%
Prescription medications	8%	19%	13%

FACT OR FICTION? ?????????????????

The Internet and e-mail have transformed the way patients use the health-care system.

Fiction: Although many people use the Internet for health information, very few report a significant impact on their health-care decisions. In a national survey, more than 90 percent of those who looked up health information online said the Internet had no impact on the number of times they called or visited a doctor. Only 6 percent used e-mail to contact a health-care professional; 5 percent or fewer used the Internet to obtain prescriptions.

Source: Laurence Baker et al. "Use of the Internet and E-Mail for Health Care Information." *Journal of the American Medical Association,* Vol. 289, No. 18, May 14, 2003, p. 2400.

---

ters with unpleasant people. Even when information is technically precise, laypeople may not know how to interpret it properly. Although peer-reviewed websites do offer high-quality information, fewer patients than clinicians reported that they looked for health information on these sites.[6]

Some doctors have set up websites for the sole purpose of selling drugs such as Viagra—a practice that state and federal regulators have deemed unethical, though not illegal. The American Medical Association has called for disciplinary action for doctors who prescribe drugs to people they have never met or examined. Other "cyberdocs" offer "virtual house calls" with board-certified physicians who engage in private chat sessions on minor illnesses and prescribe medicine (except controlled drugs like narcotics). In the future, videoconferencing may allow doctors to examine patients in cyberspace. However, there are no professional standards for doctors on the Internet, and experts advise caution. The doctor who treats your allergies may be a urologist or pathologist who is not up-to-date on new therapies or is unaware of potential side effects.

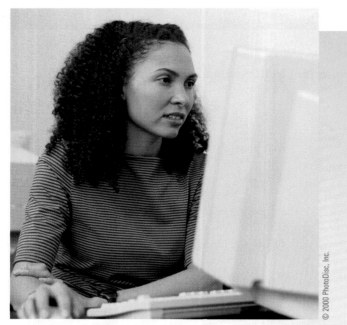

Millions of Americans go online to learn about medical problems and treatments and to chat with others who have similar questions or conditions.

Evaluating Health News

Cure! Breakthrough! Medical miracle! These words make headlines. Remember that although medical breakthroughs and cures do occur, most scientific progress is made one small step at a time. Even though medicine is considered a science, some experts estimate that no more than 15 percent of medical interventions can be supported by reliable scientific evidence.

Medical opinions invariably change over time, sometimes going from one extreme to another. For instance, several decades ago the treatment of choice for breast cancer was radical mastectomy—removal of the woman's breast, lymph nodes, and chest wall. Since then much less extensive surgery (lumpectomy), coupled with chemotherapy or radiation, or both, has proven equally effective. Once individuals who'd suffered heart attacks were advised to limit all physical activity. Today a progressive exercise program is a standard component of rehabilitation.

Health researchers are struggling to find better ways of assessing what they know and need to know in order to offer more complete and balanced information to consumers. However, sometimes the only certainty is uncertainty. Rather than putting your faith in the most recent report or the hottest trend, try to gather as much background information and as many opinions as you can. Weigh them carefully—ideally with a trusted physician—and make the decision that seems best for you.

When reading a newspaper or magazine story or listening to a radio or television report about a medical advance, look for answers to the following questions:

Here are some specific guidelines for evaluating online health sites:

:: Check the creator. Websites are produced by health agencies, health support groups, school health programs, health-product advertisers, health educators, and health-education organizations. Read site headers and footers carefully to distinguish biased commercial advertisements from unbiased sites created by scientists and health agencies.

:: If you are looking for the most recent research, check the date the page was created and last updated as well as the links. Several nonworking links signal that the site isn't carefully maintained or updated.

:: Check the references. As with other health-education materials, web documents should provide the reader with references. Unreferenced suggestions may be scientifically unsound and possibly unsafe.

:: Consider the author. Is he or she recognized in the field of health education or otherwise qualified to publish a health-information web document? Does the author list his or her occupation, experience, and education?

:: Look for possible bias. Websites may be attempting to provide healthful information to consumers, but they also may be attempting to sell a product. Many sites are merely disguised advertisements.

:: Who are the scientists involved? Are they recognized, legitimate health professionals? What are their credentials? Are they affiliated with respected medical or scientific institutions? Be wary of individuals whose degrees or affiliations are from institutions you've never heard of, and be sure that the person's educational background is in a discipline related to the area of research reported.

:: Where did the scientists report their findings? The best research is published in peer-reviewed professional journals, such as the *New England Journal of Medicine.* Research developments also may be reported at meetings of professional societies.

:: Is the information based on personal observations? Does the report include testimonials from cured patients or satisfied customers? If the answer to either question is yes, be wary.

:: Does the article, report, or advertisement include words like *amazing, secret,* or *quick?* Does it claim to be something the public has never seen or been offered before? Such sensationalized language is often a tip-off to a dubious treatment.

:: Is someone trying to sell you something? Manufacturers who cite studies to sell a product have been known to embellish the truth.

Reprinted with special permission of King Features Syndicate.

:: Does the information defy all common sense? Be skeptical. If something sounds too good to be true, it probably is.

Making Sense of Medical Research

Medical research is the only way that anyone, physician or consumer, can assess the quality of diagnostic methods, medications, or surgical treatments. The principal rule of science is that nothing works until it's been proven.

Researchers rely on a variety of studies to determine whether a new approach to prevention, diagnosis, or treatment works. These include:

:: *Epidemiological studies,* in which scientists assess the health status of a large, defined group of people, such as the population of a country or region. They may look at various health habits, such as alcohol consumption, to determine whether those who practice these habits have a higher likelihood of developing certain diseases.

:: *Animal studies,* or *preclinical trials,* in which scientists administer a drug or try a procedure on various laboratory animals to assess its safety and determine its effects.

:: *Clinical trials,* in which volunteers agree to act as test subjects—"human guinea pigs," as it were. Patients must give written permission in order to participate. Clinical trials generate data for the purpose of evaluating one or more diagnostic or therapeutic approaches in a population. Well-designed clinical trials, which must have strict eligibility criteria, a standardized

intervention, follow-up, and measures of outcome, set the "gold standard" for new diagnostic tests or medical or surgical treatments.

In *controlled studies,* the group receiving an experimental drug or treatment is compared with a group receiving no treatment or standard therapy. In *single-blind studies,* the subjects don't know whether they're receiving the experimental drug or treatment, or an inactive substance. In *double-blind studies,* neither the subjects nor the researchers have this information. In *prospective studies,* patients are selected, assessed, participate in the trial, and are then followed for a preset period. In *retrospective studies,* investigators look back at their past experiences with a certain group of patients.

The results of even the most careful studies aren't considered conclusive in and of themselves. The FDA reviews every new drug, as well as the research methods used to test it, before it's allowed on the market. And a new therapy is widely accepted (or rejected) only after publication of study results in a *peer-reviewed* journal (one in which scientists in the same field critique the research methods before accepting the paper) and after *replication* (the repetition of the same investigation by other researchers with similar results). In recent years, a technique called **meta-analysis,** which summarizes and reviews research in a particular area, has been used to evaluate the results of several large trials in a uniform manner.

One reason why study results must be confirmed is that, no matter what treatment patients receive, one-third to one-half of all patients improve temporarily. This well-documented but little-understood phenomenon is called the *placebo effect.* Scientific trials of a new treatment must show that the patients receiving the experimental medication or therapy improve *more* than those receiving a sugar pill or mock procedure (the placebo).

Evidence-Based Medicine

One of the ways in which physicians are working to improve the quality of care is by basing diagnostic testing and treatments on solid evidence produced by rigorous research studies (usually randomized controlled trials).[7] Evidence-based medicine is not an entirely new concept of medical care but a methodical approach that establishes a solid and conscientious scientific basis for decision-making about health care.[8] Evidence-based medicine pays particular attention to **outcomes,** that is, the impact that a specific medication or treatment has on a patient's condition, overall health, and quality of life.[9]

Outcomes research is designed to answer questions such as: Is treatment better or worse than no treatment? Is one treatment better than another? If a treatment is effective, is a little just as good as a lot? Does quality of life change because of treatment? Are the benefits of treatment worth the cost or the risks to the patient?

Studies of outcomes look at how patients fared with or without a specific treatment, the costs involved, and the impact of undergoing or not undergoing treatment on the patients' quality of life. Outcomes research can help determine which of several therapies or approaches provides the best results at the most reasonable costs.

When you are diagnosed with a health problem, ask your doctor if your treatment is based on the latest evidence and clinical guidelines. The National Guideline Clearinghouse provides a comprehensive database of evidence-based clinical practice guidelines for many common health problems, available at **www.guideline.gov**.

Home health tests can be more convenient and less expensive than a trip to a clinic or doctor's office.

Self-Care

Most people do treat themselves. You probably prescribe aspirin for a headache, chicken soup or orange juice for a cold, or a weekend trip to unwind from stress. At the very least, you should know what your **vital signs** are and how they compare against normal readings. (See Table 16-1.)

Once a thermometer was the only self-testing equipment found in most American homes. Now hundreds of home tests are available to help consumers monitor everything from fertility to blood pressure to cholesterol levels. (See Table 16-2.) More convenient and less expensive than a visit to a clinic or doctor's office, the new tests are generally as accurate as those administered by a professional.

TABLE 16-1	Take Your Own Vital Signs
Vital Sign	**Normal Values**
Temperature	98.9°F in the morning or 99.9°F later in the day is upper limit of the normal oral temperature for people 40 years old or younger. • Women's temperatures are slightly higher than men's. • African-Americans' temperatures are slightly higher than white Americans. Measure your temperature with a mercury or digital thermometer.
Blood pressure	120/70 to 140/90, depending on age and gender. You can measure your own blood pressure if you want to invest in blood pressure equipment. Check your local drugstore to purchase a blood pressure cuff or digital blood pressure monitor.
Pulse	72 beats per minute. Take your pulse rate at your wrist or at the carotid artery in your neck.
Respiration rate	15–20 breaths per minute.

TABLE 16-2 Home Health Tests: A Consumer's Guide	
Type of Test	**What It Does**
Pregnancy	Determines if a woman is pregnant by detecting the presence of human chorionic gonadotropin in urine. Considered 99 percent accurate.
Fertility	Measures levels of luteinizing hormone (LH), which rise 24 to 36 hours before a woman conceives. Can help women increase their odds of conceiving.
Blood pressure	Measures blood pressure by means of an automatically inflating armband or a cuff for the finger or wrist; helps people taking hypertension medication or suffering from high blood pressure monitor their condition.
Cholesterol	Checks cholesterol in blood from a finger prick; good for anyone concerned about cholesterol.
Colon cancer	Screening test to detect hidden blood in stool; recommended for anyone over 40 or concerned about colorectal disease.
Urinary tract infection	Diagnoses infection by screening for certain white blood cells in urine; advised for women who get frequent UTIs and whose doctors will prescribe antibiotics without a visit.
HIV infection	Detects antibodies to HIV in a blood sample sent anonymously to a lab. Controversial because no face-to-face counseling is available for those who test positive.

Always follow directions precisely, and if your concerns persist, see your doctor.

Self-care also can mean getting involved in the self-help movement, which has grown into a major national trend. An estimated 20 million people participate in self-help support groups. These include groups for addictions (Alcoholics Anonymous, Gamblers Anonymous); for families (Families of the Mentally Ill, Mothers of Twins Clubs); for illness/disability (National Association of People with AIDS, Tourette Syndrome Association); for mental illness (Emotions Anonymous, National Alliance of the Mentally Ill); and for lifestyles (Single Mothers by Choice, Society for the Second Self [crossdressers]). In such groups, members exchange ideas, share similar problems, and gain a new sense of control.

The National Self-Help Clearinghouse, a not-for-profit organization founded in 1976, facilitates access to self-help groups and increases awareness of the importance of mutual support. The American Self-Help Clearinghouse offers a keyword-searchable database of over 1,100 national, international, model, and online self-help support groups and a registry for persons interested in starting national or international self-help groups.[10] (See the Hales Health Almanac at the back of the book).

Oral Health

Oral health involves more than healthy teeth—it refers to the entire mouth, including all the structures that allow us to talk, bite, chew, taste, swallow, smile, scream, or scowl. Oral health is a critical part of overall health. Research has revealed links between chronic oral infection and heart and lung diseases, stroke, low birthweight, premature births, and diabetes.[11]

Thanks to fluoridated water and toothpaste, and improved dental care, Americans' oral health is better than in the past. Today's children have far less tooth decay than their parents had, and adults are keeping their teeth longer. However, as many as 32 percent of Americans are left with none of their own teeth by age 70. Without good self-care, you probably will lose some teeth to decay and gum disease. The best way to prevent such problems is through proper and regular brushing and flossing.

Gum, or periodontal, **disease,** is an inflammation that attacks the gum and bone that hold your teeth in place. The culprit is **plaque,** the sticky film of bacteria that forms on teeth. More than 300 species of bacteria live under the gum line, and about half a dozen have been linked to serious gum problems. The early stage of gum disease is called **gingivitis.** If untreated, it develops into a more serious form known as **periodontitis,** in which

Flossing every day helps prevent gum disease and other health problems. Using a gentle sawing motion, work the floss down to your gum line. Move the floss up and down to scrape the sides of each tooth. Clean between all your teeth, using a fresh section of floss for each tooth.

© Vision/Photo Researchers, Inc.

- Brush your teeth every morning and every night. Oral bacteria reach their highest count during sleep because fluids in the mouth accumulate. Nighttime cleaning reduces the bacterial population; morning cleaning lets you reduce the buildup.

- Use a toothpaste that has the American Dental Association (ADA) seal of acceptance and a toothbrush with soft, rounded bristles. Replace your toothbrush every three months.

- Hold the brush at a 45-degree angle from your gums. Pay particular attention to the space between your teeth and gums, especially on the inside, toward your tongue. Brush for two to five minutes. Don't brush too vigorously. If you scrub as hard as you can, you may damage your teeth and gums. Abrasion—a problem for more than half of American adults—erodes tooth surfaces, weakens teeth, and increases sensitivity to hot and cold foods.

- Because brushing can't reach plaque and food trapped between teeth, daily flossing is essential. Using waxed or unwaxed floss, start behind the upper and lower molars at one side of your mouth and work toward the other side.

- See your dentist twice a year for routine cleaning and examination. To find a dentist, call a local dental school, which may have a public clinic, or check with your county dental society. Ask for information regarding fees, hours, and after-hour emergency service. Your dentist should take a complete medical history from you and update it every six months, examine your mouth for signs of cancer, and thoroughly outline all treatment options.

- Make sure that everyone who works on the inside of your mouth wears a mask and rubber gloves to reduce the risk of disease transmission (that is, bacterial and viral infections, such as hepatitis, herpes, and HIV).

- Check your family's dental insurance coverage. Many dental plans cover all costs for regular six-month checkups and cleanings and a percentage of the costs for fillings, gum treatment, root canals, and so on.

plaque moves down the tooth to the roots, which then become infected. In advanced periodontitis, the infection destroys the bone and fibers that hold teeth in place.

Symptoms of gum disease include bleeding during brushing or flossing, redness and puffiness of gums, tenderness or pain, persistent bad breath or a bad taste in the mouth, receding gums, shifted or loosened teeth, and changes in the way your teeth fit together when you bite. New treatments, which offer an alternative to traditional gum surgery, include a single antibiotic injection or the implant of a small antibiotic chip in the periodontal pockets to promote healing.

Taking care of your mouth isn't important only for dental health: It may affect how long you live. Gingivitis and periodontitis trigger an inflammatory response that causes the arteries to swell, which leads to a constriction of blood flow that can increase the incidence of cardiovascular disease. Periodontal disease also leads to a higher white blood cell count, an indicator that the immune system is under increased stress. The good news: You can prevent these problems by flossing daily and brushing your teeth and your tongue (to get rid of bacteria that can cause gum disease and bad breath).

Many Americans favor dental implants, artificial teeth attached to full or partial dentures, as an option for replacing missing teeth. According to the American Dental Association (ADA), implant procedures nearly tripled in the last ten years. Tooth brighteners also have grown in popularity, but the ADA cautions against over-the-counter whitening products. Safer and more effective are in-office "power" bleaches, in which an oxidizing agent is painted onto the teeth and activated by a special light, and night-guard bleaching, which uses a bleaching gel placed in a custom-made mold and worn at night for about two weeks. Dentists often combine these two approaches. Some dentists are using lasers to whiten teeth, but the ADA has not yet evaluated or endorsed this new approach.

Getting the Best Health Care

Once patients simply put their faith in physicians and assumed that they knew best and would make the correct medical decisions. Today health care has become far more complex and impersonal. Increasingly doctors as well as consumer advocates insist that patients need to take responsibility for their own care. Rather than assuming that health care providers will do whatever is necessary and appropriate, you must take the initiative to ensure that you get quality care.

How Good is American Health Care?

Many people assume that health care in the United States is the best in the world. It certainly is the most expensive. The United States spends more than any other nation—

13.9 percent of its Gross Domestic Product, or an esti-mated $4,887 per person—on health.[12] Yet a 2003 study—the first ever "report card" for the American health care system—gave the nation's health care system poor grades for providing preventive services and adequate treatments.[13]

In the largest and most comprehensive examination of health care quality ever conducted in the United States, doctors failed to provide recommended health care nearly half the time. The researchers described these deficiencies as "serious threats . . . that could contribute to thousands of preventable deaths in the United States each year."[14]

The study, which consisted of telephone interviews and examination of medical records of 6,700 adults in twelve metropolitan areas, examined preventive care as well as the management of 30 common health problems such as diabetes, asthma, high blood pressure, and heart disease. Underuse of care occurred far more often than overuse. Patients failed to receive recommended care approximately 46 percent of the time, compared with 11 percent of the time when they received care that was not recommended and potentially harmful. Overall, patients received 55 per-cent of recommended care—whether for prevention, screening, diagnosis, treatment, or follow-up, even when they had health insurance and access to health-care services.[15]

The Doctor-Patient Partnership

Once the family doctor was indeed part of the family. The family doctor brought babies into the world, shepherded them through childhood, comforted and counseled them, stood by their bedside in their darkest hours. Patients entrusted the doctor with their cares, their confidences, their very lives. Dramatic breakthroughs in diagnosing and treating illness shifted the focus in medicine from the fam-ily physician to the specialist, from basic caring to high-tech medical care. Patients today are more likely to be cured of a vast array of illnesses than were patients a cen-tury ago. However, they often complain of insensitive, uncaring physicians who focus on their diseases rather than on them as individuals.

As more physicians have joined managed-care organi-zations (discussed later in this chapter), which emphasize efficiency, they sometimes feel pressure to see more patients a day, to spend less time with each, and to discour-age expensive tests and treatments.[16]

In a recent survey, nearly one in three doctors reported sometimes not informing patients about "useful" medical services not covered by their health insurance companies. Physicians whose salaries are closely tied to controlling costs are more likely than other doctors to withhold information.[17] Because physicians have less time

and less autonomy, patients today must do more. Your first step should be learning more about your body, any med-ical conditions or problems you develop, and your options for treatment. You can find a great deal of information via computer online services, patient advocacy and support organizations (see the Hales Health Almanac at the end of this book for listings), and libraries.

This information can help you know what questions to ask and how to evaluate what your doctor says. But you have to be willing to speak up. Busy doctors give patients less than a minute on average during a routine visit to say what's bothering them before they interrupt. This doesn't mean your doctor isn't interested, but it does mean that you have to develop good communication skills so you can tell physicians what they need to know to help you.

How Should I Choose My Primary Care Physician?

Why does a healthy young adult need a doctor? To stay healthy as long as possible, says Munsey Wheby, M.D., of the University of Virginia, president of the American College of Physicians (ACP). "At some point in early adulthood, you want to establish a relationship with a physician who will do basic screening tests, record your family history, and help you prevent problems twenty or thirty years down the road."[18]

The primary care physicians who are playing increas-ingly important roles in American health care include fam-ily practitioners, general internists, and pediatricians. Obstetrician-gynecologists serve as the primary providers of health care for more than half of all women. If you're a woman and your gynecologist is the only physician you see, make sure that he or she performs other tests, such as measuring your blood pressure, in addition to a pelvic and breast exam. If you develop other symptoms or health concerns, ask for an appropriate referral.

At college health centers, clinics, and some health-care organizations, consumers may be assigned to a primary physician or restricted to certain doctors. Even if your choices are limited, don't suspend your critical judgment. If your assigned physician does not listen to your concerns or is not providing adequate care, you can—and should—request another physician. Your rapport with your primary physician and the feelings of mutual trust and respect that develop between you can have as much of an impact on your well-being as your doctor's technical expertise.

When consumers can freely choose their physicians, they often do so, not just on the basis of qualifications, but also because of the physician's gender, race, or ethnic back-ground. Frustrated by what they see as insensitive treat-ment by male physicians, many women have turned to female physicians—especially for gynecologic care. For other health services, women say that what matters most is having a caring physician who makes them feel comfort-able and secure and invites them to participate in treat-ment decisions. Overall, patients speak more to female

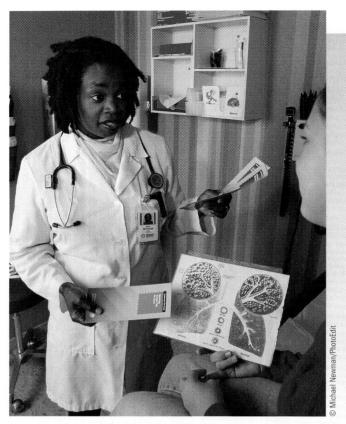

© Michael Newman/PhotoEdit

Take charge of your health by educating yourself and asking your doctor questions about your health and treatments.

physicians than male doctors, disclose more information, make more positive statements, and interrupt them more often. Female physicians also communicate higher degrees of empathy to their patients.[19]

In a study of HMO patients in California, patients who chose doctors of the opposite gender generally were more satisfied with their physicians than patients who selected doctors of the same gender. Fewer women who chose female physicians (74 percent) were satisfied with their doctors than male patients who chose female physicians (85 percent). About 79 percent of female patients of male doctors and male patients of male doctors were satisfied. The reason, the researchers theorized, may be that the women expected female doctors to provide more communication and personalized care—which may not have been possible because they were working part-time and had larger workloads.[20]

As the number of minority physicians has increased, more racial and ethnic minority group members are seeking out physicians with similar backgrounds. Often they see them as role models for their children. They may also feel that these professionals will have a natural empathy for their needs and concerns. Language also affects patient choices. Some individuals, such as Mexican-American and Puerto Rican patients, find it easier to communicate with Spanish-speaking physicians.

One key to making the health–care system work for you lies in choosing a good physician. After seeing your primary care physician, ask yourself the following questions to evaluate the quality of care you are getting.

:: Did your physician take a comprehensive history? Was the physical examination thorough?

:: Did your physician explain what he or she was doing during the exam?

:: Did he or she spend enough time with you?

:: Did you feel free to ask questions? Did your physician give you straight answers? Did he or she reassure you when you were worried?

:: Does your physician seem willing to admit that he or she doesn't know the answers to some questions?

:: Does your physician hesitate to refer you to a specialist even when you have a complex problem that warrants such care?

Look back at your answers. If they make you feel uneasy, have a talk with your physician. Or find a physician or a health plan that provides better service. (See X & Y Files: "Men and Women as Health–Care Consumers.")

the X & Y file — *Men and Women as Health-Care Consumers*

The genders differ significantly in the way they use health-care services in the United States. Women see more doctors than men, take more prescription drugs, are hospitalized more, and control the spending of three of every four health-care dollars. In a national telephone poll, 76 percent of American women—but only 60 percent of men—said they had had a health exam in the last 12 months.

Many experts believe that the need for birth control and reproductive health services gets women into the habit of making regular visits to health-care professionals, primarily gynecologists. There are no comparable specialists for men, who tend to visit urologists, specialists in male reproductive organs, only when they develop problems. Men also are conditioned to take a stoic, tough-it-out attitude to early symptoms of a disease.

Men feel they are not allowed to manifest illness unless it's overt, says family practitioner Martin Miner, M.D., who has conducted research on men and health care. One reason men die earlier than women is because of the length of time they wait to go for treatment.

The genders also differ in the symptoms and syndromes they develop. For instance, men are more prone to back problems, muscle sprains and strains, allergies, insomnia, and digestive problems. Men develop heart disease about a decade earlier in life than women. More men develop ulcers and hernias; women are more likely to get gallbladder disease and irritable bowel syndrome. An estimated 3 to 6 percent of men suffer from migraines, compared with 15 to 17 percent of women. Yet women and men spend similar proportions of their lifetimes—about 81 percent—free of disability. For men, whose lifespans are shorter, this translates into an average of 58.8 years; for women, 63.9 years.

The genders also differ in access to health services. Women are more likely than men to lack health insurance, and the lower a woman's income and education, the less her likelihood of getting important preventive services, such as an annual Pap smear or prenatal care. Women and men are about equally likely to use complementary and alternative medicine—but different types. Men outnumber women in use of chiropractic services and acupuncture, while women are more likely to try herbal medicine, mind-body remedies, folk remedies, movement and exercise techniques, and prayer or spiritual practices. Both genders turn to alternative treatments for the same reason: a desire for greater control over their health.

Your Medical Exam

Most physicians believe that you don't need annual checkups if you're young and feel well. However, certain types of screening tests should be performed periodically, particularly if you are at a higher-than-average risk of developing a particular disease, such as high blood pressure (discussed in Chapter 14) or colon cancer (discussed in Chapter 15).

Your physician will want a past **medical history,** including major illnesses, surgery, and treatments. Report any allergies you have, particularly to drugs, and the medications you take, including aspirin, antacids, sleeping pills, oral contraceptives, and recreational drugs, even if illegal. Your physician may also want to know about topics you consider private, such as sexually transmitted infections. Remember that he or she needs all this information to provide you with comprehensive treatment. Note, too, that a physician must report certain information—for example, certain sexually transmitted diseases—to health authorities.

After the physician has asked you questions about your complaints, medical history, and lifestyle, he or she will probably perform the standard tests described below. (See Figure 16-1.) During the examination, point out any pains, lumps, or skin growths you've noticed. If you feel pain when the physician palpates (feels) any part of your body, say so.

::   **Head.** Using a flashlightlike instrument called an *ophthalmoscope,* the physician will look at the lens, retina, and blood vessels of your eyes. For patients over 40, he or she may test for a treatable eye disease called *glaucoma* (a disorder characterized by increased pressure within the eye), which can cause blindness if not detected early. The physician presses against the surface of each eye a soft instrument that measures the pressure within the eye and checks to see if the reading is normal. He or she will also examine your ears, mouth, tongue, teeth, and gums.

::   **Neck.** Feeling around your neck, the physician will check for enlarged lymph glands (a sign of infection), for lumps in the thyroid gland, and for warning signs of stroke in the neck arteries.

::   **Chest.** With a *stethoscope,* the physician will listen to the sounds made by your heart, to detect heart murmurs and irregular contractions, and by your lungs, to detect asthma or emphysema. By tapping on your chest and back with his or her fingers, the physician can tell the size and shape of your heart, which may reveal some forms of heart disease, and whether any fluid has collected in your lungs. The physician will also check for abnormal lumps in a woman's breasts.

Looking into the eyes. With an ophthalmoscope, your doctor will look for changes in eye's blood vessels or the optic nerve. These can signal severe diabetes, high blood pressure, or a tumor in the brain.

Examining the throat. Your doctor will look for signs of infection and other abnormalities.

Listening to the heart, lungs, and abdomen. Your doctor will use a stethoscope to listen to the heart sounds to detect heart murmurs and other abnormalities. He or she will listen for wheezing or crackling sounds in your lungs, which could indicate asthma, bronchitis, or pneumonia. Your abdomen should make gurgling sounds. If it doesn't, the bowel may not be working properly.

Probing the abdomen. A swelling on the right side may indicate a liver problem. A swelling on the left may mean that the spleen is enlarged, which could be a sign of infection or another condition.

Figure 16-1 STANDARD TESTS PERFORMED DURING A MEDICAL CHECKUP

:: **Abdomen.** Here the physician uses his or her fingers to probe for tender spots and malformations of the liver and other organs, which may reveal signs of alcoholism, hepatitis, or hernias.

:: **Rectum and genitals.** With a gloved hand, the physician can feel in the rectum for growths and hemorrhoids. A rectal examination can also reveal enlargement of the male's prostate gland. The physician will check male testicles and spermatic cords for abnormalities.

:: **Pelvic examination.** During a pelvic examination, a woman lies on her back, with her heels in stirrups at the end of the examining table and her legs spread out to the sides. The physician inspects the labia, clitoris, and vaginal opening. Using two gloved, lubricated fingers, the physician will check for abnormalities in the vagina, uterus, fallopian tubes, and ovaries. Many physicians will also perform a rectal or rectovaginal (one finger in the rectum and one in the vagina) examination. A nurse or other health-care worker should be present throughout the exam.

The *speculum* is a medical instrument that spreads the walls of the vagina so that the inside can be seen. The physician will gently scrape cells from the cervix for a **Pap smear,** a procedure that identifies abnormal cells that may indicate an infection or, more seriously, cervical cancer, a slow-growing cancer that's usually curable if detected early (see Chapter 15). All women should start having regular Pap smears once they begin having intercourse, or at age 18. While there has been debate about how often women should have Pap smears, many health-care providers recommend Pap smears every year for women who are sexually active or have other risk factors, such as infection with the human papilloma virus (see Chapter 13).

:: **Extremities.** The physician may check your knees and other joints for reflexes, which can indicate nerve disorders, and look for tremors in outstretched hands or in the face. The color, elasticity, and wetness or dryness of your skin can alert him or her to nutritional problems, or can indicate diabetes or skin cancer. Hair and nails can give indications of internal health, such as blood disorders. Swelling of the ankles can be an indication of heart, kidney, or liver disease.

:: *Pulse and blood pressure.* Your physician may check your pulse in various places, looking for signs of poor circulation. The rhythm and speed of the heart may also signal diseases of the heart or thyroid gland. High blood pressure can be an early warning sign of possible heart attack, stroke, or kidney damage.

Medical Tests

Besides the diagnostic tests listed above, the physician may order some laboratory and other tests, including the following:

:: *Chest X ray.* A chest X ray can reveal abnormalities of the heart and lungs; if you're a smoker, the physician may insist on one.

:: *Electrocardiogram.* The *electrocardiogram,* performed while you're at rest, records the electrical activity of your heart. It can show irregularities in heart rhythm or muscle damage, as well as hardening of the arteries.

:: *Urinalysis.* Your urine may be analyzed by a medical laboratory. If sugar (glucose) is found in your urine, your physician may order a separate blood test to check for diabetes. The presence of blood cells may indicate infection of the bladder or kidneys. Abnormal amounts of albumin (protein) in the urine may also suggest kidney disease.

:: *Blood tests.* The physician or laboratory technician may draw blood to do a blood cell count. An excess of white blood cells may indicate an infection or, occasionally, leukemia. A deficiency of red blood cells may indicate anemia. Your blood may also be analyzed to measure the levels of its various components. High levels of glucose can indicate diabetes, and high levels of uric acid may mean gout or kidney stones. A high cholesterol level may indicate cardiac risk (see Chapter 14).

See the Hales Health Almanac at the back of this book for a comprehensive guide to medical tests.

Medical Decision Making

In today's high-tech health-care system, often the question is not what physicians can do medically for someone who is ill or injured, but what they should do. That is a decision only patients—or, if they are not conscious or competent, their families—can make. Good decisions require close collaboration with a doctor, reliable and relevant information, and, if possible, time to evaluate alternatives.[21]

After your exam, the physician will report his or her findings about your health and complaints, and advise you about treatment. Depending on your problem, your physician may recommend an **over-the-counter (OTC)** drug,

Many women choose female health-care practitioners to provide gynecologic services.

© Bob Daemmrich/Stock, Boston

such as aspirin or an antihistamine; prescribe a medication; or recommend more invasive treatment, such as surgery. Medications were discussed in Chapter 12 on drug use.

Once a treatment recommendation has been made, you face a decision: Do you follow the advice? Be sure you understand fully the consequences of what you do—or don't do. You may be risking harm if, for instance, you don't take the antibiotics prescribed for your strep throat, or if you stop taking them in midtreatment (strep throat can lead to heart damage). For major nonemergency procedures, get more than one physician's opinion. Eight out of ten operations are elective, meaning that they don't have to be performed to save the patient's life.

Elective Treatments

As medical technology has developed new options, millions of Americans are trying elective procedures and products that are not medically necessary but that promise to enhance health or appearance. Some are new alternatives for correcting common problems, such as poor vision, while others offer the promise of looking younger or more attractive.

Laser Vision Surgery

An estimated 1.5 million people in the United States undergo laser surgery to correct their vision every year—more than four times as many as in 1998.

In LASIK (laser-assisted in situ keratomileusis), the most common technique, a surgeon uses a razorlike instrument to lift a flap of the cornea—the clear stiff outer layer over the colored iris—and then reshapes the exposed area using a laser. The surgery alters the way the eye focuses light, correcting nearsightedness, farsightedness, and some astigmatism. Laser surgery cannot make an aging eye's lens flexible again to improve close-up vision in middle-aged adults. Numbing eye drops make the treatment painless, although burning and scratchiness are normal for a couple of hours. An estimated 10 to 30 percent of patients require additional surgery, or "enhancements," to sharpen their vision. Other complications include glare, sensitivity to bright lights, and poor night vision.

Prices have fallen, but ophthalmologists have warned consumers that some laser surgery centers have cut corners to cut prices, such as hiring inexperienced surgeons or using optometrists or technicians rather than M.D.'s for pre- and post-operative checkups. A qualified eye surgeon should have a record of 100 or more LASIK procedures and at least 25 enhancements—but on no more than 20 percent of his or her patients. Ideally, the surgeon should also be the one doing your pre- and post-procedure checks.

Cosmetic Surgery

Approximately 6.6 million Americans undergo cosmetic treatments every year; 85 percent are women. About a quarter of those undergoing plastic surgery are between the ages of 19 and 34.[22] The number of teenagers opting for cosmetic procedures—primarily liposuction, nose reshaping, and breast augmentation—is increasing.[23] Nonsurgical cosmetic procedures such as injections of synthetic collagen and botulinum toxin (Botox®) also have become more popular. Health insurance rarely covers cosmetic procedures, which range from $300 to upward of $10,000.

The most common cosmetic operation is liposuction, the removal of fatty tissue by means of a vacuum device. It can be performed on many areas of the body, from sagging jowls to midsection "love handles." The doctor first flushes the target area with a solution of lidocaine (a local anesthetic with a numbing effect), saline, and epinephrine (a drug that reduces bleeding by constricting blood vessels). Inserting a hollow wand-like cannula under the skin, the doctor breaks up fatty deposits and suctions them, along with other body fluids, with a vacuum device.

Risks and complications include infection, numbness, bleeding, discoloration, lumpiness, and, if too much tissue is removed without proper cautions, potentially fatal complications. The American Society of Plastic and Reconstructive Surgeons estimates the mortality rate is one in 5,000 liposuction patients. Several states are considering legislation to tighten restrictions on training and credentialing doctors who perform liposuction.

Breast augmentation is the second most common cosmetic procedure, and surgeons report a 300 percent increase in demand in the last six years. The Institute of Medicine, after reviewing all available evidence, has reported that there appears to be no link between breast implants and autoimmune disease, connective tissue disorders, or cancer. However, today's surgeons use implants filled with a saltwater solution. Patients still face possible complications, including rupture, scarring, infection, and leaking or hardening of their implants.

Your Medical Rights

As a consumer, you have basic rights that help ensure that you know about any potential dangers, receive competent diagnosis and treatment, and retain control and dignity in your interactions with health-care professionals. Many hospitals publish a patient's bill of rights, including your rights to know whether a procedure is experimental; to refuse to undergo a specific treatment; to designate someone else to make decisions about your care if and when you cannot; and to leave the hospital, even against your physician's advice. (See the Self-Survey: "Are You a Savvy Health-Care Consumer?" on the next page.)

You have the right to be treated with respect and dignity, including being called "Mr." or "Ms." or whatever you wish, rather than by your first name. Make clear your preferences. If you feel that health-care professionals are being condescending or inconsiderate, say so—in the same tone and manner that you would like others to use with you. If you're hospitalized, find out if there's a patient advocate or representative at your hospital. These individuals can help you communicate with physicians, make any special arrangements, and get answers to questions or complaints.

You have the right to good, safe care. More than one in five Americans or a family member have experienced a medical or prescription drug error, according to a report by the Commonwealth Fund. One in ten got sicker as a result of the mistake.[24]

You have the right to give consent to donate an organ while alive, or have your organs removed in the event of an accident, injury, or illness that leaves you brain-dead. However, you cannot agree to donate a body part for money or other compensation. Congress has prohibited the marketing of organs; any attempt to do so is a felony punishable by up to five years in jail and a $50,000 fine.

Your Right to Information

By law, a patient must give consent for hospitalization, surgery, and other major treatments. **Informed consent** is a right, not a privilege. Use this right to its fullest. Ask questions. Seek other opinions. Make sure that your expectations are realistic and that you understand the potential risks, as well as the possible benefits, of a prospective treatment. Informed consent is required for research studies, but patients often don't realize that they have the right not to participate and to get complete information on the purpose and nature of the study.

Self Survey

Are You a Savvy Health-Care Consumer?

1. You want a second opinion, but your doctor dismisses your request for other physicians' names as unnecessary. Do you:
   a. Assume that he or she is right and you would merely be wasting time.
   b. Suspect that your physician has something to hide and immediately switch doctors.
   c. Contact your health plan and request a second opinion.

2. As soon as you enter your doctor's office, you get tongue-tied. When you try to find the words to describe what's wrong, your physician keeps interrupting. When giving advice, your doctor uses such technical language that you can't understand what it means. Do you:
   a. Prepare better for your next appointment.
   b. Pretend that you understand what your doctor is talking about.
   c. Decide you'd be better off with someone who specializes in complementary/alternative therapies and seems less intimidating.

3. You feel like you're running on empty, tired all the time, worn to the bone. A friend suggests some herbal supplements that promise to boost energy and restore vitality. Do you:
   a. Immediately start taking them.
   b. Say that you think herbs are for cooking.
   c. Find out as much as you can about the herbal compounds and ask your doctor if they're safe and effective.

4. Your hometown physician's office won't give you a copy of your medical records to take with you to college. Do you:
   a. Hope you won't need them and head off without your records.
   b. Threaten to sue.
   c. Politely ask the office administrator to tell you the particular law or statute that bars you from your records.

5. Your doctor has been treating you for an infection for three weeks, and you don't seem to be getting any better. Do you:
   a. Talk to your doctor, by phone or in person, and say, "This doesn't seem to be working. Is there anything else we can try?"
   b. Stop taking the antibiotic.
   c. Try an herbal remedy that your roommate recommends.

6. Your doctor suggests a cutting-edge treatment for your condition, but your health plan or HMO refuses to pay for it. Do you:
   a. Try to get a loan to cover the costs.
   b. Settle for whatever treatment options are covered.
   c. Challenge your health plan.

7. You call for an appointment with your doctor and are told nothing is available for four months. Do you:
   a. Take whatever time you can get whenever you can get it.
   b. Explain your condition to the nurse or receptionist, detailing any symptoms and pain you're experiencing.
   c. Give up and decide you don't need to see a doctor at all.

8. Even though you've been doing sit-ups faithfully, your waist still looks flabby. When you see an ad for waist-whittling liposuction, do you:
   a. Call for an appointment.
   b. Talk to a health-care professional about a total fitness program that may help you lose excess pounds.
   c. Carefully research the risks and costs of the procedure.

9. You have a condition that you do not want anyone to know about, including your health insurer and any potential employer. Do you:
   a. Use a false name.
   b. Give your physician a written request for confidentiality about this condition.
   c. Seek help outside the health-care system.

10. Your doctor suggests a biopsy of a funny-looking mole that's sprouted on your nose. Rather than using a laboratory that specializes in skin analysis, your HMO requires that all samples be sent to a general lab, where results may not be as precise. Do you:
    a. Ask your doctor to request that a specialty pathologist at the general lab perform the analysis.
    b. Hope that in your case, the general lab will do a good-enough job.
    c. Threaten to change HMOs.

Answers:
1: c; 2: a; 3: c; 4: c; 5: a; 6: c; 7: b; 8: b and c; 9: b; 10: a

Your Health Change Plan for

Protecting Yourself from Medical Mistakes and Misdeeds

Just as physicians practice "defensive" medicine to protect themselves from legal liability, today's patients should take preventive steps to defend themselves from potentially harmful health services.

The Whats, Whys, and Hows of Medical Testing

:: Before undergoing any test, find out why you need it. Get a specific answer, not a "just in case" or "for your peace of mind." If you've had the test before, could the earlier results be used? Would a follow-up exam be just as helpful?

(Continued)

:: Get some practical information as well: Should you do specific things before the test (such as not eat for a specified period)? How long will the test take? What will the test feel like? Will you need help getting home afterward?

:: Check out the risks. Any invasive test—one that penetrates the body with a needle, tube, or viewing instrument—involves some risk of infection, bleeding, or tissue damage. Tests involving radiation also present risks, and some people develop allergic reactions to the materials used in testing.

:: Get information on the laboratory that will be evaluating the test. Ask how often **false positives** or **false negatives** occur. (False positives are abnormal results indicating that you have a particular condition when

you really don't; false negatives indicate that you don't have a particular condition when you really do.) Find out about civil or criminal **negligence** suits filed against the laboratory on charges such as failing to diagnose cervical cancer because of incorrect reading of Pap smears.

:: You'll also want to know what happens when the test indicates a problem: Will the test be repeated? Will a different test be performed? Will treatment begin immediately? Could any medications you're taking (including nonprescription drugs, like aspirin) affect the testing procedures or results?

:: If you have a test, don't assume that no news is good news. Check back to get the results.

Your Right to Privacy and Access to Medical Records

Your medical records are your property. You have the right to see them whenever you choose and to limit who else can see them. The first-ever federal standards to protect the privacy of patients' medical information took effect in 2003. They guarantee patients access to their medical records, given them more control over how personal health information is disclosed, and limit the ways that health plans, pharmacies, and hospitals can use personal medical information.

Key provisions include:

:: Access to medical records. As a patient, you should be able to see and obtain copies of your medical records and request corrections if there are errors. Health-care providers must provide these within 30 days; they may charge for the cost of copying and mailing records.

:: Notice of privacy practices. Your providers must inform you of how they use personal medical information. While doctors, nurses, and other providers can share information needed to treat their patients, they may not disclose information for purposes not related to health care.

:: Prohibition on marketing. Pharmacies, health plans, and others must obtain specific authorization before disclosing patient information for marketing.

:: Confidentiality. Patients can request that doctors take reasonable steps to ensure confidential communications, such as calling a cell phone rather than home or office.[25]

Preventing Medical Errors

Errors, which may involve diagnosis, equipment, lab reports, medications, or surgery, are more likely to occur when doctors and their patients have problems communicating. The single most important thing you can do to prevent errors is take part in every decision about your health care. Make sure you understand what may be wrong with you, which medications you are taking and why:

:: When your doctor writes you a prescription, make sure you can read it and know why and how you are to take this medication.

:: Ask for information about your medicines in terms you can understand, including explanations of possible interactions with other drugs or dietary supplements and potential side effects.

:: If you must undergo surgery and you can choose a hospital, select one at which many patients have had the procedure or surgery you need.

:: Consider asking all health-care workers who have direct contact with you whether they have washed their hands. This simple step prevents the spread of infections.

:: Speak up if you have questions or concerns. Ask a family member or friend to be your advocate and speak up for you if you can't.

Your Right to Good, Safe, Care

According to recent court rulings, patients have the right to sue health insurers that refuse to authorize medically necessary treatment. This enables patients to hold health plans accountable for their role in medical decision making.[26]

STRATEGIES FOR PREVENTION

Protecting Yourself Against Quackery

■ Arm yourself with up-to-date information about your condition or disease from appropriate organizations, such as the American Cancer Society or the Arthritis Foundation, which keep track of unproven and ineffective methods of treatment.

■ Ask for a written explanation of what a treatment does and why it works, evidence supporting all claims (not just testimonials), and published reports of the studies, including specifics on numbers treated, doses, and side effects. Be skeptical of self-styled "holistic practitioners," treatments supported by crusading groups, and endorsements from self-proclaimed experts or authorities.

■ Don't part with your money quickly. Be especially careful because insurance companies won't reimburse for unproven therapies.

■ Don't discontinue your current treatment without your physician's approval. Many physicians encourage supportive therapies—such as relaxation exercises, meditation, or visualization—as a supplement to standard treatments.

Malpractice

The essence of a **malpractice** suit is the claim that the physician failed to meet the standard of care required of a reasonably skilled and careful medical doctor. Although physicians don't have to guarantee good results to their patients and aren't held liable for unavoidable errors, they are required to use the same care and judgment in treatment that other physicians in the same specialty would use under similar circumstances. To protect themselves financially, physicians, particularly those in surgical specialties who are most likely to be sued, pay tens of thousands of dollars a year in malpractice-insurance premiums. Some of this cost is passed on to patients.

Because of fear of malpractice, many physicians practice "defensive" medicine and order more tests, refer more patients, prescribe more medications, and suggest biopsies more often than necessary for legal rather than medical reasons. In some states the cost of malpractice insurance has soared, forcing some physicians to change specialties or relocate. Health policy experts have suggested replacing the current system of handling malpractice claims with special medical courts staffed by medical experts.[27]

Most lawsuits are based on negligence and assert that a physician failed to render diagnosis and treatment with appropriate professional knowledge and skill. Other cases are brought for failure to provide information, obtain consent, or respect a patient's confidentiality. However, analysis of malpractice cases has shown that, in 70 to 80 percent, a doctor's attitude and inability to communicate effectively—by devaluing patients' views, delivering information poorly, failing to understand patients' perspectives, or displaying an air of superiority—also played a role.

The Public Citizen Health Research Group has compiled a national directory of "questionable physicians," which lists physicians disciplined by state medical boards or the federal government for offenses ranging from overprescribing drugs to sexual misconduct to negligent or substandard care. Some of these physicians committed minor misdeeds, such as failing to complete continuing medical education requirements. Consumer advocates urge patients to find out why a particular name appears on the list by calling the state licensing board. At the federal level, the agencies most involved in ensuring quality health care are the Food and Drug Administration (FDA), which approves the production and labeling of drugs; and the Federal Trade Commission (FTC), which oversees advertising and prohibits deceptive or false claims.

Medical Errors

Medical errors, which can occur whenever something goes wrong with a test or treatment, are a leading cause of injury and death. According to the Institute of Medicine, as many as 44,000 to 98,000 people die in U.S. hospitals each year as the result of medical errors—a toll greater than that of motor vehicle accidents, breast cancer, or AIDS.[28]

The Joint Commission on Accreditation of Healthcare Organizations has set national patient safety goals designed to prevent the most common errors, including misidentification of patients, miscommunication among caregivers, wrong-site surgery, and medication mix-ups. Among the steps they require are reading back medical orders given over the phone and marking the site where surgery is to be performed.[29]

When errors occur, patients and physicians differ in their responses. Patients want full disclosure of what happened and why, how the error's consequences will be mitigated, and how recurrences will be prevented. While physicians agree that harmful errors should be disclosed, they "choose their words carefully" when telling patients about errors. Often they avoid stating that an error occurred, explaining why, or offering an apology for fear of legal liability. Yet patients place a premium on a physician's emotional support and statements of regret.[30]

The risks associated with hospitalization include what health workers call the "terrible I's": infection; inactivity; incorrect actions; and the inherent risks of drugs, X rays, and false lab tests. The simplest method for preventing hospital-acquired infection—handwashing—is often ignored by health-care providers.

Surgical and medication mistakes are another hazard. In highly publicized cases, hospital physicians have amputated a patient's healthy leg, operated on the wrong side of a woman's brain, and administered deadly doses of cancer drugs. As hospitals cut back on staff and services in order to control costs, the likelihood of such errors may increase.

Quackery

Every year millions of Americans go searching for medical miracles that never happen. In all, they spend more than $10 billion on medical **quackery,** unproven health products and services. Those who lose only money are the lucky ones. Many also waste precious time, during which their conditions worsen. Some suffer needless pain, along with crushed expectations. Far too many risk their lives on a false hope—and lose.

The peddlers of such false hopes are quacks, who, by definition, promote for profit worthless or unproven treatments. The Internet has become a popular method for quacks to promote themselves and their wares. Nations have joined together in Operation Cure All, a law enforcement and public education campaign to stop Internet health fraud. It has targeted various devices, herbal products, and other dietary supplements purported to treat or cure cancer, AIDS, arthritis, hepatitis, Alzheimer's disease, diabetes, and other chronic conditions.[31] (See Savvy Consumer: "Spotting Health Hoaxes.")

Sometimes individuals with certain diseases, such as arthritis or multiple sclerosis, who try unproven remedies do indeed improve. "If someone with arthritis starts feeling better the day after getting a copper bracelet, the bracelet will get the credit," says one physician. "Yet it's just coincidence." This is one reason scientists put little stock in enthusiastic testimonials from people who genuinely believe they have been helped by a new drug or treatment. Their heartfelt stories can be persuasive but are scientifically meaningless. The satisfied patient may not actually have had the disease in the first place, may have gotten other treatments too, or may be responding to a remedy that masks the symptoms without treating the disease.

✖ Complementary and Alternative Medicine

The medical research community uses the term **complementary and alternative medicine (CAM)** to apply to all health-care approaches, practices, and treatments not widely taught in medical schools and not generally used in hospitals.[32] CAM includes many healing philosophies, approaches, and therapies, including preventive techniques designed to delay or prevent serious health problems before they start and **holistic** methods that focus on the whole person and the physical, mental, emotional, and spiritual aspects of well-being. Some approaches are based on the same physiological principles as traditional Western methods; others, such as acupuncture, are based on different healing systems.

Approximately 4 in 10 Americans use a form of complementary or alternative medicine every year. The most popular include acupuncture, chiropractic, herbal medicine, and homeopathy, which may be used in addition to or instead of the more conventional forms of medical care. Some states have mandated health insurance coverage for CAM therapies, which also are becoming more common in Canada and Europe.[33] Many medical schools now include training in CAM in their curricula.[34]

Americans make more visits to alternative practitioners than they do to primary care physicians and spend about as much in annual out-of-pocket expenditures, including money for practitioners, herbal remedies, megavitamins, diet products, and books, classes, and equipment.

Integrative medicine, which combines selected elements of both conventional and alternative medicine in a comprehensive approach to diagnosis and treatment, has gained greater acceptance within the medical community.[35]

Why People Use CAM Therapies

According to several surveys, people don't turn to CAM because they are dissatisfied with conventional care, but because they want more than conventional medicine has to offer. Those who've used CAM believed that most physicians rely too heavily on prescription drugs, don't provide enough information on nutrition and exercise, and ignore the social and spiritual aspects of care.[36] People who use CAM tend to have more education, an interest in personal and spiritual growth, and a belief that body, mind, and spirit are all involved in health. Compared to those who don't use CAM, users often report poorer health and see alternative health care as more in tune with their own values, beliefs, and philosophies about life. The main benefit they report is relief from symptoms of an illness.

Individuals with any psychiatric disorder are significantly more likely to use a CAM therapy than the general population. Those with severe depression or anxiety disorders use CAM most often. Most patients who use CAM for mental health problems also use conventional therapies. The most popular CAM therapies in mental health care are relaxation techniques and "spiritual healing." The efficacy and safety of most CAM therapies used to self-treat or treat mental health problems are not yet established.[37]

An estimated 10 to 50 percent of cancer patients try alternative treatments, many without their physicians' knowledge. These include dietary changes, antioxidant vitamins, soy, herbs, and other natural products, acupuncture, massage, exercise, and psychologic and mind-body interventions. Based on the best evidence available, cancer

Savvy Consumer

SPOTTING HEALTH HOAXES

Promoters of fraudulent health products often use similar claims and practices to trick consumers into buying their products. Be suspicious when you see:

- Claims that a product is a "scientific breakthrough," "miraculous cure," "secret ingredient," or "ancient remedy."

- Claims that the product is an effective cure for a wide range of ailments. No product can cure multiple conditions or diseases.

- Claims that use impressive-sounding medical terms. They're often covering up a lack of good science.

- Undocumented case histories of people who've had amazing results. It's too easy to make them up. And even if true, they can't be generalized to the entire population. Anecdotes are not a substitute for valid science.

- Claims that the product is available from only one source, and payment is required in advance.

- Claims of a "money-back" guarantee.

- Websites that fail to list the company's name, physical address, phone number or other contact information.

To file a complaint with the FTC or to get free information on consumer topics, call 1-877-FTC-HELP (1-877-382-4357), or use the complaint form at www.ftc.gov.

Source: Federal Trade Commission. www.ftc.gov/bcp/conline/features/healthclaims.htm

---

specialists have ranked these approaches on a continuum ranging from "recommend" to "discourage."

A reduction in dietary fat was deemed acceptable, but the use of antioxidant vitamins A, C, and E may cause more harm than benefit because of the risks of cancer progression and effects on blood clotting. Doctors discourage the use of soy supplements in women with breast cancer but accept their use by men with prostate cancer. The efficacy of shark cartilage remains unclear. Acupuncture was deemed acceptable to help control chemotherapy-related nausea and vomiting among cancer patients. Massage has not demonstrated any positive effect on cancer progression or pain relief. Psychologic and mind-body therapies such as individual and group therapy, relaxation, imagery, hypnosis, and meditation can relieve distress and pain as well as some of the physical symptoms of disease and side effects of conventional therapy.[38]

Evidence-Based CAM

Many have criticized health-care providers for giving alternative therapies "a free ride" by not demanding the same proof and regulation required of traditional treatments.[39] While many CAM treatments have been in use for a long time (sometimes for centuries), they do not have the same sort of scientific basis gained from studies of conventional medicine. Individuals who use them may be at risk for serious side effects, for example, from taking the wrong dose or using a treatment in the wrong way. Scientists are working to apply the same standards of evidence-based medicine used for conventional treatment to CAM. Recent studies that have applied rigorously scientific stan-

dards to popular alternative therapies have revealed unexpected risks, confirmed benefits from some forms of CAM, and disproved the alleged positive effects of others.[40]

What Should I Know Before I Try CAM?

You should never decide on any treatment—traditional or CAM—without fully evaluating it. Here are some key questions to ask:

:: ***Is it safe?*** The fact that a substance is "natural" or that a treatment does not require hospitalization or surgery doesn't mean it is safe. Talk to your medical doctor so you understand any particular risks to your overall health or any unknown long-term effects. Be particularly wary of unregulated products.

:: ***Is it effective?*** We know far less about the efficacy of many alternative treatments than we do about traditional therapies. You can obtain information on what is known about the effectiveness of specific treatments from the National Center for Complementary and Alternative Medicine through its website and information clearinghouse (http://nccam.nih.gov).

:: ***Will it interact with other medicines or conventional treatments?*** This is an important question to discuss with your doctor and to investigate by doing research online or in the library. Some combinations—such as the use of a prescription sleeping pill and sleep-inducing melatonin—can be dangerous, and some herbal remedies can interfere with hypertension drugs and increase the risks of anesthesia. Many widely used alternative remedies can interact with prescription medications in dangerous ways.

:: ***Is the practitioner qualified?*** Many states license practitioners who provide acupuncture, chiropractic services, naturopathy, herbal medicine, homeopathy, and other treatments. Find out if yours does, and always choose a licensed professional. You also can contact medical regulatory agencies and consumer affairs departments, which provide information about a specific practitioner's license, education, and accreditation, and will let you know if any complaints have been filed against him or her. Many organizations of specific types of practitioners have websites. However, remember that they are presenting information from an advocate's point of view.

:: ***What has been the experience of others?*** Talk to people who have used CAM for a similar problem, both recently and in the past. Keep in mind that their perspectives—positive or negative—are subjective and should not be your only criterion for selecting a therapy. Also try to find people who have been cared for by the practitioner you are considering.

:: ***Can you talk openly and easily with the practitioner?*** Your relationship with your CAM practitioner is as important as your relationship with your medical doctor. You should feel comfortable asking questions and confident in the answers you receive. What is his or her educational background, principles, and beliefs?

:: ***Are you comfortable with the CAM care setting?*** Visit the practitioner's office, clinic, or hospital. Does it put you at ease, or make you feel out-of-place or anxious? How do conditions such as cleanliness and staff professionalism compare with the health-care settings with which you are more familiar? Find out how many clients a practitioner sees every week and how much time is spent with each one.

:: ***What are the costs?*** Many CAM services are not covered by HMOs or health insurers. Find out if your plan will cover any treatments. Also check what other practitioners charge for the same service so you can decide if a fee is appropriate. Regulatory agencies and professional associations often provide cost information.

Types of CAM

The National Center for Complementary and Alternative Medicine (NCCAM) has classified CAM therapies into five categories:

:: Alternative medical systems

:: Mind-body interventions

:: Biologically based therapies

:: Manipulative and body-based methods

:: Energy therapies.

Alternative Medical Systems

Systems of theory and practice other than traditional Western medicine are included in this group. They include acupuncture, Oriental medicine, tai chi, external and internal Qi, Ayurvedic medicine, naturopathy, and unconventional Western systems, such as homeopathy and orthomolecular medicine.

Acupuncture is an ancient Chinese form of medicine, based on the philosophy that a cycle of energy circulating through the body controls health. Pain and disease are the result of a disturbance in the energy flow, which can be corrected by inserting long, thin needles at specific points along longitudinal lines, or *meridians,* throughout the body. Each point controls a different corresponding part of the body. Once inserted, the needles are rotated gently back and forth or charged with a small electric current for a short time. Western scientists aren't sure exactly how acupuncture works, but some believe that the needles alter the functioning of the nervous system.

An NIH consensus development panel that evaluated current research into acupuncture concluded that there is "clear evidence" that acupuncture can control nausea and vomiting in patients after surgery or while undergoing chemotherapy and relieve postoperative dental pain. The panel said that acupuncture is "probably" also effective in the control of nausea in early pregnancy and that there were "reasonable" studies, some using "sham" needles that make it more difficult for patients to know if they are or are not undergoing acupuncture, showing that the use of acupuncture, by itself or as an adjunct to other therapies,

The ancient Chinese practice of acupuncture produces healing through the insertion and manipulation of needles at specific points throughout the body. The procedure is not painful.

resulted in satisfactory treatment of a number of other conditions, even though there was not "firm evidence of efficacy at this time." These conditions include addiction to illicit drugs and alcohol (but not to tobacco), stroke rehabilitation, headache, menstrual cramps, tennis elbow, general muscle pain, low back pain, carpal tunnel syndrome, and asthma. Ongoing studies are evaluating its efficacy for chronic headaches and migraines.

Considered alternative here, **ayurveda** is a traditional form of medical treatment in India, where it has evolved over thousands of years. Its basic premise is that illness stems from incorrect mental attitudes, diet, and posture. Practitioners use a discipline of exercise, meditation, herbal medication, and proper nutrition to cope with such stress-induced conditions as hypertension, the desire to smoke, and obesity. The best known advocate of ayurvedic medicine is Deepak Chopra, M.D., an endocrinologist (specialist in hormone-related disorders) who has written several books on ayurveda and the intimate relationship between consciousness and health.

Homeopathy is based on three fundamental principles: "like cures like"; treatment must always be individualized; and less is more—the idea that increasing dilution (and lowering the dosage) can increase efficacy. By administering doses of animal, vegetable, or mineral substances to a large number of healthy people to see if they all develop the same symptoms, homeopaths determine which substances may be given, in small quantities, to alleviate the symptoms. Some of these substances are the same as those used in conventional medicine: nitroglycerin for certain heart conditions, for example, although the dose is minuscule.

Naturopathy emphasizes natural remedies, such as sun, water, heat, and air, as the best treatments for disease. Therapies might include dietary changes (such as more vegetables and no salt or stimulants), steam baths, and exercise. Some naturopathic physicians (who are not M.D.s) work closely with medical doctors in helping patients.

Mind-Body Interventions

Mind-body approaches include behavioral medicine techniques, such as journaling, as well as hypnosis, yoga, meditation, biofeedback, imagery, music, art and dance therapy, spiritual healing, and community-based approaches (for example, Alcoholics Anonymous and Native American sweat rituals).

Biofeedback uses machines that measure temperature or skin responses and then relays this information to the subject. In this way, people can learn to control usually involuntary functions, such as circulation to the hands and feet, tension in the jaws, and heartbeat rates. Biofeedback has been used to treat dozens of ailments, including asthma, epilepsy, pain, and Reynaud's disease (a condition in which the fingers become painful and white when exposed to cold). Many health insurers now cover biofeedback treatments.

Creative **visualization,** or imaging, helps patients, including some diagnosed as terminally ill with cancer, heal. On the premise that positive and negative beliefs and attitudes have a great deal to do with whether people get well or die of disease, patients imagine themselves getting well—they "see," for instance, immune-system cells marching to conquer cancer cells. Other patients use visualization in different ways—for example, to create a clear idea of what they want to achieve, whether the goal is weight loss or relaxation.

Biologically Based Therapies

Biologically based CAM therapies use substances such as herbs, foods, and vitamins. They include botanical medicine or phytotherapy, the use of individual herbs or combinations; special diet therapies, such as macrobiotics, Ornish, McDougall, and high fiber; Mediterranean orthomolecular medicine (use of nutritional and food supplements for preventive or therapeutic purposes); and use of other products (such as shark cartilage) and procedures applied in an unconventional manner.

Herbal medicine has become an estimated $4 billion-a-year industry, yet questions about the safety and effectiveness of herbal supplements persist.[41] Although more than 1,500 different preparations are on the U.S. market, eight herbal medications account for more than half of the single-herb preparations sold in the United States: echinacea, ephedra, garlic, ginkgo, ginseng, kava, St. John's wort, and valerian. (See Table 16-3.) Unlike medications, herbal products are exempt from the FDA's regulatory scrutiny. The ingredients and the potency of active ingredients can vary from batch to batch.

Herbal medicines are a popular form of alternative medicine.

© Kevin R. Morris/CORBIS

TABLE 16-3	Evidence-Based Evaluations of Herbal Supplements
Herb	**Evidence**
Saw Palmetto	Reduces an enlarged prostate, but the effect is small compared with prescription medication
Ginseng	No demonstrated benefits or proven effect on energy
Echinacea	No proven benefits as a cold remedy; can trigger an allergic reaction
Kava	May reduce anxiety, but can cause liver damage
Gingko biloba	No improvement in memory or thinking in the healthy elderly, but a small benefit for patients with dementia
Ephedra	Modest effect on weight loss; linked to strokes, hypertension, and deaths
Garlic	Lowers cholesterol when taken in higher doses than you would get with food, much less effective than cholesterol-lowering medications
Black Cohosh	Some studies indicate that it reduces hot flashes, long-term effects unknown

Rigorous research studies are producing the first scientific evidence on the safety and efficacy of herbal supplements.[42] Their benefits, if any, have proven modest. Ginkgo biloba, for instance, temporarily boosts memory, but no more so than eating a candy bar.[43] Other agents, such as saw palmetto or garlic, produce slight benefits, but far less than available medications.[44]

Most of the herbs tested have proven generally safe, although side effects such as headaches and nausea can occur. However, some herbs can cause serious, even fatal dangers. Echinacea, widely used as a cold remedy, may cause liver damage if taken in combination with anabolic steroids.

Several widely used herbs, including ginger, garlic, and ginkgo, are dangerous if taken prior to surgery—yet it's been estimated that more than 70 percent of patients fail to disclose their use of herbal medicine before an operation. Herbs such as ginseng and goldenseal can cause unexpected rises in blood pressure and heart rate during an operation, while St. John's Wort and Kava-kava may interact with and prolong anesthesia medications. All herbal supplements should be discontinued for periods of several days or longer prior to surgery.

The most dangerous herbal products, sold as ephedra, ma huang, sinica, and sida cordifolia, contain ephedrine, which stimulates the heart to beat faster and increases blood pressure. Ephedra has been linked with dozens of deaths and more than 1,000 adverse reactions. Products containing ephedra accounted for 64 percent of all adverse reactions to herbs in the United States.[45] The FDA has issued warnings on ephedra and other potentially dangerous herbs, including chaparral, comfrey, yohimbe, lobelia, germander, willow bark, jin bu huan, and products containing magnolia or stephania.[46]

Manipulative and Body-Based Methods

CAM therapies based on manipulation and/or movement of the body are divided into three subcategories:

:: chiropractic medicine

:: massage and body work (including osteopathic manipulation, Swedish massage, Alexander technique, reflexology, Pilates, acupressure, and rolfing)

:: unconventional physical therapies (including colonics, hydrotherapy, and light and color therapies).

Chiropractic is a treatment method based on the theory that many human diseases are caused by misalignment of the bones (subluxation). Chiropractors are licensed in all

A chiropractor can help relieve pain following an injury.

50 states, but chiropractic is considered a mainstream therapy by some and a form of CAM by others. Significant research in the last ten years has demonstrated its efficacy for acute lower-back pain. NIH is funding research on other potential benefits, including headaches, asthma, middle ear inflammation, menstrual cramps, and arthritis.

Chiropractors, who emphasize wellness and healing without drugs or surgery, may use X rays and magnetic resonance imaging (MRI) as well as orthopedic, neurological, and manual examinations in making diagnoses. However, chiropractic treatment consists solely of the manipulation of misaligned bones that may be putting pressure on nerve tissue and affecting other parts of the body. Many HMOs offer chiropractic services, which are the most widely used alternative treatment among managed care patients.

Massage therapy is the manipulation of body tissues to promote wellness and reduce pain and stress. Techniques include stroking and kneading, as in Swedish massage, and applying pressure to specific areas, as used in Shiatsu and acupuncture. It has been shown helpful in relieving pain and muscle soreness, controlling asthma, relieving constipation, and lowering stress and anxiety.

In *acupressure,* the therapist uses his or her finger and thumb to stimulate certain points, relieve pain, and relax muscles. **Reflexology** is based on the theory that massaging certain points on the foot or hand relieves stress or pain in corresponding parts of the body.

Massage appears to be an effective way to treat back pain according to a new, in-depth review of evidence from dozens of studies of alternative treatments. Spinal manipulation (commonly done by chiropractors and osteopaths) has small clinical benefits for back pain—about the same as conventional medical treatments such as over-the-counter pain relievers and various types of physical therapy.[47]

Energy Therapies

Various approaches focus on energy fields believed to exist in and around the body. Some use external energy sources, such as electromagnetic fields. Magnets are marketed to relieve pain but there is little scientific evidence of their efficacy. Others, such as therapeutic touch, use a therapist's healing energy to repair imbalances in an individual's biofield.

▉ The Health-Care System

In the past, getting health care was fairly simple. When people were sick, they went to their family physician and paid in cash. If they didn't have enough money, the physician would still provide care. Today health care involves many more people, places, and processes. As a college student, you can turn to the student health service if you get sick. There, a nurse, nurse practitioner, physician's assistant, or medical doctor may evaluate your symptoms and pro-

vide basic care. However, you may rely on a primary care physician in your hometown to perform regular checkups or manage a chronic condition like asthma. If you're injured in an accident, you probably will be treated at the nearest emergency room. If you become seriously ill and require highly specialized care, you may have to go to a university-affiliated medical center to receive state-of-the-art treatment.

Health-Care Practitioners

Fewer than 10 percent of health-care practitioners are physicians; other types of health professionals are assuming more important roles in delivering primary, or basic, health services. As a consumer, you should be aware of the range and special skills of the most common types of health-care providers.

Physicians

A medical doctor (M.D.) trained in American medical schools usually takes at least three years of premedical college courses (with an emphasis on biology, chemistry, and physics) and then completes four (but sometimes three or five) years of medical school. The first two years of medical school are devoted to the study of human anatomy, embryology, pharmacology, and similar basic subjects. During the last two years, students work directly with physicians in hospitals. Medical students who pass a series of national board examinations then enter a one-year internship in a hospital, followed by another two to five years of residency (depending on their specialty), which leads to certification in a particular field, or specialty.

About 500,000 of the nation's 700,000 physicians are specialists or subspecialists, who focus on a specific part of the body, organ system, type of disease, or type of treatment. Traditionally, they have had greater status and earned much larger incomes than primary care physicians—family practitioners, pediatricians, and internists—who provide preventive care, regular checkups, and routine treatments of uncomplicated medical conditions. However, changes in health policy (such as increases in Medicare payments to primary care physicians) and in the delivery of services have given a more prominent role to primary care physicians. They now often function as "gatekeepers" who decide whether a patient needs to see a medical specialist.

Nurses

A registered nurse (R.N.) graduates from a school of nursing approved by a state board and passes a state board examination. R.N.s may have a bachelor's or an associate degree and may specialize in certain areas, such as intensive care or nurse-midwifery. Nurse practitioners, R.N.s with advanced training and experience, may run community clinics or provide screening and preventive care at group medical practices. Some have independent practices.

Licensed practical nurses (L.P.N.s), also called licensed vocational nurses, are licensed by the state. After graduating from state-approved schools of practical nursing, they must take a board exam. They work under the supervision of R.N.s or physicians. Nursing aides and orderlies assist registered and practical nurses in providing services directly related to the comfort and well-being of hospitalized patients.

Specialized and Allied-Health Practitioners

More than 60 types of health practitioners work with physicians and nurses in providing medical services. Some, such as *occupational therapists,* have at least a bachelor's degree. Allied-health professionals may specialize in a variety of fields. *Clinical psychologists* have graduate degrees and provide a wide range of mental health services but don't prescribe medications—as do *psychiatrists. Optometrists,* trained in special schools of optometry, diagnose visual abnormalities and prescribe lenses or visual aids; however, they don't prescribe drugs, diagnose or treat eye diseases, or perform surgery—functions performed by *ophthalmologists. Podiatrists* are specially trained, licensed health-care professionals who specialize in problems of the feet.

Dentists

Most dental students earn a bachelor's degree and then complete two more years of training in the basic sciences and two years of clinical work before graduating with a degree of D.D.S. or D.M.D. (Doctor of Dental Surgery or Doctor of Medical Dentistry). To qualify for a license, graduates must pass both a written and a clinical examination. Dentists may work in general practice or choose a specialty, such as *orthodontics* (straightening teeth).

Chiropractors

Chiropractors hold the degree of Doctor of Chiropractic (D.C.), which signifies that they have had two years of college-level training, plus four years in a health-care school specializing in chiropractic, described earlier in this chapter.

Health-Care Facilities

As a prospective patient, you can choose from various options: a physician's office, a clinic, an emergency room, or a hospital. Most **primary care**—also referred to as ambulatory or outpatient care—is provided by a physician in an office, emergency room, or clinic. *Secondary care* usually is provided by specialists or subspecialists in either an

outpatient or inpatient (hospital) setting. *Tertiary care,* available at university-affiliated hospitals and regional referral centers, includes special procedures such as kidney dialysis, open-heart surgery, and organ transplants.

College Health Centers

The American College Health Association estimates that 1,500 institutions of higher learning provide direct health services. Student health centers, initially developed by departments of physical education and hygiene, range in size from small dispensaries staffed by nurses to large-scale, multispecialty clinics that provide both inpatient and outpatient care and are fully accredited by the Joint Commission on Accreditation of Healthcare Organizations.[48] Some serve only students; others provide services for faculty, staff, and family members.

On some campuses, health educators work with the student health centers to provide counseling on such topics as nutrition; tobacco, drug, and alcohol abuse; exercise and fitness; sexuality; and contraception. Some college health centers provide psychological counseling, as well as dental, pharmacy, and optometric services. Some campuses also provide sports-medicine services for student athletes. Services are paid for by various combinations of prepaid health fees, general university funds, fee-for-service charges, and health-insurance reimbursements.

Outpatient Treatment Centers

Increasingly, procedures that once required hospitalization, such as simple surgery, are being performed at outpatient centers, which may be freestanding or affiliated with a medical center. Patients have any necessary tests performed beforehand, undergo surgery or receive treatment, and return home after a few hours to recuperate. Outpatient centers can handle many common surgical procedures, including cataract removal, tonsillectomy, breast biopsy, dilation and curettage (D and C), vasectomy, and face-lifts.

Without the high overhead costs of a hospital, outpatient surgery costs run only about 30 to 50 percent of standard hospital fees. Today, 70 percent of hospitals do outpatient, or "in-and-out," surgery. To cut health-care costs, insurance companies are encouraging, or in some cases requiring, their policyholders to choose outpatient surgery. However, operations requiring prolonged general anesthesia or extensive postoperative care must still be performed on an inpatient basis.

Freestanding emergency or urgent-care centers (those not part of a hospital) claim that they deliver high-quality medical treatment with maximum convenience in minimal time. Rather than going to crowded hospital emergency rooms when they slice a finger in the kitchen, patients can go to a freestanding emergency center and receive prompt attention.

Hospitals and Medical Centers

Different types of hospitals offer different types of care. The most common type of hospital is the *private,* or community, *hospital,* which may be run on a profit or a nonprofit basis, generally contains 50 to 400 beds, and provides more personalized care than public hospitals do. The quality of care individual patients receive depends mostly on the physicians themselves. Public *hospitals* include city, county, public health service, military, and Veterans Administration hospitals. The quality of patient care depends on the overall quality of the institution.

Of the more than 6,500 hospitals nationwide, about 300 are major *academic medical centers* or teaching hospitals. Affiliated with medical schools, they generally provide the most up-to-date and experienced care, because staff physicians must stay current in order to teach their students. These centers, with the best equipment, researchers, and resources, offer high-technology care—at a price. The cost of treatment at all teaching hospitals averages approximately 20 percent higher than at nonteaching hospitals. At major teaching hospitals with large graduate training programs for physicians and other health providers, the costs are as much as 45 percent higher than those at nonteaching hospitals.

The Joint Commission on the Accreditation of Healthcare Organizations (JCAH) reviews all hospitals every three years. Eighty percent of hospitals qualify for JCAH accreditation. If you have to enter a hospital and your health insurance or plan allows a choice, try to find out as much as you can about the alternatives available to you:

:: Talk to your physician about a hospital and why he or she recommends it.

:: As a cost-cutting strategy, many hospitals have cut back on the use of registered nurses. Check with the local nursing association about the ratio of patients to nurses, and the ratio of R.N.s to L.P.N.s.

:: Find out room rates and charges for ancillary services, including tests, lab work, X rays, and medications. Check with your health plan to see whether you need preapproval for any of these costs and ask what you will be expected to pay.

:: Ask how many times in the past year the hospital has performed the procedure recommended for you, and what the success and complication rates have been. Ask about the hospital's nosocomial (hospital-caused) infection rate and accident rate. You also have the right to information on the number and types of malpractice claims filed against a hospital.

:: If possible, go on a tour of the hospital. Does the setting seem comfortable? Is the staff courteous? Does the hospital seem clean and efficiently run?

Emergency Services. Hospital emergency rooms should be used only in a true emergency. Most are overwhelmed, understaffed, and underfinanced—particularly in big cities. Patients usually see a different physician each time; he or she deals with the main complaints but doesn't have time for a full examination. Extensive tests and procedures are difficult to arrange in an emergency room, and patients who don't have truly urgent problems may have to wait for a long time. Emergency-room fees are higher than those for standard office visits and are not always covered by medical insurance.

Inpatient Care. Inpatient hospital care remains the most expensive form of health care. Health-insurance companies and health-care plans (described on pages 560–561) often demand a second opinion or make their own evaluation before approving coverage of an elective, or nonemergency, hospital admission. As another means of controlling costs, health insurers (including Medicare) may limit hospital stays or pay for hospital care on the basis of **diagnostic-related groups,** or **DRGs.** Under this system, hospitals are paid according to a patient's diagnosis—for example, a set number of dollars for every appendectomy. If the hospital can treat and discharge patients more quickly than the national average for that DRG, it makes money. On the other hand, if a patient develops unexpected complications or is slow to recover, the hospital loses money.

Because hospital stays are shorter than in the past, patients often leave "quicker and sicker"—after a shorter stay and not as far along in their recovery. Nevertheless, the benefits of shorter hospital stays, including reduced complications and more rapid resumption of normal life activities, may outweigh the slightly increased risks associated with early discharge.

Home Health Care

With hospitals discharging patients sooner, **home health care**—the provision of equipment and services to patients in the home to restore or maintain comfort, function, and health—has become a major industry. Advances in technology have made it possible for treatments once administered only in hospitals—such as kidney dialysis, chemotherapy, and traction—to be performed at home at 10 to 40 percent of the cost. The physician's house call, once considered an anachronism, has also come back in fashion. According to various surveys, the majority of primary care physicians see patients in their homes.

Hospital discharge planners usually arrange home health care for patients who've been hospitalized. Families can also contact health aides, nurses, and other needed professionals on their own. According to the Health Insurance Association of America, most private insurance policies offer some coverage for these home health-care costs.

⚙ Paying for Health Care

Health insurance did not become common as a standard benefit until World War II, when the government imposed wage controls and businesses offered free health-insurance policies to lure prospective employees. For the next 50 years, patients went to the physicians of their choice, with insurance companies usually paying part or all of their fees.

As technological breakthroughs, such as new imaging techniques and bone-marrow transplants, transformed modern medicine, subspecialists multiplied, and medical costs spiraled upward. Finally, in the 1990s, health care policymakers and the employers that had footed the bills agreed that health costs, which had grown to almost 14 percent of the gross domestic product, had to be controlled. This led to the emergence of **managed care,** a new way of delivering and paying for health-care services. Managed-care organizations provide health care or health-care insurance at lower costs to employers. The tradeoff for such savings is that a third party makes the final decision on when or if a medical visit or treatment is necessary. This differs from traditional *fee-for-service* medicine, in which patients decide when to seek care and choose which physician to see.

Both fee-for-service and managed-care systems have drawbacks. Fee-for-service medicine errs on the side of doing too much and providing unneeded tests and therapies. Managed-care organizations are more likely to do too little so they can keep costs low.

Traditional Health Insurance

In the past, most working Americans relied on conventional **indemnity** insurance policies to pay major medical expenses. Policyholders paid a percentage (generally 20 percent) of hospitalization costs and a deductible (a minimum paid out each year before the insurance company pays anything). While indemnity insurance gave patients freedom to choose physicians and hospitals, it often failed to cover routine physical exams and screening tests. Individuals with "preexisting" conditions often could not qualify for coverage or were not reimbursed for treatments related to these conditions. In the last decade, as health-care costs skyrocketed, insurers increasingly refused to pay claims, canceled groups with high medical bills, or denied coverage to people in high-risk occupations.

📠 What Is Managed Care?

Managed care has become the predominant form of health care in the United States. Managed-care organizations, which take various forms, deliver care through a network of physicians, hospitals, and other health-care professionals who agree to provide their services at fixed or discounted rates. Nine in ten physicians in the United States have contracted with managed care companies.[49]

Consumers in a managed-care group must follow certain procedures in advance of seeking care (for example, getting prior approval for a test or treatment) and must abide by a limit on reimbursement for certain services. Some procedures may be deemed unnecessary and not be covered at all. Patients who choose to see a physician who is not a participating member of the medical-insurance coverage group may have to pay the entire fee themselves.

Managed-care plans have been criticized for pressuring providers to "undertreat" patients—for example, sending them home from the hospital too soon or denying them costly tests or treatments. Members have complained of long waits, the need to switch primary physicians if their doctor leaves the plan, difficulty getting approval for needed services, and a sense that providers pay more attention to the bottom line than to the health needs of their patients.

As dissatisfaction with managed care has grown, consumers have demanded more choice of physicians, direct access to specialists, and the ability to go "out of network." In response to patients' complaints, many states have approved "patient protection acts" or "comprehensive consumer bills of rights." Federal legislators also have debated a national patients' bill of rights for years, but have disagreed over controversial provisions, such as allowing patients to sue their insurers or employers in either state or federal courts if they feel their rights have been violated.

According to the National Committee for Quality Assurance, managed-care plans have shown improvement in the delivery of care, but health-care costs continue to rise.[50] As a result, employers are cutting back coverage and asking employees to shoulder more of the burden of their health care in the belief that consumers will seek more efficient care when they are required to pay more out of pocket.[51]

Health Maintenance Organizations (HMOs)

Health maintenance organizations, or **HMOs,** are managed-care plans that emphasize routine care and prevention by providing complete medical services in exchange for a predetermined monthly payment. In a *group-model* HMO, physicians provide care in offices at a clinic run by the HMO. In an *individual practice association (IPA),* or network HMO, independent physicians provide services in their own offices. HMOs generally pay a fixed amount per patient to a physician or hospital, regardless of the type and number of services actually provided. This is called *capitation.*

Members of HMOs pay a regular, preset fee that usually includes diagnostic tests, routine physical exams, and vaccinations as well as treatment of illnesses. HMOs usually do not require a deductible, and copayments for medications or services are small. The primary drawback of standard HMOs is that the consumer is limited to a particular health-care facility and staff. Open-ended or point-of-service HMOs charge more but let members seek treatment elsewhere if they prefer. These "hybrid" plans have proven the most popular. Although some large HMOs have earned profits, the HMO industry as a whole consistently lost money in the last decade. Enrollment in HMOs rose steadily in the early 1990s but has declined in more recent years. The total number of HMOs also has dropped.

Although HMOs have been accused of undermining the quality of patient care, recent studies of the outcomes of cancer patients in HMOs and in traditional fee-for-service practices have found little difference. HMOs are, on average, more likely to detect breast cancer early and just as likely to offer breast-saving lumpectomies rather than mastectomy. Prostate cancer patients treated in HMOs also had similar ten-year survival rates as those receiving fee-for-service care.

Preferred Provider Organizations (PPOs)

In a **preferred provider organization (PPO),** a third party—a union, an insurance company, or a self-insured business—contracts with a group of physicians and hospitals to treat members at a discount. PPO members may choose any physician within the network, and usually pay a 10 percent copayment for care within the system and a higher percentage (20 to 30 percent) for care elsewhere. PPOs generally require prior approval for expensive tests or major procedures.

A *point-of-service (POS)* plan is a PPO that permits patients to use physicians outside the network. Consumers pay the difference between the preferred provider's discounted fee and the outside physician's fee. A *gatekeeper* plan requires members to choose a primary physician, as in an HMO, who must approve all referrals to specialists.

Government-Financed Insurance Plans

The government, through programs like Medicare and Medicaid, funds 45 percent of total U.S. health spending.[52] Under Medicare, the federal government pays 80 percent of most medical bills, after a deductible fee, for people over age 65. Medicare doesn't cover drugs, eyeglasses, or dental work. Seniors are more supportive of Medicare and favor its expansion, compared with those between ages 18 and 65, who tend to favor private alternatives.[53]

Medicaid, a federal and state insurance plan that protects people with very low or no incomes, is the chief source of coverage for the unemployed. However, many unemployed Americans don't qualify because their family incomes are above the poverty line. Publicly insured patients are more likely than those with private insurance to receive inadequate care and to experience adverse health outcomes.

The Uninsured

The United States is the only industrialized nation that does not have national health insurance.[54] (See Fact or Fiction? "Providing insurance . . .") As many as 41 million Americans lack health insurance. (See Figure 16-2.) Many others are underinsured, meaning that they don't have adequate coverage and are less likely to receive preventive care or routine checkups. Women, who are more likely to be caring for children or aging parents, are themselves less likely than men to have good access to health care. The number of uninsured women has grown three times faster than the number of uninsured men and, if this trend continues, will exceed that of uninsured men by the year 2005.[55]

One in three Americans younger than 65 went without insurance for all or part of the past two years. Nearly four out of five were in working families.[56] Nearly one-third of the uninsured are Latino, despite the fact that Latinos make up just 13 percent of the population. This disparity results from several factors, including citizenship issues and language barriers.[57] Nearly half of young adults between ages 18 and 24 have no health insurance—the highest proportion of any age group. (See Figure 16-2.) Some universities, such as those in the University of California system, are requiring all students to purchase insurance that can be used to cover services beyond those provided in university clinics.

Uninsured patients have shorter hospital stays, cannot undergo costly therapies, and have a greater risk of dying in the hospital than insured patients. About 85 percent of uninsured Americans are from families in which the head of the family works but can't get insurance through his or her employer. Some of these people work part-time and do not qualify for insurance. Others work for businesses too small to qualify for group insurance. The availability of

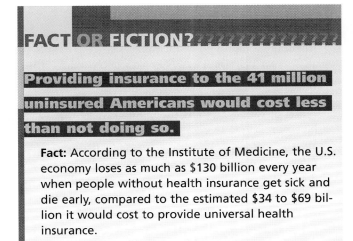

FACT OR FICTION?

Providing insurance to the 41 million uninsured Americans would cost less than not doing so.

Fact: According to the Institute of Medicine, the U.S. economy loses as much as $130 billion every year when people without health insurance get sick and die early, compared to the estimated $34 to $69 billion it would cost to provide universal health insurance.

Source: Board on Health Care Services. *Hidden Costs, Value Lost: Uninsurance in America.* Washington, DC: Institute of Medicine, 2003.

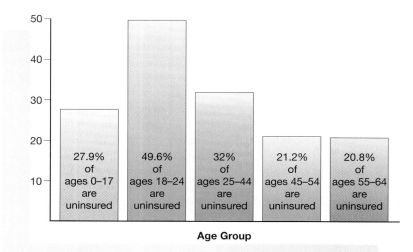

Figure 16-2 WHO ARE THE UNINSURED?

Children and younger adults account for the largest number of people without insurance. About half of college-age Americans are uninsured.

Source: Data from "Going Without Health Insurance," Robert Wood Johnson Foundation, www.rwjf.org.

insurance affects both access to care and the way care is delivered.

The Bottom Line ▼
Taking Charge of Your Health Care

You can do more to safeguard and enhance your well-being than any health care provider. Here are some recommendations to keep in mind:

:: *Trust your instincts.* You know your body better than anyone else. If something is bothering you, it deserves medical attention. Don't let your health-care provider—or your health plan administrator—dismiss it without a thorough evaluation.

:: *Do your homework.* Go to the library or online and find authoritative articles that describe what you're experiencing. The more you know about possible causes of your symptoms, the more likely you are to be taken seriously.

:: *Find a good primary care physician who listens carefully and responds to your concerns.* Look for a family doctor or general internist who takes a careful history, performs a thorough exam, and listens and responds to your concerns.

:: *See your doctor regularly.* If you're in your twenties or thirties, you may not need an annual exam, but it's important to get checkups at least every two or three years, not so much for the sake of finding hidden disease, but so you and your doctor can get to know each other and develop a trusting, mutually respectful relationship.

:: *Get a second opinion.* If you are uncertain of whether to undergo treatment or which therapy is best, see another physician and listen carefully for any doubts or hesitation about what you're considering.

:: *Challenge medical judgments based on personal circumstances.* Insist that your doctor base any diagnosis on a thorough medical evaluation, not on a value judgment about you or your lifestyle.

:: *Seek support.* Patient support and advocacy groups can offer emotional support, information on many common problems, and referral to knowledgeable physicians. (See the Hales Health Almanac at the back of the book for numbers and addresses.)

:: *If your doctor cannot or will not respond to your concerns, get another one.* Regardless of your health coverage, you have the right to replace a physician who is not meeting your health-care needs.

:: *Speak up.* If you don't understand, ask. If you feel that you're not being taken seriously or being treated with respect, say so. Sometimes the only difference between being a patient or becoming a victim is making sure your needs and rights are not forgotten or overlooked.

:: *Bring your own advocate.* If you become intimidated or anxious talking to physicians, ask a friend to accompany you, to ask questions on your behalf, and to take notes.

 After watching the CNN video segment, discuss the following question. Are patient office visits with physicians getting longer or shorter?

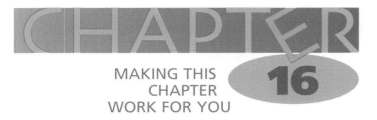

MAKING THIS CHAPTER WORK FOR YOU

16

1. Which of the following statements about health information on the Internet is true?
   a. Chat rooms are the most reliable source of accurate medical information.
   b. Physicians who have websites must adhere to a strict set of standards set by the American Medical Association.
   c. Government-sponsored sites such as that of the Centers for Disease Control and Prevention are excellent sources of accurate health-care information.
   d. The Internet is a safe and cost-effective source of prescription drugs.

2. In a preclinical trial,
   a. researchers examine the cost-effectiveness of a specific treatment.
   b. animals are used to test new medical treatments.
   c. humans are used to test new medical treatments.
   d. the health status of a large group of people who exhibit certain health habits is reviewed.

3. A good primary care physician
   a. appears to know all the answers to your questions.
   b. stays on schedule, never spending more than the allotted time with each patient.
   c. is willing to treat complex problems rather than send you to an expensive specialist.
   d. encourages you to do research about your diagnosis and answers all your questions.

4. During a medical exam, your doctor will
   a. check your cardiovascular system by listening to your heart and feeling your neck arteries.
   b. check your lungs by probing for tender spots and malformations.
   c. look into your eyes to see if you have vision problems that require glasses or contact lenses.
   d. evaluate your joints by tapping on the knees and elbows.

5. Periodontal disease
   a. results from poor eating habits.
   b. can lead to cardiovascular problems.
   c. in its early stage can be prevented by brushing alone.
   d. is caused by a variety of bacteria and viruses.

6. Patients have all the rights below *except* which of the following?
   a. access to their medical records
   b. medical care that meets accepted standards of quality
   c. to donate a body part for compensation
   d. to leave the hospital against their physician's advice

7. Examples of complementary and alternative therapies include all of the following *except*
   a. psychiatry
   b. acupuncture
   c. chiropractic
   d. homeopathy

8. Herbal remedies that have positive health effects include
   a. ayurveda for controlling asthma.
   b. acidophilus for improving memory.
   c. aloe vera for diabetes.
   d. garlic for lowering cholesterol.

9. Which of the following statements about the health-care system is true?
   a. Primary care is usually provided by specialists in a hospital.
   b. Nurses can perform some surgical procedures once they are board certified.
   c. Most hospitals in the United States are teaching hospitals and affiliated with medical schools.
   d. The length of hospital stays may be determined by a patient's diagnosis rather than the person's pace of recovery.

10. Managed care features all of the following except
    a. health maintenance organizations.
    b. a fee-for-service system of insurance.
    c. preferred provider organizations.
    d. limitations on reimbursement for certain health services.

Answers to these questions can be found on page 652.

Critical Thinking

1. Think about an experience you've had with a traditional medical practitioner. How did you feel during the physical examination? Did you trust the practitioner? Were you comfortable with the level of communication? Evaluate your experience and give your opinion of the value of the checkup.

2. Have you used any complementary or alternative approaches to health care? If so, were you satisfied with the results? How did your experience with the CAM therapist compare with your most recent experience with a traditional medical practitioner? Do you feel confident that you know the difference between alternative care and quackery?

Critical Thinking

3. If you're young and healthy, you'll have little problem getting health insurance. However, if you develop a chronic illness, sustain serious injuries in an accident, or simply get older, you may find insurance harder to get and more expensive to keep. What is your insurance coverage? Do you believe insurance companies have the right to turn down applicants with preexisting conditions, such as high blood pressure? Do they have the right to require screening for potentially serious health problems, such as HIV infection, or to cancel the policies of individuals who have run up high medical bills in the past?

Critical Thinking

4. Jocelyn has been experiencing a great deal of fatigue and frequent headaches for the past couple of months. She doesn't have health insurance and doesn't want to spend money on a doctor visit. So she did some research on the Internet about ways to relieve her symptoms and was considering taking a couple of herbal supplements that were touted as potential treatments. If she asked you for your advice, what would you tell her? Do you think that self-care is appropriate in this situation?

Profile Plus

How do you make intelligent choices about health care? Be an informed consumer with help from the guide on Profile Plus CD-ROM.

Profile Plus

- Guide to Choosing Medical Treatment

Profile Plus

Sites and Bytes

National Health Information Center
www.health.gov/nhic

This excellent site, sponsored by the National Health Information Center (NHIC) of the U.S. Office of Disease Prevention and Health Promotion, is a health information referral service providing health professionals and consumers with a database of various health organizations. The site provides a searchable database, publications, and a list of toll-free numbers for health information.

Sites and Bytes

National Center for Complementary and Alternative Medicine
http://nccam.nih.gov/

This National Institutes of Health site features a variety of fact sheets on alternative therapies and dietary supplements, research, current news, and databases for the public as well as for practitioners.

Sites and Bytes

MedicineNet
http://www.medicinenet.com/Script/Main/hp.asp

This comprehensive site is written for the consumer by board-certified physicians and contains medical news, directory of procedures, medical dictionary, pharmacy, and first aid information. You can use the information at MedicineNet.com to prepare for a doctor visit and to learn about a diagnosis or understand a prescribed treatment or procedure.

InfoTrac College Edition

Activity

Cauley, Geoffrey. "Now, Integrative Care: As Science Rigorously Examines Herbs and Acupuncture, a New Blend of Medicine Emerges." *Newsweek,* December 2, 2002, p. 46.

1. Specifically, what is integrative medical care?

2. What is the short-term goal of researchers who are studying the efficacy of alternative therapies?

InfoTrac College Edition

3. Why are increasing numbers of people using alternative/complementary forms of therapy and why is it important for them to inform their physician about their usage?

You can find additional readings related to CAM and health care with InfoTrac College Edition, an online library of more than 900 journals and publications. Follow the instructions for accessing InfoTrac College Edition

InfoTrac College Edition

that were packaged with your text-book; then search for articles using a key word search.

For additional links, resources, and suggested readings on InfoTrac College Edition, visit our Health & Wellness Resource Center at **http://health.wadsworth.com**.

Key Terms

The terms listed are used on the page indicated. Definitions of the terms are in the Glossary at the end of this book.

Key Terms

acupuncture 554
ayurveda 555
biofeedback 555
chiropractic 556
complementary and alternative medicine (CAM) 552
diagnostic-related groups (DRG) 559
false negatives 550
false positives 550
gingivitis 541
gum disease 541
health insurance organizations (HMO) 560

Key Terms

herbal medicine 555
holistic 552
home health care 559
homeopathy 555
indemnity 560
informed consent 548
integrative medicine 552
malpractice 551
managed care 560
massage therapy 557
medical history 545
meta-analysis 539
naturopathy 555
negligence 550

Key Terms

outcomes 540
over-the-counter (OTC) 547
Pap smear 546
periodontitis 541
plaque 541
preferred provider organization (PPO) 561
primary care 558
quackery 552
reflexology 557
visualization 555
vital signs 540

References

1. Rothstein, William, and Sushama Rajapaksa. "Health Beliefs of College Students Born in the United States, China, and India." *Journal of American College Health*, Vol. 51, No. 5, March 2003, p. 189.
2. Brener, Nancy, and Gowda Vani. "U.S. College Students' Reports of Receiving Health Information on College Campuses." *Journal of American College Health*, Vol. 49, No. 5, March 2001, p. 223.
3. Rothstein and Rajapaksa. "Health Beliefs of College Students Born in the United States, China, and India."

4. Baker, Laurence, et al. "Use of the Internet and E-mail for Health Care Information." *Journal of the American Medical Association*, Vol. 289, No. 18, May 14, 2003, p. 2400.
5. "Good Health Is Hard to Find on the Internet." *Medicine & Health*, Vol. 55, No. 21, May 28, 2001, p. 5.
6. Sigouin, Christopher, and Alejandro R. Jadad. "Awareness of Sources of Peer-Reviewed Research Evidence on the Internet." *Journal of the American Medical*

Association, Vol. 287, No. 21, June 5, 2002, p. 2867.
7. Mold, J. W., et al. "Evidence-Based Medicine Meets Goal-Directed Health Care." *Family Medicine*, Vol. 35, No. 5, May 2003, p. 360.
8. Smith, E. R. "Evidence-Based Decision-Making." *Canadian Journal of Cardiology*, Vol. 19, No. 6, May 2003, p. 729–730.
9. Susman, Jeff. "Practicing Evidence-Based Medicine: The Holy Grail?" *American Family Physician*, Vol. 67, No. 7, April 1, 2003, p. 1606.

References

10. www.selfhelpweb.org.

11. Satcher, David. "Surgeon General's Report on Oral Health." *Public Health Reports,* Vol. 115, No. 5, September 2000, p. 489.

12. "Global Health Spending at All-Time High," www.nlm.nih.gov.

13. Steinberg, E. P. "Improving the Quality of Care—Can We Practice What We Preach?" *New England Journal of Medicine,* Vol. 348, No. 26, June 26, 2003, p. 2681.

14. McGlynn Elizabeth, et al. "The Quality of Health Care Delivered to Adults in the United States." *New England Journal of Medicine,* Vol. 348, No. 26, June 26, 2003, p. 2635.

15. "Fact Sheet: How Good Is the Quality of Health Care in America?" Rand Fact Sheet, www.rand.org.

16. Bodenheimer, Thomas. "Innovations in Primary Care in the United States." *British Medical Journal,* Vol. 326, April 12, 2003, p. 796.

17. Wynia, Matthew, et al. "Do Physicians Not Offer Useful Services Because of Coverage Restrictions?" *Health Affairs,* Vol. 22, No. 4, July–August 2003.

18. Wheby, Munsey. Personal interview.

19. Pinn, Vivian. "Sex and Gender Factors in Medical Studies." *Journal of the American Medical Association,* Vol. 289, No. 4, 2003, p. 397.

20. "Patients' Expectations of Physicians Vary by the Gender of Patients and Doctors," *Health Care Strategic Management,* Vol. 19, No. 5, May 2001, p. 7.

21. Beers, Mark (ed.). *The Merck Manual of Medical Information, Second Home Edition.* Whitehouse Station, New York: Merck Research Laboratories, 2003.

22. "6.6 Million Americans Get a Nip, Tuck, and Lift with Cosmetic Plastic Surgery in 2002." American Society of Plastic Surgeons Reports, Press Release: April 15, 2003.

23. Weston, Pearl. "Attitudes of Adolescents about Cosmetic Surgery." *Annals of Plastic Surgery,* Vol. 50, No. 6, June 2003, p. 628.

24. Daris, Karen, et al. "Room for Improvement: Patients' Report on the Quality of Their Health Care." New York: Commonwealth Fund, April 2002.

25. "Fact Sheet: Protecting the Privacy of Patients' Health Information," Dept. of Health and Human Services, April 14, 2003.

26. Silverman, Jennifer. "A Patient's Right to Sue." *Association of Operating Room Nurses Journal,* Vol. 77, No. 6, June 2003, p. 1147.

27. "Doctors and Other Health Professionals Report That Fear of Malpractice Has a Big, and Mostly Negative, Impact on Medical Practice, Unnecessary Defensive Medicine, and Openness in Discussing Medical Errors." *Health Care News,* February 7, 2003, p. 3.

28. Agency for Healthcare Research and Quality, www.ahrq.gov/consumer/20tips.html.

29. Peters, Sally. "Health Groups Face Six New Patient Safety Goals." *Family Practice News,* Vol. 33, No. 5, March 1, 2003, p. 69.

30. Gallager, Thomas, et al. "Patients' and Physicians' Attitudes Regarding the Disclosure of Medical Errors." *Journal of the American Medical Association,* Vol. 289, No. 1, 2003, p. 1001.

31. Larkin, Marilynn. "No Cure-alls, Says US FTC." *Lancet,* Vol. 358, No. 9275, July 7, 2001, p. 80.

32. *NCCAM,* http://nccam.nih.gov.

33. Barrett, Bruce. "Alternative, Complementary, and Conventional Medicine: Is Integration Upon Us?" *Journal of Alternative and Complementary Medicine,* Vol. 9, No. 3, June 2003, p. 417.

34. Forjuoh, Samuel, et al. "Teaching Medical Students Complementary and Alternative Medicine Using Evidence-Based Principles." *Journal of Alternative and Complementary Medicine,* Vol. 9, No. 3, June 2003, p. 429.

35. Rees, Lesley, and Andrew Weil. "Integrated Medicine Imbues Orthodox Medicine with the Values of Complementary Medicine." *British Medical Journal,* Vol. 322, No. 7279, January 20, 2001, p. 119.

36. Vernarec, Emil. "Why Do Patients Turn to CAM?" *RN,* Vol. 65, No. 5, May 2002, p. 25.

37. Lake, James. "Uses of Unconventional (CAM) Treatments in U.S. Mental Health Care." Report to the Committee on Research in Psychiatric Treatments, American Psychiatric Association, May 2003.

38. Sadovsky, Richard. "Complementary and Alternative Medical Therapies for Cancer." *American Family Physician,* Vol. 67, No. 9, May 1, 2003, p. 1991.

39. Rieder, M. J. and D. Matsui. "Complementary and Alternative Medicine: How Do We Know If It Works?" *Healthcare Papers,* Vol. 3, No. 5, 2003, p. 62.

40. Giordano, James, et al. "Complementary and Alternative Medicine in Mainstream Public Health: A Role for Research in Fostering Integration." *Journal of Alternative and Complementary Medicine,* Vol. 9, No. 3, June 2003, p. 441.

41. Carey, John. "Herbal Remedies: A $4 Billion Enigma." *Business Week,* No. 3830, April 28, 2003, p. 104.

42. Zepf, Bill. "Evidence Basis for Four Commonly Used Herbs." *American Family Physician,* Vol. 67, No. 7, April 1, 2003, p. 1607.

43. Gold, Paul, et al. "The Lowdown on Ginkgo Biloba: This Popular Herbal Supplement May Slightly Improve Your Memory, But You Can Get the Same Effect by Eating a Candy Bar." *Scientific American,* Vol. 288, No. 4, April 2003, p. 86.

44. Satia-Abouta, Jessie, et al. "Dietary Supplement Use and Medical Conditions—The VITAL Study." *American Journal of Preventive Medicine,* Vol. 24, No. 1, January 2003.

45. Bent, Stephen, et al. "The Relative Safety of Ephedra Compared with Other Herbal Products." *Annals of Internal Medicine,* Vol. 138, March 2003, p. 468.

46. NCCAM Consumer Advisory on Ephedra, Revised February 28, 2003, http://nccam.nih.gov/health/alerts/ephedra/consumeradvisory.html.

47. Cherkin, D. C., et al. "A Review of the Evidence For the Effectiveness, Safety, and Cost of Acupuncture, Massage Therapy, and Spinal Manipulation for Back Pain." *Annals of Internal Medicine,* Vol. 138, No. 11, June 3, 2003, p. 898.

48. Turner, H. Spencer. "Athletic Training Services and Student Health Services on Campus: Working Together." *Journal of American College Health,* Vol. 51, No. 5, March 2003, p. 217.

49. "Managed Care Is Evolving, and Here to Stay." *Contemporary OB/GYN,* Vol. 48, No. 5, May 2003, p. 28.

50. "Managed Care Quality Makes Gains." *Business Insurance,* Vol. 36, No. 38, September 23, 2002, p. 8.

51. Iglehart, John K. "Changing Health Insurance Trends." *New England Journal of Medicine,* Vol. 347, No. 12, September 19, 2002, p. 956.

52. Bitton, Asaf, and James Kahn. "Government Share of Health Care Expenditures." *Journal of the American Medical Association,* Vol. 289, No. 9, March 5, 2003, p. 1165.

53. "New Survey Finds Most Seniors Favor Reforms That Build on Existing Medical Program, But Younger Adults Are More Favorable Toward Private Plan." Harvard School of Public Health, June 19, 2003.

54. Harrison, Bridget. "A Historical Survey of National Health Movements and Public Opinion in the United States." *Journal of the American Medical Association,* Vol. 289, No. 9, March 5, 2003, p. 1163.

55. Board on Health Care Services. *Hidden Costs, Value Lost: Uninsurance in America.* Washington, DC: Institute of Medicine, 2003.

56. Finkelstein, Joel. "Groups Come Together to Speak Up for Uninsured." *American Medical News,* March 24–31, 2003.

57. Harrell, Joseph, and Olveen Carrasquillo. "The Latino Disparity in Health Coverage," *Journal of the American Medical Association,* Vol. 289, No. 9, March 5, 2003, p. 1167.

HEALTH IN CONTEXT

PERSONAL health involves more than a single individual. We are social beings, and we live our lives as part of a network of family, friends, acquaintances, colleagues, neighbors. Our actions affect others; others' behaviors have a significant impact on our well-being.

Aging and dying are as much as part of the real world as life itself. The quest to find fulfillment in living and meaning in dying is one of the challenges of living.

For college students, staying safe is an essential part of staying healthy. Injury claims more lives of young Americans than illness. Threats such as violence and terrorism are too serious and widespread to ignore.

All of us share something else: our planet. The problems of creating a healthy environment are many and complex. They too demand our attention and commitment.

© Duomo Photography/The Image Bank/Getty Images

567

CHAPTER 17

A Lifetime of Health

Corita didn't feel old until she enrolled in a college personal health course. Formal at first, the other students—young enough to be her children—started calling her "Mom." When the professor announced that the next week's topic would be aging, Corita beamed, "I'll be the expert!"

More of us can expect to do the same. In the United States, the number of persons over age 65 is expected to increase to an estimated 71 million in 2030; the number over age 80 to 19.5 million.[1]

Although **aging**—the characteristic pattern of normal life changes that occurs as humans, plants, and animals grow older—remains inevitable, you can do a great deal to influence the impact that the passage of time has on you. Whether you're in your teens, twenties, thirties, or older, now is the time to start taking the steps that will add healthy, active, productive years to your life.

This chapter provides a preview of the changes age brings, the steps you can take to age healthfully, and the ways you can make the most of all the years of your life.

Invariably, though, no one gets out of this life alive. Death is the natural completion of things, as much a part of the real world as life itself. In time we all lose people we cherish: grandparents, aunts and uncles, parents, friends, neighbors, coworkers, siblings. With each loss, part of us may seem to die, yet each loss also reaffirms how precious life is.

This chapter explores the meaning of death, describes the process of dying, provides information on end-of-life issues, and offers advice on comforting the dying and helping their survivors.

© Dick Luria/Taxi/Getty Images

After studying the material in this chapter, you should be able to:

- **List** the benefits that older Americans can gain from physical activity.
- **Name** three memory skills that diminish with age.
- **Discuss** the issue of hormone replacement therapy for menopause symptoms.
- **Identify** some of the challenges of aging and **discuss** their risk factors and possible ways of preventing them.
- **Define** death and **explain** the stages of emotional reaction experienced in facing death.
- **Explain** the purposes of advanced directives, a living will, and a holographic will.
- **List** and **explain** factors affecting the length and intensity of grief.

✸ Living in an Aging Society

America is turning gray. People age 65 and older make up 13 percent of the U.S. population. By the year 2014, this group will grow to 15 percent.[2] By the midpoint of the twenty-first century, 80 million Americans—one in five—will be seniors (65 or older).[3]

Throughout your life, you will confront a variety of issues related not just to your age, but also to that of the aging American population. These include:

:: **Retirement costs.** Unless changes are made to decrease the demand on the Social Security system, Social Security taxes on workers may be increased.

:: **Health costs.** Health care costs for those over 65 years are three to five times greater than for younger men and women.[4]

:: **Gray-power politics.** Senior citizens go to the polls in larger numbers than younger voters. With such voting power, programs for the elderly may make up a larger share of future federal budgets.

:: **Anti-aging gimmicks.** As the population ages, health hucksters push an ever-growing number of unproven anti-aging treatments, such as melatonin or the hormone DHEA. Because some preparations have the potential to harm, consumers must be wary of all claims to turn back or slow down the biological clock. (Chapter 16 offers advice on avoiding health quackery.)

🔍 ✸ How Long Can I Expect to Live?

The answer depends on you. Statistically, you're likely to live longer than your parents or grandparents. Life expectancy has been increasing steadily over the last century, reaching an all-time high in the United States of 77.2 years. (The United States is not in the top five countries—see Table 17-1.) A newborn boy can expect to live to age 74.4 years; a girl, to age 79.8. Race also affects life expectancy, which is greater for white Americans—77.7 years—than African Americans—72.2 years.[5] A child born in the United States in 2020 should expect to live 79.25 years; one born in 2050, 82.91 years.

Women's lifespans average 5 to 10 percent longer than men's. No one knows exactly why. (See The X & Y File: "Why Do Women Live Longer Than Men?") But the gender gap in longevity narrows over time. At birth a baby boy has a life expectancy about five years shorter than a girl's. By age 65, a man can expect to live an additional 15.1 years, just 3.8 years less than a woman. By age 85, the difference in projected life expectancies is down to 1.2 years.

Contrary to common belief, heredity doesn't determine how long you'll live or how well you'll age. Genes, as studies of identical twins have revealed, influence only about 30 percent of the rate and ways in which we age.[6] "The rest is up to us," says Michael Roizen, M.D., author

TABLE 17-1	**Life Expectancies Around the World**

Top 5

Japan	81.6
Sweden	80.1
Hong Kong	79.9
Iceland	79.8
Canada	79.3

Bottom 5

Zambia	32.4
Botswana	39.7
Afghanistan	43.1
Ethiopia	45.5
Laos	54.5

the XY file *Why Do Women Live Longer Than Men?*

The gender gap in longevity has been shrinking since 1990. According to the National Center for Health Statistics, life expectancy for American women now stands at 79.8 years; for men, it is a record high of 74.4 years. Women in other developed nations—Australia, Canada, France, Greece, Italy, Japan, Netherlands, Norway, Spain, Sweden, Switzerland—live up to two years longer than those in the United States and about seven years longer than men. In the former Soviet Union, life expectancy for females is thirteen years longer than for males. By the year 2020, according to current projections for the United States, the average woman's life may increase by ten years, the average man's by six.

The gender difference in mortality rates emerges from the moment of conception. Baby girls are less likely to die in the womb or after delivery than baby boys. Once past age 30, women consistently outnumber and outlive men. By age 85, there are three women for every man.

Why do men die sooner? The female edge may begin at conception with the extra X chromosome, which provides a backup for defects on the X gene and a double dose of the genetic factors that regulate the immune system. In addition, the female hormone estrogen bolsters immunity and protects heart, bone, brain, and blood vessels.

In some cancers, estrogen may somehow protect against distant metastases. In contrast, testosterone may dampen the immune response in males—possibly to prevent attacks on sperm cells that might otherwise be mistaken as alien invaders. When the testes are removed from mice and guinea pigs, their immune systems become more active. In men, lessened immunity may lower resistance to cancer as well as infectious disease. Half of all men—compared with a third of women—develop cancer. Smoking, which for a long time was much more prevalent among men, accounts for some of this difference. However, this is changing; 23 percent of American women smoke, and lung cancer rates in women have doubled since the early 1970s.

Testosterone also has been implicated in men's risk of heart disease and stroke. Originally designed to equip men with an instantaneous burst of power—essential for survival in Stone Age times—this potent male hormone may surge so intensely that it wreaks havoc throughout the cardiovascular system.

Males also die more often as a result of intentional and nonintentional injury. Overall, men are three times more likely than women to die in accidents, mainly in cars and on the job. Men also are four times more likely to die violently. Nine in ten murderers and eight in ten murder victims are men.

---

of *RealAge,* who notes that it's possible to become healthier, fitter, and biologically younger with time. "With relatively simple changes, someone whose chronological age is 69 can have a physiological age of 45. And the most amazing thing is that it's never too late to live younger—until one foot is 6 feet under.[7]

▓ Successful Aging

The number of Americans living long enough to blow out 100 birthday candles has increased 35 percent from a decade ago. Although the proportion of people who live beyond 100 years is still very small, the worldwide number is rapidly growing. The United Nations estimates that in 2050, there will be 3.2 million centenarians, an increase of about eighteen times.[8]

Among senior citizens, the most rapid growth in the last decade has been in the oldest age groups. (See Figure 17-1.) Some 35 million persons age 65 or older live in the United States. Now 13 percent of the population, they are its fastest-growing segment. By 2030 one in five Americans—71 million men and women—will be 65 or older.[9]

Americans are living better as well as longer. (See Fact or Fiction? "The best years of life . . .") Disability decreased steadily through the 1980s and 1990s, and the rate of improvement is accelerating. Nursing home use has fallen. Senior citizens are healthier and more independent. All in all, the mortality rates of senior citizens are declining by about 1 percent a year, and their disability rates are falling by about 2 percent a year.[10] Among the factors contributing to a longer healthspan are improved medical care, diet, exercise, and public health advances.

Exercise: An Anti-aging Pill

Staying in bed for three weeks has the same effect on fitness as aging 30 years. At any age, the unexercised body—though free of the symptoms of illness—will rust out long before it could ever wear out. Inactivity can make anyone old before his or her time. Just as inactivity accelerates aging, activity slows it down. The effects of ongoing activity are so profound that gerontologists sometimes refer to exercise as "the closest thing to an antiaging pill." Exercise

FACT OR FICTION? ?????????????

The best years of life come in one's youth.

Fiction: When surveyed, about half of Americans aged 65 to 69 say "these are the best years of my life." Many people in their seventies and eighties agree. Sixty percent of older black and 57 percent of older Hispanic respondents say these are their best years. When asked about the keys to a meaningful and vital life, older adults rate having family and friends and taking care of their health as most important, followed by spiritual life.

Source: "Facts About Older Americans," National Council on Aging, www.aoa.gov.

can reverse many of the changes that occur with age, including increases in body fat and decreases in muscle strength. The bottom line: What you *don't* do may matter more than what you do do.

No one is ever too old to get in shape. Rather than telling seniors to take it easy, the American College of Sports Medicine encourages them to engage in the full range of physical activities, including aerobic conditioning. As much as 50 percent of the physiologic declines commonly attributed to aging are due to sedentary living and can be dramatically reversed. With regular conditioning,

60-year-olds can regain the fitness they had at age 40 to 45.

Adults over the age of 72 who exercise more and smoke less than their peers are most likely to enjoy long, healthy, and happy lives, according to a study that followed 1,000 seniors for nine years. Proactive health-promoting behaviors, such as exercising and not smoking, contributed to high quality throughout life regardless of when they began. Older women who start exercising after the age of 65 live longer. Newly active women had a 36 percent lower risk of heart disease and a 51 percent lower risk of cancer than those who didn't exercise.[11]

Exercise slows many changes associated with advancing age, such as loss of lean muscle tissue, increase in body fat, and decreased work capacity. It lowers the risk of heart disease and stroke in the elderly—and greatly improves general health. Male and female runners over age 50 have much lower rates of disability and much lower health-care expenses than less active seniors. Even less intense activities, such as gardening, dancing, and brisk walking, can delay chronic physical disability and cognitive decline.[12]

According to the U.S. surgeon general, physical activity offers older Americans additional benefits, including the following:

:: Greater ability to live independently.

:: Reduced risk of falling and fracturing bones.

Physical fitness can be enhanced at any age by routine activities such as gardening.

© Courtesy of Eva Chaney

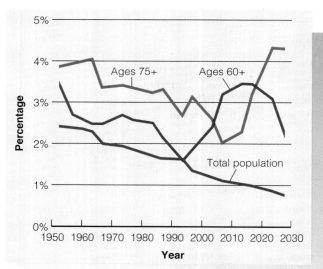

Figure 17-1 THE GRAYING OF AMERICA
The percentage of annual growth of the total U.S. population decreases as the senior population increases.

Source: National Institute on Aging.

:: Lower risk of dying from coronary heart disease and of developing high blood pressure, colon cancer, and diabetes.

:: Reduced blood pressure in some people with hypertension.

:: Fewer symptoms of anxiety and depression.

:: Improvements in mood and feelings of well-being.

Despite these potential benefits, many seniors are not active. By age 75, about one in three men and one in two women engage in no physical activity. Yet even sedentary individuals in their eighties and nineties can participate in an exercise program—and gain significant benefits. In addition to physical activity, social interactions, such as entertaining friends and getting involved with religious activities, lead to greater life satisfaction as people get older.[13]

Federal health officials recommend a moderate amount of physical activity, either in longer sessions of moderately intense activities (such as walking) or in shorter sessions of more vigorous activities (such as race-walking or stair-climbing). Seniors can gain additional health benefits by increasing the duration, intensity, or frequency of their workouts, but should avoid overdoing their training because of the risk of injury. Older adults should always consult with a physician before beginning a new physical activity program.

Changing Nutritional Needs

The most common nutritional disorder in older persons is obesity. Among Americans between 65 to 74 years old, approximately 34 percent of women and 44 percent of men are overweight; an additional 27 percent of women and 24 percent of men are obese.[14]

The Food Guide Pyramid for Older Americans was designed specifically for adults over age 70, but the USDA urges anyone age 50 or older to heed its recommendations. (See Figure 17-2.) The new guidelines advise eight or more 8-ounce glasses of water daily to reduce the risk of dehydration and constipation, which become increasing risks because of decreased thirst sensation in the elderly. The Pyramid also calls for dietary supplements of calcium and vitamins B_{12} and D.

In a four-year study of more than 22,000 Greek adults, those who most closely adhered to the Mediterranean diet (described in Chapter 5) had a 25 percent lower rate of death from both heart disease and cancer. Furthermore, the higher the level of physical activity and education, the lower the rate of death within the four-year study period.[15] Older men and women who consume more cereal fiber also have lower rates of cardiovascular disease than those with less fiber in their diets.[16]

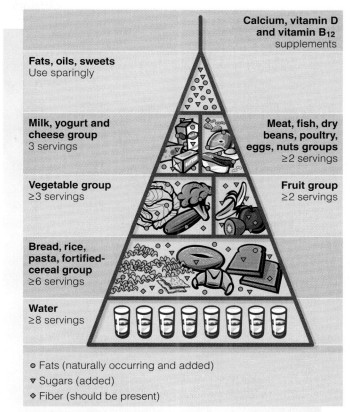

Figure 17-2 FOOD GUIDE PYRAMID FOR OLDER ADULTS

The Pyramid shows the USDA-recommended daily servings for adults 70 or older.

As many as 40 percent of elderly people who live independently do not get adequate amounts of one or more essential nutrients. The reasons are many: limited income, difficulty getting to stores, chronic illness, medications that interfere with the metabolism of nutrients, problems chewing or digesting, poor appetite, inactivity, illness, depression. Nutritionists urge the elderly, like other Americans, to concentrate on eating healthful foods; many also recommend daily nutritional supplements, which may provide the added benefit of improving cognitive function in healthy people over 65.

Does Body Composition Change with Age?

Both weight and body fat percentage typically increase in adulthood. (See Figure 17-3.) Starting in their twenties, American men and women put on an average of 1 pound of weight a year. By age 65, they have gained about 40 pounds. Because activity levels decline with age, the average individual also loses half a pound of lean body mass a year. The result is a dramatic change in body composition over time: a 20-pound loss of lean tissue and a 40-pound gain in body fat.

Figure 17-3 IDEAL BODY FAT PERCENTAGES
As we grow older, body fat percentages tend to increase about 5 to 10 percent every decade. An individual whose body fat percentages are outside the ideal range may have a weight problem.

Source: American College of Sports Medicine.

Body composition can affect how well older individuals function. In a study of women between the ages of 68 and 75, muscle strength was related to lean mass. The women with the greatest level of disability had higher BMIs and a higher percentage of body fat. Changes in body composition over time are not inevitable. Researchers have documented that physical activity—both aerobic workouts and resistance exercise—can increase and maintain lean body tissue.

The Aging Brain

Scientists used to think that the aging brain, once worn out, could never be fixed. Now they know that the brain can and does repair itself. When neurons (brain cells) die, the surrounding cells develop "fingers" to fill the gaps and establish new connections, or synapses, between surviving neurons. Although self-repair occurs more quickly in young brains, the process continues in older brains. Even victims of Alzheimer's disease, the most devastating form of senility, have enough healthy cells in the diseased brain to regrow synapses. Scientists hope to develop drugs that someday may help the brain repair itself.

Mental ability does not decline along with physical vigor. Researchers have been able to reverse the supposedly normal intellectual declines of 60- to 80-year-olds by tutoring them in problem solving. Reaction time, intellectual speed and efficiency, nonverbal intelligence, and maximum work rate for short periods may diminish by age 75. However, understanding, vocabulary, ability to remember

THE CUTTING EDGE

Time in a Bottle?

Researchers at Harvard Medical School have discovered that an ingredient in red wine extends lifespan by 70 percent—in yeast, at least. The chemical, resveratrol, boosts the ability of microscopic cells to fend off the ravages of time. In laboratory experiments with baker's yeast, resveratrol mimicked the age-extending effects of calorie restriction on fruit-flies as well as yeast. Rather than the normal lifespan of 30 days, fruit flies given a fresh grape extract lived an extra ten days.

Could red wine have similar effects on humans? While researchers caution that development of a drug or dietary supplement for humans might be a decade or more away, they predict that the discovery of resveratrol could provide major clues into slowing the aging process. It also may explain the so-called "French paradox": why the French, who often smoke and eat high-fat foods but regularly drink red wine, live longer than people in many other countries.

Resveratrol, one of a group of chemicals called polyphenols, boosts levels of an enzyme called Sir2, which is thought to extend lifespan by stabilizing DNA. Previous research has suggested that polyphenols, also found in tea, fruit, and vegetables, can protect against heart disease and osteoporosis.

Source: K. T. Howitz. "Small Molecule Activators of Sirtuins Extend Saccharomyces Cerevisiae Lifespan." *Nature,* published online, doi:10.1038/nature01960 (2003).

key information, and verbal intelligence remain about the same.

Thinking Young

The healthiest seniors are actively engaged in life, resilient, optimistic, productive, and socially involved. While seniors are not immune to life's slings and arrows, successful agers bounce back after a setback and have a can-do attitude about the challenges they face. People who have a positive perception of aging live seven-and-a-half years longer than those who don't. The reason may be a better response to stress or a stronger will to live.[17] They also tend to be life-long learners who may take up entirely new hobbies late in life—pursuits that stimulate production of more connections between neurons and that may slow aging within the brain.

Just as with muscles, the best advice for keeping your brain healthy as you age is "use it or lose it." Some memory loss among healthy older people is normal, but this is reversible with training in simple methods, such as word associations, that improve recall. The National Institute on Aging has launched a study of Vitamin E and an experimental medication, Aricept (donepezil), as potential treatments for age-related mild cognitive impairment.

Memory

Between the ages of 30 and 90, the brain loses about 10 percent of its volume. Forgetfulness isn't an automatic result, however. Scientists have recently found that loss of brain cells due to aging isn't as steep as once thought. In fact, memory problems may not be a natural part of growing older. In some studies, people with bad memories as older adults had the same deficiency when they were younger. Crossword puzzles, practicing the piano, and playing chess exercise the brain and can counteract natural changes in memory. Exercise also helps cognitive function.

Older subjects score higher on memory tests if they aren't explicitly told that the study is about memory. Elderly subjects score 20 to 30 percent worse on memory tests after reading a pessimistic newspaper account about aging and memory than those who read a cheerful article about growing older.

Some memory skills, particularly the ability to retrieve names and quickly process information, inevitably diminish over time. What normal changes should you expect? Here is a preview:

:: ***Recalling information takes longer.*** As individuals reach their mid- to late sixties, the brain slows down, but usually just by a matter of milliseconds. As long as they're not rushed, older adults eventually adapt and perform just as well as younger ones.

:: ***Distractions become more disruptive.*** College students can study and listen to the stereo at the same time. Thirty-something moms can soothe the baby, field questions about homework, and prepare dinner all at once. But as individuals pass age 50, they find it much more difficult to divide their attention or to remember details of a story after having switched their attention to something else.

:: ***"Accessing" names gets harder.*** The ability to remember names, especially those you don't use frequently, diminishes by as much as 50 percent between ages 25 and 65. Preventive strategies can help, such as repeating a person's name when introduced, writing down the name as soon as possible, and making obvious associations (the Golden Gate for a man named Bridges).

:: ***Learning new information is harder.*** The quality of memory doesn't change, just the speed at which we receive, absorb, and react to information. That's why strategies like taking notes or outlining material become critical for older students, especially when learning new skills. However, adding to existing knowledge remains as easy as ever.

:: ***Wisdom matters.*** In any memory test involving knowledge of the world, vocabulary, or judgment, older people outperform their younger counterparts.

Women at Midlife

The major changes that occur during a woman's middle years are more evident than those in men. In the next decade, the number of women between the ages of 45 and 54 will increase by half, from 13 million to 19 million. Thus, a large segment of the population will be entering **perimenopause,** the period from a woman's first irregular cycles to her last menstruation.

PET Scan of 20-year-old Brain   **PET Scan of 80-year-old Brain**

In these PET scans, the red and yellow show greater neuron activity in the young adult. The brain of the older person shows less activity and more dark areas, indicating that the fluid-filled ventricles have grown larger.

Alzheimer's Disease Education & Referral Center (both)

Self Survey

What Is Your Aging I.Q.?

Answer true or false.

1. Everyone becomes "senile" sooner or later, if he or she lives long enough.
2. American families have by and large abandoned their older members.
3. Depression is a serious problem for older people.
4. The numbers of older people are growing.
5. The vast majority of older people are self-sufficient.
6. Mental confusion is an inevitable, incurable consequence of old age.
7. Intelligence declines with age.
8. Sexual urges and activity normally cease around age 55–60.
9. If a person has been smoking for 30 or 40 years, it does no good to quit.
10. Older people should stop exercising and rest.
11. As you grow older, you need more vitamins and minerals to stay healthy.
12. Only children need to be concerned about calcium for strong bones and teeth.
13. Extremes of heat and cold can be particularly dangerous to old people.
14. Many older people are hurt in accidents that could have been prevented.
15. More men than women survive to old age.
16. Death from stroke and heart disease are declining.
17. Older people on the average take more medications than younger people.
18. Snake oil salesmen are as common today as they were on the frontier.
19. Personality changes with age, just like hair color and skin texture.
20. Sight declines with age.

Scoring

1. False. Even among those who live to be 80 or older, only 20–25 percent develop Alzheimer's disease or some other incurable form of brain disease. "Senility" is a meaningless term that should be discarded.
2. False. The American family is still the number one caretaker of older Americans. Most older people live close to their children and see them often; many live with their spouses. In all, 8 out of 10 men and 6 out of 10 women live in family settings.
3. True. Depression, loss of self-esteem, loneliness, and anxiety can become more common as older people

face retirement, the deaths of relatives and friends, and other such crises—often at the same time. Fortunately, depression is treatable.

4. True. Today, 12 percent of the U.S. population are 65 or older. By the year 2030, one in five people will be over 65 years of age.
5. True. Only 5 percent of the older population live in nursing homes; the rest are basically healthy and self-sufficient.
6. False. Mental confusion and serious forgetfulness in old age can be caused by Alzheimer's disease or other conditions that cause incurable damage to the brain, but some 100 other problems can cause the same symptoms. A minor head injury, a high fever, poor nutrition, adverse drug reactions, and depression can all be treated and the confusion will be cured.
7. False. Intelligence per se does not decline without reason. Most people maintain their intellect or improve as they grow older.
8. False. Most older people can lead an active, satisfying sex life.
9. False. Stopping smoking at any age not only reduces the risk of cancer and heart disease, it also leads to healthier lungs.
10. False. Many older people enjoy—and benefit from—exercises such as walking, swimming, and bicycle riding. Exercise at any age can help strengthen the heart and lungs, and lower blood pressure. See your physician before beginning a new exercise program.
11. False. Although certain requirements, such as that for "sunshine" vitamin D, may increase slightly with age, older people need the same amounts of most vitamins and minerals as younger people. Older people in particular should eat nutritious food and cut down on sweets, salty snack foods, high-calorie drinks, and alcohol.
12. False. Older people require fewer calories, but adequate intake of calcium for strong bones can become more important as you grow older. This is particularly true for women, whose risk of osteoporosis increases after menopause. Milk and cheese are rich in calcium as are cooked dried beans, collards, and broccoli. Some people need calcium supplements as well.
13. True. The body's thermostat tends to function less efficiently with age and the older person's body may be less able to adapt to heat or cold.

Perimenopause

During this time, the egg cells, or oocytes, in a woman's ovaries start to *senesce* or die off at a faster rate. Eventually, the number of egg cells drops to a tiny fraction of the estimated 2 million packed into her ovaries at birth. Trying to coax some of the remaining oocytes to ripen, the pituitary

gland churns out extra follicle-stimulating hormone (FSH). This surge is the earliest harbinger of menopause, occurring six to ten years before a woman's final periods. Eventually the other menstrual messenger, luteinizing hormone (LH), also increases, but at a slower rate.

Self Survey

14. True. Falls are the most common cause of injuries among the elderly. Good safety habits, including proper lighting, nonskid carpets, and keeping living areas free of obstacles, can help prevent serious accidents.
15. False. Women tend to outlive men by an average of 8 years. There are 150 women for every 100 men over age 65, and nearly 250 women for every 100 men over 85.
16. True. Fewer men and women are dying of stroke or heart disease.
17. True. The elderly consume 25 percent of all medications and, as a result, have many more problems with adverse drug reactions.

18. True. Medical quackery is a $10 billion business in the United States. People of all ages are commonly duped into "quick cures" for aging, arthritis, and cancer.
19. False. Personality doesn't change with age. Therefore, all old people can't be described as rigid and cantankerous. You are what you are for as long as you live. But you can change what you do to help yourself to good health.
20. False. Although changes in vision become more common with age, any change in vision, regardless of age, is related to a specific disease. If you are having problems with your vision, see your doctor.

Source: National Institute on Aging, www.counselingnotes.com/seniors/age/age_iq.htm

Your Health Change Plan

for Preparing for a Medical Crisis in an Aging Relative

"Medical crises are more common and more likely to lead to serious complications after age 60," says Kenneth Brummel-Smith, M.D., former president of the American Geriatrics Society. As your parents, grandparents, and other relatives get older, here is what you can do in advance:

:: **Watch for warning signals.** If your relative begins stumbling or having near-misses on the highway, make sure he or she sees a doctor before a serious fall or accident occurs. There may be a cure or, if not a cure, a way to improve functioning.

:: **Suggest a surrogate.** Even if a couple has been married for 40 years, neither has the legal right to make medical decisions for a spouse. The same is true for children and other relatives. The only way to get that right is to fill out a form, usually called an advance directive or legal power of attorney (discussed on page 587).

:: **Talk to loved ones.** "Waiting for something bad to happen doesn't make it any easier to talk about," says Dr. Brummel-Smith, who suggests sitting down for a formal discussion at some point after a relative reaches age 65 "but definitely before age 75."

:: **Focus on values.** "You don't have to discuss every possible drug or surgery or intervention," says Dr. Brummel-Smith. "What's important is that you under-

stand the older person's values. What are fates worse than death? Independence may be more important than living a longer life." Many families use the "Five Wishes" form (available online at www.agingwithdignity.org and described on page 587) to discuss preferences for medical, personal, emotional, and spiritual care.

:: **Involve the person's primary physician.** Often it's not a question of what doctors can do medically in a crisis, but of what they should do, which is the patient's decision. Encourage loved ones to discuss "what ifs" with their doctors and make their desires clear. For instance, a primary physician should know which treatments patients want (such as resuscitation during surgery) as well as those they don't want (such as remaining on a ventilator if unable to breathe on their own.)

:: **Investigate alternative living options.** Aging parents should visit retirement communities or nursing homes while they're still healthy, not with the idea of moving into them, but of knowing what's available. They also should find out if their health plan or HMO provides services for seniors after a medical crisis.

:: **Make sure you know where to find key documents.** An easily accessible folder with copies of the latest lab reports, consultations, and advance directives helps avoid unnecessary tests and get faster treatment when a crisis does occur.

These hormonal shifts can trigger an array of symptoms. The most common are night sweats (a *subdromal hot flash,* in medical terms), which can be just intense enough to disrupt sleep. About 10 to 20 percent of perimenopausal women also experience daytime hot flashes, a symptom that becomes more prevalent with the more drastic and enduring hormonal changes of menopause itself.

Menopause

Menopause, defined as the complete cessation of menstrual periods for 12 consecutive months, generally arrives at age 51 or 52. Women with a lifelong history of depression are more likely to experience early perimenopause and menopause.[18] About 1 percent of women enter menopause before age 40.[19]

About 10 to 15 percent of women breeze through this transition with only trivial symptoms. Another 10 to 15 percent are virtually disabled. The majority fall somewhere in between these extremes. Women who undergo surgical or medical menopause (the result of removal of their ovaries or chemotherapy) often experience abrupt symptoms, including flushing, sweating, sleeplessness, early morning awakenings, involuntary urination, changes in libido, mood swings, perception of memory loss, and changes in cognitive function.

Dwindling levels of estrogen subtly affect many aspects of a woman's health, from her mouth (where dryness, unusual tastes, burning, and gum problems can develop) to her skin (which may become drier, itchier, and overly sensitive to touch). The drop in estrogen levels also may cause hot flashes (bursts of perspiration that last from a few seconds to 15 minutes), which often happen at night, disturbing sleep and causing fatigue. With less estrogen to block them, a woman's androgens, or male hormones, may have a greater impact, causing acne, hair loss, and, according to some anecdotal reports, surges in sexual appetite. (Other women, however, report a drop in sexual desire.)

At the same time, a woman's clitoris, vulva, and vaginal lining begin to shrivel, sometimes resulting in pain or bleeding during intercourse. Since the thinner genital tissues are less effective in keeping out bacteria and other pathogens, urinary tract infections may become more common. Some women develop breast or ovarian cysts, which usually go away on their own. Eventually, a woman's ovaries don't respond at all to her pituitary hormones. After the last ovulatory cycle, progesterone is no longer secreted, and estrogen levels decrease rapidly. A woman's testerone level also falls.[20]

In the United States, the average woman who reaches menopause has a life expectancy of about 30 more years. However, she faces risks of various diseases, including an increased risk of obesity, metabolic syndrome, heart disease, stroke, and breast cancer.[21] Women can reduce these risks by exercise, good nutrition, and controlling weight both before and after menopause.[22]

Hormone Replacement Therapy

Many people, including physicians, believed that **hormone replacement therapy (HRT)** would prevent heart disease and strokes and help women live longer.[23] Medical thinking on HRT, particularly a combination of estrogen and progestin, has changed completely in recent years. Contrary to what once was standard practice, HRT is no longer recommended for any reason other than short-term relief of hot flashes and night sweats.[24]

For decades middle-aged women typically began taking combinations of estrogen and progestin to ease hot flashes and other miseries of menopause.[25] Many continued to take the hormones, often into their 60s and 70s, believing the drugs were good for their health and wellbeing. Landmark longitudinal studies, including the Women's Health Initiative, a federally sponsored study of 16,608 postmenopausal women ages 50 to 79, have found that combination HRT increases the risk of heart attacks, blood clots, stroke, breast cancer, and dementia.[26] In addition, it does not safeguard a woman's memory, boost her mental outlook, or improve quality of life, energy, sexual function, or memory.[27] HRT's only proven benefits are decreases in hip fractures and colon cancer.[28] The Food and Drug Administration urges that even low-dose HRT be taken for the shortest possible duration.[29]

How could so many people have been so wrong about a therapy used by millions of women? Even though HRT has been around for half a century, rigorous scientific evidence on its benefits and risks emerged only in the last few years.[30] Studies that used "evidence-based medicine"—that is, treatments tested in controlled trials in which patients were assigned at random to either HRT or a placebo—challenged the findings from observational studies, in which women themselves decided to take HRT. Many health benefits that women had reported from hormone replacement have not held up in evidence-based trials. The reason, researchers say, may be that women who opted for HRT were healthier and had better habits than women who did not choose HRT.

Other non-hormonal medications have been used to relieve hot flashes, including antihypertensive and anticonvulsant drugs. However, only one or two small, short-term studies have tested most of these options.[31] Certain antidepressants, including Prozac and Paxil, have proven beneficial for some, but not all, women.[32] Limited controlled data so far suggest that mean hot flash scores (the frequency multiplied by the average severity) decline approximately 80 percent with hormone replacement, 60 percent with antidepressants, 40 percent with the antihypertensive drug clonidine, and 25 percent with placebo.[33]

Women who exercise regularly are less likely to have hot flashes.[34] Taking slow, deep breaths when a hot flash is coming on may halt or diminish the flash. Alternative medicines have recently undergone more rigorous testing. Most, such as red clover extract, have shown little or no benefit.[35] The most promising has been black cohosh.[36] (See Savvy Consumer: "Alternative Treatments for Menopausal Symptoms.")

Men at Midlife

Although men don't experience the dramatic hormonal upheaval that women do, they do experience a decline by as much as 30 to 40 percent in their primary sex hormone, testosterone, between the ages of 48 and 70. This change, sometimes called *andropause,* may cause a range of

Savvy Consumer

ALTERNATIVE TREATMENTS FOR MENOPAUSAL SYMPTOMS

Many women who once used hormone replacement therapy (HRT) discontinued its use following reports of increased risk of heart disease, breast cancer, and dementia (discussed on page 578). Some have turned to complementary and alternative medicines, including herbal preparations, dietary supplements, and foods containing phytoestrogens, for relief of menopausal symptoms such as hot flashes, joint pain, sleep problems, forgetfulness, and fatigue. Do these alternatives work? A review of randomized, controlled clinical trials of alternative therapies for menopausal symptoms—a total of 29 from different countries—attempted to answer this question.

Trials of herbs were small, and the results were not conclusive. In three of four trials, black cohosh, the most studied herb, relieved hot flashes, but none of the trials lasted more than six months. Its mechanism of action and active ingredients are not known, and its safety has not been demonstrated for longer use. Because it may act like estrogen on the lining of the uterus, some doctors recommend that women using black cohosh on a long-term basis take progesterone as well to lower the risk of endometrial cancer.

Red clover, an herb containing phytoestrogens, failed to relieve hot flashes in two short trials. Dong quai did not relieve hot flashes and contains coumarins that can cause bleeding when administered with the blood-thinner warfarin. In the only study available, oil of evening primrose posed no risks but provided no benefits. Ginseng, which is associated with postmenopausal bleeding, failed to relieve menopausal symptoms better than placebo.

Results were conflicting in the 11 trials that studied the effects of soy or isoflavone supplements on hot flashes. Benefits were modest and generally disappeared after six weeks. Vitamin E was not more effective than a placebo in managing menopausal symptoms.

Topical wild yam preparations did not relieve menopausal symptoms. Progesterone skin cream improved hot flashes in a small group of women treated for one year, but almost one-fourth of the women had vaginal bleeding, requiring biopsies. Acupuncture had inconclusive results. Biofeedback and progressive muscle relaxation training demonstrated some decrease in hot flashes.

The researchers concluded that most complementary and alternative therapies are ineffective for hot flashes, the main menopausal symptom that women try to relieve. Behavioral approaches, such as regular exercise and relaxation techniques, have shown some success.

Source: Sadovsky, Richard. "Alternative Medicines for Menopausal Symptoms." *American Family Physician*, Vol. 67, No. 7, April 1, 2003, p. 1586.

symptoms, including decreased muscle mass, greater body fat, loss of bone density, flagging energy, lowered fertility, and impaired virility. Some researchers are experimenting with testosterone supplements, which, in tests with young men, have been shown to increase lean body mass and decrease body fat—at least temporarily. However, other researchers warn that, particularly in older men, excess testosterone might raise the risk of prostate cancer and heart disease.[37]

After age 40, the prostate gland, which surrounds the urethra at the base of the bladder, enlarges. This condition, called *benign prostatic hypertrophy,* occurs in every man. By

What 60 looks like.

age 50, half of all men have some enlargement of the gland; after 70, three-quarters do. As it expands, the prostate tends to pinch the urethra, decreasing urinary flow and creating a sense of urinary urgency, particularly at night. Other warning signs of prostate problems include difficult urination, blood in the urine, painful ejaculation, or constant lower-back pain.

The drug Proscar (generic name, finasteride), which shrinks an enlarged prostate, has provided an alternative to corrective surgery for many men. Other drugs are being tried experimentally. The older a man gets, the more likely he is to develop prostate cancer (discussed in Chapter 15).

Sexuality and Aging

About half of all Americans aged 60 and older are sexually active. Among sexually active seniors, most say they are satisfied or more satisfied with their sex lives, compared to when they were in their 40s.[38]

Health and sexuality interact in various ways as we age. When they are healthy and have a willing partner, a substantial number of older men remain sexually active. The fittest men and women report more frequent sexual activity.

Other research has found a relationship between sex and longevity. A Swedish study found that men, but not women, who had discontinued intercourse had higher death rates. A study of the entire male population of a small Welsh town found that the sexually active men had

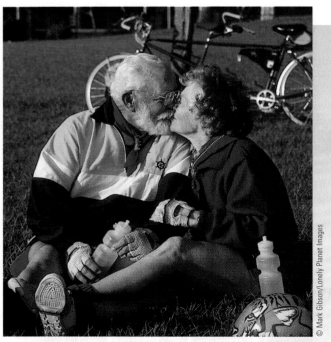

For older couples, sexual desire and pleasure can be enhanced by years of intimacy and affection.

half the mortality of the inactive group. In a Duke University study, longevity in women correlated with enjoyment of sexual intercourse, rather than with its frequency.

Aging does cause some changes in sexual response: Women produce less vaginal lubrication. An older man needs more time to achieve an erection or orgasm and to attain another erection after ejaculating. Both men and women experience fewer contractions during orgasm. However, none of these changes reduces sexual pleasure or desire.

In a poll of more than 4,000 people between the ages of 40 and 80 in the United States, Canada, Australia, and New Zealand, around 30 percent of men aged 70 to 80 reported having sex five times in the past month, although only 8 percent of women reported doing so. Most women said the lack of sex was due to the absence of a partner. Some 40 percent of men reported problems such as erectile dysfunction.[39]

◼ The Challenges of Age

No matter how well we eat, exercise, and take care of ourselves, some physical changes are inevitable as we age (see Figure 17-4). Aging brains and bodies also become vulnerable to diseases like Alzheimer's and osteoporosis. Other common life problems, such as depression, substance misuse, and safe driving, become more challenging as we age.

Alzheimer's Disease

About 15 percent of older Americans lose previous mental capabilities, a brain disorder called **dementia.** Sixty percent of these—a total of 4 million men and women over age 65—suffer from the type of dementia called **Alzheimer's disease,** a progressive deterioration of brain cells and mental capacity.

The percentage of people with Alzheimer's doubles for every five-year age group beyond 65. By age 85, nearly half of men and women have Alzheimer's. A person with the disease typically lives eight years after the onset of symptoms, but some live as long as 20 years.[40] Some 13.2 million older Americans will develop Alzheimer's disease by 2050, up from 4.5 million today. (See Figure 17-5.) The greatest increase will be among people age 85 and older.

Studies using brain imaging indicate that some cognitive deficits associated with age may be reversible. In a study that compared younger and older adults who were asked to memorize a series of words, researchers found that training may help the brains of elderly individuals function more like those of younger people.[41]

Women are more likely to develop Alzheimer's than men, and women with Alzheimer's perform significantly worse than men in various visual, spatial, and memory

Hair and nails Hair often turns gray and thins out. Men may go bald. Fingernails can thicken.

Brain The brain shrinks, but it is not known if that affects mental functions.

The senses The sensitivity of hearing, sight, taste, and smell can all decline with age.

Skin Wrinkles occur as the skin thins and the underlying fat shrinks, and age spots often develop.

Glands and hormones Levels of many hormones drop, or the body becomes less responsive to them.

Muscles Strength usually peaks in the 20s, then declines.

Immune system The body becomes less able to resist some pathogens.

Heart and blood vessels Cardiovascular problems become more common. The heart grows less efficient; buildup within arteries decreases oxygen and nutrients to cells.

Breasts Tissue degenerates after menopause, and breasts sag.

Lungs Lung capacity drops; risk of bronchitis and pneumonia grows.

Kidneys and urinary tract The kidneys become less efficient. The bladder can't hold as much, so urination is more frequent.

Digestive system Digestion slows down as the secretion of digestive enzymes decreases.

Reproductive system Women go through menopause, and testosterone levels drop for men.

Bones and joints Wear and tear can lead to arthritic joints, and osteoporosis is common, especially in women.

Figure 17-4 THE EFFECTS OF AGING ON THE BODY

tests. African Americans have higher rates of Alzheimer's disease than Africans living in Africa, according to the first study to find differences in the incidence of this illness in an industrial and a nonindustrial country.[42]

Although scientists had thought that estrogen might improve memory and delay or prevent Alzheimer's, the Women's Health Initiative found that women 65 and over taking estrogen combined with progestin had twice the rate of dementia, including Alzheimer's, as women not taking the hormones. Combination therapy also did not protect against the development of Mild Cognitive Impairment, or MCI, a form of cognitive decline less severe than dementia. According to recent studies, non-steroidal, anti-inflammatory drugs (NSAIDs) do not slow the rate of cognitive decline in people with mild to moderate Alzheimer's disease.

The early signs of dementia—insomnia, irritability, increased sensitivity to alcohol and other drugs, and decreased energy and tolerance of frustration—are usually subtle and insidious. Diagnosis requires a comprehensive assessment of an individual's medical history, physical health, and mental status, often involving brain scans and a variety of other tests.

Even though medical science cannot restore a brain that is in the process of being destroyed by an organic brain disease like Alzheimer's, medications can control difficult behavioral symptoms and enhance or partially restore cognitive ability. Often physicians find other medical or psychiatric problems, such as depression, in these patients; recognizing and treating these conditions can have a dramatic impact.

The FDA has approved several prescription drugs for people with mild to moderate Alzheimer's, including Cognex, Aricept, Exelon, and Reminyl. They all increase the level of the brain chemical acetylcholine. Researchers are studying other medications that might delay Alzheimer's or stop its progression.

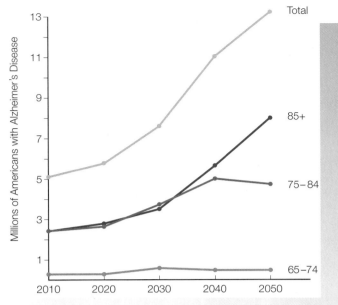

Figure 17-5 INCIDENCE OF ALZHEIMER'S DISEASE

Osteoporisis

Another age-related disease is **osteoporosis,** a condition in which losses in bone density become so severe that a bone will break after even slight trauma or injury. (See Figure 17-6.) A chronic disease, osteoporosis is silent for years or decades before a fracture occurs.

Women, who have smaller skeletons, are more vulnerable than men; in extreme cases, their spines may become so fragile that just bending causes severe pain. But although commonly seen as an illness of women, osteoporosis occurs frequently in men. One in every eight men older than 50 will suffer a hip fracture as a result of the disease.[43]

Figure 17-6 THE EFFECT OF OSTEOPOROSIS ON BONE DENSITY

(a) Section through normal bone tissue. (b) After the onset of osteoporosis, bones lose density and become hollow and brittle.

Source: © Dr. P. Motta, Department of Anatomy, University "La Sapienza," Rome/Science Photo Library/Photo Researchers, Inc.

An estimated 43.6 million men and women aged 50 and older currently have osteoporosis or low bone mass, according to the National Osteoporosis Foundation (NOF). Women make up 29.6 million of this total; 7.8 million have osteoporosis and 21.8 million have low bone mass.

By 2020 the prevalence of osteoporosis and low bone mass in the United States will rise by 41 percent to 61.4 million, according to NOF estimates. The incidence of hip fracture worldwide is expected to double in women and triple in men by 2035.[44]

Osteoporosis doesn't begin in old age. The bone weakness that increases the risk of osteoporosis may actually begin before birth. Infants undernourished in the womb are small when born, remain smaller than their age peers at age one, and have low bone mass at 25 and an increased risk of fractures in late adulthood.[45]

The ideal time to start preventing osteoporosis is adolescence. Girls achieve 42 percent of their total body bone mass between the ages of 12 and 18, yet 90 percent of girls do not get enough calcium. Beginning at age nine, children (particularly girls) should include 1,300 mg of calcium in their diet.

 Increased calcium intake, particularly during childhood and the growth spurt of adolescence, can produce a heavier, denser skeleton and reduce the risk of the complications of bone loss later in life. College-age women also can strengthen their bones and reduce their risk of osteoporosis by increasing their calcium intake and physical activity. Adequate dietary calcium and vitamin D in adulthood helps maintain bone density for years. (See Table 17-2.)

Various factors can increase a woman's risk of developing osteoporosis, including a family history (a mother, grandmother, or sister with osteoporosis, fractures, height loss, or humped shoulders); petite body structure; white or Asian background; menopause before age 40; smoking;

TABLE 17-2	Daily Calcium Requirements for Every Stage of Life
Age	**Daily Calcium Requirements**
1–3 years	500 mg
4–8 years	800 mg
9–18 years	1,300 mg
Adult women	1,000 mg
Pregnancy & lactation	1,000–1,200 mg
Post-menopause using hormones	1,200 mg
Post-menopause without hormones	1,500 mg
Adult men	
19–50 years	1,000 mg
51+ years	1,200 mg

STRATEGIES FOR PREVENTION

Lowering Your Risk of Osteoporosis

Regardless of your age and gender, you can prevent future bone problems by taking some protective steps now. The most important guidelines are as follows:

- Get adequate calcium. See Table 17-2.

- Exercise regularly. Both aerobic exercise and weight training can help preserve bone density.

- Drink alcohol only moderately. More than two or three alcoholic beverages a day impairs intestinal calcium absorption.

- Don't smoke. Smokers tend to be thin (a risk factor for osteoporosis) and enter menopause earlier, thus extending the period of jeopardy from estrogen loss.

- Let the sunshine in (but don't forget your sunscreen). Vitamin D, a vitamin produced in the skin in reaction to sunlight, boosts calcium absorption.

heavy alcohol consumption; loss of ovarian function through chemotherapy, radiation, or hysterectomy; low calcium intake; and a sedentary lifestyle.

In the past, doctors often prescribed hormone replacement therapy to protect aging bones; this is no longer the recommended practice. As many women discontinue HRT, they experience the same amount of bone loss as would occur around menopause.[46] A bisphosphonate medicine, such as alendronate or risedronate, at the time of estrogen withdrawal can protect a woman's bones.[47] Another alternative is the selective estrogen-receptor modulator (SERM) raloxifene, although it can occasionally trigger hot flashes. Few data on the long-term use of bisphosphonates and the SERMs are available.[48]

Substance Misuse and Abuse

Misuse and abuse of prescription and over-the-counter medications occur frequently among the elderly. In part this is because people over age 65 consume one-quarter of all drugs prescribed in the United States. Moreover, many older people have multiple health problems, requiring several medications at the same time. The drugs may interact and cause a confusing array of symptoms and reactions.

The most commonly misused drugs are sleeping pills, tranquilizers, pain medications, and laxatives. Sometimes a person innocently uses more than the prescribed dose or simultaneously takes several prescriptions of the same drug. Some older people are aware of their overreliance on

drugs but don't like how they feel when they don't take the pills.

Problems remembering, concentrating, and thinking are the most common psychological side effects of drugs in the elderly. As people age, their bodies take longer to metabolize drugs, so medications like sleeping pills build up in the body. Almost any amount of alcohol can make mental confusion and memory problems worse. Whenever older people become confused, forgetful, or paranoid, family members should find out which medications they've been taking.

Community surveys suggest that people older than 65 years consume less alcohol and have fewer alcohol-related problems than younger drinkers. Because of changes in body composition, older individuals have less body water, so alcohol reaches a higher concentration in their blood. Levels of a digestive enzyme that breaks down alcohol also decline, so blood alcohol levels in older people are typically 30 to 40 percent higher than in younger people consuming the same amount. Surveys conducted in health-care settings have found increasing prevalence of alcoholism among older adults. In acute-care hospitals, rates of alcohol-related admissions are similar to rates for heart attacks, and some surveys found the prevalence of problem drinking in nursing homes to be as high as 49 percent. In addition to the direct risks of alcohol, older individuals face related dangers when they drink, including falls, fractures, traffic accidents, medication interactions, depression, and cognitive changes. Brief treatment can be effective in helping the elderly overcome alcohol problems.

Is It Ever Too Late to Quit Smoking?

The sooner a smoker stops using tobacco, the greater the health benefits, and it is never too late to quit. Quitting at any age, even after age 65, can improve health and extend life—even after thirty or more years of regular smoking. A person who smokes more than 20 cigarettes a day and quits at age 65 increases life expectancy by two or three years.

Despite the well-documented benefits of quitting, an estimated 13 percent of seniors over age 65 smoke. They account for about 70 percent of the smoking-related deaths in the United States. When older people stop tobacco use, their circulation and lung function increase, they suffer less cardiovascular illness, and their quality of life improves.

Depression

Depression is a serious problem among the elderly. According to the National Institute of Mental Health, 6 percent of Americans aged 65 or older experience some form of depression. Older people face many challenges, including declining health, the loss of loved ones, social isolation, and physical limitations. However, depression is not inevitable, and the elderly are as likely to benefit from psychotherapy and medication as younger individuals.

Older individuals are less likely to seek treatment for depression than younger ones, in part because they may view depression as a weakness rather than a treatable illness. However, the elderly respond just as well to treatment.[49] More than 70 percent of the depressed elderly improve dramatically with treatment. Since loneliness and loss are often important contributing factors, psychiatrists often combine counseling, such as brief psychotherapy, with medication. Because of various physiological differences, the elderly usually respond more slowly to antidepressants than younger people, and the benefits thus may not be apparent for 6 to 12 weeks.

The consequences of not recognizing and treating depression late in life can be tragic. Older Americans have the highest suicide rate in our society, with some 8,500 elderly persons killing themselves every year. The suicide rate is five times higher for those aged 65 than for younger individuals. And depressed older men and women are also more likely to die of other causes.

Driving Risks

About a third of all drivers are over age 55; their number will increase as the baby-boom generation ages. Driving is very important to seniors, and most want to stay on the road as long as possible. While age alone is not an indicator of impairment, age-related changes can affect driving ability.

The rate of drivers involved in car accidents, including fatal ones, rises after age 70. Drivers aged 70 to 74 are twice as likely to die in an accident than those 30 to 59 years old. The risk for drivers over 80 is five times higher. Motorcycle riders 50 and older also have extremely high rates of accidents and deaths.

The most common contributing factors in accidents involving older drivers include pulling out from the side of the road or changing lanes without looking, careless backing, inaccurate turning, failure to yield the right of way, and difficulty reading traffic signs. Unlike younger drivers, older drivers' accidents seldom involve high speeds or alcohol use. Rather, problem driving in older adults involves visual, cognitive, and motor skills, which may decline with aging.

The ability of those over 85 to operate a vehicle when they have to divide their attention is half that of people under age 65. Seniors can lower their risks by limiting night driving, avoiding freeways, driving during less crowded periods of the day, making practice runs of new or difficult routes, and identifying and using alternate means of transportation.

FACT OR FICTION????????????????

Elderly people are less likely to be crime victims than teens and young adults.

Fact: Teenagers and young adults are more likely to be victims of crime than older men and women. However, this does not mean the elderly are safe. Each year, about two million older people become victims of crimes, most often robbery, personal and car theft, and burglary. Senior citizens are more likely than younger victims to face attackers who are strangers and to be attacked at or near their homes. An older victim is often more seriously hurt than a younger person.

Source: National Institute on Aging Age Page: "Crime and Older People." www.nia.nih.gov.

Death and Dying

Some 2.4 million people die in the United States each year.[50] Although most are older, death occurs in all age groups. The causes of death vary with both age and gender. Among those under age 35, intentional and nonintentional injury is the primary cause of death. (See Student Snapshot: "Dying Young.") Among older Americans, cancer and heart disease are the top killers. Men typically die at a younger age than women.

Defining Death

In our society, death isn't a part of everyday life, as it once was. Because machines can now keep people alive who, in the past, would have died, the definition of death has become more complex. Death has been broken down into the following categories:

:: *Functional death.* The end of all vital functions, such as heartbeat and respiration.

:: *Cellular death.* The gradual death of body cells after the heart stops beating. If placed in a tissue culture or, as is the case with various organs, transplanted to another body, some cells can remain alive indefinitely.

:: *Cardiac death.* The moment when the heart stops beating.

:: *Brain death.* The end of all brain activity, indicated by an absence of electrical activity (confirmed by an electroencephalogram, or EEG) and a lack of reflexes. The

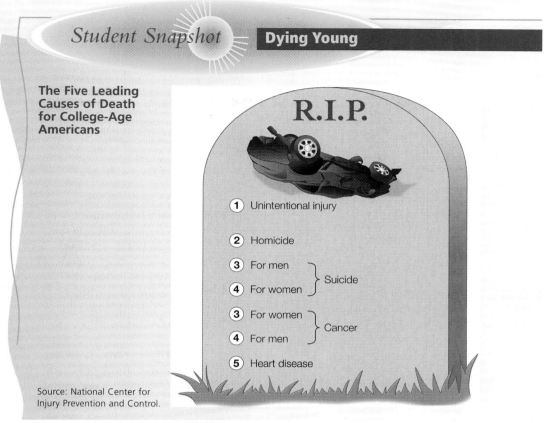

Student Snapshot — Dying Young

The Five Leading Causes of Death for College-Age Americans

R.I.P.

1. Unintentional injury
2. Homicide
3. For men
4. For women } Suicide
3. For women
4. For men } Cancer
5. Heart disease

Source: National Center for Injury Prevention and Control.

---

notion of brain death is bound up with what we consider to be the actual person, or self. The destruction of a person's brain means that his or her personality no longer exists; the lower brain centers controlling respiration and circulation no longer function.

:: **Spiritual death.** The moment when the soul, as defined by many religions, leaves the body.

When does a person actually die? The traditional legal definition of death is failure of the lungs or heart to function. However, because modern medicine is often able to maintain respiration and circulation by artificial means, most states have declared that an individual is considered dead only when the brain, including the brain stem, completely stops functioning. Brain-death laws prohibit a medical staff from "pulling the plug" if there is any hope of sustaining life.

The Meaning of Death

Death is not a mystery to those who have died. The living are the ones who struggle to find meaning in it. As far back as 60,000 years ago, prehistoric people observed special ceremonies when burying their dead. Many early cultures believed that people continued to exist after death and had the same needs that they did in life; hence they buried their loved ones with food, dishes, weapons, and

jewels. Some religions, such as Christianity, believe that the dead will rise again; to them, the burial of the body is symbolic, like the planting of a seed in the earth to await rebirth. Many Eastern religions share the belief that death marks the end only of physical existence and of the limited view of reality that human beings can grasp.

Death itself is a remote experience in most lives today, something that takes place off-stage in a hospital or nursing home. In earlier times, dying was a much more visible part of daily living. Families, friends, and other loved ones in a community would share in caring for those at the end of life. Most deaths occurred at home, often following a brief illness and unaffected by the limited medical care available. Today, the process of dying has become invisible.

Our attitudes toward dying also have changed with the development of medical technology and the extension of the human lifespan. Some people will do anything to delay aging or defeat death itself through medical science or other means. Others see death as part of a natural biological process and work toward the goal of dying well, with dignity and without undue suffering.

Denying Death

Most of us don't quite believe that we're going to die. A reasonable amount of denial helps us focus on the day-to-day realities of living. However, excessive denial can be life-threatening. Some drivers, for instance, refuse to buckle their seat belts because they refuse to acknowledge that a drunk driver might collide with them. Similarly, cigarette smokers deny that lung cancer will ever strike them, and people who eat high-fat meals deny that they'll ever suffer a heart attack.

One important factor in denial is the nature of the threat. It's easy to believe that death is at hand when someone's pointing a gun at you; it's much harder to think that cigarette smoking might cause your death 20 or 30 years down the road. Elisabeth Kübler-Ross, a psychiatrist who has extensively studied the process of dying, describes the downside of denying death in *Death: The Final Stage of Growth*.

> It is the denial of death that is partially responsible for people living empty, purposeless lives; for when you live as if you'll live forever, it becomes too easy to postpone the things you know that you must do. You live your life in preparation for tomorrow or in the remembrance of yesterday—and meanwhile, each today is lost. In contrast, when you fully understand that each day you awaken could be the last you have, you take the time that day to grow, to become more of who you really are, to reach out to other human beings.[51]

Emotional Responses to Dying

Elisabeth Kübler-Ross has identified five typical stages of reaction that a person goes through when facing death. (See Figure 17-7.)

1. **Denial ("No, not me").** At first knowledge that death is coming, a terminally ill patient rejects the news. The denial overcomes the initial shock and allows the person to begin to gather together his or her resources. Denial, at this point, is a healthy defense mechanism. It can become distressful, however, if it's reinforced by the relatives and friends of the dying patient.

2. **Anger ("Why me?").** In the second stage, the dying person begins to feel resentment and rage regarding imminent death. The anger may be directed at God or at the patient's family and caregivers, who

can do little but try to endure any expressions of anger, provide comfort, and help the patient on to the next stage.

3. **Bargaining ("Yes, me, but . . .").** In this stage, a patient may try to bargain, usually with God, for a way to reverse, or at least postpone, dying. The patient may promise, in exchange for recovery, to do good works or to see family members more often. Alternatively, the patient may say, "Let me live long enough to see my grandchild born" or "to see the spring again."

4. **Depression ("Yes, it's me").** In the fourth stage, the patient gradually realizes the full consequences of his or her condition. This may begin as grieving for health that has been lost and then become anticipatory grieving for the loss that is to come of friends, loved ones, and life itself. This stage is perhaps the most difficult: The dying person should not be left alone during this period. Neither should loved ones try to cheer up the patient, who must be allowed to grieve.

5. **Acceptance ("Yes, me; and I'm ready").** In this last stage, the person has accepted the reality of death: The moment looms as neither frightening nor painful, neither sad nor happy—only inevitable. The person who waits for the end of life may ask to see fewer visitors, to separate from other people, or perhaps to turn to just one person for support.

Several stages may occur at the same time and some may happen out of sequence. Each stage may take days or only hours or minutes. Throughout, denial may come back to assert itself unexpectedly, and hope for a medical breakthrough or a miraculous recovery is forever present.

Some experts dispute Kübler-Ross's basic five-stage theory as too simplistic and argue that not all people go through such well-defined stages in the dying process. The way a person faces death is often a mirror of the way he or she has faced other major stresses in life: Those who have had the most trouble adjusting to other crises will have the most trouble adjusting to the news of their impending death.

An individual's will to live can postpone death for a while. In a study of elderly Chinese women, researchers found that their death rate decreased before and during a holiday during which the senior women in a household play a central role; it increased after the celebration. A similar temporary drop occurs among Jews at the time of Passover. However, different events may have different effects. The prospect of an upcoming birthday postpones death in women but hastens it in men. The will to live typically fluctuates in terminal patients, varying along with depression, anxiety, shortness of breath, and a sense of well-being.[52]

The family of a dying person experiences a spectrum of often wrenching emotions. Family members, too, may deny the verdict of death, rage at the doctors and nurses who can't do more to save their loved one, bargain with God to give up their own health if necessary, sink into

Figure 17-7 KÜBLER-ROSS'S FIVE STAGES OF ADJUSTMENT TO FACING DEATH

helplessness and depression, and finally accept the reality of their anticipated loss.

One way of reducing the mystery and fear of death is to learn more about it. **Thanatology,** a term derived from the Greek god of death, Thanatos, refers to "the discipline of humanitarian caregiving for critically ill patients and their grieving family members and friends." Such care, which may be provided by physicians, nurses, social workers, psychologists, and others, helps ensure that terminally ill patients receive the compassionate, respectful care they deserve. The more we all learn about the process of dying and about what can be done to help more people die more peacefully, the better we can understand, and offer support to, the terminally ill.

✖ Preparing for Medical Crises and the End of Life

Throughout this book we have stressed the ways in which you can determine how well and how long you live. You can also make decisions about the end of your life.

The Five Wishes

An innovative document called "Five Wishes" helps the aged, the seriously ill, their loved ones, and caregivers prepare for medical crises. Written with the help of the American Bar Association's Commission on the Legal Problems of the Elderly, it enables individuals to specify:

:: which person they want to make health care decisions for them when they are no longer able to do so.

:: which kinds of medical treatments they do or don't want.

:: how comfortable they want to be.

:: how they want people to treat them.

:: what they want loved ones to know.

The Five Wishes document, available at www. agingwithdignity.org, is legally valid in 35 states. Churches, synagogues, hospices, hospitals, physicians, social service agencies, and employees also are distributing the document to help people plan for their own care or that of aging parents.[53]

You also can assure that your wishes are heeded by advance directive, such as a health-care proxy and a living will, and a holographic will.

🔳 What Are Advance Directives?

Every state and the District of Columbia have laws authorizing the use of **advance directives** to specify the kind of medical treatment individuals want in case of a medical crisis. However, few Americans have any type of advance directive. These documents are important because, without clear indications of a person's preferences, hospitals and other institutions often make decisions on an individual's behalf, particularly if family members are not available or disagree. Advance directives also help physicians, who often do not feel comfortable making these kinds of decisions about life-extending treatments for their terminally ill patients.[54]

According to the Patient Self-Determination Act, health-care facilities that receive Medicare or Medicaid reimbursements must advise patients of their right to sign advance directives for health-care decisions, including whether they want to be kept alive by artificial means. These statements allow medical professionals to know and follow an individual's wishes, or the wishes of a person to whom the patient has given authority to make decisions on his or her behalf. Figure 17-8 shows what you can include in an advance directive and the possible limitations on it because of differing state laws. Although the idea of advance directives is popular among patients and physicians, they are rarely discussed. In one study of patients who were either seriously ill or over age 70, only 2 percent had discussed advance directives with their doctors.[55]

A *health-care proxy* is an advance directive that gives someone else the power to make decisions on your behalf. (Figure 17-9 on page 589 shows the Medical Power of Attorney form for Texas.) People typically name a relative or close friend as their agent. Let family and friends know your thoughts about treatments and life support. You also should let your primary physician know about the type of care you would or wouldn't want to receive in various circumstances, such as an accident that results in an irreversible coma, but you should not designate your doctor as your agent. Many states prohibit this. Even when allowed, it is not a good idea because your doctor's primary responsibility is to administer care.

You can also sign an advance directive specifying that you want to be allowed to die naturally—you do not want to be resuscitated in case your heart stops beating. **Do-not-resuscitate (DNR)** orders apply mainly to hospitalized, terminally ill patients. However, in some states, it is possible to complete a *nonhospital DNR* form that specifies an individual's wish not to be resuscitated at home. Patients in the final stages of advanced cancer or AIDS may choose to use such forms to protect their rights in case paramedics are called to their home.

Living Wills

A **living will** isn't just for people who don't want to be kept alive by artificial means. Individuals can also use these advance directives to indicate that they want all possible medical treatments and technology used to prolong their lives. Most states recognize living wills as legally binding,

Except in California, where they must be renewed every five years, living wills are effective until they're revoked. Still, it's considered a good idea to initial and date your living will every few years to show that it still expresses your wishes.

"Imminent" is used on many living wills to express the inevitability and timing of death, but it's open to varying interpretations. A recent Virgina court decision found that it doesn't necessarily mean "immediately, at once, within a few days," and that a comatose person who's within a few months of death falls within the definition.

Except in California, Idaho, and Oregon, living wills have a space to specify treatment you do or don't want. Ask your physician what to include here. You can:

• Ask for or prohibit use of artificial feeding tubes, cardiopulmonary resuscitation, antibiotics, dialysis, and respirators.

• Ask for pain medication to keep you comfortable.

• State whether you would prefer to die in the hospital or at home.

• Designate a proxy—someone to make decisions about your treatment when you're unable.

• Donate organs or other body parts.

If your directions are contrary to state law, they'll be ignored, but the rest of the

DIRECTIVE TO PHYSICIANS

Directive made this _____day of_____ (month, year). I, _____being of sound mind, willfully and voluntarily make known my desire that my life shall not be artificially prolonged under the circumstances set forth below, and do hereby declare:

If at any time I should have an incurable condition caused by injury, disease, or illness certified to be a terminal condition by two physicians, and where the application of life-sustaining procedures would serve only to artificially prolong the moment of death and where my attending physician determines that my death is imminent whether or not life-sustaining procedures are utilized, I direct that such procedures be withheld or withdrawn, and that I be permitted to die naturally.

In the absence of my ability to give directions regarding the use of such life-sustaining procedures, it is my intention that this directive shall be honored by my family and physicians as the final expression of my legal right to refuse medical or surgical treatment and accept the consequences from such refusal.

If I have been diagnosed as pregnant and that diagnosis is known to my physician, this directive shall have no force or effect during the course of my pregnancy.

Other directions:
This directive shall be in effect until it is revoked. I understand the full import of this directive, and I am emotionally and mentally competent to make this directive. I understand that I may revoke this directive at any time.

Signed _____

City, County, and State of Residence _____

The declarant has been personally known to me and I believe him/her to be of sound mind. I am not related to the declarant by blood or marriage, nor would I be entitled to any portion of the declarant's estate on his/her decease, nor am I the attending physician of the declarant or an employee of the attending physician or a health facility in which the declarant is a patient, or a patient in the health care facility in which the declarant is a patient, or any person who has a claim against any portion of the estate of the declarant upon his/her decease.

Witness _____ Witness _____

"Life-sustaining procedures" are those that only prolong the process of dying. Most states include feeding and hydration tubes in this definition.

In some states a physician who will not carry out a patient's wishes must make a "good faith effort" to locate a doctor who will; other states require the physician to actually find someone and specify penalties—in some cases, jail terms—for failure to do so.

In some states the living will is valid for pregnant women. Others exclude women during all or part of their pregnancy, although that has been challenged on the grounds that a woman's right to privacy doesn't end when she becomes pregnant.

You can revoke or amend your living will at any time simply by making a statement to a physician, nurse, or other health-care worker.

Several states provide for the appointment of a proxy. In others decisions may be delegated through a document called a Durable Power of Attorney.

In some states, your signature must be notarized. Elsewhere, the signature of the witnesses is adequate although if you're in a hospital or nursing home in some states you may need as an additional witness the chief of staff or medical director.

Figure 17-8 PREPARING A PHYSICIAN'S DIRECTIVE

Source: "A Guide to the Living Will," *Hippocrates* (May–June, 19988).

INSTRUCTIONS

TEXAS MEDICAL POWER OF ATTORNEY — PAGE 1

TEXAS MEDICAL POWER OF ATTORNEY

DESIGNATION OF HEALTH CARE AGENT.

PRINT YOUR NAME

I, _____, appoint:
(name)

PRINT THE NAME, ADDRESS AND HOME AND WORK TELEPHONE NUMBERS OF YOUR AGENT

_____
(name of agent)

_____
(address)

_____
(work telephone number)   *(home telephone number)*

as my agent to make any and all health care decisions for me, except to the extent I state otherwise in this document. This medical power of attorney takes effect if I become unable to make my own health care decisions and this fact is certified in writing by my physician.

STATE LIMITATIONS ON YOUR AGENT'S POWER (IF ANY)

LIMITATIONS ON THE DECISION MAKING AUTHORITY OF MY AGENT ARE AS FOLLOWS.

TEXAS MEDICAL POWER OF ATTORNEY — PAGE 2

PRINT THE NAME, ADDRESS AND HOME AND WORK TELEPHONE NUMBERS OF YOUR FIRST AND SECOND ALTERNATE AGENTS

DESIGNATION OF ALTERNATE AGENT.
(You are not required to designate an alternate agent but you may do so. An alternate agent may make the same health care decisions as the designated agent if the designated agent is unable or unwilling to act as your agent. If the agent designated is your spouse, the designation is automatically revoked by law if your marriage is dissolved.)

If the person designated as my agent is unable or unwilling to make health care decisions for me, I designate the following persons to serve as my agent to make health care decisions for me as authorized by this document, who serve in the following order:

FIRST ALTERNATE

A. First Alternate Agent

_____
(name of first alternate agent)

_____
(home address)

_____
(work telephone number)   *(home telephone number)*

SECOND ALTERNATE

B. Second Alternate Agent

_____
(name of second alternate agent)

_____
(home address)

_____
(work telephone number)   *(home telephone number)*

LOCATION OF ORIGINAL

The original of this document is kept at: _____

TEXAS MEDICAL POWER OF ATTORNEY — PAGE 3

LOCATION OF COPIES

The following individuals or institutions have signed copies:

Name: _____

Address: _____

Name: _____

Address: _____

DURATION.
I understand that this power of attorney exists indefinitely from the date I execute this document unless I establish a shorter time or revoke the power of attorney. If I am unable to make health care decisions for myself when this power of attorney expires, the authority I have granted my agent continues to exist until the time I become able to make health care decisions for myself.

EXPIRATION DATE (IF ANY)

(IF APPLICABLE) This power of attorney ends on the following date: _____

PRIOR DESIGNATIONS REVOKED.
I revoke any prior medical power of attorney.

ACKNOWLEDGMENT OF DISCLOSURE STATEMENT.
I have been provided with a disclosure statement explaining the effect of this document. I have read and understood that information contained in the disclosure statement.

(YOU MUST DATE AND SIGN THIS POWER OF ATTORNEY)

PRINT THE DATE

I sign my name to this medical power of attorney on _____
(date)

PRINT YOUR LOCATION

day of _____ _____, at _____.
(month)   *(year)*   *(city and state)*

SIGN THE DOCUMENT

_____
(signature)

PRINT YOUR NAME

_____
(print name)

© 2000 PARTNERSHIP FOR CARING, INC.

TEXAS MEDICAL POWER OF ATTORNEY — PAGE 4

...ESSING ...EDURE

...R TWO ...ESSES ...IGN AND ...YOUR ...UMENT ...OW

MUST PRINT NAMES ...ND ...ESSES

...ESS #1

STATEMENT OF FIRST WITNESS.
I am not the person appointed as agent by this document. I am not related to the principal by blood or marriage. I would not be entitled to any portion of the principal's estate on the principal's death. I am not the attending physician of the principal or an employee of the attending physician. I have no claim against any portion of the principal's estate on the principal's death. Furthermore, if I am an employee of a health care facility in which the principal is a patient, I am not involved in providing direct patient care to the principal and am not an officer, director, partner or business office employee of the health care facility of any parent organization of the health care facility.

Signature: _____

Print Name: _____ Date: _____

Address: _____

...ESS #2

SIGNATURE OF SECOND WITNESS

Witness Signature: _____

Print Name: _____ Date: _____

Address: _____

© 2000 PARTNERSHIP FOR CARING, INC.

Courtesy of Partnership for Caring, Inc.   9/99
1620 Eye Street, NW, Suite 202, Washington, DC 20006 800-989-9455

Figure 17-9 HEALTH-CARE PROXY
A medical power of attorney is another advance directive. This example is from the state of Texas.

Source: Reprinted by permission of Partnership for Caring Inc., Washington D.C. 20006. 800-889-9455.

and a growing number of health-care professionals and facilities offer patients help in drafting living wills. You can obtain state-specific forms for living wills and health-care proxies free from Partnership for Caring (www.partnershipforcaring.org, 1-800-989-WILL). Computer software for preparing such documents is also available.

Once the forms are completed, make copies of your living will and other advance directives, and give them to anyone who might have input in decisions on your behalf. Also give copies to your physician or health-care organization, and ask that they be made part of your medical record.

Holographic Wills

Perhaps you think that only wealthy or older people need to write wills. However, if you're married, have children, or own property, you should either hire a lawyer to draw up a will or write a **holographic will** yourself, specifying who you wish to raise your children and who should have your property. If you die *intestate* (without a will), the state will make these decisions for you. Even a modest estate can be tied up in court for a long period of time, depriving family members of money when they need it most.

Many states will recognize a handwritten (not typed) statement by you, through which you can accomplish the following:

:: Name a family member or friend as the executor, the person who sees that your wishes are carried out.

:: List the things you own and to whom you want them to go; include addresses and telephone numbers, if possible.

:: Select a guardian for your children (if any), presumably someone whose ideas about raising children are similar to your own. Be sure that any named guardians are willing and able to accept this responsibility before writing them into your will.

:: Specify any funeral arrangements.

Be sure to keep the will in a safe place, where your executor, family members, or closest beneficiary can find it quickly and easily; tell them where it is.

Ethical Dilemmas

Modern medicine can do more to delay or defy death than was once thought possible. However, the ability to sustain life in patients with no hope of recovery has created wrenching medical and moral dilemmas. Increasingly, lawyers, ethicists, and consumer advocates are arguing that health-care providers must recognize a fundamental right of patients: the right to die.

Health economists, noting that more than half of U.S. health-care dollars are spent in the last year of life, have questioned "heroic" measures to prolong the life of chronically ill elderly patients or those with fatal diseases. Policies on such aggressive measures vary from hospital to hospital and state to state; often medical staff are not aware of patients' wishes.

Some health-care facilities require that staff members try to resuscitate any patient whose heart stops unless a do-not-resuscitate (DNR) order has been written, usually with the family's permission.

Families may demand aggressive medical care near the end of life on the basis of religious grounds, such as a conviction that every moment of life is a gift from God worth preserving at any cost. However, doctors are not obliged to provide a treatment they consider medically inappropriate or inhumane simply because of the family's religious beliefs. Ideally doctors and family members, perhaps with the aid of a chaplain, work together to reach a consensus on the appropriate limits to life-sustaining treatment.[56]

Another major ethical concern in the fate of an estimated 5,000 to 10,000 unconscious Americans who are being kept alive by artificial means. Some are in a **coma,** a state of total unconsciousness. They may have no sense of where they are, no memory, and no experience of pain. Others are in a **persistent vegetative state,** in which they're awake and yet unaware. They open their eyes; their brain waves show the characteristic patterns of waking and sleep. They can usually breathe on their own after a few weeks on artificial respiration; they can cough; the pupils of their eyes respond to light; but they do not respond to pain.

About 20 percent of deaths in the United States occur in intensive care units. The majority involve either withholding or withdrawing life-sustaining treatments.[57] The questions of when to use and when to discontinue artificial means of life support remain among the most challenging ethical dilemmas facing health-care workers and the families of critically ill patients.

The Gift of Life

If you're at least 18 years old, you can fill out a donor card (see Figure 17-10), agreeing to designate, in the event of your death, any organs or tissues needed for transplantation. Corneas may help a blind person see, for example. Kidneys, or even a heart, may be transplanted. The donation takes effect upon your death and is a generous way of giving others the possibilities for life that you have had yourself. The card should be filled out and signed; some must be signed in the presence of two witnesses. Attach the donor card to the back of your driver's license or I.D. card. (Whole-body donations may require other arrangements.)

UNIFORM DONOR CARD

OF _____
Print or type name of donor

In the hope that I may help others, I hereby make this anatomical gift, if medically acceptable, to take effect upon my death. The words and marks below indicate my desires.

I give   (a) ____ any needed organs or parts

I give   (b) ____ only the following organs or parts

_____
Specify the organ(s) or part(s)

for the purposes of transplantation, therapy, medical research, or education:

I give   (c) ____ my body for anatomical study if needed

Limitations or
special wishes, if any _____

Figure 17-10 EXAMPLE OF A UNIFORM DONOR CARD

⬢ How We Die

Life can end in very different ways. Sudden death, by accident or murder, for instance, brings an abrupt end to life in individuals who may have been in optimal health. A terminal illness, such as an aggressive and fatal cancer, can lead to a steep drop in functioning prior to death. When organs, such as the kidneys, fail, a patient's well-being tends to plummet and then recover but in a downward pattern. The frailty of old age leads to a gradual decline to ever-lower levels of functioning and eventual death.[58]

Most people who have a fatal or **terminal illness** prefer to know the truth about their health and chances for recovery. (See Table 17-3.) Even when they're not officially informed by a doctor or relative, most fatally ill people know or strongly suspect that they're dying. Dying people usually make it clear whether they want to talk about death and to what extent. The most frequent con-

cern is how much time is left. Usually physicians can give only a rough estimate, such as "several weeks or months."

Once death was a taboo topic even between doctors and patients. Filled with a zeal to heal, physicians viewed death as the enemy; it caused a sense of medical impotence and failure that often led them to pull away from dying patients. However, surveys of physicians show changes in the last decades. Today's doctors are much more open to communicating with dying patients and their families on issues concerning death. They, too, benefit from open, honest conversations with their patients.

A "Good" Death

As life expectancy has increased and high-technology interventions have multiplied, many health-care professionals as well as citizens and social organizations have begun to demand a better way of caring for those who are dying. The Center to Improve Care of the Dying, in Washington, DC, has set goals for reintegrating dying within living, thus enhancing the prospect for growth at the end of life. These experts talk of "dying well," "living while dying," and "physician-assisted living." They aim to change our way of thinking about dying so that we view the end of life as a time of love and reconciliation, and transcendence of suffering.

TABLE 17-3	Attitudes Toward the Dying	
Percent of Ethnic Group Who Believe:	**African Americans**	**European Americans**
A patient should be told a diagnosis of metastatic cancer.	89%	87%
A patient should be told of terminal prognosis.	63	69
A patient should decide about the use of life support.	60	65

Source: The University of Southern California

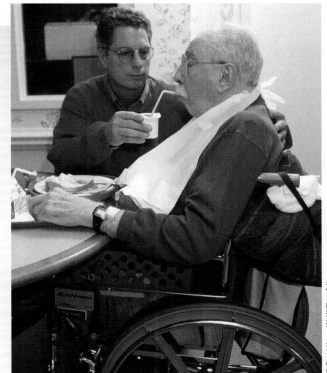

© David Young-Wolff/PhotoEdit

Humanitarian caregiving for both critically ill patients and their loved ones can take some of the fear out of death.

Physicians who care for the dying are being urged to do all that they can to eliminate pain. They are encouraged not to withhold opioid drugs, such as morphine, simply out of fear of addiction. More efforts are being made for patients to be taken care of at home, with appropriate support and well-informed guidance.

Various psychological factors can affect those at risk of dying. Elderly people who lack hope in the future are much more likely to die within the next few years. Researchers speculate that hopelessness may lead to biochemical and nervous system abnormalities or that hopeless individuals may not eat well, take medications as prescribed, or follow a doctor's recommendations.

Some terminally ill patients choose to stop eating and drinking because they are ready to die, see continued existence as pointless, and consider their quality of life poor. In a recent survey, hospice nurses reported that 85 percent of such patients die within 15 days after stopping food and fluids. On a scale from 0 (a very bad death) to 9 (a very good death), the median score for the quality of these deaths, as rated by the nurses, was 8.[59] The Oregon study found that patients choose to end their own lives by refusing food twice as often as they opt for physician-assisted suicide, which is legal only in that state.[60]

Spirituality also plays a major role. In various surveys, 41 to 94 percent of patients say they want their doctors and nurses to address their spiritual concerns. In one survey, even 45 percent of nonreligious patients thought physicians should inquire politely about patients' spiritual needs. However, some worry that such queries may be inappropriate or detract from a doctor's primary mission.

There are few data on the impact of spiritual approaches on the dying. In a survey of relatives of deceased patients, 63 percent thought that their loved one's faith was of help at the time of death. In a study of nursing home residents, traditional religious beliefs and values affected acceptance, endurance, coping, and security in the face of impending death.[61]

Caregiving

When someone becomes terminally ill, a woman—usually the patient's wife, daughter, or sister—is most likely to provide day-to-day care, often for periods longer than a year. Caregiving takes a different toll on men and women. In one study of adult daughters and husbands caring for terminally ill breast cancer patients, the daughters experienced more symptoms of anxiety and depression and greater family strain.

The impact of caregiving continues even after the death of an ill spouse. In one study, the health of older caregivers who had experienced strain prior to a spouse's death did not deteriorate. They showed no increase in depressive symptoms or use of antidepressant drugs and did not lose weight. Those who had not been caregivers were more likely to experience depression and weight loss.[62]

Hospice: Caring When Curing Isn't Possible

A **hospice** is a homelike health-care facility or program that helps dying men and women who can afford such care to live their final days to the fullest, as free as possible from disabling pain and mental anguish. Hospice workers generally work in teams, usually consisting of a nurse, physician, social worker, chaplain, and trained volunteers. Other professionals, such as a physical therapist, may join the team when needed. These workers provide the comfort, support, and care dying patients need until they do die.

Hospice programs offer a combination of medical and emotional care that involves not only the patient but also the family members or others concerned with caring for the patient. Most hospice patients have life expectancies of six months or less, and are no longer receiving treatments aimed at curing their diseases. When someone is available to provide care, patients remain in their own homes. Hospice nurses regularly visit all home patients and are available around the clock.

For patients requiring care that the family cannot provide, round-the-clock care is available at the hospice facility. Unlike a traditional hospital, where the focus is on diagnosis, cure, and treatment, a hospice works to make what is left of life pain-free and comfortable. Visiting hours for relatives and friends are flexible, with no restrictions on visits by children and grandchildren. Hospice services are covered, in full or in part, by most major insurance companies.

What Do We Know About Near-Death Experiences?

Reports of **near-death experiences** have grown, thanks largely to advances in emergency medical care. Most are remarkably similar, whether they occur in children or

A hospice provides care and support and helps people die with comfort and dignity.

adults, whether they're the result of accidents or illnesses, even whether the individuals actually are near death or only think they are. Some individuals who have survived a close brush with death report **autoscopy** (watching, from several feet in the air, resuscitation attempts on their own bodies) or **transcendence** (the sense of passing into a foreign region or dimension). Some see light, often at the end of a tunnel. Their vision seems clearer; their hearing, sharper. Some recall scenes from their lives or feel the presence of loved ones who have died. Many report profound feelings of joy, calm, and peace. Fewer than 1 percent of those who've reported near-death experiences described them as frightening or distressing, although a larger number recall transitory feelings of fear or confusion.

Many near-death experiences occur in individuals who've been sedated or given other medications; however, many others do not. Several studies have shown that individuals who received medication or anesthesia were actually less likely to remember near-death experiences than those who hadn't had any drugs. Some scientists have speculated that lack of oxygen, changes in blood gases, altered brain functioning, or the release of neurotransmitters (messenger chemicals in the brain) may play a role in near-death experiences. However, there's little solid evidence that physiological events are responsible. There's also no proof that wishful thinking, cultural conditioning, posttraumatic stress, or other psychological mechanisms may be at work. For now, the most that scientists can say for sure about this medical mystery is that it needs further study.

◐ Suicide

Suicide is among the ten leading causes of death in the United States; each year 25,000 to 55,000 people kill themselves. And for every completed suicide, there are 10 to 40 unsuccessful attempts. (Chapter 2 presents a detailed discussion of the risk factors and warning signs of suicide.)

One of the main factors leading to suicide is illness, especially terminal illness. A great deal of debate centers on quality of life, yet there is no reliable or consistent way to measure this. Patients who are dying may feel some quality of life, even when others do not recognize it, or their evaluations of the quality of their lives may fluctuate. Dying patients who say their lives are not worth living may be suffering from depression; hopelessness is one of its characteristic symptoms.

Approximately three-fourths of those who commit suicide consult a physician, most with medical complaints, within the six-month period prior to their deaths. Disease, medication, and the fear of pain or of being a burden to one's family can breed depression; treatment can make a difference. Only 10 to 14 percent of those who survive a suicide attempt take their lives in the next ten years. Fatally ill individuals who talk about suicide should be taken seriously; family physicians can arrange for them to talk with

psychotherapists. (Physician-assisted suicide is discussed below.)

"Rational" Suicide

An elderly widow suffering from advanced cancer takes a lethal overdose of sleeping pills. A young man with several AIDS-related illnesses shoots himself. A woman in her fifties, diagnosed as having Alzheimer's disease, asks a doctor to help her end her life. Are these suicides "rational" because these individuals used logical reasoning in deciding to end their lives?

The question is intensely controversial. Advocates of the right to "self-deliverance" argue that individuals in great pain or faced with the prospect of a debilitating, hopeless battle against an incurable disease can and should be able to decide to end their lives. As legislatures and the legal system tackle the thorny questions of an individual's right to die, mental health professionals worry that, even in those with fatal diseases, suicidal wishes often stem from undiagnosed depression.

In one classic study of 44 terminally ill individuals, 34 had never been suicidal or wished for death. The remaining ten (seven who did desire early death and three who specifically considered suicide) all had severe depression. Their despair and preoccupation with dying may well have contributed to their willingness to consider suicide. Numerous studies have indicated that most patients with painful, progressive, or terminal illnesses do not want to kill themselves. The percentage of those who report thinking about suicide ranges from 5 to 20 percent; most of these have major depressions. Many mental health professionals argue that what makes patients with severe illnesses suicidal is depression, not their physical condition.

Because depression may indeed warp the ability to make a rational decision about suicide, mental health professionals urge physicians and family members to make sure individuals with chronic or fatal illnesses are evaluated for depression and given medication, psychotherapy, or both. It is also important for everyone to allow enough time—an average of three to eight weeks—to see if treatment for depression will make a difference in their desire to keep living.

Physician-Assisted Suicide

According to U.S. surveys, there is greater support for physician-assisted suicide and euthanasia among patients and the general public than among physicians.[63] More Caucasians support these practices than members of ethnic minority groups.[64]

If patients have a right to die, should doctors help them end their lives? Physicians could stop any extraordinary efforts to sustain life (for example, by withholding oxygen or ending intravenous feedings); such actions are referred to as passive **euthanasia,** or **dyathanasia.** Euthanasia, the active form of so-called mercy killing, has generally been viewed as illegal and unethical. Euthanasia is tolerated and legally pardoned in the Netherlands but remains illegal in all European countries.[65] The demand for physician-assisted death in the Netherlands has not risen; and patients and physicians have become more reluctant to ask for or offer this option over the past few years.[66]

Oregon has passed the "Death with Dignity" act and is the first state to legalize physician-assisted suicide for terminally ill patients. Legal challenges to it continue. This law bars suicide assistance for anyone whose judgment may be impaired by a mental disorder.

In the 1990s Jack Kevorkian, M.D., a Michigan pathologist, stirred public debate by using a "suicide machine" to help end the life (at their request) of dozens of people suffering from chronic, but not necessarily fatal, illnesses. He is serving a prison sentence for murder. Some medical groups, such as the American Medical Association, oppose as unethical any physician's involvement in euthanasia. Others argue that individuals have the right to end their own lives and that physicians who provide prescriptions for lethal doses of certain drugs are acting out of compassion and respect for patients' wishes.[67]

▶◀ The Practicalities of Death

At a time of great emotional pain, grieving family members must cope with medical, legal, and practical concerns, including obtaining a medical certificate of the cause of death, registering the death, and making funeral arrangements. They may also want to arrange for organ donations and, in some circumstances, an autopsy.

Funeral Arrangements

A body can be either buried or cremated. Burial requires the purchase of a cemetery plot, which many families do decades before death. A burial is typically the third most expensive purchase of a lifetime, behind the cost of a house and car. The average national costs range as high as $6,000, although they vary considerably. Memorial societies are voluntary groups that help people plan in advance for death. They obtain services at moderate cost, keep the arrangements simple and dignified, and—most important, perhaps—ease the emotional and financial burden on the rest of the family when death finally does come.

If the body is to be cremated, you must comply with some additional formalities, with which the funeral director can help you. After a *cremation* (incineration of the remains), you can either collect the ashes to keep, bury, or scatter yourself, or ask the crematorium to dispose of them.

The tradition of a funeral may help survivors come to terms with the death, enabling them to mourn their loss and to celebrate the dead person's life. Funerals are usually held two to four days after the death. Many have two parts: a religious ceremony at a church or funeral home, and a burial ceremony at the grave site.

Alternatively, the body may be disposed of immediately, through burial, cremation, or bequeathal to a medical school, and a memorial service held later. In a memorial

Funerals and memorial services allow those in mourning to honor the deceased and to come to terms with their loss.

service, the body is not present, which may change the focus of the service from the person's death to his or her life.

Autopsies

An autopsy is a detailed examination of a body after death, also called a postmortem exam. There are two types:

:: **Medicolegal.** This type of autopsy is performed to establish the cause of death and to gather information about the death for use as evidence in any legal proceedings. It is done to detect any crimes and to help identify the proper person for prosecution, to investigate possible industrial hazards or contagious diseases that may endanger the public health, or to establish the cause of death for insurance purposes.

:: **Medical/educational.** This type of autopsy is performed, usually in the hospital where the person died, to increase medical knowledge and to determine a more exact cause of death. It may be requested by the attending physician or the family, but it cannot be performed without the family's permission.

Autopsies can be extremely valuable in establishing an accurate cause of death, revealing a different diagnosis that might have led to a change in therapy and prolonged survival in about 10 percent of cases. Thirty years ago about 50 percent of patients who died in hospitals were autopsied. However, the autopsy rate in the United States has been steadily declining, and today about 10 to 20 percent of deaths in teaching hospitals are autopsied.

Physicians are arguing for an increase in autopsies as the best method for establishing the cause of death, helping to spot infectious diseases, aiding medical education, and helping assure the high quality of medical practice. Between 8 and 24 percent of autopsies pick up a condition that a patient's doctor missed and that may have been the actual cause of death. Between 4 and 7 percent may detect the most serious type of medical error—meaning that, if the doctor had properly diagnosed the condition, the patient might have lived.[68]

◘ Grief

An estimated 8 million Americans lose a member of their immediate family each year. The death of a loved one may be the single most upsetting and feared event in a person's life. It produces a wide range of reactions, including anxiety, guilt, anger, and financial concern. Many may see the death of an old person as less tragic than the death of a child or young person. A sudden death is more of a shock than one following a long illness. A suicide can be particularly devastating, because family members may wonder

whether they could have done anything to prevent it. The cause of death can also affect the reactions of friends and acquaintances. Some people express less sympathy and support when individuals are murdered or take their own lives.

Encountering death can make us feel alone and vulnerable. The most common and one of the most painful experiences is the death of a parent. When both parents die, individuals may feel like orphaned children. They mourn not just for the father and mother who are gone, but also for their lost role of being someone's child.

The death of a child can be even more devastating. Grieving may continue for many years. Eventually parents may be able to resolve their grief and accept the death as "God's will" or as "something that happens." Time erases their pain and they feel a desire to get on with their lives, consciously putting the loss behind them. Others deal with their grief by keeping busy, or by substituting other problems or situations to take their minds off their loss. Yet many parents who lose a child continue to grieve for many years. Although the pain of their loss diminishes with time, they view it as part of themselves and describe an emptiness inside—even though most have rich, meaningful, and happy daily lives.

The loss of a mate can also have a profound impact, although men's and women's responses to the death—and their subsequent health risks—may depend on how their spouses died. Men whose wives die suddenly face a much greater risk of dying themselves than those whose wives die after a long illness. On the other hand, women whose husbands die after a long illness face greater risk of dying than other widows. The reason may be that men whose wives were chronically ill learned how to cope with the

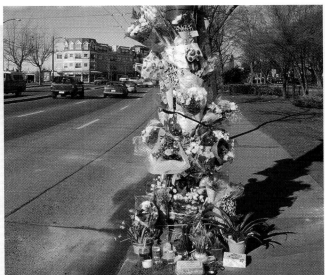

Some friends and relatives place flowers and mementoes at the accident site where a loved one died.

loss of their nurturers, while women who spend a long time caring for an ill husband may be at greater risk because of the combined burdens of caregiving and loss of financial support.

 Bereavement is not a rare occurrence on college campuses, but it is largely an ignored problem. Counselors have called upon universities to help students who have lost a loved one through initiatives such as training nonbereaved students to provide peer support and raising consciousness about bereavement.[69]

Grief's Effects on Health

Men and women who lose partners, parents, or children endure so much stress that they're at increased risk of serious physical and mental illness, and even of premature death. Studies of the health effects of grief have found the following:

:: Grief produces changes in the respiratory, hormonal, and central nervous systems, and may affect functions of the heart, blood, and immune systems.

:: Grieving adults may experience mood swings between sadness and anger, guilt and anxiety.

:: They may feel physically sick, lose their appetite, sleep poorly, or fear that they're going crazy because they "see" the deceased person in different places.

:: Friendships and remarriage offer the greatest protection against health problems.

:: Some widows may have increased rates of depression, suicide, and death from cirrhosis of the liver. The greatest risk factors are poor previous mental and physical health and a lack of social support.

:: Grieving parents, partners, and adult children are at increased risk of serious physical and mental illness, suicide, and premature death.

Methods of Mourning

Grief is a psychological necessity, not self-indulgence. Psychotherapists refer to grief as work, and it is—slow, tedious, and painful. Yet only by working through grief—dealing with feelings of anger and despair, and adjusting emotionally and intellectually to the loss—can bereaved individuals make their way back to the living world of hope and love.

Some widows and widowers move through the grieving process without experiencing extreme distress. Others stop somewhere in the midst of normal grieving and continue to pine for the deceased, become overly reliant on others, or show signs of denial, avoidance, or anxiety. Individuals who lose children or spouses in car accidents are particularly likely to remain depressed and anxious years later. One of the most devastating losses is the death

STRATEGIES FOR CHANGE

Coping with Grief

■ *Accept your feelings*—sorrow, fear, emptiness, whatever—as normal. Don't try to deny emotions such as anger, guilt, despair, or relief.

■ *Let others help you*—by bringing you food, by taking care of daily necessities, by providing companionship and comfort. (It will make them feel better, too.)

■ *Face each day as it comes.* Let yourself live in the here-and-now until you're ready to face the future. Give yourself time—perhaps more than you ever imagined—for the pain to ebb, the scars to heal, and your life to move on.

■ *Don't think there's a right or wrong way to grieve.* Mourning takes many forms, and there's no set timetable for working through the various stages of grief.

■ *Seek professional counseling* if you remain intensely distressed for more than six months or your grief does not ease over time. Therapy can help prevent potentially serious physical and psychological problems.

of a child killed by a drunk driver. Many years afterward parents often cannot find any meaning in what happened.

How Can You Help Survivors of a Loss?

Although we grieve for the dead, the living are the ones who need our help. Bereavement is such an intense state that survivors may be too numb or too stunned to ask for help. Family and friends must take the initiative and spend time with those who are mourning the loss of a loved one, even if that means sitting together silently. Offer empathy and support, and let the grieving person know with verbal and nonverbal expressions that you care and wish to help. Simply being there is enough to let your friend know you care.

You may also wish to write a simple note expressing your sympathy. "I want to let you know I'm thinking of you and praying for you" can mean a great deal. A small gift, such as a book or plant, is also thoughtful. Or you can invite your friend to do something with you. Choose something you know your friend might enjoy—a walk in the country or a concert. And don't just give your help over the first few days or weeks and then withdraw. Grieving people continue to need support for many months. The first anniversary of a death or the first holiday spent alone can be particularly difficult.

Most bereaved people don't need professional psychological counseling. In most instances, sharing their feelings with friends is all that's needed. However, you should urge a friend or relative to seek help if he or she shows no sign of grieving, or exhibits as much distress a year after the loss as during the first months. The family members of a suicide victim are those most likely to need, and benefit from, professional help in sorting out their feelings of failure, anger, and sorrow. Therapy and medication can be enormously helpful—and potentially life-saving.

The Bottom Line ▼
Living Long and Well

"Every man desires to live long," writes Jonathan Swift, "but no man would be old." We all wish for long lives, yet we want to avoid the disease and disability that can tarnish our golden years. Here are the best ways to do so.

:: ***Exercise regularly.*** By improving blood flow, staving off depression, warding off heart disease, and enhancing well-being, regular workouts help keep mind and body in top form.

:: ***Don't smoke.*** Every cigarette you puff can snuff out seven minutes of your life, according to the Centers for Disease Control and Prevention.

:: ***Watch your weight and blood pressure.*** Increases in these vital statistics can increase your risk of hypertension, cardiovascular disease, and other health problems.

:: ***Eat more fruits and vegetables.*** These foods, rich in vitamins and protective antioxidants, can reduce your risk of cancer and damage from destructive free radicals. (See Chapter 15.)

:: ***Cut down on fat.*** Fatty foods can clog the arteries (Chapter 14) and contribute to various cancers. (See Chapter 15.)

:: ***Limit drinking.*** Alcohol can undermine physical health and sabotage mental acuity. (See Chapter 11.)

:: ***Cultivate stimulating interests.*** Elderly individuals with complex and interesting lifestyles are most likely to retain sharp minds and memories beyond age 70.

:: ***Don't worry; be happy.*** At any age, emotional turmoil can undermine well-being. Relaxation techniques, such as meditation, help by reducing stress.

:: ***Reach out.*** Try to keep in contact with other people of all ages and experiences. Make the effort to invite them to your home or go out with them. On a regular basis, do something to help another person.

:: ***Make the most of your time.*** Greet each day with a specific goal—to take a walk, write letters, visit a friend.

 After watching the CNN video segment, discuss the following question. What are the stages of emotional response to dying?

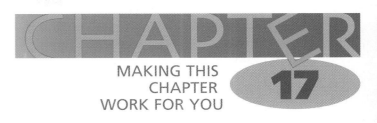

MAKING THIS CHAPTER WORK FOR YOU — 17

1. Factors that contribute to a long life and successful aging include all of the following except
   a. healthy weight.
   b. moderate smoking.
   c. regular exercise.
   d. social involvement.

2. Physically fit people over age 60
   a. have lower risk of dying from chronic heart disease.
   b. can regain the fitness level of a 25-year-old.
   c. show no difference in levels of anxiety and depression.
   d. have higher body-fat percentages.

3 Which statement about the aging brain is *false*?
   a. When brain cells die, surrounding cells can fill the gaps to maintain cognitive function.
   b. Remembering names and recalling information may take longer.
   c. "Use it or lose it."
   d. Mental ability and physically ability both decline with age.

4. Which statement about aging is false?
   a. People over age 70 who take vitamin supplements showed improvement in short-term memory and problem-solving ability.
   b. Fitness and frequency of sexual activity are linked.
   c. Hormone replacement therapy reduces the risk of heart disease in menopausal women.
   d. Seniors who take up new hobbies late in life may slow aging within the brain.

5. Which statement about age-related problems is correct?
   a. Osteoporosis affects only women.
   b. Alzheimer's disease is a form of dementia.
   c. Depression is no more prevalent in the older population.
   d. Drug interactions do not occur in the elderly.

6. When should concern change to intervention?
   a. Uncle Charlie is 85 and continues to drive himself to the grocery store and to the Senior Center during the daytime.

b. Nana takes pills at breakfast, lunch, and dinner, but sometimes mixes them up.

c. Mom's hot flashes have become a family joke.

d. Your older brother can never remember where he put his car keys.

7. According to Elisabeth Kübler-Ross, an individual facing death goes through all of the following emotional stages except

a. bargaining.

b. acceptance.

c. denial.

d. repression.

8. The gender gap related to longevity

a. is due to deficiencies in the Y chromosome.

b. results from the presence of a mutant gene.

c. may be due to the X chromosome and its hormonal influences on the immune system.

d. is about 13 years in the United States.

9. An advance directive

a. indicates who should have your property in the event you die.

b. may authorize which individuals may not participate in your health care if you are unable to care for yourself.

c. can specify your desires related to the use of medical treatments and technology to prolong your life.

d. should specify which physician you designate to be your health-care proxy.

10. You can best help a friend who is bereaved by

a. encouraging him to have a few drinks to forget his pain.

b. simply spending time with her.

c. avoiding talking about his loss because it is awkward.

d. reminding her about all she still has in her life.

Answers to these questions can be found on page 652.

Critical Thinking

1. How are your parents or other mentors staying fit and alert as they age? Do you think you might use similar strategies?

2. Do you think that coming to terms with mortality allows an individual to live each day to its fullest, rather than putting off what he or she would like to do until tomorrow? How does this concept affect your own life? Explain. Do you believe in a next life? How does this affect your view of life and death?

Critical Thinking

3. Have your living parents and grandparents written advanced directives or a living will? Have you discussed with them their preferences regarding treatment in the event of a medical crisis? If you haven't had this discussion with your family, how can you begin the process of helping your parents or grandparents communicate their wishes?

Critical Thinking

4. As many as 10,000 people in this country are chronically unconscious, kept alive by artificial respirators and feeding tubes. If you were in an accident that left you in a vegetative state, would you want doctors to do everything possible to fight for your life? Would you want to spend months or even years totally unaware of your surroundings? Should health-care professionals have the right to declare that anyone is too old, too ill, or too frail to try to save? Should they have the right to insist that someone live on even if that person isn't experiencing much of a life?

Profile Plus

Life has only one inevitable conclusion. Explore your responses to death with this activity on your Profile Plus CD-ROM:

Profile Plus

• How Do You Feel About Death?

Profile Plus

Sites and Bytes

U.S. Administration on Aging
www.aoa.gov

This site, part of the Department of Health and Human Services, has information for seniors and their families on promoting healthy lifestyles and general aging topics.

Sites and Bytes

National Institute on Aging
www.nia.nih.gov

This governmental site features a comprehensive array of resources on aging, including publications on a variety of geriatric health topics, current news events, and a resource directory for older people.

Sites and Bytes

The End of Life
www.npr.org/programs/death

This site, sponsored by National Public Radio, focuses on how Americans deal with death and dying. Features include transcripts of personal stories, a place where you can tell your story, and a comprehensive list of organizations that can help families who are coping with death, dying, and the diseases of old age.

InfoTrac College Edition

Activity

Couper, Donna R., and Fran Pratt. "Preparing Young People for Longer Lives in an Aging Society." *Social Education,* Vol. 66, No. 5, September 2002, p. M2(1).

1. How can older adults help enrich the education of young people?
2. What is a major objective of intergenerational educational programs?

InfoTrac College Edition

3. How can a reciprocal learning and teaching arrangement between generations be used to help illustrate to young people how to adopt attitudes and habits that promote wellness into later life?

You can find additional readings related to psychological health with InfoTrac College Edition, an online library of more than 900 journals and

InfoTrac College Edition

publications. Follow the instructions for accessing InfoTrac College Edition that were packaged with your textbook; then search for articles using a key word search.

For additional links, resources, and suggested readings on InfoTrac College Edition, visit our Health & Wellness Resource Center at **http://health.wadsworth.com**.

Key Terms

The terms listed are used on the page indicated. Definitions of the terms are in the Glossary at the end of this book.

Key Terms

advance directives 587
aging 568
Alzheimer's disease 580
autoscopy 593
coma 590
dementia 580
do-not-resuscitate
 (DNR) 587

Key Terms

dyathanasia 594
euthanasia 594
holographic will 590
hormone replacement
 therapy (HRT) 578
hospice 592
living will 587
menopause 577

Key Terms

osteoporosis 582
perimenopause 575
persistent vegetative
 state 590
terminal illness 591
thanatology 587
transcendence 593

References

1. Dausch, Judith. "Aging Issues Moving Mainstream." *Research Quarterly for Exercise and Sport,* Vol. 74, No. 2, June 2003, p. 136.
2. National Institute of Aging, www.nia.nih.gov/health.
3. U.S. Census Bureau.
4. Dausch, "Aging Issues Moving Mainstream."
5. National Center for Health Statistics.
6. "Scientists Find What Type of Genes Affect Longevity." *Genomics & Genetics Weekly,* August 1, 2003, p. 4.
7. Roizen, Michael. Personal interview.
8. "Facts About Older Americans," National Council on Aging, www.aoa.gov.
9. Mozaffarian, Dariush, et al. "Cereal, Fruit, and Vegetable Fiber Intake and the Risk of Cardiovascular Disease in Elderly Individuals." *Journal of the American Medical Association,* Vol. 289, No. 13, April 2, 2003, p. 1659.
10. "Studies Offer Good News on Longevity and Disability." *The Lancet,* Vol. 361, No. 9354, January 25, 2003, p. 32.
11. Gregg, Edward, et al. "Relationship of Changes in Physical Activity and Mortality Among Older Women." *Journal of the American Medical Association,* Vol. 289, No. 18, May 14, 2003, p. 2379.
12. Christensen, Carol. "Physical Activity Physiological, and Psychomotor Performance: A Study of Variously Active Older Adult Men." *American Family Physician,* Vol. 68, No. 4, August 15, 2003, p. 606.
13. Gibson, Heather. "UF Study: Healthy Aging Depends on Social As Well As Physical Activity." University of Florida News Office, January 29, 2002.
14. Dausch, "Aging Issues Moving Mainstream."
15. Trichopoulou, A. "Mediterranean Diet May Improve Longevity." *Journal of the American Dietetic Association,* Vol. 103, No. 6, June 2003, p. 683.
16. Mozaffarian et al., "Cereal, Fruit, and Vegetable Fiber Intake and the Risk of Cardiovascular Disease in Elderly Individuals."
17. Lovett, Richard. "Menopause: Four Links to Depression, Libido and Memory Loss." *Psychology Today,* Vol. 36, No. 2, March–April 2003, p. 26.
18. Ibid.
19. Andrews, Gilly. "The Menopause." *Practice Nurse,* Vol. 25, No. 12, June 27, 2003, p. 37.
20. "Study Shows Measurable Drop in Testosterone in Women Approaching Menopause." *Women's Health Weekly,* July 24, 2003, p. 36.

21. "Women Urged to Reduce Risk Before Menopause." *Women's Health Weekly,* April 3, 2003, p. 30.
22. "Aerobic Exercise Better at Reducing Heart Disease Risk After Menopause." *Heart Disease Weekly,* August 3, 2003, p. 36.
23. Hodis H. N. "Hormone Therapy and the Progression of Coronary-Artery Atherosclerosis in Postmenopausal Women." *New England Journal of Medicine,* Vol. 349, No. 6, August 7, 2003, p. 535.
24. Zuger, Abigail. "A Big Study Yields Big Questions." *New England Journal of Medicine,* Vol. 349, No. 3, July 17, 2003, p. 213.
25. Chlebowski, Rowan, et al. "Influence of Estrogen Plus Progestin on Breast Cancer and Mammography in Healthy Postmenopausal Women." *Journal of the American Medical Association,* Vol. 289, No. 24, June 25, 2003, p. 3243.
26. Manson, Joann, et al. "Estrogen Plus Progestin and the Risk of Coronary Heart Disease." *New England Journal of Medicine,* Vol. 349, No. 6, August 7, 2003, p. 523; Li, Christopher, et al. "Relationship Between Long Durations and Different Regimens of Hormone Therapy and Risk of Breast Cancer." *Journal of the American Medical Association,* Vol. 289, No. 24, June 25, 2003, p. 3254.
27. Hays, J., et al. "QOL Benefits Lacking for Long-Term Estrogen-Progestin Therapy in Postmenopausal Women." *New England Journal of Medicine,* Vol. 348, No. 19, May 8, 2003, p. 1839.
28. Nelson, Heidi. "Postmenopausal Osteoporosis and Estrogen." *American Family Physician,* Vol. 68, No. 4, August 15, 2003, p. 742.
29. Johnson, Kate. "FDA Questions Estrogen/Androgen Combination." *HealthFacts,* Vol. 28, No. 6, June 2003, p. 6.
30. Gann, Peter, and Monica Morrow. "A Single-Edged Sword." *Journal of the American Medical Association,* Vol. 289, No. 24, June 25, 2003, pp. 3304–3306.
31. Cerrato, Paul. "A Critical Look at CAM Remedies for Menopause." *Contemporary OB/GYN,* Vol. 48, No. 2, February 2003, p. 112.
32. Stearns, V., et al. "Paroxetine Shows Some Efficacy in Reducing Hot Flashes." *Journal of the American Medical Association,* Vol. 289, No. 21, June 4, 2003, p. 2827.

33. Zoler, Mitchel, and Sherry Boschert. "Drug-Update: Treating Menopausal Vasomotor Symptoms Without Hormones." *Family Practice News,* Vol. 33, No. 13, July 1, 2003, p. 46.
34. Sadovsky, Richard. "Alternative Medicines for Menopausal Symptoms." *American Family Physician,* Vol. 67, No. 7, April 1, 2003, p. 1586.
35. Tice, J. A., et al. "Phytoestrogen Supplements for the Treatment of Hot Flashes: The Isoflavone Clover Extract (ICE) Study." *Journal of the American Medical Association,* Vol. 290, No. 2, July 9, 2003, p. 207.
36. Kligler, Benjamin. "Black Cohosh." *American Family Physician,* Vol. 68, No. 1, July 1, 2003, p. 114.
37. Channer, K. S., and T. H. Jones. "Cardiovascular Effects of Testosterone: Implications of the 'Male Menopause'?" *Heart,* Vol. 89, No. 2, February 2003, p. 121.
38. "Facts About Older Americans," National Council on Aging, www.aoa.gov.
39. Lovett, "Menopause."
40. Bren, Linda. "Alzheimer's: Searching for a Cure." *cFDA Consumer,* Vol. 37, No. 4, July–August 2003, p. 18.
41. Logan, Jessica, et al. "Under-Recruitment and Nonselective Recruitment: Dissociable Neural Mechanisms Associated with Aging." *Neuron,* Vol. 33, No. 5, February 28, 2002, p. 827.
42. Josefson, Deborah. "African Americans More At Risk Than Africans from Alzheimer's Disease." *British Medical Journal,* Vol. 322, No. 7286, March 10, 2001, p. 574.
43. "More Men at Osteoporosis Risk Than Commonly Believed." *Tufts University Health and Nutrition Letter,* Vol. 21, No. 6, August 2003, p. 8(1).
44. Wehren, Lois, and Ethel Siris. "Managing Bone Loss." *Internal Medicine News,* Vol. 36, No. 13, July 1, 2003, p. 13.
45. "Increasing Evidence That Osteoporosis Begins in the Womb." *Medical Letter on the CDC and FDA,* June 29, 2003, p. 32.
46. Saag, Kenneth. "The HRT Switch in Osteoporosis." *Women's Health Weekly,* June 19, 2003, p. 30.
47. "Alendronate Prevents Bone Loss in Women Who Quit HRT." *Contemporary OB/GYN,* Vol. 48, No. 7, July 2003, p. 18.

References

48. "Update on the Treatment of Osteoporosis." *Geriatrics—Myths and Perspectives, from Medscape Psychiatry & Mental Health,* February 2003. www. medscape. com.

49. "Treating Depression at Older Ages." *On the Brain,* Spring–Summer 2002, p. 5.

50. Institute of Medicine. *Describing Death in America: What We Need to Know.* Washington, DC: National Academy of Sciences, 2003.

51. Kübler-Ross, Elisabeth. *Death: The Final Stage of Growth.* Englewood Cliffs, NJ: Prentice Hall, 1975.

52. Carpenter, E. "The End of Life Odyssey." *Gerontologist,* October 15, 2001, p. 51.

53. www.agingwithdignity.org.

54. Landers, Susan. "Decisions on End-of-Life Care Shouldn't Be Left to the End." *American Medical News,* September 2, 2002.

55. Tierney, William, et al. "Discussion of Advance Care Directives." *Journal of General Interest Medicine,* January 2001.

56. van der Heide, Agnes. "End of Life Decision-Making in Six European Countries." *The Lancet,* Vol. 362, No. 9381, August 2, 2003.

57. Rocker, Graeme, and J. Randall Curis. "Caring for the Dying in the Intensive Care Unit." *Journal of the American Medical Association,* Vol. 290, No. 16, August 13, 2003, p. 820.

References

58. Lunney, June. "Patterns of Functional Decline at the End of Life." *Journal of the American Medical Association,* Vol. 289, No. 18, May 14, 2003, p. 2387.

59. Ganzini, Linda. "Nurses' Experiences with Hospice Patients Who Refuse Food and Fluids to Hasten Death." *New England Journal of Medicine,* Vol. 349, No. 4, July 24, 2003, p. 359–365.

60. Jacobs, Sandra. "Death by Voluntary Dehydration—What the Caregivers Say." *New England Journal of Medicine,* Vol. 349, No. 4, July 24, 2003, p. 325.

61. Gibson, D., et al. "Impact of Spirituality on the Living-Dying of Terminally Ill Black and White Nursing Home Residents." *Gerontologist,* October 15, 2001, p. 338.

62. Schulz, Richard, et al. "*Involvement in Caregiving and Adjustment to Death of a Spouse." *Journal of the American Medical Association,* Vol. 285, June 27, 2001, p. 3123.

63. Kayashima, R., and K. L. Braun. "Examining the Variance in Support for Assisted Death Among Physicians, Patients, and the General Public." *Gerontologist,* October 15, 2001, p. 166.

References

64. Braun, Kathryn, et al. "Support for Physician-Assisted Suicide: Exploring the Impact of Ethnicity and Attitudes Toward Planning for Death." *Gerontologist,* Vol. 41, No. 1, February 2001, p. 51.

65. Sprung, Charles, et al. "End-of-Life Practices in European Intensive Care Units." *Journal of the American Medical Association,* Vol. 290, No. 16, August 13, 2003, p. 790.

66. van der Heide, Agnes. "'Inappropriate' Treatment Near the End of Life." *Archives of Internal Medicine,* Vol. 163, 2003, pp. 1645–1649.

67. Batlle, Juan Carlos. "Legal Status of Physician-Assisted Suicide." *Journal of the American Medical Association,* Vol. 289, No. 17, May 7, 2003, p. 2279.

68. Shojania, Kaveh, et al. "Changes in Rates of Autopsy-Detected Diagnostic Errors Over Time: A Systematic Review." *Journal of the American Medical Association,* Vol. 289, No. 21, June 4, 2003, p. 2849.

69. Balk, David. "College Student Bereavement, Scholarship, and the University." *Death Studies,* Vol. 25, No. 1, January 2001, p. 67.

Staying Safe: Preventing Injury, Violence, and Victimization

"This can't be happening to me!" This was the phrase that first ran through Parker's mind when the car swerved out of control. He kept repeating it to himself as he heard the sickening sound of metal hitting metal and felt a terrible crushing pain shoot up through his legs. Later at the hospital, when he woke up after surgery, it was his first thought. And all through the long months of rehabilitation, on the days when he thought life would never go back to normal, he'd try to tell himself that this too couldn't be happening to him.

Most young people think the same way. Accidents, injuries, assaults, crimes—all seem like things that happen only to other people, only in other places. But no one, regardless of how young, healthy, or strong, is immune from danger. The risks to college students include alcohol-associated injuries and illnesses, traffic accidents, and physical and sexual assaults.[1]

Recognizing the threat of intentional and unintentional injury is the first step to ensuring your personal safety. You may think that the risk of something bad happening is simply a matter of chance, of being in the wrong place at the wrong time. That's not the case. Certain behaviors, such as using alcohol or drugs or not buckling your seat belt, greatly increase the risk of harm. Ultimately, you have more control over your safety than anyone or anything else in your life.

This chapter is a primer in self-protection that could help safeguard—perhaps even save—your life. Included are recommendations for common sense safety on the road, at home, and outdoors. This chapter also explores other serious threats to personal safety in our society: violence and sexual victimization.

© Jim Cummins/Taxi/Getty Images

After studying the material in this chapter, you should be able to:

- **List** and **explain** factors that increase the likelihood of an accident.
- **Describe** procedures for safety on the road, at work, at home, and at play.
- **Discuss** the factors contributing to aggression and violence.
- **Define** sexual victimization, sexual harassment, and sexual coercion.
- **List** the different types of rape, and describe recommended actions for preventing rape.
- **Explain** the consequences of sexual violence.

603

⚡ Unintentional Injury: Why Accidents Happen

The major threat to the lives of college students isn't illness but injury. Almost 75 percent of deaths among Americans 15 to 24 years old are caused by "unintentional injuries" (a term public health officials prefer), suicides, and homicides.[2] The odds of dying from an injury in any given year are about one in 765; over a lifetime they rise to one in 23.[3] In all, injuries—intentional and unintentional—claim almost 150,000 lives a year. Accidents, especially motor vehicle crashes, kill more college-age men and women than all other causes combined; the greatest number of lives lost to accidents is among those 25 years of age.

Many factors influence an individual's risk of accident or injury, including age, alcohol and drug use, stress, inherently dangerous situations, and thrill seeking.

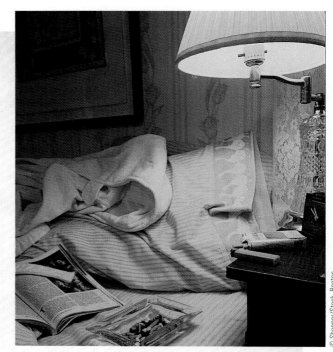

Home is a dangerous place. Many accidents happen at home—perhaps because we let down our guard there.

Age

Injury is the leading cause of death in the United States during the first four decades of life. Each year violence and unintentional injuries cause more than 146,000 deaths and cost more than $260 billion.[4] Most victims of fatal accidents are males, often in their teens and twenties. Feeling full of life and energy, they may take dangerous risks because they think they're invulnerable.

Alcohol and Drugs

An estimated 40 percent of Americans are involved in an alcohol-related accident sometime during their lives. Alcohol plays a role in about a quarter of fatal motor vehicle accidents and half of fatal motorcycle crashes.[5]

Stress

In times of tension and anxiety, we all pay less attention to what we're doing. One common result is an increase in accidents. If you find yourself having a series of small mishaps or near-misses, do something to lower your stress level, rather than wait for something more harmful to happen. (See Chapter 3 on stress.)

Situational Factors

Some situations—such as driving on a curvy, wet road in a car with worn tires—are so inherently dangerous that they greatly increase the odds of an accident. But even when

there's greater risk, you can lower the danger: For instance, you can make sure your tires and brakes are in good condition.

Thrill Seeking

To some people, activities that others might find terrifying—such as skydiving or parachute jumping—are stimulating. These thrill seekers may have lower-than-normal levels of the brain chemicals that regulate excitement. Because the stress of potentially hazardous sports may increase the levels of these chemicals, they feel pleasantly aroused rather than scared.

⚡ What Should I Do in an Emergency Situation?

Life-threatening situations rarely happen more than once or twice in any person's life. When they do, you must think and act quickly to prevent disastrous consequences.

:: ***Don't panic.*** Your immediate response to an emergency may be overwhelming fear and anxiety. Take several deep breaths. Start by assessing the circumstances. Shout for help if you're in a public place. Look for any possible dangers to you or the victim, such as a live electrical wire or a fire. Seek medical assistance as quickly as possible. Don't attempt rescue techniques, such as cardiopulmonary resuscitation (CPR), unless you're trained.

:: ***Don't wait for symptoms to go away or get worse.*** If you suspect that someone is having a heart attack or stroke, or has ingested something poisonous, *phone for help immediately.* A delay could jeopardize the person's life. Stay on the line long enough to give your name, address, and a brief description of the emergency.

:: ***Don't move a victim.*** The person may have a broken neck or back, and attempting to move him or her could cause extensive damage or even death.

:: ***Don't drive.*** Even if the hospital is just ten minutes away, you're better off waiting for a well-equipped ambulance with trained paramedics who can deliver emergency care on the spot. People rushing to emergency rooms are more likely to get into accidents themselves.

:: ***Don't do too much.*** Often well-intentioned Good Samaritans make injuries worse by trying to tie tourniquets, wash cuts, or splint broken limbs. Also, don't give an injured person anything to eat or drink. (See "Emergency!" in the Hales Health Almanac at the back of this book for more on first-aid and emergency care.)

:: ***At home, keep a supply of basic first-aid items in a convenient place.*** Beyond the emergency number 911, make sure that telephone numbers for your doctor and neighbors are handy.

❖ Safety on the Road

With more drivers and more vehicles on the roads than ever before, the fatality rate per 100 million vehicle miles of travel has fallen to an all-time low of 1.51.[6] However, despite the progress that has been made, our streets and highways remain dangerous. Every 14 seconds someone in America is injured in a traffic crash; every 12 minutes someone is killed. Motor vehicle accidents in the United States annually claim about 42,800 lives and injure almost three million people, more than any other form of unintentional injury. They are the leading cause of all deaths for people ages 2 to 33; only cancer and heart attacks claim more American lives.[7]

According to the National Highway Traffic Safety Administration (NHTSA), motor vehicle crashes on America's roadways cost $230.6 billion per year—an average of $820 for every person in the United States. This is based on an estimated cost of $977,000 for a fatality and $1.1 million for a critically injured crash survivor.[8]

In various studies, posttraumatic stress disorder (PTSD), discussed in Chapter 3, has developed in 8 to 39 percent of individuals injured in motor vehicle crashes or other accidents. It is more likely to develop after a motor

vehicle accident when other distressing events occur at the same time, when the victim feared death, when the accident was extremely serious, or when the victim was socially isolated afterward. Children injured in traffic accidents and their parents are at high risk of stress-related symptoms, particularly immediately after a crash.[9]

Safe Drivers and Vehicles

 Race, gender, and education affect a person's risk on the road. African-Americans, particularly men, are at increased risk of dying compared to whites. Hispanic men, but not Hispanic women, are at greater risk of dying than whites, but less so than blacks.[10] However, education has a strong influence. Whites without high school degrees have the highest death rates per 10 million road trips. People with no education beyond high school are less likely to use seat belts and more likely to drink and drive. College students aren't necessarily safer drivers than others their age. According to national data, full-time college students drink and drive more often than part-time students and other young adults, but they also are more likely to wear seat belts while driving and riding in cars.[11] (See Student Snapshot: "Risky Driving.")

Young drivers, particularly the newly licensed, are more likely to be in a car crash than any other age group. The risk is highest among 16 and 17-year-olds during their first six months and 500 miles on the road. In addition to inexperience, risky driving behaviors, alcohol use, not buckling up, driver distraction, fatigue, and vehicle choice all increase the danger. Restrictions that forbid nighttime driving and limit the number of passengers in a teenager's vehicle, adopted by many states, keep young drivers out of some hazardous situations but do not eliminate other risks—or risky behavior.[12]

The vehicles drivers choose affect their safety. Equipment such as air bags, padded dashboards, safety glass windows, a steel frame, and side-impact bags help protect against fatal injuries. Size and make also matter—to those in a vehicle and those in other vehicles. Per vehicle mile, motorcyclists are 26 times as likely as passenger car occupants to die in a traffic crash.

Is bigger and heavier safer? On the basis of analysis of crash studies, sports utility vehicles (SUVs), vans and pickups appear to be more crashworthy than cars. Drivers in pickups face less risk of serious injury than car drivers.[13] SUV drivers are safer in crashes but at greater risk of serious injuries in rollovers. The occupants of passenger cars that collide with pickups or SUVs experience more than twice the risk than those who collide with another car.[14]

Student Snapshot **Risky Driving**

Data from interviews with 11,549 18- to 25-year-olds nationwide.

Source: M. J. Paschall. "College Attendance and Risk-Related Driving Behavior in a National Sample of Young Adults." *Journal of Studies of Alcohol*, Vol. 64, No. 1, January 2003, p. 43.

Who admits drinking and driving in the last year?

Full-time college students   34.2%

Part-time college students   32.8%

Other young adults   27.9%

Who always wears a seat belt while driving?

Full-time college students   76.1%

Part-time college students   71.8%

Other young adults   62.7%

Unsafe Driving Behaviors

Most road accidents don't just happen. A variety of factors—alcohol, speed, aggressive driving, age, and inexperience—increase the danger. Drunk driving is the number one cause of serious motor vehicle accidents. In recent years, there has been a decline in the number of fatalities caused by drunk driving, particularly among young people. The NHTSA attributes this decline to increases in the drinking age, to educational programs aimed at reducing nighttime driving by teens, to the formation of Students Against Destructive Decisions (SADD) and similar groups, and to changes in state laws that penalize drivers younger than age 21 for driving with even lower blood–alcohol concentration levels than were previously acceptable (from 0.01 to 0.05 percent). (See Chapter 11 for more information on blood–alcohol concentrations and drunk driving.)

Falling asleep at the wheel is second only to alcohol as a cause of serious motor-vehicle accidents. About half of drivers in the United States drive while drowsy. Nearly 14 million have fallen asleep at the wheel in the past year, according to the National Sleep Foundation. Men and young adults between the ages of 18 and 29 are at the highest risk for driving while drowsy or falling asleep at the wheel.[15] Each year 200,000 sleep-related motor vehicle accidents claim more than 5,000 lives, cause hundreds of thousands of injuries, and lead to billions of dollars in indirect costs. Too little sleep, recent research suggests, may be as detrimental to driving skills as drinking too much. Employees who work night shifts, long hours, or more than one job run an increased risk of falling asleep at the wheel and being in a sleep-induced crash.

Speed literally kills, claiming more than 12,000 lives a year. Among male drivers 15 to 20 years old, 39 percent of those involved in fatal crashes were speeding.[16]

Aggressive driving behaviors endanger everyone on the road. With traffic deaths rising, states nationwide are cracking down on all types of aggressive drivers, from illegal street racers to tailgating commuters. Psychological tests of college students reveal correlations between aggressive driving and aggressive impulses toward one's self and others.[17]

Seat Belts

Seat belt use has reached an all-time high, with three in four Americans buckling up. States with seat belt laws have even higher rates of use: 80 percent.[18] However, young people are less likely to use seat belts. By official estimates, two-thirds of 15- to 20-year-olds killed in motor vehicle accidents were not wearing seat belts.[19]

Seat belts save an estimated 9,500 lives in the United States each year. When lap-shoulder belts are used properly, they reduce the risk of fatal injury to front-seat passengers by 45 percent and the risk of moderate-to-critical injury by 50 percent. The risk of death or severe injury increases nearly fivefold for front-seat passengers when backseat passengers aren't wearing seat belts. In a collision, unbelted backseat passengers may be thrown forward, pushing the front-seat passengers into the dashboard and the windshield.[20]

Seat belts save lives in several ways. When a crash occurs, occupants continue to travel at the vehicle's original speed at the moment of impact. After the vehicle comes to a complete stop, unbelted occupants slam into the steering wheel, windshield, or into another part of the car. Seat belts reduce injuries from this second collision and also prevent ejection from the car.[21]

Air Bags

An air bag, either with or without a seat belt, has proven the most effective means of preventing adult death, somewhat more so for women than for men. However, they do not lower the risk of serious injury.[22] (See Fact or Fiction? "An air bag won't keep you from being injured . . .") Because there is controversy over the potential hazard they pose to children, the American Academy of Pediatrics recommends that children be placed in the backseat, whether or not the car is equipped with a passenger air bag.

Road Rage

The emotional outbursts known as road rage are a factor in as many as two-thirds of all fatal car crashes and one-third of nonfatal accidents, according to the NHTSA. Psychologist Arnold Nerenberg of Whittier, California, a specialist in motorway mayhem, estimates 1.78 billion episodes of road rage a year, resulting in more than 28,000 deaths and 1 million injuries.[23]

Some strategies for reducing road rage include the following:

:: **Lower the stress in your life.** Take a few moments to breathe deeply and relax your shoulders before putting the key in the ignition.

:: **Consciously decide not to let other drivers get to you.** Decide that whatever happens, it's not going to make your blood pressure go up.

:: **Slow down.** If you're going five or ten miles over the speed limit, you won't have the time you need to react to anything that happens.

:: **Modify bad driving habits one at a time.** If you tend to tailgate slow drivers, spend a week driving at twice your usual following distance. If you're a habitual horn honker, silence yourself.

:: **Be courteous—even if other drivers aren't.** Don't dawdle in the passing lane. Never tailgate or switch lanes

© 2000 PhotoDisc, Inc.

Buckling up is one of the simplest and most effective ways of protecting yourself from injury.

FACT OR FICTION?

An air bag won't keep you from being injured in a serious car accident.

Fact: An air bag may keep you alive in a motor vehicle collision, but it will not protect you from injury. A study of 15 million people involved in crashes found that seat belts provided the most protection. Air bags used in conjunction with seat belts did not significantly reduce the risk of injury; without seat belts, they increased the risk of injury, particularly to the head and legs.

Source: Sherry Melton et al. "Emphasizing Mechanism of Injury and Therapeutic Management." *The Journal of Trauma: Injury, Infection, and Critical Care*, Vol. 54, No. 4, April 2003, p. 781.

without signaling. Don't use your horn or high beams unless absolutely necessary.

:: **Never retaliate.** Whatever another driver does, keep your cool. Count to ten. Take a deep breath. If you yell or gesture at someone who's upset with you, the conflict may well escalate.

:: **If you do something stupid, show that you're sorry.** On its website, the AAA Foundation for Traffic Safety solicited suggestions for automotive apologies. The most popular: slapping yourself on your forehead or the top of your head to indicate that you know you goofed. Such gestures can soothe a miffed motorist—and make the roads a slightly safer place for all of us.

STRATEGIES FOR PREVENTION

How to Drive Safely

- Don't drive while under the influence of alcohol or other drugs, including medications that may impair your reflexes, cause drowsiness, or affect your judgment. Never get into a car if you suspect the driver may be intoxicated or affected by a drug.

- Remain calm when dealing with drivers who are reckless or rude. Be alert and anticipate possible hazards. Don't let yourself be distracted by conversations, children's questions, arguments, food or drink, or scenic views.

- Don't get too comfortable. Alertness matters. Use the rearview mirror often. Don't let passengers or packages obstruct your view. Use turn signals when changing lanes or making a turn. If someone cuts you off, back off to a safe distance.

- Watch out for warning signs of fatigue, such as difficulty focusing, frequent blinking or heavy eyelids, trouble keeping one's head up; repeated yawning; trouble remembering the last few miles driven; and drifting from the lane or hitting the shoulder rumble strip.

- Drive more slowly if weather conditions are bad. Avoid driving at all during heavy rain, snow, or other conditions that affect visibility and road conditions. If you must drive in hazardous conditions, make sure that your car has the proper equipment, such as chains or snow tires, and that you know how to respond in case of a skid.

- Maintain your car properly, replacing windshield wipers, tires, and brakes when necessary. Keep flares and a fire extinguisher in your car for use in emergencies.

Is It Safe to Use a Car Phone While Driving?

According to the National Highway Traffic Safety Administration, driver distraction from various causes plays a role in 20 to 30 percent of all motor vehicle crashes. An estimated 80 to 90 percent of mobile-phone owners use their phones while driving at least some of the time; about 30 percent regularly use their phones and drive at the same time. (In some states, it is now illegal to talk on a cell phone while driving.) An average of 3 percent of American motorists—500,000 people—are talking on the phone at any given time. Women use mobile phones twice as much as men.[24]

A person using a cell phone while driving increases the probability of dying in a motor vehicle crash by about 15 chances in a million per year. The annual risk for another motorist, a bicyclist, or a pedestrian being killed by a driver using a mobile phone is four in a million. These numbers add up to approximately 2,600 deaths and 330,000 injuries a year, 12,000 of them serious.[25]

Although many believe that hands-free car phones are less hazardous, researchers have shown this is not the case. Talking on a wireless phone while driving a car is just as dangerous with a hands-free or a handheld phone. The reason is that talking while driving distracts the brain as well as the eyes—much more so than talking to another person in the vehicle. Conversation on any type of phone disrupts a driver's attention to the visual environment, leading to what researchers call "inattention blindness," the inability to recognize objects encountered in the driver's visual field. This form of cognitive impairment may distract drivers for up to two minutes after the phone conversation has ended.[26]

STRATEGIES FOR PREVENTION

Car Phone Safety Tips

- Find out if cell phone use while driving is legal in your state.

- Do not dial new calls until you're stopped or in a safe low-traffic environment.

- Keep calls short, less than 1 or 2 minutes.

- When you're on the phone, avoid difficult maneuvers, such as changing lanes, that require a lot of attention.

- Have a passenger send or receive calls.

- Invest in a hands-free model, especially if you use your phone regularly. While the cognitive distraction is the same, it helps to avoid the mechanical distraction.

On the other hand, car phones are helpful in alerting authorities to road hazards, congestion, or problem drivers and in summoning help in case of a breakdown or another emergency.

Safe Cycling

Mile for mile, motorcycling is far more risky than automobile driving. The most common motorcycle injury is head trauma, which can lead to physical disability, including paralysis and general weakness, as well as problems reading and thinking. It can also cause personality changes and psychiatric problems, such as depression, anxiety, uncontrollable mood swings, and anger. Complete recovery from head trauma can take four to six years, and the costs can be staggering. Head injury can also result in permanent disability, coma, and death. To prevent head trauma, motorcycle helmets are required in most states.

Approximately 80.6 million people ride bicycles. Each year, bicycle crashes kill about 900 of these individuals; about 200 of those killed are children under age 15. Men are more likely to suffer cycling injuries. Bicycle injuries are the most common cause of serious head injury in children, and most of these injuries are preventable.[27] The risk increases with high speed; collisions with motor vehicles are most likely to be fatal.[28]

According to a national survey, 50 percent of all bicycle riders in the United States regularly wear bike helmets—43 percent every time they ride and 7 percent

In the states with motorcycle helmet laws, motorcyclist deaths and injuries have decreased drastically.

more than half the time. Safety is the primary reason that 98 percent of those surveyed gave for wearing a helmet, followed by the insistence of a parent or spouse. The reasons for not wearing a bike helmet included riding only a short distance, forgetting to put it on, or feeling that the helmet was uncomfortable. (See Savvy Consumer: "Buying a Bicycle Helmet.")

✖ Safety at Work

The workplace is second only to the home as the most frequent site of accidents. More than 5,500 injury deaths occur on the job every year.[29] The industries with the highest fatality rates are mining; transportation, communication, and public utilities; construction; and agriculture, forestry, and fishing. Whatever your job, find out about potential hazards and learn the proper safety regulations. (Chapter 19 discusses some potential environmental hazards at work, including noise, toxic substances, and video display terminals.)

According to a report by the National Research Council and Institute of Medicine, about one million workers annually suffer musculoskeletal disorders of the lower back and upper extremities as a result of their "particular jobs and working conditions—including heavy lifting, repetitive and forceful motions, and stressful working conditions." Many can be prevented.[30]

▣ Can My Computer Be a Health Hazard?

As computers have become part of daily life for everyone from preschoolers to seniors, health professionals have learned a great deal about potential health problems, including repetitive motion injuries and vision-related difficulties.

Repetitive Motion Injuries

Repetitive motion injuries (RMI) have surpassed back and neck injuries as the number one claim for workers compensation injuries. Repeated motions—such as the hand and arm movements made while using a computer keyboard—all day, every day, can result in muscle and tendon strain and inflammation. About 20 percent of people with pain, tingling, or numbness in the hands may have carpal tunnel syndrome, an overuse injury caused by repetitive motions in the hands and wrists. Symptoms include pain, swelling, and numbness and weakness in the hands or the arms. If these problems are identified early, permanent damage can generally be avoided by altering the work environment and allowing for more breaks during the day.

Savvy Consumer

BUYING A BICYCLE HELMET

What should you look for when buying a helmet? Here are some basic guidelines:

- A government regulation requires all helmets produced after 1999 to meet the Consumer Product Safety Commission standard; look for a CPSC sticker inside the helmet. The ASTM standard is comparable to CPSC. The Snell Memorial Foundation's B-90 standard is even better.

- Check the fit. The helmet should sit level on your head, touching all around, comfortably snug but not tight. The helmet should not move more than about an inch in any direction, regardless of how hard you tug at it.

- Pick a bright color for visibility. Avoid dark colors, thin straps, or a rigid visor that could snag in a fall.

- Look for a smooth plastic outer shell, not one with alternating strips of plastic and foam.

- Watch out for excessive vents, which put less protective foam in contact with your head in a crash.

- Mirrors should have a breakaway mount; the wire type mounted on eyeglasses can gouge an eye in a fall.

The slope and height of a computer keyboard can affect the likelihood of repetitive motion injuries. If you work at a computer, good posture and correct positioning of the computer screen and keyboard can help prevent repetitive motion injuries, eyestrain, and back strain. (See Figure 18-1.) Here are some additional tips:

:: Place the keyboard so that your elbows are bent at a 90° angle and you don't have to bend your wrists to type.

:: Use a chair that provides ample back support. Keep your thighs parallel to the floor and your feet on the floor. If your feet don't reach the floor, use a footrest.

:: If you experience neck strain, place a document holder next to your screen so that you can view the materials more easily.

:: Every 15 minutes take a 30-second break, stretch your arms, and walk around the office. Take a 15-minute break at least once every two hours.

Vision Problems

Computer vision syndrome is a condition marked by tired and sore eyes, blurred vision, headaches and neck, shoulder, and back pain. The American Optometric Association estimates that it afflicts nearly 90 percent of workers who use computers and also is common among children and students of all ages. The symptoms result from repeatedly stressing some aspect of the visual system, but they often disappear as soon as the person stops working at the computer.

The eye focuses on a computer image differently from the way it focuses on a printed one. The pixels that appear on a computer screen, unlike printed characters, are bright in the center and gradually fade away into the background color. This makes it difficult for the eye to sustain focus. Optometrists have developed a specific method, called a PRIO examination, that simulates how the eye responds to

Figure 18-1 SAFE COMPUTING
By paying attention to your posture and your computer's position, you can help protect yourself from repetitive motion injury, back strain, and eyestrain.

The screen should be at eye level (22–26 inches higher than your seat).

Position the keyboard so that your elbows are bent at a 90° angle and your hands and wrists are straight.

Sit straight in your chair; for extra back support, place a rolled-up towel behind you.

Keep your hands and wrists relaxed.

pixels on a computer screen. It can determine the need and proper prescription for computer-only eyeglasses.

▣ Safety at Home

Every year home accidents cause nearly 25 million injuries. Poison poses the greatest threat, causing more than 17,000 deaths every year. Half a million children swallow poisonous materials each year; 90 percent are under age 5.

Adults may also be poisoned by mistakenly taking someone else's prescription drugs or taking medicines in the dark and swallowing the wrong one. In most cities, you can call a poison control center for advice.

Falls

Falls of all kinds are the second leading cause of death from unintentional injury in the United States. High heels or worn footgear, poor lighting, slippery or uneven walkways, broken stairs and handrails, loose or worn rugs, and objects left where people walk all increase the likelihood of a slip.

Fires

You can prevent fires by making sure that the three ingredients of fire—fuel, a heat source, and oxygen—don't get a chance to mix. Almost anything can act as fuel for fire, including paper, wood, and flammable liquids such as oils, gasoline, and some paints. A heat source can be a spark from a lighted match, a pilot light, or an electrical wire. Oxygen is necessary for the chemical reaction between the fuel and heat source that causes combustion.

If a fire starts and it's small, you may be able to put it out with a portable fire extinguisher before it spreads. However, if the fire does get out of control, you might have only two to five minutes to get out of the house or building alive. A fire-escape plan can save time and lives. Sketch a plan of your house, apartment building, dormitory, or fraternity or sorority house. Identify two ways out of each room or apartment. Make sure everyone is familiar with these escape routes. Designate an area outside where

Your home first-aid kit should include (at minimum) bandages, sterile gauze pads, adhesive tape, scissors, cotton, antibiotic ointment, a needle, safety pins, calamine lotion, syrup of ipecac to induce vomiting, and a thermometer.

all family members or dorm residents should meet after escaping from a fire.

In a national survey, 67 percent of colleges had at least one dorm without a sprinkler system.[31] If a fire breaks out in your dorm room, get out as quickly as possible, but don't run. Before opening a room door, place your hand on it. If it's hot, don't open it. If the door feels cool, open it slightly to check for smoke; if there's none, leave by your planned escape route. If you're on an upper floor and your escape routes are blocked, open a window (top and bottom, if possible) and wait or signal from the window for help. Never try to use an elevator in a fire.

⚫ Safety at Play

According to a study by the Johns Hopkins School of Public Health, every year 750,000 Americans are injured during recreational activities such as horseback riding, skiing, sledding, skating, and playground activities; 82,000 suffer head injuries requiring emergency room or hospital treatment.

Handling Heat

Each year as many as 1,000 Americans die from heat-caused illnesses that are almost always preventable. Two common heat-related maladies are **heat cramps** and **heat stress.** Heat cramps are caused by hard work and heavy sweating in the heat. Heat stress may occur simultaneously or afterward, as the blood vessels try to keep body temperature down. **Heat exhaustion,** a third such malady, is the result of prolonged sweating with inadequate fluid replacement. (See Table 18-1.)

The first step in treating these conditions is to stop exercising, move to a cool place, and drink plenty of water. Don't resume work or activity until all the symptoms have disappeared; see a doctor if you're suffering from heat exhaustion. **Heat stroke** is a life-threatening medical emergency caused by the breakdown of the body's mechanism for cooling itself. The treatment is to cool the body down: Move to a cooler environment; sponge down with cool water, and apply ice to the back of the neck, armpits, and groin. Immersion in cold water could cause shock. Get medical help immediately.

Coping with Cold

The tips of the toes, fingers, ears, nose, chin, and cheeks are most vulnerable to exposure to high wind speeds and low temperatures, which can result in **frostnip.** Because frostnip is painless, you may not even be aware of it occurring. Watch for a sudden blanching or lightening of your skin.

TABLE 18-1	Heat Dangers	
Illness	**Symptoms**	**Treatment**
Heat cramps	Muscle twitching or cramping; muscle spasms in arms, legs, and abdomen	Stop exercising; cool off; drink water.
Heat stress	Fatigue, pale skin, blurred vision, dizziness, low blood pressure	Stop exercising; cool off; drink water.
Heat exhaustion	Excessive thirst, fatigue, lack of coordination, increased sweating, elevated body temperature	Stop exercising; cool off; drink water. See a doctor.
Heat stroke	Lack of perspiration, high body temperature (over 105°F), dry skin, rapid breathing, coma, seizures, high pulse	Cool the body; sponge down with cool water; apply ice to the back of the neck, the armpits, and the groin. Get immediate medical help.

The best early treatment is warming the area by firm, steady pressure with a warm hand; blowing on it with hot breath; holding it against your body; or immersing it in warm (not hot) water. As the skin thaws, it becomes red and starts to tingle. Be careful to protect it from further damage. Don't rub the skin vigorously or with snow, as you could damage the tissue.

More severe is **frostbite,** which can be either superficial or deep. *Superficial frostbite,* the freezing of the skin and tissues just below the skin, is characterized by a waxy look and firmness of the skin, although the tissue below is soft. Initial treatment should be to slowly rewarm the area. As the area thaws, it will be numb and bluish or purple, and blisters may form. Cover the area with a dry, sterile dressing, and protect the skin from further exposure to cold. See a doctor for further treatment. *Deep frostbite,* the freezing of skin, muscle, and even bone, requires medical treatment. It usually involves the tissues of the hands and feet, which appear pale and feel frozen. Keep the victim dry and as warm as possible on the way to a medical facility. Cover the frostbitten area with a dry, sterile dressing.

The gradual cooling of the center of the body may occur at temperatures above, as well as below, freezing—usually in wet, windy weather. When body temperature falls below 95° Fahrenheit, the body is incapable of rewarming itself because of the breakdown of the internal system that regulates its temperature. This state is known as **hypothermia.** The first sign of hypothermia is severe shivering. Then the victim becomes uncoordinated, drowsy, listless, confused, and is unable to speak properly. Symptoms become more severe as body temperature continues to drop, and coma or death can result.

Hypothermia requires emergency medical treatment. Try to prevent any further heat loss: Move the victim to a warm place, cover him or her with blankets, remove wet clothing, and replace it with dry garments. If the victim is conscious, administer warm liquids, not alcohol.

Drowning

Over the last few decades, deaths from drowning have declined. Possible reasons include less use of alcohol by swimmers and boaters, and an increase in body fat, which makes floating easier. Toddlers under age 4 and teenage boys between 15 and 19 remain at greatest risk. Among young children, 90 percent of drownings occur in residential swimming pools.

Drowning is a leading cause of injury-related death in children, claiming the lives of more than 1,400 children younger than 20 years every year. For each drowning death, at least one to four children suffer a serious near-drowning, which often causes permanent disabilities.[32] Among young adults the risk factors for drowning and near-drowning include lack of knowledge about the water being entered and alcohol consumption.[33]

The causes of drowning, in order of frequency, are becoming exhausted, being swept into deep water, losing support, becoming trapped or entangled, having a cramp or other attack, and striking an underwater object. Many drowning victims were strong swimmers. Most drownings occur at unorganized facilities, such as ponds or pools with no lifeguard present.

© Lew Merrim/Photo Researchers, Inc.

Water safety training can begin in early childhood. Swimming, treading water, and engaging in safe water practices are all important to preventing drownings.

⚫ Intentional Injury: Living in a Dangerous World

Although the United States remains the most violent country in the Western world, the rate of violent crime is going down. The World Health Organization (WHO) defines violence as "the intentional use of physical force or power, threatened or actual, against oneself, another person, or a group or community, that either results in, or has a high likelihood of resulting in, injury, death, psychological harm, maldevelopment, or deprivation."[34] Record numbers of children around the world have witnessed violence and are at risk for post-traumatic stress disorder (discussed in Chapter 3).[35]

In the Americas, more than 300,000 people die each year as a result of violence, suicide, or accidental injury. Interpersonal violence is the third-leading cause of death among people 15 to 44 years old. Some studies show that a third of women age 16 to 49 have, at some point in their lives, been victims of sexual abuse. In the last decade, rates of armed urban violence have increased along with the number of youth gangs.[36]

Coping with the Threat of Violence and Terrorism

Uncertainty can be the most difficult aspect of living in a dangerous world. While you cannot eliminate risk, the following strategies can help you deal with it:

:: Focus on the here-and-now. Make a daily to-do list. Check off each chore as you complete it. Break down large projects into a series of manageable steps.

:: Act despite fear. Take that first step even if you are anxious, trusting that the second will be easier.

:: Adjust your attitude. The way you appraise a situation—as a threat that endangers your life or as a challenge that can be overcome—has a tremendous impact on your psychological and physical responses.

:: Draw on your spiritual beliefs. Faith and values provide a bridge over the unknown.

:: Dare to hope. This may be the most life-affirming coping strategy of all.

Violence in the United States

Gun-related injuries and deaths have declined, but guns remain the second-leading cause of injury-related death in the United States after car accidents. About 260 Americans are injured by firearms every day; one-third die from their wounds.[37] Despite the decline in crime, gun violence annually takes the lives of nearly 30,000 Americans, includ-

ing 10 children every day. The proportion of youth involved in crime has actually risen. Almost half the victims of violent crime are under 25 years of age.[38]

Although men commit nine times more violent crimes than women, the rates are getting closer. (See The X & Y File: "Which Gender Is at Greater Risk?") Individuals with mental illness are somewhat more likely to become violent than others. In people with no psychiatric disorder, the prevalence of violence is 2 percent, compared with 8 percent in those with schizophrenia. The risk of violence is highest in people with alcohol or drug misuse or dependence disorders.[39]

There are ethnic and racial differences in patterns of violence. African Americans are at greater risk of victimization by violent crime than whites or persons of other racial groupings. Hispanics are at greater risk of violent victimization than non-Hispanics. There is little difference between white women and nonwhite women in rape, physical assault, or stalking. Native American and Alaska Native women are significantly more likely than white women or African-American women to report being raped. Mixed-race women also have a significantly higher incidence of rape than white women. Native American and Alaska Native men report significantly more physical assaults than Asian and Pacific Islander men.

Alcohol availability increases the rates of total crime, violent crime, property crime, and homicides.

The Roots of Aggression and Violence

While anger is considered a normal, sometimes inevitable emotion, aggression—behavior with the intent to control or dominate—is a threat to individuals and to society. Angry people may *want* to push or punch someone; aggressive people carry through on such impulses and become violent. Why? The reasons, discussed in the following sections, are complex.

Biological Causes

Traumatic brain injury, which can lead to violent outbursts of explosive anger, is one of many medical factors associated with violence. As many as 70 percent of those who suffer head injuries report some degree of irritability or explosive rage. The use of alcohol or drugs before or after a head injury may increase the likelihood of such problems. Illnesses that affect the brain—stroke and neurologic diseases, brain tumors, infectious illnesses, epilepsy, metabolic disorders (such as hyperthyroidism or hypothyroidism), multiple sclerosis, and systemic lupus erythematosus—can also lead to aggressive behavior.

Certain medications—painkillers, antianxiety agents, steroids, antidepressants, and over-the-counter sedatives (which may produce delirium)—can trigger aggression.

the **X & Y** *file* — *Which Gender Is at Greater Risk?*

Just like illness, injury doesn't discriminate against either gender. Both men and women can find themselves in harm's way—but for different reasons. Here are some gender differences in vulnerability:

- Men are ten times more likely to die of an occupational injury than women.
- Males are most often the victims and the perpetrators of homicides in the United States. In about 68 percent of cases reported by the Bureau of Justice Statistics, both the offender and the victim were male.
- Overall, men are 3.6 times more likely than women to be murdered and 9 times more likely to commit murder. Both men and women are more likely to kill or attempt to kill male victims than female victims.

- Men are 1.5 times more likely than women to be assaulted as an adult. Each year 3.2 million men, compared with 1.9 million women, are physically attacked.
- Women are more often the targets of partner violence. Approximately 1.3 million women and 835,000 men are annually assaulted by an intimate partner. At some point in their lifetime, 22.1 percent of women—compared with 7.4 percent of men—report a physical attack by a spouse, partner, boyfriend or girlfriend, or date.
- Physical assaults are more likely to injure women than men. Of female assault victims, 39 percent—compared with 24.8 percent of male assault victims—reported being injured during their most recent attack.
- Thunderstorms kill twice as many men as women, according to the CDC. When lightning strikes, 85 percent of those killed are men. Men also are more likely to die from floods, tornados, and high winds.

Alcohol abuse, which lowers inhibitions against violent behavior and interferes with judgment, and many street drugs, including amphetamines, cocaine, and hallucinogens, are also associated with violence.

In searching for other biological abnormalities that may be linked with violence, neuroscientists have noted low levels of the neurotransmitter serotonin in men convicted of homicide. Serotonin is involved in the control of impulses, particularly toward violent or self-destructive acts. Other neurotransmitters also may play important roles in aggression, and the relations among these chemicals ultimately may prove more critical than the levels of any single one of them.

Sex chromosome abnormalities have been investigated but do not seem to lead to a greater tendency toward vio-

lence in, for example, men with an extra Y chromosome. The role of the male sex hormone testosterone also has been investigated. The highly competitive men most likely to dominate a situation or group—whether it's a seminar or a street gang—tend to have higher testosterone levels than other men. But testosterone in itself does not make men aggressive. Rather, scientists explain, it is only one of many contributing factors.

Individuals with serious mental disorders may be somewhat more violent than the general population, especially immediately after discharge from the hospital. Individuals with a serious mental illness (such as schizophrenia) report having been violent much more often than those with no mental disorder. However, alcohol and drug users are, as a group, more violent than individuals with serious mental illnesses.[40]

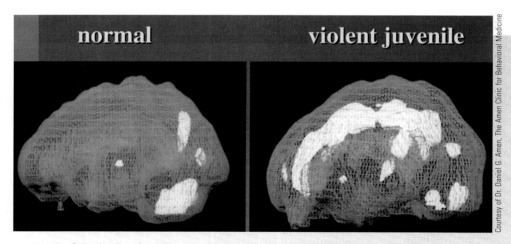

normal — **violent juvenile**

Courtesy of Dr. Daniel G. Amen, The Amen Clinic for Behavioral Medicine

Scans of the brain of a 16-year-old who assaulted another teen show several abnormalities compared with a normal brain. They may reflect some combination of early head injuries, depression, and exposure to violence as a child.

Developmental Factors

For years, experts have debated whether some individuals are violent from a very young age or whether they "learn" violent behavior as they grow. According to current research, teen violence can develop in either way.

Most children who are highly aggressive or have behavioral disorders early in life do not become serious violent offenders. However, some offenders follow the "early onset" path and commit their first serious violent act before puberty. Early-onset offenders commit more and more serious crimes in adolescence and are more likely to remain violent throughout their lives.

Teens who develop "late-onset" violence—the majority of male adolescent offenders—do not become violent until puberty, at about age 13. As children, they show few or no signs of problem behavior, aggression, or behavioral disorders. As teenagers, their offenses tend to be less frequent and less serious. Most give up their violent behavior as they reach adulthood.

While some risk factors for violence, such as simply being born male, are biological, most come from a child's environment or ability to respond to his or her environment. Children of violent parents who become violent themselves are more likely to have learned this behavior than to have inherited a tendency to act this way.

The strongest risk factor during childhood are involvement in serious, but not necessarily violent, criminal behavior, substance use, physical aggression, poverty, and parents who are violent or criminal. During adolescence, when peers become more influential, the strongest risk factors are weak ties to conventional teens, relationships with antisocial or delinquent peers, gang membership, and involvement in other criminal acts.

Being "at risk" does not doom any child to become violent. Most children whose childhoods are shadowed by abuse or poverty do not turn to violence. And some children with no risk factors in their early lives become ensnared in dangerous lifestyles that include not only violence, but drugs, alcohol, and other risky behaviors. There is no one single underlying trigger for teen violence, but a combination of factors that may all play a role.

Exposure to violence in the media may have some effect on violent behavior. Early viewing of violent TV programs has been linked to later aggression, including violent crimes, spousal abuse, and child abuse. Sensationalized news reports that exaggerate or romanticize danger also can desensitize youngsters to the loss and horror violence cause—and can inspire "copycats," who imitate kids who receive intense attention after committing a crime.

Adding to this volatile mix are drugs and weapons. In numerous analyses, school violence has been linked with tobacco, alcohol, and marijuana use and with the availability of illegal drugs on school property. In one study of teen mass murders, the majority used a variety of legal and illegal drugs as well as alcohol.

Both fights and revenge fantasies are more likely to become deadly when guns are readily available. Firearms are the most commonly used weapons in mass murders by teens. In some cases, school shooters took guns from a parent's or relative's home. Some became fascinated with firearms at early ages.

Some school districts and national advocacy groups are offering violence prevention programs to children as young as age 4, using techniques such as taking turns and dealing with angry feelings.

Teen Violence

Today's adolescents, according to federal statistics, seem the least violent generation in decades. Fewer teens are being arrested for murder, robbery, and rape. America's schools are reporting fewer serious crimes, both violent and nonviolent.

Yet the reality behind the numbers is complex. Teen violence—though less prevalent than during the 1980s—remains "an ongoing, startlingly pervasive problem," according to the Office of the Surgeon General. Homicide is the second leading cause of death (after accidents) for young people between the ages of 15 and 20. Murder rates for young people in the United States remain the highest in the world—10 times higher than in Canada, 15 times higher than in Australia, 28 times higher than in France or Germany. American teenagers are more likely to die of gunshot wounds than of all natural causes combined.

Experts offer a host of explanations for the high rates of violence in American adolescents: the breakdown of families, violence-saturated media, easy access to guns, bullying and harassment in schools, undiagnosed mental disorders, abuse of alcohol and drugs. Teenagers involved in violent crime weren't necessarily victimized as children. They often show no early signs of aggressive behavior, and they aren't more likely to belong to any one racial or ethnic group.[41]

 ## Hate Crimes

Recent years have seen the emergence of violent crimes motivated by hatred of a particular person's (or group of persons') race, religion, sexual orientation, or political values. These hate crimes have included the dragging death of a young African-American man, the beating death of a young gay man, the shooting of children and teachers at a Jewish community center, and the vandalizing of Muslim-owned businesses after the terrorist attacks of September 11, 2001. Politicians and government leaders have called for an expansion of hate-crime laws that would inflict especially severe sentences on those who commit violence on the basis of racism, sexism, homophobia, anti-Semitism, or other forms of prejudice.

 ## Crime on Campus

Once considered havens from the meanness of America's streets, colleges and universities have seen a dramatic rise in crime in recent years. However, crime rates in these institutions are lower than in

A peaceful scene like this doesn't mean there is no crime on a campus. Do you know the crime statistics for your college?

the general community. Property crimes, such as burglary and theft, account for most crimes in campus. However, the rates of murder and of hate crimes have risen in recent years.[42] According to the U.S. Department of Education, the criminal homicide rate on campus is 0.07 per 100,000 students—compared with a criminal homicide rate of 5.7 per 100,000 persons overall in the United States and of 14.1 per 100,000 for young people ages 17 to 29.[43]

Colleges must compile annual security reports with statistics on violent crime, as well as drug and alcohol violations.[44] The most recent crime statistics for the nation's 6,269 colleges, universities, and career schools are posted on the Internet at http://ope.ed.gov/security. Under the Federal Student Right to Know and Campus Security Act, all colleges and universities receiving federal funds must publish and make readily available the number of campus killings, assaults, sexual assaults, robberies, burglaries, and other crimes, and their security policies.[45] (See Self-Survey:"How Safe Is Your School?")

In a random sample of more than 10,000 undergraduates at four-year schools, 4.3 percent of the students reported that they have a working firearm at college; 1.6 percent had been threatened with a gun. The students most likely to own or to be threatened with a gun are male, live off campus, binge drink, and engage in other risky behavior after drinking.[46]

Because of concerns about safety on campus, more schools are taking tougher stands on student behavior. Many have established codes of conduct barring the use of alcohol and drugs, fighting, and sexual harassment. Many also have instituted policies requiring suspension or expulsion for students who violate this code.

According to new guidance from the federal government, victims of violent crime on college campuses no longer have to worry about a student privacy law if they publicly share the final results of disciplinary action taken against their assailants. Responding to concerns raised by Security On Campus, Inc., a national nonprofit victim assistance organization, the U.S. Department of Education clarified regulations that some schools have used to justify policies keeping victims from talking about their cases, often subjecting the victim to disciplinary action themselves if they talk.[47]

As a preventive measure, many campuses have set up public safety programs, which include late-night shuttle buses and escorts, student bicycle patrols, outdoor emergency phones, and increased numbers of police and security guards. Sexual-assault services provide counseling, crisis intervention, and educational programs. Students are urged to walk in groups, lock their doors and windows, and limit alcohol consumption. Freshman orientation often includes mandatory sessions on campus safety and sexual assault.

Family Violence

Violence doesn't stop at the front door of America's homes. According to the Federal Bureau of Investigation, the most common and least-reported violent crime is an attack in which the victim and the perpetrator knew each other at the time of or before the incident. One-third of all murders occur within families. Physical violence may occur in 20 to 30 percent of all American households. As with other forms of violent crime, there has been a decline in assaults and murders by intimates.

Partner Abuse

During their lifetime, at least one of every five women will be assaulted by a partner or ex-partner. Domestic violence is the single most common cause of injury to women— more common than car accidents, muggings, and rapes combined—and accounts for 42 percent of female murders.

Battered women (who outnumber battered men ten to one) are victims of severe, deliberate, and repeated physical assaults, often accompanied by psychological abuse and threats on their lives. A significant proportion of women who visit emergency departments seek help for symptoms related to ongoing abuse, yet only 5 percent are identified as victims of domestic violence by the physicians who treat them.

The primary factors contributing to physical abuse are the degree of frustration and stress a man is under, his use of alcohol (involved in up to 60 percent of battering cases), and whether he was raised in an abusive home. Only one in twenty men who beat their partners is violent outside the home; nine in ten refuse to admit that

Self Survey   **How Safe Is Your School?**

DORMITORY SECURITY

YES   NO   STUDENTS:

____ ____ Card swipe (like hotels)
____ ____ Patented keys
____ ____ Standard keys
____ ____ Propped doors
____ ____ Doors locked at night
____ ____ Doors never locked
____ ____ Doors always locked
____ ____ Guards on duty (24 hrs.)

VISITORS:

____ ____ Intercom at entrance
____ ____ Show ID
____ ____ Sign-in guests

DORM FEATURES:

____ ____ Single sex dorms
____ ____ Freshman dorms
____ ____ Coed dorms
____ ____ Senior dorms
____ ____ Alcohol prohibited
____ ____ Drugs prohibited
____ ____ Substance-free
____ ____ Propped door alarms
____ ____ Fire sprinklers
____ ____ Peep hole in room door
____ ____ Dead bolt in room door
____ ____ Safety chain on room door
____ ____ Toilet in room
____ ____ Shower in room
____ ____ Bathrooms down hallway
____ ____ Single sex bathrooms
____ ____ Female hall bathrooms locked
____ ____ Single sex floors locked
____ ____ Secure windows (1st & 2nd floors)
____ ____ Panic alarms in rooms

SECURITY PATROLS IN DORMS:

____ ____ By police nightly
____ ____ By security nightly
____ ____ By students (unreliable)
____ ____ By no one

**ROOMMATES QUICKLY
TRANSFERRED BY DEAN FOR:**

____ ____ Using illegal drugs
____ ____ Having sex
____ ____ Underage drinking
____ ____ Throwing up after drinking
____ ____ Noisy parties
____ ____ Hate speech
____ ____ Physical abuse
____ ____ You have to move out instead!!

CAMPUS SECURITY

YES   NO   CAMPUS SECURITY FORCE:

____ ____ Sworn police
____ ____ Arrest power
____ ____ Patrolling day
____ ____ Patrolling night
____ ____ Carry fire arms
____ ____ Security guards
____ ____ Bicycle patrols
____ ____ Surveillance cameras
____ ____ Emergency phones
____ ____ Student amateurs
____ ____ Escort services
____ ____ Shuttle services

HEALTH SERVICES:

____ ____ Rape crisis center
____ ____ Alcohol – drug counselors
____ ____ AA meetings on campus

PARENTAL INVOLVEMENT

PARENTAL NOTIFICATION:

____ ____ For underage drinkers
____ ____ For alcohol poisoning
____ ____ For illegal drug use
____ ____ For acts of violence
____ ____ For public drunkenness
____ ____ For housing fire arms
____ ____ For sexual assault
____ ____ For hate crimes or speech
____ ____ For academic probation
____ ____ For disciplinary probation
____ ____ For residence hall violations
____ ____ For DUI convictions

CAMPUS JUDICIAL SYSTEM:

____ ____ Open campus judicial hearings
____ ____ Reveal names of campus sex offenders

Get campus crime statistics for the last 3 years from admissions office:

CRIMINAL OFFENSES

Murder ____
Forcible sex offenses ____
Nonforcible sex offenses ____
Robbery ____
Aggravated assault ____
Burglary ____
Arson ____
Motor vehicle theft ____
Hate crimes ____
Total criminal offenses ____
Per student crime ratio ____

(continued)

Self Survey | How Safe Is Your School? (continued)

CAMPUS ARRESTS

Liquor law violations ____

Drug law violations ____

Weapons violations ____

TOTAL CAMPUS ARRESTS ____

Calculate campus crimes per thousand students and compare them with other schools. Also, attempt a balanced evaluation by combining your subjective impressions with any calculations.

Source: Security on Campus, Inc. www.securityoncampus.org

Your Health Change Plan

for Personal Safety on Campus

FUNDAMENTALS

- Freshmen should "respectfully decline" to have photo and personal information published for distribution to the campus community. Fraternities and upperclassmen have abused this type of publication to "target" naive freshmen.
- Study the campus and neighborhood with respect to routes between your residence and class/activities schedule. Know where emergency phones are located.
- Share your class/activities schedule with parents and a network of close friends, effectively creating a type of "buddy" system. Give network telephone numbers to your parents, advisors, and friends.
- Always travel in groups. Use a shuttle service after dark. Never walk alone at night. Avoid shortcuts.
- Survey the campus, academic buildings, residence halls, and other facilities while classes are in session and after dark to see that buildings, walkways, quadrangles, and parking lots are adequately secured, lit, and patrolled. Are emergency phones, escorts, and shuttle services adequate?
- To gauge the social scene, drive down fraternity row on weekend nights and stroll through the student hangouts. Are people behaving responsibly, or does the situation seem reckless and potentially dangerous? Remember, alcohol and/or drug abuse is involved in about 90 percent of campus crime. Carefully evaluate off-campus student apartment complexes and fraternity houses if you plan to live off-campus.

RESIDENCE

- Doors and windows to your residence hall should be equipped with quality locking mechanisms. Room doors should be equipped with peep holes and deadbolts.

Always lock them when you are absent. Do not loan out your key. Rekey locks when a key is lost or stolen.

- Card access systems are far superior to standard metal key and lock systems. Card access enables immediate lock changes when keys are lost, stolen, or when housing arrangements change. Most hotels and hospitals have changed to card access systems for safety reasons. Higher education institutions need to adopt similar safety features.
- Always lock your doors and 1st and 2nd floor windows at night. Never compromise your safety for a roommate who asks you to leave the door unlocked.
- Dormitories should have a central entrance/exit lobby where nighttime access is monitored, as well as an outside telephone which visitors must use to gain access.
- Dormitory residents should insist that residential assistants and security patrols routinely check for propped doors— day and night.
- Do not leave your identification, wallets, checkbooks, jewelry, cameras, and other valuables in open view.
- Program your phone's speed dial memory with emergency numbers that include family and friends.
- Know your neighbors and don't be reluctant to report illegal activities and suspicious loitering.

OFF-CAMPUS RESIDENTS

Off-campus residents should contact their student legal aid representative to draft leases that stipulate minimum standards of security and responsibility. Students and parents should also consult any "Neighborhood Watch" association active in the community or the municipal police regarding local crime rates.

Source: Reprinted with permission by Security on Campus, Inc. www.securityoncampus.org. Security on Campus assists victims of campus crime.

---

they have a problem. In homes where a wife is beaten, children also may be abused. The primary risk factors for domestic murder are poverty and household crowding; the lower a family's socioeconomic status—regardless of its racial or ethnic background—the greater the risk of deadly violence.

Abused wives and children are often trapped in terror. Wives may stay with abusive husbands because of love, financial dependence, shame, guilt, fear of being pursued, harmed, or killed if they leave, or a sense of responsibility to their children.[48] The incidence of alcoholism, substance abuse, depression, and suicide attempts is higher in battered women than others.

Emotional violence causes a variety of physical problems, including chronic neck and back pain, migraine, high blood pressure, and ulcers.[49] In one study of more than 1,000 women, those who'd experienced only emotional battering were 70 percent more likely than the average woman to have poor physical as well as mental health.[50]

Social support can help women recover and move on with their lives.[51]

⬛ Sexual Victimization and Violence

Sexual victimization refers to any situation in which a person is deprived of free choice and forced to comply with sexual acts. This is not only a woman's issue; in fact, men are also victimized. In recent years, researchers have come to view acts of sexual victimization along a continuum, ranging from street hassling, stalking, and obscene telephone calls to rape, battering, and incest.

⬛ What Is Sexual Harassment?

All forms of sexual harassment or unwanted sexual attention—from the display of pornographic photos to the use of sexual obscenities to a demand for sex by anyone in a position of power or authority—are illegal.

Sexual Harassment on the Job

As defined by the Equal Employment Opportunity Commission, sexual harassment takes two basic forms: in **quid pro quo** harassment, a person in power or authority makes unwanted sexual advances as a condition for receiving a job, a promotion, or another type of favor; in harassment by means of a **hostile or offensive environment,** supervisors or coworkers engage in persistent inappropriate behaviors that make the workplace hostile, abusive, or otherwise unbearable.

"There's a spectrum of verbal, nonverbal and physical acts, ranging from making off-color remarks to grabbing someone's breast or buttocks," says consultant Susan L. Webb of Seattle, author of *Step Forward: Sexual Harassment in the Workplace.* "But sexual harassment always involves behavior that is related to or based on sex, that is deliberate or repeated, and that is not welcome, not asked for, and not returned."[52] Sexual comments, propositions, dirty jokes, suggestive looks or remarks, displays of pinups or pornography, "accidental" touches, pats, squeezes, pinches, fondling, and ogling are all potentially offensive.

"There isn't always a clear line," says Webb. "Each sexual harassment case has to be considered in its own context." The standard the courts use is whether a reasonable person would consider the behavior or environment abusive or hostile. Since most targets of sexual harassment are women, that usually translates into what a reasonable *woman* would think—which may be quite different from a man's view.

Sexual harassment can affect employees in many ways—financially, psychologically, even physically. If they are fired because they refuse to endure sexual harassment, they may jeopardize their own and their family's economic security. Common psychological effects include crying spells, loss of self-esteem, anger, humiliation, shame, alienation, helplessness, and degradation. Many victims also suffer physical symptoms that stem directly from pressures associated with sexual harassment, including headache, stomach ailments, decreased appetite, weight loss, back and neck pain, decreased sleep, and other stress-related problems.[53]

Workers who feel victimized by sexual harassment should document their complaints by writing down specific incidents (including dates, times, places, and what happened). It sometimes helps initially to confront the harasser, either in person or by writing a note, and state that you're not interested in his or her attention. Many companies have established grievance procedures for handling sexual harassment complaints. The courts have awarded substantial payments of both punitive and compensatory damage to victims of physical and verbal harassment and have held companies liable for failing to halt offensive actions.

Sexual harassment has taken a new turn in the 21st century: "e-harassment," the use of electronic mail and the Internet. An increasing number of compliants brought against employers are based on inappropriate e-mail or viewing of sexual material on the Internet while at work. Most employers have adopted policies stating that employees who use company property, including e-mail, for personal use in violation of company policy are subject to discipline.[54]

Sexual Harassment on Campus

As many as 30 to almost 50 percent of female undergraduates and 12 to 18 percent of male undergraduates have experienced some form of sexual harassment.[55] Professors or supervisors may pressure students into sexual involvement for the sake of a grade, recommendation, or special opportunity. If a student tries to end a sexual relationship, the professor or supervisor may threaten reprisals. Most harassment comes from male faculty members, but both men and women report having been harassed by either male or female faculty. In a University of Washington study, college men were almost as likely as women to report unwanted sexual contact and coercion.

Sexual harassment can undermine students' well-being and academic performance. Its effects include diminished ambition and self-confidence, reduced ability to concentrate, sleeplessness, depression, physical aches, and numerous other ailments. Some students avoid classes or other contact with certain faculty members because of the risk of sexual advances. However, few victims of sexual harassment file official grievances.

Sexual harassment can take many forms, ranging from suggestive comments to physical touching, and can occur in classrooms as well as offices and other workplaces.

Because college administrations can be held legally responsible for allowing a hostile or offensive sexual environment, many schools have set up committees to handle student complaints and to take action against faculty members. Universities also are discouraging and, in some cases, restricting consensual relationships between teachers and students, especially any dating of students by their academic professors or advisers. Although such relationships may seem consensual, in reality they may not be because of the power faculty members have to determine students' grades and futures. In some cases, students have sued their universities for failing to protect them from professors who pressured them into sexual liaisons.

If you encounter sexual harassment as a student, report it to the department chair or dean. If you don't receive an adequate response to your complaint, talk with the campus representatives who handle matters involving affirmative action or civil rights. Federal guidelines prevent any discrimination against you in terms of grades or the loss of a job or scholarship if you report harassment. Schools that do not take measures to remedy harassment could lose federal funds.

Sexual harassment is not always directed at students. Recent research has documented that students of both sexes admit to harassing faculty members. In one survey, a third of undergraduates reported harassing a professor with uninvited gender-based remarks and, more rarely, unwanted sexual attention. Over two-thirds of professors reported having been targets of sexual harassment during their careers.[56] (See Fact or Fiction? "Students are always victims . . .")

Researchers theorize that "contrapower" harassment on college campuses may stem from gender-stereotyped notions of male dominance. Although a female faculty member has more organizational power than a male student, she lacks power in terms of her status as female. This may explain why male students are far more likely than female students to engage in behaviors that could be perceived as sexually harassing. Women, whether students or faculty, perceive sexually harassing behaviors as more threatening, inappropriate, and bothersome than men do.

Sexual Victimization on Campus

As the nation has become more aware of issues such as sexual harassment and coercion, there has been growing recognition that college campuses are not ivory towers isolated from these dangers. Federal legislation now requires colleges and universities to report crimes of all sorts, including sexual victimization.

A national survey found that the most common forms of sexual victimization on campus involved sexual or sexist remarks, catcalls, and whistles. One in five women reported obscene phone calls or being asked intrusive questions about her sex or romantic life. One in ten had false rumors spread about her sex life. About 6 percent confronted

FACT OR FICTION?????????????

Students are always victims, not perpetrators, of campus sexual harassment.

Fiction: In a survey of 158 college students, almost one-third reported having sexually harassed a professor at least once. Male students were much more likely than female students to harass a faculty member. The students were equally likely to harass professors of the same or opposite sex. In a separate survey of 209 professors, more than half said they had encountered sexual harassment—in language, behavior, unwanted sexual attention or sexual coercion—by students at least once. Male professors reported unwanted sexual attention from students of both sexes more often than did female professors.

Source: Eros DeSouza and A. Gigi Fansler. "Contrapower Sexual Harassment: A Survey of Students and Faculty Members." *Sex Roles: A Journal of Research,* June 2003, p. 529.

Model mugging courses train women to actively resist assault and rape.

pornographic pictures, while 5 percent encountered a man exposing his sexual organs.[57]

Sexual Violence on Campus

Over the course of five years (the national average for a college career), including summers and vacations, one of every four or five female students is raped. In a single academic year, 2.7 percent of coeds are raped—35 rapes for every 1,000 women. According to the Department of Justice, a campus with 6000 coeds averages one rape a day every day for the entire school year.[58] College women are twice as likely to be stalked as women in the general population; as many as one woman in eight is stalked each year.[59]

In nine surveys of male university students, between 3 and 6 percent had been raped by other men; up to 25 percent had been sexually assaulted. Like female rape victims, male victims suffer long term psychological problems, physical injuries, and are at risk of contracting a sexually transmitted infection.[60]

☒ Sexual Coercion and Rape

At a bar on a weekend night, a group of intoxicated young men grab a woman and squeeze her breasts as she struggles to get free. At a party, a man offers his date drugs and alcohol in the hope of lowering her resistance to sex. Although some people don't realize it, such actions are forms of sexual coercion (forced sexual activity), which is very common on and off college campuses. In fact, about one in five college women report being forced to have sexual intercourse.

Sexual coercion can take many forms, including exerting peer pressure, taking advantage of one's desire for

popularity, threatening an end to a relationship, getting someone intoxicated, stimulating a partner against his or her wishes, or insinuating an obligation based on the time or money one has expended. Men may feel that they need to live up to the sexual stereotype of taking advantage of every opportunity for sex. Women are far more likely than men to encounter physical force.

Rape refers to sexual intercourse with an unconsenting partner under actual or threatened force. Sexual intercourse between a male over the age of 16 and a female under the age of consent (which ranges from 12 to 21 in different states) is called *statutory rape.* In *acquaintance rape,* or *date rape,* discussed in depth later in this chapter, the victim knows the rapist. In *stranger rape,* the rapist is an unknown assailant. Both stranger and acquaintance rapes are serious crimes that can have a devastating impact on their victims.

According to the National Violence Against Women survey, more than half of all women in the United States report an attempted or completed rape and/or physical assault. One in six women, compared with one in 33 men, has experienced an attempted or completed rape in the course of a lifetime.[61] In the previous 12 months, according to the survey, 0.3 percent of the women and 0.1 percent of the men had been raped. These findings indicate that some 302,091 women and 92,748 men are forcibly raped in the United States every year.

The motives of rapists vary. Those who attack strangers often have problems establishing intimate relationships, have poor self-esteem, feel inadequate, and may have been sexually abused as children. Some rapists report a long history of fantasizing about rape and violence, generally while masturbating. Others commit rape out of anger that they can't express toward a wife or girlfriend. The more sexually aggressive men have been, the more likely they are to see such aggression and violence as normal and to believe rape myths, such as that it's impossible to rape a woman who doesn't really want sex. Sexually violent and degrading photographs, films, books, magazines, and videos may contribute to some rapists' assaultive behaviors. Hard-core pornography depicting violent rape has been strongly associated with judging oneself capable of sexual coercion and aggression, and with engaging in such acts.

Alcohol and drugs also play a major role. About 25 percent of both men and women report unwanted sexual experiences as a result of alcohol use. Many rapists drink prior to an assault, and alcohol may interfere with a victim's ability to avoid danger or resist attack.

For many years, the victims of rape were blamed for doing something to bring on the attack. Researchers have since shown that women are raped because they encounter sexually aggressive men, not because they look or act a certain way. Although no woman is immune to attack, many rape victims are children or adolescents. Women who were sexually abused or raped as children are at greater risk than others. Scientists are exploring the reasons for this greater vulnerability.

Women who successfully escape rape attempts do so by resisting verbally and physically, usually by yelling and fleeing. Women who use forceful verbal or physical resistance (screaming, hitting, kicking, biting, and running) are more likely to avoid rape than women who try pleading, crying, or offering no resistance.

Types of Rape

Although rape has long been viewed as an act of violence and domination, recent studies indicate that not all rapes fit into a single pattern. Within the broad category of rape are specific, but not mutually exclusive, subcategories of the crime, including anger rape, power rape, sadistic rape, gang rape, and sexual gratification rape.

Anger rape, usually on a total stranger, is motivated by hatred and a desire for revenge for the rejection the rapist feels he's suffered from women. Anger rapists often harbor long-standing hostility toward women, use far more physical violence than is needed for submission, and usually don't find the rape sexually gratifying.

Power rape is a generally premeditated attack motivated by a desire to dominate and control another person. Power rapists, unable to deal with stress and their sense of failure, may rape to regain a sense of power. They use only as much force as needed to make their victims submit and may find the rape sexually gratifying, even though that's not their primary motive.

Sadistic rape is a premeditated assault that often involves bondage, torture, or sexual abuse. Sadistic rapists find power and anger sexually arousing and may subject victims to rituals of humiliation or torture. They're often preoccupied with violent pornography; their motives are more complex and difficult to understand than those of other types of rapists.

Gang rape involves three or more rapists. Men in close groups that drink and party together—such as fraternities or athletic teams—are more likely to participate in such assaults. The reasons may go beyond aggression and sexual gratification to the excitement and camaraderie the men feel while sharing the experience.

Sexual gratification rape is usually an impulsive attack by someone willing to use physical coercion for the sake of sex. These rapists generally use no more force than needed to get a partner to submit and may stop the attack if it becomes clear they'll have to use extreme violence to overcome resistance. Many acquaintance rapes fit into this category.

Certain myths can contribute to rape and reactions to it. One is the myth of female precipitation, which blames the victim, often for dressing or behaving provocatively. Others are the myths of male pathology, which views the rapist as mentally ill, and of male's supposedly uncontrollable sexuality. In research with college students, women were more likely to see male hostility and dominance in society as causes of rape while men believed more strongly in female provocation.

Acquaintance or Date Rape

Most rapes are committed by someone who is known to the victim. Both women and men report having been forced into sexual activity by someone they know. Many college students are in the age group most likely to face this threat: women aged 16 to 25 and men under 25. Women are most vulnerable and men are most likely to commit assaults during their senior year of high school and their first year of college.

Women who describe incidents of sexual coercion that meet the legal definition of rape often don't label it as such. They may have a preconceived notion that true rape consists of a blitzlike attack by a stranger. Or they may blame themselves for getting into a situation in which they couldn't escape. They may feel some genuine concern for others who would be devastated if they knew the truth (for example, if the rapist were the brother of a good friend or the son of a neighbor).

 According to various studies, 25 to 60 percent of college men have engaged in some form of sexual coercion. Most often these men simply ignored a woman when she said no or protested. In addition, many college men reported engaging in sexual activity against their own wishes, most often because of male peer pressure or a desire to be popular.

The same factors that lead to other forms of sexual victimization can set the stage for date rape. Socialization into an aggressive role, acceptance of rape myths, and a view that force is justified in certain situations increase the likelihood of a man's committing date rape. Other factors can also play a role, including the following:

:: ***Personality and early sexual experiences.*** Certain factors may predispose individuals to sexual aggression, including first sexual experience at a very young age, earlier and more frequent than usual childhood sexual experiences (both forced and voluntary), hostility toward women, irresponsibility, lack of social consciousness, and a need for dominance over sexual partners.

:: ***Situational variables (what happens during the date).*** Men who initiate a date, pay all expenses, and provide transportation are more likely to be sexually aggressive, perhaps because they feel they can call all the shots.

:: ***Acceptance of sexual coercion.*** Some social groups, such as fraternities and athletic teams, may encourage the use of alcohol; reinforce stereotypes about masculinity; and emphasize violence, force, and competition. The group's shared values, including an acceptance of sexual coercion, may keep individuals from questioning their behavior.

Acquaintance rape and alcohol use are very closely linked. Both men and women may find their judgment impaired or their communications unclear as a result of drinking.

© 2000 PhotoDisc, Inc.

:: **Drinking.** Alcohol use is one of the strongest predictors of acquaintance rape. Men who've been drinking may not react to subtle signals, may misinterpret a woman's behavior as a come-on, and may feel more sexually aroused. At the same time, drinking may impair a woman's ability to effectively communicate her wishes and to cope with a man's aggressiveness.

:: **Date rape drugs.** Drugs such as Rohypnol (roofie, La Rocha, rope, Mexican Valium, Rib Roche, R-2), a tranquilizer used overseas, and gamma hydroxybutrate (GHB), a depressant with potential benefits for people with narcolepsy, have been implicated in cases of acquaintance or date rape. Since both are odorless and tasteless, victims have no way of knowing whether their drink has been tampered with. The subsequent loss of memory leaves victims with no explanation for where they've been or what's happened.

Rohypnol—which can cause impaired motor skills and judgment, lack of inhibitions, dizziness, confusion, lethargy, very low blood pressure, coma, and death— has been outlawed in this country. Deaths also have been attributed to GHB overdoses.

:: **Gender differences in interpreting sexual cues.** In research comparing college men and women, the men typically overestimated the woman's sexual availability and interest, seeing friendliness, revealing clothing, and attractiveness as deliberately seductive. In one study of date rape, the men reported feeling "led on," in part

because their female partners seemed to be dressed more suggestively than usual.

How Can I Prevent Date Rape?

For men:

:: Remember that it's okay not to "score" on a date.

:: Don't assume that a sexy dress or casual flirting is an invitation to sex.

:: Be aware of your partner's actions. If she pulls away or tries to get up, understand that she's sending you a message—one you should acknowledge and respect.

:: Restrict drinking, drug use, or other behaviors (such as hanging out with a group known to be sexually aggressive in certain situations) that could affect your judgment and ability to act responsibly.

:: Think of the way you'd want your sister or a close woman friend to be treated by her date. Behave in the same manner.

For women:

:: If the man pays for all expenses, he may think he's justified in using force to get "what he paid for." If you cover some of the costs, he may be less aggressive.

:: Back away from a man who pressures you into other activities you don't want to engage in on a date, such as chugging beer or drag racing with his friends.

:: Avoid misleading messages and avoid behavior that may be interpreted as sexual teasing. Don't tell him to stop touching you, talk for a few minutes, and then resume petting.

:: Despite your clearly stated intentions, if your date behaves in a sexually coercive manner, use a strategy of escalating forcefulness—direct refusal, vehement verbal refusal, and, if necessary, physical force.

:: Avoid using alcohol or other drugs when you definitely do not wish to be sexually intimate with your date.

For additional advice, see the no-nonsense Dating Guide in Figure 18-2.

Male Nonconsensual Sex and Rape

In one recent study of 247 young heterosexual men (mean age 18 years), one in four reported at least once incident of nonconsensual sex (kissing/petting, sexual intercourse, or oral sex) with a woman or attempts by women to make them engage in nonconsensual sexual activity. In another study of 153 heterosexual men (mean age of 22 years), 30 percent reported nonconsensual sexual interactions and

Women

Beware of possible implied obligations for sex if a man appears interested in you, and offers to buy you a drink.

At parties, mix your own drinks. At bars, watch when a bartender makes your drink. Use alcohol responsibly. 80 to 90 percent of acquaintance rapes involve alcohol and/or drugs. You are more at risk.

Know that sex is not a male entitlement. **You can say "no" at any time.**

Beware of men who are hostile if you say no, who threaten, bully, or try to control you, try to make you feel guilty, accuse you of being uptight, put you down, or talk negatively about women.

If you feel preasured, afraid, or uncomfortable, leave, get help, or protest loudly.

Be clear about your desires, limits, and expectations. Ask and tell.

Don't listen to persuasion. You don't have to give reasons. Be assertive. State clearly what you want and do not want. Do not be afraid to set limits.

Consent to some sexual activity (kissing, touching, ect.) does NOT imply consent to all kinds of sexual activity.

Many women are in denial about what rape is. Get clear.

Threats, force, and coercion make it rape.

Getting drunk does not make rape OK. If you are too drunk to say no, it's rape, automatically.

Men

Be interested in women because you are truly interested, not as a means to getting sex.

Do not use alcohol as a means to increase the likelihood of sex. Make sure that non-alcoholic beverages are available. If you see a women in trouble at a party, don't be afraid to intervene.

Know that sex is not a male entitlement. **It's safer and better to ask.**

Never force, pressure, or coerce anyone to have sex. Don't take silence as consent. Don't make or laugh at degrading jokes about women. Challenge abusive behavior when you witness it.

If you see a women in trouble at a party, don't be afraid to intervene.

Be clear about your desires, limits, and expectations. Ask. Tell. No secret agenda. No LIES!

 Don't try to persuade or argue. Respect her "No" whether it is verbal or physical. Stop.

Consent to some sexual activity (kissing, touching, etc.) does NOT imply consent to all kinds of sexual activity.

Many men are in denial about what rape is. Get clear.

Threats, force, and coercion make it rape.

Don't have sex with someone who is too drunk to make responsible decisions, has passed out, or is asleep. Legally, It's rape.

Figure 18-2 DATING GUIDE TO RAPE-FREE SEX

Source: http://webits3.appstate.edu/apples/life/Rape/dating_guide.htm

23.5 percent attempts at making them engage in nonconsensual sex. In both samples, women exploited the man's inability to offer resistance. Kissing/petting was the most frequently reported unwanted sexual activity, followed by sexual intercourse and oral sex. Men were more likely to engage in nonconsensual sex with an (ex-) partner or friend than with an unknown woman. They described the experiences as moderately upsetting.[62]

No one knows how common male rape is because men are less likely to report such assaults than women. In a recent survey in England, nearly 3 percent of men reported nonconsensual sexual experiences as adults. Other researchers estimate that the victims in about 10 percent of acquaintance rape cases are men. These hidden victims often keep silent because of embarrassment, shame, or humiliation, as well as their own feelings and fears about homosexuality and conforming to conventional sex roles.

Although many people think men who rape other men are always homosexuals, most male rapists consider themselves to be heterosexual. Young boys aren't the only victims. The average age of male rape victims is 24. Rape is a serious problem in prison, where men may experience brutal assaults by men who usually resume sexual relations with women once they're released.

Impact of Rape

Rape-related injuries include unexplained vaginal discharge, bleeding, infections, multiple bruises, and fractured ribs. Victims of sexual violence often develop chronic symptoms, such as headaches, backaches, high blood pressure, sleep disorders, pelvic pain, and sexual fertility problems. But sexual violence has both a physical and a psychological impact. The psychological scars of a sexual assault take a long time to heal. Therapists have linked sexual victimization with hopelessness, low self-esteem, high levels of self-criticism, and self-defeating relationships. An estimated 30 to 50 percent of women develop posttraumatic stress disorder following a rape. Many do not seek counseling until a year or more after an attack, when their symptoms have become chronic or intensified.[63]

Acquaintance rape may cause fewer physical injuries but greater psychological torment. Often too ashamed to tell anyone what happened, victims may suffer alone, without skilled therapists or sympathetic friends to reassure them. Women raped by acquaintances blame themselves more, see themselves less positively, question their judgment, have greater difficulty trusting others, and have higher levels of psychological distress. Nightmares, anxiety, and flashbacks are common. The women may avoid others, become less capable of protecting themselves, and continue to be haunted by sexual violence for years. A therapist can help these victims begin the slow process of healing.

Counseling from a trained professional can help ease the trauma suffered by a rape victim.

What to Do in Case of Rape

If a woman has been raped, she will have to decide whether to report the attack to the police. Even an unsuccessful rape attempt should be reported because the information a woman may provide about the attack—the assaulter's physical characteristics, voice, clothes, car, even an unusual smell—may prevent another woman from being raped.

Only a small percentage of college women who are raped report their assault to police; many don't even tell a close friend or relative about the assault. Women who are raped should call a friend or a rape crisis center. A rape victim should not bathe or change her clothes before calling the police. Semen, hair, and material under her fingernails or on her apparel all may be useful in identifying the man who raped her.

A rape victim who chooses to go to a doctor or hospital should remember that she may not necessarily have to talk to police. However, a doctor can collect the necessary evidence, which will then be available if she later decides to report the rape to police. All rape victims should talk with a doctor or health-care worker about testing and treatment for sexually transmitted infections and postintercourse conception.

Many rape victims find it very helpful to contact a rape crisis center, where qualified staff members assist in dealing with the trauma. They can also put victims in touch with other survivors of rape and support groups. Many colleges, universities, and large urban communities in the United States have such programs. Friends and family members should remember that many women mistakenly blame themselves for the rape. However, the victim hasn't committed a crime—the man who raped her has.

STRATEGIES FOR PREVENTION

Reducing the Risk of Stranger Rape

Rape prevention consists primarily of making it as difficult as possible for a rapist to make you his victim:

- Don't advertise that you're a woman living alone. Use initials on your mailbox. Install and use secure locks on doors and windows, changing door locks after losing keys or moving into a new residence.

- Don't open your door to strangers. If a repairman or public official is at your door, ask him to identify himself and call his office to verify that he is a reputable person on legitimate business.

- Lock your car when it is parked, and drive with locked car doors. Should your car break down, attach a white cloth to the antenna and lock yourself in. If someone other than a uniformed officer stops to offer help, ask this person to call the police or a garage but do not open your locked car door.

- Avoid dark and deserted areas, and be aware of the surroundings where you're walking. Should a driver ask for directions when you're a pedestrian, avoid approaching his car. Instead, call out your reply from a safe distance.

- Have house or car keys in hand as you approach the door. Check the back seat before getting into your car.

- Carry a device for making a loud noise, like a whistle or, even better, a small pint-sized compressed air horn available in many sporting goods and boat supply stores. Sound the noise alarm at the first sign of danger.

- Take a self-defense class to learn techniques of physical resistance that can injure the attacker or distract him long enough for you to escape.

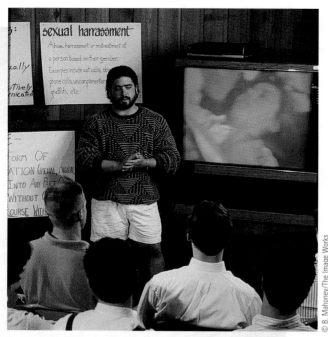

All-male workshops can generate discussions about gender roles and violence, and may also provide positive pressure against rape and other forms of aggression against women.

Halting Sexual Violence

Sexual violence has its roots in social attitudes and beliefs that demean women and condone aggression. According to international research, much sexual violence takes place within families, marriage, and dating relationships. In many settings, rape is a culturally approved strategy to control and discipline women. In these places, laws and policies to improve women's status are critical to ending sexual coercion.[64]

As colleges and universities have become more aware of the different forms of sexual danger, many have taken the lead in setting up primary prevention programs (including newspaper articles; seminars in dormitories, fraternities, and sororities; and lectures) to help students examine their attitudes and values, understand cultural influences, and develop skills for avoiding or escaping from dangerous situations. All men and women should recognize misleading rape myths and develop effective ways of communicating to avoid misinterpretation of sexual cues. Students should also know to whom they can turn to learn more about and seek help for sexual victimization: counselors, campus police, deans of student affairs, fraternity or sorority representatives, and campus ministers.

While most campuses provide self-defense seminars for potential female victims of rape and general campus safety measures, some have tried innovative approaches, such as Men Against Violence, a peer-education program that confronts male students' conceptions of manhood and appropriate gender roles to reduce their likelihood of sexual or physical violence.[65] Such all-male, peer-guided approaches that challenge myths about rape and rape victims also have proven effective with college fraternity men.

In addition, practical institutional steps—such as providing adequate lighting, escort services, and clear policies against both violence and drug and alcohol abuse—can help. Self-defense classes teach women how to avoid becoming victims either by escaping or protecting themselves. Follow-up studies of college women have found that self-defense training increased their sense of control over their life, confidence, security, independence, and physical prowess. (See "Your Health Change Plan.")

Campuses are also providing secondary prevention by getting help to victims of sexual violence as soon as possible through rape-crisis teams and emergency mental-health services, and tertiary prevention by working with victims to ameliorate the long-term effects of their experience through psychotherapy, educational services, and medical care.

The Bottom Line ▼
Helping the Victims
of Violence

As their numbers have grown and their anguish has been recognized, the victims of violence have received greater attention. Hundreds of shelters for battered wives and their children have been set up across the country. They offer physical and psychological treatment, and a haven where women can begin to rebuild their shattered self-esteem, as well as their daily lives. Rape counseling and crisis centers on college campuses and in the community provide various forms of assistance to victims of rape. In many cities, the telephone directory lists hot lines and resources. More than 400 victims' advocacy groups have been set up across the country to advise those hurt by crime. Support organizations help many survivors deal with the emotional aftermath of their experiences. (See "Your Health Almanac" at the back of this book for listings.)

Sometimes well-intentioned friends and relatives add to the stress felt by the victims of violence. Here's how to offer comfort without implying criticism:

:: ***Don't blame the victim.*** Even when no one doubts that the victim is completely innocent, individuals may be plagued by regrets and self-accusation: Why didn't I lock the windows? Why did I park on that dark street? Any second-guessing or implied criticism adds to this burden of blame and shame.

:: ***Don't try to deny that it happened.*** Although it may be hard to talk about—or even listen to—what happened, the reality of the event must not be ignored. Denial makes victims doubt their own experience and question themselves at a time when they crave reassurance.

:: ***Don't pressure the victim to talk***—or not to talk. Some individuals need to go over every detail of what happened, again and again, until they work out their feelings of outrage and become ready to get on with their lives. Others find going into details too humiliating. Let the victim set the tone and limits for disclosure. Don't pry or prod.

:: ***Don't try to rush the victim to leave the past behind and get on with his or her life.*** Recovery from any traumatic event takes time, and only the victim knows the appropriate pace. If, however, months pass without any lessening of symptoms or improvement in day-to-

day functioning, family members and friends shouldn't hesitate to recommend that their loved one see a mental health professional.

 After watching the CNN video segment, discuss the following question. Are courses in conflict management and peace studies a solution to preventing school violence?

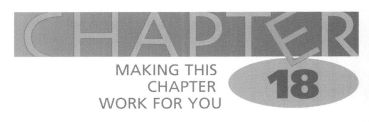

MAKING THIS
CHAPTER
WORK FOR YOU

18

1. You can help keep yourself safe by doing all of the following *except*
   a. using seatbelts when driving or a passenger.
   b. wearing pajamas made of nonflammable materials.
   c. removing or fixing loose carpets.
   d. allowing a spilled liquid to dry on a slippery floor before cleaning it up.

2. Which of the following factors affects an individual's risk of accident or injury?
   a. hunger level
   b. stress level
   c. amount of automobile insurance coverage
   d. knowledge of CPR

3. Safe-driving tips include all of the following *except*
   a. Avoid driving at night for the first year after getting a license.
   b. Make sure your car has snow tires or chains before driving in hazardous snowy conditions.
   c. If riding with an intoxicated driver, keep talking to him so that he doesn't fall asleep at the wheel.
   d. Don't let packages or people obstruct the rear or side windows.

4. Which of the following statements about home safety is true?
   a. Falls pose the greatest threat of injury in the home, followed by poison.
   b. The three ingredients of fire are fuel, a heat source, and oxygen.
   c. The risk of falls is lowest in the elderly.
   d. When using cleaning products, make sure that windows are tightly closed.

5. Which of the following statements about recreational safety hazards is true?
   a. Hypothermia is a life-threatening medical emergency caused by the inability of the body to cool itself.

b. The most common heat-related conditions are heat stroke and heat exhaustion.

c. Most drownings occur at organized facilities.

d. Frostbite usually affects the tissues of the hands and feet.

6. Which of the following statements about violence in the United States is *false*?

a. Almost half the victims of violent crime are under 25 years of age.

b. Risk of violence is highest in people with alcohol or drug misuse or dependence disorders.

c. Gun-related deaths are the leading cause of death in the United States, followed by car accidents.

d. Boys and men are most likely to be the perpetrators of homicide, domestic abuse, and hate-related crimes.

7. Which statement about violence on college campuses is *false*?

a. Property crimes account for most crimes on campus.

b. Crime rates at colleges and universities are higher than in the general community.

c. Students most likely to own a gun are male, live off campus, and binge drink.

d. Crime statistics for colleges and universities are posted on the Internet.

8. Sexual victimization

a. includes sexual harassment, sexual coercion, and rape.

b. is gender-specific, affecting women who are violated emotionally or physically by men.

c. is rare in academic environments such as college campuses.

d. most commonly takes the form of physical assault and stalking.

9. Which of the following statements about rape is true?

a. When a person is sexually attacked by a stranger, it is referred to as *rape*. When a person is sexually attacked by an acquaintance, it is referred to as *sexual coercion*.

b. Statutory rape is defined as sexual intercourse initiated by a woman under the age of consent.

c. Men who rape other men usually consider themselves heterosexuals.

d. Women who flirt and dress provocatively are typically more willing to participate in aggressive sex than women who dress conservatively and do not flirt.

10. Ways to protect or prevent rape include:

a. Use alcohol and drugs only in familiar surroundings.

b. Take a self-defense class.

c. To avoid angering a sexually aggressive person, become passive and quiet.

d. Do not discuss your sexual limits on a first or second date because just talking about sex will encourage your date to think you are interested in a sexual relationship.

Answers to these questions can be found on page 652.

Critical Thinking

1. Can you name two risk factors in your daily life that might increase the likelihood of accidental injury? What actions have you taken to keep yourself safe? Are there other risk factors you could minimize or eliminate? What might you do about them?

2. A friend of yours, Eric, frequently makes crude or derogatory comments about women. When you finally call him on this, his response

Critical Thinking

is, "I didn't say anything wrong. I like women." What might you say to him?

3. At one college, women raped by acquaintances or dates scrawled the names of their assailants on the walls of women's restrooms on campus. Several young men whose names appeared on the list objected, protesting that they were innocent and were being unfairly accused. How do you feel about

Critical Thinking

this method of fighting back against date rape? Do you think it violates the rights of men? How do you feel about naming women who've been raped in news reports? Are there circumstances in which a woman's identity should be revealed? Would fewer women report a rape if not assured of privacy?

Profile Plus

Can your world be a safer place? Discover strategies to lessen the risk of injury with the information found on your Profile Plus CD-ROM.

Profile Plus

• Injury Prevention and Control

Profile Plus

Sites and Bytes

National Safety Council
www.nsc.org

This site provides resources and fact sheets on issues related to public safety, the environment, the community, and the workplace. Topics include auto safety, first aid, air quality, lead poisoning, sun safety, and disaster recovery.

Sites and Bytes

Occupational Safety and Health (OSHA)

www.osha.gov

This U.S. Department of Labor site features a wealth of information on occupational safety and accident prevention, as well as a searchable database. Included is a section on ergonomics.

Sites and Bytes

The Rape Crisis Center
www.rapecrisis.com

This private nonprofit organization provides support to victims of sexual violence and their families, including a 24/7 crisis hotline and several advocacy programs.

InfoTrac College Edition

Activity

Holcomb, Derek R., et al. "A Mixed-Gender Date Rape Prevention Intervention Targeting Freshmen College Athletes." *College Student Journal*, Vol. 36, No. 2, June 2002, p. 165(15).

1. Describe eight factors that may contribute to the complexity concerning the problems of date or

InfoTrac College Edition

acquaintance rape among college athletes?

2. Why are men and women athletes considered to be a "high risk" population requiring special attention regarding the issue of sexual abuse?

3. List four goals of a rape prevention intervention program that targets college athletes.

InfoTrac College Edition

You can find additional readings relating to injury and violence with InfoTrac College Edition, an online library of more than 900 journals and publications. Follow the instructions for accessing InfoTrac that were packaged with your textbook; then search for articles using a keyword search.

For additional links, resources, and suggested readings on InfoTrac College Edition, visit our Health & Wellness Resource Center at **http://health.wadsworth.com**.

Key Terms

The terms listed are on the page indicated. Definitions of the terms are in the Glossary at the end of this book.

Key Terms

computer vision syndrome 610
frostbite 612
frostnip 611
heat cramps 611
heat exhaustion 611

Key Terms

heat stress 611
heat stroke 611
hostile or offensive environment 619
hypothermia 612
quid pro quo 619

Key Terms

rape 621
repetitive motion injury (RMI) 609
sexual coercion 621

References

1. Keeling, Richard. "Risks to Students' Lives: Setting Priorities." *Journal of American College Health*, Vol. 51, No. 2, September 2002, p. 53.
2. Grossman, David. "Adolescent Injury Prevention and Clinicians: Time for Instant Messaging." *Western Journal of Medicine*, Vol. 172, No. 3, March 2000, p. 151.

References

3. National Safety Council. www.nsc.org.
4. "CDC to Launch New Injury Research Agenda." *Medical Letter on the CDC and FDA*, July 21, 2002, p. 9.
5. Villaveces, A. "Association of Alcohol-Related Laws with Deaths Due to Motor Vehicle and Motorcycle Crashes in the United States, 1980–1997." *American Journal of Epidemiology*, Vol. 157, No. 2, January 15, 2003, p. 131.

References

6. National Highway Traffic Safety Administration. www.nhtsa.dot.gov/.
7. Ibid.
8. "Study Shows Economic Impact of U.S. Vehicle Crashes Reaches $230.6 Billion." *Public Roads*, Vol. 66, No. 1, July–August 2002, p. 52.
9. Winston, Flaura Koplin, et al. "Acute Stress Disorder Symptoms in Children

References

and Their Parents after Pediatric Traffic Injury." *Pediatrics,* Vol. 109, No. 6, June 2002, p. 1163.

10. Braver, E. R. "Race, Hispanic Origin, and Socioeconomic Status in Relation to Motor Vehicle Occupant Death Rates and Risk Factors Among Adults." *Accident Analysis and Prevention,* Vol. 35, No. 3, May 2003, p. 295.

11. Paschall, M. J. "College Attendance and Risk-Related Driving Behavior in a National Sample of Young Adults," *Journal of Studies of Alcohol,* Vol. 64, No. 1, January 2003, p. 43.

12. Ferguson, Susan. "Other High-Risk Factors for Young Drivers—How Graduated Licensing Does, Doesn't, or Could Address Them." *Journal of Safety Research,* Vol. 34, No. 1, January 2003, p. 71.

13. Henary, B. Y. "Child and Adult Pedestrian Impact: The Influence of Vehicle Type on Injury Severity." *Annual Proceedings/Association for the Advancement of Automotive Medicine,* Vol. 47, September 2003, p. 105.

14. Kweon, Y. J., and K. M. Kockelman. "Overall Injury Risk to Different Drivers: Combining Exposure, Frequency, and Severity Models." *Accident Analysis and Prevention,* Vol. 35, No. 4, July 2003, p. 441.

15. "Poll Finds Many U.S. Drivers Are Falling Asleep at the Wheel." *AORN (Association of Operating Room Nurses) Journal,* Vol. 77, No. 3, March 2003, p. 654.

16. National Highway Traffic Safety Administration.

17. Mihura, J. L., et al. "Rorschach Measures of Aggressive Drive Derivatives: A College Student Sample." *Journal of Personality Assessment,* Vol. 80, No. 1, February 2003, p. 41.

18. "U.S. Seatbelt Use at 75%." *Injury Prevention,* Vol. 9, No. 1, March 2003, p. 8.

19. "Young Americans Still Shunning Seat Belts." *Health and Medicine Week,* August 25, 2003, p. 638.

20. Stephenson, Joan. "Backseat Seat Belts." *Journal of the American Medical Association,* Vol. 287, No. 6, February 13, 2002, p. 706.

21. Melton, Sherry, et al. "Emphasizing Mechanism of Injury and Therapeutic Management." *The Journal of Trauma: Injury, Infection, and Critical Care,* Vol. 54, No. 4, April 2003, p. 781.

22. Ferguson, Susan. "The Blue Ribbon Panel on Depowered and Advanced Airbags—Status Report on Airbag Performance." *Annual Proceedings/Association for the Advancement of Automotive Medicine,* Vol. 47, September 2003, p. 79.

23. Nerenberg, Arnold. Personal interview.

24. "Cell Phones Distract Drivers, Hands Down." *Science News,* Vol. 163, No. 6, February 8, 2003, p. 94.

25. Ropeik, David, and George Gray. "Cell Phones and Driving: How Risky?" *Consumers' Research Magazine,* Vol. 86, No. 1, January 2003, p. 14.

26. Strayer, David, et al. "Cell Phone Use Can Lead to Inattention Blindness Behind the Wheel." *Injury Insight,* February/March 2003.

27. Coffman S. "Bicycle Injuries and Safety Helmets in Children. Review of Research." *Orthopedic Nursing,* Vol. 22, No. 1, January–February 2003, p. 9.

28. Thompson, Matthew, and Fredrick Rivara. "Bicycle-Related Injuries." *American Family Physician,* Vol. 63, No. 10, May 15, 2001, p. 2007.

29. National Center for Health Statistics (NCHS).

30. Reichard, John. "Report Cites One Million Annual Ergonomics Injuries." *Medicine and Health,* Vol. 55, No. 5, January 29, 2001, p. 3.

31. Fitzgerald, Nancy. "Safety on Campus." *Careers & Colleges,* Vol. 22, No. 18, March 2002, p. 18.

32. Brenner, R. A. "Prevention of Drowning in Infants, Children, and Adolescents." *Pediatrics,* Vol. 112, No. 2, August 2003, p. 440.

33. Chalmers, D., and L. Morrison. "Epidemiology of Non-Submersion Injuries in Aquatic Sporting and Recreational Activities." *Sports Medicine,* Vol. 33, No. 10, 2003, p. 745.

34. Heath, Iona. "Treating Violence As a Public Health Problem: The Approach Has Advantages But Diminishes the Human Rights Perspective." *British Medical Journal,* Vol. 325, No. 7367, October 5, 2002, p. 726.

35. "Violence Report Highlights Ubiquity of PTSD in United States." *Health and Medicine Week,* August 25, 2003, p. 604.

36. "Impact of Violence and Prevention Strategies Discussed at Symposium." *Medical Letter on the CDC and FDA,* July 6, 2003, p. 44.

37. Centers for Disease Control and Prevention (CDC).

38. Purugganan, Ruth, et al. "Exposure to Violence Among Urban School-Aged Children: Is It Only on Television?" *Pediatrics,* Vol. 106, No. 4, October 2000, p. 949.

39. Walsh, Elizabeth, and Thomas Fahy. "Violence in Society: Contribution of Mental Illness Is Low." *British Medical Journal,* Vol. 325, No. 7363, September 7, 2002, p. 507.

40. Tardiff, Kenneth. *"Violence." Textbook of Clinical Psychiatry (4th edition).* Washington, DC; American Psychiatric Publishing, Inc., 2003, p. 1485.

41. Hales, Dianne. "Teen Violence." *Worldbook Annual,* 2002.

42. Fitzgerald. "Safety on Campus."

43. U.S. Department of Education.

44. Dervarics, Charles. "College Groups Battle Safety Advocates over Reform Plan." Community *College Week,* Vol. 13, No. 26, August 6, 2001, p. 3.

45. "Database Will List Campus Crime Figures." *Black Issues in Higher Education,* Vol. 17, No. 11, July 20, 2000.

46. Millder, Matthew, et al. "Guns and Gun Threats at College." *Journal of American College Health,* Vol. 51, No. 2, p. 57.

47. "Campus Crime Victims Can Redisclose Disciplinary Results." U.S. Department Of Education News Release, March 19, 2003.

48. Battaglia, T. A. "Survivors of Intimate Partner Violence Speak Out." *Journal of General Internal Medicine,* Vol. 18, No. 8, August 2003, p. 617.

49. Coggins, M., and L. F. Bullock. "The Wavering Line in the Sand: The Effects of Domestic Violence and Sexual Coercion." *Issues in Mental Health Nursing,* Vol. 24, No. 6–7, September–November 2003, p. 723.

50. "Some Physical Effects of Emotional Violence." *Harvard Mental Health Letter,* Vol. 17, No. 10, April 2001.

51. Coker, A. L. "Social Support Reduces the Impact of Partner Violence on Health: Application of Structural Equation Models." *Preventive Medicine,* Vol. 37, No. 3, September 2003, p. 259.

52. Webb, Susan. Personal interview.

53. Kibeom, Lee, et al. "Personality and the Likelihood to Sexually Harass." *Sex Roles: A Journal of Research,* July 2003, p. 59.

References

54. Towns, Douglas, and Mark Johnson. "Sexual Harassment in the 21st Century: E-Harassment in the Workplace." *Employee Relations Law Journal,* Vol. 29, No. 1, Summer 2003, p. 7.

55. Murnen, Sarah, and Linda Smolak. "The Experience of Sexual Harassment Among Grade-School Students: Early Socialization of Female Subordination?" *Sex Roles: A Journal of Research,* July 2000.

56. DeSouza, Eros, and A. Gigi Fansler. "Contrapower Sexual Harassment: A Survey of Students and Faculty Members." *Sex Roles: A Journal of Research,* June 2003, p. 529.

57. Fisher, Bonnie, et al. *The Sexual Victimization of College Women.* Washington, DC: U.S. Department of Justice, December 2000.

58. Hughes, Patricia, et al. "Self-Defense and Martial Arts Evaluation for College Women: Preliminary Validation of

References

Perceptions of Dangerous Situations Scale." *Research Quarterly for Exercise and Sport,* Vol. 74, No. 2, June 2003, p. 153.

59. Dye, M. L., and K. E. Davis. "Stalking and Psychological Abuse: Common Factors and Relationship-Specific Characteristics." *Violence and Victims,* Vol. 18, No. 2, April 2003, p. 163.

60. Isely, P. J. "Sexual Assault of Men: College Age Victims." *National Association of Student Personnel Administrators Journal,* Vol. 35, No. 4, pp. 305–317. (Reported at webits3.appstate.edu.)

61. Hensley, Laura. "Treatment for Survivors of Rape: Issues and Interventions." *Journal of Mental Health Counseling,* Vol. 24, No. 4, October 2002, p. 330.

62. Krahe, Barbara, et al. "Men's Reports of Nonconsensual Sexual Interactions with Women: Prevalence and Impact." *Archives*

References

of Sexual Behavior, Vol. 32, No. 2, April 2003, p. 165.

63. Hensley. "Treatment for Survivors of Rape."

64. Jewkes, Rachel. "Preventing Sexual Violence: A Rights-Based Approach." *Lancet,* Vol. 360, No. 9339, October 5, 2002, p. 1092.

65. Hong, Luoluo. "Toward a Transformed Approach to Prevention: Breaking the Link Between Masculinity and Violence." *Journal of American College Health,* Vol. 48, No. 6, May 2000, p. 269.

Working Toward a Healthy Environment

As a teenager, Ocean Robbins wanted to change the world. At age 16, he founded Youth for Environmental Sanity (YES!) to mobilize his generation to save the planet. Now in his late twenties, Robbins has seen his California-based organization grow into what *Time* magazine describes as "a mini-movement that spans environmental consciousness raising, leadership training and community building." Over the last eleven years, more than 600,000 students in seven countries have taken part in YES! events in schools, summer camps,

and workshops. "Part of my mandate is to help my generation see the power we have," says Robbins.[1]

No one has more stake in the future of the planet than the young. Environmental concerns may seem so enormous that nothing any individual can do will have an effect. This is not the case. Some individuals, like Ocean Robbins, become international advocates. But all of us, as citizens of the world, can help

find solutions to the challenges confronting our planet. The first step is realizing that you have a personal responsibility for safeguarding the health of your environment and, thereby, your own well-being.

This chapter explores the complex interrelationships between your world and your well-being. It discusses major threats to the environment—including atmospheric changes; air, water, and noise pollution; chemical risks; and radiation—and provides specific guidance on what you can do about them.

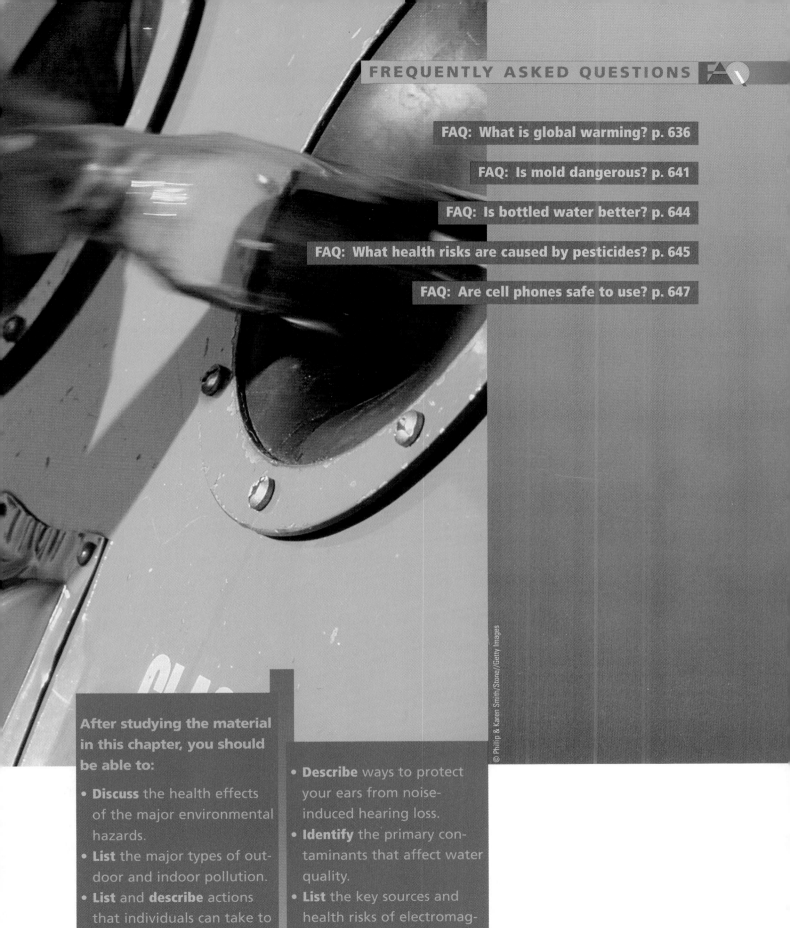

© Phillip & Karen Smith/Stone//Getty Images

After studying the material in this chapter, you should be able to:

- **Discuss** the health effects of the major environmental hazards.
- **List** the major types of outdoor and indoor pollution.
- **List** and **describe** actions that individuals can take to protect the environment.

- **Describe** ways to protect your ears from noise-induced hearing loss.
- **Identify** the primary contaminants that affect water quality.
- **List** the key sources and health risks of electromagnetic fields.

633

The State of the Environment

Ours is a planet in peril. A recent report by the United Nations documented increasing dangers to the planet Earth and its inhabitants. Sea levels are rising. Forests are being destroyed. Droughts in Asia and Africa have become more frequent and more intense. Despite some recent improvements, more than 3 million people die every year from the effects of air pollution while 2.2 million people die from contaminated water.[2]

However, there has been significant progress. Levels of many contaminants, including lead and DDT, have decreased in the environment by as much as 90 percent over the last quarter of a century.[3] As a result of these large decreases, levels of environmental chemicals in the general population are well below those considered to be a risk to public health.[4]

Our Planet, Our Health

The planet Earth—once taken for granted as a ball of rock and water that existed for our use for all time—now is seen as a single, fragile **ecosystem** (a community of organisms that share a physical and chemical environment). Our environment is a closed ecosystem, powered by the sun. The materials needed for the survival of this planet must be recycled over and over again. Increasingly, we're realizing just how important the health of this ecosystem is to our own well-being and survival. However, as shown in Student Snapshot: "Do Students Care About the Environment?" the majority of undergraduates do not share this concern.

Students at all-black colleges are more likely to express environmental concerns.[5]

Our environment affects our well-being both directly and indirectly. Changes in temperature and rainfall patterns disturb ecological processes in ways that can be hazardous to health. The environment may account for 25 to 40 percent of diseases worldwide. Children are the most vulnerable because of their greater sensitivity to toxic threats. In response to this trend, Congress has approved funding to create a nationwide system to track environmental links to chronic diseases.

No individual is immune to environmental health threats. Depletion of the ozone layer has already been implicated in the increase in skin cancers and cataracts. Global warming, according to some theorists, might lead to changes in one-third to one-half of the world's vegetation types and to the extinction of many plant and animal species. A warmer world is expected to produce more severe flooding in some places and more severe droughts in others, jeopardizing natural resources and the safety of our water supply. Warmer weather—a consequence of changes in atmospheric gases and climate—worsens urban-industrial air pollution and, if the air also is moist, increases concentrations of allergenic pollens and fungal spores. These are truly problems without borders.

For good or for ill, we cannot separate our individual health from that of the environment in which we live. The air we breathe, the water we drink, the chemicals we use all have an impact on the quality of our lives. At the same time, the lifestyle choices we make, the products we use, the efforts we undertake to clean up a beach or save wetlands affect the quality of our environment.

Multiple Chemical Sensitivity

The proliferation of chemicals in modern society has led to an entirely new disease, **multiple chemical sensitivity (MCS),** also called environmentally triggered illness, universal allergy, or chemical AIDS. MCS was first described almost a half century ago when a Chicago allergist treated a number of patients who reported becoming ill after being exposed to various petrochemicals. Since that time, many more cases of MCS have been reported, yet there is no agreed-upon definition for the condition, no medical test that can diagnose it, and no proven treatment.

According to medical theory, people become chemically sensitive in a two-step process: First, they experience a major exposure to a chemical, such as a pesticide, a solvent, or a combustion product. The sensitized person then begins to react to low-level chemical exposures from ordinary substances, such as perfumes and tobacco smoke. In other words, these low-level exposures trigger a physiological response. Over time, chemically unrelated substances may induce symptoms such as chest pain, depression, difficulty remembering, dizziness, fatigue, headache, inability to concentrate, nausea, and aches and pains in muscles and joints.

Glenn M. Oliver/Visuals Unlimited

Environmental factors may be to blame for a rise in the number of deformed frogs, toads, and salamanders that have been discovered in recent years.

Student Snapshot   **Do Students Care About the Environment?**

Freshman who say that "becoming involved in programs to clean up the environment" is essential or very important:

All students 17.1%

Men   16.9%

Women   17.2%

Source: Linda Sax et al. *The American Freshman: National Norms for Fall 2002.* Los Angeles: Higher Education Research Institute, UCLA, 2002.

Individuals who may be at risk of MCS include Persian Gulf veterans, industrial workers, occupants of "sick buildings" with high levels of indoor pollutants, and people who live near contaminated sites. Because of the variety of racial, ethnic, and socioeconomic groups affected, medical professionals have become convinced that MCS is a real and serious health problem that requires investigation.

Pollution

Any change in the air, water, or soil that could reduce its ability to support life is a form of **pollution.** Natural events, such as smoke from fires triggered by lightning, can cause pollution. The effects of pollution depend on the concentration (amount per unit of air, water, or soil) of the **pollutant,** how long it remains in the environment, and its chemical nature. An *acute effect* is a severe immediate reaction, usually after a single, large exposure. For example, pesticide poisoning can cause nausea and dizziness, even death. A *chronic effect* may take years to develop or may be a recurrent or continuous reaction, usually after repeated exposures. The development of cancer after repeated exposure to a pollutant such as asbestos is an example of a chronic effect.

Environmental agents that trigger changes, or **mutations,** in the genetic material (the DNA) of living cells are called **mutagens.** The changes that result can lead to the development of cancer. A substance or agent that causes cancer is a *carcinogen:* All carcinogens are mutagens; most mutagens are carcinogens. Furthermore, when a mutagen affects an egg or a sperm cell, its effects can be passed on

to future generations. Mutagens that can cross the placenta of a pregnant woman and cause a spontaneous abortion or birth defects in the fetus are called **teratogens.**

Pollution is a hazard to all who breathe. Deaths caused by air pollution exceed those from motor vehicle injuries, according to research in Austria, France, and Switzerland.[6] Those with respiratory illnesses are at greatest risk during days when smog or allergen counts are high. However, even healthy joggers are affected; carbon monoxide has been shown to impair their exercise performance. The effects of carbon monoxide are much worse in smokers, who already have higher levels of the gas in their blood.

Toxic substances in polluted air can enter the human body in three ways: through the skin, through the digestive system, and through the lungs. The combined interaction of two or more hazards can produce an effect greater than that of either one alone. Pollutants can affect an organ or organ system directly or indirectly.

Among the health problems that have been linked with pollution are the following:

:: Headaches and dizziness.

:: Eye irritation and impaired vision.

:: Nasal discharge.

:: Cough, shortness of breath, and sore throat.

:: Constricted airways.

:: Constriction of blood vessels and increased risk of heart disease.[7]

:: Chest pains and aggravation of the symptoms of colds, pneumonia, bronchial asthma, emphysema, chronic bronchitis, lung cancer, and other respiratory problems.

:: Birth defects and reproductive problems.

:: Nausea, vomiting, and stomach cancer.

:: Allergy and asthma from diesel fumes in polluted air.[8]

What Is Global Warming?

In the last century Earth's average surface temperature has risen by an estimated 0.6 to 1.2 degrees Fahrenheit.[9] More of the warming has occurred over land than over water, more at night than during the day, and more in winter than in summer. No one can predict exactly the long-term impact of a continuing temperature rise, but experts believe that recent droughts and increases in carbon dioxide are early effects of global warming.[10]

Why is our planet getting warmer? Global warming may have many causes, including natural processes like volcanic activity, but most of the warming over the last 50 years is attributable to human activities.[11] Our activities have increased the amount of greenhouse gases in our atmosphere—primarily carbon dioxide, methane, and nitrous oxide. These atmospheric gases trap some of the sun's energy, retaining heat somewhat like the glass panels of a greenhouse.

When fossil fuels (oil, natural gas, and coal), and wood and wood products are burned, carbon dioxide is released into the atmosphere. The production of coal, natural gas, and oil, the decomposition of organic wastes in municipal solid waste landfills, and livestock all emit methane. Nitrous oxide is emitted during agricultural and industrial activities. These greenhouse gases have increased worldwide. (See Figure 19-1.) The Intergovernmental Panel on Climate Change projects a global average warming of 2.5 to 10.4°F (1.4 to 5.8°C) by the year 2100, compared with the global average temperature in 1990. (See Figure 19-2.)

The consequences of global warming are many and even include planetary motion. According to French scientists, higher temperatures may be slowing Earth's daily spin by around half a millisecond every century. A more visible consequence is the melting of the Antarctic ice shelves, flat expanses of ice up to 1,000 feet thick, which extend into the ocean from opposite sides of the Antarctic Peninsula. Satellite imagery shows that chunks of ice, some the size of aircraft carriers, are breaking off the shelves and drifting into the sea. The shelves themselves will probably disappear within a few years, but most scientists do not now think they will raise sea levels since they are already displacing ocean water in their frozen state. Within the next century, though, if global warming continues, the sea level will probably creep up more modestly, by about a foot or two, enough to endanger beachfront property and cost billions of dollars of damage.

Rising temperature during the summer on the arctic tundra may increase both snowfall and the emission of carbon dioxide. This may further contribute to atmospheric changes. However, farms, forests, and grasslands—if protected from development—may help counterbalance this trend. According to scientists' calculations, agricultural lands could remove from 40 to 80 billion metric tons of carbon from the atmosphere over the next 50 to 100 years and store it in the soil.

In addition to significant climate changes, global warming is affecting both plants and animals, with some species dying off.[12] Altered temperatures, extremes of precipitation (floods and droughts), and increased air pollution will all have a direct impact on health.[13]

For the last ten years, world leaders have been focusing on global warming and its potential consequences. In 2001, 165 countries—not including the United States—signed the first international treaty to fight global warming by implementing the rules known as the Kyoto Protocol. The treaty calls on about 40 industrialized nations to limit carbon emissions or reduce them to levels below those of 1990. The United States, which is responsible for 23 percent of greenhouse-gas emissions,[14] rejected the accord as harmful to the U.S. economy and unfair because it excused heavily polluting nations, such as India and China, from any obligation.

Clearing the Air

In most places in the United States, you can breathe easier today than you would have a quarter century ago. Smog has declined by about a third, although there are now 85 percent more vehicles being driven 105 percent more miles a year. Current model automobiles emit an average of 80 percent less pollution per mile than was emitted by new cars in 1970. However, tailpipe emissions from cars and trucks still account for almost a third of the air pollution in the United States.[15] California remains the smoggiest state.[16]

According to the Harvard School of Public Health, living in a city with even moderately sooty air may shorten your lifespan by about a year. In fact, air pollution can be as harmful to breathing capacity as smoking. Residents of polluted cities are exposed to some of the same toxic gases, such as nitrogen oxide and carbon monoxide, found in cigarettes.

Air pollution of any sort can cause numerous ill effects. As pollutants destroy the hairlike cilia that remove irritants from the lungs, individuals may suffer chronic bronchitis, characterized by excessive mucus flow and continuous coughing. Emphysema may develop or worsen, as pollutants constrict the bronchial tubes and destroy the air sacs in the lungs, making breathing more difficult. In addition to respiratory diseases, air pollution also contributes to heart disease, cancer, and weakened immunity. For the elderly and people with asthma or heart disease, polluted air can be life-threatening. Even healthy individuals can be affected, particularly if they exercise outdoors during high-pollution periods.

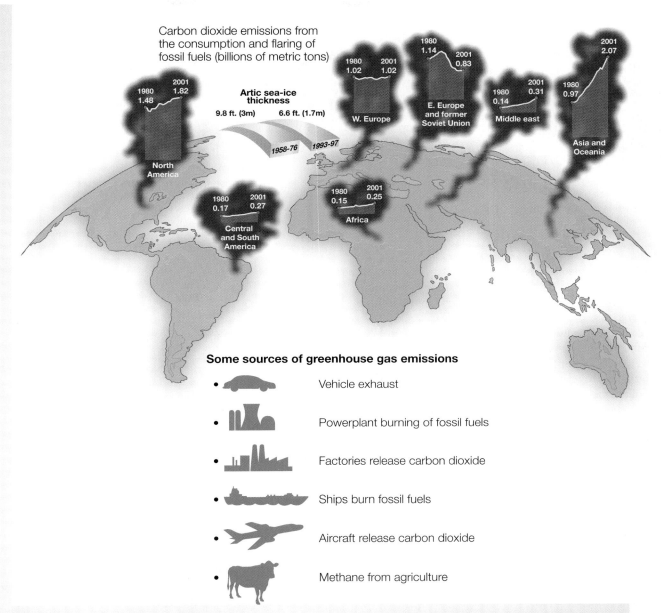

Figure 19-1 WHY THE WORLD IS HEATING UP

The buildup of carbon dioxide and other greenhouse gases in the atmosphere could result in great climate change. A combination of factors, including the burning of fossil fuels and deforestation, is causing the atmosphere to retain heat.

Source: Data from Energy Information Administration, Department of Energy (www.eia.doe.gov).

Smog

A combination of smoke and fog, **smog** is made up of chemical vapors from auto exhaust, industrial and commercial pollutants (volatile organic compounds, carbon monoxide, nitrogen oxides, sulfur oxides, particulates), and ozone. The most obvious sources of these pollutants are motor vehicles, industrial factories, electric utility plants, and wood-burning stoves.[17]

Gray-air, or *sulfur-dioxide,* smog, often seen in Europe and much of the eastern United States, is produced by burning oil of high sulfur content. Among the cities that must deal with gray-air smog are Chicago, Baltimore, Detroit, and Philadelphia. Like cigarette smoke, gray-air smog affects the cilia in the respiratory passages; the lungs are unable to expel particulates, such as soot, ash, and dust,

Global annual average temperature (Fahrenheit)

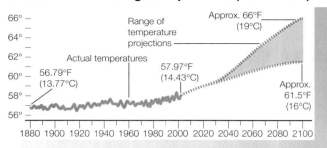

Figure 19-2 GLOBAL ANNUAL AVERAGE TEMPERATURE

The graph shows actual temperatures from 1880 to 2001 and range of temperature projections to 2100, depending on assumptions and models used for projections.

Source: Intergovernmental Panel on Climate Change (http://yosemite.epa.gov/oar/globalwarming.nsf/content/ClimateFutureClimateGlobalTemperature.html).

which remain and irritate the tissues. This condition is hazardous to people with chronic respiratory problems.

Brown-air, or *photochemical,* smog is found in large traffic centers such as Los Angeles, Salt Lake City, Denver, Mexico City, and Tokyo. This type of smog results principally from nitric oxide in car exhaust reacting with oxygen in the air, forming nitrogen dioxide, which produces a brownish haze and, when exposed to sunlight, other pollutants.

One of these, *ozone,* the most widespread pollutant, can impair the body's immune system and cause long-term lung damage. (Ozone in the upper atmosphere protects us by repelling harmful ultraviolet radiation from the sun, but ozone in the lower atmosphere is a harmful component of air pollution.) Automobiles also produce carbon monoxide, a colorless and odorless gas that diminishes the ability of red blood cells to carry oxygen. The resulting oxygen deficiency can affect breathing, hearing, and vision in humans and stunt the growth of plants and trees.[18] (See Fact or Fiction? "Ozone levels are higher . . .")

The effects of acid rain on a forest.

FACT OR FICTION?????????????????

Ozone levels are higher in rural areas than in cities.

Fact: In a surprising study, scientists discovered that the chemical precursors of ozone are blown out of urban areas to the countryside, where ozone forms and remains in the atmosphere. Many trees in an asphalt jungle like New York City grow twice as large as those in farming communities an hour away because the higher ozone levels in rural areas stunt their growth.

Source: Jillian Gregg et al. "Urbanization Effects on Tree Growth in the Vicinity of New York City." *Nature*, Vol. 10, No. 424, July 2003, p. 183.

Acid Rain

The burning of fossil fuels, such as oil and gas, and the smelting of certain ores, such as copper and nickel, can produce **acid rain**—rain, sleet, snow, mist, fog, and clouds containing sulfuric acid and nitric acid. These pollutants are carried through the atmosphere long distances from their sources and fan to Earth when it rains. Acid rain, which is believed to be declining in some regions, has damaged buildings, monuments, and other structures.

During the last 30 years, acid rain has contributed to the death of more than half of certain trees, including red spruce and sugar maples, in the Northeast.[19] More than a decade after the passage of the Clean Air Act in 1990, habitats in the northeastern states have not yet recovered from acid rain damage.[20]

STRATEGIES FOR CHANGE

Doing Your Part for Cleaner Air

- Drive a car that gets high gas mileage and produces low emissions. Keep your speed at or below the speed limit.

- Keep your tires inflated and your engine tuned. Recycle old batteries and tires. (Most stores that sell new ones will take back old ones.)

- Turn off your engine if you're going to be stopped for more than a minute.

- Collect all fluids that you drain from your car (motor oil, antifreeze) and recycle or properly dispose of them.

Self Survey

Are You Doing Your Part for the Planet?

You may think that there is little you can do, as an individual, to save Earth. But everyday acts can add up and make a difference in helping or harming the planet on which we live.

	Almost Never	Sometimes	Always
1. Do you walk, cycle, carpool, or use public transportation as much as possible to get around?	_____	_____	_____
2. Do you recycle?	_____	_____	_____
3. Do you reuse plastic and paper bags?	_____	_____	_____
4. Do you try to conserve water by not running the tap as you shampoo or brush your teeth?	_____	_____	_____
5. Do you use products made of recycled materials?	_____	_____	_____
6. Do you drive a car that gets good fuel mileage and has up-to-date emission control equipment?	_____	_____	_____
7. Do you turn off lights, televisions, and appliances when you're not using them?	_____	_____	_____
8. Do you avoid buying products that are elaborately packaged?	_____	_____	_____
9. Do you use glass jars and waxed paper rather than plastic wrap for storing food?	_____	_____	_____
10. Do you take brief showers rather than baths?	_____	_____	_____
11. Do you use cloth towels and napkins rather than paper products?	_____	_____	_____
12. When listening to music, do you keep the volume low?	_____	_____	_____
13. Do you try to avoid any potential carcinogens, such as asbestos, mercury, or benzene?	_____	_____	_____
14. Are you careful to dispose of hazardous materials (such as automobile oil or antifreeze) at appropriate sites?	_____	_____	_____
15. Do you follow environmental issues in your community and write your state or federal representative to support "green" legislation?	_____	_____	_____

Count the number of items you've checked in each column. If you've circled 10 or more in the "always" column, you're definitely helping to make a difference. If you've circled 10 or more in the "never" column, read this chapter carefully and "Your Health Change Plan for Protecting the Planet" to find out what you can do. If you've mainly circled "sometimes," you're moving in the right direction, but you need to be more consistent and more conscientious.

Your Health Change Plan

for Protecting the Planet

By the choices you make and the actions you take, you can improve the state of the world. No one expects you to sacrifice every comfort or spend great amounts of money. However, for almost everyone, there's plenty of room for improvement. If enough people make small individual changes, they can have an enormous impact.

One basic environmental action is **precycling:** buying products packaged in recycled materials. According to Earthworks, a consumer group, packaging makes up a third of what people in the United States throw away. When you precycle, you consider how you're going to dispose of a product and the packaging materials before purchasing it. For example, you might choose eggs in recyclable cardboard packages rather than in plastic cartons, and look for juice and milk in refillable bottles.

Recycling—collecting, reprocessing, marketing, and using materials once considered trash—has become a necessity for several reasons: We've run out of space for all the garbage we produce; waste sites are often health and safety hazards; recycling is cheaper than landfill storage or incineration (a major source of air pollution); and recycling helps save energy and natural resources. Different communities take different approaches to recycling. Many provide regular curbside pickup of recyclables, which is so convenient that a majority of those eligible for such services participate. Most programs pick up bottles, cans, and newspapers—either separated or mixed together. Other communities have drop-off centers where consumers can leave recyclables. Conveniently located and sponsored by community organizations (such as charities or schools), these centers accept beverage containers, newspapers, cardboard, metals, and other items.

(continued)

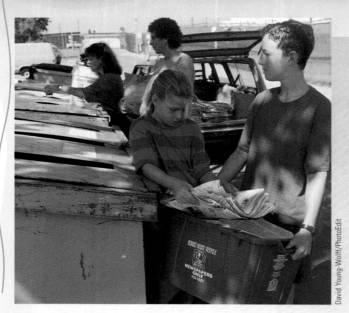

David Young-Wolff/PhotoEdit

Recycling helps save energy and conserve resources.

Buyback centers, usually run by private companies, pay for recyclables. Many centers specialize in aluminum cans, which offer the most profit. Some operate in supermarket parking lots; other centers have regular hours and staff members who carefully weigh and evaluate recyclables. In some places, reverse vending machines accept returned beverage containers and provide deposit refunds, in the form of either cash or vouchers.

Discarded computers and other electronic devices should also be recycled, by donating them to schools or charitable organizations. "Tech trash" buried in landfills is creating a new hazard because trace amounts of potentially hazardous agents, such as lead and mercury, can leak into the ground and water.

With *composting*—which some people describe as nature's way of recycling—the benefits can be seen as close as your backyard. Organic products, such as leftover food and vegetable peels, are mixed with straw or other dry material and kept damp. Bacteria eat the organic material and turn it into a rich soil. Some people keep a compost pile (which should be stirred every few days) in their backyard; others take their organic garbage (including mowed grass and dead leaves) to community gardens or municipal composting sites.

Indoor Pollutants

Because people in industrialized nations spend more than 90 percent of their time in buildings, the quality of the air they breathe inside can have an even greater impact on their well-being than outdoor pollution. The most hazardous form of indoor air pollution is cigarette smoke. Passive smoking—inhaling others' cigarette smoke—may rank behind active smoking and alcohol use as the third-leading preventable cause of death. Each year secondhand cigarette smoke kills 53,000 nonsmokers.

Formaldehyde

Unlike outdoor contaminants from exhaust pipes or smokestacks, indoor pollutants come from the very materials the buildings are made of and from the appliances inside them. For instance, formaldehyde, commonly used in building materials, carpet backing, furniture, foam insulation, plywood, and particle board, can cause nausea, dizziness, headaches, heart palpitations, stinging eyes, and burning lungs. Formaldehyde gas, which is colorless and odorless, has been shown to cause cancer in animals.[21] Most manufacturers have voluntarily quit using it, but many homes already contain materials made with urea-formaldehyde, which can seep into the air. To avoid formaldehyde exposure, buy solid wood or nonwood products whenever possible, and ask about the formaldehyde content of building products, cabinets, and furniture before purchasing them.

Asbestos

Asbestos, a mineral widely used for building insulation, has been linked to lung and gastrointestinal cancer among asbestos workers and their families, although it may take 20 to 30 years for such cancer to develop. Fibers from asbestos home insulation or fireproofing that become airborne can cause progressive and deadly lung diseases, including cancer. More than 200,000 lawsuits have been filed for asbestos-related injuries, and as many as 300,000 American workers may have died from asbestos-linked diseases, including lung cancer. The danger may be greatest for those who smoke and are also exposed to asbestos.

If you're concerned about asbestos in your home, don't waste money searching for asbestos in the air. The results of such tests are meaningless. To check a building material for asbestos, put three small pieces in a film canister and send it to a laboratory approved by the U.S. Environmental Protection Agency (EPA). The cost for testing is usually $25 to $75 per sample. If you find asbestos in your house, sealing the source (for example, an old linoleum floor) may be safer than removing it. Contact

Savvy Consumer

"GOING GREEN"

Simple steps can help save energy, lower carbon dioxide (CO_2) emissions, and cut down on energy costs. Here are some recommendations from the Environmental Defense and World Wildlife Fund:

- Wash laundry in warm or cold water, not hot. *Average annual CO_2 reduction: up to 500 pounds for two loads of laundry a week.*

- Buy products sold in the simplest possible packaging. Carry a tote bag or recycle shopping bags. *Average annual CO_2 reduction: 1,000 pounds because garbage is reduced 25 percent.*

- Switch from standard light bulbs to energy-efficient fluorescent ones. *Average annual CO_2 reduction: about 500 pounds per bulb.*

- Set room thermostats lower in winter and higher in summer. *Average annual CO_2 reduction: about 500 pounds for each two-degree reduction.*

- Run dishwashers only when full, and choose the energy-saving mode rather than the regular setting. *Average annual CO_2 reduction: 200 pounds.*

- Bike, carpool, or take mass transit whenever possible. *Average annual CO_2 reduction: 20 pounds for each gallon of gasoline saved.*

---

your state or city health department for advice. If asbestos must be removed, have it done by professionals.

Lead

A danger both inside and outside our homes is lead, which lurks in some 57 million American homes, most built before 1960, with walls, windows, doors, and banisters coated with more than 3 million metric tons of lead-based paint. The percentage of children aged one to five with elevated levels of lead in their blood has dropped to 2.2 percent, half of what it was in the early 1990s.[22]

Fetuses and children under age 7 are particularly vulnerable to lead because their nervous systems are still developing and because their body mass is so small that they ingest and absorb more lead per pound than adults. Even 10 micrograms (millionths of a gram) of lead per deciliter of blood—the CDC standard for lead poison-ing—can kill a child's brain cells and cause poor concentration, reduced short-term memory, slower reaction times, and learning disabilities.

Adults exposed to low levels of lead (which once were thought to be safe) may develop headaches, high blood pressure, irritability, tremors, and insomnia. Health effects increase with exposure to higher levels and include anemia, stomach pain, vomiting, diarrhea, and constipation. Long-term exposure can impair fertility and damage the kidneys. Workers exposed to lead may become sterile or suffer irreversible kidney disease, damage to their central nervous system, stillbirths, or miscarriages.

The CDC and the American Academy of Pediatrics recommend annual testing of blood levels of lead in all children from age 9 months to 6 years, regardless of where they live. High-risk youngsters—those who live or play in older housing (especially if a building is in poor condition or undergoing renovation), those who live with someone who uses lead for a job or hobby, and those who live near a lead smelter, a processing plant, or a heavily traveled road or highway—should be screened every two or three months until age 3 and every six months until age 6. High levels of ascorbic acid (vitamin C) have been associated with a lower rate of elevated blood lead levels.

Lead-based paint poses a hazard, especially to children, who can be poisoned even by ingesting small amounts of paint chips.

© Tony Freeman/PhotoEdit

Is Mold Dangerous?

One of the oldest and most widespread substances on earth, mold—a type of fungus that decomposes organic matter and provides plants with nutrients—has emerged as a major health concern. Common molds include *Aspergillus, Penicillium,* and *Stachybotrys,* a slimy, dark green mold that has been blamed for infant deaths and various illnesses, from Alzheimer's disease to cancer, in adults that breathe in its spores. Faulty ventilation systems and airtight buildings have been implicated as contributing to the increased mold problem.[23]

Experts agree that mold may trigger or worsen a number of health problems, including allergic reactions, dizziness, breathing problems, nausea, and asthma attacks. Individuals with preexisting health conditions or suppressed immunity are at greater risk.[24] In the last decade, high-profile lawsuits have resulted in multimillion dollar judgments, despite minimal scientific evidence linking mold exposure and cancer or brain damage. An estimated 10,000 cases are currently pending.

Mold problems can range from small patches to large infestations of entire rooms or even a whole building. The first step to reduce mold exposure is moisture control, which may require new methods of keeping rainwater and ground water away from the interior and maintaining the heating ventilation and air conditioning systems appropriately. Bleach or soap and water can clean up small infestations. Larger ones may require appropriate protective respiratory equipment or professionally trained, licensed and experienced contractors.[25]

Mercury

While free of lead, some popular, easy-to-use latex paints may contain potentially hazardous mercury, which manufacturers routinely added, until a 1990 ban, to prevent the growth of mold and mildew. The threat of mercury poisoning is greatest during painting and immediately after. Even mercury in medical devices, such as sphygmomanometers that measure blood pressure, can be a hazard. Symptoms of mercury poisoning include a racing heartbeat, sweating, aching limbs, kidney problems, hand tremors, peeling skin, and emotional problems. Levels of mercury in children and women of childbearing age have fallen in recent years.[26]

Carbon Monoxide and Nitrogen Dioxide

Carbon monoxide (CO) gas, which is tasteless, odorless, colorless, and nonirritating, can be deadly. Produced by the incomplete combustion of fuel in space heaters, furnaces, water heaters, and engines, it reduces the delivery of oxygen in the blood. Every year an estimated 10,000 Americans seek treatment for CO inhalation; at least 250 die because of this silent killer. Those most at risk are the chronically ill, the elderly, pregnant women, and infants. Typical symptoms of CO poisoning which is most common in winter, are headache, nausea, vomiting, fatigue, and dizziness. More severe poisoning can damage the heart and cause respiratory distress, confusion, and coma.[27] A blood test can measure CO levels; inhaling pure oxygen speeds removal of the gas from the body. Most people who don't lose consciousness as a result of CO poisoning recover completely.

Another dangerous gas, nitrogen dioxide, can reach very high levels if you use a natural gas or propane stove in a poorly ventilated kitchen. This gas may lead to respiratory illnesses. Pilot lights are a steady source of nitrogen dioxide; to reduce exposure, switch to spark ignition.

Radon

Radioactive radon—which diffuses from rock, brick, concrete building materials, and natural soil deposits under some homes—produces charged decay products that cling to dust particles. Once trapped inside a building, radon can reach levels that may increase the risk of lung cancer. The EPA estimates that the inhalation of indoor radon is responsible for approximately 14,000 lung cancer deaths per year. Radon levels tend to be highest in areas with granite and black shale topped with porous soil.

An estimated 10 million homes and over 30 million people are at risk from high levels of radon.[28] If you live in a high-radon area, don't panic. Your hypothetical risk of dying from radon-caused lung cancer is about equal to the known risk of dying in a home fire or fall. Check with the geology department at the nearest university or with your state health department to find out if they've performed radon tests in your area. If there may be danger, you can buy a radon detector. In most homes, the readings turn out to be low. If not, your state health department can provide guidelines for bringing them down.

❖ Your Hearing Health

Hearing loss is the third most common chronic health problem, after high blood pressure and arthritis, among older Americans.[29] Approximately 25 to 40 percent of adults older than age 65 have some degree of hearing loss, as do 40 to 66 percent of people age 75 and older.[30] Loud noises cause hearing loss in an estimated 10 million Americans every year.

Most hearing loss occurs on the job. The people at highest risk are firefighters, police, military personnel, construction and factory workers, musicians, farmers, and truck drivers. Other sources of danger include live or recorded high-volume music, recreational vehicles, airplanes, lawn-care equipment, woodworking tools, some appliances, and chain saws.

How Loud Is That Noise?

Loudness, or the intensity of a sound, is measured in **decibels (dB).** A whisper is 20 decibels; a conversation in a living room is about 50 decibels. On this scale, 50 isn't two and a half times louder than 20, but 1,000 times louder: Each 10-dB rise in the scale represents a tenfold increase in the intensity of the sound. Very loud but short bursts of sounds (such as gunshots and fireworks) and quieter but longer-lasting sounds (such as power tools) can induce hearing loss.

Sounds under 75 dB don't seem harmful. However, prolonged exposure to any sound over 85 dB (the equivalent of a power mower or food blender) or brief exposure to louder sounds can harm hearing. The noise level at rock concerts can reach 110 to 140 dB, about as loud as an air raid siren. Personal sound systems (boom boxes) can blast sounds of up to 115 dB. Cars with extremely loud music systems, known as boom cars, can produce an earsplitting 145 dB—louder than a jet engine or thunderclap. (See Figure 19-3.)

Common "sound offenders" are nightclubs (with sustained levels of well over 100 decibels), restaurants (with levels of 80 to 96 decibels), and street traffic (80 decibels or more).[31] However, even low-level office noise can undermine well-being and increase health risks.[32]

Effects of Noise

Noise-induced hearing loss is 100 percent preventable—and irreversible. Hearing aids are the only treatment, but they do not correct the problem; they just amplify sound to compensate for hearing loss.

The healthy human ear can hear sounds within a wide range of frequencies (measured in hertz), from the low-frequency rumble of thunder at 50 hertz to the high-frequency overtones of a piccolo at nearly 20,000 hertz. High-frequency noise damages the delicate hair cells that serve as sound receptors in the inner ear. Damage first begins as a diminished sensitivity to frequencies around 4,000 hertz, the highest notes of a piano.

Early symptoms of hearing loss include difficulty understanding speech and *tinnitus* (ringing in the ears). Brief, very loud sounds, such as an explosion or gunfire, can produce immediate, severe, and permanent hearing loss. Longer exposure to less intense but still hazardous sounds, such as those common at work or in public places, can gradually impair hearing, often without the individual's awareness.

Conductive hearing loss, often caused by ear infections, cuts down on perception of low-pitched sounds. Sensorineural loss involves damage or destruction of the sensory cells in the inner ear that convert sound waves to nerve signals.

Noise can harm more than our ears: High-volume sound has been linked to high blood pressure and other stress-related problems that can lead to heart disease, insomnia, anxiety, headaches, colitis, and ulcers. Noise frays the nerves; people tend to be more anxious, irritable, and angry when their ears are constantly barraged with sound.

Chronic airport noise can affect children's physical and mental health. Even unborn babies respond to sounds; some researchers speculate that noise, particularly if it stresses the mother, may be hazardous to the fetus. As a result of exposure to damaging noise levels, 12.5 percent of

Decibels	Example	Zone
0	The softest sound a typical ear can hear	Safe
10	Just audible	
20	Watch ticking; leaves rustling	
30	Soft whisper at 16 feet	
40	Quiet office; suburban street (no traffic)	
50	Interior of typical urban home; rushing stream	
60	Normal conversation; busy office	
70	Vacuum cleaner at 10 feet; hair dryer	
80	Alarm clock at 2 feet; loud music; average city traffic	
90*	Motorcycle at 25 feet; jet 4 miles after takeoff	Risk of injury
100*	Video arcade; loud factory; subway train	
110*	Car horn at 3 feet; symphony orchestra; chain saw	
120	Jackhammer at 3 feet; boom box; nearby thunderclap	Injury
130	Rock concert; jet engine at 100 feet	
140	Jet engine nearby; amplified car stereo; firearms	

*Note: The maximum exposure allowed on the job by federal law, in hours per day: 90 decibels, 8 hours; 100 decibels, 2 hours; 110 decibels, 1/2 hour.

Figure 19-3 LOUD AND LOUDER
The human ear perceives a 10-decibel increase as a doubling of loudness. Thus, the 100 decibels of a subway train sound much more than twice as loud as the 50 decibels of a rushing stream.

Besides listening to the music at your next concert, tune in to the noise level and how your ears are feeling.

young Americans, an estimated 5.2 million, between ages 6 and 19 have incurred permanent damage to the hair cells within the ear. Take the online hearing test at www.onlinehearing.org to check out your hearing.

The Quality of Our Drinking Water

According to a survey by the Water Quality Association, some 86 percent of the people in the United States are concerned about the quality of their tap water, while 32 percent think their water is not as safe as it should be. About two-thirds take steps to drink purer water, either by using filtration and distillation methods or by drinking bottled water.[33] Fears about the public water supply have led many Americans to turn off their taps. However, Consumer Union, a nonprofit advocacy group, maintains that the United States has the safest water supply in the world. The Environmental Protection Agency has set standards for some 80 contaminants. These include many toxic chemicals and heavy metals—including lead, mercury, cadmium, and chromium—that can cause kidney and nervous system damage and birth defects.

Each year the CDC reports an average of 7,400 cases of illness related to the water people drink. The most common culprits include parasites, bacteria, viruses, chemicals, and lead. Health officials suggest having your water tested

STRATEGIES FOR CHANGE

Protecting Your Ears

- If you must live or work in a noisy area, wear hearing protectors to prevent exposure to blasts of very loud noise. Don't think cotton or facial tissue stuck in your ears can protect you; foam or soft plastic earplugs are more effective. Wear them when operating lawn mowers, weed trimmers, or power tools.

- Soundproof your home by using draperies, carpets, and bulky furniture. Put rubber mats under washing machines, blenders, and other noisy appliances. Seal cracks around windows and doors.

- When you hear a sudden loud noise, press your fingers against your ears. Limit your exposure to loud noise. Several brief periods of noise seem less damaging than one long exposure.

- Be careful if you wear Walkman-type stereos. The volume is too high if you can feel the vibrations.

- Beware of large doses of aspirin. Researchers have found that eight aspirin tablets a day can aggravate the damage caused by loud noise; twelve a day can cause ringing in the ears (tinnitus).

- Don't drink in noisy environments. Alcohol intensifies the impact of noise and increases the risk of lifelong hearing damage.

if you live near a hazardous waste dump or industrial park, if the pipes in your house are made of lead or joined together with lead solder, if your water comes from a well, or if you purchase water from a private company. Check to see if your state health department or local water supplier will provide free testing. If not, use a state-certified laboratory that tests water in accordance with EPA standards.

Is Bottled Water Better?

Is bottled water better? That's what consumers have often assumed. Bottled water sales have tripled in the past ten years. Women and college-age Americans make up the majority of bottled-water drinkers.[34] Yet in the past, the Food and Drug Administration (FDA) simply defined bottled water as "sealed in bottles or other containers and intended for human consumption." Bottled water wasn't required to be "pure" or even to be tested for toxic chemicals. One survey found chemical contaminants associated with cancer in 22 of 100 brands tested.

The FDA has called for federal monitoring of the purity of bottled water. Some states, including California and New York, have their own bottled-water safety standards to ensure that bottled water is at least as safe as drinking water. In cases where public drinking water has been contaminated (for instance, by a toxic spill) and health authorities advise using bottled waters, check the label to make sure that the brand you purchase has been tested or undergone purification treatment. Health experts also caution against bottled waters "fortified" with vitamins or minerals, which you can—and should—get from a healthful diet.

Flouride

About half (53 percent) of Americans drink water containing fluoride, an additive to water and toothpaste that helps teeth resist decay. According to the American Dental Association, the incidence of tooth decay is 50 to 70 percent lower in areas with fluoridated water. However, laboratory rats given fluoridated water have shown a high rate of bone cancer. The more fluoride they drank in their water, the more likely they were to develop this cancer. But this type of cancer is extremely rare in humans, and the estimated lifetime risk to any individual from drinking fluoridated water is less than one in 5,000.

Federal health officials have found no evidence that fluoride causes cancer in humans and have concluded that its benefits far outweigh any risks. However, excessive fluoride can increase bone loss and fractures in pre- and postmenopausal women. Health professionals advise consumers to use only small amounts of fluoridated toothpaste, rinse thoroughly after brushing, and use fluoride supplements only when the home water supply is known to be deficient.

Chlorine

Three-quarters of the population of the United States drinks water treated with chlorine to kill disease-causing bacteria. The Council on Environmental Quality has warned that people drinking chlorinated water have a 53 percent greater risk of getting colon and bladder cancer and a 13 to 93 percent greater risk of getting rectal cancer than those not drinking chlorinated water. There may even be a link between soft water and a higher rate of cardiovascular disease, perhaps because soft water in some areas tends to have more sodium in it.

Lead

Long recognized as a hazard in paint and dust, lead can also leach into the drinking supply from pipes made of or soldered with lead. The highest risk exists in cities with older housing and with lead pipes or water lines.

Chemical Risks

According to the CDC, there have been declines of levels of potentially harmful chemicals, including pesticides and lead, in the country's blood.[35] (See Fact or Fiction? "Levels of lead . . .") No relationship has been found between fertility, as measured by time to pregnancy (that is, the time taken for a couple to conceive once they decide they want to), and male exposure to pesticides. Exposure to pesticides may, however, pose a risk to pregnant women and their unborn children. Exposure to toxic chemicals causes about 3 percent of developmental defects.

An estimated 50,000 to 70,000 U.S. workers die each year of chronic diseases related to past exposure to toxic substances, including lung cancer, bladder cancer, leukemia, lymphoma, chronic bronchitis, and disorders of the nervous system. **Endocrine disruptors,** chemicals that act as or interfere with human hormones, particularly estrogen, may pose a different threat. Scientists are investigating their impact on fertility, falling sperm counts, and cancers of the reproductive organs.

What Health Risks Are Caused by Pesticides?

The FDA estimates that 33 to 39 percent of our food supply contains residues of pesticides that may pose a long-term danger to our health. Scientists have detected traces of pesticides in groundwater in both urban and rural areas.

FACT OR FICTION?

Levels of lead, pesticides, and other chemicals in the blood and bodies of Americans have risen sharply in the last decade.

Fiction: According to the largest study to date on human exposure to environmental chemicals in the United States, levels of potentially toxic chemicals have declined over the past decade. Lead levels, which have been linked to developmental delays and lower IQs in children, have dropped since the early 1990s. Other potentially harmful substances, including mercury, cadmium, dioxins, herbicides, pest repellents, and disinfectants, also are lower. However, blood or urine levels of metabolites of tobacco smoke are substantially higher in children than in adults.

Source: *Second National Report on Human Exposure to Environmental Chemicals.* Atlanta, GA: CDC, 2003. Available online at www.cdc.gov/exposurereport.

Pesticides protect crops from harmful insects, plants, and fungi but may endanger human health.

Various chemicals, including benzene, asbestos, and arsenic, have been shown to cause cancer in humans. Probable carcinogens include DDT and PCB. Risks can be greatly increased with simultaneous exposures to more than one carcinogen, for example, tobacco smoke and asbestos.[36] No link to pesticides has been found with clusters of breast cancer.[37] Men whose jobs routinely expose them to pesticide may be at increased risk of prostate cancer.[38] Parental exposure does not increase the likelihood of childhood brain cancer.[39]

Chlorinated hydrocarbons include several high-risk substances—such as DDT, kepone, and chlordane—that have been restricted or banned because they may cause cancer, birth defects, neurological disorders, and damage to wildlife and the environment. They are extremely resistant to breakdown.

Organic phosphates, including chemicals such as malathion, break down more rapidly than the chlorinated hydrocarbons. Most are highly toxic, causing cramps, confusion, diarrhea, vomiting, headaches, and breathing difficulties. Higher levels in the blood can lead to convulsions, paralysis, coma, and death.

Farmworkers and those in the communities surrounding agricultural land are at greatest risk for pesticide exposure. However, even city dwellers aren't out of range. About half (52 percent) of the nation uses insect repellents, including some made with potent insecticides.

✷ Possible Invisible Dangers

Among the unseen threats to health are various forms of *radiation,* energy radiated in the form of waves or particles.

Electromagnetic Fields

Any electrically charged conductor generates two kinds of invisible fields: electric and magnetic. Together they're called **electromagnetic fields (EMFs).** For years, these fields, produced by household appliances, home wiring, lighting fixtures, electric blankets, and overhead power lines, were considered harmless. However, epidemiological studies have revealed a link between exposure to high-voltage lines and cancer (especially leukemia, a blood cancer) in electrical workers and children.

Laboratory studies on animals have shown that alternating current, which changes strength and direction 60 times a second (and electrifies most of North America), emits EMFs that may interfere with the normal functioning of human cell membranes, which have their own electromagnetic fields. The result may be mood disorders, changes in circadian rhythms (our inner sense of time), miscarriage, developmental problems, or cancer. Researchers have documented an increase in breast cancer deaths in women who worked as electrical engineers, electricians, or in other high-exposure jobs, and a link between EMF exposure and an increased risk of leukemia and possibly brain cancer.[40]

After six years of congressionally mandated research, the National Institute of Environmental Health Sciences concluded that the evidence of a risk of cancer and other human disease from the electric and magnetic fields around power lines is "weak." This finding applies to the extremely low frequency electric and magnetic fields surrounding both the big power lines that distribute power and the smaller but closer electric lines in homes and

Although laboratory studies on animals show that EMFs affect human cell membranes, research on human populations shows only a weak connection between EMFs and human disease.

appliances. However, the researchers also noted that EMF exposure "cannot be recognized as entirely safe."

Appliances that are used only briefly, such as hair dryers, are probably less dangerous than electric blankets, which people sleep under for an entire night. Expectant mothers who often use electric blankets or heated water beds during winter have a higher miscarriage rate than nonusers. Babies conceived in the winter by electric blanket-users grow more slowly in the womb and tend to have a lower birthweight than others. Federal officials urge "prudent avoidance" of electric blankets for women who are pregnant or hoping to conceive.

Microwaves

Microwaves (extremely high frequency electromagnetic waves) increase the rate at which molecules vibrate; this vibration generates heat. There's no evidence that existing levels of microwave radiation encountered in the environment pose a health risk to people, and all home microwave ovens must meet safety standards for leakage.

Another concern about the safety of microwave ovens stems from the chemicals in plastic wrapping and plastic containers used in microwave ovens. Chemicals may leak into food. In high concentrations, some of the chemicals (such as DEHA, which makes plastic more pliable) can cause cancer in mice. Consumers should be cautious about using clingy plastic wrap when reheating leftovers, and plastic-encased metal "heat susceptors" included in convenience foods such as popcorn and pizza. Although these materials seem safe when tested in conventional ovens at temperatures of 300° to 350° Fahrenheit, microwave ovens can boost temperatures to 500° Fahrenheit.

Are Cell Phones Safe to Use?

Since cellular phone service was introduced in the United States in 1984, mobile and handheld phones have become ubiquitous. More than 86 million people use cell phones, and concern has grown about their possible health risks. The federal government sets upper exposure limits to electromagnetic energy from cell phones known as the specific absorption rate, or SAR. A phone emits the most radiation during a call, but it also emits small amounts periodically whenever it's turned on.

Can exposure to low levels of electromagnetic energy that the body absorbs from a cell phone be harmful? More than 70 research papers on the potentially harmful effects of cell phone use have raised concerns about cancer, neurological disorders, sleep problems, or headaches; others have shown no association or were inconclusive. The Food and Drug Administration (FDA) and Federal Communications Commission (FCC) have stated that "the available scientific evidence does not show that any health problems are associated with using wireless phones. There

is no proof, however, that wireless phones are absolutely safe." Additional studies are underway.

Swedish and Finnish researchers have found no "consistent evidence" of increased risk of cancer from use for up to five years, but they did document protein changes in human cells exposed to cell phone radiation and an increased rate of benign brain tumors. Health experts in Britain, France, and Germany have discouraged children from using cell phones largely because of concerns that their developing nervous system may be especially vulnerable.

A headset can keep the phone's antenna away from your head and body. Shields that claim to reduce exposure generally don't work as advertised, say the FDA and FCC.[41]

Irradiated Foods

The use of radiation on food, from either radioactive substances or devices that produce X rays, is known as **irradiation.** It doesn't make the food radioactive—its primary benefit is to prolong the food's useful life. Like the heat in canning, irradiation can kill all the microorganisms that might grow in food; the sterilized food can then be stored for years in sealed containers at room temperature without spoiling. In addition, low-dose irradiation can inhibit the sprouting of vegetables such as potatoes and onions, and delay the ripening of some fruits, such as bananas, mangoes, tomatoes, pears, and avocados—cost-saving benefits of great appeal to the food industry.

Irradiated foods are believed to be safe to eat, and the federal government has approved their distribution. Most research has focused on low-dose irradiation to delay ripening and destroy insects. Nutritional studies have shown no significant decreases in the quality of the foods, but high-dose treatments may cause vitamin losses similar to those that occur during canning. It's also possible that the ionizing effect of radiation creates new compounds in foods that may be mutagenic or carcinogenic. In meats, irradiation proved less effective than cooking in destroying bacteria.[42]

Ionizing Radiation

Radiation that possesses enough energy to separate electrons from their atoms, leaving charged ions, is called **ionizing radiation.** Its effects on health depend on many factors, including the amount, length of exposure, type, part of the body exposed, and the health and age of the individual.

We're surrounded by low-level ionizing radiation every day. Most comes from cosmic rays and radioactive minerals, which vary according to geography. (Denver has more than Atlanta, for instance, because of its altitude.)

Man-made sources, including medical and dental X rays, account for approximately 18 percent of the average person's lifetime exposure.

Radiation exposure in humans is measured in units called rads and rems. A *rad (radiation absorbed dose)* is a measure of the energy deposited by ionizing radiation when it's absorbed by an object. A *rem (roentgen equivalent man)* is a measure of the biological effect of ionizing radiation. Different types of radiation cause different amounts of damage. The rem measurement takes this into account. For X rays, rads and rems are equivalent. A quantity of 1 rad or 1 rem is a substantial dose of radiation. Smaller doses are measured in *millirads* (thousandths of a rad) or *millirems* (thousandths of a rem). The average annual radiation exposure for a person in the United States is about one-tenth of a rem.

Virtually any part of the body can be affected by ionizing radiation, although bone marrow and the thyroid are especially vulnerable. Radon exposures in homes can increase the risk of lung cancer. Although high levels of radiation are most dangerous, even low-level radiation can be harmful to health. According to the National Research Council, the risk of getting cancer from small amounts of radiation is four times more than had been previously estimated, and there's much greater danger of mental retardation among babies exposed to radiation in the womb from eight to fifteen weeks after conception.

Diagnostic X Rays

The EPA estimates that 30 to 50 percent of the 700 million X rays taken every year in the United States are unnecessary. However, doctors sometimes prescribe X rays or newer imaging techniques involving radiation, such as CT scans, to protect themselves from malpractice suits, and hospitals benefit financially from the heavy use of X-ray equipment.

Dental X rays involve little radiation, but many people receive so many so often that they're second only to chest examinations in frequency. Dentists typically obtain radiographs of all the teeth at the beginning of a patient's care, and again every three to five years. However, you can cut down on total X rays by bringing previous films with you or having your dentist forward copies when you switch dentists.

Always ask why an X ray is being ordered. Don't give your consent unless there's a clear need. Keep a record of the date and location of every X-ray exam. Some of these X rays may someday provide information that would make more X rays unnecessary. Ask the radiologist to explain specifically how much radiation you'll be exposed to, and be sure to wear a protective leaded apron. There's no sense in refusing a needed medical X ray just because you're afraid of the radiation exposure. Under certain circumstances, the benefits far outweigh the risks.

The Bottom Line ▼
Taking Care of Mother Earth

Environmental problems can seem so complex that you may think there's little you can do about them. That's not the case. This world can be made better instead of worse. The job isn't easy, and all of us have to do our part. Just as many diseases of the previous century have been eradicated, so, in time, we may be able to remove or reduce many environmental threats. Your future—and our planet's future—may depend on it.

:: *Plant a tree.* Even a single tree helps absorb carbon dioxide and produces cooling that can reduce the need for air-conditioning.

:: *Look for simply packaged items.* Whenever possible, choose items packed in recycled materials or something recyclable.

:: *Bring your own bag.* Whenever possible, avoid using plastic or paper bags for items you could carry in a cloth or string carryall.

:: *Hit the switch.* Turn off all electrical appliances (TVs, CD players, radios, lights) when you're not in the room or paying attention to them.

:: *Avoid disposables.* Use a mug instead of a paper or Styrofoam cup, a sponge instead of a paper towel, a cloth napkin instead of a paper one.

:: *Be water wise.* Turn off the tap while you shave or brush your teeth. Install water-efficient faucets and shower heads. Wash clothes in cold water.

:: *Cancel junk mail.* It consumes 100 million trees a year. To get off mailing lists, write: Direct Mail Association, Mail Preference Service, P.O. Box 9008, Farmingdale, NY 11735-9008

:: *Spare the seas.* If you live near the coast or are picnicking or hiking near the ocean, don't use plastic bags (which are often blown into the water) or plastic six-pack holders (which can get caught around the necks of sea birds).

:: *Don't buy products made of endangered substances.* Examples include coral, ivory, tortoise shell, or wood from endangered forests (teak, mahogany, ebony, rosewood).

:: *Speak out.* E-mail your senators and congressional representatives, who vote on pollution controls, budgets for the enforcement of safety regulations, and the preservation of forests and wildlife. Identify the particular bill or issue you're addressing. Be as specific, brief, and to the point as possible. Go to www.senate.gov and click on "Senators" to find the e-mail addresses. To find your congressional representative, go to www.house.gov and click on "Write Your Representative."

After watching the CNN video segment, discuss the following question. Can the sights and smells of nature improve your health?

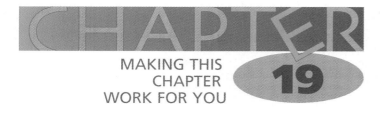

MAKING THIS CHAPTER WORK FOR YOU

19

1. Threats to the environment include
   a. an open ecosystem
   b. depletion of the oxygen layer
   c. ecological processes
   d. global warming

2. Mutagens
   a. are caused by birth defects.
   b. result in changes to the DNA of body cells.
   c. are agents that trigger changes in the DNA of body cells.
   d. are caused by repeated exposure to pollutants.

3. Which of the following statements about global warming is true?
   a. In 2001, the United States signed the first international treaty to fight global warming.
   b. Global warming may result in severe drought and a rise in ocean levels.
   c. Increasing tree cover and agricultural lands will contribute to global warming.
   d. Increasing carbon dioxide production will slow the progress of global warming.

4. One of the most important things you can do to help protect the environment is
   a. recycle paper, bottles, cans, and unwanted food.
   b. use as much water as possible to help lower the ocean water levels.
   c. avoid energy-depleting fluorescent bulbs.
   d. use plastic storage containers and plastic wrap to save trees from being cut down.

5. Which of the following statements about air pollution is false?
   a. Current model automobiles emit much less pollution per mile than new cars in 1970.
   b. The three types of smog include sulfur-dioxide smog, produced by burning oil; photochemical smog, resulting from car exhaust; and carbon-monoxide smog, caused by fossil fuels.
   c. Ozone in the upper atmosphere protects us from harmful ultraviolet radiation from the sun, but in the lower atmosphere, it is a harmful air pollutant.

   d. Air pollution can cause the same types of respiratory health problems as smoking.

6. Indoor pollutants include
   a. lead, which is often found in paint and can result in nervous system damage in adults and impaired fertility and kidney damage in children.
   b. radon, which is found in building materials and can cause heart disease.
   c. asbestos, which may be found in building insulation and can cause lung diseases.
   d. carbon monoxide, which can be produced by furnaces and engines and can result in chronic illnesses such as emphysema.

7. You can protect your hearing by
   a. avoiding prolonged exposure to sounds under 75 decibels.
   b. using foam earplugs when operating noisy tools or attending rock concerts.
   c. limiting noise exposure to short bursts of loud sounds such as fireworks.
   d. drinking alcohol in noisy environments to mute the sounds.

8. Drinking water safety
   a. may be compromised if your water comes from a well.
   b. is high in the United States because of the use of sodium chloride to kill disease-causing bacteria.
   c. can be guaranteed by using bottled water, which is completely free of chemical contaminants.
   d. has been significantly decreased in those communities that add fluoride to the water.

9. Which of the following statements about electromagnetic fields is true?
   a. Overwhelming evidence indicates a strong link between electromagnetic fields around power lines and cancer and other diseases.
   b. The electromagnetic fields emitted by electric blankets are probably less dangerous than those from hair dryers.
   c. The amount of radiation from video display terminals exceeds present standards for safe occupational exposure.
   d. Electrical engineers and electricians who have high exposure to EMFs may be at greater risk for developing leukemia.

10. Which statement about radiation usage is false?
    a. Chemicals in plastic wrap may leak into foods heated in microwave ovens.
    b. Radio frequency signals from cell phones cause brain cancer.
    c. Irradiation can be used to kill microorganisms in food.
    d. Irradiation can delay the ripening of fruits.

Answers to these questions can be found on page 652.

Critical Thinking

1. How do you contribute to environmental pollution? How might you change your habits to protect the environment?

2. An excerpt from a recent newspaper article stated, "Children living in a public housing project near a local refinery suffer from a high rate of asthma and allergies, and an environmental group says the plant may be to blame." The refinery has met all the local air quality standards, employs hundreds in the community, and pays substantial

Critical Thinking

city taxes, which support police, fire, and social services. If you were a city council member, how would you balance health and environmental concerns with the need for industry in your community? What actions would you recommend in this particular situation?

3. In one Harris poll, 84 percent of Americans said that, given a choice between a high standard of living (but with hazardous air and water pollution and the depletion of natural resources) and a lower stan-

Critical Thinking

dard of living (but with clean air and drinking water), they would prefer clean air and drinking water and a lower standard of living. What about you? What exactly would you be willing to give up: air conditioning, convenience packaging and products, driving your own car rather than using public transportation? Do you think most people are willing to change their lifestyles to preserve the environment?

Profile Plus

The health of the planet contributes to the health and well-being of all its inhabitants. Discover how you can contribute to a healthy environment with this activity on your Profile Plus CD-ROM.

Profile Plus

• Are You Doing Your Part for the Planet?

Profile Plus

Sites and Bytes

Environmental Protection Agency
www.epa.gov

This comprehensive government site features environmental topics including ecosystems, global warming, air and water pollution, compliance and enforcement, pesticides and toxins, accident prevention, and treatment.

Sites and Bytes

National Center for Environmental Health (NCEH)
www.cdc.gov/nceh

This site, sponsored by the U.S. Centers for Disease Control and Prevention, features a searchable database as well as fact sheets and brochures on a variety of environmental topics, from emergency preparedness and public health tracking to environmental hazards and lead poisoning prevention.

Sites and Bytes

EnviroLink
www.envirolink.org

This nonprofit organization maintains a comprehensive database of environmental resources, including current news events as well as information on agriculture, air quality, ecosystems, environmental ethics, environmental legislation, and much more.

InfoTrac College Edition

Activity

Shearman, David. "Time and Tide Wait For No Man: Global Warming Presents a New Hazard to Human Health (Troubled Planet)." *British Medical Journal,* Vol. 325, No. 7378, December 21, 2002, p. 1466(3).

1. Describe how global warming can adversely affect one's health.

InfoTrac College Edition

2. How do Darwinian and psychological mechanisms make strategies to curb global warming difficult to enact?

3. According to the authors, what should be done to help decrease the effects of global warming?

You can find additional readings relating to safeguarding the environment with InfoTrac College Edition, an

InfoTrac College Edition

online library of more than 900 journals and publications. Follow the instructions that were packaged with your textbook; then search for articles using a keyword search.

For additional links, resources, and suggested readings on InfoTrac College Edition, visit our Health & Wellness Resource Center at **http://health.wadsworth.com**.

Key Terms

The terms listed are used on the page indicated. Definitions of the terms are in the Glossary at the end of this book.

acid rain 638
chlorinated hydrocarbons 646
decibel (dB) 642
ecosystem 634
electromagnetic fields (EMFs) 646
endocrine disruptors 645

ionizing radiation 647
irradiation 647
microwaves 647
multiple chemical sensitivity (MCS) 634
mutagen 635
mutation 635
organic phosphates 646

pollutant 635
pollution 635
precycling 639
recycling 639
smog 637
teratogen 635

References

1. "Ocean Robbins: Youth for Environmental Sanity." *Time International*, Vol. 153, No. 16, October 22, 2001, p. 71.
2. U.N. Department for Economic and Social Affairs. *Global Outlook 3*. New York: United Nations, 2002.
3. *Second National Report on Human Exposure to Environmental Chemicals*. Atlanta, GA: Centers for Disease Control and Prevention, 2003. Available online at www.cdc.gov/exposurereport.
4. Kamin, Michael. *Traces of Environmental Chemicals in the Human Body: Are They a Risk to Health?* American Council on Science and Health, May 2003.
5. Sax, Linda. *The American Freshman: National Norms for Fall 2002*. Los Angeles, CA: UCLA Higher Education Research Institute, 2002.
6. Richter, Elihu, and Tamar Berman. "Speed, Air Pollution, and Health: A Neglected Issue." *Archives of Environmental Health*, Vol. 56, No. 4, July 2001, p. 296.
7. Brook, Robert, et al. "Inhalation of Fine Particulate Air Pollution and Ozone Causes Acute Arterial Vasoconstriction in Healthy Adults." *Circulation*, Vol. 105, No. 10, March 2002, p. 1534.
8. "Diesel Fumes in Particulate Air Pollution Linked to Increased Atopy and Allergy." *Health and Medicine Week*, September 1, 2003, p. 652.
9. Environmental Protection Agency's website on global warming: www.epa.gov/globalwarming/.
10. "Risks of Global Warming Are Here Already." *Occupational Hazards*, Vol. 65, No. 7, July 2003, p. 14(1).
11. Environmental Protection Agency, www.epa.gov/globalwarming/.
12. Stolzenburg, William. "Nature Feels the Heat: As Climate Goes Awry, Wildlife Goes Away." *Nature Conservancy*, Vol. 51, No. 5, September–October, 2001, p. 12.
13. Patz, Jonathan, and R. Sari Kovats. "Hotspots in Climate Change and Human Health." *British Medical Journal*, Vol. 325, No. 7372, November 9, 2002, p. 1094.
14. "A Wake-Up Call for Environmental Health." *The Lancet*, Vol. 362, No. 9384, August 23, 2003, p. 587.
15. Environmental Protection Agency, www.epa.gov.
16. American Lung Association, www.ala.com.
17. "State of Smog." *Journal of Property Management*, Vol. 68, No. 4, July–August 2003, p. 11.
18. Gregg, Jillian, et al. "Urbanization Effects on Tree Growth in the Vicinity of New York City." *Nature*, Vol. 10, No. 424, July 2003, p. 183.
19. "Hard Rain Keeps Falling." *National Wildlife*, August–September 2001.
20. "EPA's Acid Rain Program Progress Report." *Air Pollution Consultant*, Vol. 13, No. 2, February 2003, p. 1.
21. "The Facts on Formaldehyde." *Safety Compliance Letter*, June 15, 2003, p. 9.
22. *Second National Report on Human Exposure to Environmental Chemicals*.
23. Brown, Ray. "Mold: The New Asbestos?" *Architecture*, Vol. 92, No. 7, July 2003, p. 32.
24. Fung, F. and W. G. Hughson. "Health Effects on Indoor Fungal Bioaerosol Exposure." *Applied Occupational and Environmental Hygiene*, Vol. 18, No. 7, July 2003, p. 535.
25. Eggleston, P. A. "Environmental Control for Fungal Allergen Exposure." *Current Allergy and Asthma Reports*, Vol. 3, No. 5, September 2003, p. 424.
26. Schober, Susan, et al. "Blood Mercury Levels in U.S. Children and Women of Childbearing Age, 1999–2000." *Journal of the American Medical Association*, Vol. 289, No. 11, April 2, 2003, p. 1667.
27. "Carbon Monoxide Poisoning Guides." *GP*, February 3, 2003, p. 78.
28. "American Radon Scientists Call on EPA to Act on Radon Exposure." *Health and Medicine Week*, June 9, 2003, p. 36.
29. Parmer, Sharon. "Adult Hearing Loss." *Journal of the American Medical Association*, Vol. 289, No. 15, April 16, 2003, p. 2020.
30. Yueh, Bevan, et al. "Screening and Management of Adult Hearing Loss in Primary Care." *Journal of the American Medical Association*, Vol. 289, No. 15, April 16, 2003, p. 1976.
31. "Recent Findings Suggest Urban Setting Means More Noise Exposure and More Hearing Loss." *Facts of Life: Issue Briefing for Health Reporters*, Vol. 6, No. 5, July–August 2001.
32. Lang, Susan. "Even Low-Level Office Noise Can Increase Health Risks." Cornell University News Office, January 22, 2001.
33. "Water, Water, Everywhere." *American Demographics*, October 1, 2001, p. 50.
34. Ibid.
35. Stephenson, Joan. "CDC Report on Environmental Toxins." *Journal of the American Medical Association*, Vol. 289, No. 10, March 12, 2003, p. 1230.
36. "Environmental Cancer Risks." *Cancer Facts & Figures 2003*, American Cancer Society, 2003.
37. "U.S. Study Shows No Link to Pollution." *Medical Devices and Surgical Technology Week*, September 8, 2002, p. 11.
38. "Occupational Use of Pesticides May Be Implicated in Prostate Cancer." *Health and Medicine Week*, September 8, 2003, p. 669.
39. "Parental Exposure to Pesticides Is Not Likely Linked to Childhood Brain Cancer." *Health and Medicine Week*, August 18, 2003, p. 64.
40. Doube, Clare. "Electromagnetic Exposure: Real Risks or Paranoia?" *New Internationalist*, July 2002, p. 7.
41. "Are Cell Phones Safe? Research Hasn't Proved Any Hazards, But There May Be Cause for Concern." *Consumer Reports*, Vol. 68, No. 2, February 2003, p. 24(1).
42. "Radiation Benefits Are Disputed." *Food Ingredient News*, Vol. 11, No. 8, August 2003.

Making this chapter work for you

Answers to multiple choice questions

Chapter 1
1. b; 2. a; 3. d; 4. c; 5. a; 6. d; 7. b; 8. c; 9. d; 10. a

Chapter 2
1. b; 2. d; 3. a; 4. c; 5. c; 6. a; 7. b; 8. a; 9. d; 10. b

Chapter 3
1. b; 2. d; 3. a; 4. a; 5. c; 6. c; 7. b; 8. a; 9. c; 10. d

Chapter 4
1. c; 2. c; 3. b; 4. a; 5. d; 6. c; 7. b; 8. b; 9. a; 10. d

Chapter 5
1. c; 2. a; 3. d; 4. d; 5. b; 6. a; 7. c; 8. a; 9. d; 10. b

Chapter 6
1. d; 2. b; 3. c; 4. c; 5. a; 6. c; 7. d; 8. a; 9. c; 10. b

Chapter 7
1. d; 2. c; 3. b; 4. a; 5. d; 6. a; 7. d; 8. c; 9. c; 10. b

Chapter 8
1. b; 2. d; 3. c; 4. d; 5. d; 6. b; 7. d; 8. c; 9. a; 10. a

Chapter 9
1. c; 2. d; 3. a; 4. c; 5. c; 6. b; 7. d; 8. a; 9. b; 10. d

Chapter 10
1. a; 2. c; 3. d; 4. b; 5. c; 6. c; 7. d; 8. a; 9. b; 10. d

Chapter 11
1. c; 2. b; 3. d; 4. a; 5. b; 6. c; 7. a; 8. d; 9. b; 10. d

Chapter 12
1. a; 2. c; 3. d; 4. b; 5. c; 6. a; 7. d; 8. b; 9. c; 10. d

Chapter 13
1. a; 2. c; 3. d; 4. b; 5. c; 6. a; 7. a; 8. d; 9. b; 10. c

Chapter 14
1. b; 2. c; 3. d; 4. a; 5. a; 6. b; 7. c; 8. d; 9. c; 10. b

Chapter 15
1. d; 2. b; 3. a; 4. d; 5. a; 6. d; 7. b; 8. c; 9. d; 10. a

Chapter 16
1. c; 2. b; 3. d; 4. a; 5. b; 6. c; 7. a; 8. d; 9. d; 10. b

Chapter 17
1. b; 2. a; 3. d; 4. c; 5. b; 6. b; 7. d; 8. c; 9. c; 10. b

Chapter 18
1. d; 2. b; 3. c; 4. b; 5. d; 6. c; 7. b; 8. a; 9. c; 10. b

Chapter 19
1. d; 2. c; 3. b; 4. a; 5. b; 6. c; 7. b; 8. a; 9. d; 10. b

HALES HEALTH

ALMANAC

Contract for Change

Health Information on the Internet

Your Health Directory

Emergency!

A Consumer's Guide to Medical Tests

Counting Your Calories and Fat Grams

My Contract For Change

Date: _____

Personal Goal: _____

_____

Motivating Factors: _____

_____

Change(s) I Promise to Make to Reach This Goal:

_____

Plan for Making This Change: _____

_____

_____

Start Date: _____

Assessment Plan: _____

_____

_____

_____

If I Need Help: _____

_____

_____

Target Date for Reaching Goal: _____

Reward for Achieving Goal: _____

Penalty for Failing to Achieve Goal: _____

_____

Signed: _____

Witnessed By: _____

◼ Using the Internet

What are the very latest statistics on the incidence of AIDS? Are any new drugs in the works for the treatment of diabetes? How can I get in touch with others who suffer from asthma? Is it possible to make a low-fat chocolate cake? You can answer these kinds of questions from your home or computer lab, with the help of the Internet. A gold mine of information for the student of health, the Internet can help you with research for your schoolwork and also with personal questions and concerns about your own health. But the Internet is not comprehensively catalogued, and finding information can be daunting. This guide will introduce you to health resources on the Internet and how to find them.

What are the practical uses of the Internet for the student of health and the health care consumer?

- **Research.** The Internet is a repository for many health journals, government statistics, archives, and other sources of scholarly information. Subscribing to a mailing list or posting to a newsgroup in an area of interest can yield new sources of information that would be hard to get elsewhere.
- **Self-help and support.** Dozens of newsgroups and mailing lists offer support and advice for people dealing with all kinds of health-related issues, from Alzheimer's caregivers to people with eating disorders to athletes comparing training programs.
- **Goods and services.** Online shopping for health-related products is easy.
- **Graduate school and career information.** If you are interested in a career in a health-related field, most graduate schools have websites that list their programs, entrance requirements, faculty profiles, and other information of interest to prospective students. And you can consult online listings of jobs available in many areas of health care.

The World Wide Web

The World Wide Web is an information retrieval system with a user-friendly graphic interface with the Internet. You can surf the Web using any one of a number of different browsers, such as Netscape or Internet Explorer. Each website has its own unique address, or URL. To go to a website, type its URL into the box at the top of your browser or click on a hyperlink from another page that will take you to the new site. Hyperlinks often appear as color or underlined text and offer links to other websites. (If you want more information or further definitions for web-related terms, go to www.webopedia.com.)

Thousands of websites are related to health and wellness. As a starting point, go to any of the sources listed in the Sites & Bytes in this book or at this book's website at http://health.wadsworth.com. Or you can look for specific information by doing a web search.

Bookmarks

When you find a website you will want to return to again, "bookmark" it. To bookmark a site, go to that site and choose "bookmark" from your menu bar. Your browser will record the address of that site in your bookmark folder. Anytime you want to return to that site, you simply open the bookmark folder and click on the title of that website.

Tips for Using the World Wide Web

- **Be patient.** Accessing a website can take time depending on how elaborate the site is, how fast your connection is, and what time of day you are surfing. You can speed things up a bit by not showing images (check your browser Preferences).
- **Keep in mind that glitches can occur in the transfer process.** Sometimes the server of the website you are trying to reach may be down, there may be a lot of activity on that site, or there may be line noise. Try again later.
- **Sites and links change every day.** Links won't work if the link has moved to a new server or address.
- **Remember that not everything on the web is true.** It is up to you to evaluate the information you get from the Web; see the section on Thinking Critically about Health Information on the Internet.

Searching the Web

One way to find websites of interest to you is to use a search engine. A search engine allows you to type in key words on the topic you are interested in, and it will retrieve sites that contain those words. Some of the larger and more popular search engines are:

- **Google**   www.google.com
- **Yahoo!**   www.yahoo.com

- **AltaVista**   www.altavista.com
- **Excite**   www.excite.com
- **Lycos**   www.lycos.com
- **WebCrawler**   webcrawler.com

To use a search engine, type in one of the URLs listed above. When the home page for the site comes up, type one or more key words or phrases into the "search" box. The engine will then search all the sites in its index and return a list to you, with hyperlinks and sometimes short descriptions, of those that contain your key words.

No single search engine contains all the contents of the Internet. After connecting to a search engine for the first time, it is a good idea to read the tool's description, search options, and rules and restrictions. Each engine offers a different "view" of the Web and you'll want to tailor your query to make the best use of that system.

The key to an effective search is picking the right key words. Commonly used words make poor search key words; try to find distinctive words or combinations of words. If you use several key words, check your search engine's searching tips—in most cases you can use the plus sign, the minus sign, quotation marks and the word OR to make your search more precise. For example, the word "OR" broadens the search results. You may try searching "pregnancy teen OR adolescent," to find sites that refer to teen or adolescent pregnancy.

Your search may turn up hundreds or even thousands of results—or only a few. If you have more results than you can handle, try making the key words in your search more precise or go to your search engine's advanced search section. If you have too few results, try another search engine, using synonyms or variations on your key words, or be less specific in your query.

News Groups/Discussion Forums

News groups and discussion forums are ways of discussing topics over the Internet with other people who share the same interests or concerns. They are a popular way to establish an online community, share information, and give and receive support. For example, a person suffering from a relatively rare disorder may not know anyone else with the same problems and concerns on campus or in town, but he or she can frequent a news group specifically for people with that disorder to learn about other peoples' experiences, the latest treatments, and just to commiserate. Or a person who is trying to quit smoking can participate in a news group to share frustrations, tips, and successes. But, as always, be aware that not everything posted to a news group is necessarily true; you must be a critical thinker.

Many commercial online services offer members-only news groups to their subscribers, but many other news groups are available to anyone. To find a news group on a topic of interest to you, try going to http://groups.google.com.

News group addresses are grouped into several broad categories called hierarchies. Listed below are some of the standard hierarchies that relate to health.

- **alt**   groups generally alternative in nature (i.e., alt.sex)
- **bionet**   groups discussing biology and biological sciences (i.e., bionet.immunology)
- **misc**   groups that don't fit into other categories (i.e., misc.fitness)
- **rec**   groups discussing hobbies, sports, music, and art (i.e., rec.food)
- **sci**   groups discussing subjects related to the science and scientific research (i.e., sci.epidemiology)
- **soc**   groups discussing social issues including politics, social programs, etc. (i.e., soc.college)
- **talk**   public debating forums on controversial issues (i.e., talk.abortion)

Before you make a posting to a news group, you may want to "lurk" for awhile, that is, read the discussion without contributing your own posting. Lurking will give you a sense of the kinds of postings that are appropriate for that news group and what the news group culture is like. Read the news group's "FAQ," or list of answers to frequently asked questions before joining the discussion.

Postings to many news groups are updated frequently, so if an item is of interest to you, you should print it or save it to your computer since it may be gone the next day. After lurking for awhile, you can join in the discussion by posting a message to the news group. You may also want to reply only to the originator of a certain message. You may want to join in on the discussion of an already-existing topic, or start your own "thread."

Be cautious when providing your e-mail address to a site or news group. Spam is junk e-mail, and spammers scoop up e-mail addresses in news groups and chat rooms.

Mailing Lists

You are probably already on a few mailing lists—they are used by retailers, organizations, politicians, educational institutions, and many other groups who e-mail large numbers of people. But mailing lists (or list serves) are also groups of people who "get together" via e-mail to discuss a specific topic. Mailing lists offer a way to participate in lively discussions, stay up on current research, or find out answers to burning questions. There are mailing lists on nearly every topic imaginable. Mailing lists are similar to news groups in that they are forums for discussion, but the messages are delivered to your e-mail account instead of to a public bulletin board. Here's how it works:

- First, find a mailing list dealing with a subject you are interested in discussing with others (i.e., attention deficit disorder).
- Then, you have to subscribe: send an e-mail to that mailing list's "subscribe" address with the word "sub-

scribe" in the subject line and in the main body of the text.

- Usually, the mailing list will then subscribe you to the list and send you instructions on how to "post" to the group. "Posting" means that you send out a comment to the entire mailing list that you have subscribed to.
- Every time any member posts to the list serve, all the subscribers get that posting as an e-mail message.
- Once you have subscribed you will begin to receive e-mail messages from the mailing list. Be careful though: Some discussion groups have a large following and you may find your mailbox filling up faster than you can read the messages.
- Again, evaluate carefully any information you get from a mailing list to make sure it is accurate.

Thinking Critically About Health Information on the Internet

Unlike information in most books and journals, anyone can post information or advice on the Internet. Some of this information can be misleading or downright harmful, so it is important to use your best critical thinking skills to evaluate health information you find on the Internet. Ask yourself the following questions:

- *Who is the author or sponsor of the information?* The author of the site is usually listed at the top or bottom of a site's home page. Be very wary of any anonymous site. Sites that are maintained by established schools or universities, government agencies, professional organizations, or other established organizations like the American Cancer Society are probably trustworthy. Sites created by individuals or other groups may or may not contain valid information; see if you can verify their information in other places.
- *Is it current?* Many sites post the date of their last update. Look for sites where you can determine when the information was created or modified; many of the best sites are updated weekly or even daily.
- *What is the purpose of the site?* The hidden purpose of some health websites is to sell products or act as a vehicle for advertisements. Be wary of any site that tries to sell you things or get your money. Also beware of sites that seem to be trying to persuade you of things, promote "miracle cures" or anything that seems too good to be true. Some people also use news groups and other chat forums to sell or persuade. Be skeptical and use your common sense.
- *Who is the intended audience?* Some Internet information is intended for doctors and other health-care professionals; although the information may be accurate, it may be too difficult for a layperson to interpret. Other web-

sites or Internet forums are targeted toward people with specific problems or disorders, students, or the general public.

- *Is the information verifiable?* To get a better perspective on information from the Internet, see if you can verify it with other sources. Before you follow any health advice you get from the Net, check it out with your physician.

Health Resources on the Internet

"Your Health Directory" (next pages) contains web addresses for many health-related organizations. And hundreds of health-related Internet addresses can be found at http://health.wadsworth.com.

In *An Invitation to Health,* I emphasize that you shoulder a great deal of responsibility for your health and the quality of your life. Given the complexity of our minds and bodies and the many social and environmental factors that affect us, this responsibility can be a very heavy burden. But your load can be made lighter if you know where to turn for health information, services, and support.

In this directory, you will find more than 100 health-related topics and about 250 resources, including addresses, phone numbers, and websites for government agencies, community organizations, professional associations, recovery groups, and Internet sources. Many of these organizations and groups have toll-free 800 or 888 phone numbers, and most have websites (one caution: as you may have experienced, website addresses—like street addresses and phone numbers—change on occasion). Much of the material available from these groups is free.

Also included in Your Health Directory are clearinghouses and information centers that are especially rich sources of health knowledge. Their main purpose is to collect, help manage, and disseminate information. Clearinghouses often perform other services as well, such as creating original publications and providing tailored responses to individual requests. These organizations also may provide referrals to other groups that can help you.

Many of the groups listed here have local offices or chapters. You can call, write, or visit the websites of these organizations to find out if there is a branch in your vicinity, or you can check your local telephone directory.

The purpose of this directory is to help you be in control of your health. If you know where to turn for answers to your questions and if you know what choices you have, you may find that you have more control over your life.

Resources by Topic

Abortion

National Abortion Federation
(provides information about abortion and referral for abortion services)
1755 Massachusetts Ave., N.W. Suite #600
Washington, DC 20036
(202) 667-5881
(800) 772-9100
www.prochoice.org

Accident Prevention

Centers for Disease Control and Prevention
1600 Clifton Rd. N.E.
Atlanta, GA 30333
(404) 639-3311
www.cdc.gov

National Safety Council
1121 Spring Lake Dr.
Itasca, IL 60143-3201
(630) 285-1121
(800) 621-7619
www.nsc.org

Adoption

AASK (Adopt a Special Kid)
(provides assistance to families who adopt older and handicapped children)
1025 N. Reynolds Rd.
Toledo, OH 43615
(800) 246-1731
(419) 534-3350
www.adoptamerica.org

Aging

Administration on Aging
U.S. Department of Health and Human Services
200 Independence Ave., S.W.
Washington, DC 20201
(800) 677-1116 (Eldercare Locator—to find services for an older person in his or her locality)
(202) 619-0724 (AoA's National Aging Information Center)
Fax: (202) 260-1012
E-mail: aoainfo@aoa.gov
www.aoa.gov

American Association of Retired Persons
601 E St., N.W.
Washington, DC 20049
(800) 424-3410
(202) 434-2277
www.aarp.org

Gray Panthers
733 15th St., N.W., Suite 437
Washington, DC 20005
(800) 280-5362
(202) 737-6637
www.graypanthers.org

AIDS (Acquired Immunodeficiency Syndrome)

National Center for HIV, STD, and TB Prevention (NCHSTP)

Centers for Disease Control and Prevention
1600 Clifton Rd. N.E.
Atlanta, GA 30333
(800) 311-3435
(404) 639-3311
www.cdc.gov/hiv/dhap.htm

University of California at San Francisco HIV Insite
4150 Clement St., Bldg. 16 VAMC 111V-UCSF
San Francisco, CA 94121
Fax: (415) 379-5547
E-mail: info@hivinsite.ucsf.edu
www.hivinsite.ucsf.edu

Gay Men's Health Crisis
119 West 24th St.
New York, NY 10011
(800) 243-7692
(212) 807-6664
www.gmhc.org

National AIDS Hotline
(800) 342-2437

San Francisco AIDS Foundation
995 Market St. #200
San Francisco, CA 94103
(415) 487-3000
www.sfaf.org

Alcohol Abuse and Alcoholism

Al-Anon and Alateen
(support groups for friends and relatives of alcoholics)
1600 Corporate Landing Pkwy.

Virginia Beach, VA 23454
(888) 425-2666
(757) 499-1443
www.al-anon-alateen.org
See also white pages of telephone directory
for listing of local chapter

Alcohol Hotline
(800) ALCOHOL

Alcoholics Anonymous
475 Riverside Dr., 11th Floor
New York, NY 10115
(212) 647-1680
www.alcoholics-anonymous.org
See also white pages or telephone directory
for listing of local chapter

National Association of Children of Alcoholics
11426 Rockville Pike, Suite 100
Rockville, MD 20852
(888) 554-COAS (554-2627)
(301) 468-0985
www.nacoa.org

National Clearinghouse for Alcohol and Drug Information
P.O. Box 2345
Rockville, MD 20847-2345
(800) 729-6686
(301) 468-2600
www.health.org/

National Institute on Alcohol Abuse and Alcoholism
6000 Executive Blvd.
Willco Building
Bethesda, MD 20892-7003
(301) 443-3860
www.niaaa.nih.gov
See also Drug Abuse; Drinking & Driving
Groups

Allopathic Medicine

American Medical Association
515 N. State St.
Chicago, IL 60610
(312) 464-5000
www.ama-assn.org

Alternative Medicine

National Center for Complementary and Alternative Medicine (NCCAM)
P.O. Box 7923
Gaithersburg, MD 20898
(888) 644-6226
International: (301) 519-3153
TTY: (866) 464-3615 (toll-free)
www.nccam.nih.gov

Alzheimer's Disease

Alzheimer's Association
National Office
919 N. Michigan Ave., Suite 1000

Chicago, IL 60611-1676
(800) 272-3900
(312) 335-8700
www.alz.org

Arthritis

Arthritis Foundation
1330 West Peachtree St.
Atlanta, GA 30309
(800) 283-7800
(404) 872-7100
www.arthritis.org

National Institute of Arthritis and Musculoskeletal and Skin Diseases
National Institutes of Health
1 Ams Circle
Bethesda, MD 20892-3675
(301) 495-4484
(877) 22-NIAMS (226-4267)
E-mail: NIAMSInfo@mail.nih.gov
www.nih.gov/niams

Asthma

Asthma and Allergy Foundation of America
1233 20th St., N.W., Suite 402
Washington, DC 20036
(800) 7-ASTHMA (727-8462)
(202) 466-7643
Fax: (202) 466-8940
www.aafa.org

Lung Line
National Jewish Medical Research Center
(information and referral service)
1400 Jackson St.
Denver, CO 80206
(800) 222-5864
(303) 388-4461
www.njc.org

Attention Deficit Disorder

National Attention Deficit Disorder Association (National ADDA)
1788 Second St., Suite 200
Highland Park, IL 60035
(847) 432-ADDA
www.add.org

Children and Adults with Attention Deficit Disorder (CHADD)
8181 Professional Place, Suite 201
Landover, MD 20785
(800) 233-4050
(301) 306-7070
www.chadd.org/

Automobile Safety

American Automobile Association (AAA)
1000 AAA Dr. #28
Heathrow, FL 32746-5080
(407) 444-4240

www.aaa.com
See also white or yellow pages of telephone directory for listing of local
chapter

Insurance Institute for Highway Safety
1005 North Glebe Rd., Suite 800
Arlington, VA 22201
(703) 247-1500
www.highwaysafety.org/

National Highway Traffic Safety Administration
Office of Publications
400 7th St., S.W.
Washington, DC 20590
(888) 327-4236
(202) 366-0123
www.nhtsa.dot.gov

Auto Safety Hotline
(for consumer complaints about auto safety and child safety seats, and requests for
information on recalls)
(800) 424-9393

Birth Control and Family Planning

Advocates for Youth
(develops programs and material to educate youth on sex and sexual
responsibility)
1025 Vermont Ave. N.W., Suite 200
Washington, DC 20005
(202) 347-5700
Fax: (202) 347-2263
E-mail: info@advocatesforyouth.org
www.advocatesforyouth.org

American College of Obstetricians and Gynecologists
(provides literature and contraceptive
information)
409 12th Street, S.W.
P.O. Box 96920
Washington, DC 20090-6920
(202) 638-5577
www.acog.com

Engender Health
(provides information and referrals to individuals considering tubal ligation or
vasectomy)
440 Ninth Ave.
New York, NY 10001
(212) 561-8000
www.engenderhealth.org

Planned Parenthood Federation of America (PPFA)
434 West 33rd St.
New York, NY 10001
(212) 541-7800
www.plannedparenthood.org
See also white or yellow pages of telephone directory for listing of local
chapter

Birth Defects

Cystic Fibrosis Foundation (CFF)
6931 Arlington Rd.
Bethesda, MD 20814
(800) FIGHT-CF (344-4823)
(301) 951-4422
Fax: (301) 951-6378
www.cff.org

**March of Dimes Birth Defects
Foundation**
1275 Mamaroneck Ave.
White Plains, NY 10605
(888) 663-4637
(914) 428-7100
www.modimes.org

Blindness

American Foundation for the Blind
11 Penn Plaza, Suite 300
New York, NY 10001
(800) AFB-LINE (232-5463)
(212) 502-7600
www.afb.org

National Federation of the Blind
1800 Johnson St.
Baltimore, MD 21230
(800) 638-7518
(410) 659-9314
www.nfb.org

**National Library Service for the
Blind and Physically Handicapped**
Library of Congress
1291 Taylor St., N.W.
Washington, DC 20011
(800) 424-8567
(202) 707-5100
www.loc.gov/nls

Blood Banks

American Red Cross
431 18th St., N.W.
Washington, DC 20006
(202) 639-3520
www.redcross.org
See also white or yellow pages of telephone directory for listing of local
chapter

Breast Cancer

Reach to Recovery
(support program for women who have
undergone mastectomies as a result of
breast cancer)
American Cancer Society
2200 Lake Blvd.
Atlanta, GA 30319
(800) 227-2345
(404) 816-7800
www.cancer.org

Cancer

American Cancer Society
American Cancer Society
2200 Lake Blvd.
Atlanta, GA 30319
(800) 227-2345
(404) 816-7800
www.cancer.org

Cancer Information Service
National Cancer Institute
Suite 3036A
6116 Executive Blvd.
Bethesda, MD 20892
(800) 4-CANCER (422-6237)
(301) 435-3848
www.cis.nci.nih.gov/

**Leukemia & Lymphoma Society of
America**
1311 Mamaroneck Ave.
White Plains, NY 10605
(914) 949-5213
Fax: (914) 949-6691
www.leukemia.org

**National Coalition for Cancer
Survivorship**
1010 Wayne Ave., Suite 770
Silver Spring, MD 20910-5600
(301) 650-9127
(877) NCCS-YES (622-7937)
Fax: (301) 565-9670
www.canceradvocacy.org

**R. A. Bloch Cancer Foundation
(Cancer Connection)**
(support group that matches cancer
patients with volunteers who are cured,
in remission, or being treated for same
type of cancer)
4400 Main St.
Kansas City, MO 64111
(800) 433-0464
(816) 932-8453
www.blochcancer.org

Child Abuse

National Child Assault Prevention
(provides services to children, adolescents,
mentally retarded adults, and elderly)
606 Delsea Drive
Sewell, NJ 08080
(800) 258-3189
www.ncap.org

National Child Abuse Hotline
(800) 422-4453

**National Committee for the
Prevention of Child Abuse**
(provides literature on child abuse prevention programs)
200 S. Michigan Ave., 17th Floor
Chicago, IL 60604-2404
(312) 663-3520
www.preventchildabuse.org

Parents Anonymous
(self-help group for abusive parents)
675 W. Foothill Blvd., Suite 220
Claremont, CA 91711-3475
(909) 621-6184
Fax: (909) 625-6304
www.parentsanonymous.org

Childbirth

American College of Nurse-Midwives
(R.N.s who provide services through the
maternity cycle)
818 Connecticut Ave., N.W.
Suite 900
Washington, DC 20006
(202) 728-9860
www.midwife.org

**American College of Obstetricians
and Gynecologists**
409 12th St., S.W.
P.O. Box 96920
Washington, DC 20090-6920
(202) 638-5577
www.acog.com

Lamaze International
2025 M St., Suite 800
Washington, DC 20036-3309
(800) 368-4404
(202) 367-1128
Fax: (202) 367-2128
www.lamaze-childbirth.com

**International Childbirth Education
Association**
P.O. Box 20048
Minneapolis, MN 55420
(952) 854-8660
Fax: (952) 854-8772
www.icea.org

Child Health and Development

**National Center for Education in
Maternal and Child Health**
Georgetown University
Box 571272
Washington, DC 20007-2292
(202) 784-9770
Fax: (202) 784-9777
www.ncemch.org

**National Institute of Child Health &
Human Development**
Bldg. 31, Rm. 2A32, MSC 2425
31 Center Dr.
Bethesda, MD 20892-2425
(800) 370-2943
www.nichd.nih.gov

Chiropractic

American Chiropractic Association
1701 Clarendon Blvd.
Arlington, VA 22209

(800) 986-4632
Fax: (703) 243-2593
www.amerchiro.org

Consumer Information

Federal Consumer Information Center
(catalog of publications developed by federal agencies for consumers)
Department WWW
Pueblo, CO 81009
(888) 878-3256
www.pueblo.gsa.gov

U.S. Consumer Product Safety Commission
Office of Information Services
4330 East-West Highway
Bethesda, MD 20814-4408
(800) 638-2772
(301) 504-6816
Fax: (301) 504-0124 and (301) 504-0025
E-mail: info@cpsc.gov
www.cpsc.gov

Consumers Union of United States
(tests quality and safety of consumer products: publishes *Consumer Reports* magazine)
101 Truman Ave.
Yonkers, NY 10703
(914) 378-2000
www.consumerreports.org

Council of Better Business Bureaus
4200 Wilson Blvd., Suite 800
Arlington, VA 22203-1804
(703) 276-0100
Fax: (703) 525-8277
www.bbb.org
See also white or yellow pages of telephone directory for listing of local chapter

Food and Drug Administration (FDA)
Office of Consumer Affairs
Consumer Inquiries
5600 Fishers Lane
Rockville, MD 20857
(888) INFO-FDA (463-6332)
www.fda.gov

Crime Victims

Crisis Prevention Institute, Inc.
(offers programs on nonviolent physical crisis interventions)
3315-K North 124th St.
Brookfield, WI 53005
(800) 558-8976 (U.S. and Canada)
(262) 783-5787
www.crisisprevention.com

National Center for Victims of Crime
2000 M Street, N.W., Suite 480
Washington, DC 20010

(202) 467-8700
Fax: (202) 467-8701
www.ncvc.org

Death and Grieving

Share
(support group for parents who have lost a newborn)
c/o St. Joseph's Health Center
300 First Capitol Dr.
St. Charles, MO 63301-2893
(800) 821-6819
(636) 947-6164
www.nationalshareoffice.com

Dental Health

American Dental Association (ADA)
211 E. Chicago Ave.
Chicago, IL 60611
(312) 440-2500
www.ada.org

National Institute of Dental Research
Public Information & Liaison Branch
45 Center Dr., MSC 6400
Bethesda, MD 20892-6400
(301) 496-4261
www.nidr.nih.gov

Depressive Disorders

American Psychiatric Association
1000 Wilson Blvd., Suite 1825
Arlington, VA 22209-3901
(888) 357-7924
(703) 907-7300
E-mail: apa@psych.org
www.psych.org

American Psychological Association
750 First St., N.E.
Washington, DC 20002-4242
(800) 374-2721
(202) 336-5510
TDD/TTY: (202) 336-6123
www.apa.org

Depression & Bipolar Support Alliance
730 N. Franklin, Suite 501
Chicago, IL 60610-7204
(800) 826-3632
(312) 642-0049
Fax: (312) 642-7243
www.dbsalliance.org

DES (Diethylstibestrol)

DES Action, USA
(support group for persons exposed to DES)
610 16th St., Suite 301
Oakland, CA 94612
(510) 465-4011
Fax: (510) 465-4815
www.desaction.org

Diabetes

American Diabetes Association
National Center
1701 North Beauregard St.
Alexandria, VA 22311
(800) DIABETES (342-2383)
(703) 549-1500
www.diabetes.org

Juvenile Diabetes Research Foundation International (JDRFI)
120 Wall St.
New York, NY 10005-4001
(800) JDF-CURE (533-2873)
(212) 785-9500
Fax: (212) 785-9595
www.jdfcure.org

National Diabetes Information Clearinghouse
1 Information Way
Bethesda, MD 20892-3560
(800) 860-8747
(301) 654-3327
E-mail: ndic@info.niddk.nih.gov
www.niddk.nih.gov/health/diabetes/ndic.htm

Digestive Diseases

National Institute of Diabetes & Digestive & Kidney Diseases (NIDDK)
Office of Communication & Public Liaison
NIDDK, NIH, Building 31
Room 9A04 Center Dr., MSC 2560
Bethesda, MD 20892-2560
(301) 654-3810
www.niddk.nih.gov

Disabled Services

American Alliance for Health, Physical Education, Recreation & Dance (AAHPERD)
(provides information about recreation and fitness opportunities for the disabled)
1900 Association Drive
Reston, VA 20191-1598
(800) 213-7193
Fax: (703) 476-9527
www.aahperd.org

National Library Service for the Blind and Physically Handicapped
Library of Congress
1291 Taylor St., N.W.
Washington, DC 20011
(800) 424-8567
(202) 707-5100
TDD: (202) 707-0744
Fax: (202) 707-0712
www.loc.gov/nls

Special Olympics International (SOI)
1325 G St., N.W.
Suite 500
Washington, DC 20005
(202) 628-3630
Fax: (202) 824-0200
www.specialolympics.org

Domestic Violence

National Coalition Against Domestic Violence (NCADV)
P.O. Box 18749
Denver, CO 80218
(303) 839-1852
Fax: (303) 831-9851
www.ncadv.org

National Domestic Violence Hotline
(800) 799-SAFE (799-7233)

National Network to End Domestic Violence
660 Pennsylvania, SE, Suite 303
Washington, DC 20003
(202) 543-5566
www.nnedv.org

Down Syndrome

National Association for Down Syndrome (NADS)
P.O. Box 4542
Oak Brook, IL 60522-4542
(630) 325-9112
www.nads.org

National Down Syndrome Society
666 Broadway, 8th Floor
New York, NY 10012-2317
(800) 221-4602
(212) 460-9330
www.ndss.org

Drug Abuse

Cocaine Anonymous World Services
P.O. Box 2000
Los Angeles, CA 90049-8000 or
3740 Overland Ave., Ste. C
Los Angeles, CA 90034
(800) 347-8998
(310) 559-5833
www.ca.org

Narcotics Anonymous (NA)
(support group for recovering narcotics
   addicts)
P.O. Box 9999
Van Nuys, CA 91409
(818) 773-9999
Fax: (818) 700-0700
www.na.org
See also white or yellow pages of telephone directory for local chapter

National Cocaine Hotline
(800) COCAINE (262-2463)

National Institute on Drug Abuse
6001 Executive Blvd., Room 5213
Bethesda, MD 20892-9651
(301) 443-1124
Helpline: (800) 662-4357
www.nida.nih.gov

National Parents Resource Institute for Drug Education (PRIDE)
166 St. Charles St.
Bowling Green, KY 42101
(800) 279-6361
Fax: (270) 746-9598
www.prideusa.org

Center for Substance Abuse Prevention (CSAP)
Substance Abuse and Mental Health
   Administration
5600 Fishers Lane
Rockwall 2 Bldg.
Rockville, MD 20857
(301) 443-8956
www.prevention.samhsa.gov

Drinking and Driving Groups

Mothers Against Drunk Driving
511 E. John Carpenter Frwy., Suite 700
Irving, TX 75062
(800) GET-MADD (438-6233)
(214) 744-6233
www.madd.org
See also white or yellow pages of telephone directory for local chapter

Students Against Destructive Decisions (also Students Against Driving Drunk (SADD))
Box 800
Marlboro, MA 01752
(877) SADD-INC (723-3462)
(508) 481-3568
Fax: (508) 481-5759
www.saddonline.com

Eating Disorders

National Eating Disorders Association (NEDA)
(self-help groups that provide information
   and referrals to physicians and therapists)
603 Stewart St., Suite 803
Seattle, WA 98101
(800) 931-2237
(206) 382-3587
www.nationaleatingdisorders.org

Anorexia Nervosa and Related Eating Disorders (ANRED)
(provides information and referrals for
   people with eating disorders)
P.O. Box 5102
Eugene, OR 97405
(541) 344-1144
www.anred.com

Environment

U.S. Environmental Protection Agency (EPA)
Ariel Rios Bldg.
1200 Pennsylvania Ave., N.W.
Washington, DC 20460
(202) 260-2090
www.epa.gov

Greenpeace, USA
702 H St. N.W.
Washington, DC 20001
(800) 326-0959
(202) 462-1177
www.greenpeaceusa.org

Natural Resources Defense Council
40 West 20th St.
New York, NY 10011
(212) 727-2700
Fax: (212) 727-1773
www.nrdc.org

Sierra Club
85 2nd St., 2nd Floor
San Francisco, CA 94105-3441
(415) 977-5500
(415) 977-5799
www.sierraclub.org

World Wildlife Fund
1250 24th St., N.W.
P.O. Box 97180
Washington, DC 20090-7180
(800) CALL-WWF (225-5993)
(202) 293-4800
Fax: (202) 293-2911
www.wwfus.org

Epilepsy

Epilepsy Foundation of America
4351 Garden City Drive
Landover, MD 20785-7223
(800) EFA-1000 (332-1000)
(301) 459-3700
www.efa.org

Gay and Lesbian Organizations and Services

Human Rights Campaign
919 18th St., N.W., Suite 800
Washington, DC 20006
(202) 628-4160
Fax: (202) 347-5323
www.hrc.org

National Gay and Lesbian Task Force (NGLTF)
1325 Massachusetts Ave., N.W., Suite 600
Washington, DC, 20005
(202) 393-5177
Fax: (202) 393-2241
www.ngltf.org

Parents, Families, and Friends of Lesbians and Gays (PFLAG)
1726 M St., N.W., Suite 400
Washington, DC 20036
(202) 467-8180
Fax: (202) 467-8194
www.pflag.org

Genetics

American College of Medical Genetics
9650 Rockville Pike
Bethesda, MD 20814-3998
(301) 634-7127
Fax: (301) 571-0677
E-mail: acmg@faseb.org
www.acmg.net

The Human Genome Organization
HUGO Americas
Laboratory of Genetics
National Institute on Aging
NIH/NIA-IRP. GRC, Box 31
5600 Nathan Shock Dr.
Baltimore, MD 21224-6825
(410) 558-8337
Fax: (410) 558-8331
E-mail: schlessingerd@grc.nia.nih.gov

GeneTests—GeneClinics
(a database of information for patients and families with genetic disorders, providing access to support groups)
University of Washington School of Medicine
Seattle, WA
www.genetests.org

Hazardous Waste

Environmental Protection Agency (EPA)
Ariel Rios Bldg.
1200 Pennsylvania Ave., N.W.
Washington, DC 20460
(202) 260-2090
www.epa.gov

Hazardous Waste Hotline Information
(800) 424-9346

Health Care

Association for Applied and Therapeutic Humor (AATH)
(publishes a newsletter and sponsors seminars for people in the helping professions)
1951 W. Camelback Rd., Suite 445
Phoenix, AZ 85015
(602) 995-1454
FAX: (602) 995-1449
www.aath.org

American Medical Association
515 N. State St.
Chicago, IL 60610
(312) 464-5000
www.ama-assn.org

American Nurses Association
600 Maryland Ave., S.W.
Suite 100 West
Washington, DC 20024-2571
(800) 274-4ANA (274-4262)
(202) 651-7000
www.ana.org

Health Education

National Center for Chronic Disease Prevention and Health Promotion
Centers for Disease Control and Prevention
Mail Stop A34
1600 Clifton Rd., N.E.
Atlanta, GA 30333
(404) 639-3534
(800) 311-3435
www.cdc.gov/nccdphp

Hearing Impairment

American Society for Deaf Children
(resource group for parents of hard of hearing and deaf children)
P.O. Box 3355
Gettysburg, PA 17325
(717) 334-7922
Fax: (717) 334-8808
(800) 942-ASDC (Parent Hotline)
www.deafchildren.org

Better Hearing Institute (BHI)
(provides educational and resource materials on deafness)
Better Hearing Institute
515 King St., Suite 420
Alexandria, VA 22314
(703) 684-3391
www.betterhearing.org

Heart Disease

American Heart Association (AHA)
7272 Greenville Ave.
Dallas, TX 75231
(800) 242-8721
(214) 373-6300
www.americanheart.org

National Heart, Lung, and Blood Institute
(provides information on cardiovascular risk factors and disease)
Bldg. 31, Room 5A52
31 Center Dr., MSC 2486
Bethesda, MD 20892
(800) 575-9355
(301) 592-8573
www.nhlbi.nih.gov/index.htm

Helping Others

United Way of America
701 N. Fairfax St.
Alexandria, VA 22314-2045
(703) 836-7100
www.unitedway.org

Hospice

The National Hospice and Palliative Care Organization
1700 Diagonal Rd., Suite 625
Alexandria, VA 22314
(703) 837-1500
(800) 646-6460
www.nhpco.org

Immunization

National Immunization Program
Centers for Disease Control
Mail Stop E-05
1600 Clifton Rd., N.E.
Atlanta, GA 30333
(404) 639-3311
(800) 232-2522
www.cdc.gov/nip/diseases/adult-vpd.htm

Immunization Action Coalition
(information for children, adolescents, and adults)
1573 Selby Ave., Suite 234
St. Paul, MN 55104
(651) 647-9009
Fax: (651) 647-9131
www.immunize.org

Infant Care

La Leche League International
(provides information and support to women interested in breast-feeding)
1400 N. Meacham Rd.
Schaumburg, IL 60168-4079
(800) LA-LECHE (525-3243)
(847) 519-7730
www.lalecheleague.org

Infectious Diseases

Centers for Disease Control and Prevention
1600 Clifton Rd., N.E.
Atlanta, GA 30333
(800) 311-3435
(404) 639-3534
www.cdc.gov

Infertility

Resolve: The National Infertility Association
(offers counseling, information, and support to people with problems of infertility)

1310 Broadway
Somerville, MA 02144-1779
(888) 623-0744
(617) 623-0744
www.resolve.org

Kidney Disease

American Kidney Fund (AKF)
(provides information on financial aid to
patients, organ transplants, and kidney-
related diseases)
6110 Executive Blvd., Suite 1010
Rockville, MD 20852
(800) 638-8299
(301) 881-3052
www.akfinc.org

**American Association of Kidney
Patients (AAKP)**
3505 E. Frontage Rd., Suite 315
Tampa, FL 33607
(800) 749-2257
Fax: (813) 636-8122
www.aakp.org

National Kidney Foundation (NKF)
30 East 33rd St., Suite 1100
New York, NY 10016
(800) 622-9010
(212) 889-2210
Fax: (212) 689-9261
www.kidney.org

Liver Disease

American Liver Foundation (ALF)
75 Maiden, Suite 603
New York, NY 10038
(800) 465-4837
(212) 668-1000
www.liverfoundation.org/

Lung Disease

American Lung Association
61 Broadway, 6th Floor
New York, NY 10006
(212) 315-8700
www.lungusa.org

**National Heart, Lung, and Blood
Institute**
(provides information on cardiovascular
risk factors and disease)
Bldg. 31, Room 5A52
31 Center Dr., MSC 2486
Bethesda, MD 20892
(800) 575-9355
www.nhlbi.nih.gov/index.htm

Lupus Erythematosus

Lupus Foundation of America (LPA)
1300 Piccard Dr., Suite 200
Rockville, MD 20850-4303
(301) 670-9292

(800) 558-0121
www.lupus.org/lupus/index.html

Marriage and Family

**Women Work! The National Network
for Women's Employment**
(national advocacy group for women over
35 who have lost their primary means
of support through death, divorce, or
disabling of spouse)
1625 K St. N.W., Suite 300
Washington, DC 20006
(202) 467-6346
www.womenwork.org

Alliance for Children & Families
11700 West Lake Park Dr.
Milwaukee, WI 53224-3099
(414) 359-1040
Fax: (414) 359-1074
E-mail: info@alliance1.org
www.alliance1.org

Stepfamily Association of America
(provides information and publishes quarterly newsletter)
650 J St., Suite 205
Lincoln, NE 68508
(800) 735-0329
(402) 477-7837
Fax: (402) 477-8317
www.stepfam.org

Medications

(Prescriptions and Over-the-Counter)

**Food and Drug Administration
(FDA)**
Office of Consumer Affairs Public
Inquiries
5600 Fishers Lane (HFE-88)
Rockville, MD 20857-0001
(888) 463-6332 (INFO-FDA)
www.fda.gov

Mental Health

American Psychiatric Association
1000 Wilson Blvd., Suite 125
Arlington, VA 22209
(888) 357-7924
(703) 907-7300
E-mail: apa@psych.org
www.psych.org

American Psychological Association
750 First St., N.E.
Washington, DC 20002-4242
(800) 374-2721
(202) 336-5510
TDD/TTY: (202) 336-6123
www.apa.org

American Psychoanalytic Foundation
9 Breakers Isle
Dana Point, CA 92629

(503) 244-5700
E-mail: APF@cyberpsych.org
www.cyberpsych.org/apf

**National Alliance for the Mentally Ill
(NAMI)**
(self-help advocacy organization for persons with schizophrenia and depressive
disorders and their families)
Colonial Place Three
2107 Wilson Blvd., Suite 300
Arlington, VA 22201
(703) 524-7600
HelpLine: (800) 950-NAMI (950-6264)
www.nami.org/

National Institute of Mental Health
Information Resources and Inquiries
Branch
6001 Executive Blvd., Room 8184
MSC 9663
Bethesda, MD 20892-9663
(301) 443-4513
Fax: (301) 443-4279
TTY: (301) 443-8431
E-mail: nimhinfo@nih.gov
www.nimh.nih.gov/

**National Mental Health Association
(NMHA)**
2001 N. Beauregard St., 12 Floor
Alexandria, VA 22311
(800) 969-NMHA (969-6642)
(703) 684-7722
Fax: (703) 684-5968
www.nmha.org

Mental Retardation

**Association for Retarded Citizens
(ARC)**
1010 Wayne Ave., Suite 650
Silver Spring, MD 20910
(301) 565-3842
E-mail: info@thearc.org
www.thearc.org

Missing and Runaway Children

Child Find of America
(800) I-AM-LOST (426-5678)
Runaway Hotline
(800) 621-4000
www.childfindofamerica.org

**National Center for Missing and
Exploited Children (NCMEC)**
699 Prince St., Suite 550
Alexandria, VA 22314
(703) 274-3900
Fax: (703) 274-2200
24-hour Hotline:
(800) THE-LOST (843-5678)
www.missingkids.org

Neurological Disorders

National Institute of Neurological Disorders and Stroke
National Institutes of Health
31 Center Dr., Room 8A18
Bethesda, MD 20892-2540
(800) 352-9424
(301) 496-5751
Fax: (301) 402-2186
E-mail: braininfo@ninds.nih.gov
www.ninds.nih.gov

Nutrition

American Dietetic Association
120 South Riverside Plaza, Suite 2000
Chicago, IL 60606-6995
(312) 899-0040
www.eatright.org

American Society for Nutritional Sciences
9650 Rockville Pike, Suite 4500
Bethesda, MD 20814-3990
(301) 530-7050
Fax: (301) 571-1892
www.asns.org

Food and Drug Administration (FDA)
Office of Consumer Affairs
Public Inquiries
5600 Fishers Lane (HFE-88)
Rockville, MD 20857
(888) 463-6332 (INFO-FDA)
www.fda.gov

Food and Nutrition Information Center
U.S. Dept. of Agriculture
National Agricultural Library
10301 Baltimore Ave.
Beltsville, MD 20705-2351
(301) 504-5719
Fax: (301) 504-6409
TTY: (301) 504-6856
E-mail:fnic@nal.usda.gov
www.nal.usda.gov/fnic

Center for Nutrition in Sport and Human Performance
206A Chenoweth Lab
University of Massachusetts
Amherst, MA 01002
(413) 545-1076
Fax: (413) 545-1074
E-mail: volpe@nutrition.umass.edu
www.umass.edu/cnshp/

National Dairy Council
10255 W. Higgins Rd., Suite 900
Rosemont, IL 60018-5616
(800) 426-8271
www.nationaldairycouncil.org

Occupational Safety and Health

Occupational Safety and Health Administration (OSHA)
U.S. Dept. of Labor
Office of Public Affairs, Room N3647
200 Constitution Ave.
Washington, DC 20210
(202) 693-1999
(800) 321-OSHA (6742)
TTY: (877) 889-5627
www.osha.gov

Organ Donations

The Living Bank (TLB)
(provides information and acts as registry and referral service for people wanting to donate organs for research or transplantation)
P.O. Box 6725
Houston, TX 77265
(800) 528-2971
www.livingbank.org

Osteopathic Medicine

American Osteopathic Association (AOA)
142 East Ontario St.
Chicago, IL 60611
(800) 621-1773
(312) 202-8000
Fax: (312) 202-8200
E-mail: info@aoa-net.org
www.aoa-net.org

Parent Support Groups

National Organization of Mothers of Twins Clubs (NOMOTC)
P.O. Box 438
Thompson Station, TN 37179-0438
(877) 540-2200
(615) 595-0936
www.nomotc.org

Parents Anonymous
(self-help group for abusive parents)
675 W. Foothill Blvd., Suite 220
Claremont, CA 91711-3475
(909) 621-6184
Fax: (909) 625-6304
E-mail: parentsanonymous@parentsanonymous.org
www.parentsanonymous.org

Parents Without Partners, Inc.
1650 South Dixie Highway, Suite 510
Boca Raton, FL 33432
(561) 391-8833
Fax: (561) 395-8557
E-mail: pwp@jti.net
www.parentswithoutpartners.org

Parenting

National Parent Information Network
ERIC Clearinghouse on Elementary and Early Childhood Education
University of Illinois at Urbana-Champaign
Children's Research Center
51 Gerty Dr.
Champaign, IL 61820-7469
(800) 583-4135
(217) 333-1386
Fax: (217) 333-3767
www.npin.org

Phobias

Anxiety Disorders Association of America (ADAA)
(provides information about phobias and referrals to therapists and support groups)
8730 Georgia Ave., Suite 600
Silver Spring, MD 20910
(240) 485-1001
Fax: (240) 485-1035
www.adaa.org

TERRAP Programs
(headquarters for national network of treatment clinics for agoraphobia)
932 Evelyn St.
Menlo Park, CA 94025
(415) 327-1312
(800) 2-PHOBIA (274-6242)
www.terrap.com

Physical Fitness

See local yellow and white pages of telephone directory for listing of local health clubs and YMCAs, YWCAs, and Jewish Community Centers

Cooper Institutes for Aerobics Research
12330 Preston Rd.
Dallas, TX 75230
(972) 341-3200
Fax: (972) 341-3227
E-mail: courses@cooperinst.org
www.cooperinst.org

President's Council on Physical Fitness and Sports
Dept. W 200 Independence Ave., S.W.
Room 738 H
Washington, DC 20201
(202) 690-9000
Fax: (202) 690-5211
www.fitness.gov

American College of Sports Medicine
ACSM National Center
P.O. Box 1440

Indianapolis, IN 46206-1440
(317) 637-9200
www.acsm.org

Center for Nutrition in Sport and Human Performance
206A Chenoweth Lab
University of Massachusetts
Amherst, MA 01002
(413) 545-1076
Fax: (413) 545-1074
E-mail: volpe@nutrition.umass.edu
www.umass.edu/cnshp/

Poisoning

See emergency numbers listed in the front of your local phone directory

National Poison Hotline
(800) 962-1253

Pregnancy

National Institute of Child Health & Human Development
Bldg. 31, Room 2A32, MSC 2425
31 Center Dr.
Bethesda, MD 20892-2425
(800) 370-2943
www.nichd.nih.gov

Product Safety

U.S. Consumer Product Safety Commission
4330 East-West Highway
Bethesda, MD 20814-4408
(800) 638-CPSC (638-2772)
(301) 504-6816
www.cpsc.gov

Radiation Control and Safety

Center for Devices and Radiological Health

U.S. Food and Drug Administration
Office of Consumer Affairs
1350 Piccard Drive, HFZ-210
Rockville, MD 20850
(888) 463-6332
(301) 827-3990
www.fda.gov/cdrh/index.html

National Institute of Environmental Health Sciences

National Institutes of Health
P.O. Box 12233
Research Triangle Park, NC 27709
(919) 541-3345
www.niehs.nih.gov

Rape, Victimization

See white pages of telephone directory for listing of local rape crisis and counseling centers

National Center for Victims of Crime
2000 M St., N.W., Suite 480
Washington, DC 20010
(202) 467-8700
Fax: (202) 467-8701
www.ncvc.org

National Coalition Against Sexual Assault
125 N. Enola Dr.
Enola, PA 17025
(717) 728-9764
Fax: (717) 728-9781
www.dreamingdesigns.com/other/
indexncasa.html

National Organization for Victim Assistance (NOVA)
1730 Park Rd. N.W.
Washington, DC 20010
(800) TRY-NOVA (879-6682)
(202) 232-6682
Fax: (202) 462-2255
www.try-nova.org

National Sexual Violence Resource Center
123 North Enola Dr.
Enola, PA 17025
(877) 739-3895
(717) 909-0710
Fax: (717) 909-0714
TTY: (717) 909-0715
E-mail: resources@nsvrc.org
www.nsvrc.org

Reye's Syndrome

National Reye's Syndrome Foundation
P.O. Box 829
Bryan, OH 43506-0829
(800) 233-7393 (U.S. only)
(419) 636-2679
Fax: (419) 636-9897
E-mail: nrsf@reyessyndrome.org
www.reyessyndrome.org

Self-Care/Self-Help

National Self-Help Clearinghouse (NSHC)
(provides information about self-help groups)
365 5th Ave., Suite 3300
New York, NY 10016
(212) 817-1822
http://selfhelpweb.org

Sex Education

American Association of Sex Educators, Counselors and Therapists (AASECT)
P.O. Box 5488
Richmond, VA 23220-0488

E-mail: AASECT@mediaone.net
www.aasect.org

Advocates for Youth
(develops programs and material to educate youth on sex and sexual responsibility)
1025 Vermont Ave. N.W., Suite 200
Washington, DC 20005
(202) 347-5700
Fax: (202) 347-2263
E-mail: info@advocatesforyouth.org
www.advocatesforyouth.org

Planned Parenthood Federation of America (PPFA)
434 West 33rd St.
New York, NY 10001
(212) 541-7800
www.plannedparenthood.org

Sexuality Information and Education Council of the U.S. (SIECUS)
(maintains an information clearinghouse on all aspects of human sexuality)
130 West 42nd St., Suite 350
New York, NY 10036-7802
(212) 819-9770
Fax: (212) 819-9776
E-mail: siecus@siecus.org
www.siecus.org

Sexual Abuse and Assault

National Center for Assault Prevention
(provides services to children, adolescents, mentally retarded adults, and elderly)
606 Delsea Dr.
Sewell, NJ 08080
(800) 258-3189
(908) 369-8972
www.ncap.org/aboutncap.htm

Prevent Child Abuse America
200 S. Michigan Ave., Suite 1700
Chicago, IL 60604
(312) 663-3520
Fax: (312) 939-8962
www.preventchildabuse.org

Sexually Transmitted Diseases

Centers for Disease Control and Prevention
1600 Clifton Rd. N.E.
Atlanta, GA 30333
(404) 639-3311
www.cdc.gov

American Social Health Association
P.O. Box 13827
Research Triangle Park, NC 27709
(919) 361-8400
Fax: (919) 361-8425
www.ashastd.org

National Herpes Resource Center
American Social Health Association
P.O. Box 13827
Research Triangle Park, NC 27709-3827
(919) 361-8488
www.ashastd.org/hrc/index.html

National STD Hotline
(800) 227-8922

Sexuality Information and Education Council of the U.S. (SIECUS)
(maintains an information clearinghouse on all aspects of human sexuality)
130 West 42nd St., Suite 350
New York, NY 10036-7802
(212) 819-9770
Fax: (212) 819-9776
E-mail: siecus@siecus.org
www.siecus.org

Sickle-Cell Disease

Sickle Cell Disease Association of America
200 Corporate Pointe, Suite 495
Culver City, CA 90230-7633
(800) 421-8453
(310) 216-6363
www.sicklecelldisease.org

The Sickle Cell Information Center
The Georgia Comprehensive Sickle Cell Center at Grady Health System
P.O. Box 109, Grady Memorial Hospital, 80 Jesse Hill Jr. Dr.
Atlanta, GA 30303
(404) 616-3572
Fax: (404) 616-5998
E-mail: aplatt@emory.edu
www.emory.edu/peds/sickle

Skin Diseases

American Academy of Dermatology
P.O. Box 4014
Schaumburg, IL 60168-4014
(888) 462-DERM (3376)
(847) 330-0230
Fax: (847) 330-0050
www.aad.org

University of Iowa Hospitals and Clinics

Department of Dermatology
200 Hawkins Drive BT 2045-1
Iowa City, IA 52242-1090
(319) 356-7500 (appointments only)
(319) 356-2274 (business only)
Fax: (319) 356-8317 (business only)
www.tray.dermatology.uiowa.edu

National Psoriasis Foundation
6600 SW 92nd Ave., Suite 300
Portland, OR 97223-7195
(800) 723-9166
(503) 244-7404

Fax: (503) 245-0626
getinfo@npfusa.org
www.psoriasis.org

Sleep and Sleep Disorders

American Sleep Apnea Association
1424 K St., N.W., Suite 302
Washington, DC 20005
(202) 293-3650
Fax: (202) 293-3656
E-mail: asaa@sleepapnea.org
www.sleepapnea.org

American Academy of Sleep Medicine
One Westbrook Corporate Center, Suite 920
West Chester, IL 60154
(708) 492-0930
Fax: (708) 492-0943
www.aasmnet.org

Better Sleep Council
501 Wythe St.
Alexandria, VA 22314
(703) 683-8371
www.bettersleep.org/

National Sleep Foundation
1522 K St., N.W., Suite 500
Washington, DC 20005
(202) 347-3471
Fax: (202) 347-3472
www.sleepfoundation.org

Smoking and Tobacco

Action on Smoking and Health (ASH)
(provides information on nonsmokers' rights and related subjects)
2013 H St., N.W.
Washington, DC 20006
(202) 659-4310
http://ash.org

American Cancer Society
(provides information about quitting smoking and smoking cessation programs)
2200 Lake Blvd.
Atlanta, GA 30319
(800) 227-2345
(404) 816-7800
www.cancer.org

American Heart Association
(provides information about quitting smoking and smoking cessation programs)
7272 Greenville Ave.
Dallas, TX 75231
(800) 242-8721
(214) 373-6300
www.americanheart.org

American Lung Association
(provides information about quitting smoking and smoking cessation programs)
61 Broadway, 6th Floor
New York, NY 10006
(212) 315-8700
To reach your local American Lung Association: (800) LUNG-USA (586-4872)
www.lungusa.org

Americans for Nonsmokers' Rights
2530 San Pablo Ave., Suite J
Berkeley, CA 94702
(510) 841-3032
Fax: (510) 841-3060
E-mail: anr@no-smoke.org
www.no-smoke.org

Stress Reduction

American Institute of Stress
124 Park Ave.
Yonkers, NY 10703
(914) 963-1200
Fax: (914) 965-6267
E-mail: stress124@earthlink.net
www.stress.org

American Psychological Association
750 First St., N.E.
Washington, DC 20002-4242
(800) 374-2721
(202) 336-5510
TDD/TTY: 202-336-6123
www.apa.org

Association for Applied Psychophysiology and Biofeedback
10200 W. 44th Ave., Suite 304
Wheat Ridge, CO 80033
www.aapb.org

Stroke

Council on Stroke
American Heart Association
7272 Greenville Ave.
Dallas, TX 75231
(214) 373-6300
www.americanheart.org

National Institute of Neurological Disorders and Stroke
National Institutes of Health
P.O. Box 5801
Bethesda, MD 20824
(800) 352-9424
(301) 496-5751
www.ninds.nih.gov/

Stuttering

National Center for Stuttering
200 East 33rd St.
New York, NY 10016

Hotline: (800) 221-2483
(212) 532-1460
www.stuttering.com

Sudden Infant Death Syndrome (SIDS)

SIDS Alliance
(provides information and referrals to families who have lost an infant because of SIDS)
1314 Bedford Ave., Suite 210
Baltimore, MD 21208
(800) 221-7437
(410) 653-8226
Fax: (410) 653-8709
E-mail: info@sidsalliance.org
www.sidsalliance.org

Suicide Prevention

American Association of Suicidology (AAS)
4201 Connecticut Ave., N.W., Suite 408
Washington, DC 20008
(202) 237-2280
National Hopeline: (800) SUICIDE
Fax: (202) 237-2282
E-mail: ajkulp@suicidology.org
www.suicidology.org

American Psychoanalytic Foundation
9 Breakers Isle
Dana Point, CA 92629
(503) 244-5700
www.cyberpsych.org/apf

Terminal Illness

Make-A-Wish Foundation of America (MAWFA)
(dedicated to granting the special wishes of terminally ill children)
3550 North Central Ave., Suite 300
Phoenix, AZ 85012-2127
(800) 722-WISH (722-9474)
(602) 279-WISH (279-9474)
Fax: (602) 279-0855
E-mail: mawfa@wish.org
www.wish.org

Make Today Count (MTC)
(self-help group for persons with terminal illness)
St. Johns Hospital
1235 E. Cherokee St.
Springfield, MO 65804
(800) 432-2273
(417) 885-3324

Victimization

National Center for Victims of Crime
2000 M St., N.W., Suite 480
Washington, DC 20036

(202) 467-8700
Fax: (202) 467-8701
www.ncvc.org

National Coalition Against Domestic Violence
P.O. Box 18749
Denver, CO 80218
(303) 839-1852
Fax: (303) 831-9251
www.ncadv.org

National Coalition Against Sexual Assault
125 N. Enola Dr.
Enola, PA 17025
(717) 728-9764
Fax: (717) 728-9781
http://dreamingdesigns.com/other/indexncasa.html

National Organization for Victim Assistance (NOVA)
1730 Park Rd., N.W.
Washington, DC 20010
(800) Try-NOVA (879-6682)
(202) 232-6682
Fax: (202) 462-2255
www.try-nova.org

Weight Control

Overeaters Anonymous (OA)
P.O. Box 44020
Rio Rancho, NM 87174-4020
(505) 891-2664
Fax: (505) 891-2664
E-mail: info@overeatersanonymous.org
www.oa.org

Weight-Control Information Network (WIN)
National Institute of Diabetes and Digestive and Kidney Diseases
1 WIN Way
Bethesda, MD 20892-3665
(877) 946-4627
(202) 828-1025
Fax: (202) 828-1028
E-mail: win@info.niddk.nih.gov
www.niddk.nih.gov/health/nutrit/win.htm

Take Off Pounds Sensibly (TOPS)
P.O. Box 07360
4575 S. Fifth St.
Milwaukee, WI 53207-0360
(800) 932-8677
(414) 482-4620
www.tops.org

Weight Watchers International
175 Crossways Park West
Woodbury, NY 11797
(516) 390-1657
www.weight-watchers.com

Wellness

National Wellness Institute, Inc.
1300 College Court
P.O. Box 827
Stevens Point, WI 54481-0827
(800) 243-8694
(715) 342-2969
Fax: (715) 342-2979
E-mail: nwi@nationalwellness.org
www.nationalwellness.org

Wellness Associates of Chicago
(publishes *The Wellness Inventory*)
4250 Marine Dr., Suite 200
Chicago, IL 60613
(773) 935-6377
Fax: (773) 929-4446
E-mail: info@wellnessofchicago.com
www.wellness-associates.com

Women's Health

National Women's Health Network (NWHN)
514 10th St., N.W., Suite 400
Washington, DC 20004
(202) 347-1140
Health Info: (202) 628-7814
Fax: (202) 347-1168
www.womenshealthnetwork.org

National Women's Health Information Center

U.S. Public Health Service on Women's Health
8550 Arlington Blvd., Suite 300
Fairfax, VA 22031
(800) 994-WOMAN (994-9662)
www.4women.gov

GenneX Healthcare Technologies, Inc.

Estronaut: A Forum for Women's Health
GenneX Healthcare Technologies, Inc.
207 E. Ohio, 186
Chicago, IL 60611
(312) 335-0095
E-mail: ask@gennexhealth.com
www.estronaut.com

Planned Parenthood
434 West 33rd St.
New York, NY 10001
(212) 541-7800
Fax: (212) 245-1845
www.plannedparenthood.org
See also white or yellow pages of telephone directory for listing of local chapter

By definition, an emergency is a situation in which you have to think and act fast. Start by assessing the circumstances. Shout for help if you're in a public place. Look for any possible dangers to you or the victim, such as a live electrical wire or a fire. Seek medical assistance as quickly as possible. Dial 911 or a local emergency phone number. Don't attempt rescue techniques, such as cardiopulmonary resuscitation (CPR), unless you are trained. If you have a car, be sure you know the shortest route from your home to the nearest 24-hour hospital emergency department.

Supplies

Every home should have a kit of basic first aid supplies kept in a convenient location out of the reach of children. Stock it with the following:

- Bandages and sterile gauze pads
- Adhesive tape
- Scissors
- Cotton balls or absorbent cotton
- Cotton swabs
- Thermometer
- Antibiotic ointment
- Sharp needle
- Safety pins
- Calamine lotion

Keep a similar kit in your car or boat. You might want to add some extra items from your home, such as a flashlight, soap, blanket, paper cups, and any special equipment that a family member with a chronic illness may need.

Bleeding

Blood loss is frightening and dangerous. Direct pressure stops external bleeding. Since internal bleeding can also be life-threatening, you must be aware of the warning signs.

For an Open Wound

1. Apply direct pressure over the site of the wound. Cover the entire wound.
2. Use sterile gauze, a sanitary napkin, a clean towel, sheet, or handkerchief or, if necessary, your washed bare hand. Ice or cold water in a pad will help stop bleeding and decrease swelling.
3. Apply firm, steady pressure for five to fifteen minutes. Most wounds stop bleeding within a few minutes.
4. If the wound is on a foot, hand, leg, or arm, use gravity to help slow the flow of blood. Elevate the limb so that it is higher than the victim's heart.
5. If the bleeding doesn't stop, press harder.
6. Seek medical attention if the bleeding was caused by a serious injury, if stitches will be needed to keep the wound closed, or if the victim has not had a tetanus booster within the last ten years.

For Internal Bleeding

1. Suspect internal bleeding if a person coughs up blood, vomits red or brown material that looks like coffee grounds, passes blood in urine or stool, or has black, tarlike bowel movements.
2. Do not let the victim take any medication or fluids by mouth until seen by a doctor, because surgery may be necessary.
3. Have the victim lie flat. Cover him or her lightly.
4. Seek immediate medical attention.

For a Bloody Nose

1. Have the victim sit down, leaning slightly forward so the blood does not run down his or her throat. The person should spit out any blood in his or her mouth.
2. Use the thumb and forefingers to pinch the nose. If the victim can do the pinching, apply a cold compress to the nose and surrounding area.
3. Apply pressure for ten minutes without interruption.
4. If pinching does not work, gently pack the nostril with gauze or a clean strip of cloth. Do not use absorbent cotton, which will stick. Let the ends hang out so you can remove the packing easily later. Pinch the nose, with the packing in place, for five minutes.
5. If a foreign object is in the nose, do not attempt to remove it. Ask the person to blow gently. If that does not work, seek medical attention.
6. The nose should not be blown or irritated for several hours after a nosebleed stops.

◆ Breathing Problems

If a person appears to be unconscious, approach carefully. The victim may be in contact with electrical current. If so, make sure the electricity is shut off before touching the victim. The first function you should check is respiration. Tap or shake the victim's shoulder gently, shouting, "Are you all right?" Look for any signs of breathing: Can you hear breath sounds? Can you feel breath on your cheek? If the person is breathing, do not perform mouth-to-mouth resuscitation.

If you aren't certain if the victim is breathing, or if there are no signs of breath, follow these steps:

1. Lay the person on his or her back on the floor or ground. Roll the victim over if necessary, being careful to turn the head with the remainder of the body as a unit to avoid possible neck injury. Loosen any tight clothing around the neck or chest.
2. Check for any foreign material in the mouth or throat and remove it quickly.
3. Open the airway by tilting the head back and lifting the chin up.
4. Pinch the nostrils shut with your thumb and index finger.
5. Take a deep breath, open your mouth wide and place it securely over the victim's, and give two slow breaths, each lasting 1 to 10 seconds. Remove your mouth, turn your head, and check to see if the victim's chest rises and falls. If you hear air escaping from the victim's mouth and see the chest fall, you know that you are getting air into the lungs.
6. Repeat once every five seconds (twelve breaths per minute) until professional help takes over, or the victim begins breathing on his or her own. It may take several hours to revive someone. If you stop, the victim may not be able to breathe on his or her own. Once the person does begin to breathe independently, always get professional help.
7. If air doesn't seem to be entering the chest, or the chest doesn't fall between breaths, tilt the head further back. If that doesn't work, follow the directions for choking emergencies later in this section.
8. If the victim is a child, do not pinch the nose shut. Cover both the mouth and nose with your mouth, and place your free hand very lightly on the child's chest. Use small puffs of air rather than big breaths. Feel the chest inflate as you blow, and listen for exhaled air. Repeat once every three seconds (twenty breaths per minute).

◆ Broken Bones

If you suspect that a person has broken a leg, do not move him or her unless there is immediate danger.

1. Check for signs of breathing. If there is none or breathing is very weak, administer mouth-to-mouth resuscitation.
2. If the person is bleeding, apply direct pressure on the site of the wound.
3. Try to keep the victim warm and calm.
4. Do not try to push a broken bone back into place if it is sticking out of the skin. You can apply a moist dressing to prevent it from drying out.
5. Do not try to straighten out a fracture.
6. Do not allow the victim to walk.
7. Splint unstable fractures to prevent painful motion.

◆ Burns

1. If fire caused the burn, cool the affected area with water to stop the burning process.
2. Remove the victim's garments and jewelry and cover him or her with clean sheets or towels.
3. Call for help immediately.
4. If chemicals caused the burn, wash the affected area with cool water for at least 20 minutes. Chemical burns of the eye require immediate medical attention after flushing with water for 20 minutes.

◆ Choking

A person with anything stuck in the throat and blocking the airway can stop breathing, lose consciousness, and die within four to six minutes. A universal signal of distress because of choking is clasping the throat with one or both hands. Other signs are an inability to talk and noisy, difficult breathing. You need to take immediate action, but NEVER slap the victim's back. This could make the obstruction worse.

If the victim can speak, cough, or breathe, do not interfere. Coughing alone may dislodge the foreign object. If the choking continues without lessening, call for medical help.

If the victim cannot speak, cough, or breathe but is conscious, use the Heimlich maneuver, as follows

1. Stand behind the victim (who may be seated or standing) and wrap your arms around his or her waist.
2. Make a fist with one hand and place the thumb side of your fist against the victim's abdomen, just above the navel. Grasp your fist with your other hand and press into his or her abdomen with a quick, upward thrust.

Do not exert any pressure against the rib cage with your forearms.

3. Repeat this procedure until the victim is no longer choking or loses consciousness.

4. If the person is lying face down, roll the victim over. Facing the person, kneel with your legs astride his or her hips. Put the heel of one hand below the rib cage and place your other hand on top. Press into the abdomen with a quick, upward thrust. Repeat thrusts as needed.

5. If you start choking when you're by yourself, place your fist below your rib cage and above your navel. Grasp this fist with your other hand and press into your abdomen with a quick, upward thrust. You also can lean over a fixed, horizontal object, such as a table edge or chair back, and press your upper abdomen against it with a quick, upward thrust. Repeat as needed until you dislodge the object.

If the Victim Is Unconscious

1. Place him or her on the ground and give mouth-to-mouth resuscitation as described earlier.

2. If the victim does not start breathing and air does not seem to be going into his or her lungs, roll the victim onto his or her back and give one or more manual thrusts: Place one of your hands on top of the other with the heel of the bottom hand in the middle of the abdomen, slightly above the navel and below the rib cage. Press into the abdomen with a quick, upward thrust. Do not push to either side. Repeat six to ten times as needed.

3. Clear the airway. Hold the victim's mouth open with one hand and use your thumb to depress the tongue. Make a hook with the index finger of your other hand and, using a gentle, sweeping motion, reach into the victim's throat and feel for a swallowed foreign object in the airway.

4. Repeat the following steps in this sequence:
   - Six to ten abdominal thrusts
   - Probe in mouth
   - Try to inflate lungs
   - Repeat

5. If the victim suddenly seems okay, but no foreign material has been removed, take him or her directly to the hospital. A foreign object, such as a fish or chicken bone or other jagged object, could do internal damage as it passes through the victim's system.

If the Victim Is a Child

1. If the child is coughing, do nothing. The coughing alone may dislodge the object.

2. If the airway is blocked and the child is panicky and fighting for breath, do *NOT* probe the airway with your fingers to clear an unseen foreign object. You might push the material back into the airway, worsening the obstruction.

3. For an infant younger than a year, hang the child over your arm so that the head is lower than the trunk. Using the heel of your hand, administer four firm blows high on the back between the shoulder blades. For a bigger child, follow the same procedure, but invert the child over your knee rather than your arm.

4. After four back blows, perform four chest thrusts (the Heimlich maneuver as described above).

Drowning

A person can die of drowning four to six minutes after breathing stops. Although prevention is the wisest course, follow these steps in case of a drowning emergency:

1. Get the victim out of the water fast. Be extremely cautious, because a drowning person may panic and grasp at a rescuer, endangering that individual as well. If possible, push a branch or pole within the victim's reach.

2. If the victim is unconscious, use a flotation device if at all possible. Carefully place the person on the device. Once out of the water, place the victim on his or her back.

3. If the victim is not breathing, start mouth-to-mouth resuscitation. Continue until the person can breathe unassisted or help arrives. (Note that it may take an hour or two for a drowning victim to resume independent breathing.) Do not leave the victim alone for any reason.

4. Once the person is breathing without assistance, even if he or she is still coughing, you need only stay nearby until professional help arrives.

Electrical Shock

1. If you suspect that an electrical shock has knocked a person unconscious, approach very carefully. Do not touch the victim unless the electricity has been turned off.

2. Shut off the power at the plug, circuit breaker, or fuse box. Simply shutting off an appliance does not remove the shock hazard. Use a dry stick to move a wire or downed power line from the victim. Keep in mind that you also are in danger until the power is off.

3. If the person's breathing is weak or has stopped, follow the steps for mouth-to-mouth resuscitation.

4. Even if the victim returns to consciousness, call for medical help. While waiting, cover the victim with a blanket or coat to keep him or her warm. Place a blanket underneath the body if the surface is cold. Be sure

the person lies flat if conscious, with legs raised. If the victim is unconscious, place him or her on one side, with a pillow supporting the head. Do not give the victim anything to eat or drink.

5. Electrical burns can extend deep into the tissue, even when they appear minor. Do not put butter, household remedies, or sprays on burns without a doctor's instruction. Do not use ice or cold water on an electrical burn that is more than 2 inches across.

Heart Attack

Chest pain can be caused by indigestion, strained muscles, or lung infections. The warning signs of a heart attack are:

- Intense pain that lasts for more than two minutes, produces a tight or crushing feeling, is centered in the chest, or spreads to the neck, jaw, shoulder, or arm
- Shortness of breath that is worse when the person lies flat and improves when the person sits
- Heavy sweating
- Nausea or vomiting
- Irregular pulse
- Pale or bluish skin or lips
- Weakness
- Severe anxiety, feeling of doom

If an individual develops these symptoms:

1. Call for emergency medical help immediately.
2. Have the person sit up or lie in a semi-reclining position. Loosen tight clothing. Keep him or her comfortably warm.
3. If the person loses consciousness, turn on his or her back and check for breathing and pulse. If vomiting occurs, turn the victim's head to one side and clean the mouth.
4. If the person has medicine for angina pectoris (chest pain) and is conscious, help him or her take it.
5. If the person is unconscious, and you are trained to perform cardiopulmonary resuscitation (CPR), check for a pulse at the wrist or neck. If there is none, beginCPR in conjunction with mouth-to-mouth resuscitation. Do not attempt CPR unless you are trained. It is not a technique you can learn from a book.

Poisoning

Many common household substances, including glue, aspirin, bleaches, and paint, can be poisonous. If you think someone has been poisoned, call the National Poison Control Center: (800) 222-1222. Be prepared to provide the following information:

- The kind of substance swallowed and how much was swallowed
- If a child or adult swallowed the substance
- Symptoms
- Whether or not vomiting has occurred
- Whether you gave the person anything to drink
- How much time it will take to get to an emergency room

The Poison Control Center will tell you whether or not to induce vomiting or neutralize a swallowed poison. Here are some additional guidelines:

1. Always assume the worst if a small child has swallowed or might have swallowed something poisonous. Keep the suspected item or container with you to answer questions.
2. Do not give any medications unless a physician or the Poison Control Center instructs you to do so.
3. Do not follow the directions for neutralizing poisons on the container unless a doctor or the Poison Control Center confirms that they are appropriate measures to take.
4. If the child is conscious, give moderate doses of water to dilute the poison.
5. If a poisoning victim is unconscious, make sure he or she is breathing. If not, give mouth-to-mouth resuscitation. Do not give anything by mouth or attempt to stimulate the person. Call for emergency help immediately.
6. If the person is vomiting, make sure he or she is in a position in which he or she cannot choke on what is brought up.
7. While vomiting is the fastest way to expel swallowed poisons from the body, never try to induce vomiting if the person has swallowed any acid or alkaline substance, which can cause burns of the face, mouth, and throat (examples include ammonia, bleach, dishwasher detergent, drain and toilet cleaners, lye, oven cleaners, or rust removers), or petroleum-like products, which produce dangerous fumes that can be inhaled during vomiting (examples include floor polish, furniture wax, gasoline, kerosene, lighter fluid, turpentine, and paint thinner).

✔ **What They Tell the Doctor**
✔ **How Often You Need Them**
✔ **What to Do About Abnormal Results**

Do you wonder what the doctor sees when he looks into your eyes with that little light or what it means when your blood or urine test is normal? In this section we cover some of the most common tests your doctor does, what they tell, and how often they should be done.

General Information

- Always ask your doctor what tests are being done, why they are being ordered, what they involve, and what the results mean.
- No test is foolproof. If a result is unexpected, whether normal or abnormal, your doctor should repeat the test before making any decisions.
- Modern X-ray machines expose you to a minuscule amount of radiation. Nevertheless, be sure to tell the physician or X-ray technician if there is even a chance you may be pregnant.
- Often a doctor orders a test because that is the only way to prove you do not have a disease.

Allergy Skin Testing

- Skin testing is still the most reliable method.
- The physician either pricks your skin 20 to 40 or more times to introduce a tiny bit of potentially allergic material or injects a small amount.
- Children who are frightened by multiple needle sticks and are unlikely to sit still for as long as necessary may have blood (RAST) tests instead.

What the results mean

If you develop redness or a hivelike bump around an area, you are probably allergic to the injected substance. Sometimes you can avoid the offending material, but things like pollen and dust are everywhere. Your allergist may recommend desensitizing shots to reduce your reac-

tion. The results of skin tests won't be reliable if you take antihistamines within 48 hours of the test.

How often to be tested

Skin tests are necessary only if you cannot get allergy relief from other measures such as over-the-counter medications, reducing mold and dust in the house, and staying away from animals.

Blood Pressure Reading

- High blood pressure, a major cause of stroke and heart attacks, usually causes no symptoms.
- The upper number in a reading—the systolic—refers to peak amount of pressure generated when your heart pumps blood, the lower number—the diastolic—measures the least amount of pressure.

What the results mean

Most doctors today think the lower the pressure the better, which means a reading of 120/80 or less. Because the mere anxiety of having your blood pressure taken can cause a mild elevation, your doctor will want to repeat an abnormal test, ideally on a different day, before diagnosing high blood pressure.

How often to be tested

Everyone—no matter how healthy—should have a blood-pressure reading taken at least once a year, more often if you have high blood pressure.

Blood Tests

- Blood may be taken from either a finger prick or, more commonly, a vein in your arm.
- See below for information on cholesterol testing, which is also done from a blood sample.

Complete Blood Count (CBC)

This is the most commonly performed of all blood tests.

What the results mean

A low red-cell count, called anemia, can be caused by something as simple as too little iron in your diet, as complex as an abnormality in your digestion, or as serious as a bone marrow problem or silent bleeding. Iron deficiency is the most frequent cause, with women who menstruate and limit their intake of red meat at the greatest risk. If your doctor diagnoses this problem, ask about making dietary changes as well as taking iron supplements.

A high white-cell count, a measure of the body's defenses against infection, usually indicates some kind of infection. Depending on the type of cell that predominates, your doctor may be able to identify whether you have a bacterial or viral infection.

Platelets, the first participants in blood clotting, may be decreased because of a viral infection, abnormal bleeding, or for no identifiable reason.

Chemistry Panels (Chem 12 or 18, SMA 12 or 24)

Kidney, bone, liver, pancreas, prostate, and some glandular functions are screened by these tests.

What the results mean

An abnormality may signal a problem that needs treatment. Because accuracy decreases when many tests are run together, any specific abnormal test should be repeated, especially if unexpected.

CAT (Computerized Axial Tomography) Scan

- A CAT scan is 100 times more sensitive than an X ray.
- You lie as motionless as possible in a large tube while an X-ray beam travels 360 degrees around you. The test takes about an hour.

What the results mean

The test can help diagnose such conditions as tumors, blood clots, cysts, and bleeding in the brain as well as in various other organs.

Cholesterol Test/ Lipoprotein Profile

- Anyone can have a high cholesterol level, but you are more apt to be at risk if there is a family history of early heart attacks, strokes, or high blood cholesterol.
- Your doctor will look at total blood cholesterol, high-density lipoprotein (HDL, the "good" cholesterol that prevents cholesterol from sticking to your blood vessels), low-density lipoprotein (LDL, the "bad" cholesterol that does the reverse), and triglycerides.

What the results mean

Experts today think optimum total cholesterol levels are below 200 mg/dL of blood. Persistently high cholesterol values will prompt your doctor to advise dietary and lifestyle changes—less fat intake, more exercise—and perhaps medication. Optimal LDL levels are less than 100 mg/dL, and optimal HDL levels are 60 mg/dL or higher.

How often to be tested

If your cholesterol level is under 200 and your LDL level is under 130, repeat the test every five years. If your test is borderline, repeat it annually. (Note that the test should be taken when you have not eaten for at least twelve hours.)

If you have a family history of cholesterol problems, have your children tested annually from age 2; if you don't, have them tested around age 10 and every few years thereafter. Children under 2 should not be given a low-cholesterol diet; they need extra fat to make brain tissue and hormones for growth.

Fundoscopy

The doctor looks into your eye with a little light.

What the results mean

The beginnings of cataracts may be visible, as well as irregularities in the blood vessels that indicate damage from high cholesterol (fatty deposits in the blood vessels), high blood pressure (narrowing and notching), diabetes, or other diseases. If the optic nerve is swollen, there may be excess pressure inside your skull.

What your doctor *cannot* see are the early signs of glaucoma, which can lead to blindness if not treated. Over age 20, have a pressure check for glaucoma from an ophthalmologist or optometrist every three years—or every year if you have a family history of glaucoma.

� Heart Tests

- The following tests are listed from the simplest through the most complicated.
- Also see listings for blood pressure readings, cholesterol tests, and pulse.

Electrocardiogram (ECG, EKG)

A machine amplifies the electrical signals from your heart and records them on paper.

What the results mean

An EKG can detect such things as an enlarged heart, abnormal levels of potassium or calcium, disease of the small vessels of the heart, or the source of an abnormal heart rhythm. It is a nonspecific test, however, and more advanced studies should be done if serious disease is suspected.

Echocardiogram

In this painless test sound waves are used to produce a picture of the heart in action on a TV-type screen.

What the results mean

The test investigates the size of the heart chambers, the thickness of the walls, how the four heart valves are working, and the condition of the membrane surrounding the heart. Mitral valve prolapse, a common minor abnormality, often shows up on this test, as well as more serious problems.

Stress Test

Your heart rate, blood pressure, and EKG are constantly monitored as you exercise on a treadmill that goes faster and faster with a steeper and steeper incline. This test—also called an exercise tolerance test or treadmill test—should be performed in the presence of a cardiologist and in or near a hospital in case the strain causes heart problems that need emergency treatment. The test should be stopped immediately if you experience any light-headedness, chest pain, nausea, or palpitations.

What the results mean

The increasing strain on the heart causes changes that can tell your doctor if you are at risk of a heart attack. This is because a blockage in the coronary arteries—the blood vessels that feed your heart muscle—may show up only during exercise.

Angiography

A dye is injected into various arteries, and X rays are taken.

What the results mean

The doctor can detect blockages in the blood vessels that can lead to heart attack or stroke, as well as aneurysms (weakened spots in the blood-vessel walls). The test carries some risk of causing stroke.

☐ Kidney Tests

The two tests listed here involve taking X rays. Ultrasound (similar to an echocardiogram) can also be used to outline the kidneys.

Intravenous Pyelogram (IVP)

After an iodine-containing substance is injected into a vein, X rays are taken at five-minute intervals to show the outlines of the kidney, ureter, and bladder.

What the results mean

Tumors, kidney stones, and swelling of the kidney tissue can be seen, as well as blockage to urine flow or a mass that may be pressing on the kidney. A kidney that is not functioning will not appear on the X ray, and one in an abnormal position can be found.

Voiding Cystourethrogram (VCUG)

A technician will fill your bladder with a dye injected through a catheter and take X rays while you urinate.

What the results mean

If you have recurrent urinary-tract infections, the test will show if there is a significant backup of urine from the bladder into the ureter, in which case daily antibiotics may be needed to prevent infection. Investigating recurrent urinary tract infections is particularly important for children.

Magnetic Resonance Imaging (MRI)

MRI uses no radiation but produces pictures of the brain that are much more detailed than those of a CAT scan.

What the results mean

In addition to locating bleeding or tumors, as a CAT scan does, the test picks up subtle signs such as those of Parkinson's disease and multiple sclerosis in the brain or a herniated disc in the spinal column.

Mammography

- Only a small amount of radiation is used to take the mammogram. You usually stand up and put your breast on a photographic plate where it is compressed with a plastic shield or balloonlike device. It shouldn't hurt. If your breasts are tender at certain times in your menstrual cycle, schedule your mammogram when they are least sensitive.
- Mammograms can detect breast abnormalities at easily treated stages before you can feel them, but they are not foolproof. Examine your breasts monthly.

What the results mean

Mammograms can detect cysts, abscesses, and tumors. Whether a mass is benign or malignant is hard to tell in the early stages, so abnormalities usually need to be biopsied or removed totally to determine treatment.

How often to be tested

Although there is controversy over the benefits of mammography for women under 50, many experts still recommend having a first mammogram between ages 35 and 40, followed by one every two years between 40 and 50, and yearly thereafter. If your mother or sister has had breast cancer, consult your doctor for an appropriate schedule. And if you have a lump, pain, or nipple discharge, have a mammogram right away, no matter what your age.

You also should have a breast examination by a doctor at least every three years between ages 20 and 40, and every year after 40.

Pap Smear

- A routine part of every gynecological examination.
- Your doctor takes a painless swab from the cervix and vaginal walls and sends it to a lab for analysis.

What the results mean

Pap smears can detect not only cervical cancer but also inflammation and many infections, minor and more serious; they also provide important information about the state of your female hormones. A normal test is termed class I, and abnormal results are graded by degree into four classifications, with only the most severe—a class V test—signifying outright cancer. Treatment depends on the diagnosis and may range from doing nothing for a minor inflammation to, in rare cases, a hysterectomy for cancer. Because the error rate of Pap smears is high, the doctor should always repeat an abnormal test.

How often to be tested

Women who are on birth control pills and are sexually active should have a Pap smear every six months; other women should be checked every year.

Physical Examination

The routine physical exam generally includes a pulse and blood-pressure reading, measure of height and weight, blood tests (including a lipoprotein profile), fundoscopy, and sometimes other tests as well, such as a fecal occult blood test.

What the results mean

A physical exam serves as a general measure of health and sometimes picks up early signs of disease.

How often to have a physical exam

Most doctors no longer recommend yearly physicals for everybody. A good schedule to follow instead is to have a complete checkup every four or five years under age 40, every three years between 40 and 50, every two years between 50 and 60, and every year after that. At any age, you should have more frequent examinations if you have chronic medical problems such as diabetes or high blood pressure, are obese, or smoke cigarettes.

Pulse

To take your own pulse, press two fingertips over the artery in your wrist, just below the base of the thumb. Count the beats in 20 seconds, then multiply by 3.

What the results mean

The normal pulse rate—the speed at which your heart pumps blood—is 60–80 beats a minute; it should be regular, without skipped or extra beats. Abnormal rates can be due to thyroid problems (too high causes a fast rate, too low a slow one), heart problems, anxiety (even the stress of a physical exam), or weakness from an illness such as the flu or other problems.

The character of your pulse is also important. A discrepancy between the strength of the pulse on one side of the neck and the other may mean you are in danger of a stroke. A pulse that is abnormally strong and bounding can signal a problem with a heart valve. If the pulse is weak, you may have blockages in your blood vessels from diabetes, atherosclerosis (hardening of the arteries), or a variety of other disorders.

Stomach and Intestinal Tests

Though most of these tests are uncomfortable, they generally are not painful.

Barium Enema

Barium, a radioactive material, is instilled in your large intestine through a tube inserted into your anus. Because barium is constipating, drink fluids afterward. Don't be alarmed if you have white stools for a day or two.

What the results mean

The doctor will be able to see tumors or polyps, any obstructions, and other abnormalities.

Colonoscopy and Sigmoidoscopy

In colonoscopy, for which you will be sedated, the doctor looks into the colon with a flexible tube inserted into your anus. The procedure is essentially the same for sigmoidoscopy, except that the doctor looks only into the lower third of the intestine.

What the results mean

Your doctor can see where bleeding comes from, remove a polyp, or biopsy a mass.

Upper GI Series

You will be asked to down a drink of barium so that X rays can be taken of the esophagus, stomach, duodenum, and sometimes the small intestine.

What the results mean

Your doctor can diagnose swallowing disorders, hiatus hernias, ulcers, tumors, and some inflammations of the stomach and small bowel.

Fecal Occult Blood Test (FOBT)

A small sample of stool that remains on the doctor's glove after a rectal exam or that is collected by you at home is tested for blood that is invisible to the eye.

What the results mean

This test is done routinely as part of a regular checkup to detect the earliest sign of cancer of the colon. It is also part of an investigation of anemia or abdominal pain. If your test is positive, tell your doctor if you recently ate radishes, turnips, or red meat, took large doses of vitamin C or iron pills, or had a nosebleed. All of these things can produce misleading results.

Urinalysis

Urine can tell about the health not only of the kidneys but also of other organ systems.

What the results mean

Specific gravity is the degree to which your urine is concentrated or diluted. If it is persistently too dilute, your doctor may ask for a first morning sample to see how well your kidneys concentrate your urine overnight. Urine that is too concentrated may indicate poor fluid intake, decreased kidney function, or dehydration from vomiting and diarrhea.

Acidity or alkalinity (pH) is useful information when there is a history or possibility of kidney stones, urinary tract infection, or kidney disease.

Glucose or sugar in the urine may mean you have diabetes. You will need a blood test to confirm the diagnosis, as some families filter sugar easily through their kidneys but do not have any disease. Inflammation of the pancreas and thyroid problems also may cause sugar in the urine.

Blood in the urine may mean infection, a stone, or an inflammation of the kidney. Excessive exertion such as running sometimes causes some blood to leak into the urine; this usually disappears after resting.

Protein molecules are large and under normal conditions should not filter into the urine. However, they may appear in small amounts in the urine after strenuous exercise or an illness, especially one with a fever. In large amounts, protein in the urine warrants a search for an underlying kidney problem.

Nitrites, substances produced when bacteria multiply, may be the earliest or only sign of an infection.

White blood cells may be present because of a urinary tract or vaginal infection.

X Ray

The simple X ray is a nonspecific test that is being replaced more and more by CAT scans, magnetic resonance imaging, and other tests.

What the results mean

An X ray can detect such things as an enlarged heart, a broken bone, a sinus infection, or pneumonia.

Total calorie values for each item in this table were rounded to the nearest 5 calories (calories from fat and fat grams were not). The portion sizes are given in common household units and in grams. The portion size shown may not be the amount that you eat. If you choose larger or smaller portions than listed, increase or decrease the calorie and fat counts accordingly. Check nutrition labels on foods for additional information, including saturated fat, cholesterol, and sodium content.

Breads, Cereals, and Other Grain Products

Breads	Calories	Fat grams	Calories from fat
Bagel			
plain, 1, 3½" diam.	195	1	10
oat bran, 1, 3½"	180	1	8
poppy seed, 1, Sara Lee	190	1	9
Cracked-wheat bread, 1, 25 g slice	65	1	9
French bread, 1, 25 g slice	70	1	7
Pita bread			
white, 1, 6½" diam.	165		6
whole wheat, 1, 6½" diam.	170		15
Pumpernickel, 1, 32 g slice	80	1	9
Raisin, 1, 26 g slice	70	1	10
Rye, 1, 32 g slice	85	1	10
White			
regular, 1, 25 g slice	65	1	8
Wonder bread light, 2 slices, 45 g	80	1	9
Whole wheat			
regular, 1, 25 g slice	70	1	11
Wonder bread, 2 slices, 45 g	80	<1	14
Rolls			
Croissant, prepared w/butter, 1, 57 g	230	12	108
Dinner, 1, 28 g	85	2	19
Frankfurter or hamburger, 1, 43 g	125	2	20
French, 1, 38 g	105	2	15
Hard, 1 3½", 57 g	165	2	22
Quick breads, Biscuits, Muffins, Breakfast Pastries			
Biscuit			
plain, 2½" diam., 60 g	210	10	88
from dry mix, 3" diam., 57 g	190	7	62
from refrig. dough, 2½" diam., 27 g	95	4	36
Banana bread, 1 slice, 60 g	195		57
Coffee cake			
cinnamon w/crumb topping, 63 g	265	15	132
butter streusel, Sara Lee, 41 g	160	7	63
Danish			
cheese, Sara Lee, individual, 36 g	130	8	72

	Calories	Fat grams	Calories from fat
cheese-filled, Entenmann's, fat-free 54 g	130	0	0
Doughnuts			
plain cake, 1, 47 g	200	11	97
glazed, 1, 45 g	190	10	93
English muffin, plain, 1, 57 g	135	1	9
Muffin			
blueberry, 1, 2½", 57 g	160	4	33
bran w/raisins, Dunkin' Donuts 1, 104 g	310	9	81
Pancake			
plain, from dry mix, 1, 56 g	200	1	9
plain, frozen Aunt Jemima, 3, 114 g	185	2	22
Waffle			
plain, 7" diam., 75 g	220	11	95
blueberry, frozen, Eggo, 2, 78 g	220	8	72
Breakfast Cereal			
All-Bran, ½ cup, 30 g	80	1	9
Bran flakes, ¾ cup, 28 g	100	1	9
Cheerios, 1¼ cup, 28 g	110	2	18
Corn flakes, 1 cup, 30 g	110	0	0
Cream of Wheat			
regular or instant, cooked, ⅔ cup, 168 g	100	0	0
instant, cooked, ⅔ cup, 161 g	100	<1	0
mix'n eat, 1 pkg., 28 g	100	0	0
Frosted Flakes, ¾ cup, 30 g	120	0	0
Frosted Mini-Wheats, 1 cup, 55 g	190	1	9
Grape-Nut Flakes, 1 cup, 28 g	100	1	9
Granola, date nut, Erewhon, ¼ cup, 28 g	130	6	50
Oatmeal			
reg., quick, or instant, cooked, 1 cup, 234 g	145	2	21
cinnamon & spice, instant , 1 pkg., 46 g	170	2	18
Raisin bran, 1 cup, 55 g	170	1	9
Rice Chex, 1 cup, 31 g	120	0	0
Rice Krispies, 1¼ cup, 30 g	110	0	0
Shredded wheat, Quaker	220	2	14
Special K, 1 cup, 30 g	110	0	0
Total, 1 cup, 28 g	100	1	9
Wheaties, 1 cup, 28 g	100	1	9
Pasta and Rice			
Macaroni			
cooked, plain, ½ cup, 65 g	95	<1	3
spinach, cooked, Ronzoni, ½ cup, 67 g	105	<1	4
Pasta			
fresh, cooked, plain, 1 cup, 170 g	225	2	16
homemade w/egg, cooked, 1 cup, 170 g	220	3	27
Ravioli, cheese, cooked, Contadina, ⅓ container, 190 g	270	11	99
Rice, cooked, 1/2 cup			
Brown, medium grain, 98 g	110	1	7
White, glutinous, 120 g	115	<1	2
White, long grain instant, 82 g	80	<1	1

White, medium grain, 93 g	120	<1	2
Wild rice, 82 g	85	<1	3
Spaghetti, cooked, plain, 1 cup, 140 g	155	<1	4

Crackers

Cheez-it, Sunshine, 24 crackers, 32 g	140	8	72
Finn-Crisp dark, 3 crackers, 15 g	60	0	0
Matzo, plain, 1, 28 g	110	<1	4
Ritz, Nabisco, 4 crackers, 14 g	70	4	36
Saltine, 10 crackers, 28 g	120	4	36
Soup or oyster, 4 crackers, 14 g	70	4	36
Triscuit, Nabisco, 6 crackers, 28 g	120	4	36

Fruits

Fruits

(calories in cooked and canned
    fruit include both fruit and liquid)

Apple, raw, sliced, ½ cup, 55 g	30	<1	2
Applesauce, ½ cup			
sweetened, 128 g	95	<1	2
unsweetened, 122 g	50	<1	1
Apricots			
canned, heavy syrup, 3 halves, 85 g	70	<1	1
canned, light syrup pack, 3 halves, 85 g	55	<1	0
dried, cooked without sugar, ½ cup, 125 g	105	<1	2
raw, 4 halves, 78 g	35	<1	3
Avocados			
California, 3", ½, 86 g	155	15	135
Florida, 3⅜", ½, 152 g	170	13	121
Banana, medium, 114 g	105	1	5
Blueberries, ½ cup			
frozen, unsweetened, 78 g	40	<1	4
frozen, sweetened, 115 g	95	1	5
raw, 72 g	40	<1	3
Cherries, ½ cup			
raw, sweet, 72 g	50	1	6
sweet, frozen, sweetened, 130 g	115	<1	2
sour red, frozen, unsweetened, 78 g	35	<1	3
Cranberry sauce, sweetened, ¼ cup, 70 g	110	0	0
Dates, dried, 10, 83 g	230	<1	3
Fruit cocktail, canned, ½ cup			
juice pack, 124 g	55	<1	0
heavy syrup, 128 g	95	<1	1
Grapefruit, raw, 3¾", ½, 118 g	40	<1	1
Melon, honeydew, cubed, ½ cup, 85 g	30	<1	1
Oranges, ½ cup			
mandarin, canned, light syrup, 122 g	80	0	0
raw, sections, 90 g	40	<1	1
Peaches			
canned, in juice, ½ cup, 77 g	55	0	0
canned, in light syrup, ½ cup, 77 g	70	<1	1
Pears			
canned, in light syrup, 1 half, 77 g	35	<1	1
dried, without added sugar, ½ cup, 128 g	165	<1	4
Pineapple			
canned, juice pack, ½ cup, 125 g	75	<1	1
raw, diced, ½ cup, 78 g	40	<1	3
Plums			
canned, juice pack, 3, 95 g	55	<1	0

raw, 2⅛" diam., 66 g	35	<1	4
Prunes			
dried, cooked, without sugar, ½ cup, 106 g	115	<1	2
dried, uncooked, 10, 84 g	200	<1	4
Raisins, seedless, ¼ cup, 41 g	125	<1	2
Raspberries, ½ cup			
frozen, unsweetened, 125 g	61	1	6
raw, 62 g	30	<1	3
Rhubarb, cooked, sweetened, ½ cup, 120 g	140	<1	1
Tangerines, sections, ½ cup, 98 g	45	<1	2
Watermelon, 10" x 1", 480 g	155	2	19

Juices

Apple juice or cider, 1 cup, 249 g	120	0	0
Apricot nectar, canned, ¾ cup, 188 g	105	<1	2
Cranberry juice cocktail, ¾ cup, 190 g	110	<1	2
Grape juice			
bottled, ¾ cup, 188 g	110	0	0
from frozen concentrate, ¾ cup, 188 g	96	<1	2
Lemonade, ¾ cup			
homemade, prepared w/sugar, 186 g	90	0	0
from frozen concentrate, 186 g	75	<1	0
Orange juice, ¾ cup			
fresh, 186 g	85	<1	3
from frozen concentrate, 187 g	85	<1	1
Pineapple juice, canned, ¾ cup, 188 g	105	<1	1
Prune juice, canned, ¾ cup, 192 g	135	<1	1
Snapple, 1 bottle			
Dixie Peach, 295 g	140	0	0
Lemonade, 240 g	110	0	0
Passion Supreme, 309 g	160	0	0
Pink Grapefruit Cocktail, 249 g	120	0	0
V-8 juice, canned, ¾ cup, 182 g	35	0	0

Vegetables

Alfalfa sprouts, raw, 1 cup, 33 g	10	<1	2
Artichoke, cooked, medium, 120 g	60	<1	2
Asparagus, ½ cup			
canned, drained, 120 g	25	1	7
cooked, drained, 90 g	20	<1	3
Bean sprouts, Mung, raw, ½ cup, 52 g	15	<1	1
Beet greens, cooked, drained, ½ cup, 72 g	20	<1	1
Beets, ½ cup			
canned, sliced, drained, 85 g	25	<1	1
cooked, sliced, drained, 85 g	35	<1	1
Broccoli, ½ cup			
frozen florets, cooked, 71 g	20	0	0
raw, chopped, 44 g	10	<1	1
Brussels sprouts, cooked, drained, ½ cup, 78 g	30	<1	4
Cabbage, ½ cup			
Chinese bok choy, shredded, raw, 35 g	5	<1	1
shredded, raw, 35 g	10	<1	1
shredded, cooked, drained, 75 g	15	<1	3
Carrots			
frozen, sliced, cooked, drained, ½ cup, 73 g	25	<1	1
raw, 7½" x 1⅛", 72 g	30	<1	1
Cauliflower, ½ cup			
frozen, cooked, drained, 90 g	15	<1	2
raw, 1" pieces, 50 g	10	<1	1
Celery, raw			
cooked, drained, ½ cup, 75 g	15	<1	1
raw, 7½ in x 1¼", 40 g	5	<1	1

Corn, cooked			
canned, yellow, cream style, ½ cup, 128 g	90	1	5
canned, solids & liquid, ½ cup, 128 g	80	1	5
frozen, white, cooked, drained, ½ cup, 82 g	65	<1	1
on the cob, drained, 1 ear, 140 g	85	1	9
Cucumber, raw, sliced, ½ cup, 52 g	10	<1	1
Eggplant			
cooked, drained, 1" pieces, ½ cup, 48 g	15	<1	1
in tomato sauce, 1 cup, 231 g	75	<1	3
Green beans, ½ cup			
canned, drained, 68 g	25	0	0
cooked, drained, 62 g	20	<1	2
frozen, French style 85 g	25	0	0
raw, snap, 55 g	15	<1	1
Kale, cooked, drained, ½ cup, 65 g	20	<1	2
Lettuce			
iceberg, ¼ of a 6" head, 135 g	20	<1	2
looseleaf, shredded, ½ cup, 28 g	5	<1	1
romaine, shredded, ½ cup, 28 g	5	<1	4
Lima beans, cooked, drained, ½ cup, 85 g	105	<1	2
Mushrooms			
canned, pieces, drained, ½ cup, 78 g	20	<1	2
raw, whole, 1, 18 g	5	<1	1
shiitake, cooked, ½ cup, 73 g	40	<1	1
Onions			
canned, solids & liquid, 1", 63 g	10	<1	1
raw, chopped, ½ cup, 80 g	30	<1	1
Peas, green, ½ cup			
frozen, cooked, drained, 80 g	60	<1	2
raw, 72 g	50	<1	3
Peppers, sweet, red or green, ½ cup			
cooked, drained, 68 g	20	<1	1
raw, 50 g	15	<1	1
Potatoes			
baked, w/skin, 4¾" x 2⅓", 156 g	220	<1	2
boiled, no skin, 2½ inch diameter, 135 g	115	<1	1
hash browns, Ore-Ida frozen, 1 patty, 85 g	70	<1	0
mashed, w/whole milk, ½ cup, 105 g	80	1	6
scalloped, frozen, Stouffer's, ½ pkg., 165 g	135	6	52
Tater Tots, frozen, Ore-Ida, 1¼ cup, 85 g	160	7	63
Spinach, ½ cup			
frozen, cooked, drained, 95 g	25	<1	2
raw, chopped, 28 g	5	<1	1
Squash, ½ cup			
summer, cooked, drained, 90 g	20	<1	3
winter, baked cubes, 102 g	40	1	6
Sweet potatoes			
baked in skin, 5" x 2", 114 g	115	<1	1
canned, mashed, 128 g	130	<1	2
Tomato sauce, canned, ½ cup, 112 g	35	<1	2
Tomatoes, ½ cup			
canned, stewed, 103 g	35	0	0
raw, chopped, 90 g	20	<1	3
Turnip greens, cooked, drained, ½ cup, 72 g	15	<1	2
Turnips, cooked, mashed, ½ cup, 115 g	20	<1	1

Meat, Poultry, Fish, and Alternates

(Serving sizes are cooked, edible parts.)

Beef

Beef liver, 3 oz., 85 g			
braised	135	4	37
pan-fried	185	7	61
Corned beef, canned, 1 oz., 28 g	70	4	38
Ground beef, broiled, medium, 3 oz., 85 g			
extra lean	220	14	125
ground chuck	230	16	141
regular	245	18	158
Roast beef, 3 oz., 85 g			
bottom round, lean & fat	160	6	56
eye of round, lean & fat	195	11	98
pot roast, lean & fat	280	20	182
rib, lean & fat	300	24	216
tip round, lean & fat	160	7	60
Sirloin, broiled, lean & fat, 3 oz., 85 g	165	6	55
Veal, loin, lean only, roasted, 3 oz., 85 g	150	6	53

Lamb

Ground lamb, broiled, 3 oz., 85 g	240	17	150
Leg of lamb, lean & fat roasted, 3 oz., 85 g	250	18	158
Shoulder chop, lean & fat, braised, 3 oz., 85 g	295	20	185

Pork

Bacon, thick, broiled, 1 slice, 10 g	55	4	40
Bacon, Canadian, grilled, 1 slice, 23 g	45	2	18
Ham			
center slice, 3 oz., 85 g	170	11	99
canned, lean, 3 oz., 85 g	100	4	35
canned, regular, 3 oz., 85 g	190	13	116
Pork chop, loin, broiled, 3 oz., 85 g	205	11	100
Pork loin ribs, braised, 3 oz., 85 g	250	18	165
Pork roast, center loin, 3 oz., 85 g	200	11	103
Pork roast, sirloin, 3 oz., 85 g	175	8	72
Pork shoulder, roasted, 3 oz., 85 g	245	20	180

Sausage and Luncheon Meats

Bologna, 1 slice, 28 g			
beef & pork	90	8	72
turkey	55	4	40
Braunschweiger, 1 slice, 18 g	65	6	52
Chicken breast			
Oscar Mayer, roasted, 1 slice, 28 g	25	<1	3
Healthy Choice, roasted, 3 slices, 28 g	30	<1	4
Ham, boiled, 1 slice, 21 g	20	1	9
Salami			
beef, 1 slice, 23 g	60	5	43
turkey, 10% fat, 1 oz., 28 g	45	3	24
Sausage, summer, beef, 1 slice, 23 g	70	6	54
Turkey			
Oscar Mayer, roasted, 1 slice, 28 g	25	1	7
Oscar Mayer, fat-free, smoked, 4 slices, 52 g	40	<1	3

Poultry

Chicken breast, ½ breast			
boneless, w/out skin, roasted, 86 g	140	3	28
boneless, w/skin, flour fried, 98 g	220	9	78
Chicken drumstick, 1			
w/out skin, roasted, 72 g	75	2	22
w/skin, roasted, 81 g	110	6	52
Chicken liver, simmered, ½ cup, 70 g	110	4	34
Chicken, thigh, 1			
w/out skin, roasted, 71 g	110	6	51
w/skin, roasted, 81 g	155	10	86
Turkey, ground, cooked, 1 patty, 82 g	195	11	97

COUNTING YOUR CALORIES AND FAT GRAMS

Turkey, roasted			
dark meat w/out skin, diced, ½ cup, 64 g	120	5	42
dark meat w/skin, 3 oz., 85 g	190	10	88
light meat w/out skin diced, ½ cup, 64g	100	2	19
light meat w/skin, 3 oz., 85 g	170	7	64
Turkey liver, simmered, ½ cup, 70 g	120	4	38

Fish and Shellfish

Anchovies, canned in oil, drained, 5, 20 g	45	2	17
Clams, canned, drained, ½ cup, 80 g	120	2	14
Fish fillets			
breaded, frozen, 2, 99 g	280	19	171
breaded, Healthy Choice, 1, 99 g	160	5	45
Flounder, cooked, dry heat, 3 oz., 85 g	100	1	12
Halibut, cooked, dry heat, 3 oz., 85 g	120	2	22
Salmon 3 oz., 85 g			
Chinook, cooked, dry heat	195	11	102
Chum, cooked, dry heat	130	4	37
Coho, cooked, moist heat	155	6	57
Sardines, Atlantic, canned in oil, drained solids, 2, 24 g	50	3	25
Sea Bass, cooked, dry heat, 3 oz., 85 g	105	2	20
Shrimp, cooked			
breaded & fried, 4, 30 g	75	4	33
moist heat, large, 4 22 g	20	<1	2
Tuna, light, canned in water, ½ cup, 74 g	85	1	5

Eggs

Fried, whole, 1, 46 g	90	7	62
Hard-cooked, whole, 1, 50 g	80	5	48
Poached, 1 whole, , 50 g	75	5	45
Scrambled, w/marg. & whole milk, 1, 64 g	105	8	7
Soft-boiled, whole, 1, 50 g	80	6	50
Whites, raw, 1, 33 g	15	0	0

Beans and Peas

Baked beans, canned			
pork & beans, tomato sauce, ½ cup, 114 g	100	1	13
w/pork, molasses & sugar, ½ cup, 126 g	190	6	58
Black-eyed peas, ½ cup			
canned, solids & liquid, 120 g	90	1	6
cooked, drained, ½ cup, 82 g	80	<1	3
Chickpeas (garbanzos), canned, ½ cup, 120 g	145	1	12
Black beans, cooked, ½ cup, 86 g	115	<1	4
Kidney beans, cooked, ½ cup, 88 g	110	<1	4
Lima beans, cooked, drained, ½ cup, 85 g	105	<1	2
Navy beans, cooked, ½ cup, 91 g	130	1	5
Refried beans, canned, ½ cup, 126 g	135	1	12

Nuts and Seeds

Almonds, unblanched			
dried, 3 Tbs., 28 g	165	15	133
dry roasted, 3 Tbs., 26 g	150	13	119
Cashews, dry roasted, 3 Tbs., 28 g	165	13	118
Coconut, dried, sweetened, flaked, 2 Tbs., 9 g	45	3	27
Peanut butter, 2 Tbs., 32 g	190	14	126
Peanuts, roasted			
dry roasted, 3 Tbs., 28 g	165	14	125
honey roasted, 3 Tbs., 28 g	170	14	126
Pecans, dried, ½ cup, 28 g	190	19	173
Pine nuts, dried, 1 Tbs., 10 g	50	5	46

Pistachios, dry roasted, 3 Tbs., 28 g	170	15	135
Sesame seeds			
Tahini, raw kernels, 1 Tbs., 15 g	85	7	65
dried, kernels, 1 Tbs., 8 g	45	4	39
Sunflower seeds, dry roasted, 3 Tbs., 28 g	165	14	127
Walnuts, dried, ¼ cup, 28 g	180	18	158

Meat Substitutes

Burger, vegetarian			
Vege burger, Natural Touch, 1, 64 g	140	6	54
Veggie Sizzler, nonfat, Soy Boy, 1, 85 g	90	0	0
Hot dog, Not Dogs, 1, 43 g	105	5	45
Tofu			
fried, 2¾ x 1 x ½", 29 g	80	6	53
regular, ½ cup, 124 g	95	6	53

Dairy Products

Cheese

American, light, 1 slice, 28g	70	4	36
Blue, crumbled (not packed), ¼ cup, 34 g	120	10	87
Brie, 1 oz., 28 g	95	8	70
Cheddar			
1″ cube, 17 g	70	6	51
light, 1 slice, 28 g	70	4	36
Colby, 10 oz., 28 g	110	9	79
Cottage cheese, ½ cup			
creamed, large curd, 113 g	115	5	46
dry curd, 73 g	60	<1	3
low-fat, 1% fat, 113 g	80	1	10
Cream cheese, 2 Tbs.			
light, Philadelphia brand, 28 g	60	5	45
regular, 30 g	105	10	94
whipped, Philadelphia brand, 28 g	100	10	90
Feta, 1 oz., 28 g	75	6	54
Mozzarella, 1 oz., 28 g			
regular	80	6	54
part skim	70	4	40
Parmesan, grated, 1 Tbs., 5 g	25	2	14
Swiss			
1″ cube, 15 g	55	4	37
light, 1 slice, 28 g	70	3	27

Cream

Half & half, 1 Tbs., 15 g	20	2	16
Heavy, whipping, 1 Tbs., 15 g	50	6	48
Sour cream			
cultured, 2 Tbs., 24 g	50	5	45
light, 50% less fat, 2 Tbs., 30 g	40	2	22
Whipped cream, pressurized, 1 Tbs., 3 g	10	1	6

Imitation Cream Products

Coffee creamers			
nondairy, liquid, Coffee Rich, 1 Tbs., 14 g	25	1	13
nondairy, liquid, Int'l Delight, 1 Tbs., 15 g	45	2	14
Sour cream			
imitation, cultured, nondairy, 2 Tbs., 28 g	60	5	49
imitation, nonbutterfat, 2 Tbs., 24 g	45	4	36
powdered, Coffee-Mate, 1 tsp., 2 g	10	1	6
Whipped topping			
nondairy, pressurized, 2 Tbs., 9 g	25	2	19
nondairy, frozen, Cool Whip, 1 Tbs., 4 g	10	1	7

Milk

Buttermilk, 1% fat, 1 cup, 245 g	100	2	19
Chocolate milk, 1 cup, 250 g			
low-fat, 1% fat	160	2	22
whole	210	8	76
Condensed, sweetened, 2 Tbs., 38 g	125	3	30
Evaporated, canned, 2 Tbs., 32 g			
low-fat	30	1	5
skim	25	<1	1
whole	40	2	21
Low-fat, 1% fat, 1 cup, 244 g	100	3	23
Skim, 1 cup, 245 g	85	<1	4
Whole, 3.3% fat, 1 cup, 244 g	150	8	73

Yogurt

Fruit flavors, custard, Yoplait, 1 cont., 170 g	190	4	36
Fruit-on-the-bottom, low-fat, 1 cont., 226 g	230	3	27
Plain, 1 cont., 226 g			
low-fat	145	4	32
nonfat	125	<1	4

Soups

Canned Soups

(Canned, condensed soups are prepared with water, unless otherwise noted.)

Bean & ham, Healthy Choice, ½ can, 228 g	220	4	36
Beef broth, ready-to-serve, 1 cup, 240 g	15	1	5
Black bean, Healthy Valley, 1 cup, 240 g	110	0	0
Chicken broth, ready-to-serve, ½ can, 249 g	30	3	27
Chicken noodle, Campbell's, 1 cup, 226 g	60	2	18
Chicken rice, 1 cup, 241 g	60	2	17
Clam chowder, New England			
frozen, Stouffer's 1 cup, 227 g	180	9	81
prepared w/skim milk, 1 cup, 233 g	100	2	18
prepared w/water, Campbell's, 1 cup, 224 g	80	2	20
Cream of Chicken, 1 cup, 244 g	110	7	62
Cream of mushroom, 1 cup			
prepared w/water, 244 g	130	9	81
prepared w/whole milk, 248 g	205	14	122
Minestrone			
prepared w/water, 1 cup, 241 g	80	3	23
ready-to-serve, Hain, ½ can, 270 g	160	3	27
Tomato, 1 cup			
prepared w/water, 244 g	85	2	17
prepared w/whole milk, 248 g	160	6	54
Vegetable			
prepared w/water, 1 cup, 241 g	90	1	9
ready-to-serve, Pritikin, ½ can, 209 g	70	0	0

Dried or Dehydrated Soups

Black bean, Nile Spice, 1 container, 309 g	180	1	5
Chicken vegetable, 1 cup, 251 g	50	1	7
Cream of chicken, 1 cup, 261 g	105	5	48
Mushroom, 1 cup, 253 g	95	1	44
Onion, 1 pkg., 7 g	20	<1	4
Split pea, 1 cup, 271 g	135	2	14
Tomato, 1 cup, 265 g	105	2	22

Desserts, Snack Foods, and Candy

Cakes

Angel food, ½ of 10" tube, 50 g	130	<1	1
Boston Cream Pie, ⅛ of 20 oz., 92 g	230	8	70
Carrot cake, Sara Lee, snack size, 1, 52 g	180	7	63
Cheesecake, plain, ⅙ of 17 oz., 80 g	255	18	160
Cupcake, 1			
chocolate, Hostess, 46 g	170	5	45
yellow, w/icing, 36 g	130	4	34
Devil's food, w/icing, ⅙ of 9", 69 g	235	8	72
Fruitcake, 1 slice, 34 g	140	4	35
Pound cake, Sara Lee, ¹⁄₁₀ of cake, 30 g	130	7	63
Yellow cake, w/icing, ⅛ of 8 oz., 64 g	240	9	84

Cookies and Bars

Brownies, chocolate			
frozen, Weight-Watchers, 1, 36 g	100	3	27
from mix, 2" square, 33 g	140	7	59
Chocolate chip			
Chips Ahoy!, 3, 32 g	160	8	72
refrigerated, Pillsbury, 2, 31 g	140	7	59
Creme sandwich, Nabisco, 2, 28 g	140	6	54
Fig bar, 2, 31 g	110	2	21
Gingersnaps, Sunshine, 6, 28 g	120	4	36
Graham crackers, 4, 1½" squares, 28 g	120	2	18
Oatmeal raisin, Barbara's, 2, 38 g	160	7	63
Oreo, Nabisco, 2, 28 g	100	4	36
Shortbread, 1⅝" square, 4, 32 g	160	8	69
Vanilla wafers, Nabisco, 7, 28 g	120	4	36

Pies

Apple, ⅛ of 9" pie, 155 g	410	19	175
Blueberry, ⅛ of 9" pie, 147 g	360	17	157
Cherry, ⅛ of 9" pie, 180 g	485	22	198
Chocolate cream, ⅛ of 9" pie, 142 g	400	23	206
Custard, ⅛ of 9" pie, 127 g	260	11	102
Lemon meringue, ⅛ of 9" pie, 127 g	360	16	147
Pumpkin, ⅛ of 9" pie, 155 g	315	14	130

Other Desserts

Custard, baked, ½ cup, 141 g	150	7	60
Frozen yogurt, vanilla, ½ cup			
Häagen-Dazs, 98 g	160	2	22
Yoplait, soft, 72 g	90	3	27
Gelatin, Jell-O, ½ cup, 140 g	80	0	0
Ice cream, vanilla, ½ cup			
regular, 10% fat, 66 g	135	7	65
Häagen-Dazs, 106 g	260	17	153
Ice cream, chocolate, ½ cup			
regular, 10% fat, 66 g	145	7	65
Häagen-Dazs, 106 g	270	17	153
Ice milk sandwich, Weight Watchers, 78 g	160	4	36
Juice bars			
Strawberry, Fruit'n Juice, Dole, 74 g	70	0	0
Strawberry, Welch's, 85 g	80	0	0
Puddings, from mix, prepared w/2% milk			
butterscotch, ½ cup, 148 g	150	2	20
chocolate, ½ cup, 147 g	150	2	20

tapioca, ½ cup, 141 g	145	2	22
vanilla, ½ cup, 144 g	140	2	20
Sherbet, ½ cup, 87 g	135	2	17

Snack Foods

Corn chips, ¾ cup, 28 g	155	9	85
Crackers (see Crackers)			
Nuts (see Nuts and Seeds)			
Popcorn			
air-popped, 1 cup, 8 g	30	<1	3
microwave, natural flavor, 1 cup, 8 g	35	2	18
Potato chips, 1 cup, 28 g	150	10	90
Pretzels			
Dutch, twisted, 2¾", 2, 32 g	120	1	10
Sticks, 2½ x ⅛", 60, 30 g	115	1	9
Twists, thin, Rold Gold, 10, 28 g	110	1	9

Candy

Caramel, plain, ¾ inch, 8 g	30	1	6
Fudge, chocolate, 1 cu inch, 17 g	65	1	13
Gum drops, 8, 28 g	110	0	0
Hard candy, 5, 28 g	105	0	0
Jellybeans, 10 large or 26 small, 28 g	105	<1	1
Hershey's Kisses, 6, 28 g	150	9	81
Lollipops, 1, 28 g	110	0	0

Beverages

(Milk and juices are in Dairy Products and Fruits sections.)

Carbonated Sodas

Cola, 1½ cup, 370 g	150	<1	0
Diet cola, w/aspartame, 1½ cup, 355 g	4	0	0
Gingerale, 1½ cup, 366 g	125	0	0
Grape soda, 1½ cup, 372 g	160	0	0
Lemon-lime, 1½ cup, 368 g	145	0	0
Orange soda, 1½ cup, 372 g	180	0	0
Root beer, 1½ cup, 370 g	150	0	0

Coffee and Tea

Coffee			
brewed, 1 cup, 235 g	5	<1	0
brewed, decaffeinated, 1 cup, 240 g	3	0	0
instant, 1 cup, 240 g	5	0	0
Tea, brewed, 1 cup 237 g	2	<1	0
Tea, brewed herb, unflavored, 1 cup, 236 g	2	<1	0
Tea, iced, instant, lemon flavored			
sweetened w/aspartame, 1 cup, 259 g	2	0	0
sweetened w/sugar, made w/4 tsp., 23 g	85	<1	0

Alcoholic Beverages

Beer, 1½ cup, 355 g			
light	100	0	0
regular	145	0	0
nonalcoholic	50	0	0
Gin, Rum, Whiskey, or Vodka,			
80 proof, 1 jigger, 42 g	95	0	0
Wine, 1 glass			
red, 147 g	105	0	0
white, 147 g	100	0	0
Wine cooler, 1 glass, 360 g	175	<1	0

Wine, dessert, 1 glass			
dry, 59 g	75	0	0
sweet, 59 g	90	0	0

Fats, Oils, and Condiments

Fats and Oils

Butter			
regular or unsalted, 1 tsp., 5 g	35	4	37
whipped, 1 Tbs., 11 g	80	9	80
Margarine			
spread, tub, 1 Tbs., 14 g	75	9	75
stick, 1 Tbs., 14 g	100	11	100
Oil			
corn, 1 Tbs., 14 g	120	14	122
olive, 1 Tbs., 14 g	120	14	122
vegetable spray, 1¼ seconds, 1 g	5	1	5
Salad dressing			
blue cheese, 1 Tbs., 15 g	75	8	72
French 1 Tbs., 16 g	65	6	57
French, low-calorie, 1 Tbs., 16 g	20	1	9
Italian, 1 Tbs., 15 g	70	7	64
Italian, low calorie, 1 Tbs., 16 g	15	1	12
mayonnaise-like, 1 Tbs., 15 g	55	5	43
thousand island, 1 Tbs., 16 g	60	6	50
Barbecue sauce, 1 Tbs., 15g	15	<1	3
Catsup, 1 Tbs., 15 g	15	<1	0
Gravy, canned			
au jus, ¼ cup, 60 g	10	<1	1
beef, ¼ cup, 58 g	30	1	12
chicken, ¼ cup, 60 g	45	3	30
turkey, ¼ cup, 60 g	30	1	11
Horseradish, prepared, 1 tsp., 5 g	2	<1	0
Mustard, prepared, 1 tsp., 5 g	4	<1	2
Olives			
black, canned, small, 3, 10 g	10	1	9
green, medium, 4, 13 g	15	2	14
green, stuffed, 10, 34 g	35	4	34
Pickles			
dill, kosher spears, 1, 28 g	5	0	0
sweet, gherkins, small, 2½", 2, 30 g	40	<1	0
Relish, sweet pickle, 2 Tbs., 30 g	40	<1	1
Soy sauce, tamari, 1 Tbs., 18 g	10	<1	0
Tartar sauce, 1 Tbs., 14 g	75	8	68

Sugar, Jams, and Jellies

Chocolate syrup			
fudge-type, 2 Tbs., 42 g	145	6	51
thin-type, 2 Tbs., 38 g	82	<1	3
Honey, 1 Tbs., 21 g	65	0	0
Jams and preserves, 1 Tbs., 20 g	50	<1	0
Jellies, 1 Tbs., 19 g	50	<1	0
Maple syrup, 2 Tbs., 40 g	105	<1	1
Sugar			
brown, unpacked, 1 cup, 145 g	545	0	0
white, granulated, 1 tsp., 4 g	15	0	0

Fast Foods

Burgers and Sandwiches

Burger King

Big Fish	700	41	370
Broiler Chicken	550	29	260
Double Cheeseburger with Bacon	640	39	350
Hamburger	330	15	140
Whopper	640	39	350

McDonald's

Big Mac	530	28	250
Filet-O-Fish	360	16	150
Hamburger	270	10	90
McChicken	570	30	270
McGrilled Chicken	510	30	270

Wendy's

Big Bacon Classic	610	33	290
Chicken Club	500	23	200
Grilled Chicken Sandwich	310	8	70
Hamburger, with everything	420	20	180

Salads, Fries, and Miscellaneous

(Salad values are given for salads without dressing.)

Burger King

Broiled Chicken Salad	200	10	90
French fries, medium	370	20	180
Garden Salad	100	5	45
Salad dressing, 30 g, thousand island	140	12	110
Salad dressing, 30 g, ranch	180	19	170
Salad dressing, 30 g, reduced-calorie Italian	15	<1	5

McDonald's

Chef Salad	210	11	100
Fajita Chicken Salad	160	6	60
French fries, large	450	22	200
French fries, small	210	10	90
Salad dressing, 1 pkg., blue cheese	190	17	150
Salad dressing, 1 pkg., lite vinaigrette	50	2	20
Salad dressing, 1 pkg., ranch	180	19	170

Pizza Hut

Breadsticks, 5	770	25	223
Buffalo wings, 12	565	35	310
Cheese pizza, ⅛ of med., thin crust	205	8	75
Cheese pizza, ⅛ of med., pan pizza	260	11	98
Pepperoni pizza, ⅛ of med., thin crust	215	10	69
Veggie Lover's, ⅛ of med., thin crust	185	7	61

Wendy's

Baked potato, plain	310	0	0
Baked potato w/chili and cheese	620	24	220
Baked potato w/sour cream and chives	380	6	60
Deluxe Garden Salad	110	6	50
Salad dressing, 2 Tbs., blue cheese	170	19	170
Salad dressing, 2 Tbs., fat-free French	30	0	0
Salad dressing, 2 Tbs., ranch	90	10	90

Desserts

Burger King

Dutch apple pie	300	15	140

McDonald's

Baked apple pie	260	13	120
Cookies	260	9	80

Pizza Hut

Dessert pizza, ⅛ of med.	245	5	46

Wendy's

Chocolate chip cookies, 1, 57 g	270	11	100

abscess A localized accumulation of pus and disintegrating tissue.

absorption The passage of substances into or across membranes or tissues.

abstinence Voluntary refrainment from sexual intercourse.

acid rain Rain with a high concentration of acids produced by air pollutants emitted during the combustion of fossil fuels and the smelting of ores; damages plant and animal life and buildings.

acquired immune deficiency syndrome (AIDS) The final stages of HIV infection, characterized by a variety of severe illnesses and decreased levels of certain immune cells.

active stretching A technique that involves stretching a muscle by contracting the opposing muscle.

acupuncture A Chinese medical practice of puncturing the body with needles inserted at specific points to relieve pain or cure disease.

acute injuries Physical injuries, such as sprains, bruises, and pulled muscles, which result from sudden traumas, such as falls or collisions.

adaptive response The body's attempt to reestablish homeostasis or stability.

addiction A behavioral pattern characterized by compulsion, loss of control, and continued repetition of a behavior or activity in spite of adverse consequences.

additive Characterized by a combined effect that is equal to the sum of the individual effects.

additives Substances added to foods to enhance certain qualities, such as appearance, taste, or freshness.

adoption The legal process for becoming the parent to a child of other biological parents.

advance directives Documents that specify individual's preferences regarding treatment in a medical crisis.

aerobic circuit training Combining aerobic and strength exercises to build both cardiorespiratory fitness and muscular strength and endurance.

aerobic exercise Physical activity in which sufficient or excess oxygen is continually supplied to the body.

aging The characteristic pattern of normal life changes that occur as humans grow older.

alcohol abuse Continued use of alcohol despite awareness of social, occupational, psychological, or physical problems related to its use, or use of alcohol in dangerous ways or situations, such as before driving.

alcohol dependence Development of a strong craving for alcohol due to the pleasurable feelings or relief of stress or anxiety produced by drinking.

alcoholism A chronic, progressive, potentially fatal disease characterized by impaired control of drinking, a preoccupation with alcohol, continued use of alcohol despite adverse consequences, and distorted thinking, most notably denial.

allergy A hypersensitivity to a particular substance in one's environment or diet.

allopathic medicine Conventional or orthodox Western medicine.

allostasis The body's ability to adapt to constantly changing environments.

altruism Acts of helping or giving to others without thought of self-benefit.

Alzheimer's disease A progressive deterioration of intellectual powers due to physiological changes within the brain; symptoms include diminishing ability to concentrate and reason, disorientation, depression, apathy, and paranoia.

amenorrhea The absence or suppression of menstruation.

amino acids Organic compounds containing nitrogen, carbon, hydrogen, and oxygen; the essential building blocks of proteins.

amnion The innermost membrane of the sac enclosing the embryo or fetus.

amphetamine Any of a class of stimulants that trigger the release of epinephrine, which stimulates the central nervous system; users experience a state of hyper-alertness and energy, followed by a crash as the drug wears off.

anabolic steroids Drugs derived from testosterone and approved for medical use, but often used by athletes to increase their musculature and weight.

anaerobic exercise Physical activity in which the body develops an oxygen deficit.

androgyny The expression of both masculine and feminine traits.

anemia A condition characterized by a marked reduction in the number of circulating red blood cells or in hemoglobin, the oxygen-carrying component of red blood cells.

angina pectoris A severe, suffocating chest pain caused by a brief lack of oxygen to the heart.

angioplasty Surgical repair of an obstructed artery by passing a balloon catheter through the blood vessel to the area of disease and then inflating the catheter to compress the plaque against the vessel wall.

anorexia nervosa A psychological disorder in which refusal to eat and/or an extreme loss of appetite leads to malnutrition, severe weight loss, and possibly death.

antagonistic Opposing or counteracting.

antibiotics Substances produced by microorganisms, or synthetic agents, that are toxic to other types of microorganisms; in dilute solutions, used to treat infectious diseases.

antidepressant A drug used primarily to treat symptoms of depression.

antioxidants Substances that prevent the damaging effects of oxidation in cells.

antiviral drug A substance that decreases the severity and duration of a viral infection if taken prior to or soon after onset of the infection.

anxiety A feeling of apprehension and dread, with or without a known cause; may range from mild to severe and may be accompanied by physical symptoms.

anxiety disorders A group of psychological disorders involving episodes of apprehension, tension, or uneasiness, stemming from the anticipation of danger and sometimes accompanied by physical symptoms, which cause significant distress and impairment to an individual.

aorta The main artery of the body, arising from the left ventricle of the heart.

appetite A desire for food, stimulated by anticipated hunger, physiological changes within the brain and body, the availability of food, and other environmental and psychological factors.

arrhythmia Any irregularity in the rhythm of the heartbeat.

arteriosclerosis Any of a number of chronic diseases characterized by degeneration of the arteries and hardening and thickening of arterial walls.

arthritis Inflammation of the joints.

artificial insemination The introduction of viable sperm into the vagina by artificial means for the purpose of inducing conception.

assertive Behaving in a confident manner to make your needs and desires clear to others in a nonhostile way.

asthma A disease or allergic response characterized by bronchial spasms and difficult breathing.

atherosclerosis A form of arteriosclerosis in which fatty substances (plaque) are deposited on the inner walls of arteries.

atrial fibrillation A condition characterized by an irregular, abnormally rapid heartbeat.

atrium (plural **atria**) Either of the two upper chambers of the heart, which receive blood from the veins.

attention deficit/hyperactivity disorder (ADHD) A spectrum of difficulties in controlling motion and sustaining attention, including hyperactivity, impulsivity, and distractibility.

autoimmune disorder Resulting from the attack on body tissue by an immune system that fails to recognize the tissue as self.

autonomy The ability to draw on internal resources; independence from familial and societal influences.

autoscopy The sensation of one's self being outside its body, often experienced by individuals in near-death medical crises.

aversion therapy A treatment that attempts to help a person overcome a dependence or bad habit by making the person feel disgusted or repulsed by that habit.

axon The long fiber that conducts impulses from the neuron's nucleus to its dendrites.

axon terminal The ending of an axon, from which impulses are transmitted to a dendrite of another neuron.

ayurveda A traditional Indian medical treatment involving meditation, exercise, herbal medications, and nutrition.

bacteria (singular, **bacterium**) One-celled microscopic organisms; the most plentiful pathogens.

bacterial vaginosis A vaginal infection caused by overgrowth and depletion of various microorganisms living in the vagina, resulting in a malodorous white or gray vaginal discharge.

ballistic stretching Rapid bouncing movements.

barbiturates Antianxiety drugs that depress the central nervous system, reduce activity and induce relaxation, drowsiness, or sleep; often prescribed to relieve tension and treat epileptic seizures or as a general anesthetic.

barrier contraceptives Birth-control devices that block the meeting of egg and sperm, either by physical barriers, such as condoms, diaphragms, or cervical caps, or by chemical barriers, such as spermicide, or both.

basal body temperature The body temperature upon waking, before any activity.

basal metabolic rate (BMR) The number of calories required to sustain the body at rest.

behavior therapy Psychotherapy that emphasizes application of the principles of learning to substitute desirable responses and behavior patterns for undesirable ones.

benign prostatic hypertrophy Enlargement of the prostate gland, resulting in a pinching of the urethra.

benzodiazepines Antianxiety drugs that depress the central nervous system, reduce activity and induce relaxation, drowsiness, or sleep; often prescribed to relieve tension, muscular strain, sleep problems, anxiety, and panic attacks; also used as an anesthetic and in the treatment of alcohol withdrawal.

bidis Skinny, sweet-flavored cigarettes.

binge drinking For a man, having five or more alcoholic drinks at a single sitting; for a woman, having four drinks or more at a single sitting.

binge eating The rapid consumption of an abnormally large amount of food in a relatively short time.

biofeedback A technique of becoming aware, with the aid of external monitoring devices, of internal physiological activities in order to develop the capability of altering them.

bipolar disorder Severe depression alternating with periods of manic activity and elation.

bisexual Sexually oriented toward both sexes.

blended family A family formed when one or both of the partners bring children from a previous union to the new marriage.

blood-alcohol concentration (BAC) The amount of alcohol in the blood, expressed as a percentage.

body composition The relative amounts of fat and lean tissue (bone, muscle, organs, water) in the body.

body mass index (BMI) A mathematical formula that correlates with body fat; the ratio of weight to height squared.

bone-marrow transplantation A cancer treatment involving high doses of radiation or chemotherapy during which the marrow is destroyed and then replaced with healthy bone marrow.

botulism Possibly fatal food poisoning, caused by a type of bacterium that grows and produces its toxin in the absence of air and is found in improperly canned food.

bradycardia An abnormally slow heart rate, under 60 beats per minute.

breech birth A birth in which the infant's buttocks or feet pass through the birth canal first.

bulimia nervosa Episodic binge eating, often followed by forced vomiting or laxative abuse, and accompanied by a persistent preoccupation with body shape and weight.

bupropion A drug, also known as Zyban, for treating nicotine addiction that is an alternative to the nicotine patch.

burnout A state of physical, emotional, and mental exhaustion resulting from constant or repeated emotional pressure.

caesarean delivery The surgical procedure in which an infant is delivered through an incision made in the abdominal wall and uterus.

calorie The amount of energy required to raise the temperature of 1 gram of water by 1 degree Celsius. In everyday usage related to the energy content of foods and the energy expended in activities, a calorie is actually the equivalent of a thousand such calories, or a kilocalorie.

candidiasis An infection of the yeast *Candida albicans,* commonly occurring in the vagina, vulva, penis, and mouth and causing burning, itching, and a whitish discharge.

capillary A minute blood vessel that connects an artery to a vein.

carbohydrates Organic compounds, such as starches, sugars, and glycogen, that are composed of carbon, hydrogen, and oxygen, and are sources of bodily energy.

carbon monoxide A colorless, odorless gas produced by the burning of gasoline or tobacco; displaces oxygen in the hemoglobin molecules of red blood cells.

carcinogen A substance that produces cancerous cells or enhances their development and growth.

cardiopulmonary resuscitation (CPR) A method of artificial stimulation of the heart and lungs; a combination of mouth-to-mouth breathing and chest compression.

cardiorespiratory fitness The ability of the heart and blood vessels to circulate blood through the body efficiently.

celibacy Abstention from sexual activity; can be partial or complete, permanent or temporary.

cell-mediated The portion of the immune response that protects against parasites, fungi, cancer cells, and foreign tissue, primarily by means of T cells, or lymphocytes.

certified social worker A person who has completed a two-year graduate program in counseling people with mental problems.

cervical cap A thimble-sized rubber or plastic cap that is inserted into the vagina to fit over the cervix and prevent the passage of sperm into the uterus during sexual intercourse; used with a spermicidal foam or jelly, it serves as both a chemical and a physical barrier to sperm.

cervix The narrow, lower end of the uterus that opens into the vagina.

chanchroid A soft, painful sore or localized infection usually acquired through sexual contact.

chemoprevention The use of natural or synthetic substances to reduce the risk of developing cancer.

chiropractic A method of treating disease, primarily through manipulating the bones and joints to restore normal nerve function.

chlamydial infections A sexually transmitted disease caused by the bacterium *Chlamydia trachomatis,* often asymptomatic in women, but sometimes characterized by urinary pain; if undetected and untreated, may result in pelvic inflammatory disease (PID).

chlorinated hydrocarbons Highly toxic pesticides, such as DDT and chlordane, that are extremely resistant to breakdown; may cause cancer, birth defects, neurological disorders, and damage to wildlife and the environment.

cholesterol An organic substance found in animal fats; linked to cardiovascular disease, particularly atherosclerosis.

chronic fatigue syndrome (CFS) A cluster of symptoms whose cause is not yet known; a primary symptom is debilitating fatigue.

chronic obstructive lung disease (COLD) Any one of several lung diseases characterized by obstruction of breathing, including emphysema and chronic bronchitis.

circumcision The surgical removal of the foreskin of the penis.

cirrhosis A chronic disease, especially of the liver, characterized by a degeneration of cells and excessive scarring.

clitoris A small erectile structure on the female, corresponding to the penis on the male.

club drugs Illegally manufactured psychoactive drugs that have dangerous physical and psychological effects.

cocaine A white crystalline powder extracted from the leaves of the coca plant which stimulates the central nervous system and produces a brief period of euphoria followed by a depression.

codependence An emotional and psychological behavioral pattern in which the spouses, partners, parents, children, and friends of individuals with addictive behaviors allow or enable their loved ones to continue their self-destructive habits.

cognitive therapy A technique used to identify an individual's beliefs and attitudes, recognize negative thought patterns, and educate in alternative ways of thinking.

cohabitation Two people living together as a couple, without official ties such as marriage.

coitus interruptus The removal of the penis from the vagina before ejaculation.

colpotomy Surgical sterilization by cutting or blocking the fallopian tubes through an incision made in the wall of the vagina.

coma A state of total unconsciousness.

companion-oriented marriage A marital relationship in which the partners share interests, activities, and domestic responsibilities.

complementary and alternative medicine (CAM) A term used to apply to all health-care approaches, practices, and treatments not widely taught in medical schools, not generally used in hospitals, and not usually reimbursed by medical insurance companies.

complementary proteins Incomplete proteins that, when combined, provide all the amino acids essential for protein synthesis.

complete proteins Proteins that contain all the amino acids needed by the body for growth and maintenance.

complex carbohydrates Starches, including cereals, fruits, and vegetables.

computer vision syndrome A condition caused by computer use marked by tired and sore eyes, blurred vision, headaches, and neck, shoulder, and back pain.

conception The merging of a sperm and an ovum.

conditioning The gradual building up of the body to enhance one or more of the three main components of physical fitness: flexibility, cardiorespiratory or aerobic fitness, and muscular strength and endurance.

condom A latex sheath worn over the penis during sexual acts to prevent conception and/or the transmission of disease; some condoms contain a spermicidal lubricant.

congestive heart failure Inability of the heart to pump at normal capacity, resulting in decreased blood flow throughout the body, collection of blood fluids in the lungs, and pulmonary congestion.

constant-dose combination pill An oral contraceptive that releases synthetic estrogen and progestin at constant levels throughout the menstrual cycle.

contraception The prevention of conception; birth control.

coronary angiography A diagnostic test in which a thin tube is threaded through the blood vessels of the heart, a dye is injected, and X rays are taken to detect blockage of the arteries.

coronary bypass Surgical correction of a blockage in a coronary artery by grafting an artery from the patient's leg or chest wall onto the damaged artery to detour blood around the blockage.

corpus luteum A yellowish mass of tissue that is formed, immediately after ovulation, from the remaining cells of the follicle; it secretes estrogen and progesterone for the remainder of the menstrual cycle.

Cowper's glands Two small glands that discharge into the male urethra; also called bulbourethral glands.

crib death *See* sudden infant death syndrome (SIDS).

cross-training Alternating two or more different types of fitness activities.

crucifers Plants, including broccoli, cabbage, and cauliflower, that contain large amounts of fiber, proteins, and indoles.

culture The set of shared attitudes, values, goals, and practices of a group that are internalized by an individual within the group.

cunnilingus Sexual stimulation of a woman's genitals by means of oral manipulation.

cystitis Inflammation of the urinary bladder.

daily values (DV) Reference values developed by the FDA specifically for use on food labels.

decibel (dB) A unit for measuring the intensity of sounds.

defense mechanism A psychological process that alleviates anxiety and eliminates mental conflict; includes denial, displacement, projection, rationalization, reaction formation, and repression.

deleriants Chemicals, such as solvents, aerosols, glue, cleaning fluids, petroleum products, and some anesthetics, that produce vapors with psychoactive effects when inhaled.

delirium tremens (DTs) The delusions, hallucinations, and agitated behavior following withdrawal from long-term chronic alcohol abuse.

dementia Deterioration of mental capability.

dendrites Branching fibers of a neuron that receive impulses from axon terminals of other neurons and conduct these impulses toward the nucleus.

dental dam A small sheet of latex used as a barrier between the vagina and the mouth during cunnilingus to prevent transmission of STIs.

depression In general, feelings of unhappiness and despair; as a mental illness, also characterized by an inability to function normally.

depressive disorders A group of psychological disorders involving pervasive and sustained depression.

dermatitis Any inflammation of the skin.

detoxification The supervised removal of a poisonous or harmful substance (such as a drug) from the body; a therapy for alcoholics in which they are denied alcohol in a controlled environment.

diabetes mellitus A disease in which the inadequate production of insulin leads to failure of the body tissues to break down carbohydrates at a normal rate.

diagnostic-related group (DRG) A category of conditions requiring hospitalization for which the cost of care has been determined prior to a client's hospitalization.

diaphragm A bowl-like rubber cup with a flexible rim that is inserted into the vagina to cover the cervix and prevent the passage of sperm into the uterus during sexual intercourse; used with a spermicidal foam or jelly, it serves as both a chemical and a physical barrier to sperm.

diastole The period between contractions in the cardiac cycle, during which the heart relaxes and dilates as it fills with blood.

dietary fiber The nondigestible form of carbohydrates found in plant foods, such as leaves, stems, skins, seeds, and hulls.

dilation and evacuation (D and E) A medical procedure in which the contents of the uterus are removed through the use of instruments.

distress A negative stress that may result in illness.

do-not-resuscitate (DNR) An advance directive expressing an individual's preference that resuscitation efforts not be made during a medical crisis.

drug Any substance, other than food, that affects bodily functions and structures when taken into the body.

drug abuse The excessive use of a drug in a manner inconsistent with accepted medical practice.

drug misuse The use of a drug for a purpose (or person) other than that for which it was medically intended.

dyathanasia The act of permitting death by the removal or ending of any extraordinary efforts to sustain life; passive euthanasia.

dynamic flexibility The ability to move a joint quickly and fluidly through its entire range of motion with little resistance.

dysfunctional Characterized by negative and destructive patterns of behavior between partners or between parents and children.

dysmenorrhea Painful menstruation.

dyspareunia A sexual difficulty in which a woman experiences pain during sexual intercourse.

dysthymia Frequent, prolonged mild depression.

eating disorders Bizarre, often dangerous patterns of food consumption, including anorexia nervosa and bulimia nervosa.

ecosystem A community of organisms sharing a physical and chemical environment and interacting with each other.

ecstasy (MDMA) A synthetic compound, also known as methylenedioxymethamphetamine, that is similar in structure to methamphetamine and has both stimulant and hallucinogenic effects.

ectopic pregnancy A pregnancy in which the fertilized egg has implanted itself outside the uterine cavity, usually in the fallopian tube.

ejaculation The expulsion of semen from the penis.

ejaculatory duct The canal connecting the seminal vesicles and vas deferens.

electrocardiogram (ECG, EKG) A graphic record of the electric current associated with heartbeats.

electromagnetic fields (EMFs) The invisible electric and magnetic fields generated by an electrically charged conductor.

embryo An organism in its early stage of development; in humans, the embryonic period lasts from the second to the eighth week of pregnancy.

emergency contraception Types of oral contraceptive pills usually taken within 72 hours after intercourse that can prevent pregnancy.

emotional health The ability to express and acknowledge one's feelings and moods.

emotional intelligence A term used by some psychologists to evaluate the capacity of people to understand themselves and relate well with others.

enabling To unwittingly contribute to a person's addictive or abusive behavior. Components of enabling include shielding or covering up for an abuser/addict; controlling them; taking over responsibilities; rationalizing addictive behavior; or cooperating with them.

endocrine disruptors Synthetic chemicals that interfere with the ways that hormones work in humans and wildlife.

endocrine system The group of ductless glands that produce hormones and secrete them directly into the blood for transport to target organs.

endometrium The mucous membrane lining the uterus.

endorphins Mood-elevating, pain-killing chemicals produced by the brain.

endurance The ability to withstand the stress of continued physical exertion.

environmental tobacco smoke Secondhand cigarette smoke; the third leading preventable cause of death.

epididymis That portion of the male duct system in which sperm mature.

epidural block An injection of anesthesia into the membrane surrounding the spinal cord to numb the lower body during labor and childbirth.

epilepsy A variety of neurological disorders characterized by sudden attacks (seizures) of violent muscle contractions and unconsciousness.

erectile dysfunction The consistent inability to maintain a penile erection sufficient for adequate sexual relations.

ergogenic aids Dietary supplements that purport to boost strength and enhance athletic performance, such as androstenedione and creatine.

erogenous Sexually sensitive.

essential nutrients Nutrients that the body cannot manufacture for itself and must obtain from food.

estrogen The female sex hormone that stimulates female secondary sex characteristics.

ethyl alcohol The intoxicating agent in alcoholic beverages; also called ethanol.

eustress Positive stress, which stimulates a person to function properly.

euthanasia Any method of painlessly causing death for a terminally ill person.

failure rate The number of pregnancies that occur per year for every 100 women using a particular method of birth control.

fallopian tubes The pair of channels that transport ova from the ovaries to the uterus; the usual site of fertilization.

false negative A diagnostic test result that falsely indicates the absence of a particular condition.

false positive A diagnostic test result that falsely indicates the presence of a particular condition.

family A group of people united by marriage, blood, or adoption, residing in the same household, maintaining a common culture, and interacting with one another on the basis of their roles within the group.

fellatio Sexual stimulation of a man's genitals by means of oral manipulation.

fertilization The fusion of the sperm and egg nuclei.

fetal alcohol effects (FAE) Milder forms of FAS, including low birthweight, irritability as newborns, and permanent mental impairment as a result of the mother's alcohol consumption during pregnancy.

fetal alcohol syndrome (FAS) A cluster of physical and mental defects in the newborn, including low birthweight, smaller-than-normal head circumference, intrauterine growth retardation, and permanent mental impairment caused by the mother's alcohol consumption during pregnancy.

fetus The human organism developing in the uterus from the ninth week until birth.

fiber Indigestible materials in food that lower blood cholesterol or facilitate digestion and elimination.

FITT A formula that describes the frequency, intensity, type, and length of time for physical activity.

flexibility The range of motion allowed by one's joints; determined by the length of muscles, tendons, and ligaments attached to the joints.

folate Various chemical forms of a water-soluble B vitamin that can be obtained from a diet high in vegetables and citrus fruit.

folic acid A form of folate used in vitamin supplements and fortified foods.

food allergies Hypersensitivities to particular foods.

food toxicologists Specialists who detect toxins in food and treat the conditions toxins produce.

frostbite The freezing or partial freezing of skin and tissue just below the skin, or even muscle and bone; more severe than frostnip.

frostnip Sudden blanching or lightening of the skin on hands, feet, and face, resulting from exposure to high wind speeds and low temperatures.

functional fiber Isolated, nondigestible carbohydrates with beneficial effects in humans.

fungi (singular, **fungus**) Organisms that reproduce by means of spores.

gallstones Clumps of solid material, usually cholesterol, that form in bile stored in the gallbladder.

gamma globulin The antibody-containing portion of the blood fluid (plasma).

GBL gamma butyrolactone The main ingredient in gamma hydroxybutyrate (GHB), also known as the "date rape drug"; once ingested, GBL converts to GHB and can cause the ingestor to lose consciousness.

gender Maleness or femaleness, as determined by a combination of anatomical and physiological factors, psychological factors, and learned behaviors.

gene therapy A cancer treatment involving the insertion of genes into a patient.

general adaptation syndrome (GAS) The sequenced physiological response to a stressful situation; consists of three stages: alarm, resistance, and exhaustion.

generalized anxiety disorder (GAD) An anxiety disorder characterized as chronic distress.

generic Refers to products without trade names that are equivalent to other products protected by trademark registration.

GHB gamma hydroxybutyrate A brain messenger chemical that stimulates the release of human growth hormone; commonly abused for its high and its alleged ability to trim fat and build muscles. Also known as "blue nitro" or the "date rape drug."

gingivitis Inflammation of the gums.

glia Support cells for neurons in the brain and spinal cord that separate the brain from the bloodstream, assist in the growth of neurons, speed transmission of nerve impulses, and eliminate damaged neurons.

gonadotropins Gonad-stimulating hormones produced by the pituitary gland.

gonorrhea A sexually transmitted disease caused by the bacterium *Neisseria gonorrhoeae;* symptoms include discharge from the penis; women are generally asymptomatic.

guided imagery An approach to stress control, self-healing, or motivating life changes by means of visualizing oneself in the state of calmness, wellness, or change.

gum disease Inflammation of the gum and bones that hold teeth in place.

hallucinogen A drug that causes hallucinations.

hashish A concentrated form of a drug, derived from the cannabis plant, containing the psychoactive ingredient TCH, which causes a sense of euphoria when inhaled or eaten.

health A state of complete well-being, including physical, psychological, spiritual, social, intellectual, and environmental components.

health maintenance organization (HMO) An organization that provides health services on a fixed-contract basis.

health promotion An educational and informational process in which people are helped to change attitudes and behaviors in an effort to improve their health.

heat cramps Painful muscle spasms caused by vigorous exercise accompanied by heavy sweating in the heat.

heat exhaustion Faintness, rapid heart beat, low blood pressure, an ashen appearance, cold and clammy skin, and nausea, resulting from prolonged sweating with inadequate fluid replacement.

heat stress Physical response to prolonged exposure to high temperature; occurs simultaneously with or after heat cramps.

heat stroke A medical emergency consisting of a fever of at least 105°F, hot dry skin, rapid heartbeat, rapid and shallow breathing, and elevated or lowered blood pressure, caused by the breakdown of the body's cooling mechanism.

helminth A parasitic roundworm or flatworm.

hemoglobin The oxygen-transporting component of red blood cells; composed of heme and globin.

hepatitis An inflammation and/or infection of the liver caused by a virus, often accompanied by jaundice.

herbal medicine An ancient form of medical treatment using substances derived from trees, flowers, ferns, seaweeds, and lichens to treat disease.

hernia The abnormal protrusion of an organ or body part through the tissues of the walls containing it.

herpes simplex A condition caused by one of the herpes viruses and characterized by lesions of the skin or mucous membranes; herpes virus type 2 is sexually transmitted and causes genital blisters or sores.

heterosexual Primary sexual orientation toward members of the other sex.

holistic An approach to medicine that takes into account body, mind, emotions, and spirit.

holographic will A will wholly in the handwriting of its author.

home health care Provision of medical services and equipment to patients in the home to restore or maintain comfort, function, and health.

homeopathy A system of medical practice that treats a disease by administering dosages of substances that would in healthy persons produce symptoms similar to those of the disease.

homeostasis The body's natural state of balance or stability.

homocysteine A naturally occurring amino acid that has recently been identified as a risk factor for heart disease.

homosexual Primary sexual orientation toward members of the same sex.

hormone Substance released in the blood that regulates specific bodily functions.

hormone replacement therapy (HRT) The use of supplemental hormones during and after menopause.

hospice A homelike health-care facility or program committed to supportive care for terminally ill people.

host A person or population that contracts one or more pathogenic agents in an environment.

hostile or offensive environment A workplace made hostile, abusive, or unbearable by persistent inappropriate behaviors of coworkers or supervisors.

human immunodeficiency virus (HIV) A type of virus that causes a spectrum of health problems, ranging from a symptomless infection to changes in the immune system, to the development of life-threatening diseases because of impaired immunity.

human papilloma virus (HPV) A pathogen that causes genital warts and increases the risk of cervical cancer.

humoral A portion of the immune response that provides lifelong protection against bacterial or viral infections, such as mumps, by means of antibodies whose production is triggered by the release of antigens upon first exposure to the infectious agent.

hunger The physiological drive to consume food.

hypertension High blood pressure occurring when the blood exerts excessive pressure against the arterial walls.

hypothermia An abnormally low body temperature; if not treated appropriately, coma or death could result.

hysterectomy The surgical removal of the uterus.

hysterotomy A procedure in which the uterus is surgically opened and the fetus inside it removed.

immune deficiency Partial or complete inability of the immune system to respond to pathogens.

immunity Protection from infectious diseases.

immunotherapy A series of injections of small but increasing doses of an allergen, used to treating allergies.

implantation The embedding of the fertilized ovum in the uterine lining.

impotence A sexual difficulty in which a man is unable to achieve or maintain an erection.

incomplete proteins Proteins that lack one or more of the amino acids essential for protein synthesis.

incubation period The time between a pathogen's entrance into the body and the first symptom.

indemnity A form of insurance that pays a major portion of medical expenses after a deductible amount is paid by the insured person.

indoles Naturally occurring chemicals found in foods such as winter squash, carrots, and crucifers; may help lower cancer risk.

infertility The inability to conceive a child.

infiltration A gradual penetration or invasion.

inflammation A localized response by the body to tissue injury, characterized by swelling and the dilation of the blood vessels.

inflammatory bowel disease (IBD) A digestive disease that causes frequent and intense diarrhea, abdominal pain, gas, fever, and rectal bleeding. Crohn's disease is an inflammation anywhere in the digestive tract, and ulcerative colitis causes severe ulcers in the inner lining of the colon and rectum.

informed consent Permission (to undergo or receive a medical procedure or treatment) given voluntarily, with full knowledge and understanding of the procedure or treatment and its possible consequences.

inhalants Substances that produce vapors having psychoactive effects when sniffed.

integrative medicine An approach that combines traditional medicine with alternative/complementary therapies.

intercourse Sexual stimulation by means of entry of the penis into the vagina; coitus.

interpersonal therapy (IPT) A technique used to develop communication skills and relationships.

intimacy A state of closeness between two people, characterized by the desire and ability to share one's innermost thoughts and feelings with each other either verbally or nonverbally.

intoxication Maladaptive behavioral, psychological, and physiologic changes that occur as a result of substance abuse.

intramuscular Into or within a muscle.

intrauterine device (IUD) A device inserted into the uterus through the cervix to prevent pregnancy by interfering with implantation.

intravenous Into a vein.

ionizing radiation A form of energy emitted from atoms as they undergo internal change.

irradiation Exposure to or treatment by some form of radiation.

irritable bowel syndrome A digestive disease caused by intestinal spasms, resulting in frequent need to defecate, nausea, cramping, pain, gas, and a continual sensation of rectal fullness.

isokinetic Having the same force; exercise with specialized equipment that provides resistance equal to the force applied by the user throughout the entire range of motion.

isometric Of the same length; exercise in which muscles increase their tension without shortening in length, such as when pushing an immovable object.

isotonic Having the same tension or tone; exercise requiring the repetition of an action that creates tension, such as weight lifting or calisthenics.

kidney stones Formations of calcium salts or minerals that form in the kidneys; may be passed out of the body in urine, surgically removed, or decomposed by high-frequency sound waves.

labia majora The fleshy outer folds that border the female genital area.

labia minora The fleshy inner folds that border the female genital area.

labor The process leading up to birth: effacement and dilation of the cervix; the movement of the baby into and through the birth canal, accompanied by strong contractions; and contraction of the uterus and expulsion of the placenta after the birth.

lacto-vegetarians People who eat dairy products as well as fruits and vegetables (but not meat, poultry, or fish).

Lamaze method A method of childbirth preparation taught to expectant parents to help the woman cope with the discomfort of labor; combines breathing and psychological techniques.

laparoscopy A surgical sterilization procedure in which the fallopian tubes are observed with a laparoscope inserted through a small incision, and then cut or blocked.

laparotomy A surgical sterilization procedure in which the fallopian tubes are cut or blocked through an incision made in the abdomen.

licensed clinical social worker (LCSW) *See* certified social worker.

lipoprotein A compound in blood that is made up of proteins and fat; a high-density lipoprotein (HDL) picks up excess cholesterol in the blood; a low-density lipoprotein (LDL) carries more cholesterol and deposits it on the walls of arteries.

listeria A bacterium commonly found in deli meats, hot dogs, and soft cheeses that can cause an infection called listeriosis.

living will A written statement providing instructions for the use of life-sustaining procedures in the event of terminal illness or injury.

lochia The vaginal discharge of blood, mucus, and uterine tissue that occurs after birth.

locus of control An individual's belief about the source of power and influence over his or her life.

lumpectomy The surgical removal of a breast tumor and its surrounding tissue.

Lyme disease A disease caused by a bacterium carried by a tick; it may cause heart arrhythmias, neurological problems, and arthritis symptoms.

lymph nodes Small tissue masses in which some immune cells are stored.

macronutrients Nutrients required by the human body in the greatest amounts, including water, carbohydrates, proteins, and fats.

mainstream smoke The smoke inhaled directly by smoking a cigarette.

major depression Sadness that does not end.

male pattern baldness The loss of hair at the vertex, or top, of the head.

malpractice The failure of a doctor or other health-care professional to provide appropriate and skillful medical or surgical treatment.

mammography A diagnostic X-ray exam used to detect breast cancer.

managed care Health-care services and reimbursement predetermined by third-party insurers.

marijuana The drug derived from the cannabis plant, containing the psychoactive ingredient THC, which causes a mild sense of euphoria when inhaled or eaten.

marriage and family therapist A psychiatrist, psychologist, or social worker who specializes in marriage and family counseling.

massage therapy A therapeutic method of using the hands to rub, stroke, or knead the body to produce positive effects on an individual's health and well-being.

mastectomy The surgical removal of an entire breast.

masturbation Manual (or nonmanual) self-stimulation of the genitals, often resulting in orgasm.

medical abortion Method of ending a pregnancy within 9 weeks of conception using hormonal medications that cause expulsion of the fertilized egg.

medical history The health-related information collected during the interview of a client by a health-care professional.

meditation A group of approaches that use quiet sitting, breathing techniques, and/or chanting to relax, improve concentration, and become attuned to one's inner self.

menarche The onset of menstruation at puberty.

meningitis An extremely serious, potentially fatal illness that attacks the membranes around the brain and spinal cord; caused by the bacterium *Neisseria meningitis.*

menopause The complete cessation of ovulation and menstruation for twelve consecutive months.

menstruation Discharge of blood from the vagina as a result of the shedding of the uterine lining at the end of the menstrual cycle.

mental disorder Behavioral or psychological syndrome associated with distress or disability or with a significantly increased risk of suffering death, pain, disability, or loss of freedom.

mental health The ability to perceive reality as it is, to respond to its challenges, and to develop rational strategies for living.

meta-analysis Summarization and review of research in a particular area to evaluate the results of several large clinical trials in a uniform manner.

metastasize To spread to other parts of the body via the bloodstream or lymphatic system.

micronutrients Vitamins and minerals needed by the body in very small amounts.

microwaves Extremely high frequency electromagnetic waves that increase the rate at which molecules vibrate, thereby generating heat.

migraine headache Severe headache resulting from the constriction, then dilation of blood vessels within the brain; sometimes accompanied by vomiting and nausea.

mindfulness A method of stress reduction that involves experiencing the physical and mental sensations of the present moment.

minerals Naturally occurring inorganic substances, small amounts of some being essential in metabolism and nutrition.

minilaparotomy A surgical sterilization procedure in which the fallopian tubes are cut or sealed by electrical coagulation through a small incision just above the pubic hairline.

minipill An oral contraceptive containing a small amount of progestin and no estrogen, which prevents contraception by making the mucus in the cervix so thick that sperm cannot enter the uterus.

miscarriage A pregnancy that terminates before the twentieth week of gestation; also called spontaneous abortion.

mitral valve prolapse A condition in which a valve in the heart is abnormally long and floppy, which can cause heart murmurs.

mononucleosis An infectious viral disease characterized by an excess of white blood cells in the blood, fever, bodily discomfort, a sore throat, and kidney and liver complications.

monophasic pill *See* constant-dose combination pill.

mons pubis The rounded, fleshy area over the junction of the female pubic bones.

mood A sustained emotional state that colors one's view of the world for hours or days.

multiphasic pill An oral contraceptive that releases different levels of estrogen and progestin to mimic the hormonal fluctuations of the natural menstrual cycle.

multiple chemical sensitivity (MCS) A sensitivity to low-level chemical exposures from ordinary substances, such as perfumes and tobacco smoke, that results in physiological responses such as chest pain, depression, dizziness, fatigue, and nausea. Also known as environmentally triggered illness.

muscular fitness The amount of strength and level of endurance in the body's muscles.

mutagen An agent that causes alterations in the genetic material of living cells.

mutation A change in the genetic material of a cell or cells that is brought about by radiation, chemicals, or natural causes.

myocardial infarction (MI) A condition characterized by the dying of tissue areas in the myocardium, caused by interruption of the blood supply to those areas; the medical name for a heart attack.

naturopathy An alternative system of treatment of disease that emphasizes the use of natural remedies such as sun, water, heat, and air. Therapies may include dietary changes, steam baths, and exercise.

near-death experiences *See* autoscopy *and* transcendence.

negligence The failure to act in a way that a reasonable person would act.

neoplasm Any tumor, whether benign or malignant.

nephrosis A cluster of symptoms indicating chronic damage to the kidneys.

neuron The basic working unit of the brain, which transmits information from the senses to the brain and from the brain to specific body parts; each nerve cell consists of an axon, an axon terminal, and dendrites.

neuropsychiatry The study of the brain and mind.

neurotransmitters Chemicals released by neurons that stimulate or inhibit the action of other neurons.

nicotine The addictive substance in tobacco; one of the most toxic of all poisons.

nocturnal emissions Ejaculations while dreaming; wet dreams.

nongonococcal urethritis (NGU) Inflammation of the urethra caused by organisms other than the gonococcus bacterium.

nonopioids Chemically synthesized drugs that have sleep-inducing and pain-relieving properties similar to those of opium and its derivatives.

norms The unwritten rules regarding behavior and conduct expected or accepted by a group.

nucleus The central part of a cell, contained in the cell body of a neuron.

nutrition The science devoted to the study of dietary needs for food and the effects of food on organisms.

obesity The excessive accumulation of fat in the body; a condition of having a BMI of 30 or above.

obsessive-compulsive disorder (OCD) An anxiety disorder characterized by obsessions and/or compulsions that impair one's ability to function and form relationships.

oncogene A gene that, when activated by radiation or a virus, may cause a normal cell to become cancerous.

opioids Drugs that have sleep-inducing and pain-relieving properties, including opium and its derivatives and nonopioid, synthetic drugs.

optimism The tendency to seek out, remember, and expect pleasurable experiences.

oral contraceptives Preparations of synthetic hormones that inhibit ovulation; also referred to as birth control pills or simply the pill.

organic Term designating food produced with, or production based on the use of, fertilizer originating from plants or animals, without the use of pesticides or chemically formulated fertilizers.

organic phosphates Toxic pesticides that may cause cancer, birth defects, neurological disorders, and damage to wildlife and the environment.

orgasm A series of contractions of the pelvic muscles occurring at the peak of sexual arousal.

osteopathy The manipulation of the spine and other structural parts of the body to treat disorders.

osteoporosis A condition common in older people in which the bones become increasingly soft and porous, making them susceptible to injury.

outcomes The ultimate impacts of particular treatments or absence of treatment.

ovary The female sex organ that produces egg cells, estrogen, and progesterone.

over-the-counter (OTC) drugs Medications that can be obtained legally without a prescription from a medical professional.

overload principle Providing a greater stress or demand on the body than it is normally accustomed to handling.

overloading Method of physical training involving increasing the number of repetitions or the amount of resistance gradually to work the muscle to temporary fatigue.

overtrain Working muscles too intensely or too frequently, resulting in persistent muscle soreness, injuries, unintended weight loss, nervousness, and an inability to relax.

overuse injuries Physical injuries to joints or muscles, such as strains, fractures, and tendinitis, which result from overdoing a repetitive activity.

overweight A condition of having a BMI between 25.0 and 29.9.

ovo-lacto-vegetarians People who eat eggs, dairy products, and fruits and vegetables (but not meat, poultry, or fish).

ovulation The release of a mature ovum from an ovary approximately 14 days prior to the onset of menstruation.

ovulation method A method of birth control based on the observation of changes in the consistency of the mucus in the vagina to predict ovulation.

ovum (plural, **ova**) The female gamete (egg cell).

oxytocin A hormone that has been linked to one's ability to bond with others; also plays a key role in inducing labor during childbirth.

panic attack A short episode characterized by physical sensations of light-headedness, dizziness, hyperventilation, and numbness

of extremities, accompanied by an inexplicable terror, usually of a physical disaster such as death.

panic disorder An anxiety disorder in which the apprehension or experience of recurring panic attacks is so intense that normal functioning is impaired.

Pap smear A test in which cells removed from the cervix are examined under a microscope for signs of cancer; also called a Pap test.

passive stretching A stretching technique in which an external force or resistance (your body, a partner, gravity, or a weight) helps the joints move through their range of motion.

pathogen A microorganism that produces disease.

PCP (phencyclidine) A synthetic psychoactive substance that produces effects similar to other psychoactive drugs when swallowed, smoked, sniffed, or injected, but may also trigger unpredictable behavioral changes.

pelvic inflammatory disease (PID) An inflammation of the internal female genital tract, characterized by abdominal pain, fever, and tenderness of the cervix.

penis The male organ of sex and urination.

percutaneous transluminal coronary angioplasty (PTCA) A procedure for unclogging arteries; also called balloon angioplasty.

perimenopause The period from a woman's first irregular cycles to her last menstruation.

perinatology The medical specialty concerned with the diagnosis and treatment of pregnant women with high-risk conditions and their fetuses.

perineum The area between the anus and vagina in the female and between the anus and scrotum in the male.

periodontitis Severe gum disease in which the tooth root becomes infected.

persistent vegetative state A state of being awake and capable of reacting to physical stimuli, such as light, while being unaware of pain or other environmental stimuli.

phobia An anxiety disorder marked by an inordinate fear of an object, a class of objects, or a situation, resulting in extreme avoidance behaviors.

physical dependence The physiological attachment to, and need for, a drug.

physical fitness The ability to respond to routine physical demands, with enough reserve energy to cope with a sudden challenge.

phytochemicals Chemicals such as indoles, coumarins, and capsaicin, which exist naturally in plants and have disease-fighting properties.

placenta An organ that develops after implantation and to which the embryo attaches, via the umbilical cord, for nourishment and waste removal.

plaque The sludgelike substance that builds up on the inner walls of arteries; the sticky film of bacteria that forms on teeth.

pneumonia An inflammation of the lungs caused by infection or irritants.

pollutant A substance or agent in the environment, usually the by-product of human industry or activity, that is injurious to human, animal, or plant life.

pollution The presence of pollutants in the environment.

polyabuse The misuse or abuse of more than one drug.

postpartum depression The emotional downswing that occurs after having a baby due to hormonal changes, physical exhaustion, and psychological pressures.

posttraumatic stress disorder (PTSD) The repeated reliving of a trauma through nightmares or recollection.

potentiating Making more effective or powerful.

preconception care Health care to prepare for pregnancy.

precycling The use of products that are packaged in recycled or recyclable material.

preferred provider organization (PPO) A group of physicians contracted to provide health care to members at a discounted price.

prehypertension A condition of slightly elevated blood pressure, which is likely to worsen in time.

premature ejaculation A sexual difficulty in which a man ejaculates so rapidly that his partner's satisfaction is impaired.

premature labor Labor that occurs after the twentieth week but before the thirty-seventh week of pregnancy.

premenstrual dysphoric disorder (PMDD) A disorder that causes symptoms of psychological depression during the last week of the menstrual cycle.

premenstrual syndrome (PMS) A disorder that causes physical discomfort and psychological distress prior to a woman's menstrual period.

prevention Information and support offered to help healthy people identify their health risks, reduce stressors, prevent potential medical problems, and enhance their well-being.

primary care Ambulatory or outpatient care provided by a physician in an office, emergency room, or clinic.

progesterone The female sex hormone that stimulates the uterus, preparing it for the arrival of a fertilized egg.

progestin-only pill See minipill.

progressive overloading Gradually increasing physical challenges once the body adapts to the stress placed upon it to produce maximum benefits.

progressive relaxation A method of reducing muscle tension by contracting, then relaxing certain areas of the body.

proof The alcoholic strength of a distilled spirit, expressed as twice the percentage of alcohol present.

prostate gland A structure surrounding the male urethra that produces a secretion that helps liquefy the semen from the testes.

prostatitis Inflammation of the prostate gland.

protection Measures that an individual can take when participating in risky behavior to prevent injury or unwanted risks.

protein A substance that is basically a compound of amino acids; one of the essential nutrients.

protozoa Microscopic animals made up of one cell or a group of similar cells.

psoriasis A chronic skin disorder caused by stress, skin damage, or illness and resulting in scaly, deep-pink, raised patches on the skin.

psychiatric drugs Medications that regulate a person's mental, emotional, and physical functions to facilitate normal functioning.

psychiatric nurse A nurse with special training and experience in mental health care.

psychiatrist Licensed medical doctor with additional training in psychotherapy, psychopharmacology, and treatment of mental disorders.

psychoactive Mood-altering.

psychodynamic Interpreting behaviors in terms of early experiences and unconscious influences.

psychological dependence The emotional or mental attachment to the use of a drug.

psychologists Mental health-care professionals who have completed doctoral or graduate programs in psychology and are trained in a variety of psychotherapeutic techniques, but who are not medically trained and do not prescribe medications.

psychoneuroimmunology A scientific field that explores the relationships between and among the mind, the central nervous system, and the immune system.

psychoprophylaxis See Lamaze method.

psychotherapy Treatment designed to produce a response by psychological rather than physical means, such as suggestion, persuasion, reassurance, and support.

psychotropic Mind-affecting.

pyelonephritis Inflammation of the kidney.

quackery Medical fakery; unproven practices claiming to cure diseases or solve health problems.

quid pro quo A form of harassment in which a person in power or authority makes unwanted sexual advances as a condition for receiving a job, promotion, or favor.

rape Sexual penetration of a female or a male by means of intimidation, force, or fraud.

rapid-eye-movement (REM) sleep Regularly occurring periods of sleep during which the most active dreaming takes place.

receptors Molecules on the surface of neurons on which neurotransmitters bind after their release from other neurons.

recycling The processing or reuse of manufactured materials to reduce consumption of raw materials.

reflexology A treatment based on the theory that massaging certain points on the foot or hand relieves stress or pain in corresponding parts of the body.

refractory period The period of time following orgasm during which the male cannot experience another orgasm.

rehabilitation medicine The use of surgical procedures, medication, and physical therapy to improve the condition of patients with disabling conditions such as blindness, deafness, and arthritis.

reinforcement Reward or punishment for a behavior that will increase or decrease one's likelihood of repeating the behavior.

relapse prevention An alcohol recovery treatment method that focuses on social skills training to develop ways of preventing or minimizing a relapse.

relative risk The risk of developing cancer in persons with a certain exposure or trait compared to the risk in persons who do not have the same exposure or trait.

rep (or repetition) In weight training, a single performance of a movement or exercise.

repetitive motion injury (RMI) Inflammation of or damage to a part of the body due to repetition of the same movements.

rescue marriage A marital relationship in which one partner has had a traumatic childhood and views marriage as a way of healing the past.

resting heart rate The number of heartbeats per minute during inactivity.

reuptake Reabsorption by the originating cell of neurotransmitters that have not connected with receptors and have been left in synapses.

reversibility principle The physical benefits of exercise are lost through disuse or inactivity.

rhythm method A birth-control method in which sexual intercourse is avoided during those days of the menstrual cycle in which fertilization is most likely to occur.

romantic marriage A marital relationship in which sexual passion never fades.

rubella An infectious disease that may cause birth defects if contracted by a pregnant woman; also called German measles.

satiety A feeling of fullness after eating.

saturated fat A chemical term indicating that a fat molecule contains as many hydrogen atoms as its carbon skeleton can hold. These fats are normally solid at room temperature.

schizophrenia A general term for a group of mental disorders with characteristic psychotic symptoms, such as delusions, hallucinations, and disordered thought patterns during the active phase of the illness, and a duration of at least six months.

scrotum The external sac or pouch that holds the testes.

secondary sex characteristics Physical changes associated with maleness or femaleness, induced by the sex hormones.

self-actualization A state of wellness and fulfillment that can be achieved once certain human needs are satisfied; living to one's full potential.

self-efficacy Belief in one's ability to accomplish a goal or change a behavior.

self-esteem Confidence and satisfaction in oneself.

self-talk Repetition of positive messages about one's self-worth to learn more optimistic patterns of thought, feeling, and behavior.

semen The viscous whitish fluid that is the complete male ejaculate; a combination of sperm and secretions from the prostate gland, seminal vesicles, and other glands.

seminal vesicles Glands in the male reproductive system that produce the major portion of the fluid of semen.

set-point theory The proposition that every person has an unconscious control system for keeping body fat (and therefore weight) at a predetermined level, or set point.

sets In weight training, the number of repetitions of the same movement or exercise.

sex Maleness or femaleness, resulting from genetic, structural, and functional factors.

sexual addiction A preoccupation with sex so intense and chronic that an individual cannot have a normal sexual relationship with a spouse or lover; sexual compulsion.

sexual coercion Sexual activity forced upon a person by the exertion of psychological pressure by another person.

sexual compulsion *See* sexual addiction.

sexual dysfunction The inability to react emotionally and/or physically to sexual stimulation in a way expected of the average healthy person or according to one's own standards.

sexual health The integration of the physical, emotional, intellectual, and social aspects of sexual being in ways that are positively enriching and that enhance personality, communication, and love.

sexuality The behaviors, instincts, and attitudes associated with being sexual.

sexually transmitted infections (STIs) Any of a number of diseases that are acquired through sexual contact.

sidestream smoke The smoke emitted by a burning cigarette and breathed by everyone in a closed room, including the smoker; contains more tar and nicotine than mainstream smoke.

simple carbohydrates Sugars; like all carbohydrates, they provide the body with glucose.

smog A grayish or brownish fog caused by the presence of smoke and/or chemical pollutants in the air.

social isolation A feeling of unconnectedness with others caused by and reinforced by infrequency of social contacts.

social phobia A severe form of social anxiety marked by extreme fears and avoidance of social situations.

specificity principle Each part of the body adapts to a particular type and amount of stress placed upon it.

sperm The male gamete produced by the testes and transported outside the body through ejaculation.

spermatogenesis The process by which sperm cells are produced.

spinal block An injection of anesthesia directly into the spinal cord to numb the lower body during labor and childbirth.

spiritual health The ability to identify one's basic purpose in life and to achieve one's full potential; the sense of connectedness to a greater power.

spiritual intelligence The capacity to sense, understand, and tap into ourselves, others, and the world around us.

static flexibility The ability to assume and maintain an extended position at one end point in a joint's range of motion.

static stretching A gradual stretch held for a short time of 10 to 30 seconds.

sterilization A surgical procedure to end a person's reproductive capability.

stimulant An agent, such as a drug, that temporarily relieves drowsiness, helps in the performance of repetitive tasks, and improves capacity for work.

strength Physical power; the maximum weight one can lift, push, or press in one effort.

stress The nonspecific response of the body to any demands made upon it; may be characterized by muscle tension and acute anxiety, or may be a positive force for action.

stressor Specific or nonspecific agents or situations that cause the stress response in a body.

stroke A cerebrovascular event in which the blood supply to a portion of the brain is blocked.

subcutaneous Under the skin.

suction curettage A procedure in which the contents of the uterus are removed by means of suction and scraping.

sudden infant death syndrome (SIDS) The unexplained death of an apparently healthy baby under one year of age during sleep.

synapse A specialized site at which electrical impulses are transmitted from the axon terminal of one neuron to a dendrite of another.

synergistic Characterized by a combined effect that is greater than the sum of the individual effects.

syphilis A sexually transmitted disease caused by the bacterium *Treponema pallidum,* and characterized by early sores, a latent period, and a final period of life-threatening symptoms including brain damage and heart failure.

systemic disease A pathologic condition that spreads throughout the body.

systole The contraction phase of the cardiac cycle.

tachycardia An abnormally rapid heart rate, over 100 beats per minute.

tamoxifen An estrogen-based medication that can help reduce the likelihood of developing cancer.

tar A thick, sticky dark fluid produced by the burning of tobacco, made up of several hundred different chemicals, many of them poisonous, some of them carcinogenic.

target heart rate Sixty to eighty-five percent of the maximum heart rate; the heart rate at which one derives maximum cardiovascular benefit from aerobic exercise.

teratogen Any agent that causes spontaneous abortion or defects or malformations in a fetus.

terminal illness An illness in which death is inevitable.

testes (singular, **testis**) The male sex organs that produce sperm and testosterone.

testosterone The male sex hormone that stimulates male secondary sex characteristics.

thallium scintigraphy A diagnostic test in which radioactive isotopes are injected into the bloodstream, and images of the rays emitted by the isotopes are captured and then translated into images of the heart as it pumps.

thanatology The discipline of humanitarian caregiving for critically ill patients and their grieving family members and friends.

toxic shock syndrome (TSS) A disease characterized by fever, vomiting, diarrhea, and often shock, caused by a bacterium that releases toxic waste products into the bloodstream.

toxicity Poisonousness; the dosage level at which a drug becomes poisonous to the body, causing either temporary or permanent damage.

traditional marriage A marital relationship in which the roles of the partners are distinct; defined by gender-based cultural norms and expectations.

trans-fatty acids Fats formed when liquid vegetable oils are processed to make table spreads or cooking fats, and also found in dairy and beef products; considered to be especially dangerous dietary fats.

transcendence The sense of passing into a foreign region or dimension, often experienced by a person near death.

transgendered Having a gender identity opposite one's biological sex; transsexual.

transient ischemic attack (TIA) A cerebrovascular event in which the blood supply to a portion of the brain is blocked temporarily; repeated attacks are predictors of more severe strokes.

trichomoniasis An infection of the protozoan *Trichomonas vaginalis;* females experience vaginal burning, itching, and discharge, but male carriers may be asymptomatic.

triglyceride A blood fat that flows through the blood after meals and is linked to increased risk of coronary artery disease.

tubal ligation The suturing or tying shut of the fallopian tubes to prevent pregnancy.

tubal occlusion The blocking of the fallopian tubes to prevent pregnancy.

tuberculosis A highly infectious bacterial disease that primarily affects the lungs and is often fatal.

tumor suppressor gene Gene that normally controls cell growth. Many cancers are linked to defects in a tumor suppressor gene.

twelve-step programs Self-help group programs based on the principles of Alcoholics Anonymous.

ulcer A lesion in, or an erosion of, the mucous membrane of an organ.

unsaturated fat A chemical term indicating that a fat molecule contains fewer hydrogen atoms than its carbon skeleton can hold. These fats are normally liquid at room temperature.

urethra The canal through which urine from the bladder leaves the body; in the male, also serves as the channel for seminal fluid.

urethral opening The outer opening of the thin tube that carries urine from the bladder.

urethritis Infection of the urethra.

uterus The female organ that houses the developing fetus until birth.

vagina The canal leading from the exterior opening in the female genital area to the uterus.

vaginal contraceptive film (VCF) A small dissolvable sheet saturated with spermicide that can be inserted into the vagina and placed over the cervix.

vaginal spermicide A substance that kills or neutralizes sperm, inserted into the vagina in the form of a foam, cream, jelly, or suppository.

vaginismus A sexual difficulty in which a woman experiences painful spasms of the vagina during sexual intercourse.

values The criteria by which one makes choices about one's thoughts and actions and goals and ideals.

vas deferens Two tubes that carry sperm from the epididymis into the urethra.

vasectomy A surgical sterilization procedure in which each vas deferens is cut and tied shut to stop the passage of sperm to the urethra for ejaculation.

vector A biological or physical vehicle that carries the agent of infection to the host.

vegans People who eat only plant foods.

ventricle Either of the two lower chambers of the heart, which pump blood out of the heart and into the arteries.

video display terminal (VDT) A screen or monitor that emits electromagnetic fields from all sides; these fields may lead to increased reproductive problems, miscarriages, low birthweights, and cataracts.

virus A submicroscopic infectious agent; the most primitive form of life.

visualization An approach to stress control, self-healing, or motivating life changes by means of guided, or directed, imagery.

vital signs Measurements of physiological functioning; specifically, temperature, blood pressure, pulse rate, and respiration rate.

vitamins Organic substances that are needed in very small amounts by the body and carry out a variety of functions in metabolism and nutrition.

waist-hip ratio The proportion of one's waist circumference to one's hip circumference.

wellness A state of optimal health.

withdrawal Development of symptoms that cause significant psychological and physical distress when an individual reduces or stops drug use.

zygote A fertilized egg.

Section I

p. 1, © Gary Buss/Taxi/Getty Images.

Chapter 1

p. 3, © Zephyr Picture/Index Stock Imagery. **p. 4,** © David H. Wells/CORBIS; © Walter Hodges/CORBIS; © Kelly Harriger/CORBIS. **p. 6,** © SW Production/Index Stock Imagery. **p. 7,** © Bob Daemmerich/Stock, Boston. **p. 10,** © Chet Gordon/The Image Works. **p. 12,** © Dex Images/CORBIS. **p. 19,** © Michael Keller/Index Stock Imagery. **p. 20,** © Neil Rabinowitz/CORBIS. **p. 21,** Geri Engberg Photography.

Chapter 2

p. 37, © Marac Romanelli/The Image Bank/Getty Images. **p. 38,** © Tom Stewart/CORBIS; © Bob Daemmerich/Stock, Boston. **p. 43,** © Bob Torrez/Stone/Getty Images. **p. 44,** © Stockbyte/PictureQuest. **p. 46,** © Bob Schatz/Getty Images. **p. 47,** © Robert W. Ginn/PhotoEdit. **p. 49,** © Mark Richards/PhotoEdit. **p. 53,** © Secchi-Lecaque/Roussel-UCLA/CNRI/Photo Researchers, Inc. **p. 56,** © 2000 PhotoDisc, Inc. **p. 57,** © David Young-Wolff/PhotoEdit. **p. 59,** Paul Avis/Getty Image. **p. 61,** Mary Kate Denny/PhotoEdit. **p. 64,** "My Head is Going Round and Round" from *Art as Healing* by Edward Adamson/Coventure, Limited. **p. 66,** © Tony Latham/Stone/Getty Images. **p. 67,** © Pierre Perrin/CORBIS Sygma.

Chapter 3

p. 75, © Paul Thomas/The Image Bank/Getty Images. **p. 76,** © CORBIS; © 2000 PhotoDisc. **p. 81,** © Bill Aron/PhotoEdit. **p. 83,** © Ulrike Welsch. **p. 85,** Geri Engberg Photography; © SuperStock, Inc. **p. 86,** © Anthony Redpath/CORBIS. **p. 88,** © Will and Deni McIntyre/Photo Researchers, Inc. **p. 89,** AP/Wide World Photos. **p. 91,** © CORBIS. **p. 92,** © Richard T. Nowitz/Photo Researchers, Inc.; © James Schnepf/Getty Images. **p. 94,** © AFP/CORBIS. **p. 95,** © CORBIS.

Section II

p. 101, © ZEFA/Masterfile

Chapter 4

p. 103, © Peter Correz/Stone/Getty Images. **p. 104,** clockwise, left to right © Lori Adamski Peek/Stone/Getty Images; © Jurgen Reisch/Stone/Getty Images; © 2000 PhotoDisc, Inc.; © Fitness & Wellness, Boise, Idaho. **p. 107,** © PhotoDisc, Inc. **p. 113,** © 2001 PhotoDisc; © David Hanover; © David Hanover. **p. 118,** © Jim Cummins/Taxi/Getty Images. **p. 121,** © 2000 PhotoDisc, Inc. **p. 125,** (all) © David Madison. **p. 128,** © David Young-Wolff/PhotoEdit; © Photo courtesy of Hologic, Inc. **p. 129,** © 2002 PhotoDisc, Inc.

Chapter 5

p. 141, © Chris Cole/The Image Bank/Getty Images. **p. 142,** © 2000 PhotoDisc, Inc. **p. 143,** © Polara Studios Inc. **p. 147,** © Polara Studios, Inc. **p. 149,** © 2000 PhotoDisc, Inc. **p. 152,** © PhotoDisc, Inc. **p. 157,** © 2002 PhotoDisc/Getty Images. **p. 159,** © Polara Studios, Inc. **p. 160,** Polara Studios, Inc. **p. 161,** (both) © Polara Studios, Inc. **p. 162,** (both) © Polara Studios, Inc. **p. 166,** Source: Journal of THE AMERICAN DIETETIC ASSOCIATION. April 2002, pp.484–485. **p. 169,** Felicia Martinez/PhotoEdit; © Allan Montaine. **p. 172,** © Marc Alcarez/Index Stock Imagery.

Chapter 6

p. 181, © David Oliver/Taxi/Getty Images. **p. 182,** © Christie's Images, London/SuperStock. **p. 191,** © William Thompson/Index Stock Imagery. **p. 192,** © Michael Newman/PhotoEdit. **p. 193,** © Bruce Ayres/Stone/Getty Images. **p. 194,** (both) © Tony Freeman/PhotoEdit. **p. 199,** © Great American Stock/Index Stock

Imagery; © Polara Studios, Inc.; Polara Studios, Inc. **p. 203,** © Michael Newman/PhotoEdit.

Section III

p. 209, © Alyson Aliano/Stone/Getty Images.

Chapter 7

p. 211, © JFB/Stone/Getty Images. **p. 212,** © 2000 David Roth/Stone/Getty Images; © 2000 PhotoDisc, Inc. **p. 218,** © David Hanover/Stone/Getty Images. **p. 220,** © Art Wolfe/Stone/Getty Images; © Patrick N. Lucero/SuperStock; © David Hanson/Stone/Getty Images; © Carl & Ann Purcell/CORBIS; © Art Wolfe/Stone/Getty Images; © Robin Smith/Stone/Getty Images. **p. 226,** Photo used with permission of Sylvia Chaney; © 2000 PhotoDisc, Inc.; Photo used with permission of Sylvia Chaney; © 2000 PhotoDisc, Inc. **p. 227,** © Jon Riley/Stone/Getty Images. **p. 228,** © Tony May/Stone/Getty Images. **p. 231,** Bill Bachmann/Stock, Boston/Picture Quest.

Chapter 8

p. 239, © Michael Jang/Stone/Getty Images. **p. 240,** © Custom Medical Stock. **p. 242,** AP/Wide World Photos; © Laura Dwight/CORBIS. **p. 253,** © Marc Dolphin/Stone/Getty Images. **p. 255,** © Deborah Davis/PhotoEdit. **p. 259,** © Rob Lewine/CORBIS. **p. 263,** © Carol Ford/Stone/Getty Images. **p. 267,** © Gail Mooney/CORBIS.

Chapter 9

p. 275, © Stephen Simpson/Taxi/Getty Images. **p. 281,** © Michael Dwyer/Stock, Boston. **p. 284,** © Joel Gordon Photography. **p. 286,** © Joel Gordon Photography; Ortho-McNeil Pharmaceutical, ORGANON Communications. **p. 287,** © Saturn Stills/Photo Researchers, Inc. **p. 288,** Courtesy © Berlex Laboratories, Inc.; © Joel Gordon Photography. **p. 290,** © Joel Gordon Photography. **p. 291,** Courtesy of FemCap, Inc., and Alfred Shihata, MD. **p. 294,** © Joel Gordon Photography. **p. 295,** Courtesy of Allendale Pharmaceuticals; © Joel Gordon Photography. **p. 296,** © Joel Gordeon Photography. **p. 297,** Cycle Technologies and Institute for Reproductive Health, Georgetown University. **p. 304,** AP/Wide World Photos. **p. 307,** © Petit Format/Nestle/ScienceSource/Photo Researchers, Inc. **p. 308,** © Lisa M. McGoody/CORBIS. **p. 311,** © SIU/Peter Arnold, Inc. **p. 314,** © Dana Fineman/CORBIS-Sygma. **p. 315,** Mike Greenlar/The Image Works.

Section IV

p. 321, © Network Productions/Index Stock Imagery.

Chapter 10

p. 323, © Gary S. and Vivian Chapman /The Image Bank/Getty Images. **p. 326,** Geri Engberg Photography. **p. 330,** © CORBIS. **p. 335,** © Lon C. Diehl/PhotoEdit. **p. 342,** National Institute on Drug Abuse, www.clubdrugs.org; © Scott Houston/CORBIS. **p. 343,** © TekImage/SPL/Photo Researchers, Inc. **p. 344,** DEA/Office of Forensic Sciences **p. 348,** © Oscar Burriel/Latin Stock/Photo Researchers, Inc. **p. 349,** © Roy Morsch/CORBIS. **p. 350,** Mimi Forsyth Photography. **p. 353,** Hank Morgan/Science Source/Photo Researchers, Inc.

Chapter 11

p. 361, © DTF Productions/The Image Bank/Getty Images. **p. 369,** © 2000 PhotoDisc, Inc. **p. 370,** © Uwe Krejci/Taxi/Getty Images. **p. 373,** © Evan Schneider Photography. **p. 377,** © Tony Freeman/PhotoEdit. **p. 378,** © Mark Richards/PhotoEdit. **p. 379,** © K. L. Jones/LLR Research. **p. 380,** © SuperStock, Inc. **p. 384,** (both) Mark Nielsen.

Chapter 12

p. 395, © Peter Dokus/Stone/Getty Images. **p. 398,** © Spencer Grant/PhotoEdit, Inc. **p. 399,** © Science VU/Visuals Unlimited. **p. 400,** © Peter Poulides/Stone/Getty Images. **p. 408,** AP/Wide World Photos. **p. 409,** Leonard Morse/Medical Images. **p. 410,** Felicia Martinez/PhotoEdit. **p. 412,** Courtesy of Non-Smoker's Rights Association. **p. 414,** © Michael Newman/PhotoEdit. **p. 415,** © Billy E. Barnes/Stock, Boston.

Section V

p. 421, © Lori Adamski Peek/Stone/Getty Images.

Chapter 13

p. 423, Steve Allen/Brand X Pictures/Getty Images. **p. 425,** (a) © Omikron/Photo Researchers, Inc.; (b) © John Durham/SPL/Photo Researchers, Inc.; (c) © David Philips/Visuals Unlimited; (d) © Howard Sochurek/Medichrome; (e) © Biophoto Associates/Photo Researchers, Inc. **p. 428,** © Boehringer Ingelheim International GmbH, photo by Lennart Nilsson/Bonnier Alba AB; © Boehringer Ingelheim International GmbH, photo by Lennart Nilsson. **p. 432,** © F. Hoffman/The Image Works. **p. 435,** © Myrleen Ferguson Cate/PhotoEdit. **p. 441,** © Scott Camazine/Photo Researchers, Inc. **p. 443,** © Reuters NewMedia Inc./CORBIS. **p. 447,** © LWA/CORBIS. **p. 453,** © Science VU/Visuals Unlimited. **p. 455,** (a) St. Bartholomew's Hospital/Science Photo Library/Photo Researchers, Inc.; (b) Biophoto Associates/Photo Researchers, Inc. **p. 456,** © Marazzi/Photo Researchers, Inc. **p. 457,** © E. Gray/Photo Researchers, Inc. **p. 459,** Lennart Nilsson © Boehringer Ingelheim International GmbH.

Chapter 14

p. 469, © Peter Beavis/Taxi/Getty Images. **p. 471,** © Charles Gupton/Stock, Boston. **p. 474,** © Bonnie Kamin/PhotoEdit. **p. 483,** © Will & Deni McIntyre/Photo Researchers, Inc. **p. 486,** (both) © Cabisco/Visuals Unlimited. **p. 491,** © Robert Llewellyn/SuperStock, Inc. **p. 492,** © Bruce Ayres/Stone/Getty Images. **p. 494,** © Will & Deni McIntyre/Photo Researchers, Inc.

Chapter 15

p. 503, © Steve Smith/Taxi/Getty Images. **p. 506,** © Michael Doolittle/The Image Works. **p. 507,** © 2000 PhotoDisc, Inc. **p. 509,** © 2001 PhotoDisc, Inc.; (bottom) Courtesy of the Skin Cancer Foundation. **p. 510,** © Bill Crump/Brand X Pictures/PictureQuest. **p. 511,** © 2001 PhotoDisc, Inc.; © Corbis Images; © 2001 PhotoDisc, Inc.; © Corbis Images. **p. 517,** © Lawrence Migdale. **p. 521,** © Damien Lovegrove/Science Photo Library/Photo Researchers, Inc. **p. 524,** (both) Biological Photo Service. **p. 525,** © A. B. Dowsett/Science Photo Library/Photo Researchers, Inc. **p. 526,** David Young-Wolff/PhotoEdit.

Chapter 16

p. 535, © Lightscapes Photography, Inc./CORBIS. **p. 538,** © 2000 PhotoDisc, Inc. **p. 540,** © Geri Engberg. **p. 541,** © Vision/Photo Researchers, Inc. **p. 544,** Michael Newman/PhotoEdit. **p. 547,** © Bob Daemmrich/Stock, Boston. **p. 554,** © Tim Malyon & Paul Biddle/Photo Researchers, Inc. **p. 555,** © Kevin R. Morris/CORBIS. **p. 556,** © 2000 PhotoDisc, Inc.

Section VI

p. 567, © Duomo Photography/The Image Bank/Getty Images.

Chapter 17

p. 569, © Dick Luria/Taxi/Getty Images. **p. 572,** © Courtesy of Eva Chaney. **p. 575,** (both) Alzheimer's Disease Education & Referral Center. **p. 579,** Jo Hale/Getty Images; © 2002 Glenn Weiner/Zuma Press; Bob Foy/Newsmakers/Getty Images. **p. 580,** © Mark Gibson/Lonely Planet Images. **p. 582,** (both) P. Motta, Department of Anatomy, University "La Sapienza," Rome/Science Photo Library/Photo Researchers, Inc. **p. 591,** © David Young-Wolff/PhotoEdit. **p. 592,** Al Campanie, © The Syracuse Newspaper/The Image Works. **p. 594,** A. Ramey/PhotoEdit. **p. 595,** © Gunter Marx Photography/CORBIS.

Chapter 18

p. 603, © Jim Cummins/Taxi/Getty Images. **p. 604,** © Shopper/Stock, Boston. **p. 607,** © 2000 PhotoDisc, Inc. **p. 609,** © Robert W. Ginn/PhotoEdit. **p. 611,** © Tony Freeman/PhotoEdit. **p. 612,** © Lew Merrim/Photo Researchers, Inc. **p. 614,** Courtesy of Dr. Daniel G. Amen, The Amen Clinic for Behavioral Medicine. **p. 616,** © Bob Krist/CORBIS. **p. 620,** © Image Source/SuperStock. **p. 621,** © Yvonne Hemsey/Liaison/Getty Images. **p. 623,** © 2000 PhotoDisc, Inc. **p. 625,** © Rhoda Sidney/PhotoEdit. **p. 626,** © B. Mahoney/The Image Works.

Chapter 19

p. 633, © Phillip & Karen Smith/Stone//Getty Images. **p. 634,** Glenn M. Oliver/Visuals Unlimited. **p. 638,** © David Woodfall/Stone/Getty Images. **p. 640,** David Young-Wolff/PhotoEdit. **p. 641,** © Tony Freeman/PhotoEdit. **p. 644,** © Rune Hellestad/CORBIS. **p. 646,** © Paul Grebliunas/Stone/Getty Images; © Tony Freeman/PhotoEdit.